Life Care Planning and Case Management Across the Lifespan

Celebrating 25 years since its first publication, the fifth edition of this best-selling text is the most up-to-date and complete resource available on what a life care planner does, how the life care planner does it, and issues that affect the day-to-day role of a life care planner.

Now featuring new material on pediatric life care planning and case management, including brachial plexus injuries and neurodevelopmental disorders, this new edition provides guidance and planning for cases across the lifespan. It begins with a series of chapters examining ten different professional specializations that often contribute to a life care plan, before providing critical information for developing life care plans for individuals with different physical, mental, and cognitive conditions including spinal cord injury, brain injury, and chronic pain. Uniquely comprehensive, the book also includes chapters on the forensic and legal context of life care planning, as well as equipment/technology, evidence-based literature/resources, and special education/special needs planning relevant to pediatric life care planning.

Also including chapters dedicated to life care planning methodology and life care planning research, this is an essential resource for anyone practicing or studying life care planning or managing the needs of those requiring chronic medical care over the lifespan.

Tanya Rutherford-Owen, PhD, CRC, CLCP, CDMS, LPC, FIALCP is a certified rehabilitation counselor, certified life care planner, and life care planning fellow. She has over 25 years of experience providing rehabilitation services and forensic work in various states. She has served as an adjunct professor at the University of Arkansas in the Department of Rehabilitation Education and Research and is currently an adjunct faculty member of Capital University Law School. She has served on the Board of Directors for the Foundation for Life Care Planning & Rehabilitation Research and served as a work group member in the development of the fourth edition of the Standards of Practice for Life Care Planners. She has independently researched and published articles in peer-reviewed journals including *Journal of Life Care Planning*, *The Rehabilitation Professional* and the *Journal of Rehabilitation*. She worked as the editor of the *Journal of Life Care Planning* (JLCP) from 2016 to 2020, prior to assuming the managing editor role for both the *Journal of Life Care Planning* and *The Rehabilitation Professional*. Dr. Owen earned a PhD in Rehabilitation in 2011 and a Master's degree in Counseling Psychology in 1996. In 1993, she graduated Magna Cum Laude and Phi Beta Kappa from Millsaps College. She has provided testimony in various state and federal courts and in Social Security disability adjudication hearings for 20 years. In the course of her work, she has received various awards including the Sherry Jasper Memorial Award (2022) by the Foundation for Life Care Planning & Rehabilitation Research; Outstanding Life

Care Planning Educator Award (2018); a President's Commendation Award from the International Association of Rehabilitation Professionals (IARP, 2017 & 2018); Best Student Paper Award by the Foundation for Life Care Planning Research & International Academy of Life Care Planners (2011); the Outstanding Rehabilitation Education & Research Doctoral Student at the University of Arkansas (2010); the Russell Baxter Award at the University of Arkansas (2010–2011); and was a Doctoral Academy Fellow at the University of Arkansas (2009–2011).

Mary Barros-Bailey, PhD, CRC, CLCP, NCC, ABVE/AE, CVE, CCC is a Multilingual Rehabilitation Counselor (Spanish/English/Portuguese), Vocational Expert, Life Care Planner, and principle with Intermountain Vocational Services, Inc. She is a practitioner-scientist with a national, sometimes international, caseload. Dr. Barros-Bailey is adjunct faculty at Capital University Law School's graduate certificate in life care planning and has taught with a variety of graduate programs in rehabilitation counseling. She serves as a peer reviewer or on editorial boards of peer-review publications, has presented over 200 times nationally and internationally, and authored over 130 publications such as a book, textbook chapters, and peer-reviewed journal articles. Recent awards are: Best Article, *The Advocate*, Idaho State/Idaho Bar Foundation, Inc. (2018); Alumni Achievement Award, Middlebury Institute of International Studies (2018); Outstanding Educator Award, Foundation for Life Care Planning Research (2017); and Lifetime Achievement Award, International Association of Rehabilitation Professionals (2016). Dr. Barros-Bailey is currently a Fulbright Specialist working with the largest rehabilitation counseling organization in Australia and rehabilitation counseling credentialing organization in the world to establish the first credential in forensic vocational rehabilitation in the southern hemisphere.

Roger O. Weed, PhD, CRC/R, LPC/Ret, CCM/R, CDMS/R, FNRCA, FIALCP/R, Professor Emeritus, and Fellow Emeritus, International Academy of Life Care Planning, is retired as professor and graduate rehabilitation counseling coordinator at Georgia State University. He also held doctoral student graduate faculty status in Counseling Psychology as well as Counselor Education and Practice doctoral programs. He has authored or co-authored approximately 200 books, reviews, articles, and book chapters, more than 80 of which were specific to life care planning. Prior to achieving the PhD, Dr. Weed practiced rehabilitation counseling and consulting for 15 years in Alaska. During his more than 42 years in the profession, Dr. Weed was honored several times for his work including the Distinguished Professor Award (2006) from Georgia State University's Alumni Association (sole recipient), Lifetime Appreciation Award from the International Commission on Health Care Certification (2011), Larry Huggins Lifetime Achievement Award (2009) from the Private Rehabilitation Specialists of Georgia, Lifetime Achievement Award (2005), from the sponsors of the International Life Care Planning Conference, Lifetime Achievement Award from the International Association of Rehabilitation Professionals (2004) (as well as recognition in 1997 and 1991 as the Outstanding Educator), the National Professional Services Award from the American Rehabilitation Counseling Association (1993), and Research Excellence Award (2003) from the College of Education at Georgia State University. Dr. Weed is the creator and senior editor for the first four editions of the *Life Care Planning and Case Management Handbook*. He is one of the five founders of the original, nationwide training program leading to life care planning certification. He is also past-chair of the Georgia State Licensing Board for professional counselors, marriage and family therapists, and social workers, as well as past-president of the International Association of Rehabilitation Professionals.

Life Care Planning and Case Management Across the Lifespan

Fifth Edition

Edited by
Tanya Rutherford-Owen,
Mary Barros-Bailey,
and Roger O. Weed

Routledge
Taylor & Francis Group
NEW YORK AND LONDON

Fifth edition published 2024
by Routledge
605 Third Avenue, New York, NY 10158

and by Routledge
4 Park Square, Milton Park, Abingdon, Oxon, OX14 4RN

Routledge is an imprint of the Taylor & Francis Group, an informa business

© 2024 selection and editorial matter, Tanya Rutherford-Owen, Mary Barros-Bailey and Roger O. Weed; individual chapters, the contributors

The right of Tanya Rutherford-Owen, Mary Barros-Bailey and Roger O. Weed to be identified as the authors of the editorial material, and of the authors for their individual chapters, has been asserted in accordance with sections 77 and 78 of the Copyright, Designs and Patents Act 1988.

All rights reserved. No part of this book may be reprinted or reproduced or utilised in any form or by any electronic, mechanical, or other means, now known or hereafter invented, including photocopying and recording, or in any information storage or retrieval system, without permission in writing from the publishers.

Trademark notice: Product or corporate names may be trademarks or registered trademarks, and are used only for identification and explanation without intent to infringe.

First edition published by July 2nd, 1998 by CRC Press
Fourth edition published September 11, 2018 by Routledge

Library of Congress Cataloging-in-Publication Data
Names: Rutherford-Owen, Tanya, editor. | Barros-Bailey, Mary, editor. | Weed, Roger O., editor.
Title: Life care planning and case management across the lifespan /
edited by Tanya Rutherford-Owen, Mary Barros-Bailey, and Roger O. Weed.
Other titles: Life care planning and case management handbook.
Description: Fifth edition. | New York : Routledge, an imprint of the Taylor & Francis Group, an informa business, 2023. | Revised edition of: Life care planning and case management handbook / edited by Debra Berens and Roger Weed. Fourth edition. 2018. |
Includes bibliographical references and index.
Identifiers: LCCN 2023004516 (print) | LCCN 2023004517 (ebook) |
ISBN 9781032192338 (hardback) | ISBN 9781032483207 (paperback) |
ISBN 9781003388456 (ebook)
Subjects: LCSH: Life care planning.
Classification: LCC RM930.7 .L54 2023 (print) | LCC RM930.7 (ebook) |
DDC 362.61–dc23/eng/20230428
LC record available at https://lccn.loc.gov/2023004516
LC ebook record available at https://lccn.loc.gov/2023004517

ISBN: 978-1-032-19233-8 (hbk)
ISBN: 978-1-032-48320-7 (pbk)
ISBN: 978-1-003-38845-6 (ebk)

DOI: 10.4324/9781003388456

Typeset in Garamond Pro
by Newgen Publishing UK

Contents

Lists of Figures ix
List of Tables xi
List of Contributors xiii
Foreword xxix
Acknowledgements xxxi

PART ONE HISTORICAL, METHODOLOGICAL, AND PROFESSIONAL ISSUES AND RESEARCH IN LIFE CARE PLANNING

1   Life Care Planning: Past, Present, and Future 3
       Roger O. Weed and Tanya Rutherford-Owen

2   Methodology, Scope of Practice, Standards of Practice, and Consensus in Life Care Planning 25
       Mary Barros-Bailey, Tanya Rutherford-Owen, and Karen Preston

3   Research in Life Care Planning 81
       Aaron Mertes and Christine Reid

4   Credentialing in Life Care Planning 107
       Sherry A. Latham

5   Ethics in Life Care Planning 123
       Mary Barros-Bailey

6   Multicultural and Cross-Cultural Considerations for Life Care Planning 157
       Mary Barros-Bailey

PART TWO LIFE CARE PLANNING ACROSS THE LIFESPAN

7   Pediatric Care Management in Life Care Planning 171
       Kristi B. Bagnell and Elizabeth Moberg-Wolff

8   Elder Care Management in Life Care Planning 209
       Jennifer Crowley and Shanna Huber

PART THREE THE TRANSDISCIPLINARY TEAM

9 The Role of the Physiatrist in Life Care Planning 233
Richard Paul Bonfiglio and Debbe Marcinko

10 The Role of the Rehabilitation Nurse in Life Care Planning 253
Amy M. Sutton

11 The Role of the Rehabilitation Counselor in Life Care Planning 267
Debra E. Berens and Ann T. Neulicht

12 The Role of the Neuropsychologist in Life Care Planning 319
Carol P. Walker

13 The Role of the Neurologist in Life Care Planning 361
Stephen L. Nelson

14 The Role of the Occupational Therapist in Life Care Planning 369
Sarah Brown, Amy Thompson, and Sarah Malloy

15 The Role of the Physical Therapist in Life Care Planning 389
Diana Bubanja

16 The Role of the Speech-Language Pathologist and Audiologist in
Life Care Planning 409
Carolyn Wiles Higdon

17 The Role of the Prosthetist in Life Care Planning 467
LeRoy Oddie

18 The Role of the Economist in Life Care Planning 483
Frederick A. Raffa and Matthew B. Raffa

PART FOUR SELECTED DIAGNOSES, FORENSIC, LEGAL, AND OTHER ISSUES

19 Life Care Planning for the Patient with an Amputation 501
Robert H. Meier, Liesl Meier Rose, and Christian D. Meier

20 Life Care Planning for Acquired Brain Injury 533
David L. Ripley

21 Life Care Planning for the Patient with Burns 569
Ruth B. Rimmer and Kevin N. Foster

22 Life Care Planning for the Patient with a Mental Health Disorder 607
Alexander Amit Missner and Shani Cohen Missner

23 Life Care Planning for the Patient with Chronic Pain 645
Jarna R. Shah, Carrie Hyde, Gregory Lawson Smith, Jaleesa Jackson,
Chiedozie Uwandu, and Johnathan H. Goree

24 Life Care Planning for the Patient with Spinal Cord Injury 661
David Altman and Dan Bagwell

25	**Life Care Planning for People with Visual Impairment** 697	
	Christine Reid and Sandra Bullins	
26	**Life Care Planning for the Patient with a Brachial Plexus Injury**.............................737	
	Scott H. Kozin and Mona Goldman Yudkoff	
27	**Forensic Issues in Life Care Planning** 765	
	Rick H. Robinson	
28	**Admissibility Considerations in Life Care Planning** 793	
	Timothy F. Field	
29	**A Plaintiff's Attorney's Perspective on Life Care Planning**..811	
	Bruce H. Stern	
30	**A Defense Attorney's Perspective on Life Care Planning** 835	
	Aubrey Lyon and Simão Ávila	
31	**Special Education Law and Practices for the Pediatric Life Care Planner** 853	
	Brenda Eagan-Johnson and Margaret Lockovich	
32	**Special Needs Planning**..883	
	Benji Rubin	
33	**Assistive Technology, Durable Medical Equipment, and Transportation in Life Care Planning**..897	
	Irmo Marini and Laura Villarreal	
34	**A Personal Perspective of Life Care Planning** 913	
	Various Authors	
35	**Life Care Planning Costing, Literature, and Summary of Resources**........................935	
	Mary Barros-Bailey	

Index.. 1005

Figures

2.1	Ecological Model-ICF Model for Life Care Planning	35
2.2	Initial Standards to Determine Qualifications for Life Care Planning Training	41
2.3	Progression From Standards for Training to Standards for Being a Life Care Planner	41
2.4	Standards of Practice Evolve From Defining Who the Life Care Planner is to Using a Process of Steps for Life Care Planning	42
2.5	Complex Intertwining of Standards of Practice Within the Specialty Practice	44
3.1	Hierarchy of Evidence Pyramid	82
7.1	Life Care Planner and Team Collaboration	198
15.1	Hip Flexion	399
15.2	Knee Extension: Right Knee Extension (ibid.)	400
15.3	Ankle Plantar Flexion (Knee Neutral)	400
16.1	Audiogram	427
16.2	Tympanograms	428
17.1	U.S. Map of Licensure, Accreditation, and Certification Requirements by State	470
19.1	X-Ray Showing Extremely Short Above-Elbow Amputation Post Electrical Burn With Nothing Remaining Other Than Humeral Head	505
19.2	X-Ray Showing Same Arm With lengthening Using Allograft Bone Plated into the Residual Humeral Head. A Pedicle Graft of Latissimus Dorsi Muscle and Overlying Soft Tissue Were Used to Cover the Added Bone Length. Amputee is Now Able to Wear and Use an Above-Elbow Prosthesis	506
19.3	Traumatic Amputations of the Ring and Little Fingers with Cosmetic Deformity	515
19.4	Finger Amputations now Covered with a Passive Cosmetic Glove Replacing the Ring and Little Fingers that Permits use of the Residual Thumb, Index, and Long Digits	515
19.5	"I-Hand" Without Coverage of a Cosmetic Glove. Individual Fingers Move Using Myoelectric Signals	516
20.1	Cerebrum, Lateral Views	536
20.2	Cerebrum, Medial Views	538
23.1	Transforaminal Epidural Steroid Injection	650
23.2	Sacroiliac Joint Injections	651
23.3	Lumbar Facet Injections	652
24.1	Vertebrae Surrounding Spinal Cord and Other Neural Elements	663
24.2	Cross Section of Vertebra Surrounding Spinal Cord and Other Neural Elements	664
24.3	Cross Section of Spinal Cord	664
24.4	International Standards for Neurological Classification of Spinal Cord Injury	667

List of Figures

25.1	Example Life Care Planning Tables for Betty Williams	723
26.1	Anatomy of the Brachial Plexus	738
26.2	A Variety of Toys, Props, and Games Are Used to Examine Children	742
26.3	Modified Mallet Classification for Shoulder Motion	743
26.4	Proper Stretching Exercises Are Necessary to Prevent Joint Contracture	744
26.5A	Fabricated Splint to Place the Arm Hand in a More Functional Position	745
26.5B	MRI with Meningeal Pouch Filled with Cerebrospinal Fluid	746
26.6	Five-Month-Old Female Child with Right Global Brachial Plexus Injury	749
26.7	Fabricated Splint Consists of a Trunk Portion and a Posterior Elbow Splint With Elbow Flexion	751
26.8	Nerve Transfer for Bicep's Function	751
26.9	Isolation of a Group Fascicle from the Ulnar Nerve (left loop) for Transfer to the Musculocutaneous Branch to the Biceps Muscle (right loop)	752
26.10	Tendon Transfer to Improve Shoulder Motion	753
26.11	Humeral Fracture Brace to Protect Humeral Osteotomy and to Allow Elbow Motion	753
26.12	Tendon Transfer for Elbow Flexion. Bipolar Latissimus Dorsi Muscle Harvested from Flank for Elbow Flexorplasty	754
26.13	Pronation Deficiency Leads to Difficulty With Many More Bimanual Tasks Such As Keyboarding, Writing, and Tabletop Activities	756

Tables

1.1	Life Care Planning Timeline of Selected Historical Events	13
2.1	Phases of the Life Care Planning Method	30
2.2	Scopes of Practice in Life Care Planning	38
2.3	Reasons for Standards of Practice	40
2.4	Planning Process Language Used by Healthcare Professions	43
2.5	Steps Used in the Life Care Planning Process as a Foundation for Standards of Practice	43
2.6	Consensus Research Methods and Their Processes, Advantages, and Disadvantages	45
2.7	Work Product Peer Review Method	49
5.1	Dual or Multiple Roles	129
5.2	Welfare of Those Served	131
5.3	Respecting Diversity	132
5.4	Termination and Referral	133
5.5	Competency	135
5.6	Qualifications	137
5.7	Respecting Colleagues	139
5.8	Confidentiality, Privilege, and Privacy	141
5.9	Records	144
5.10	Remote Assessment	145
5.11	Legal Issues in Forensic Ethics	147
5.12	Research and Publications	148
5.13	Fees	149
5.14	Reporting Ethical Violations	150
7.1	Pediatric Life Care Plan Checklist	199
8.1	Age-Related Changes	214
8.2	Areas of the Assessment	217
8.3	Sample Basic Care Plan	219
9.1	JLCP Vol 17 No1 (2019) Appendix B Table 3	238
10.1	Desirable Traits for Rehabilitation Nurse Life Care Planners	258
10.2	Additional Roles and Expectations of the Rehabilitation Nurse Life Care Planner	261
10.3	Questions for the Attorney: Life Care Planner Qualifications and Expertise	262
10.4	Questions the Nurse Life Care Planner Should Ask the Vocational Expert	262
11.1	Checklist for Selecting a Rehabilitation Counselor in Life Care Planning	277
11.2	Life Care Planning Questions Regarding Vocational Needs	278
11.3	Three Stages in the Occupational Choice Process	283

11.4	Development of Self-Concept and Formalized Vocational Development Stages	283
11.5	Developmental Tasks	284
11.6	Example Excerpts for Vocationally-Related Recommendations from a Life Care Plan	293
11.7	Sources of Information by Age Group for Earnings Capacity Opinion	298
12.1	Piaget's Stages of Development	324
14.1	Occupational Therapist Contributions to Life Care Plan Recommendations	376
15.1	Lumbar ROM	399
15.2	Lower Extremity Muscle Tests	399
15.3	PT Article Tables Adult	400
15.4	PT Tables Pediatric	404
16.1	ASHA Special Interest Groups (SIGs)	413
16.2	Comprehensive List of SLP Billing Resources	418
16.3	Risk Factors for Hearing Loss in Infants and Young Children	425
16.4	Birth to 24 Months: Red Flags	430
16.5	Cochlear Implant Candidacy Criteria	437
16.6	Comprehensive List of Audiology Billing Resources	441
17.1	Medicare Functional Classification Levels (MFCLs)/K Levels	477
18.1	Categories Used by Most Economists	486
18.2	Summary of the Yields on U.S. Treasury Bonds from November 2021 to April 2022	489
18.3	Life Care Plan for Mr. Doe	491
18.4	Economist's Present Value Table	493
19.1	Medical and Rehabilitation Progression of Amputation	507
19.2	Functional Expectations for the Below-Knee Amputee	509
19.3	Functional Expectations for the Above- and Below-Elbow Amputee	510
19.4	Advantages and Disadvantages of Various Upper Limb Prostheses	514
20.1	The Glasgow Coma Scale	540
20.2	Potential Cognitive Problems after TBI	546
20.3	Rancho Los Amigos Scale of Cognitive Functioning: Variable Outcomes Dependent on Nature and Severity of Injury	546
20.4	Neuropsychologist Questions	550
21.1	Complications Commonly Associated with Burn Injury	581
22.1	The Scope of Mental Health care Professionals in the Life Care Plan	632
22.2	Example Entries for a Life Care Plan for an individual with Schizophrenia	635
22.3	Life Care Plan Checklist for Mental Health	637
24.1	Life Care Cost Analysis	686
26.1	Etiology of Brachial Plexus Injuries	740
26.2	Patterns of Brachial Plexus Injuries	740
26.3	Practical Anatomy for Brachial Plexus Injury Pattern	741
26.4	Muscle Grading Chart	744
26.5	Active Movement Scale and Toronto Score	747
28.1	Admissibility Related Topics Checklist	806
33.1	Replacement Values	906

Contributors

David Altman, MD, CLCP is a physician specializing in neurology with an active clinical practice in San Antonio, Texas. Dr. Altman completed his undergraduate training at Brandeis University in 1992, after which he attended medical school at the University of Connecticut, receiving his medical degree in 1996. After completing his internship at Hartford Hospital in 1997, Dr. Altman completed his neurology residency at the University of Texas Health Science Center in San Antonio, Texas in 2000. He also completed a fellowship in Clinical Neurophysiology at Brown University in 2001 before returning to San Antonio to begin his clinical practice in neurology. Dr. Altman provides inpatient clinical services as a neuro-hospitalist for the Methodist Healthcare System. In this capacity, he provides neurology consultation services for diagnosis, emergency management and follow-up inpatient care of patients who have suffered stroke, brain injury, spinal cord injury, peripheral nerve injury, and other neurologic injuries or diseases in all departments at this Level I Trauma Center and Joint Commission Certified Stroke Center, as well as other hospitals within this system of care throughout south Texas. He has taken an active role in developing and building the stroke program for the Methodist Healthcare System. Dr. Altman has served as the Regional Neurology Advisor for the Warm Springs Healthcare System in San Antonio. He has also served as the Medical Director for Global Rehabilitation Hospital in San Antonio and partner with the Neurology Center of San Antonio, as well as the Neurology Director of Access Quality Therapy Services. In addition to his clinical neurology practice, Dr. Altman is a certified life care planner and provides life care planning services as a consultant with Rehabilitation Professional Consultants, Inc., in San Antonio.

Sim Ávila, JD is Deputy General Counsel at St. Luke's Health System in Boise, Idaho. Prior to joining the Legal Department at St. Luke's, Sim was Senior Counsel, Office of the General Counsel for Kaiser Permanente in Oakland, California. He was part of the Labor and Employment team and served as liaison counsel for Kaiser's Colorado and Northwest Regions. Among his duties, Sim advised human resources personnel and labor relations consultants on representational and labor relations issues pertaining to contracts with unions. He also counseled clients on preventative steps to avoid claims of negligent hiring, supervision and retention, claims of discrimination and harassment, (sex, sexual orientation, race, color, age, medical condition and disability, national origin, ancestry, religious creed, marital status), wrongful discharge, breaches of contract and implied covenants, employment compliance issues and immigration matters. Prior to joining Kaiser Permanente, Sim was labor and employment counsel for seven years in the Office of General Counsel, University of California. He was previously a partner with Littler Mendelson for 14 years where he represented private and public sector clients on nearly all aspects of employment and labor law. Sim lectured at Stanford University, Law School (Gould Center), at University of California – Boalt Hall and, more recently, at University of Idaho Law School on negotiations and ADR. Sim obtained his JD from the University of Santa Clara School of Law in 1983. Sim has presented on various subjects at professional conferences and speaks regularly on pertinent labor and employment issues dealing with the complexities of today's diverse work force. Sim co-authored a handbook entitled, *Terror and Violence in the Workplace* and was also a co-author in *A Litigator's Guide to Effective Use of ADR in California* published by Continuing Education of the Bar (CEB).

Kristi B. Bagnell, MD, FAAP, CLCP attended Indiana University School of Medicine and completed her pediatric residency at Indiana University Medical Center and James Whitcomb Riley Hospital for Children in 1995. She is board-certified by the American Board of Pediatrics. Dr. Bagnell has over 27 years of extensive private practice experience treating newborn through young adult patients in both inpatient and outpatient settings. She has participated on multiple boards and committees serving hospital and community needs and has given presentations on a variety of topics to numerous groups of professionals, parents, and children throughout her clinical years of practice. Dr. Bagnell is a certified life care planner and has developed a wide range of life care plans concerning individuals in the pediatric age group, from birth to 21 years. She has served on the Board of the International Academy of Life Care Planners (IALCP) and is actively involved in the promotion of education for life care planners. Dr. Bagnell presented at the annual IALCP Symposium and has published in the *Journal of Life Care Planning* regarding life care planning for persons diagnosed with autism spectrum disorder.

Dan Bagwell, RN, CCM, CDMS, CLCP is chief executive officer of Rehabilitation Professional Consultants, Inc. in San Antonio, Texas. Mr. Bagwell is a registered nurse, licensed in the state of Texas. He received a Bachelor of Science in Nursing in 1978 from the University of Mississippi School of Nursing. He is a certified life care planner, certified case manager, and certified disability management specialist. Mr. Bagwell provides adult and pediatric catastrophic case management and life care planning services for individuals in Texas and throughout the United States. His clinical nursing experience spans 42 years, 38 of which have been dedicated primarily to the rehabilitation field and medical case management. His clinical experience has also included critical care nursing and service as an officer in the United States Air Force Nurse Corps and Air Force Reserves. Mr. Bagwell completed the USAF Flight Nurse School in 1979 and performed duties as a medical crew director and flight nurse in Tactical Aeromedical Evacuation. He previously served as president and co-founder of Life Care Personal Living Centers and vice-president and co-founder of MediSys Rehabilitation, Inc. Mr. Bagwell has given presentations, lectures and symposiums concerning life care planning at regional, national and international conferences. He has authored and coauthored numerous peer-reviewed articles and textbook chapters in life care planning.

Mary Barros-Bailey, PhD, CRC, CLCP, NCC, ABVE/AE, CVE, CCC is a Multilingual Rehabilitation Counselor (Spanish/English/Portuguese), Vocational Expert, Life Care Planner, and principle with Intermountain Vocational Services, Inc. She is a practitioner-scientist with a national, sometimes international, caseload. Dr. Barros-Bailey is adjunct faculty at Capital University Law School's graduate certificate in life care planning and has taught with a variety of graduate programs in rehabilitation counseling. She serves as a peer reviewer or on editorial boards of peer-review publications, has presented over 200 times nationally and internationally, and authored over 130 publications such as a book, textbook chapters, and peer-reviewed journal articles. Recent awards are: Best Article, *The Advocate*, Idaho State/Idaho Bar Foundation, Inc. (2018); Alumni Achievement Award, Middlebury Institute of International Studies (2018); Outstanding Educator Award, Foundation for Life Care Planning Research (2017); and, Lifetime Achievement

Award, International Association of Rehabilitation Professionals (2016). Dr. Barros-Bailey is currently a Fulbright Specialist working with the largest rehabilitation counseling organization in Australia and rehabilitation counseling credentialing organization in the world to establish the first credential in forensic vocational rehabilitation in the southern hemisphere.

Debra E. Berens, PhD, CRC, CCM, CLCP is a nationally certified life care planner, case manager, and rehabilitation counselor with a nationwide consulting practice since 1989. Specializing in life care planning and rehabilitation consulting for both children and adults with catastrophic injuries and disabilities, Dr. Berens has authored or co-authored chapters in several texts including *Rehabilitation Consultants Handbook* (2012), *Brain Injury Medicine: Principles and Practice* (2007, 2012, 2021), *Manual of Traumatic Brain Injury* (2011, 2016, 2021), *Pediatric Life Care Planning and Case Management* (2004, 2011), and is a contributing author and co-editor of the third and fourth editions of the *Life Care Planning and Case Management Handbook* (2010, 2018). Having taught in the graduate Clinical Rehabilitation Counseling program at Georgia State University in Atlanta, Georgia for 23 years, Dr. Berens has written over 50 publications and is a frequent invited speaker at national, state, and local conferences in the areas of life care planning, rehabilitation consulting, rehabilitation ethics, and case management. She served on the Editorial Board of the peer-reviewed *Journal of Life Care Planning* from its inception in 2001 to 2011 and was a familiar face as moderator of the annual Life Care Planning Symposium for over 15 years. Dr. Berens served on the Board of Directors for the Foundation for Life Care Planning Research (FLCPR) from 2007 to 2020, serving as president from 2016 to 2020, and was instrumental in the successful affiliation of the Foundation with IARP where she continues to serve on the Board of the newly expanded Foundation for Life Care Planning and Rehabilitation Research (FLCPRR). In recognition of her service and leadership in the rehabilitation and life care planning professions, Dr. Berens is recipient of industry awards including the 2013 Lifetime Achievement Award in Life Care Planning, 2010 Outstanding Life Care Planning Educator Award, 2009 Chi Sigma Iota International Outstanding Practitioner Award, and the inaugural Paul Deutsch Professional Development Award presented in 2021 at the annual life care planning symposium.

Richard Paul Bonfiglio, MD is board certified by the American Board of Physical Medicine and Rehabilitation. Dr. Bonfiglio has previously served as the medical director of several nationally recognized rehabilitation facilities, including the Lake Erie Institute of Rehabilitation and the Bryn Mawr Rehabilitation Hospital. He has also maintained close academic ties, including having served as residency program director at the Schwab Rehabilitation Center. Dr. Bonfiglio's clinical practice within the field of physical medicine and rehabilitation has included providing care to children and adults with traumatic brain injuries, spinal cord injuries, amputations, and acute and chronic pain problems. He is an internationally recognized speaker on rehabilitation topics. Dr. Bonfiglio has been involved for years in the review and critical analysis of life care plans. His interests include the development of a strong medical foundation to enhance the accuracy and reliability of these plans. He is also an expert in life expectancy determinations for individuals following catastrophic illnesses and injuries. Historically, he was one of the five founders who designed the original multi-modules training program leading to certification and was a faculty member of the Rehabilitation Training Institute and MediPro Seminars for life care planning. Dr. Bonfiglio has sustained a strong clinical practice within the field of physical medicine and rehabilitation, providing care to children with a variety of physical and cognitive impairments, and children and adults with traumatic brain injuries, spinal cord injuries, amputations, and acute and chronic pain problems.

Sarah Brown, MS, OTR/L, BCP, CLCP is the founder and owner of Building Blocks Therapy, Inc. She received her Master's degree in Occupational Therapy from Colorado State University in 2002. In 2021, she earned her Board Certification in Pediatrics through the American Occupational Therapy Association. Sarah became a Certified Life Care Planner in 2019. She was designated as a member of the Editorial Board for both the *Journal of Life Care Planning* and *The Rehabilitation Professional*.

Diana Bubanja, DPT, CLCP, CFCE, CEAS is a Licensed Physical Therapist, a Certified Life Care Planner and Certified Functional Capacity Evaluator. She has owned and operated physical therapy clinics in Oakland and Richmond, California and possesses more than 30 years of experience in inpatient, outpatient, and home-based physical therapy, specializing in orthopedic and neurological physical rehabilitation. She earned her Doctorate in Physical Therapy at Boston Sargent University. Dr. Bubanja has acted as a retained expert in personal injury, medical malpractice, Workers' Compensation, Maritime, and Long-Term Disability cases involving Functional Capacity and Life Care Plan development. She has worked with attorneys and clients to provide Functional Capacity Evaluations and Life Care Plans for a wide range of injury conditions for both the plaintiff and defense. Dr. Bubanja has also provided expert witness services related to the Standards of Care in the field of Physical Therapy. Dr. Bubanja is a member of the American Physical Therapy Association and International Association of Rehabilitation Professionals.

Sandra Bullins, PhD, CRC is the Assistant Director for Student Accessibility and Accommodations at Piedmont Virginia Community College. She has a Master's degree in Rehabilitation Counseling, and a doctoral degree in Counselor Education; she completed a postdoctoral research fellowship at Virginia Commonwealth University. She has published multiple journal articles and book chapters and her chapter is informed by her lived experience as a blind person.

Jennifer Crowley, BSN, RN, CLCP, CADDCT, CDP, CMC is the founder of Eagleview West Life Care Planning. Jennifer completed training to become a Certified Life Care Planner in 2009. Jennifer diversified her life care planning practice to include life care management, helping individuals and their loved ones during life transitions. Jennifer published the guidebook *7 Steps to Long-term Care Planning* to help individuals and families design a roadmap for aging. Jennifer is also the co-author of *The Life Care Management Handbook*, a desk reference for care managers. She co-founded the Life Care Management Institute with colleague Shanna Huber in 2019. The Life Care Management Institute is an educational business that provides classes and membership to care managers in order to start and grow a successful care management practice. Jennifer has been a registered nurse for 29 years. Jennifer is a Certified Life Care Planner, Certified Alzheimer's Disease & Dementia Care Trainer, Certified Dementia Practitioner and Care Manager Certified.

Brenda Eagan-Johnson, EdD, CBIST has over two decades' experience in the field of pediatric brain injury and neurodevelopmental/special education issues. As a legal expert witness in pediatric acquired brain injury cases, she investigates pre/post injury changes and makes education/transition recommendations into adulthood. Dr. Eagan-Johnson is State Director of Pennsylvania's BrainSTEPS Brain Injury School Consulting Program (since 2007). She is also involved in multiple research projects and serves as a consultant for a CDC-funded study.

Timothy F. Field, PhD, a former educator in rehabilitation counseling at the University of Georgia, is Founder and President of Elliott and Fitzpatrick, Inc, a consulting and publishing company in Athens, GA. E & F produces resources (books, journals, and related materials) for the practicing forensic rehabilitation consultant and life care planner. Dr. Field has been a frequent conference speaker on forensic topics including transferable skills, estimating lost earning, admissible expert testimony, and the law, and more recently, the *Affordable Care Act*, collateral sources and implications for the life care planners. Dr. Field continues to author manuscripts and pamphlets related to the above topics.

Kevin N. Foster, MD, MBA, FACS is the Director of the Arizona Burn Center, and the Director of Surgical Research for Valleywise Medical Center. The Arizona Burn Center is the state's only nationally verified burn center, treating more than 5,000 children and adults each year with a survival rate of 97 percent. Dr. Foster is a graduate of the Medical College of Ohio at the University of Toledo Medical School. He completed a general surgery residency at the University of Wisconsin, followed by burn surgery and trauma research fellowships at the University of Washington. He also completed an MBA at the Indiana University School of Business. Dr. Foster has served on multiple committees for the American Burn Association and has been influential in acute burn care and surgery research nationally and internationally. He is also a professor of surgery at the University of Arizona and Creighton University Schools of Medicine.

Johnathan Goree, MD is an Associate Professor of Anesthesiology at the University of Arkansas for Medical Sciences where he is the Director of the Chronic Pain Division, Program Director of the Pain Medicine Fellowship, and Chief of Staff-Elect at UAMS Health. He completed medical school and anesthesia residency at the Weill College of Medicine at Cornell University and chronic pain medicine fellowship at Emory University. He joined the faculty at the University of Arkansas for Medical Sciences in 2014 where he continues to practice today. Dr. Goree considers himself a "quality of life" specialist who focuses on patient-led goals instead of pathology. He has published over 30 peer-reviewed manuscripts and given hundreds of national and international lectures. His research interests include novel implantable technologies for complex pain care, implementation of chronic pain education, racial disparities in chronic pain care, and complex regional pain syndrome.

Shanna Huber, MSN/Ed, BSN, RN, CCM, CMC, CLCP, CNLCP is the founder of Ripple Life Care Planning providing care management, helping seniors and their loved ones during life transitions, and life care planning services. Shanna had a need for a client management system for her business and developed software to track clients, time, invoicing and resources. She began selling her software, My Junna, to other businesses in 2018 and it is now nationwide. My Junna helps other professionals efficiently run their small businesses. Shanna is the co-author of the *Life Care Management Handbook*, a desk reference for care managers. She is also the co-founder of the Life Care Management Institute, an educational business that provides classes and memberships to care managers in order to help start and grow a successful care management practice. Shanna has been a registered nurse for 25 years. Shanna is a Certified Case Manager (CCM), Certified Life Care Planner, and Care Manager Certified.

Carrie Hyde, MD attended the University of Arkansas for Medical Sciences, completed Internal Medicine Residency, and Hospice and Palliative Care fellowship there also. She is board certified by the American Board of Internal Medicine as well as Hospice and Palliative Medicine. During her academic career, she decided to pursue acupuncture training and completed the Medical Acupuncture for Physicians course through Helms Medical Institute in Berkeley California. She now works in corporate medicine for a startup company, developing and providing palliative telemedicine services to chronic kidney disease patients across the United States. She continues to see and provide acupuncture services to her local community, focusing on holistic wellness for her patients. She actively lectures on topics about pain, communication, and complementary therapies at regional and national levels.

Jaleesa Jackson, MD attended medical school at the Johns Hopkins University School of Medicine. She then completed an anesthesiology residency and interventional pain fellowship at Harvard Medical School/Massachusetts General Hospital program. She is board certified by the American Board of Anesthesiology. She is an assistant professor at the University of Arkansas for Medical Sciences, where she also serves as the director of Diversity, Equity, and Inclusion for the Department of Anesthesia.

Scott H. Kozin, MD is currently the chief of staff at Shriners Children's Philadelphia. Dr. Kozin graduated from Duke University in 1982 with a degree in computer science, medical school at Hahnemann University in Philadelphia, and an orthopedic residency at Albert Einstein Medical Center. In 1992, he completed a fellowship at the Mayo Clinic focusing on hand and microvascular surgery. Dr. Kozin cared for both adults and children until 2000, when he devoted his practice and research to children at Shriners Children's Philadelphia. Since that time, Dr. Kozin has been an advocate for improving the lives of children via research, education and patient care. He has published over 100 peer-reviewed papers, mainly on the care of children with various diagnoses, including brachial plexus injury, spinal cord injury and congenital differences. He routinely travels to developing countries to operate on children in need. Dr. Kozin received the Weiland Metal from the American Society for Surgery of the Hand in 2010, which honors a hand surgeon/scientist who has contributed a body of research that advances the field.

Sherry A. Latham, BSN, RN, CLCP, MSCC, CNLCP, FIALCP is the founder of Oklahoma Medical Legal Consulting Services LLC, which transitioned to Sherry Latham & Associates in 2019. She is an experienced Certified Life Care Planner and Certified Nurse Life Care Planner (CNLCP). Ms. Latham was designated a Fellow of International Academy of Life Care Planners, (FIALCP), in June of 2019. She serves on the International Academy of Life Care Planners Advisory Committee for the Standards of Life Care Planning. Ms. Latham began teaching as Adjunct Faculty for Capital Law School Life Care Planning Program in 2018. She was designated as a member of the Editorial Board for both the *Journal of Life Care Planning* and *The Rehabilitation Professional*. Ms. Latham served as a Commissioner of the Certified Life Care Planner Board of the International Commission on Health Care Certification (ICHCC™) from 2007 to 2019. She served as Chair of ICHCC™ of the CLCP Board of Commissioners, as well as the Executive Board of the ICHCC™ from 2015 to 2019.

Margaret Lockovich, MA, CCC/SLP, CLCP, CBIS is a Speech Language Pathologist and Certified Brain Injury Specialist with over 20 years of experience working with children with disabilities. Maggie holds a certificate as Special Education Supervisor in Pennsylvania and has administered education programs in public schools including Early Intervention, Hearing Impaired, and Speech Therapy. Maggie is a team facilitator for BrainSTEPS. Maggie earned her Certified Life Care Planner credential and is owner of Lockovich Life Care, LLC.

Aubrey Lyon, JD is an attorney with St. Luke's Health System, Ltd. in Boise, Idaho. His practice with St. Luke's focuses on general litigation and health care regulation. Prior to joining St. Luke's,

Aubrey spent more than ten years in a litigation practice primarily involving professional liability defense, insurance law, and transportation liability matters. Aubrey is a member of the Idaho and Oregon State Bars and while in private practice was selected as a Super Lawyers Mountain States Rising Star. Aubrey attended undergraduate school at Lewis & Clark College in Portland, Oregon. Between college and law school, Aubrey worked with a Taiwanese trading company sourcing bicycles and parts for European and American clients and ran a bicycle distribution business in Portland, Oregon. Aubrey graduated from Lewis & Clark Law School in 2009.

Sarah Malloy, MS, OTR, CCM, CLCP is the owner of Malloy Life Care Planning based in Massachusetts. She obtained her Bachelor of Science degree in occupational therapy from University of Western Ontario in London, Ontario and her Master of Science in occupational therapy through Mount Mary University. She holds certifications as a Certified Life Care Planner, Certified Case Manager, and an occupational therapist. Ms. Malloy is an active member in the International Association of Rehabilitation Professionals, the New England Chapter of the International Association of Rehabilitation Professionals, the International Academy of Life Care Planners as well as the American Occupational Therapy Association.

Debbe Marcinko, BSN, RN, MA, CRRN, CCM, CRC, CLCP, CNLCP, LPC is a rehabilitation nurse, case manager, and life care planner located in Pittsburgh, PA providing adult and pediatric catastrophic case management and life care planning. She is a registered nurse licensed to practice in Pennsylvania and Ohio. She received her Bachelor of Science in nursing, and Master of Arts in rehabilitation counseling. She is a Certified Rehabilitation Registered Nurse, Certified Life Care Planner, Certified Nurse Life Care Planner, Certified Case Manager, Certified Rehabilitation Counselor, and Licensed Professional Counselor. Her clinical nursing experience spanning over 45 years includes general nursing practice, critical care, long-term care and administration, school nursing, private case management, U.S. Department of Labor Office of Worker's Compensation field nursing, and life care planning. She is active in several professional organizations and has held offices in the Association of Rehabilitation Nurses and International Association of Rehabilitation Professionals and International Academy of Life Care Planners. She has published and presented on case management and life care planning. She was awarded the International Association of Rehabilitation Professionals' President's Commendation in 2015, and the International Academy of Life Care Planners' Sheri Jasper Award in 2017. She is currently serving as President of the Foundation for Life Care Planning and Rehabilitation Research.

Irmo Marini, PhD, CRC, CLCP is a professor in the School of Rehabilitation at the University of Texas- Rio Grande Valley in Edinburg Texas. Dr. Marini has been involved in forensic rehabilitation consulting as well as in academe for 27+ years. In that time, he has published over 100 peer-reviewed journal articles, completed eight books, and 70+ book chapters. He is the former Chair of the Commission on Rehabilitation Counselor Certification, and former president of the American Rehabilitation Counseling Association. Dr. Marini has won numerous University in national awards in teaching and research, including three distinguished career awards from various national associations.

Christian D. Meier, CPO received his BA in Integrative Physiology from University of Colorado, Boulder and subsequently earned a postgraduate certificate from California State University Dominguez Hills in 2011. He has 11 years of experience working as a Prosthetist/Orthotist and is affiliated with Achilles Prosthetics & Orthotics.

Robert H. Meier, III, MD is a physiatrist who has practiced in the Specialty of Physical Medicine and Rehabilitation for more than 50 years. He completed his medical school and residency training in Physical Medicine and Rehabilitation at the Temple University School of Medicine in Philadelphia, Pennsylvania. Dr. Meier began his professional career at the Institute for Rehabilitation and Research (TIRR) and at the Baylor College of Medicine in 1973 where he provided comprehensive rehabilitation services for persons with spinal cord injury, amputation, burn injury, and brachial plexus injuries. He moved to Denver, Colorado and the University of Colorado Health Sciences Center in 1986. He was Chairman of the Department of Rehabilitation Medicine until 1996. He has served as the President of both the American Congress of Rehabilitation Medicine and the Association of Academic Physiatrists. In 1996, he entered private practice to concentrate on developing a comprehensive center of excellence for persons with amputations, now called the Amputee Services of America. In 2005, he moved his practice to the Presbyterian/St. Luke's Medical Center in Denver to focus on the rehabilitation needs of complex limb dysfunction including amputation nerve injury, burns and tumors. He is the physiatric consultant for the Institute for Limb Preservation that deals with complex extremity injuries, vascular problems and tumors that threaten the function of an extremity. In this setting, he has every level and type of rehabilitation, acute medical and surgical service that a person would need to regain function of a threatened or damaged extremity. During his extensive career, Dr. Meier has provided comprehensive rehabilitation services for over 4,000 adults and children with amputations and limb deficiencies. Dr. Meier has also been involved with life care planning for persons with amputation, burns and neurologic injury. He actively participated in the teaching of Life Care Planners and in their summit meetings for education and development of the field of Life Care Planning. In the past, Dr. Meier has been a surveyor for the Commission on the Accreditation of Rehabilitation Facilities and, in 2011, he became a Paradigm Medical Director for Amputee Care. In March 2012, Dr. Meier was the President of the Active Medical Staff for the Spalding Rehabilitation Hospital, a CARF-accredited facility in Denver, Colorado.

Aaron Mertes, PhD, CRC, CLCP, IPEC, PCLC served as chair of the International Academy of Life Care Planners and is also the editor-in-chief of the *Journal of Life Care Planning*. He has worked with people with disabilities in independent living, special education, job coaching, higher education, workers' compensation, and career placement for over 18 years. He has also provided mental health counseling services in private practice, as a community crisis counselor, in an inpatient psychiatric facility, and outpatient day treatment. He received his PhD in Counselor Education and Supervision from the University of Iowa in 2019 and is a professor at Montana State University Billings in the Rehabilitation and Mental Health Counseling program. He was awarded a faculty excellence award in 2020 and has served in various supportive leadership roles to the Commission on Rehabilitation Counseling Certification.

Alexander Amit Missner, BS is a medical student in the class of 2025 at Georgetown University School of Medicine. Mr. Missner earned a Bachelor of Science in neurobiology from Georgetown University where he graduated as a Sweeny Scholar and earned the distinction of Summa Cum Laude. During his undergraduate education, he performed research and gained clinical experience in the Department of Neurology at Georgetown University Medical Center. His research was in the Laboratory for Dementia and Parkinsonism where he studied novel therapeutics for Parkinson's disease, and he has published in this field.

Shani Cohen Missner, MD, PhD, LMSW, CLCP's main areas of practice are in life care planning and psychotherapy. She works in private practice where she serves as an expert witness in life care planning on numerous complex health care needs and injuries. She completed the life care planning certification through the University of Florida. Dr. Missner also works as a psychotherapist for children, adolescents, and adults with various mental health needs. Dr. Missner integrates her current work with medical and pharmacological understanding for the personalized care of each client. She earned her LMSW from the Catholic University of America, her PhD in Pharmacology from Georgetown University, and her MD from Georgetown University School of Medicine. She has performed research and published in the fields of life care planning, drug development, and medicine.

Elizabeth Moberg-Wolff, MD, FAAPMR attended the University of Wisconsin Medical School, completed the Physical Medicine & Rehabilitation (PM&R) residency at the Medical College of Wisconsin, and then a Pediatric PM&R fellowship at the University of Colorado Children's Hospital. She is board certified by the American Board of Physical Medicine & Rehabilitation, as well as in Pediatric Rehabilitation Medicine and Brain Injury Medicine. After practicing in academic medicine for over 20 years, Dr. Moberg-Wolff has practiced independently for the last decade, which has allowed her to follow her patients into adulthood. She has served in a variety of leadership positions for the American Academy of Physical Medicine & Rehabilitation, actively lectures nationally, and teaches medical and therapy students. She also volunteers on several boards of local non-profit organizations serving children with disabilities. Dr. Moberg-Wolff has been assisting in preparing life care plans for both adults and pediatric patients for 20 years.

Stephen L. Nelson, MD, PhD is a triple board-certified pediatric neurologist with more than 15 years of experience. He holds board certifications from the American Board of Psychiatry and Neurology in epilepsy and neurology, and in general pediatrics from the American Board of Pediatrics. Dr. Nelson is widely published and a member of more than dozen professional medical associations. He has been the recipient of numerous honors and awards throughout his distinguished career. In addition to this practice as a pediatric neurologist, Dr. Nelson is a subject matter expert, educator, and consultant in the fields of child neurology, adult neurology, psychiatry, pediatrics and epilepsy.

Ann T. Neulicht, PhD, CRC, CLCP, CVE, CDMS, LCMHC, ABVE/D earned her doctorate in Rehabilitation Research and has worked in private sector rehabilitation for over 38 years. Based in Raleigh NC, her nationwide consulting practice focuses on Life Care Planning, Vocational/Earnings Capacity Assessment, Labor Market Analysis, and Case Management. She has been a Vocational Expert for the Social Security Administration since 1990 and has qualified as a Rehabilitation and/or Life Care Planning Expert in multiple court settings. Dr. Neulicht has held multiple leadership positions within the International Association of Rehabilitation Professionals (IARP) and the Commission on Rehabilitation Counselor Certification (CRCC). She is a principal investigator for the Life Care Plan Surveys (2001, 2009, 2022) and Labor Market Research Survey (2006). Dr. Neulicht is the recipient of the Lifetime Achievement Award (2021, International Academy of Life Care Planners), Outstanding Life Care Planning Educator Award (2016, Foundation for Life Care Planning Research), and Outstanding Individual Professional Member Award (2004, IARP). She also received the 1995 Distinguished Service and Harley B. Reger Awards from the National Rehabilitation Counseling Association for her research contributions, creative activity, dedication to consumers, and commitment to professional organizations. Her interest in ethics and rehabilitation/life care plan protocols has led to multiple publications and presentations at local, regional, and national conferences.

LeRoy Oddie, CP, MBA, CLCP is a Certified Prosthetist and Certified Life Care Planner. Since the age of 19, Oddie has served amputees as a clinician, researcher, technician, and prosthetic consultant. Oddie is a published author of numerous chapters and has traveled to over 20 countries as a prosthetic expert and invited speaker. Mr. Oddie is a guest lecturer of the life care planning program at Capital University.

Karen Preston, PHN, MS, CRRN, FIALCP, FARN is owner of RNS HealthCare Consultants, a consulting company providing case management, life care planning, education, and consulting services. Her clinical background is in rehabilitation, including spinal cord injury and brain injury. She has experience as a practicing clinician in acute care and home care settings. Currently she focuses on case management and life care planning for catastrophic pediatric and adult cases. She teaches case management and life care planning in the Masters of Nursing program at Samuel Merritt University. She is past-President of the Association of Rehabilitation Nurses. She is past-Chairperson of the International Academy of Life Care Planners. She is past-President of Association of Workers' Compensation Professionals. She has published in peer-reviewed journals and regularly presents at various conferences. She is on the editorial board of the *Journal of Life Care Planning*. She was the chairperson of the Standards of Practice for Life Care Planners revision committee for the third and fourth editions. She is a certified rehabilitation nurse, Fellow of the Association of Rehabilitation Nurses, and Fellow of the International Academy of Life Care Planners. She was awarded the Lifetime Achievement Award for the Foundation for Life Care Planning and Research in 2014, the Distinguished Service Award for the Association of Rehabilitation Nurses in 2022, and the Lifetime Achievement Award for the International Association of Rehabilitation Professionals in 2022.

Frederick A. Raffa, PhD and **Matthew B. Raffa**, PhD have been engaged as forensic economists for a combined 75 years. Both father (Fred) and son (Matt) obtained their PhDs in Economics from Florida State University, and both taught at the University of Central Florida prior to entering the forensic economic consulting field. Together, the Raffas head up the firm Raffa Consulting Economists (RCE), a ten-person firm that specializes in forensic economic consulting. RCE evaluates the present value of over 200 life care plans per year for both the plaintiff and the defendant. Fred Raffa is the author of three volumes of the Lexis-Nexis Damages in Tort Actions series, titled *Evaluation and Proof of Economic Loss*.

Christine Reid, PhD, CRC, CLCP, LAP is a Full Professor at Virginia Commonwealth University, in the Rehabilitation and Mental Health Counseling Department. She also maintains a private practice in life care planning, vocational analysis, and research consultation. Dr. Reid has over 30 years of experience as an educator, researcher, and service provider. She has served as project director for multiple training grants for the US Rehabilitation Services Administration, and as an affiliate of Helen Keller National Center. Dr. Reid has served on journal editorial boards and in leadership roles for several national organizations, including the Commission on Rehabilitation Counselor Certification, Council on Rehabilitation Education, and Foundation for Life Care Planning Research. She is a past-president and fellow of the National Rehabilitation Counseling Association and was presented a Lifetime Achievement Award by the sponsoring organizations of the International Symposium on Life Care Planning.

Ruth B. Rimmer, PhD, CLCP is President & CEO of Care Plans for Life and has been working in the field of burn injury for over 28 years. She received her PhD in Lifespan Developmental

Psychology and a Certification in Gerontology from Arizona State University. During her tenure at the Arizona Burn Center at Valleywise she served as the Family Service Director and as the Director of Psycho/Social and Prevention Research. Dr. Rimmer was responsible for assisting victims and their families with their rehabilitative needs. She also developed multiple research protocols and published and lectured regarding the psycho/social and pain management issues of burn injury on a national and international level. She continues to do pro bono research in these areas. Rimmer has been providing life care plans for pediatric and adult burn, electrical, amputation, and polytrauma-injured individuals for the past 19 years and has authored and lectured extensively on the critical aspects of burn and electrical injury recovery. Dr. Rimmer is fluent in Spanish.

David L. Ripley, MD, MS, CRC, FAAPM&R is Chief Medical Officer of HealthBridge Complex Care & Rehabilitation. He has been actively involved in the care of persons with brain and spinal cord injuries for over 20 years. He holds an academic appointment as Adjunct Associate Professor in the Department of Physical Medicine & Rehabilitation at Northwestern University's Feinberg School of Medicine. He is board certified in Physical Medicine and Rehabilitation and Brain Injury Medicine. He is a fellow of the American Academy of Physical Medicine and Rehabilitation. Prior to entering medical school, Dr. Ripley worked as a vocational rehabilitation counselor.

Rick H. Robinson, PhD, MBA, LMHC, CRC, D-ABVE, CLCP has nearly 30 years' work experience in various vocational & disability settings. He has extensive experience as an expert in both civil and administrative settings, having provided expert testimony in several hundred hearings, trials and depositions related to vocational rehabilitation and life care planning issues. Dr. Robinson is nationally credentialed in rehabilitation counseling, vocational evaluation and life care planning. He is state licensed in Florida as a Mental Health Counselor. He is board certified by the National Board for Certified Counselors and as a Diplomate by the American Board of Vocational Experts. He holds doctoral a degree in Rehabilitation Science from the University of Florida. His research focus is on forensic rehabilitation analysis methodologies and models. He is the president of Robinson Work Rehabilitation Services, Co., a private vocational, life care planning, and rehabilitation consulting firm in Jacksonville, FL. He formerly held academic appointments at Florida State College at Jacksonville and in the college of public health and health professions at the University of Florida.

Liesl Rose, RN is the owner of Rosebud Consulting LLC, an independent case management firm assisting insurers, attorneys and accountable organizations with providing care to catastrophically injured workers. Drawing on her years as an emergency department nurse in Level I trauma centers of excellence, she has expertise working with acquired brain injury, spinal cord, injury, burns, multiple trauma and amputations. She collaborates with employers and insurance carriers to facilitate medical rehabilitation, improved function and an improved quality of life. Her practice is located in Greenwood Village, Colorado.

Benjamin (Benji) Rubin, JD graduated from the University of Illinois College of Law, Magna Cum Laude, received his undergraduate degree in Economics from Northwestern University, and his Graduate Law Degree, an LLM (Tax), with honors, also from Northwestern University. Benji is a member of the national Board of Directors of the Special Needs Alliance, the national, non-profit, association of experienced special needs planning attorneys (membership is by invitation only), is Vice-Chair, American Bar Association Elder Law and Special Needs Planning, Prior

Chairman of the American Bar Association Special Needs Planning Committee, serves as the President of SIBS (Supporting Illinois Brothers and Sisters), the Illinois chapter of the national Sibling Leadership Network, an organization of adult siblings of individuals with intellectual disabilities, developmental disabilities and/or mental illness. Benji is also a member of the board of directors of SEDOL Foundation (the Special Education District of Lake County), as well as the board of directors for NSSRA Foundation (Northern Suburban Special Recreation Association). Benji is also a Faculty Member for the Illinois Institute for Continuing Legal Education on the topic of special needs planning, as well as a Speaker for the American Bar Association and the Illinois State Bar Association on those topics. Having Mitchell as a brother profoundly shaped who Benji is today, and thus the type of law he chose to practice. His firsthand experiences as a sibling offer a unique perspective into the responsibilities that come with caring for a sibling with special needs. Now as an adult, those sometimes present and future responsibilities he has regarding his brother's care are a concern that he shares with all brothers and sisters of individuals with special needs.

Tanya Rutherford-Owen, PhD, CRC, CLCP, CDMS, LPC, FIALCP is a certified rehabilitation counselor, certified life care planner, and life care planning fellow. She has over 25 years of experience providing rehabilitation services and forensic work in various states. She has served as an adjunct professor at the University of Arkansas in the Department of Rehabilitation Education and Research and is currently an adjunct faculty member of Capital University Law School. She has served on the Board of Directors for the Foundation for Life Care Planning & Rehabilitation Research and served as a work group member in the development of the fourth edition of the Standards of Practice for Life Care Planners. She has independently researched and published articles in peer-reviewed journals including *Journal of Life Care Planning, The Rehabilitation Professional* and the *Journal of Rehabilitation*. She worked as the editor of the *Journal of Life Care Planning* from 2016 to 2020, prior to assuming the managing editor role for both the *Journal of Life Care Planning* and *The Rehabilitation Professional*. Dr. Owen earned a PhD in Rehabilitation in 2011 and a Master's degree in Counseling Psychology in 1996. In 1993, she graduated Magna Cum Laude and Phi Beta Kappa from Millsaps College. She has provided testimony in various state and federal courts and in Social Security disability adjudication hearings for 20 years. In the course of her work, she has received various awards including the Sherry Jasper Memorial Award (2022) from the Foundation for Life Care Planning & Rehabilitation Research; Outstanding Life Care Planning Educator Award (2018); a President's Commendation Award from the International Association of Rehabilitation Professionals (IARP, 2017 & 2018); Best Student Paper Award by the Foundation for Life Care Planning Research & International Academy of Life Care Planners (2011); the Outstanding Rehabilitation Education & Research Doctoral Student at the University of Arkansas (2010); the Russell Baxter Award at the University of Arkansas (2010–2011); and was a Doctoral Academy Fellow at the University of Arkansas (2009–2011).

Jarna Shah, MD is an assistant professor in the division of anesthesiology and pain medicine at the University of Arkansas Medical Sciences in Little Rock. She is a board certified anesthesiologist and interventional pain physician. She completed her bachelors, medical degree, and anesthesiology residency at the University of Illinois at Chicago. Dr. Shah then completed her fellowship in interventional pain medicine at Johns Hopkins in Baltimore, MD. She has authored a number of peer-reviewed publications and book chapters, and her research interests are focused on neuromodulation, medical education, and obstetric-related chronic pain.

Gregory Lawson Smith, MD attended the University of Arkansas Medical School (UAMS), completed an Anesthesiology residency at UAMS, and then a Pain Fellowship at the UAMS. He is double board certified by the American Board of Anesthesiology in Anesthesiology and Pain Medicine. He currently is an Assistant Professor at UAMS where he works to develop treatment plans for patients with chronic pain. He has special research interests in neuromodulation and peripheral nerve stimulation. He is actively involved in the education of medical students, residents, and fellows. He is actively involved as a member of the Opioid Stewardship Committee at UAMS.

Bruce H. Stern is certified as a Certified Civil Trial Attorney by both the New Jersey Supreme Court and the National Board of Trial Advocacy. Mr. Stern specializes his practice in representing the victims of traumatic brain and spinal cord injuries and wrongful death. In July 2004, Bruce began publishing the *Traumatic Brain Injury Law* blog as a way to share his knowledge as a brain injury lawyer. Additionally, he is the author of numerous articles and a frequent lecturer on the subject of traumatic brain injury litigation, evidence and trial techniques. He also co-authored a book entitled *Litigating Brain Injuries* published by Thomson Reuters and a chapter entitled "Brain Injuries" which is included in AAJ's Litigation Tort Case Series, published by AAJ Press. Bruce served as the President of the American Association for Justice (AAJ) from 2019 to 2020. He is a past chair of the Traumatic Brain Injury Litigation Group and a past chair of AAJ's Motor Vehicle Collision, Highway and Premises Section. Bruce is a past president of the New Jersey Association for Justice (formerly ATLA-NJ) and recipient of its highest award, the Gold Medal for Distinguished Service and the NJAJ Gerald B. O'Conner Award for Trial Skill. He is also a fellow of the International Academy of Trial Lawyers and has been selected a fellow in the International Society of Barristers. He is the Treasurer of the International Brain Injury Association and the North American Brain Injury Society. He has been listed in Best Lawyers in America 2003–2023.

Amy M. Sutton, PhD, RN, BSN, MA, CLCP is a certified life care planner and counseling psychologist in private practice. She has her doctorate in counseling psychology from Georgia State University, has received two bachelor's degrees in psychology and nursing from Purdue University and Indiana University and a Master's degree in psychology from Ludwig Maximillian's University in Munich, Germany. Amy lived and worked as a home health nurse in Germany for four years. During her graduate studies in Germany, Amy conducted a six-week internship/research project in South Africa on AIDS education in the public school system. During her graduate studies in Georgia, Amy published several articles and textbook chapters in life care planning as well as publishing the first life care plan validation study. As a registered nurse, Amy has worked in pediatric critical care, pediatric and adult home health, and inpatient pediatric rehabilitation. Amy is currently working as a life care planner in southern California.

Amy Thompson, MS, OTR/L, BCP, CLCP is the owner of Momentum Life Care Planning, based in Rapid City, SD, and a practicing occupational therapist in local school districts. She received her Bachelor of Science degree in Occupational Therapy from St Louis University in 1997 and her Master of Science degree in Rehabilitation Sciences from the University of Oklahoma Health Sciences Center in 2008. Ms. Thompson became a Certified Life Care Planner in 2019 and earned her board certification in Pediatrics from the American Occupational Therapy Association in 2022.

Chiedozie Uwandu, MD is a graduate of the Johns Hopkins University School of Medicine. He completed an Anesthesiology residency and fellowship in Interventional Pain at Harvard Medical School/Beth Israel Deaconess Medical Center. He is board certified by the American Board of Anesthesiology. He is currently in private practice in Little Rock, Arkansas.

Laura Villarreal, MS, CRC is a PhD student in Rehabilitation Counseling at the University of Texas at Rio Grande Valley. She is a Certified Rehabilitation Counselor and currently works as an ADA Accommodation Specialist for Sedgwick. She is also a research and teaching assistant at the university. She has a special interest in forensic rehabilitation work and has provided consulting work as a rehabilitation expert in litigated cases involving personal injury for over five years.

Carol Walker, PhD, ABPP-CN, CLCP completed her PhD in Clinical/Medical Psychology at the University of Alabama at Birmingham mentored by Thomas J. Boll, PhD, ABPP, who is a nationally recognized leader in the field of Neuropsychology. Her primary interests in her graduate training were Neuropsychology, Chronic Pain, and Cardiovascular Disease. Dr. Walker completed an internship at the Medical College of Georgia in Augusta, Georgia, where she received specialized training in Post-Traumatic Stress Disorder. Her postdoctoral training was completed in an acute rehabilitation hospital setting under the supervision of Dr. Boll. Dr. Walker is Board Certified in Clinical Neuropsychology by the American Board of Professional Psychology. She received specialized training in Life Care Planning from the University of Florida/Intelicus, which is known as the most extensive and comprehensive training program for life care planning in the nation. She is a Certified Life Care Planner, and past board member of the Foundation for Life Care Planning Research. She has 27 years of combined experience as a clinician treating patients with Traumatic Brain Injury, Spinal Cord Injury, and other catastrophic injuries in an acute rehab setting and currently in full-time private practice. She also provides treatment to patients suffering from Cardiovascular Accidents, Alzheimer's Disease, and other neurological conditions. Dr. Walker also has an active Chronic Pain Program and furnishes Independent Medical Examinations for patients, insurance companies, and attorneys. She has given numerous invited lectures to a variety of audiences in professional communities locally and nationally. She is also a lecturer for the University of Florida's online life care planning curriculum, offering specialized expertise to life care planners in the University of Florida's online training program; proceeds of which Dr. Walker donates to the Foundation for Life Care Planning Research.

Roger O. Weed, Professor Emeritus, and Fellow Emeritus, International Academy of Life Care Planning, is retired as professor and graduate rehabilitation counseling coordinator at Georgia State University. He also held doctoral student graduate faculty status in Counseling Psychology as well as Counselor Education and Practice doctoral programs. He has authored or co-authored approximately 200 books, reviews, articles, and book chapters, more than 80 of which were specific to life care planning. Prior to achieving the PhD, Dr. Weed practiced rehabilitation counseling and consulting for 15 years in Alaska. During his more than 42 years in the profession, Dr. Weed was honored several times for his work including the Distinguished Professor Award (2006) from Georgia State University's Alumni Association (sole recipient), Lifetime Appreciation Award from the International Commission on Health Care Certification (2011), Larry Huggins Lifetime Achievement Award (2009) from the Private Rehabilitation Specialists of Georgia, Lifetime Achievement Award (2005), from the sponsors of the International Life Care Planning Conference, Lifetime Achievement Award from the International Association of Rehabilitation

Professionals (2004) (as well as recognition in 1997 and 1991 as the Outstanding Educator), the National Professional Services Award from the American Rehabilitation Counseling Association (1993), and Research Excellence Award (2003) from the College of Education at Georgia State University. Dr. Weed is the creator and senior editor for the first four editions of the *Life Care Planning and Case Management Handbook*. He is one of the five founders of the original, nationwide training program leading to life care planning certification. He is also past-chair of the Georgia State Licensing Board for professional counselors, marriage and family therapists, and social workers, as well as past-president of the International Association of Rehabilitation Professionals.

Carolyn Wiles Higdon, PhD, CCC-SLP owns and operates a national/international private practice in assistive technology and speech-language pathology services, based in Georgia, licensed in multiple states. Her practice includes assistive technology for all ages, as well as educational consulting, forensics and life care planning, catastrophic health care of acquired brain injury and trach- and ventilator-dependent patients, tele-practice/tele-supervision and mediation and legal consulting. Dr. Higdon testifies as an expert witness in all areas of communication sciences and disorders (hearing, speech, language, swallowing, technology) for all ages, is a past chair of the Georgia Board of Examiners for Speech Pathology and Audiology, and is a past chair of Special Interest Group 12 of American Speech-Language-Hearing Association (ASHA), the AAC SIG. Dr. Higdon is a Fellow of the ASHA, a Fellow of the National Academies of Practice, is active in multiple professional organizations, and has taught/consulted in Russia, eastern Europe, Hong Kong, China, Costa Rica, Kenya, Guyana and Thailand. Dr. Higdon is an ASHA consultant to the American Medical Association in the areas of augmentative and alternative communication and current procedural terminology codes. Dr. Higdon is the past chair of the Department of Communicative Disorders and the past director of the Center for Speech and Hearing Research in the School of Applied Sciences at the University of Mississippi (Oxford, MS), and is an adjunct clinical associate professor at the University of Mississippi Medical Center in Jackson, MS. Dr. Higdon is a past Vice President of Finances on the American Speech-Language and Hearing Association's Board of Directors (2011–2014), has received the Mississippi Speech and Hearing (MSHA) Honors of the Association with recognition as MSHA Clinician of the Year in 2017. She teaches to the PAHO/ASHA CSD Program in Guyana. Dr. Higdon is active in developing universal licensure for speech-language pathology and audiology, is past Chair of the Council of Academic Programs Committee on Inter-Professional Practice and Inter-Professional Education and is currently on the American Board of AAC, to establish specialty credentialing in AAC. She has extensive experience in accreditation as well as working with several accreditation agencies. Dr. Higdon's publications and research are directed to technology, neurogenics, and telehealth. She is the recipient of the ASHA 2022 Certificate for Outstanding Contributions in International Achievement.

Mona Goldman Yudkoff, BSN, MPH, CRRN, CCM, CLCP received a bachelor's degree in nursing from the University of Pennsylvania in 1971 and a master's in public health from Hebrew University in Jerusalem in 1978. She has taken numerous continuing education courses and has achieved certification in rehabilitation nursing, case management, and life care planning. Ms. Yudkoff has more than 35 years of pediatric and rehabilitation nursing experience, including three years as the assistant director of nursing at Children's Seashore House in Philadelphia, Pennsylvania. Mona Yudkoff Rehab Consultants, established in 1989, offers private case management services for catastrophically injured clients and provides life care plans for both plaintiff and defense law firms. Ms. Yudkoff has authored more than 2,500 life care plans. She has testified in more than 500 trials and depositions in more than 20 states. She is a nationally recognized leader in the field of life care planning. She has authored chapters on life care planning in two textbooks and has been invited to speak about this to healthcare providers, parent groups, and attorneys. Ms. Yudkoff was a founding member of the Philadelphia Chapter of the American Association of Legal Nurse Consultants and has served as president and treasurer of that chapter.

Foreword

Life Care Planning and Case Management Across the Lifespan is the first text to address the medical, social, vocational, and financial challenges faced by children and adults with disabilities. Editors Drs. Rutherford-Owen, Barros-Bailey, and Weed have successfully brought together contributions in medicine, research, life care planning, case management, and ethics to discuss the wide-ranging issues that impact people with disabilities throughout their lives.

Since its initial publication in 1999, *Life Care Planning and Case Management Handbook*, created and edited by Dr. Roger Weed, has been used as a textbook by students and practitioners in various disciplines entering the specialty practice of life care planning. It has also served as a professional reference for life care planners, attorneys, and trust managers. The fourth edition in 2018 provided the most recent updates to aid life care planners in adult plan development.

As a young professional coming into the field of life care planning in the 1980s, I was highly motivated by the vision and mission of helping improve the lives of people with disabilities. The field of life care planning met that need, and I was privileged to be mentored by Drs. Paul Deutsch and Roger Weed. With their support and guidance, I went on to become a writer, lecturer, and teacher in the field of life care planning. With their encouragement, I created and edited the first book (two editions) addressing pediatric life care planning issues. *Pediatric Life Care Planning and Case Management* (2004, 2011) provided a comprehensive overview of the essential issues in care coordination and case management for children with disabilities.

Life Care Planning and Case Management Across the Lifespan combines adult and pediatric chapters by bringing together authors with specialized knowledge and experiences in pediatric and adult planning.

The first six chapters discuss the historical, methodological, and professional issues and research in life care planning. In the past few years, the field has been impacted by COVID-19, changes in healthcare delivery services, cost of care issues, and access to home supports. The reader will want to review these chapters to understand how the community of life care planners addressed these contemporary issues.

The text offers a pediatric-specific chapter that examines how the life care plan establishes an integrated continuum that can result in improved outcomes, a reduction in complications, and appropriate use of resources for children with chronic illnesses and catastrophic injuries. Separate chapters discuss special education and special needs planning. At the other end of the life span spectrum, the chapter on elder care focuses on the needs and services of aging individuals.

The text continues with several chapters defining the roles played by each key team member working with the life care planner. It provides life care planners with insights critical to successful interaction with medical, health-related professionals, and economic team members they are likely to encounter as they work to build an objective life care plan with a solid foundation.

Building on prior publications, this text provides the reader with up-to-date information on disabilities most frequently encountered by the life care planner. Given the complexities in the medical management of these disabilities, coupled with advancements in medical research, therapy, and rehabilitative technologies, the chapters provide the current information and a myriad of resources to be considered in developing a lifelong care plan. Separate chapters address medical equipment, assistive technology, and transportation.

Life care planners are instrumental in personal injury/medical malpractice cases. The rules, regulations, and case decisions impacting the expert testimony of life care planners have changed over time. The forensic chapters discuss admissibility considerations and other topics that life care planners need to know.

This text will be foundational in helping to advance the specialized practice of life care planning. Drs. Rutherford-Owen, Barros-Bailey, and Weed are to be commended for their leadership and contribution to the field. A special thank you to the authors for sharing their unique knowledge and experiences.

Last, it is essential to acknowledge that the true beneficiaries of this educational resource will be individuals and families living with a disability.

Susan Grisham-Riddick, BA, RN, CLCP
Creator and editor, Pediatric Life Care Planning and Case Management Handbook (2 editions)
Founder (one of five) life care planning training modules leading to certification
Past Chair, Foundation for Life Care Planning Research
Past Chair, International Academy of Life Care Planners section
Past Board of Directors International Association of Rehabilitation Professionals
Founder, Care Planner Network
2006 Lifetime Achievement Award IALCP
2011 Lifetime Achievement Award ICHCC

Acknowledgements

From Tanya Rutherford-Owen

Years ago, in an effort to digitize my office, I enlisted the assistance of my then teenage son to scan articles. Midway through the project, he commented, "Roger Weed really published a lot". He could not have captured more perfectly in one sentence what any student of life care planning knows – that is, we all owe so much to the tireless efforts of Dr. Roger Weed. But for Dr. Weed, this text, in all of its editions, would not exist. I am beyond grateful that Dr. Weed entrusted Mary and me with the responsibility of the fifth edition of this text and it has been my great honor to work with both Drs. Weed and Barros-Bailey in this process.

Although known to me by reputation, but not by any personal connection prior to 2020, Dr. Mary Barros-Bailey has somehow proven to be even more impressive than I originally imagined. Dr. Barros-Bailey's assiduous pursuit of the highest forms of knowledge has resulted in this text providing unparalleled quality materials to the rehabilitation community. Without a doubt, her contributions to this process will be both frequently cited and widely revered as the gold standard for life care planning work. Mary, I remain in awe of the scope of your expertise in topics ranging from life care planning, to travel, to historic building construction, and cannot express my gratitude enough for you agreeing to endeavor in this process with me.

In 2011, I wrote in my dissertation acknowledgement to my husband, Ben, that I would "never take on a project like this again" and likely believed it at the time. Because he has known me since I was 17 years old, however, he wisely knew that I would. So, this time, I will not make promises that I cannot keep but, like I did in 2011, and in 1999, and in 1990, I will profess my love and gratitude for you in my life. Your quiet and unassuming manner has always allowed me to be out front taking risks, because I knew I had the safety, security, and support that you have always provided.

Finally, it is well known that my work ethic, commitment to lifelong learning, and my sense of giving back are not of my making but are a direct result of the loving inspiration of my mother, Beverly Rutherford. Like my husband, her quiet and unassuming nature prevents her taking any credit but rather it allows me to shine. Like many women of her generation, she was not given the opportunities that I was, so she made sure that her daughters found their own voice and learned to use it. I have always preferred using my voice in writing over speaking and hope that the text that Dr. Weed, Dr. Barros-Bailey and I offer here will be helpful to current and future life care planners.

From Mary Barros-Bailey

For over 25 years, I have been a life care planner. From my early practice until today, I have been formed by the insights, processes, and practices of those who have developed and advanced the field. A book does not enter its fifth edition if it is not an important publication to those flipping through its pages. Therefore, it was humbling to be asked by a leader in the field, Dr. Roger Weed, to take over the co-editorship of this edition. Dr. Weed and Susan Riddick-Grisham entrusted us to join their texts into a single lifespan book, a mission we took on with gusto and care. Thank you both for your incalculable contributions to life care planning and for that trust.

It has truly been a pleasure to work, write, and wonder with Dr. Rutherford-Owen, my co-editor. This is the first project I have completed with her. Dr. Rutherford-Owen's reputation as a skillful author, visionary, and "cat herder" of very busy professionals ultimately resulted in the successful delivery of the text ahead of schedule; it was remarkable to watch her as I sat along with her in the front seat and buckled in. As the lead editor, she went beyond her role taking on a significant burden in the development of the fifth edition, a responsibility for which I am grateful.

To the other three Barros-Baileys – Bob, Teresa, and Rachel – you know the drill: My successes are not my own. Without your forever support, love, and ability to distract me so I don't take myself too seriously, you have brought levity and balance into my life all the while cheering me on. Por isso, estou muito agradecida. Muito obrigada!

Finally, to life care planners new and seasoned, thank you for serving those who come across your practices. I hope that the words and resources in this edition will make your task lighter.

From Roger Weed

As mentioned in previous editions, my parents encouraged me to pursue higher education even though one high school administrator told me that I was not "college material". My parents lived to see me graduate with a master's in rehabilitation counseling in 1969, a goal no other person in my family tree had accomplished. That same year, I was offered an exciting adventurous job as a state rehabilitation counselor based in Anchorage, Alaska (primarily serving Kenai peninsula, Kodiak Island and the Aleutian chain and "camping out" in some villages) by supervisor Dale Reeves who was exceptionally supportive during my two-year tenure working for the state. Over time, a few other work opportunities eventually led me to open an Alaskan private practice specializing in workers compensation at a time no other such occupation existed in the state. By the time I sold my interest in a rehabilitation consulting practice in Alaska in 1984 to pursue the doctorate, my father passed on – but his advice to pursue *my* dreams lived on.

I met Dr. Timothy Field, professor at the University of Georgia, in the late 1970s or very early 1980s by attending one of his conferences on VDARE/transferability of skills. Through many interactions at conferences as well as personal contacts, it became clear that he could be instrumental in my professional growth. In about 1983, I approached him with the proposal that if he would agree to be my PhD academic advisor, I would sell my private practice based in Anchorage and Paula and I would move to Georgia. He agreed. From 1984 to my retirement, I can report that the decision was a phenomenal boost to my career. He invited me to share the stage at many conferences, co-author many publications and generally encouraged me to seek higher horizons. Dr. Field was outstanding mentor and is a wonderful friend.

Dr. Paul Deutsch, the founder of the life care planning movement, was a speaker at a university-sponsored conference in 1986. I instantly recognized the value of life care planning as an enhancement to my forensic practice. A relationship was cultivated and he enthusiastically encouraged my participation in promoting the specialty practice by inviting me to assist with conferences and contribute to the *Guide to Rehabilitation*, a seminal publication at the time. The collaborative relationship continued to the day of his retirement. The personal relationship lives on. When this publication was in development (2022), we visited on his birthday and reminisced about the early days of life care planning.

My wife, Paula, has always encouraged me to pursue professionally whatever I wanted. This support resulted in moves and job changes for her, but she never complained. Although we had planned to return to Alaska, the moves eventually unveiled dream career opportunities for *both* of us in the Atlanta metro area. Being invited to assume the leadership of the graduate rehabilitation counseling program at Georgia State University launched an incredible new opportunity. In the fourth edition I wrote, "looking back over an amazing career of teaching and consulting reminds me that what unfolded surpassed all expectations."

Finally, it is with great pleasure that Dr. Tanya Rutherford-Owen and Dr. Mary Barros-Bailey, exceptional professionals, talented authors and popular speakers, agreed to assume editorship roles for this fifth edition.

HISTORICAL, METHODOLOGICAL, AND PROFESSIONAL ISSUES AND RESEARCH IN LIFE CARE PLANNING

Chapter 1

Life Care Planning: Past, Present, and Future

Roger O. Weed and Tanya Rutherford-Owen

Author Note

This chapter, although updated for the fifth edition, includes information contained in Weed, R. (2019) A brief history of life care planning. *Journal of Life Care Planning 17*(3), 5–14, as well as Weed (2018) Life care planning: Past, present, and future. In R. Weed & D. Berens (Eds.), *Life Care Planning and Case Management Handbook* (4th ed., pp. 3–20). Routledge.

History of Life Care Planning

In 1999, when the first edition of the *Life Care Planning and Case Management Handbook* was published, the concept of a life care plan was well-established but life care planning, as a specialty practice area, was still relatively new. By 2022 and the fifth edition of this text, we have 23 additional years of growth in this practice area and thousands of life care planners practicing worldwide.

Life care planning tenets and methodologies emerged from a combination of case management practices and catastrophic disability research from the mid-1970s (Deutsch, et al., 2003a; Weed, 1995; Weed & Riddick, 1992). Although life care planning as a concept evolved within the context of the litigation system, in the 40+ years that this field has existed, multiple entities (many of which do not involve litigation) have used life care planning as a tool. Historically, it is important to understand that the specialty practice of life care planning exists today due to the tireless efforts of those in the field who have endeavored in professional development activities for over 40 years. The history of life care planning could not be written without individuals including, but not limited to Paul Deutsch, PhD, Richard Bonfiglio, MD, Ms. Susan Riddick-Grisham, Ms. Julie Kitchen, Ms. Patricia McCollum, Frederick Raffa, PhD, Horace Sawyer, PhD, and Roger Weed, PhD. Others who were instrumental in supporting the spread of life care planning during the early days were Terry Winkler, MD (speaker and author with an emphasis on spinal cord injury), Timothy Field, PhD (publisher), Robert Meier, III, MD (speaker and author with an emphasis on amputation), and Tyron Elliott, Esq. (speaker and author on forensic applications).

As this discipline evolves, it is important that current and future practitioners understand the rich history that exists in the specialty practice area of life care planning. This chapter outlines the history of life care planning and provides insight into the areas of growth that lie ahead. As with previous editions, it is helpful to review the roots of the specialty practice of life care planning as a foundation for this book.

The 1970s

In the 1970s, Dr. Frederick (Fred) Raffa, a Florida-based economist and faculty member at what is now the University of Central Florida, was often retained to opine about economic damages in personal injury lawsuits and wrongful death cases (F. Raffa, personal communication, April 26, 2019). On one of these occasions, the attorney had also retained the services of a vocational expert, Mr. Paul Deutsch (Note: Dr. Deutsch received his PhD in January 1983). Dr. Raffa was asked to meet the attorney at Deutsch's office for a deposition. Dr. Raffa reported that he and "Paul hit it off right away," and several mutual cases led to discussions regarding the process of evaluation of damages in litigation (personal communication, April 26, 2019; P. Deutsch, personal communication, May 23, 2022). In the late 1970s, Dr. Raffa mentioned that he had been referred a case to determine future medical needs and associated costs and asked Deutsch to assist by compiling future needed medical services and products. Dr. Raffa provided the structure for economic projections and developed a reporting format that was initially titled *Catastrophic Summary Profile Sheet* (J. Kitchen, personal communication, April 27 & 28, 2019). The categories and interview worksheets were designed to capture the required data for an economist to comprehensively assess future care needs and associated costs in litigated matters (P. Deutsch, personal communication, April 22, 2019, May 23, 2022). In a 1995 interview, Dr. Deutsch noted that the first use of an organized life care planning format occurred in 1978 (Inside Life Care Planning, 1995). To streamline the process, a revised format, which became known as the *Life Care Plan*, was developed shortly thereafter (J. Kitchen, personal communication, April 28, 2019).

The 1980s

An opportunity to author a textbook and educate attorneys about life care planning was presented when publisher Matthew Bender agreed to a contract regarding economic damages in litigation (P. Deutsch, personal communication, April 22, 2019, May 23, 2022). Deutsch and Raffa committed to an extensive treatise on the topic that appeared in volumes eight and nine of the legal publication *Damages in Tort Actions* (Deutsch & Raffa, 1982), a text that established the guidelines for determining damages in civil litigation cases. It was here that the term "life care plan" was first seen in a text (Neulicht et al., 2010). The original definition, in the early 1980s, of life care planning was:

> A consistent methodology for analyzing all of the needs dictated by the onset of a catastrophic disability through to the end-of-life expectancy. Consistency means that the methods of analysis remain the same from case to case and does not mean that the same services are provided to like disabilities.
> (Deutsch & Raffa, 1982; Deutsch & Sawyer, 2002 as cited in Deutsch et al., 2003b, p. 5–7)

In the fall of 1983, the newly minted PhD, Dr. Paul Deutsch, was speaking to a class of students in the rehabilitation counseling program at the University of Florida where he met Dr. Horace Sawyer, the chair of the department (H. Sawyer, personal communication, May 1, 2019; P. Deutsch, personal communication, May 23, 2022). They enjoyed a lunch together and an association began that would lay the foundation for introducing the concept of life care planning to the rehabilitation consulting discipline. Deutsch urged Sawyer to join him as co-author of a new Matthew Bender publication titled the *Guide to Rehabilitation* (Deutsch & Sawyer, 1985). Although initially reluctant, Sawyer reported that he eventually joined Deutsch in promoting life care planning concepts as a co-author of the *Guide* and facilitator of conference presentations (H. Sawyer, personal communication, May 1, 2019). During 1984, he and Deutsch, along with Julie Kitchen (who was also a driving force; H. Sawyer, personal communication, May 1, 2019) created the seminal text on life care planning. In 1985, the life care plan was introduced to the healthcare profession in the *Guide to Rehabilitation* (Deutsch & Sawyer, 1985).

With the 1985 publication of the *Guide*, Sawyer, as an academic leader in the rehabilitation profession, was instrumental in adding Deutsch to the agendas of state rehabilitation conferences, university rehabilitation counselor training programs, established health professional groups, and national rehabilitation conferences, among others. According to Sawyer:

> Paul was always ready to go anyplace at any time that I was scheduling for us. In the early days, it was exciting to introduce life care planning to so many different state and national groups with the pretense of national exposure to life care planning and the promotion of the *Guide to Rehabilitation*
>
> (personal communication, May 1, 2019).

Dr. Paul Deutsch was the first rehabilitation professional to formally teach "life care planning" concepts and methodology. He is considered the founder of the life care planning process and was the first person to publish on the topic in the rehabilitation literature with Dr. Raffa. The *Guide to Rehabilitation* (co-authored with Dr. Horace Sawyer) remained in publication with yearly updates until 2005.

As the concept received ever-widening acceptance Dr. Deutsch offered more extensive training in life care planning in several states titled Life Care Planning—The Basics in Boston, August 1987; Atlanta, September 1987; St. Louis, October 1987; Orlando, November 1987; and Richmond, May 1988 (Deutsch, n.d.b.). On September 16–17, 1988, (editor's note: In previous editions, the year was reported as 1986) one of the first *nationwide* attendee life care planning "start to finish" rehabilitation professional training programs (J. Kitchen personal communication, May 29, 2022) was organized by Dr. Deutsch and Julie Kitchen. More than 100 rehabilitation professionals from throughout the United States assembled in Hilton Head, South Carolina, to begin the process of learning about life care planning from beginning to end format as published in the *Guide to Rehabilitation*. Deutsch's tireless efforts to educate rehabilitation professionals, combined with the enthusiasm of attendees for life care planning, led to what some believe to be the turning point in the development of the practice of life care planning. It also became evident that many people were practicing what they identified as life care planning in a variety of ways, some of which appeared to be inconsistent with the intended goals and purposes of ethical rehabilitation practice. In addition, some used the term *life care planning* as it became more popular while having little or no awareness of the appropriate uses or practices associated with this emerging industry. In an interview on his birthday on May 23, 2022, Dr. Deutsch reflected that, although he had expected life care planning to expand, it is impressive to look back and see how much of an effect the practice has had on the profession: "It was a gratifying career and I had a lot of fun too."

In 1986, the first issue of the *Journal of Private Sector Rehabilitation*, the peer-reviewed journal of the National Association of Rehabilitation Professionals in the Private Sector (now known as the International Association of Rehabilitation Professionals—IARP), included a description of the process pertaining to life care planning (Deutsch et al., 1986). In 1989, a series of "step-by-step" booklets were published to help train life care planners by offering prepared life care plans for individuals with certain diagnoses. In 1989, *Life Care Facts*, a life care planning-specific publication was published quarterly by Paul M. Deutsch Press, Inc. This publication covered topics including medical aspects of disability and life care planning resources and was edited by Dr. Roger Weed, Dr. Horace Sawyer, Dr. Paul Deutsch, Ms. Julie Kitchen, and Mr. Earl Mezhoff.

The 1990s

Between 1986 and 1992, sporadic life care planning training programs took place. In 1990, The Rehabilitation Training Institute, Inc. (RTI), another brainchild by Dr. Deutsch, offered nine nationwide seminars on topics including life care planning for pediatrics, head injury, and spinal cord injury, as well as practice management seminars focused on building and managing a rehabilitation practice. In 1990, *The Rehab Consultant*, a quarterly newsletter for the practitioner in vocational rehabilitation, case management, and life care planning was also published by Paul M. Deutsch Press with editors Ann Groom and Myrene O'Connor. In a 1991 edition of the newsletter, articles spoke specifically to life care planning, including an article titled "Life Care Planning Resource Tips" by Julie Kitchen.

In 1991, RTI continued to offer nationwide training seminars on topics including advanced life care planning for head injury, life care planning basics, and rehabilitation testimony. Through the training, professional networking, and distribution of life care planning publications, it became evident that demand for a consistent, methodical, and organized approach to life care planning was growing.

In the fall of 1992, five rehabilitation professionals, Dr. Richard (Rick) Bonfiglio, Dr. Paul Deutsch, Ms. Julie Kitchen, Ms. Susan Riddick, and Dr. Roger Weed, met to discuss the apparent problems associated with some life care planning practices. The group was concerned that fragmentation and poor standardization would result in the overall decline of the specialty practice. As a result, they decided to develop a concentrated training program consisting of eight modules, each module being two and a half days in length, to provide standardized training on the various aspects of life care planning. On February 18, 1993, the founders of the comprehensive training met and outlined eight modules (also known as tracks) with assignments of speakers.

Module I: Basic overview of life care planning process methods, standards, and formats (presenter: Julie Kitchen, CDMS, CCM)
Module II: Vocational aspects of clients/evaluees (presenter: Dr. Roger Weed)
Module III: Effective case management strategies within the complex medical environment (presenter: Susan Grisham, RN, BA)
Module IV: Forensic rehabilitation issues (presenter: Dr. Paul Deutsch)
Module V: Spinal cord injury (presenters: Dr. Paul Deutsch, Dr. Rick Bonfiglio, and Ms. Julie Kitchen)
Module VI: Brain injury (presenters: Dr. Rick Bonfiglio and Susan Grisham, RN, BA)

Module VII: Long-term care issues for other physical and emotional disabilities and disease processes (presenters: Dr. Rick Bonfiglio and Dr. Roger Weed)

Module VIII: Business and ethical practices and the use of technology in life care planning (presenters: Dr. Paul Deutsch and Dr. Roger Weed)

Following this process, the Rehabilitation Training Institute, a management company, was contracted to establish training programs throughout the United States. Before the flyers were fully distributed, the first of the organized modules, which was scheduled for November 1993 and limited to 100 attendees, was filled. Two introductory courses were developed—one on the west and one on the east coast. It was obvious that many rehabilitation professionals were interested in pursuing additional education related to life care planning. Several participants requested official recognition for their educational efforts. Dr. Horace Sawyer of the University of Florida and co-author/editor of the *Guide to Rehabilitation* was approached, and he agreed to pursue an official certificate of completion through the University of Florida's Continuing Education Department, which was approved in November 1993.

To better manage life care planning training, a private-public partnership between the Rehabilitation Training Institute and the University of Florida formed in 1994 and was named Intelicus. The five founders donated the program content to Intelicus effective January 1994, which was purchased by Medipro Seminars in 2003. Until their retirement, three of the founders (i.e., Paul Deutsch, Julie Kitchen, and Roger Weed) continued to donate time and services in support of online training through the University of Florida and/or the annual life care planning symposium. As of 2022, Susan Riddick-Grisham and Dr. Bonfiglio remain active in the specialty practice.

In July 1995, the newsletter *Inside Life Care Planning* was published by St. Lucie Press. This publication was published bimonthly starting in July-August 1995, with volume 1, number 1 and focused on topics including objectivity in life care planning, technology in life care planning, and practice issues in life care planning. The editorial advisory board included nine individuals, one attorney (J. Sherrod Taylor), two physicians (Richard Bonfiglio, MD and Nathan Zasler, MD), one nurse (Jan Roughan, PhN), and five PhD trained practitioners (Patricia Murphy, PhD, Donald Shrey, PhD, Randall Thomas, PhD, Robert Voogt, PhD, and Roger Weed, PhD). In the 1995 July-August edition of *Inside Life Care Planning*, it was noted that 115 individuals had graduated from the eight-part life care planning course offered in 1994 and 1995. Dr. Deutsch recalls (personal communication, May 23, 2022) the celebration organized in Orlando for the first group who completed all of the modules (see "Track 9" below). He recalls that the attendees were enthusiastic proponents of the specialty practice, which motivated him to continue the promotion of life care planning.

Although the certificate of completion from programs such as the University of Florida or Kaplan University (which offered training beginning in 2003) (Deutsch, n.d.b) underscored the value of obtaining education specific to this specialized practice, it did not provide the assurance of ethical practice nor a professional identity that was desired by founding professionals who invested time and monetary resources in this field's development. Several certification boards were contacted, with three indicating an interest in leading the way to life care planning certification. Eventually, through facilitation by Dr. Sawyer, the Commission on Disability Examiner Certification (now known as the International Commission on Health Care Certification, or ICHCC) based in Midlothian, Virginia, and owned by V. Robert May, PhD, assumed responsibility of developing a credential. The first certifications in life care planning were offered in spring 1996, and within five months, 130 individuals were certified in life care planning (May, n.d.). Beginning in October

2005, the ICHCC began issuing a Canadian Life Care Planning credential (CCLCP™) (K. May, personal communication October 19, 2021).

Starting in 1996, the first life care planning conference was held. The first conference was labeled "Track 9" and was offered to individuals who had previously completed the first eight life care planning tracks outlined above (Fawber, 2019). The goal of the conference was to update life care planners on developments in disciplines that affected life care planning including medicine, law, etc. Between 1992 and 2002, Annual Life Care Planning Conferences were offered but by 2003, the meeting name was changed to the "International Conference on Life Care Planning" (Fawber, 2019). This name remained for the 2004, 2005, and 2006 conferences, but was renamed the International Symposium on Life Care Planning in 2007. This name has remained intact through to the date of this publication. The goal of the life care planning symposia is to continue educating attendees on current and future life care planning trends by providing life care planning-specific training and education (McCollom & Weed, 2002). Between 1996 and 2022, these annual in-person meetings occurred in various locations throughout the United States, with two meetings offered online (2020–2021) due to the COVID-19 pandemic. Since 2016, the symposia have been offered through the IARP usually several days prior to the annual IARP conference. This training, as of 2022, is offered yearly in the fall and includes two full days of life care planning training. For a full discussion of locations and topics presented at each meeting, as well as a list of the many supporters of the annual meetings, the reader is referred to *25 Years of the International Symposium of Life Care Planning* (Fawber, 2019).

As noted in Patricia "Patti" McCollom's 2006 vitae, another significant development, which took place in October 1996, was the formation of the American *Academy* [emphasis added] of Nurse Life Care Planners by Patricia "Patti" McCollom (IALCP, 2000). This was the first life care planning-specific professional organization in existence. McCollom (1997) stated that she initially began the group as a mechanism for additional education and networking for nurses. In January 1997, the professional group consisted of approximately 60 (all-nurse) members (McCollom, 1997), but in December of 1997, after meeting with life care planning leaders beyond RNs, membership in the group was opened to all professional life care planners (K. Preston, personal communication, May 6, 2019). The name of the group was changed to the International Academy of Life Care Planners (IALCP). In June 2000, there were 157 members (IALCP, 2000). By 2002, the membership was estimated at 240 members (McCollom, 2002). This multidisciplinary group has remained intact for approximately 25 years, with a current membership estimate of 549 members as of April 2022 (K. Bailey, personal communication, April 18, 2022). From 2005 until present, the group has been recognized as a special interest group with IARP (Berens, 2006).

A second nurses-only life care planning professional group was founded by Kelly Lance in 1997. This group, the American *Association* of Nurse Life Care Planners (AANLCP®), was created for nurse life care planners who wished to affiliate with an organization that certified only nurses as life care planners. This group has remained intact until the date of this publication. Over time, the group began allowing non-nurses to join and they can currently join at "associate" status (K. Nebel personal communication April 15, 2022; K. Nebel personal communication May 29, 2022). The AANLCP® has an estimated membership of 270 professionals as of May 2022 (A. Nebel personal communication May 12, 2022).

Publications at standards intervals were published by the professional organizations. In January 1997, the AANLCP® began publishing a two-page *Newsletter* that provided news about the field of life care planning and membership in the group. The *Newsletters* were published in 1997 and 1998. On May 15, 1998, the *Academy Letter* was published by the IALCP. These *Academy Letters* were typically between four and eight pages in length with contributions for individuals in life care planning and related fields on topics including durable medical equipment, standards of practice, costing, etc. and remained in publication until 2001 when the *Journal of Life Care Planning* debuted.

According to the January 1997 AANLCP® *Newsletter*, the Inaugural American Academy of Nurse Life Care Planners educational program was to be held in Des Moines, Iowa on April 4–5, 1997. This same publication notes that a June (1997) pediatric-specific program was also being planned.

As life care planning interest spread, encompassing an ever-widening group of professions and professionals, it became evident that the definition offered in 1982 by Deutsch and Raffa in *Damages in Tort Action* needed revision. Dr. Roger Weed took the lead on this task at a 1998 national conference which was a large group primarily comprised of rehabilitation consultants and nurses engaged in life care planning. The goal was to reach consensus on the definition of life care planning as defined by a diverse assembly of professionals. These consensus events expanded and came to be known as life care planning summits. The result of these efforts are *Majority and Consensus Statements* that continue to be refined and used in life care planning to this day (Johnson et al., 2018; Weed & Berens, 2018). Through this consensus activity, the definition of the term "life care plan" was established in 1998 and remains the accepted definition of a life care plan at the time of this publication. Although the initial description of life care planning was offered by Drs. Deutsch and Raffa in *Damages in Tort Action* (1982), collaboration with leaders and organizations resulted in an agreed upon definition, as follows:

> A Life Care Plan is a dynamic document based upon published standards of practice, comprehensive assessment, data analysis, and research, which provides an organized concise plan for current and future needs with associated costs, for individuals who have experienced catastrophic injury or have chronic health care needs.
>
> (Combined definition of the University of Florida and Intelicus annual life care planning conference and the American Academy of Nurse Life Care Planners (now known as the International Academy of Life Care Planners) presented at the Forensic Section meeting, National Association of Rehabilitation Professionals in the Private Sector [NARPPS] annual conference, Colorado Springs, Colorado, and agreed upon April 3, 1998)

In November 1998, the first edition of the *Journal of Nurse Life Care Planning* was published, with Joan Schoefield, RN, BSN, MBA serving as editor. Wendi Howland, MN RN-BC CRRN CCM CNLCP® LNCC became editor in spring 2009 and served in that capacity through to 2017 (W. Howland personal communication April 15, 2022).

In 1999, the seminal publication, *Life Care Planning and Case Management Handbook* was published with Dr. Roger Weed serving as editor. This text provided the foundation for future life care planning training and sought input from a diverse collection of authors including physicians, psychologists, nurses, rehabilitation counselors, occupational therapists, speech language pathologists, physical therapists, and attorneys, among others. The publication highlights the transdisciplinary nature of life care planning as early as 1999. This 1999 publication has now been updated five times over 23 years.

Life Care Planning in the 2000s

The first life care planning summit, a meeting for life care planners designed to develop a consensus on critical life care planning topics, took place in 2000. The first summit was attended by a group of 100 experienced life care planners (66 were certified life care planners), as well as several significant life care planning organizations. The results of the meeting were memorialized by Drs. Roger Weed and Debbie Berens in a seminal publication of the process along with letters from several organizations endorsing the results (Weed & Berens, 2000). In 2009, Karen Preston and Cloie Johnson collected, analyzed, and presented all *Consensus and Majority Statements* developed at summits since 2000 (Johnson & Preston, 2009).

Historically, these summits were limited to approximately 100 active professionals belonging to significant life care planning-related organizations. Since 2000, life care planning summits have occurred in the United States in 2002, 2004, 2006, 2008, 2010, 2012, 2015, 2017, 2022, and in 2011 in Canada. Over the years, hundreds of transdisciplinary and transorganizational life care planners have participated in these life care planning summits (Johnson, 2018).

Outcomes from the summits have led to transdisciplinary and transorganizational consensus and majority views on over 100 statements (Johnson, 2015). After the 2012 summit, these statements were codified and published as life care planning's first set of *Consensus and Majority Statements* derived from life care planning summits held in 2000, 2002, 2004, 2006, 2008, 2010, and 2012 (Johnson & Preston, 2012).

Following the 2017 summit, a multi-association systemic review was conducted of the 102 statements with Johnson et al. (2018) finding that 33 of the 102 statements had 75% or greater acceptance; 74 of the 102 statements had 60% or greater acceptance; and 87 of the 102 statements had 51% or greater acceptance. Based upon a review made by 139 life care planners, 96 of the original 102 consensus statements were retained through a Delphi analysis and were published in 2018 (Johnson et al., 2018). For detailed information about summit locations and number of attendees, the reader is referred to the 2018 *Journal of Life Care Planning*, 16(4) and 2019 *Journal of Life Care Planning* 17(3) issues.

In 2000, the first life care planning role and function study was published (Turner et al., 2000). This and subsequent studies sought to identify job tasks and competencies specific to life care planning service delivery (May & MoradiRekabdarkolee, 2020). This process was updated by Pomeranz et al. (2010). The most recent role and function study was published in the *Journal of Life Care Planning* (May & MoradiRekabdarkolee, 2020). In this study, the transdisciplinary nature of life care planning was demonstrated once again by survey respondents who held 21 different licenses and certifications and had earned 15 different academic degrees (May & MoradiRekabdarkolee, 2020).

In addition to role and function studies, practitioners were seeking confirmation that life care planning tenets, methods, and processes were reliable. The first such study by Sutton, Deutsch, Weed, and Berens (2002) supported the worth of life care planning practice. Others were to follow and most are listed with the Foundation for Life Care Planning Research.

As early as 1997, the idea of developing a life care planning "Fellow" designation was discussed to recognize professionals who not only possessed a certain level of experience, knowledge, and skill in life care planning, but also promoted the advancement of life care planning (Albee, 2019; Shahnasarian, 2015). In October 1997, the AANLCP® announced levels of membership, one of which being Fellow within the organization (AANLCP®, 1997). By 2000, the life care planning Fellow Program was officially introduced through the IALCP. To qualify for Fellow designation, the applicant was required to achieve 80% of the possible 120 criterion points, which was decided through blind review of applications and sample work products. The Fellow Program was evaluated between 2012–2014 by a task force and changes in the criteria for awarding the Fellow designation were made. In 2017, the College of Life Care Planning Excellence was created as the entity through which Fellows would be designated (Albee, 2019). By 2019, there were 21 life care planners who had earned the Fellow designation, 17 of whom were actively practicing (Albee, 2019), and as of May 20, 2022, 23 life care planners who had earned the Fellow designation, 16 of whom were practicing (IARP, 2022). In addition, on January 25, 2019, the board announced the establishment of a Fellow Emeritus, awarding the first two to retired life care planners Dr. Paul Deutsch and Dr. Roger Weed.

In 2000, the first edition of the IALCP life care planning *Standards of Practice* which was founded on survey research and comments by practitioners, was published (Preston, 2019). The origins of life care planning practice standards, however, began much earlier as noted in the first volume of the *Academy Letter* in an editorial by Patricia McCollom (IALCP, 1998) which documented the beginning of a "national dialogue about Standards of Practice for Life Care Planners" (McCollom, p. 3). As life care planning is transdisciplinary and professionals involved in life care planning are bound by standards of practice in their primary disciplines (Preston, 2019), standards for governing life care planning practices could not be created by an association of a single profession. Standards of practice are typically created by people who practice in the field (Preston, 2019). In 1997, to achieve consistency in the performance of life care planning, Dr. Roger Weed began soliciting comments from approximately 200 practicing life care planners regarding life care planning standards (Preston, 2019). The result of his efforts was the publication of the first edition of the IALCP Life Care Planning *Standards of Practice* (Reavis, 2000). Since 2001, life care planning standards of practice have been updated by the IALCP in 2006 (IALCP, 2006), 2015 (Preston & Reid, 2015), and 2022 (IALCP, 2022).

In December 2001, the articles of incorporation for the Foundation for Life Care Planning Research (FLCPR) were filed, creating the first life care planning research foundation (Berens, 2019). The foundation was created by Dr. Paul Deutsch in coordination with the University of Florida, Georgia State University, and the Medical College of Virginia, Virginia Commonwealth University. The mission of the foundation was to support life care planning-related research as well as bestowing annual awards in several categories. The foundation funded multiple research projects related to life care planning with over 30 of these published in peer-reviewed journals between 2002 and 2019. One such supported publication was the first study on reliability (Sutton et al., 2002). The Foundation for Life Care Planning Research was reincorporated as the Foundation for Life Care Planning and Rehabilitation Research in 2021, with the goal of expanding the focus of the foundation to include rehabilitation-related research outside of the singular focus on life care planning. The foundation, since 2019, has been affiliated with IARP. More information on the foundation can be found at https://connect.rehabpro.org/flcprr/home.

In the spring of 2002 (T. Field, personal communication November 3, 2021), the premier peer-reviewed life care planning journal, *Journal of Life Care Planning*, began publication. In the inaugural publication, the objectives of the journal were to: 1) publish materials that add to the growing life care planning literature base; 2) provide the field with information about life care planning events; 3) provide a forum to discuss practice issues; 4) promote professional practice by addressing certification, ethics, standards, and research methodology; and 5) publish continuing education articles (Berens, 2019). The journal has been published, typically on a quarterly schedule, from 2002 through to the date of this text. The roots of the journal are seen in early life care planning publications including *Life Care Facts* published by Paul M. Deutsch Press starting in 1989, *The Rehab Consultant*, published quarterly between 1990–1992, *Inside Life Care Planning* (published 1995–1996), *Newsletters* published by the American Academy of Nurse Life Care Planners in 1997–1998, and *Academy Letters* published by IALCP in 1998–2001 (Paul Deutsch & Associates, P.A., n.d.a). While the vision for the *Journal* was shared by many, bringing the publication to fruition resulted directly from the efforts of Dr. Tim Field, founder (along with his wife Janet) of

Elliott and Fitzpatrick, Inc., experienced publisher, journal editor, author, and popular conference speaker. He provided funding, as well as technical and publisher services, to bring the journal to the profession. He gifted the journal to the IALCP section of IARP in late 2006 (Field, 2006) where it continues to thrive.

In 2004, another life care planning text, dedicated specifically to pediatric issues, the *Pediatric Life Care Planning and Case Management Handbook*, edited by Susan Grisham, RN, BA, CCM, CLCP™ was published. A second edition of the text was published and edited by Susan Grisham, RN, BA, CCM, CLCP and Laura Deming, MS, RN, PNP-BC, CCM, CLCP in 2011.

Prior to 2005, the IALCP (which had existed since 1996) was a standalone entity. However, on August 1, 2005, IALCP merged with the IARP. Since that time, IALCP has operated as the life care planning section of IARP, retaining a board of directors and continuing to offer annual symposia.

In 2006, the second edition of the *Standards of Practice for Life Care Planners* was published.

In 2009, Leahy et al. published a survey of 648 certified rehabilitation counselors about knowledge domains essential to effective rehabilitation counseling practice. In that survey, life care planning was identified as a knowledge domain. It was again acknowledged in 2018 (Leahy et al., 2018)

In 2010, Pomeranz et al. published the second role and function study of life care planners, which surveyed 160 life care planners.

2011–2022

In 2013, a third professional faction of life care planners was formed when a group of physicians formed the American Academy of Physician Life Care Planners (AAPLCP™). This assembly held their inaugural conference in San Antonio in April 2016, chaired by Joe Gonzales, MD (AAPLCP™, 2014–2022). Reportedly, this physician-focused group is a professional organization of board-certified physicians *and* other qualified clinical and forensic professionals dedicated to the practice and advancement of life care planning. According to their website, only life care planning certified physicians (CPLCP™) will be members with the Fellow designation. Qualified physicians and non-physicians may join as a member, associate member, or resident member (see www.physicianlcp.com/ for criteria).

In 2015, the third edition of the academy's *Standards of Practice for Life Care Planners* (IALCP, 2015) was published.

Beginning its exam administration in October 2017, the Commission on Rehabilitation Counselor Certification included life care planning as one of its knowledge domain areas under the category of Community Resources and Partnerships for which applicants would be tested (Commission on Rehabilitation Counselor Certification, 2021). Life care planning tenets and methodologies have been included in the curricula of accredited rehabilitation counseling programs (Marini et al., 2004), with a 2003 unpublished study of accredited graduate rehabilitation counselor training programs revealing that two-thirds offered training in life care planning (Isom et al., 2003). As life care planning has become a component of rehabilitation-related education, some universities are developing graduate-level programs to endorse or encompass life care planning procedures and methods.

Continuing the desire to provide a foundation for the validity of the CLCP™ examination, in 2020, May and MoradiRekabdarkolee published the third role and function study of life care planners, which surveyed 212 life care planners.

In 2022, the fourth edition of the academy's *Standards of Practice for Life Care Planners* (IALCP, 2022) was published.

Table 1.1 outlines a timeline of selected historical events in the practice of life care planning.

Table 1.1 Life Care Planning Timeline of Selected Historical Events

Year	Event
1970s	Paul Deutsch meets economist Frederick (Fred) Raffa who was instrumental in designing the format to provide data needed for projecting future cost of needs.
1979	Julie Kitchen joins Paul Deutsch in May; an association that will endure nearly four decades.
1982	Life care planning concepts first appeared in the legal literature in *Damages in Tort Action*, Volumes 8 & 9 by Deutsch and Raffa. Damages texts were be updated yearly to 2019.
January 1983	Paul Deutsch awarded PhD from the University of Florida.
Fall 1983	Deutsch meets Horace Sawyer, PhD, chair of the rehabilitation counseling program at U of FL, after speaking to rehabilitation counseling class at the U of FL.
1984 +	Sawyer was instrumental in introducing life care planning to rehabilitation professionals and students via arranging conferences for Deutsch nationwide.
1985 +	Life care planning introduced to the rehabilitation literature in the book *Guide to Rehabilitation* by Deutsch & Sawyer. This seminal text was updated yearly for decades until publisher ceased operation in 2005.
1986	Widely believed to be the "turning point" comprehensive conference held at Hilton Head Island, September 16 & 17. Organized by Paul Deutsch, Julie Kitchen, and Horace Sawyer. First peer-reviewed life care planning article appeared in rehabilitation literature in the *Journal of Private Sector Rehabilitation*, *1*(1), 13–27 Life care planning in catastrophic case management by Deutsch, Paul M., Sawyer, Horace W., Jenkins, William M., Kitchen, Julie A.
1989–1990, 2007, 2018	Series of "step-by-step" booklets published for training (adult and pediatric brain injury, spinal cord injury, amputations, and general procedures).
1992	Initial preparation for coordinated nationwide training initiated by five professionals representing physician, nursing, and rehabilitation consulting. Founders were Paul Deutsch, PhD, Richard (Rick) Bonfiglio, MD, Susan Riddick-Grisham, RN, Julie Kitchen, BS, and Roger Weed, PhD.
1993	February, the founders completed the first comprehensive curriculum consisting of 8 tracks, which were 2 ½ days each. Instructors for each track identified. Training initiated, fall 1993. Dr. Horace Sawyer associated with U of FL on November 14 agrees to offer a certificate in life care planning to professionals who successfully complete the eight-track program from the Rehabilitation Training Institute*.
1994	U of FL assumes responsibility for curriculum via public private partnership which is known as Intelicus.
1996	The Commission on Disability Examiner Certification (led by V. Robert May, PhD) administers the first certification exam in March leading to Certified Life Care Planner designation. Certificates first mailed in July 1996. First annual Life Care Planning symposium is held November in Atlanta.

(Continued)

Table 1.1 (Continued)   Life Care Planning Timeline of Selected Historical Events

Year	Event
	First association specific to life care planning formed—American *Academy* for Nurse Life Care Planners (not to be confused with the American *Association* of Nurse Life Care Planners).
	Fellow designation (FIALCP) was first established through the International Academy of Life Care Planners (IALCP).
1997	The American *Academy* of Nurse Life Care Planners (led by Patti McCollom) evolved into the IALCP and professional membership expanded beyond nursing. Approved December 12 and announced to association members 1/28/98.
	The American *Association* of Nurse Life Care Planners was formed.
	The previously offered 8-track life care planning certificate program through Intelicus changed to six seminars and two distance learning modules.
1998	Life care planning definition agreed upon by U of FL, IALCP, and NARPPS (now IARP) Forensic Section members Colorado Springs, CO, April 3, 1998.
1999	*Life Care Planning and Case Management Handbook* edited by Roger Weed published (first of 5 editions).
2000	First life care planning summit held on April 12, Dallas, TX, invited experts and affiliations consisted of Rick Bonfiglio (Medical), Patti Costantini (AALNC), Paul Deutsch (Founder), Tyron Elliott (Legal), Tim Field (Publications), Don Lawson (Legal), Anne Llewellyn (CMSA), Bob May (CLCP™), Patti McCollom (IALCP), Ann Neulicht (IARP), Fred Raffa (Economist), Horace Sawyer (U of FL), Linda Shaw (Intelicus), Roger Weed (Georgia State Univ.) The results were endorsed by *all* organizations invited.
	First, role and function study published [Turner, T., Taylor, D., Rubin, S., & May, V.R. (2000). Job functions associated with the development of life care plans. *Journal of Legal Nurse Consultants, 11*(3), 3–7].
2000	First life care planning *Standards of Practice* published.
2002	Paul Deutsch forms the 501(c)3 Foundation for Life Care Planning Research. Initial board members Paul Deutsch, Roger Weed, Patti McCollom, Susan Riddick-Grisham, Chris Reid, Terry Winkler, and Bernie Kleinman.
	Journal of Life Care Planning is launched. Patti McCollom founding editor, Dr. Roger Weed, associate editor. Dr. Tim Field, through Elliott & Fitzpatrick publishing, underwrites the launch.
	Second life care planning summit May 19 (Summits occur approximately every two years).
2004	*Pediatric Life Care Planning and Case Management Handbook* by Susan Grisham published (first of 2 editions).
2005	IALCP merges with IARP effective August 1.
2006	IALCP Standards of Practice revised 2nd ed.

(Continued)

Table 1.1 (Continued)   Life Care Planning Timeline of Selected Historical Events

Year	Event
2007	Patti McCollom, Founder of IALCP, loses battle with cancer October 6.
2010	Second CLCP™ role and function study published. [Pomeranz, J., Yu, N., & Reid, C. (2010). Role and function study of life care planners. *Journal of Life Care Planning*, 9(3), 57–106].
2013	American Academy of Physician Life Care Planners formed.
2015	IALCP *Standards of Practice* revised 3rd ed.
2020	CLCP™ role and function study updated. The International Commission on Health Care Certification Life Care Planner Role and Function Investigation (2020). *Journal of Life Care Planning*, 18(2), 3–67.
* NOTE	Initial training of tracks developed by the five founders was offered through the Rehabilitation Training Institute (RTI). RTI became Intelicus (U of FL/private partnership), then Medipro (Bernie Kleinman, AHAB Press). For a time there also was a Paul M. Deutsch Press (PMD Press).

Source: Weed (2019). Reprinted with permission from IARP.

Current Life Care Planning Training

To teach skills associated with being a life care planner in 2022, multiple life care planning training programs exist. A brief description of the available life care planning training programs (in alphabetical order) is included in the next sections.

Capital University Law School

Capital University Law School offers a 16-credit graduate-level certificate in life care planning (Barros-Bailey & Latham, 2021). The program's format includes synchronous and face-to-face learning and is designed to be completed within eight months. The program includes 224-hours of life care planning, offered within eight modules as follows:

Module I: Introduction: History, professional issues, evidence-based standards, life care plan, medical cost projection assessment
Module II: Adult: Amputation, brain injury, burns, polytrauma, sensory, spinal cord injury, transplants
Module III: Pediatric: Brachial plexus, cerebral palsy, childhood sexual abuse, epilepsy, respiratory
Module IV: Advanced and Special Issues: Aging, chronic pain and conditions, mental health, premorbid and co-morbid conditions
Module V: Pricing, collateral sources, critique/rebuttal of a life care plan
Module VI: Vocational, avocational, educational issues; economic & structured settlements
Module VII: Life care plan development and report practicum
Module VIII: Life care planning litigation capstone

FIG Services, Inc.

Life care plan training is offered through FIG Services, Inc. (2017). This 120-credit hour program was founded by Shelene Giles, MS, BSN, BA, RN, CRC, CNLCP*, LNCC, LCP-C in 2010. This program is offered in an online format and consists of 24 lessons, each of five hours in length, which are designed to be completed within 6–12 months. The 24 lessons include:

Rehabilitation/case management foundation
Life care planning certification and standards
Life care planning process
Spinal cord injury
Traumatic brain injury
Amputation
Burns
Chronic pain
Pediatrics
Cerebral palsy
Aging
Referral, review, and summary
Life care plan assessment and medical diagnosis
Collaboration
Medical research
Recommendations
Coding and costing
Costing research
Goals of life care planning and report writing
Catastrophic case management and vocational rehabilitation
Anatomy of lawsuit
Quality as an expert witness
Prepare as an expert witness
Testify as an expert witness (S. Giles personal communication April 11, 2022).

More information can be found at www.figeducation.com/life-care-planning/.

Institute of Rehabilitation and Training (IRET)

Training is offered through the IRET based in Florida. This 120-credit hour program was developed by Dr. Jamie Pomeranz and colleagues at the University of Florida. In 2015, the program was transferred to IRET and is now owned and operated by Dr. Pomeranz and Dr. Nami Yu. This program is offered in a hybrid format with five online training modules (i.e., professional orientation of life care planning; medical and psychosocial aspects of life care planning with spinal cord injury; medical and psychosocial aspects of life care planning with brain injury; medical and psychosocial aspects of life care planning with amputations; medical and psychosocial aspects of life care planning with multiple disabilities) and one on-site training module (forensic aspects of life care planning). Students also complete a work sample in which they develop a complete life care plan based on a real clinical case (J. Pomeranz personal communication April 11, 2022). More information can be found at www.iretprograms.com.

Thomas Jefferson University

Life care planning training is offered by Thomas Jefferson University, through the College of Rehabilitation Sciences. This program is 12 months (4 semesters) in duration and offers a graduate certificate upon completion of the required 12 credit hours. The Life Care Planning Graduate Certificate at Thomas Jefferson University is comprised of four graduate-level courses, three credits each. The 12 graduate credits are "stackable," meaning they can be transferred as graduate credits into other master's and doctoral degree programs within and external to Thomas Jefferson University. The courses are offered in an online format, using a combination of synchronous and asynchronous formats and include the following:

- JCRS 730: Introduction to Life Care Planning
- JCRS 731: Primer on Catastrophic Injuries and Chronic Diseases
- JCRS 732: Specialty Topics in Life Care Planning (understanding research literature, litigation, civil procedure, laws, courtroom simulation, delve deeper into methods to project costs)
- JCRS 733: Practicum (critique an existing life care plan, create a life care plan) (M. J. Mulcahey personal communication April 13, 2022).

Additional information can be found at www.jefferson.edu/academics/colleges-schools-institutes/rehabilitation-sciences/departments/outcomes-measurement/education/life-care-planning-graduate-certificate.html.

Upon completion of a life care planning training program, interested individuals may choose to pursue certification in life care planning. In 2022, there were approximately 1200 individuals holding the CLCP™ credential in the United States and 195 Canadian certified life care planners (K. May personal communication May 2, 2022).

Current Topics of Interest in Life Care Planning

In 2017, researchers inquired of 31 participants in a life care planning training program in Canada about the three biggest challenges they faced in their life care planning work. Through a qualitative research process, six essential themes were identified as barriers, including collaboration for recommendations; practice challenges; research and training; referral constraints; attendant care; and future care costs (Fischer & Wilkins, 2017). Two years later, similar research was conducted with 52 life care planners in the United States who held certifications including CLCP™, CRC, and CCM and reported diverse educational backgrounds including nursing degrees, master's degrees, and doctoral (PhD) degrees (Owen & Wilkins, 2019). In that research, life care planners identified eight areas of concern as being collaboration for recommendations; business challenges; evolution of field of life care planning; referral constraints; attorney concerns; future care costs; case development and legal proceedings. Specifically identified concerns about the evolution of the field of life care planning included concerns about fracturing of the field and some life care planners who were observed to not be following life care planning standards of practice and/or consensus and majority statements in their work (Owen & Wilkins, 2019). These are concepts that are seen in some of the earliest life care planning writings and were discussed as early as 1986 in the first life care planning training program, yet they remain relevant today. These concepts may provide insight into areas of development in the future of life care planning.

Life Care Planner Qualifications

Even 25 years after the establishment of life care planning as a transdisciplinary practice, some continue to assert that individuals with certain academic backgrounds are uniquely qualified to be life care planners. In these authors' opinion, this assertion fails to consider the entire transdisciplinary history of life care planning, which was established in the 1980s and has continued for four decades. Acceptance of this proposition would also require someone to ignore the transdisciplinary backgrounds of many of the founders of life care planning who had earned PhDs, RNs, MDs, and master's degrees from backgrounds including nursing, rehabilitation, medicine, etc. It was the cross-discipline richness of this specialty practice that makes it unique from other homogenous practices and the training by early educators with different backgrounds was likely the key to the development of one product that successfully incorporated economics, medicine, case management, rehabilitation, and behavioral psychology into one cogent document, the life care plan. The practice of life care planning has roots in case management. In 1992, Weed and Riddick wrote, "Effective case management is interdisciplinary in nature involving all members of the treatment team, the client, and often, family members" (p. 26). Life care planning, as a specialty area of practice, was developed through the work of an economist and a rehabilitation counselor and quickly attracted practitioners from the disciplines of nursing, rehabilitation counseling, physical/occupational/speech therapy, psychology, and medicine. The proposition that life care planning is only within the purview of one discipline is devoid of face validity when reviewing any of the four prior life care planning textbooks (Weed, 1998; Weed, 2004; Weed & Berens, 2010; Weed & Berens, 2019) where one finds life care planning-related chapters authored by nurses, rehabilitation counselors, physical therapists, psychologists, audiologists, physicians, etc., many of whom have made significant contributions to the field of life care planning. By 2022, any student of life care planning history will note that the argument that life care planning is best performed by any one homogenous group was abandoned almost three decades ago when the first life care planning professional association, the American Academy of Nurse Life Care Planners, voted to become a transdisciplinary organization. Their vision was codified in the third volume of the *Academy Letter* (June 13, 2000, p. 2), which stated that: "During the developmental months, contact was maintained with various other professionals who were not nurses. These colleagues continued to voice one concern: 'Life care planners need one organization.'" In November 1997, Roger Weed hosted a meeting in Dallas, including the Commission on Disability Examiner Certification (CDEC), Inteleicus, and the academy, to openly discuss commonalities and conflicts and to determine avenues for collaboration. The outcome of the session was that the academy became the IALCP, with full membership open to all [appropriately qualified] practitioners. The advisory panel believed the practice, indeed, was/is transdisciplinary—as is case management—and that working toward the good of the whole was critical to successful practice for all.

Perhaps to rebut the spread of the erroneous assertion that life care planning is monodisciplinary, in 2019, the IALCP reiterated the position that life care planning has always been and should always be transdisciplinary. They issued a position paper authored by nine practicing life care planners and endorsed by an additional 14 life care planners of diverse backgrounds. The full paper, which can be found in a 2019 issue of the *Journal of Life Care Planning*, volume *17*(2), states in part that: "There is no single profession that can claim to be the most qualified to do this" and "that means that it is, and has been, the position of this community that life care planning is a practice open to all those who demonstrate the appropriate qualifications, experience, and skill to author life care plans" (p. 3).

As life care planners come from a heterogenous mix of professional disciplines, each individual life care planner brings with them specialized skills to contribute to a life care plan (IALCP, 2019; Weed, 2002). For example, the life care planner first trained in audiology may be particularly well-suited to opine on needs replacement of a cochlear implant but less well-suited to opine on mental health needs. A psychologist life care planner, by contrast, may be well-suited to independently opine on psychologically related needs but unable to independently opine about the need for a future hip surgery. It is expected that life care planning members are part of a team, and it is further expected that team members will remain within their scope of practice and their knowledge area. For a complete discussion of the scope of practice responsibilities and limitations by primary disciplines involved in life care planning, the reader is referred to the *Journal of Life Care Planning*, *17*(1) published in 2019.

Current Uses of Life Care Plans

Over the years, life care planning has morphed from an almost entirely litigation-oriented tool to one used in a wide variety of venues. Since its inception, many organizations and hospitals have adopted life care planning procedures for discharge planning (Riddick & Weed, 1996; Weed & Field, 2001; Weed & Field, 2012; Weed & Riddick, 1992). In civil litigation, both plaintiff and defense attorneys have increasingly turned to rehabilitation professionals to consult on life care planning issues. Venues utilizing life care plans include, but are not limited to, workers' compensation, medical malpractice, special needs trusts, family trusts, insurance reserve settings, wounded warrior support, elder care, discharge planning, and more. Life care plans have been used in government-funded programs including the Vaccine Injury Compensation Program (Owen & Henry, 2019; Voogt, 1995) and other programs administrated through special masters including the 9/11 victim fund (E. Provder personal communication May 21, 2022) and the Gulf oil spill. Life care planners participate in the development of Medicare set-aside plans (ICHCC, 2022). At least one nationwide case management firm adopted the basic life care planning procedure to work with insurance companies for catastrophic injury claims to assist them with overall rehabilitation planning and projection of costs (Weed, 2001). Structured settlement companies use life care plans to develop proposals for settlements and estate planning. Another area that appears on the horizon but slow to catch on is provision for the care of children who have complex healthcare needs and who are in the foster care system, or are adopted (Buckles et al., 2008).

Another exceptionally ripe specialty area has to do with the care of wounded warriors. Leskin et al. (2007) constructed life care plans for 20 survivors of combat related polytrauma within the Department of Veterans Affairs system. Their goal was to evaluate feasibility of using life care plans to facility identifications of need and coordination of lifelong care across institutions and geographic locations. The researchers noted that life care planning's use in medicolegal areas has "clouded perception regarding the intrinsic value of several core components of the life care planning process" (p. xxiv) and concluded that life care planning methods could be used within existing VA healthcare systems to support complex case management and care delivery. By 2021, a request for proposal

(RFP) was being distributed to life care planners to potentially participate in construction of life care plans for wounded warriors (S. Grisham personal communication May 20, 2021).

Current Sources of Life Care Planning Data

The very definition of a life care plan consists of essentially two elements—the needs of an individual and the costs. Inherent in the process of life care plan development, therefore, is the identification of healthcare costs. As healthcare pricing has become increasing complex (Busch, 2017), the acquisition of healthcare costs as incorporated in a life care plan remains challenging. As identified in the 2017 and 2019 surveys of life care planners (Fischer & Wilkins, 2017; Owen & Wilkins, 2019), life care planners, like most Americans, continue to be challenged by the complexity in healthcare pricing. This is clearly not a problem specific to the practice of life care planning, as noted in the national discourse around transparency in healthcare pricing. One answer to this was the H.R. 3029 Health Care Price Transparency Act which went into effect in early 2021. This legislation, designed to make healthcare pricing more transparent to the consumer, required certain hospitals to disclose the prices for 300 shoppable services or face a $300 per day penalty for non-compliance. However, by June 2021, Nikpay et al. (2021) reported that of the 470 hospitals surveyed, fewer than 25% met the price transparency information requirements of the rule. As healthcare costing remains difficult to ascertain, this is likely to remain a hot topic in life care planning in the coming years.

Many life care planners have acquired knowledge and expertise in medical coding procedures for determining medical charges. Other life care planners rely upon healthcare cost databases as a source of these data, a tool not available in earlier years in life care planning. Proficiency in the use of costing databases and similar tools will also continue to be relevant to the practice of life care planners.

Legal Decisions Impacting Life Care Planning

As of 2022, legal decisions continue to impact the admissibility of expert witness work, including those working in the specialty practice of life care planning. More information on this topic can be found in the chapters in this text titled, "Forensic Issues in Life Care Planning", "Admissibility Consideration in Life Care Planning", "A Plaintiff's Attorney's Perspective on life Care Planning," and "A Defense Attorney's Perspective on Life Care Planning." Recent decisions concerning hearsay and the Collateral Source Rule have been topics of conversation in life care planning venues. Following the passage of the Patient Protection and Affordable Care Act of 2010 many life care planners in litigation venues have been challenged to consider the collateral source and financially offset appropriate categories (Field & Weed, 2015). By 2022, legal decisions, including the 2017 California decision in *Cuevas v. Contra Costa County*, have required that life care planners in California consider various factors historically excluded from admissibility due to the Collateral Source Rule. With the changing and undetermined future of healthcare insurance in the United States, life care planning professionals should be prepared to answer challenging questions regarding cost of future care needs.

The Future of Life Care Planning

Life care planning has emerged as an effective method for identifying and outlining future care needs and costs. The specialty practice continues to grow and evolve. It is specifically of importance that a coordinated effort with standardized approaches be promoted so that the practice progresses and becomes useful in an ever-increasing number of venues. As more professionals become involved in this process, the specialty practice will mature and develop more effective outcome measurements.

The original definition of life care planning promulgated in the 1980s lacked the word "dynamic," but by 1998, the word appeared in what is now the commonly agreed upon definition of life care planning. While the life care plan document itself must be dynamic, so, too must the field of individuals currently involved in life care planning. As such, the following topics in life care planning are identified as areas of emerging interest in the specialty practice of life care planning.

In the 2015 publication of the AANLCP *Scope and Standards of Practice* (1st edition) various trends were identified as potential areas of growth in life care planning. These include:

1. Costing accountability and transparency
2. Medicare set-aside arrangements
3. Tort reform
4. Elder care (p. 51)

In 2022, the following topics in life care planning remain of interest and are identified as areas of potential growth:

- Promoting relevant educational opportunities for new and existing life care planners to promote the understanding of the history of life care planning and the historical methods of life care planning, to combat any spread of misinformation
- Funding and supporting research in life care planning including implementation, costing methods, and the role of technology
- Clarifying the role of certifying bodies versus life care planning associations in formulating standards of practice and ensuring that life care planning certifying bodies meet professional standards
- Seeking consensus among various life care planning associations, training programs, and certification bodies, to promote the specialty practice as a whole
- Understanding the influence of changing jurisdictional requirements and new legal decisions on the work of life care planners
- Identifying new applications for life care planning methods and tools in the context of changing healthcare costing, technological advances, and identification of inequity in healthcare access

Conclusion

Since the life care plan first emerged in rehabilitation literature in the early 1980s, the concept has grown immensely (Weed, 1994) to now represent a highly effective case management method, particularly regarding complex, medically challenging cases (Blackwell et al., 1997; Deutsch et al., 1989; Kitchen et al., 1989; Weed & Sluis, 1990, Weed & Owen, 2018; Weed, 2019). In the early years, life care planning services were offered by only a few professionals but between the years of 1986 and 2022, the specialty practice of life care planning exploded into a major force of its own. Life care planners have been called upon to contribute their expertise in times of national crisis, such as post-9/11as well as with increasing frequency by government agencies including the

Department of Veterans Affairs. Life care plans have been useful in assessing the needs of thousands of individuals with disabilities, not only in the United States, but also internationally.

To meet these challenges, life care planners continue to develop educational tools. While initially publications related to life care planning were few and far between, currently, life care planning literature can be found in thousands of professional books, chapters, and articles in professional disciplines of nursing, medicine, economics, neuropsychology, rehabilitation counseling, occupational/speech/physical therapy, veterans' rehabilitation, legal decisions, insurance, and more. The life care plan methodology is well-established and will continue to be a valuable tool within many venues for years to come.

References

Albee, T. (2019). A historical look at the fellow of the International Association of Life Care Planning (FIALCP) designation. *Journal of Life Care Planning*, *17*(3), 53–56.

American Academy of Nurse Life Care Planners. (1997). *Newsletter*, *1*(4).

Barros-Bailey, M., & Latham, S. (2021). Life care planning education: Evidence-based curriculum design using contemporary standards. *Journal of Life Care Planning*, *19*(1), 59–64.

Berens, D. (2006). Are you a joiner? *Journal of Life Care Planning*, *4*(4), 157–158.

Berens, D. (2019). A journey through the history of life care planning research: The Journal of Life Care Planning and the Foundation for Life Care Planning Research. *Journal of Life Care Planning*, *17*(3), 61–69.

Blackwell, T., Kitchen, J., & Thomas, R. (1997). *Life Care Planning for the Spinal Cord Injured*. E & F Vocational Services.

Buckles, V., Pomeranz, J., & Young, M. E. (2008). The applicability of the life care plan for adopted children with disabilities: What will Medicaid pay? *Journal of Life Care Planning*, *75*(3), 107–122.

Busch, R. (2017). Managing the notion of UCR in a life care plan. *Journal of Life Care Planning*, *15*(3), 3–14.

Commission on Rehabilitation Counselor Certification. (2021). https://crccertification.com/get-certified/crc-exam-overview/

Congratulations…(1995, July-August). *Inside Life Care Planning*, *1*(1), 12. St. Lucie Press.

Cuevas v. Contra Costa County (2017). 11 cal. App. 163, 217 cal. Rptr 3d 519.

Deutsch, P. (n.d.b). *Paul Deutsch Curriculum Vitae*. http://paulmdeutsch.com/CVs-deutsch.htm

Deutsch, P. M., Sawyer, H. W., Jenkins, W. M., & Kitchen, J. (1986) Life care planning in catastrophic case management. *Journal of Private Sector Rehabilitation*, *1*(1), 13–27.

Deutsch, P., & Raffa, F. (1982). *Damages in Tort Action* (Vols. 8 & 9). Matthew Bender.

Deutsch, P., & Sawyer, H. (1985). *Guide to Rehabilitation*. Matthew Bender.

Deutsch, P., Allison, K., & Reid, C. (2003a). *Guide to Rehabilitation* 5–1. AHAB Press.

Deutsch, P., Allison, K., & Reid, C. (2003b). *Guide to Rehabilitation* 5–7. AHAB Press.

Deutsch, P., Weed, R., Kitchen, J., & Sluis, A. (1989). *Life Care Plans for the Spinal Cord Injured: A Step by Step Guide*. Elliott & Fitzpatrick.

Fawber, H. (2019). 25 years of the international symposium of life care planning. *Journal of Life Care Planning*, *17*(3), 15–22.

Field, T. (2006). To our subscribers. *Journal of Life Care Planning*, *4*(4), 158.

Field, T., & Weed R. (2015). Will the Affordable Care Act and tort reform render the Collateral Source Doctrine obsolete in resolving the issue of damages in cases involving personal injury and life care planning? *The Rehabilitation Professional*, *23*(3), 133–148.

FIG Services. (2017). www.figeducation.com/

Fischer, J., & Wilkins, M. J. (2017). Challenges and practice issues faced by Canadian life care planners. *Journal of Life Care Planning*, *15*(3), 31–36.

International Academy of Life Care Planners. (1998). *Academy Letter*, *1*(1), 1–6.

International Academy of Life Care Planners. (2000). *Academy Letter*, *3*(1), 1–4.

International Academy of Life Care Planners. (2006). *Standards of Practice*. International Association of Rehabilitation Professionals.
International Academy of Life Care Planners. (2015). *Standards of Practice for Life Care Planners* (3rd ed). www.rehabpro.org/sections/ialcp/life-care-planning/standards
International Academy of Life Care Planners. (2019). Transdisciplinary practice position paper. *Journal of Life Care Planning*, *17*(2), 3–4.
International Academy of Life Care Planners. (2022). *Standards of Practice for Life Care Planners* (4th ed). https://rehabpro.org/general/custom.asp?page=ialcp-standards-of-practice
International Association of Rehabilitation Professionals. (2022). *Current Fellows*. https://connect.rehabpro.org/lcp/fellow/current-fellows
International Commission for Health Care Certification. (2022). *Certification Programs*. http://ichcc.org/index.htm
Interview. (1995, July-August). *Inside Life Care Planning*, *1*(1), 6–7. St. Lucie Press.
Isom, R., Marini, I., & Reid, C. (2003). Life care planning: Rehabilitation education curricula and faculty needs. *Journal of Life Care Planning*, *2*, 171–174.
Johnson C., & Preston, K. (2012). Consensus and majority statements derived from life care planning summits held in 2000, 2002, 2004, 2006, 2010 and 2012. *Journal of Life Care Planning*, *11*(2), 9–14.
Johnson, C. (2015). Life care planning consensus statements. *Journal of Life Care Planning*, *13*(4), 35–38.
Johnson, C. (2018). A historical review of life care planning summits since 2000. *Journal of Life Care Planning*, *17*(3), 37–51.
Johnson, C., & Preston, K. (2009, September 26). *Life Care Planning Summits: An Analysis of Results and Relevancy for the Future*. International Symposium of Life Care Planning, Chicago, IL.
Johnson, C., Pomeranz, J., & Stetten, N. (2018). Life care planning consensus and majority statements, 2000–2018: Are they still relevant and reliable? A Delphi study. *Journal of Life Care Planning*, *16*(4), 5–13.
Journal of Life Care Planning. (2019). *17*(1). International Association of Rehabilitation Professionals.
Kitchen, J., Cody, L., & Deutsch, P. (1989). *Life Care Plans for the Brain Damaged Baby: A Step by Step Guide*. Paul M. Deutsch Press.
Leahy, M. J., Chan, F., Iwanga, K., Umucu, E., Sung, C., Bishop, M., & Strauser, D. (2018). Empirically derived test specifications for the Certified Rehabilitation Counselor examination: Revising the essential competencies of rehabilitation counselors. *Rehabilitation Counseling Bulletin*, *00*(0), 1–15.
Leahy, M. J., Muenzen, P., Saunders, J. L., & Strauser, D. (2009). Essential knowledge domains underlying effective rehabilitation counseling practice. *Rehabilitation Counseling Bulletin*, *52*(2), 95–106.
Leskin, G., Lew, H., Queen, H., Reeves, D., & Bleiberg, J. (2007). Adaptation of life care planning to patients with polytrauma in a VA inpatient setting: Implications for seamless care coordination. *Journal of Rehabilitation Research & Development*, *44*(7), xxiii–xxvi.
Marini, I., Isom, R., & Reid, C. (2004). Integrating life care planning and expert testimony into rehabilitation education. *Rehabilitation Education*, *17*(4), 248–255.
May V., & MoradiRekabdarkolee, H. (2020). The International Commission on Health Care Certification life care planner role and function investigation. *Journal of Life Care Planning*, *18*(2), 3–67.
May, V. R. (n.d.). Commission reports on first five months of certifying life care planners. *Inside Life Care Planning*, *1*(6), 5,12.
McCollom, P. (1998, May 15). Dialogue for tomorrow. *American Academy of Nurse Life Care Planners' Newsletter*, *1*(1), 3.
McCollom, P. (1997, January 28). Membership status. *American Academy of Nurse Life Care Planners' Newsletter*, *1*(1), 1.
McCollom, P. (2002, December). *International Academy of Life Care Planning Academy Letter, Year of 2002 in review*, 2.
McCollom, P., & Weed, R. (2002). Life care planning: Yesterday, and today. *Journal of Life Care Planning*, *1*(1), 3–7.
Neulicht, A. T., Riddick-Grisham, S., & Goodrich, W. R. (2010). Life care plan survey 2009: Process, methods, and protocols. *Journal of Life Care Planning*, *9*(4), 131–200.

Nikpay, S., Golberstein, E., Neprash, H. T., Carroll, C., & Abraham, J. M. (2021). Taking the pulse of hospitals' response to the New Price Transparency Rule. *Medical Care Research & Review*, *79*(3), 428–434. https://doi.org/10.1177/10775587211024786

Owen, T. R., & Henry, E. K. (2019). Evaluation of reasonableness of fees for life care plan services in Vaccine Act cases. *Journal of Life Care Planning*, *17*(4), 31–37.

Owen. T. R., & Wilkins, M. J. (2019). Practice challenges identified by life care planners in the United States. *Journal of Life Care Planning*, *17*(2), 33–39.

Patient Protection and Affordable Care Act of 2010, Pub. L. No. 111-148, 124 Stat. 119 (2010). www.congress.gov/111/plaws/publ148/PLAW-111publ148.pdf

Paul Deustch & Associates, P. A. (n.d.a). www.paulmdeutsch.com/other-publications.htm

Pomeranz, J., Yu, N., & Reid, C. (2010). Role and function study of life care planners. *Journal of Life Care Planning*, *9*(3), 57–106.

Preston, K. (2019). Standards of practice for life care planners: A 25-year history. *Journal of Life Care Planning*, *17*(3), 57–60.

Preston, K., & Reid, C. (2015). Revision process for the standards of practice for life care planners. *Journal of Life Care Planning*, *13*(3), 21–29.

Reavis, S. (2000). *Standards of Practice*. International Academy of Life Care Planners Standards Committee.

Riddick, S., & Weed, R. (1996). The life care planning process for managing catastrophically impaired patients. In *Case Studies in Nursing Case Management* (pp. 61–91). Aspen.

Shahnasarian, M. (2015). Insights into the International Association of Life Care Planning Fellow Program: Questions and answers from program developers. *Journal of Life Care Planning*, *13*(4), 21–25.

Sutton, A., Deutsch, P., Weed, R., & Berens, D. (2002). Reliability of life care plans: A comparison of original and updated plans. *Journal of Life Care Planning*, *1*, 187–194.

Turner, R. N., Taylor, D. W., Rubin, S. E., & May, V. R., III. (2000). Job functions associated with the development of life care plans. *Journal of Legal Nurse Consulting*, *11*(3), 3–7.

Voogt, R. D. (1995, July-August). Controversial issues in life care planning. *Inside Life Care Planning*, *1*(1), 9.

Weed, R. (1989). Life care planning questions and answers. *Life Care Facts*, *1*, 5–6.

Weed, R. (1994). Life care plans: Expanding the horizons. *Journal of Private Sector Rehabilitation*, *9*, 47–50.

Weed, R. (1995). Life care plans as a managed care tool. *Medical Interface*, *8*, 111–118.

Weed, R. (2001). Life care planning: Past, present, and future. In Guide to Injury Management Vol, III, 3–9. General RE Corporation.

Weed, R. (2002). Life care plan development. *Topics in Spinal Cord Injury* *7*(4), 5–20.

Weed, R. (2004). *Life Care Planning and Case Management Handbook*, 2nd edition. CRC Press.

Weed, R. (2019). A brief history of life care planning. *Journal of Life Care Planning*, *17*(3), 5–14.

Weed, R., & Berens, D. (Eds.) (2000, April 12). *Life Care Planning Summit 2000 Proceedings*. Sponsored by Intelicus, International Academy of Life Care Planners, International Association of Rehabilitation Professionals, and the Commission on Disability Examiner Certification, Dallas, TX. Elliott & Fitzpatrick, Inc.

Weed, R., & Berens, D. (Eds.) (2018). *Life Care Planning and Case Management Handbook* (4th ed.). Routledge Press.

Weed, R., & Berens, D. (Eds.). (2010). *Life Care Planning and Case Management Handbook* (3rd ed.). St. Lucie/CRC Press.

Weed, R. & Field, T. (2001). *The Rehabilitation Consultant's Handbook* (3rd ed.). E & F Vocational Services

Weed, R. & Field, T. (2012). *The Rehabilitation Consultant's Handbook* (4th ed.). E & F Vocational Services

Weed, R., & Owen, T. (2018). *Life Care Planning: A Step-by-Step Guide*. E & F Vocational Services.

Weed, R., & Riddick, S. (1992). Life care plans as a case management tool. *The Individual Case Manager Journal*, *3*, 26–35.

Weed, R., & Sluis, A. (1990). *Life Care Plans for the Amputee: A Step-by-Step Guide*. CRC Press.

Chapter 2

Methodology, Scope of Practice, Standards of Practice, and Consensus in Life Care Planning

Mary Barros-Bailey, Tanya Rutherford-Owen, and Karen Preston

The authors would like to thank Dr. Penelope Caragonne, Dr. Chris Reid, and Dr. Roger Weed for their reviews and feedback to this first chapter in the literature on life care planning methodology.

The purpose of this chapter is to bring together the contemporary information about life care planning methodology, scope of practice, standards of practice, and consensus statements into one source. Written for novice and seasoned life care planners, this chapter bridges the history of the discipline (see chapter titled Life Care Planning: Past, Present, and Future in this text) into a contemporary and emerging application. As life care planning is honed, melded, and changed by the reality of evolving and vibrant healthcare, as well as legal, economical, and technological environments in which it dwells, our hope is that this chapter will present life care planners with a marquis to practice as performed in the 2020s and be fodder for advancements in core practices in the field.

Life Care Planning Foundations

Life care planning was developed as a solution to the problem that rehabilitation researchers experienced when trying to effectively communicate to families the complex needs of children diagnosed with cerebral palsy. This problem presented the need for a "structured, systematic reference tool" to provide a roadmap to future care (Deutsch et al., 2003, p. 5–4). From this need, emerged the product of the life care plan, and along with it, the specialty practice of life care planning as a discipline.

As with any specialty practice, life care planning methods must be built upon a foundation, which is defined as "a basis (such as a tenet, principle, or axiom) upon which something stands or is supported" (Merriam-Webster, n.d.-a, para. 1). Therefore, the foundations of life care planning in rehabilitation are traced to case management, applied behavior analysis (informed in part through experimental psychology), and developmental psychology (Deutsch et al., 2003).

Underlying Principles in Life Care Planning

In the early 1970s, case management emerged to meet the need for service coordination for individuals with long-term healthcare needs. The Commission for Case Manager Certification (2022, para 1) defines case management as, "… a professional and collaborative process that assesses, plans, implements, coordinates, monitors, and evaluates the options and services required to meet an individual's health needs." By the early 1990s, the Individual Case Management Association and a certification in case management (Certified Case Manager) were formed (Case Management Society of America, 2021; Weed & Field, 2012). Elements of case management are seen in the tool of the life care plan as it creates for the reader an integrated, coordinated plan of care for an individual with a disability. Sorenson (1995, p. 73) wrote, "In case management, long- or short-term care activities are coordinated into blocks of time. In life care plans, these blocks are reorganized, divided, and subcategorized for optimum definition." This subdivision rested in part on the field of applied behavior analysis.

The influence of applied behavior analysis is evident in the component of life care planning that addresses an individual's behavioral change over time. Through counting and charting discrete behaviors, experimental psychologists and applied behavior analysts are able to break down human behavior and measure behavioral change over time (Paul M. Deutsch & Associates, n.d.). Relying upon patient-specific behavior and research literature, life care planners can reliably determine patient-specific needs to achieve rehabilitation goals.

The influence of developmental psychology in life care planning is seen in the components of social, cognitive, and physical changes that occur within an individual over their lifespan. This lifespan approach is foundational to a life care plan because prior to the emergence of life care planning, no method existed whereby healthcare professionals could methodically organize, evaluate, and project needs over one's lifetime. With the convergence of behavioral analysis, developmental psychology, and case management, the foundation for life care planning was laid.

By the 1990s, pioneers in life care planning began to acknowledge the need for a specialty-wide consensus on a life care planning methodology. Establishing a methodology to prepare life care plans was dependent, as noted by Deutsch et al. (2003) on several factors, namely:

1. The need for a summative statement
2. A tool of communication
3. Forethought of planning
4. Analysis of complex concerns into basic components
5. Plans are individualized to meet the unique needs of each [evaluee/client/patient]
6. Needs, rather than funding sources, drive the planning process

Life care planning is not a title, it is a practice. In licensing, the terms title and practice make a difference such that:

> ... title acts refer to those licensure laws that restrict the use of a specific title to only those individuals meeting education, training, and examination standards ... Practice acts refer to those licensure laws that prohibit [a professional practice] without licensure. (American Counseling Association, 2022, para. 6)

Regardless of what someone calls themselves or their work product, if they are using methods and techniques that are easily found in the life care planning literature, they are engaging in the specialty practice of life care planning. Deutsch (2011, p. 846) stated:

> There are many reasons that require our specialty practice to reach a similar consensus on the required foundations for the development of a life care plan and within those foundations to agree on guidelines on the steps that should be taken to accomplish the completion of tasks in multiple areas of plan development.
> Deutsch (2011, p. 846)

It is clear that over 20 years ago, Dr. Deutsch recognized the need for life care planning methodology to be properly grounded in clearly established standards based upon a proper foundation. As early as 2000, the life care planning community devised a process, which became known as the Life Care Planning Summit, to address this need.

In 2011, Paul M. Deutsch, who is widely considered to be the father of life care planning wrote:

> Although there are always those outliers who only follow their own approach to this specialty practice, the majority seems to have accepted the areas to cover within the life care plan regardless of the format within which they present these areas.
> (Deutsch, 2011, p. 845)

In 2003, Deutsch and Reid outlined the following basic tenets of life care planning:

1. First and foremost, life care planners are rehabilitation professionals and educators
2. All plan recommendations should clearly relate to patient-specific evaluation data
3. Assume the probability of success of recommendations
4. Life care plans are designed to answer questions, not raise them
5. Life care plans specify provisions throughout life expectancy and cannot depend on any one individual, service, or supplier for fulfilling plan recommendations
6. Recommendations must consider disability, individual, family, and regional factors
7. Attend to details
8. Recommendations are proactive, not reactive
9. Recognize the benefits of maximizing patient potential
10. Life care planning is multidimensional
11. Consider the entire cost of each recommendation
12. The costs provided in a life care plan do not include two important categories: potential complications and future technology
13. Consider the psychological effects of the injury or disability
14. Disability interacts with age to produce additional concerns (pp. 5-14–5-19)

Operational Definitions

A chapter about methodologies and foundational sources serves as a guideline for life care planners. To ensure clarity in terminology, a few definitions are necessary.

Methodology

To start with the basics: What is a method? It is simply "a systematic procedure, technique, or mode of inquiry employed by or proper to a particular discipline of art" (Merriam-Webster, n.d.-b, para. 2). Probably the most known process that has existed for over 400 years is the scientific method developed by Sir Francis Bacon (Online Library of Liberty, 2022) that has five steps:

1. Make an observation
2. Ask a question
3. Form a hypothesis, or testable explanation
4. Make a prediction based on the hypothesis
5. Test the prediction (The Kahn Academy, 2022)

However recognizable these steps may be over the last four centuries, conceivably the greatest contribution of the method is a final feedback step that is not formally part of the method, but a consequence of it; the step places an iterative loop-back expectation into the method, suggesting that the results of one study will spring thought resulting in further observations, questions, hypotheses, predictions, and tests, and so on (The Khan Academy, 2022). Like the scientific method, a process does not have to be complicated to endure and be impactful.

Scope of Practice

Another operational definition is a scope of practice. The American Medical Association (2022) describes a scope of practice as "those activities that a person licensed to practice as a health professional is permitted to perform" (para. 1). Each life care planner comes from a profession that has educational standards and assessment of that practitioner's competencies to meet the minimum requirements for that discipline's general scope of practice. Although life care planners have a general scope of practice from their professional discipline, through additional knowledge, training, and experience specific to life care planning, they also develop an individualized scope of practice that is defined as:

> … more specialized than the professional scope. An individual scope of practice is based on one's own knowledge of the abilities and skills that have been gained through a program of education and professional experience. A person is ethically bound to limit [their] practice to that individual scope of practice.
> (Commission on Rehabilitation Counselor ., 2022, para. 3)

Standards of Practice

After defining the boundaries of what a life care planner does comes the standards of *how* practices are performed within those boundaries. Thus, the third definition is of a standard (specifically applied to practice) as "something established by authority, custom, or general consent as a model or example" (Merriam-Webster, n.d.-c, para. 3). The most recent standards contained within this chapter have regularly been reviewed and refined with changes in the specialty practice.

Consensus Statements

Lastly, professional consensus statements are generally described as "developed by an independent panel of experts, usually multidisciplinary, convened to review the research literature in an evidence-based manner for the purpose of advancing the understanding of an issue, procedure[,] and method" (Jacobs et al., 2014, para. 5). Such is the case with consensus statements in life care planning, which will be explored further.

Methodology in Life Care Planning

The agreed-upon definition of a life care plan that has been in existence for nearly 25 years is:

> A life care plan is a dynamic document based upon published standards of practice, comprehensive assessment, data analysis, and research, which provides an organized concise plan for current and future needs with associated costs, for individuals who have experienced catastrophic injury or have chronic health care needs.
>
> (Combined definition of the University of Florida and Intelicus annual life care planning conference and the American Academy of Nurse Life Care Planners (now known as the International Academy of Life Care Planners) presented at the Forensic Section meeting, NARPPS annual conference, Colorado Springs, Colorado, and agreed upon April 3, 1998)

The definition itself has several components that could be considered methodological.

Further, Weed and Grisham (Weed, 2018), in their Step-by-Step Procedure for Life Care Planning identify what is likely the closest detailed process to the dictionary definition of a methodology currently existing in life care planning. This exhaustive procedure has the following steps:

1. Case Intake Details
2. Medical Records
3. Supporting Documentation
4. Initial Interview Arrangements
5. Initial Interview Materials
6. Consulting with Therapeutic Team Members
7. Preparing Life Care Planning Options
8. Filling in the Holes
9. Research Costs and Sources
10. Finalizing the Life Care Plan
11. Distribution of Life Care Plan

Like the scientific method and the detailed steps by Weed and Grisham, the definition of life care planning, and the standards of practice from across the field can be consolidated into a five-part multi-phasic methodology with a feedback phase as detailed in Table 2.1.

Table 2.1 Phases of the Life Care Planning Method

Phase	Description
1	**Determine Purpose**: Identify the purpose of the life care plan.
2	**Review Secondary Data and Conceptualize Case**: Review all secondary data provided and develop a conceptualization of the case to guide the life care planning process for the evaluee/client/patient.[1]
3	**Collect Primary Data**: Collect primary data.
4	**Research and Data Analysis**: Determine relevant categories, costs, and support for current and future needs.
5	**Report Findings**: Provide a narrative and tabular report of findings, conclusions, and recommendations.
6	**Re-Evaluation**: Returning to any phase of the life care planning method depending on the dynamic need of the case.

[1] Although much of life care planning is performed in forensic practice where the standard of care is not the provision of clinical services, it can also be used in a clinical setting (e.g., case management); therefore, where the concepts used in this chapter equally apply to those settings, the "evaluee/client/patient" terminology is used, unless it is within a quote from another source.

Each of the phases can have a multitude of steps, checklists, categories, techniques, degrees of detail, etc. depending on the purpose of the assignment, details of the case, and/or the resources available (e.g., time). This methodology is not only anchored in current life care planning literature, but also in the case study research process (Yin, 2018).

Phase 1: Determine Purpose

Akin to Weed and Grisham's Case Intake Details or the Case Initiation or Forensic Application steps in the International Academy of Life Care Planners ([IALCP], 2022) *Standards of Practice*, determining the purpose of the life care plan, or the case, drives all other activities within the case (Yin, 2018). For example, if the purpose is not to provide a comprehensive assessment of the individual—an inherent component of life care planning—but to list the likely future costs of a single treatment option (e.g., revision of a total knee arthroplasty), a life care plan is likely not warranted. In this situation, an alternative work product that may or may not require all the phases in the life care planning methodology could be undertaken. The result of this process is what some life care planners may call a medical cost projection.

Phase 2: Review Evidence and Conceptualize Case

Secondary data are those which the life care planner is provided, such as a comprehensive medical, legal, education, vocational, etc. set of records (all called *documents*), that may contain *archival data* not yet analyzed or interpreted by a particular professional (e.g., imaging films, list of medications, vital records), and *physical artifacts* such as pictures of the incident scene, of the evaluee/client/patient in inpatient treatment, durable medical equipment, etc. Barros-Bailey (2018) classifies these three case study categories of evidence (Yin, 2018) as secondary data, which are defined as data collected by someone other than the life care planner but viewed and reviewed by the professional to provide grounding about the case. Cross walked to the Weed and Grisham step-by-step process, this phase contains the Medical Records and Supporting Documentation steps. At the completion of this phase, the life care planner's education, training, experience, and skill results in a conceptualization of the individual, which stimulates questions and activities for the next phase of the methodology through such tasks as steps 4 and 5 of the Weed and Grisham procedures: Initial Interview Arrangements and Initial Interview Materials. The American Association of Nurse Life Care Planning (AANLCP®) *Standards of Practice* steps for Nursing Process Assessment and Diagnosis occur during Phases 2 and 3 of the Life Care Planning Method. Similarly, Phases 2 and 3 represent the collection of data and evidence best represented in the third step of the IALCP *Standards of Practice* (2022; Analysis, Synthesis to Identify Functioning, Disability, and Health).

Phase 3: Collect Primary Data

The other three types of case study data (Yin, 2018) are classified by Barros-Bailey (2018) as primary data, or data which life care planners collect themselves, and that results in a significant component of the comprehensive assessment aspect of the definition of the life care plan. That is, secondary evidence is that which someone else developed and the life care planner reviews while primary data is that which the life care planner collects for the case through *interviews* (e.g., evaluee/client/patient, family, treatment or damages team, other collateral sources), *observation* (e.g., administration of formal or informal assessments, sensorial observation of evaluee/client/patient), or by participating in an activity with the evaluee/client/patient (called *participant-observation*), such as understanding how the evaluee/client/patient performs a task by doing the task with them. This third phase is partly consistent with step 6 by Weed and Grisham, or Consulting with Therapeutic Team Members. Phases 2 and 3 are not necessarily sequential, but can be cyclical, meaning that after meeting with the evaluee/client/patient, the life care planner may learn there are records for services that were not included in records already reviewed and may need to cycle back between Phases 2 and 3 during the secondary and primary data collection phases.

Phase 4: Research and Data Analysis

As this is likely the phase of the life care planning method that takes the longest, it has the most written about it as evidenced by the development of various checklists, summits focused on one aspect of the phase (e.g., costing), and research or opinion articles about it. This stage encompasses steps 7 through 9 of the Weed and Grisham steps (Preparing Life Care Planning Options, Filling in the Holes, and Research Costs and Sources) as well as the parts of the life care plan definition involving research and data analysis and steps 3 through 5 of the IALCP *Standards of Practice* (Analysis and Synthesis to Identify Functioning, Disability, and Health; Delineating Future Care Recommendations; and Delineating Costs), and AANLCP®'s Outcomes Identification and Planning. In this phase, the life care planner classifies the needs into categories. Whatever category classification system the life care planner uses or chooses to call each category, it is important to understand that as a member of a team that may contain a forensic economist, accountant, or other professional who calculates the lifetime values of the recommended items, it is imperative that like items be clustered together by the kind of growth rate category (Dillman, 2018) as was the original intention of the categories developed by Deutsch and Raffa (1981). As demonstrated by several chapters in this text (e.g., Admissibility Considerations in Life Care Planning; A Defense Attorney's Perspective on Life Care Planning; Forensic Issues for Life Care Planners; A Plaintiff's Attorney's Perspective on Life Care Planning; Research in Life Care Planning), the bar for life care planners is rising; therefore, the inclusion of critical appraisal or other literature, clinical practice guidelines, or other secondary data and evidence at this phase is equally important as in Phase 2.

Various authors have called for evidence-based practice integration into life care planning (Caragonne, 2013; Mertes, 2018; Metekingi, 2013; Owen, 2012). Evidence-based practice is a concept that was introduced into the medical practice lexicon by Gordon Guyatt of McMaster University in 1990 (Chalmers et al., 2018). It has since spread throughout allied health, education, business, and many other disciplines. Conceptually, there are several hierarchal levels of potential quantitative, qualitative, or mixed methods data from subject matter expert opinion at the lowest level of evidence and critical appraisal literature at the top (see Research in Life Care Planning and Life Care Planning Costing, Literature, and Summary of Resources chapters in this text). A life care plan that includes not only the case-specific primary and secondary data, but also aligns the critical factors of the individualized assessment to peer-reviewed publications, clinical practice guidelines, and other evidence-based literature has the ability correlate various associated data points, thereby improving the internal consistency and validity of the life care plan.

Phase 5: Report Findings

Written—and sometimes oral—reports are common in the practice of life care planning. They are the last two steps of Weed and Grisham's procedural steps (Finalizing the Life Care Plan and Distributing the Life Care Plan) as well as steps 6 through 8 of the IALCP *Standards of Practice* (2022, Work Product Creation; Evaluation for Consistency within the Life Care Plan and Adherence to Standards of Practice; and Education of Consumers/Users of Life Care Plans) as well as AANLCP"s Implementation and Evaluation steps. This phase also includes the part of the life care plan definition about producing an organized concise plan with costs, reviewing it for internal consistency and validity, and sharing the work product with the appropriate stakeholders. How the life care plan report is written is as individualized as the life care planner and should contain content from the first four phases. Verifying inclusion of important components of the report could be accomplished with a life care plan report writing checklist (Barros-Bailey, 2020).

Phase 6: Re-Evaluation

Phase 6 in life care planning methodology provides the opportunity for the life care plan to undergo re-evaluation over time. This phase serves a different purpose than Phases 1 through 5, which are focused on the original product creation. Foundational to the life care planning definition is the concept of dynamism. As the human body and the human experience are in a constant state of change, so too is the life care plan a dynamic document that may also require changes over time. This phase allows for the evaluation of the life care plan for such change. Revision to the life care plan over time does not mean that the original plan was faulty, but rather that the forces acting upon the individual (e.g., access to care or changes in bodily function) or the environment in which they reside or receive services necessitate re-evaluation of elements of the life care plan. The accuracy of needs identification is not threatened by re-evaluation, as the threshold for including items in a plan remains "more likely than not" at the time of each evaluation or re-evaluation.

Last Word on Life Care Planning Methodology

The life care planning method is iterative, flexible, and individualized to the needs of a person. It aligns not only within the literature that has been published in the field for four decades, but also with basic methodology and design of how to research a case study (Yin, 2018). The method is reiterative like the scientific method and can be cyclical or linear depending on the dynamic nature of the process.

Lifespan Development in Life Care Planning

For the first time, this fifth edition text addresses life care planning across the lifespan by bringing together two seminal edited publications in the field–the *Life Care Planning and Case Management Handbook* (4th ed., Weed & Berens, 2018) and the *Pediatric Life Care Planning and Case Management Handbook* (2nd ed., Riddick-Grisham & Deming, 2011). By taking a lifespan approach, this text celebrates the origins of life care planning rooted in developmental psychology and the importance of human development applied to the disability process. Theoretical orientation of human development across the lifespan is important foundational knowledge regardless of the point when an evaluee/client/patient acquired a physical, mental, or cognitive condition.

Ecological Model (Bronfenbrenner) in Life Care Planning

Tethering life care planning to its foundation in developmental psychology, the evaluee/client/patient's interaction with their environment is well-represented by Bronfenbrenner's ecological model (Bronfenbrenner, 1975). This model posits that the individual simultaneously exists within a nested arrangement of structures, which Bronfenbrenner named the microsystem, mesosystem, exosystem, and macrosystem. He organized these structures by order of how much of an impact each system has on an individual. Each system is defined as follows:

- Microsystem: "… the pattern of activities, social roles, and interpersonal relations experienced by an individual in a given setting" (ScienceDirect, 2019, para. 1).
- Mesosystem: "… the interlinking system of microsystems in which a person participates – for example, linkages between family and school" (ScienceDirect, 2008a, para. 1).
- Exosystem: "… one or more settings that do not involve the … person as an active participant, but in which events occur that affect – or as affected by – what happens in the setting containing the … person" (ScienceDirect, 2018, para. 1).
- Macrosystem: "… the overarching pattern of the culture or subculture in which the micro-, meso-, and exosystems are nested" (ScienceDirect, 2008b, para. 1).

As a human development model that covers the lifespan, he also superimposed it upon a temporal system he calls the chronosystem. The original definition of a life care plan published, in the early 1980s, reflected the element of chronicity in disability, stating that life care planning was:

> A consistent methodology for analyzing all of the needs dictated by the onset of a catastrophic disability through to the end of life expectancy. Consistency means that the methods of analysis remain the same from case to case and does not mean that the same services are provided to like disabilities.
> (Deutsch & Raffa, 1981; Deutsch & Sawyer, 2002 as cited in Deutsch et al., 2003, pp. 5–7)

Bronfenbrenner's model acknowledges that the individual's systems persist through time chronologically within the chronosystem; yet, like the original definition implies, the needs of each person are individualized.

Bronfenbrenner's ecological model is a useful framework for the life care planner to conceptualize the evaluee/client/patient for whom they are developing a life care plan. Surprisingly, an all database EBSCO search of Bronfenbrenner's model applied to disability regardless of date found few publications and limited to the following areas:

- autism (Brisendine et al., 2021; Ravindran & Myers, 2012) and intellectual disabilities (Jacobs et al., 2018; Pedrinelli et al., 2018)
- cross-cultural disability issues (Melchiorre et al., 2016; Suarez-Balcaza et al., 2020)
- education and special education (Bean, 2012; Brunsting et al., 2014; Howie, 1999; Skarbek et al., 2009; Smit et al., 2020)
- health risks (Boateng et al., 2017)
- neuropsychiatry and neurodiversity (Aftab, 2022)
- testing (Úbeda-Colomer et al., 2018)
- therapeutic recreation (King et al., 2013)
- vocational, work, and rehabilitation counseling (Céspedes, 2005; Durand et al., 2003; Hershenson, 1998; Landon et al., 2019)
- youth in transitions (Boaden et al., 2021)

These publications deal with people with special needs in particular disability groups or contexts, and typically at particular points in their development. However, the literature appeared silent on the application of the ecological model across the lifespan and largely ignored the chronosystem part of the model.

The International Classification of Functioning, Disability, and Health in Life Care Planning

Since Bronfenbrenner developed his model, the World Health Organization (WHO) established the International Classification of Functioning, Disability, and Health (ICF) in 2001. Pomeranz and Shaw (2007) found strong similarities between the life care planning process and the ICF model, and the ICF framework's usefulness to life care planning and Stetten et al. (2022) recently applied the ICF model to medical marijuana use and chronic pain implications for life care planning.

When exploring the interaction of the more recent ICF system within the ecological model, the models located seemed focused on a singular cross-section period within the lifespan, typically childhood, and did not progressively consider disability across the entire lifespan (Adolfsson et al., 2018; McLinden et al., 2017; Schewcik, 2017; Simeonsson et al., 2010). Macy and Rusch (2010) published a comprehensive chapter on the integration of the ICF into life care planning that provides tools that help the life care planner in the evaluation process regardless of the evaluee/client/patient's stage of life, but do not integrate it within an ecological model that blends with the various Bronfenbrenner systems. Based on the application of the ICF to the ecological model, the authors of this chapter considered the chronosystem and developed a visual model, shown in Figure 2.1, which adapts the Bronfenbrenner ecological model with each system of impact on human development and within the temporal context of the chronosystem, to acknowledge that

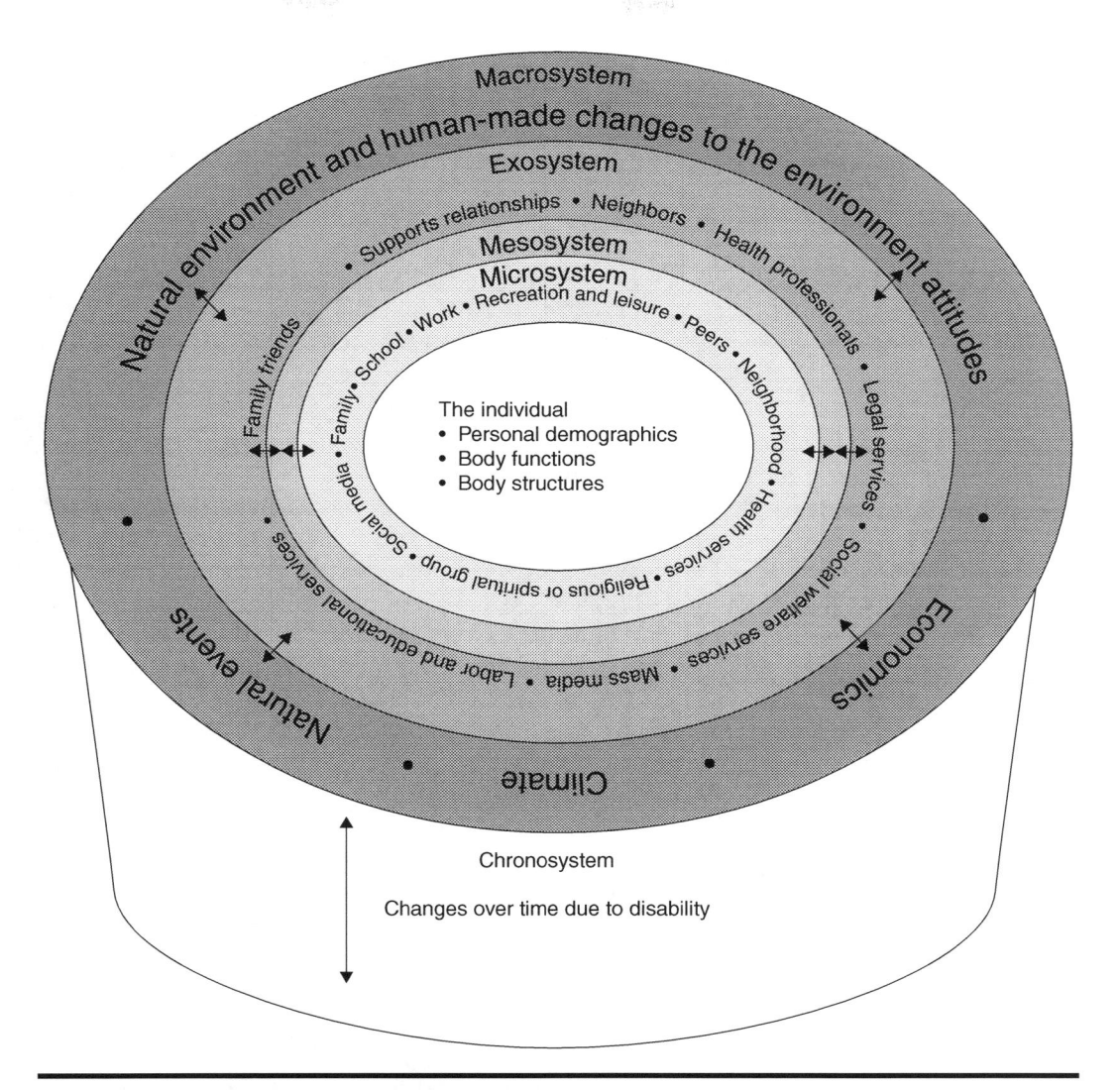

Figure 2.1 Ecological Model-ICF Model for Life Care Planning

disability can occur at any period and that future needs can endure throughout short periods or over the lifespan.

An acquired physical, mental, or cognitive condition from an incident or exposure can occur any time during the lifespan—any time after conception or late in the lifespan along the timeline represented by the chronosystem, which is defined as changes that are as:

> ... a result of the movements, events, and shifting ideologies associated with historical time. The chronosystem also includes other temporal elements of environmental change, such as sequential processes, chronological age, generational cohort, and developmental growth ....
>
> (Arnold et al., 2012, p. 83)

The disability can affect the evaluee/client/patient's body structures and functions, even their demographics if life expectancy is altered (Jokela et al., 2020; O'Leary et al., 2018; Polinder et al., 2012; Roseen et al., 2021; Seid et al., 2022; Tyrer et al., 2021). The evaluee/client/patient's interaction with the various systems in their life can likewise be transformed, changing dependencies and interdependencies as well as access to people, environments, technologies, etc. For example, a middle school child who was active in a league soccer team and an average achieving student sustains a spinal cord injury resulting in an American Spinal Injury Association (ASIA) A tetraplegia. In the ICF, core sets are "facilitate the description of functioning … by providing lists of essential categories that are relevant for specific health conditions and health care contexts …. Selected from the entire IFC" (IFC Research Branch, 2022, para. 1). At the core of the ecological model, or the individual level, a life care planner can use the comprehensive and brief ICF core sets for spinal cord injury at the early post-acute and the long-term contexts (WHO, 2017a, 2017b). These core sets can help the life care planner identify changes in body structures and body functions to detect current and future needs along the choronsystem, as well as the impact of aging and life expectancy itself along that system. The activities and participation elements of the ICF model specific to the spinal cord injury core sets can help the life care planner identify how the child interacts with the world and, for instance, what level of assistance may be needed for such activities as driving or using transportation. Other activities of daily living (ADLs) or instrumental activities of daily living (IADLs) from individuals or organizations in their microsystem (family, friends, school, religious community, health services, neighborhood, etc.) can also be identified. At the mesosystem level, which is the interaction of two microsystems (such as family and healthcare), the life care planner can explore what relationships need to be developed now and into the future for short- and long-term support as the child matures and transitions into other stages of the human development process. Such system interactions, that would not be in place but for the injury, may be attendant care and case management, which will interact between the child-turned-adult or the family at the mesosystem level. Likewise, the ICF core set elements in activities and participation can help identify future services that relate to intimate relationships, remunerative employment, economic self-sufficiency, as well as recreation and leisure. Additional elements in this area include products and technologies that allow the youth to live, thrive, and enjoy life differently, such as products and technologies for culture, recreation, and sport that allow the child to access adapted sports or similar activities. While the child in our example would not interact directly with all the entities contained within the exosystem level (e.g., a parent's employer), the parents would and this might indirectly affect the child if the parent needs to leave employment temporarily or permanently, or cut back in the amount of work they do, to care for the child because of the inability to get consistent and reliable attendant care. Although exosystem core sets are generally not as strong in their influence as the other systems within the model, they nonetheless can serve as a guide when considering elements as they relate to other system levels in their application to the mesosystem. Finally, at the macrosystem level that includes systems of individuals in society (e.g., institutions, media, governments, or other entities), the ICF core sets provide a strong and long list of considerations that might be important for the life care planner's consideration:

- Architecture and construction services, systems, and policies
- Associations and organizational services, systems, and policies
- Communication services, systems, and policies
- Education and training services, systems, and policies
- General social support services, systems, and policies
- Health services, systems, and policies

- Housing services, systems, and policies
- Labor and employment services, systems, and policies
- Legal services, systems, and policies
- Services, systems, and policies for the production of consumer goods
- Social norms, practices, and ideologies
- Social security services, systems, and policies
- Societal attitudes
- Transportations services, systems, and policies
- Utilities services, systems, and policies

The ICF also has a set of qualifiers that cover anatomical location (e.g., uni- and bilateral, front, back, proximal, distal), barrier/facilitator (e.g., no [0–4%], mild [5–24%]), capacity (same measurement levels as barrier/facilitator), extent or magnitude of impairment (same measure levels as barrier/facilitator), nature of change to body structure (e.g., no change, total absence, partial absence), and performance (same measurement levels as barrier/facilitator). The interaction between the Bronfenbrenner ecological model and the ICF can provide the life care planner with tools for a comprehensive and thorough individualized assessment and, consequently, a valid and reliable plan of care across the lifespan.

Scope of Practice in Life Care Planning

By 2022, it is well established that life care planning is transdisciplinary in nature (IALCP, 2022; Mauk, 2017). In practice this means that professionals from a variety of healthcare disciplines may engage in the specialty practice of life care planning. Those disciplines include, but are not limited to, registered nursing, medicine, occupational therapy, physical therapy, psychology, rehabilitation counseling, and speech language pathology. As life care planners are trained in a primary discipline prior to completing further training in life care planning, they work within the realm of life care planning in the scope of practice of their primary discipline. For instance, occupational therapists in their role as life care planners, must work within their scope of practice as occupational therapists to qualify as practitioners within the principles of that profession. It is with this professional foundation they dive deeper in their formation into the application of that general knowledge to life care planning and qualify as life care planners.

In 2019, the *Journal of Life Care Planning* (IARP, 2019) published a special edition outlining the scope of practice of seven primary professional disciplines within life care planning. The authors who addressed the scope of practice for each discipline were individuals involved in current practice in their discipline. The goal of this issue was to lay the "foundation for scope of practice for each profession but recognize that each life care planner needs to look at their own 'extras' and consider the 'extras' that another life care planner has when reviewing another person's life care plan" (Preston, 2019, p. 3). The reader is referred to the issue for a discussion of the scope of practice of each life care planning discipline covered including occupational therapy, physical therapy, physiatry, psychology, registered nursing, rehabilitation counseling, and speech language pathology. A summary of the tables from the publication can be found in Table 2.2. The summary table is based on the opinions of the subject matter authors of the respective articles and has not been validated through consensus or other research across the life care planning field or each profession's credentialing boards. Such consensus research may result in different opinions as to qualifications to provide opinions in each area of the table.

Table 2.2 Scopes of Practice in Life Care Planning

CARE CATEGORY	OT	PT	PM&R	PSY	RN	RC	SLP
Physician (MD, DO, DC, DDS) Referral to Evaluate/Consult	S/C	S	Y	Y	Y	N	Y
Physician (MD, DO) On-Going Visits	N	N	Y	N	Y/C	N	C
Chiropractic Visits	N	Y	C	N	C	N	N
Dentist On-Going Visits and Sedation	N	N	Y	N	C	N	N
Ancillary (non-physician professionals) Referrals	Y	S	Y	Y	Y/C	W	Y
Ancillary On-Going Visits	S	S	C	C	C	S	Y/C
Diagnostic Testing	N	C	Y	S	Y/C	N	S
Surgery	N	N	S/C	N	N	N	N
Aggressive Interventions (e.g., invasive procedures, specialty programs)	S	S	Y/C	S	Y	N	S
Wheelchairs, Including Features and Accessories	Y	Y	Y/C	N/C	S/C	C	S
Other Mobility Equipment	Y	Y	Y/C	N/C	C	C	S
Orthotics	Y	Y	Y/C	N/C	C	N	N
Prosthetics	C	C	C	S	Y/C	N	S
Other Medical Equipment	S/C	Y/C	Y/C	N/C	Y/C	Y/C	S
Adaptive Aids for Independent Function	Y	Y	Y/C	S	S	Y/C	S
Drugs Requiring Prescription	N	N	Y	O	O	N	N
Over-the-Counter Drugs	N	N	Y	O	Y	N	N
Disposable Supplies	N	Y/C	Y/C	S	Y	Y/C	S
Home Care Skill Level (to attend to person) (i.e., unlicensed aide, licensed nurse)	Y	Y	C	C	Y	Y	C
Home Care Hours	Y	Y	C	C	Y	Y	N
Household (housekeeping, yard care, house repairs) Services and Hours	Y	Y	C	C	Y	Y	C
Adapted Transportation (evaluation, training, equipment)	Y	Y	Y/C	C	Y	Y	N

(Continued)

Table 2.2 (Continued)   Scopes of Practice in Life Care Planning

CARE CATEGORY	OT	PT	PM&R	PSY	RN	RC	SLP
Alternative Transportation	Y	Y	C	C	Y	Y	N
Architectural Modification	Y	Y	Y/C	C	Y	Y	C
Home Furnishings	Y	Y	N	C	Y	Y	S
Health Maintenance	S	Y	C	C	Y	Y/C	C
Adaptive or Therapeutic Recreation	Y/C	Y	Y	C	Y	Y	S
Potential Complications	Y/C	C	Y	Y	Y	Y/C	S

Legend:

N = Outside Scope of Practice
N/C = Outside Scope of Practice or Collaborative
Y = Within Scope of Practice
Y/C = Within Scope of Practice or Collaborative
C = Collaborative
S = Some of this category is in the discipline's scope of practice
S/C = Some of this category is within the scope of practice; otherwise it is collaborative
O = Other (see footnote)

1. OT=Boniface
2. PT=Bubanja
3. PM&R= Mann
4. PSY=Jacobs
5. RN=Carey
6. RC=Mertes
7. SLP=Higdon
8. Next to the "O" in the cell of Drugs Requiring Prescription for PSY
9. Next to the "O" in the cell of Drugs Requiring Prescription for RN
10. Next to the "O" in the cell for Over-the-Counter Drugs and PSY

1 Boniface et al., 2017.
2 Bubanja & Conover, 2017.
3 Mann, 2017.
4 Jacobs & Strum, 2017.
5 Carey & Marcinko, 2017.
6 Mertes & Harden, 2017.
7 Higdon, 2017.
8 Outside scope of practice except for allowed drugs by prescribing psychologists.
9 Outside scope of practice except for allowed drugs by prescribing registered nurses.
10 Outside scope of practice except for prescribing psychologists.

Table 2.3 Reasons for Standards of Practice

- Determine desired level of performance.
- Reflect normative behavior.
- Represent a level of requirement agreed upon by members of a practice.
- Public declaration to society, consumers, and others about what constitutes quality.
- Describe the structure, process, or outcomes of professional practice.
- A reference tool to understand job requirements.
- A statement of values and priorities.
- A tool against which actual performance can be measured.

Standards of Practice in Life Care Planning

Standards related to life care planning have a complex history. Historically, professional associations were responsible for articulating standards. However, the development of standards pre-dates the existence of any professional association for life care planners. A brief review of standards' evolution will provide the context for understanding the current state of standards and how standards continue to evolve.

An important point to recognize is that standards for life care planners are an adjunct to other standards. Life care planners come from a variety of health professions (i.e., counseling, nursing, therapy, and others), each of which has its own set of standards. Those professions have licensing or regulatory authority and can use standards as part of their compliance measurement, allowing the professional to practice. Life care planning is not a profession. It is a field of specialty practice, much like case manager, academician, bedside clinician, or researcher. There is no regulating body that controls entry into life care planning practice; no professional discipline has authority over life care planning. Thus, standards for life care planners are delineated by practitioners for the purpose of self-definition, a voluntary desire to have consistency within the specialty practice, and a tool for educating others. Does this mean that a life care planner does not need to follow standards of practice? In practical application, no one can prohibit someone from doing life care plans, but market forces will certainly affect the ability to get referrals and defend work product. Some of the common reasons for delineating and following standards are shown in Table 2.3 (Fick & Preston, 2015).

The earliest standards were designed to address qualifications to become a life care planner. In 1995–1996, the concept of life care planning as a methodology for addressing future needs was being developed. Dr. Paul Deutsch and Dr. Horace Sawyer were interested in identifying necessary content for training programs. Working through the University of Florida, they identified knowledge and skills. Their initial work led to a standardized program that emphasized expertise in research, development, coordination, integration, interpretation, and management of life care plans for persons with catastrophic disabilities. Completion of the training program deemed a person to be considered a qualified life care planner (H. Sawyer, personal communication, May 20, 2022).

In 1996, the first professional association for life care planners was founded by Patricia McCollom with the initial standards to determine qualifications for life care planning training (Figure 2.2). Named the American Academy of Nurse Life Care Planners, within one year it was renamed the IALCP to be inclusive of life care planners from all disciplines. In 1998, the first *Academy Letter* was published to begin a national dialogue about standards of practice for life care planners. As a fledgling field of practice, life care planners were eager to establish some consistency

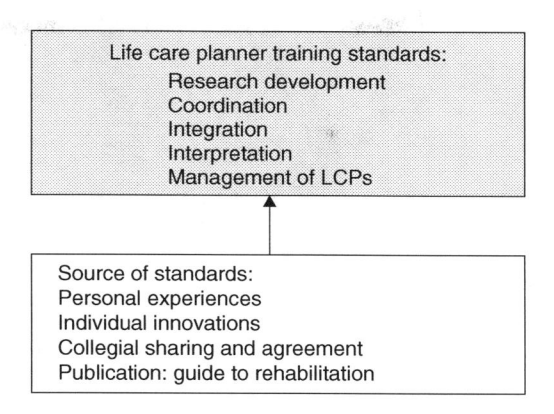

```
Life care planner training standards:
    Research development
    Coordination
    Integration
    Interpretation
    Management of LCPs
```
↑
```
Source of standards:
Personal experiences
Individual innovations
Collegial sharing and agreement
Publication: guide to rehabilitation
```

Figure 2.2 Initial Standards to Determine Qualifications for Life Care Planning Training

```
Life care planner professional standards:
    Credentialling/experience
    Qualifications
    Formal education
    Business practices
```
↑
```
Source of standards:
Collegial sharing and agreement
Training program content
Use of training standards to define the life
care planner
```

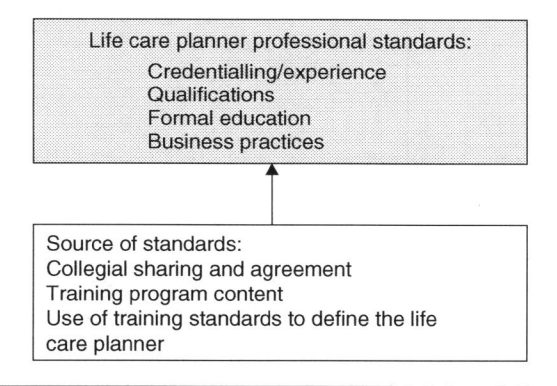

Figure 2.3 Progression From Standards for Training to Standards for Being a Life Care Planner

and credibility for practice. McCollom acknowledged the work done by Deutsch and Sawyer to standardize training. Further, she noted that the Commission on Disability Examiner Certification used this work to guide development of a certification program for life care planners. Thus, she noted, "begins the process of actual standards development by specifying parameters of skill and expertise" (McCollom, 1998, p. 3). The academy established a standards committee, chaired by Sharon Reavis.

In 1997, input on standards was obtained from over 200 participants at both the annual life care planning conference and through other educational offerings. Dr. Roger Weed compiled the first set of proposed standards. These standards addressed the educational background, training for life care planning, and some business practices. There were no standards addressing methodology (McCollom, 1998).

Figure 2.3 identifies the progression from standards for training to standards for being a life care planner. In the late 1990s, life care planning standards were also being defined by the AANLCP®, a second (nurse only) life care planning group established in 1997. The first draft of their standards, adopted in 1998, included discussion of how a life care plan is prepared. The

```
┌─────────────────────────────────────────┐
│   Nurse life care planner process standards: │
│              Assessment                 │
│   Analysis, issue identification, diagnosis │
│         Outcome identification          │
│              Planning                   │
│              Evaluation                 │
│           Quality assurance             │
│                Ethics                   │
└─────────────────────────────────────────┘
                    ▲
                    │
┌─────────────────────────────────────────┐
│ Source of standards:                    │
│ American Nurses Association framework   │
│ Collegial sharing and agreement on meaning │
│ of ANA framework                        │
│ Use of training standards to define the activity │
│ of the life care planner                │
└─────────────────────────────────────────┘
```

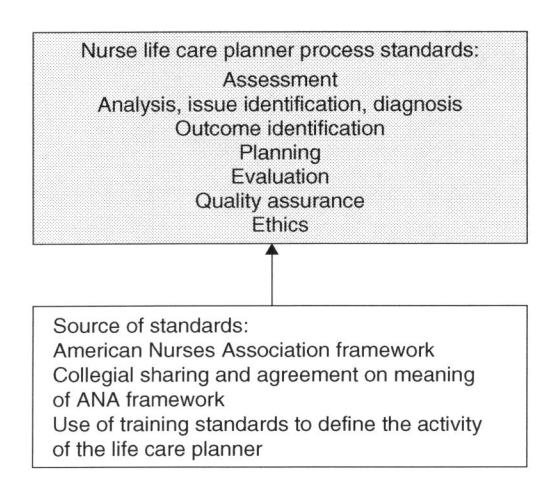

Figure 2.4   Standards of Practice Evolve From Defining Who the Life Care Planner is to Using a Process of Steps for Life Care Planning

foundation of these standards was the nursing process of assessment, diagnosis, outcome identification, planning, implementation, and evaluation (AANLCP®, 2011). The nursing process is a set of steps universally taught in registered nurse programs and is part of the standard methodology mandated by professional nursing. AANLCP® used this common nursing language as a guide for life care planner standards.

Figure 2.4 represents when the standards of practice evolved from defining who the life care planner was to using a process of steps for life care planning. As a result of these early efforts, the IALCP published the first edition of the *Standards of Practice for Life Care Planners* in 2000. As the IALCP continued to spearhead efforts to build greater unity in standards, subsequent editions, codifying standards for life care planners, were published as follows:

- 2009, second edition
- 2015, third edition
- 2022, fourth edition

A significant point of progress in defining standards has been to acknowledge that all professional disciplines use similar language that defines a process in performing their work. The 2022, fourth edition used the various terms to delineate the life care planning process in language that is familiar and relevant to all professions. This illustrates the commonalities among the professions and helps to validate the transdisciplinary nature of the specialty practice.

Tables 2.4 and 2.5 identify the planning process language used by health care professionals and the steps used in the life care planning process, respectively. Over time, the uses of life care planning standards have extended into providing a basis for research, education, peer review, and life care planning credentialing programs. Figure 2.5 shows the life care planner process, knowledge, skills, and behaviors at the center as the core of standards. As shown in the figure, standards have facilitated life care planners with the ability to establish professional self-determination, measurement and validation of work product, measurement and dissemination of the core, and the ability to establish credentials that validate knowledge and skills. While all these flow from standards, they

Table 2.4 Planning Process Language Used by Healthcare Professions

- Assessment
- Examination
- Evaluation
- Diagnoses (medical, nursing, therapy, psychology)
- Analysis and synthesis
- Interpretation
- Integration
- Interview
- Problem identification
- Goal setting
- Outcome identification
- Intervention planning
- Treatment
- Outcome measurement
- Follow-up

Table 2.5 Steps Used in the Life Care Planning Process as a Foundation for Standards of Practice

- Case initiation.
- Assessment and evaluation of an evaluee.
- Analysis and synthesis to identify functioning, disability, and health.
- Delineating future care recommendations.
- Delineating costs.
- Work product creation.
- Evaluation for consistency and adherence to standards of practice.
- Education of consumers/users of life care plans.
- Forensic applications.

simultaneously feed back into the sources for on-going standard development, creating a cyclic and symbiotic relationship for continued standard evolution.

As life care planning evolved, the focus of standards has grown beyond defining life care planning as a specialty practice to describing the process that life care planners use to conduct their work. A review of the IALCP *Standards of Practice* (4th ed.) shows how the most recent edition of life care planning standards of practice (IALCP, 2022) builds upon the early work of AANLCP® members by expanding the concept of process to all disciplines. The 2022 update of the IALCP *Standards of Practice* (4th ed.) resulted in significant expansion of life care planning standards to the most comprehensive set of existing standards at the date of the publication and are, therefore, included in Appendix A.

Consensus in Life Care Planning

In 1998, a group of professionals engaged in life care planning worked together to reach a consensus on the definition of a life care plan. Through this consensus activity was born the Life Care Planning

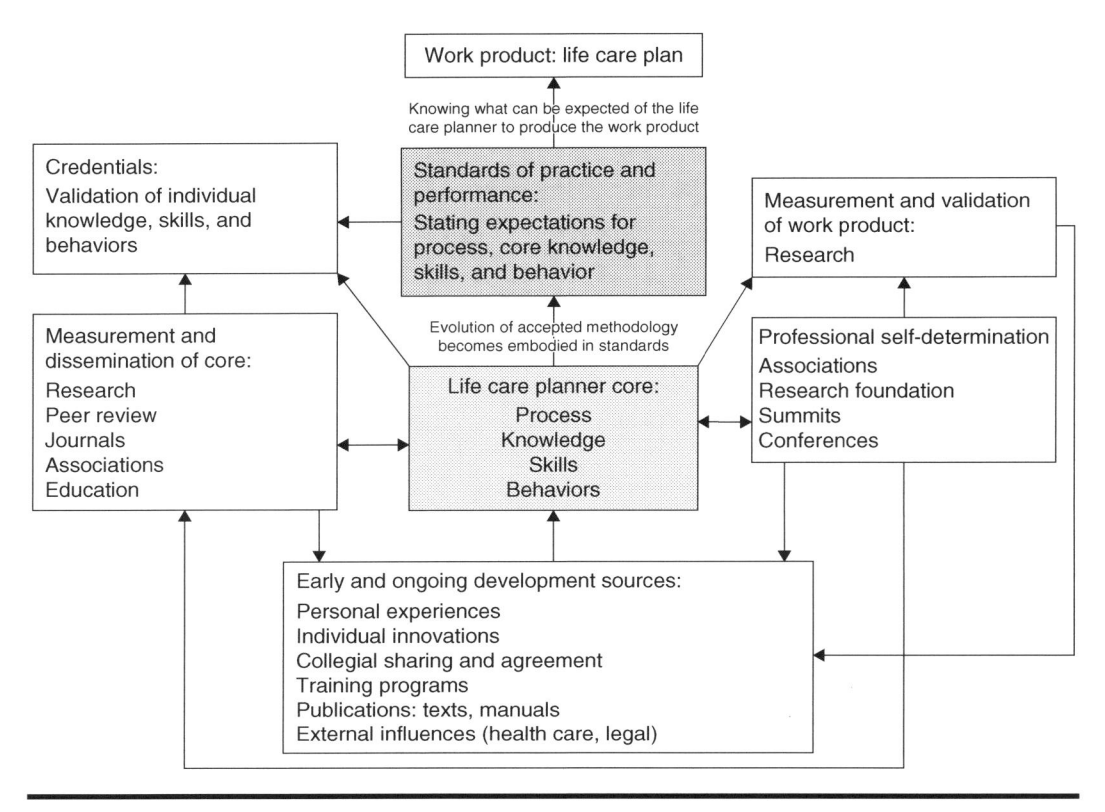

Figure 2.5 Complex Intertwining of Standards of Practice Within the Specialty Practice

Summit, a series of meetings attended by life care planners from various professional backgrounds who had a shared goal of developing consensus on critical life care planning topics. Over the course of the summits, organizations involved included: AANLCP®; American Association of Legal Nurse Consultants (AALNC); Care Planner Network; Case Management Society of America (CMSA); Commission on Disability Examiner Certification (CDEC); Commission on Health Care Certification (now, ICHCC™); Foundation of Life Care Planning Research (FLCPR); Georgia State University; Intelicus; IALCP); International Association of Rehabilitation Professionals (IARP); IARP-Canada; University of Florida; and, Vocational Rehabilitation Association of Canada (VRA). The first of these summits was held in 2000 (Weed & Berens, 2000) and as of the date of this text, nine life care planning summits have been completed, attended by an estimated 700 life care planners.

There are three types of consensus research methods: consensus development conference, nominal group technique, and the Delphi technique (James & Warren-Forward, 2015). Table 2.6 adapts the research by James and Warren-Forward (2015) into a tabular format for greater ease of understanding the three historic and existing methods of reaching consensus among groups of individuals.

In life care planning, the development of consensus statements for over two decades has arisen out of the nominal group process and, most recently, the Delphi technique. With the nominal group process, there is no participant anonymity, the participant numbers are smaller, but the costs are higher (e.g., each participant's cost to attend, facility, and other costs). A significant

Table 2.6 Consensus Research Methods and Their Processes, Advantages, and Disadvantages

Type	Processes, Advantages, and Disadvantages	Used in LCPing
Nominal Group Technique	• No participant autonomy • Small participant numbers • High costs • Short time frame	Yes
Delphi Technique	• Participant autonomy available • Variable participant numbers • Low cost • Long time frame	Yes
Consensus Development Conference	• Identify research question • Perform systematic review • If high level of evidence results from systematic review, perform consensus development conference • If low level of evidence results from systematic review, perform either a nominal group technique or a Delphi technique	No

advantage is that the shorter time frame of the process allows the ability to reach consensus rather quickly. Regarding the first 2000 summit, Dr. Weed, one of the organizers, commented:

> A significant factor is that within the nominal groups, words can be refined until true consensus is reached. I selected the in-person process to see if we could get 100 people from a variety of backgrounds to agree. That method worked GREAT in 2000.
> (R. Weed, personal communication, October 14, 2022)

The Delphi technique results in participant anonymity, has variable participant numbers, costs less, but has a longer time frame (James & Warren-Forward, 2015). This method was implemented after the last summit where consensus statements were reviewed as a method to re-evaluate nearly two decades of consensus statements, ensure their relevancy, and allow any life care planner who might not normally attend a summit to have input into the existing consensus statements in the field (Johnson et al., 2018).

The last consensus research method, the consensus development conference, asks a research question, undertakes a systematic review, and arrives at the determination of the level of evidence (James & Warren-Forward, 2015). If the systematic review's level of evidence is low, the process continues to either a nominal group or Delphi technique, depending on what the group desires for level of autonomy, number of participants, costs, and timeline. As described in the Research in Life Care Planning chapter in this text, because life care planning is a fairly new field without sufficient literature to reach the meta-analytic review level, a systematic review might be possible depending on the topic of desired consensus to engage in part of the consensus development conference process if the level of evidence is high. However, time and interest has been insufficient in the field to determine if the result of a systematic review achieves a high enough level of evidence to proceed to a consensus development conference or if the two other consensus research techniques that have been used for over two decades in life care planning continue to be the best way to achieve current and future consensus in the field.

Thus, the two consensus research techniques used to date by the life care planning community over more than two decades leading to existing consensus statements have been the most appropriate and complementary to each other. Because of the adversarial nature of the environment in which some life care planners practice, future summits could consider the impact of the anonymity of each consensus research technique and determine the feasibility of combining both methods to maximize the benefits of each and minimize the disadvantages.

Through the work of summit attendees in nominal groups refined by the Delphi research process of life care planners in the field, *Life Care Planning Consensus and Majority Statements* have been published (Johnson et al., 2018) and are available in Appendix B. These 96 updated and revised statements reflect agreed-upon best practices and, as such, are used by practicing life care planners in their daily work (Johnson et al., 2018). Overall, most of the majority statements are about life care planner practices and differences, the life care plan's content, life care planning in general (e.g., certifying bodies), or standards of practice.

Work Product Peer Review

Occasionally, life care planners are asked to review a colleague's work product and provide input regarding its contents. Although these requests may come from defense counsel in litigated cases, it may also come from any party who wants a peer's opinion on a previously developed life care plan. As noted in Phase 1 of the Life Care Planning Method, identifying the purpose for the referral is paramount to directing the activities the life care planner may take on a case. If the request is for a second opinion and the development of a life care plan, the life care planner would follow the same method, steps, standards of practice, ethical standards, and best practices as they normally would in the development of any life care plan. The colleague's life care plan is merely one of the documents of secondary data reviewed and considered in the process.

If the referral request is for a professional review and critique of another life care plan, the methodological approach is different. Two established methods of offering such a critique are embedded in the scholarly peer review method and in the replication concept within research.

Peer review is a term typically used in the publication of scholarly works. However, if we are reviewing a plan developed by another life care planner (peer) and providing a critique (sometimes referred to as a "rebuttal report"), by definition the task is called a peer review because it is the "review of work products performed by others qualified to do the same work" (International Organization for Standardization [ISO], 2017, 3.13).

In research, a direct test to reliability occurs when a secondary researcher replicates an analysis using the same methods, assumptions, and data of the first researcher and concludes that the outcome is the same or similar or can understand how the findings and conclusions were logically reached by replicating the process. If a similar outcome is attained, the analysis is considered reliable and has the potential of also being valid. If replication results in a different outcome, the reliability of the peer-reviewed life care plan is questionable and so is its validity. So too, to test the reliability of a life care plan—and, therefore, any limitations to its validity—it is important to study replication, in which a peer uses methods, systems, protocols, standards, and other tools in the field to replicate what the life care planner did in arriving at their work product. Examples of such studies are provided in the research chapter of this text.

There is virtually no published life care planning literature about how to perform a comprehensive professional peer review of a colleague's work product and offer a critique or rebut the contents of that life care plan. Dr. Roger Weed created documents used in the University of Florida/Intelicus' life care planning training modules for work product peer reviews (2003). One was a checklist of components to consider when performing such reviews and contained: 1) Read the Report; 2) Know and Understand Diagnosis; 3) Scrutinize the Details; 4) Wheel Reinvention; 5) Does the Report Contain All of the Elements? 6) Face Validity; and 7) Vocational Opinions. To assist life care planning students with the analysis, Dr. Weed also developed a comparison matrix to document and compare the recommendation contained in the life care plan with the secondary data and evidence in the case (Barros-Bailey, 2018) including: documentation (medical and psychological records, discovery documents, expert reports, etc.), archival records (raw diagnostic information, vital records, etc.), and physical artifacts (pictures or videos of the evaluee/client/patient pre- and post-incident, day-in-the-life videos, etc.). Taken together, these preliminary peer review documents assisted students to review the foundation of the recommendations within the life care plan report and whether the life care planner remained within their scope of practice in making their recommendations.

Most of the literature associated with work product peer review arose out of the 2006 Life Care Planning Summit (Riddick-Grisham, 2006). A *Sample Life Care Plan Review Form* by Paul M. Deutsch & Associates, PA was contained in an appendix to the proceedings of the 2006 Summit (Riddick-Grisham, 2006). The form contained six areas: 1) Review of Areas Covered; 2) Review of Terminology; 3) Analysis of Overlaps; 4) Additional Recommendations to be Considered by the Life Care Planner; 5) Is the Plan Easy to Understand for all Parties Concerned? and 6) Other Comments. Also included in the 2006 summit proceedings was the 2002 *Checklist for Review of Life Care Plans* developed by Berens and Weed (Riddick-Grisham, 2006) that contains the following questions: 1) Was a complete set of medical records and other relevant records provided with the referral? 2) Does life care planfollow published standards and procedures? 3) Are entries to LCP appropriate for disability/injury? 3) Overlaps? 4) In-home/Facility care? 5) Appropriate cost reductions made or noted to economist with regard to general expenses incurred without disability? 6) Are costs calculated correctly? 7) Vocationally relevant items? 8) Plan confirmation? and 9) Aesthetics? As a result of a presentation at the 2006 summit, Neulicht (2006) developed the PEERS© mnemonic to consider five issues: 1) Philosophical Focus; 2) Education & Experience; 3) Evaluation; 4) Recommendations; and 5) Standards of Performance. The PEERS© process asks a series of questions within each thematic area for consideration by the peer reviewer in the areas of review, analysis, critique, and evaluation.

In the same year as the 2006 summit, Caragonne presented a paper at the American Board of Vocational Experts' conference to help spot deficiencies in life care plans, what she called the "Red Flag" concept within an explanatory framework for life care plans presented in tort litigation, although the framework can also apply in other jurisdictions such as in administrative law settings. In general, the 12 "Red Flags" identified by Caragonne for defects in life care plans are:

1. Insufficient detail on methods and times
2. Lack of specificity on assumptions
3. Obsolete evaluee/client/patient information
4. Meeting evaluee/client/patient in public places rather than their home environment
5. No collaboration with providers
6. Service recommendations outside planner's scope of practice
7. Illegible planner records
8. Progressively increased costs with each plan revision
9. Lack of transparency in cost charts

10. Duplicated items in cost charts
11. Insufficient offsets in cost charts
12. Dependance on obsolete or undependable publications

Beyond the dozen cautionary considerations for life care plans themselves, in her paper, Caragonne also outlined another six "Red Flags" for insufficiencies in background, training, and experience:

1. Dependence on antiquated theories and dated services
2. Evaluee/client/patient not included in the planning process
3. Not protecting evaluee/client rights
4. Unsupported methodology within the planner's profession
5. Bias in opinions regarding evaluee/client/patient needs
6. Insufficient description of technology, housing, or transportation recommendations

A dozen years later, Husted (2018) described 20 "Red flags" within three categories: 1) Plan Structure (e.g., missing list of documents, no narrative); 2) Costs in Life Care Plan (e.g., unrelated, outliers, outdated, duplicated); and 3) Specific Goods & Services (e.g., not case-specific, not in geographical area, unreasonable number, frequency, costs).

Most recently, Caragonne et al. (2019) published a paper that detailed a Plan Evaluation Roadmap by criteria where each of the selected criteria contain the definition of the attribute, the tasks performed and the process, consequences of deficits in the criteria, representative review questions, and summary critique. Appendix C contains a detailed table concerning the process. The criteria are:

- Criterion 1: Comprehensive data collection (case records, depositions, medical records, any other text materials)
- Criterion 2: Comprehensive and individualized data collection (client-based)
- Criterion 3: Collaborative planning processes
- Criterion 4: Reproducible planning methods
- Criterion 5: Informed planning: General knowledge, skills, and experience base
- Criterion 6: Outcomes-based planning processes targeting the service delivery system
- Criterion 7: Factual planning processes: Resource and cost verification

Two life care planners from different professions, or even the same profession, may have different life care plan recommendations. However, in the replication process, the peer should be able to follow what primary and secondary data were used by the life care planner, how the evaluation was performed, and understand how the planner logically reached the conclusions of the life care plan based on the rules of the jurisdiction or system without taking an inferential leap.

As the existing checklists or evaluation frameworks imply, while the tasks involved with the life care planner's assignment may vary, the documents that guide their work do not. That is, life care planning work products are peer reviewed through the lens of accepted life care planning methodology as set forth in guiding documents including (but not limited to) consensus statements, peer-reviewed journals, standards of practice, textbooks, and white papers. Such documents can provide a protocol through which the informed reader can evaluate if the life care planner adhered to, or deviated from, statements set forth in the document.

Building on the known work of Weed (2003), Berens and Weed (2002), Caragonne (2006), Paul M. Deutsch and Associates .n.d., Neulicht (2006), Husted (2018), and Caragonne et al. (2019), Table 2.7 outlines a Work Product Peer Review Method for life care plans.

Table 2.7   Work Product Peer Review Method

Domain	Description
1	**Jurisdiction/System Rules**: Does the life care plan outline its purpose and follow the rules or guidelines for the system for which it was prepared? *Example*: If the life care plan is being prepared for a personal injury claim where only current and future needs associated with the incident should be included, does it include everything the person will need in the future as if it were being prepared for a special needs trust regardless of etiology?
2	**Best Practices**: Does the life care planner use best practices consistent with the consensus statements in the field? *Example*: Does the life care planner deal with divergent physician opinions or select one over another (e.g., Consensus Statement #65)?
3	**Ethical Guidelines**: Is the life care plan consistent with ethical standards in the field? *Example*: Is the life care plan performed for someone (i.e., a niece) where there may be a conflict of interest? Does the life care planner have the expertise needed and is the person appropriately credentialed to provide the life care plan? Is the plan objective and not one-sided?
4	**Standards of Practice**: Did the life care planner follow an established standard of practice in the life care planning field? *Example*: Using the list of standards in the field of life care planning, does the life care planner stay within their scope of practice?
5	**Transparency**: Is it clear what primary, secondary, and research was performed to arrive at the data analysis and subsequent conclusions? *Example*: Is the life care planner transparent in their processes? What diagnostic, functional, and healthcare assumptions were made and are they consistent with the type of analysis required for the case? Is there foundation for each plan element?
6	**Findings/Conclusions/Recommendations**: Do the findings, conclusions, and recommendations flow from the facts and research in the case, or are they nonsensical? *Example*: A series of medications are included in the life care plan without foundation in the primary or secondary data, the diagnoses, or any other material available in the case or being within the life care planner's scope of practice to recommend. Are the conclusions speculative or possible rather than probable?

Source: In part, the development of this model was adapted from Rutherford-Owen, T. M. (2022). Life care plan peer review [PowerPoint slides]. Capital University Law School, Life Care Planning Program.

The Work Product Peer Review Method is intentionally broad to fit the various systems or jurisdictions in which it might be applied. Each domain can have its own set of checklists, steps, and subdomains. In providing the work product peer review oral or written report, the peer life care planner must be professional, focusing on the review of the work product without disparaging their colleague.

Each of the domains is detailed below with corresponding inclusion of the various known checklists and evaluation frameworks and criteria in the field. Each of these peer review lists may be cross-functional across more than one domain. For example, using outdated materials and resources may be an ethical issue of competency as well as inconsistent with best practices or standards of practice. To classify the Weed (2003), Berens and Weed (2002), Caragonne (2006), Paul M. Deutsch and Associates (n.d.), Neulicht (2006), Husted (2018), and Caragonne et al. (2019) step, factor, or criteria across domains, a content analysis placed each in the domain that likely had the highest correspondence.

Domain 1: Jurisdiction/System Rules

To perform an accurate work product peer review, the life care planner should understand the context in which the life care plan was developed. This filtering domain assumes the life care planner had knowledge of the definitions, rules, and guidelines consistent to the context in which the life care plan was developed.

In clinical or forensic life care planning, understanding the system or jurisdiction where the case rests becomes the limiter or delimiter as to how the life care plan is developed, its content, and its conclusions, and the bumpers for how it should be peer reviewed. There may even be geographical or regional differences or nuances within similar jurisdictions beyond systemic variances.

Domain 2: Best Practices

There is strong consensus in life care planning across a variety of practice issues. Therefore, does the life care plan under review demonstrate adherence to best practices as identified by those statements? Domain 2 is also consistent with Neulicht's Standards of Performance, the first two factors of the Paul M. Deutsch & Associates checklist, and the Berens and Weed step 1. This domain contains Caragonne's life care plan "Red Flag" factors 1 and 5 and background, training, and experience "Red Flags" 2 and 4, as well as Caragonne et al.'s Criterion 3. Lastly, Husted's Plan Structure would likely fall into this domain.

Domain 3: Ethical Guidelines

Ethical life care planning practice requires that the life care planner demonstrates a baseline level of competency and objectivity, as well as understand that their main responsibility is to the person who is the subject of the evaluation (see Ethics in Life Care Planning chapter in this text).

Competency assumes that the life care planner has adequate training in the individualized scope of practice of life care planning, while objectivity assumes that the life care planner equitably applies that training to the facts of a case regardless of whom is paying the bill—or other factors that could impact bias. Along the ethical precept of competency, this domain contains Steps 2 and 3 of Weed's checklist, Caragonne's life care plan "Red Flags" 3, 6, and 12, the background, training, and experience "Red Flags" 1, and Caragonne et al.'s Criterion 5. Generally, Neulicht's Education and Experience issues fall into the competency ethical theme, as would Berens and Weed's third step.

The objectivity ethical expectations are consistent with the Caragonne life care plan "Red Flags" 8 and with her background, training, and experience "Red Flags" 4 and 5. Neulicht's (2006) Philosophical Focus has some consistency with objectivity, justice, and fidelity ethical principles.

Related to objectivity and the attempt to minimize bias is the bedrock understanding that while the life care plan is being developed in a particular clinical or forensic context, ultimately the life care planner's ethical responsibility is to safeguard the evaluee/client/patient's rights, which is consistent with Caragonne's background, training, and skill "Red Flag" 3.

Domain 4: Standards of Practice

Standards of practice evolve to respond to emerging needs of a professional field and are recognized in this domain as the "how" guidelines of life care planning. Sometimes these changes are substantial. Therefore, becoming and staying updated in the use of current standards of practice in the development of a life care plan becomes a checklist point of comparison in a work product peer review (Step 5 of the Weed checklist; Caragonne life care plan "Red Flag" 3, 5; background, training, and experience "Red Flag" 4). Berens and Weed's steps 2 and 8 are consistent with this domain, as is Husted's Specific Goods and Services.

Domain 5: Transparency

To perform a peer review of a colleague's life care plan assumes that the authoring life care planner provided sufficient information for the peer reviewer to replicate. Therefore, transparency is important in the peer review and replication process and the focus of this domain. This assumed transparency is inherent and consistent with Caragonne's life care plan "Red Flags" 1, 2, 7, 9 as well as her background, training, and experience "Red Flags" 6. Transparency is also a component of Criteria 1, 2, and 4 of the Caragonne et al. evaluation framework. Questions such as on the Paul M. Deutsch & Associates' "Is the plan easy to understand for all those concerned?" suggests the need for transparency in writing.

Domain 6: Findings/Conclusions/Recommendations

The bulk of the peer review comes down to the details in this pivotal domain where the life care planner takes all the primary and secondary data in their analysis and brings it to its finite conclusion on a certain date which is memorialized in a report that contains qualitative data in the form of a narrative and quantitative data including numerical frequencies, durations, and costs, usually presented in tabular form. This domain contains the Weed steps 1, 3, 4, 6, 7, and 8 as well as Caragonne's life care plan "Red Flags" 10 and 11, and Caragonne et al.'s Criteria 6 and 7. Neulicht's Evaluation and Recommendation issues would be consistent with this domain as would the Paul M. Deutsch & Associates' Recommendations step, Berens and Weeds steps 4, 5, 6, 7, and 9, and Husted's Costs in a Life Care Plan.

Emerging Issues Life Care Planning

With its rapid growth from a practice with fewer than 100 people just 25 years ago to well over 500 members of the IALCP (K. Bailey, personal communication April 18, 2022), and others through other organizations resulting in thousands of life care planners, as of the date of this publication, there are issues that have emerged and continue to emerge that will require the attention of life care planners now and into the future. Just as research was performed and articles were written when the *Daubert* decision was handed down, contemporary issues will emerge as the practice of life care planning evolves. Two of these issues, the challenges in costing items in a life care plan and the emergence of remote work are addressed here.

Costing

In life care planning research conducted with Canadian and U.S. based life care planners, each group identified costing items in a life care plan to be challenging (Fisher & Wilkins, 2017; Rutherford-Owen & Wilkins, 2019). While not a new topic, how to properly determine the cost of items contained in a life care plan has become increasingly complex as healthcare pricing has also become increasingly complex. One tool commonly used to meet this challenge is the use of a costing database. In a 2020 study of life care planners, 73% of respondents reported using costing databases to assist in the determination of costs for items in a plan (Rutherford-Owen et al., 2021). As new data sources emerge, life care planners would need to remain abreast of costing methodologies.

Assessment: Face-to-Face vs. Remote

As part of the step-by-step process a life care planner engages in to prepare a life care plan, conducting a face-to-face interview (when possible) with the evaluee/client/patient is important as was identified in the 2021 survey of life care planning practice, pandemic edition (Barros-Bailey et al., in press). Often, this interview is conducted in the evaluee/client/patient's home, which is not only more comfortable for the evaluee/client/patient, but also facilitates the life care planner's observation of current equipment and supplies as well any environmental barriers in the home (Weed & Owen, 2018). While the use of video conferencing in life care planning was mentioned well over a decade ago (Weed & Berens, 2010), arguably the catalyst for its adoption occurred in 2020 with the spread of COVID-19. A 2020 survey of life care planners revealed that 72% of survey respondents were conducting home visits or evaluee/client/patient interviews virtually while only 31.25% of respondents conducted home visits virtually prior to the COVID-19 outbreak (Rutherford-Owen et al., 2021. Such changes in how life care planners provide services was approved by the International Commission on Healthcare Certification (ICHCC™), the body that issues the Certified Life Care Planning (CLCP™) credential (B. May, personal communication, December 29, 2020) and their distribution of a "Consent to use virtual care/interaction tools" form available from www.ichcc.org/resources/research-publications.html. How the pandemic impacted the long-term distance assessment practice for life care planners is uncertain. As life care planning as a specialty practice continues to develop, there will inevitably be new developments (e.g., technology or healthcare changes) and challenges like those seen during the COVID-19 pandemic, which create the need for life care planning tools and processes to evolve.

Summary

In a 1995 interview with Dr. Paul Deutsch, he was asked to identify the biggest challenge facing life care planning (Deutsch, 1995). His response identified adherence to professional standards. It is incumbent on the life care planning professional to assure that services offered are consistent with the standards of the profession and the methodologies that have been endorsed by practitioners. Building on the work of others, rather than reinventing the wheel, will assist in achieving this goal.

This first chapter dedicated to methodology provides a brief foundation of life care planning along with underlying principles. Operational definitions for each part of the title (methodology, scope of practice, standards of practice, consensus statements) allow for clear understanding of what each term means before it is applied within a new multi-phasic model in life care planning that encompasses the various definitions and checklists, suggests steps in the process, and is tied in level and domain to the scientific method. Maintaining consistency with developmental psychology that is the theoretical foundation of life care planning, an ecological model was introduced and populated with the ICF taxonomy, along with a lifespan approach to human development. Although performing a review of a life care plan is common practice in forensic life care planning, published literature is largely moot on this point. Therefore, this chapter introduces a Work Product Peer Review Method as well as an introduction to the phases in the Life Care Planning Method. Finally, we identify contemporary issues of costing and distance service provision in life care planning as two emerging issues in the field that may result in greater future attention in research and the literature.

References

Adolfsson, M., Sjöman, M., & Björck-Åkesson, E. (2018). ICF-CY as a framework for understanding child engagement in preschool. *Frontiers in Education, Section on Special Education Needs*. www.frontiersin.org/articles/10.3389/feduc.2018.00036/full

Aftab, A. (2022). Neurodiversity and the social ecology of disability … Robert Chapman, PhD: The neurodiversity movement is a social justice movement. *Psychiatric Times, 39*(5), https://www.psychiatrictimes.com/view/neurodiversity-and-the-social-ecology-of-disability

American Association of Nurse Life Care Planners. (2011). Recreational and vocational aspects of life care planning. *Journal of Nurse Life Care Planning, 11*(2), 372.

American Counseling Association. (2022). *State counseling of professional counselors*. www.counseling.org/knowledge-center/licensure-requirements/overview-of-state-licensing-of-professional-counselors#

American Medical Association. (2022). *What is scope of practice?* www.ama-assn.org/practice-management/scope-practice/what-scope-practice

Arnold, K. D., Lu, E. C., & Armstrong, K. J. (2012). Chronosystem: The role of time in college readiness. *ASHE Higher Education Report, 38*(5), 83–89.

Barros-Bailey, M. (2018). An evidence source model for clinical and forensic practice. *The Rehabilitation Professional, 26*(3), 117–128.

Barros-Bailey, M. (2020). Life care planning report writing foundations, standards, methods, and ethics: Development of a checklist. *Journal of Life Care Planning, 18*(2), 69–79.

Barros-Bailey, M., Knott, M., Neulicht, A. T., Mitchell, N., Albee, T., Robinson, R., Grisham, S., & Marcinko, D. (in press). Results of the 2021 survey of remote life care planning practice: Pandemic edition.

Bean, K. (2012). *Ecological factors and the behavioral and educational outcomes of African American students in special education* (ED549526) [Doctoral dissertation, Arizona State University].

Boaden, N., Purcal, C., Fisher, K., & Meltzer, A. (2021). Transition experience of families with young children in the Australian National Disability Insurance System (NDIS). *Australian Social Work, 74*(3), 294–306.

Boateng, G. O., Adams, E. A., Boateng, M. O., Luginaah, I. N., & Taabazuing, M. (2017). Obesity and the burden of health risks among the elderly in Ghana: A population study. *PLoS ONE, 12*(11), e0186947. doi:10.1371/journal.pone.0186947

Boniface, G., Smith, J., Mitchell, C., & Bowles, H. L. (2017). What life are planners need to know about the professional discipline of occupational therapist. *Journal of Life Care Planning, 17*(1), 7–11.

Brisendine, A. E., O'Kelley, S. E., Preskitt, J. K., Sen, B., & Wingate, M. S. (2021). Testing a tailored social-ecological model for Autism Spectrum Disorders. *Maternal & Child Health Journal, 25*(6), 956–966. https//doi.org/1007/s10995-020-03064-5

Bronfenbrenner, U. (1975, July 13–17). *The ecology of human development in retrospect and prospect*. Conference on Ecological Factors in Human Development, International Society for the Study of Behavioral Development, Guilford, England.

Brunsting, N. C., Sreckovic, M. A., & Lane, K. L. (2014). Special education teacher burnout: A synthesis of research from 1979 to 2013. *Education and Treatment of Children, 4*, 681–712.

Bubanja, D., & Conover, S. M. (2017). What life are planners need to know about the professional discipline of physical therapy. *Journal of Life Care Planning, 17*(1), 13–17.

Caragonne, P. (2006, March 24). *How to spot deficiencies in life care plans: The "Red Flags" concept and explanatory framework* [Paper presentation]. American Board of Vocational Experts Bi-Annual Conference, Ft. Lauderdale, Florida.

Caragonne, P., Sofka, K., & Howland, W. (2019, October 9). *Frameworks For evaluating life care plans.* www.americanbar.org/groups/health_law/publications/health_lawyer_home/2019-october/life-care/

Caragonne, P. (2013, September 26). *Evidence-based practice, or the judicious use of facts and peers reviewed research, can be incorporated into the methodology you use in life care planning* [Paper presentation]. Evidence-Based Life Care Planning, International Symposium on Life Care Planning, Atlanta, Georgia.

Carey, E. M., & Marcinko, D. A. (2017). What life are planners need to know about the professional discipline of registered nurse. *Journal of Life Care Planning, 17*(1), 31–38.

Case Management Society of America. (2021). *Our history.* https://cmsa.org/about-cmsa/

Céspedes, G. M. (2005). La nueva cultura de la discapacidad y los modelos de rehabilitación. *Revista Aquichan, 5*(1), 108–113.

Chalmers, I., Guyatt, G., Haynes, B., Sackett, D., Dickerson, K., Rennie, D., Gray, M., & Glasziou, P. (2018). *Evidence-based medicine: An oral history* [video]. JAMA Network. https://files.jamanetwork.com/sdebm/index.html

Commission on Rehabilitation Counselor Certification. (2022). *Scope of practice assumptions.* https://crccertification.com/scope-of-practice/

Deutsch, P. M. (1995). Interview. *Inside Life Care Planning, 1*(1), 6–7.

Deutsch, P. M. (2011). Establishing foundations for life care plan development. In Riddick-Grisham, S. & Deming, L. M. (Eds.). (2011). *Pediatric life care planning and case management* (2nd ed., pp. 845–853). CRC Press.

Deutsch, P. M., Allison, L., & Reid, C. (2003). *An introduction to life care planning: history, tenets, methodologies, and principles. a guide to rehabilitation*, 5–1. AHAB Press, Inc.

Deutsch, P., & Raffa, F. (1981). *Damages in tort action* (Vols. 8 & 9). Matthew Bender.

Dillman, E. G. (2018). The role of the economist in life care planning. In R. O. Weed & D. E. Berens, *Life care planning and case management handbook* (4th ed., pp. 317–332). Routledge.

Durand, M. J., Vachon, B., Loisel, P., & Berthelette, D. (2003). Constructing the program impact theory for an evidence-based work rehabilitation program for workers with low back pain. *Work, 21*, 233–242.

Fick, N., & Preston, K. (2015). An attorney perspective on standards of practice: A weapon or a shield? *Journal of Life Care Planning, 13*(3), 17–20.

Fisher, J., & Wilkins, M. J. (2017). Challenges and practice issues faced by Canadian life care planners. *Journal of Life Care Planning, 15*(3), 31–36.

Hershenson, D. B. (1998). Systemic, ecological model for rehabilitation counseling. *Rehabilitation Counseling Bulletin, 42*(1), 40–50.

Higdon, C. W. (2017). What life are planners need to know about the professional discipline of speech-language pathologist. *Journal of Life Care Planning, 17*(1), 45–72.

Howie, D. (1999). Models and morals: Meanings underpinning the scientific study of special education needs. *International Journal of Disability, Development, and Education, 46*(1), 9–24.

Husted, L. (2018, November 13). *20 red flags in a life care plan/life care plan review.* [PowerPoint slides]. International Association of Rehabilitation Professionals Webinar.

ICF Research Branch. (2022). *ICF core sets.* www.icf-core-sets.org/

International Association of Rehabilitation Professionals, International Academy of Life Care Planners. (2022). Standards of practice for life care planners (4th ed.). *Journal of Life Care Planning, 20*(3), 7–23.

International Organization for Standardization. (2017). *Work product reviews: 3.13 Peer review.* www.iso.org/obp/ui/fr/#iso:std:67407:en

Jacobs, H. E., & Strum, K. (2017). What life are planners need to know about the professional discipline of psychologist. *Journal of Life Care Planning, 17*(1), 23–29.

Jacobs, C., Graham, I. D., Makarski, J., Chassé, M., Fergusson, D., Hutton, B., & Clemons, M. (2014). Clinical practice guidelines and consensus statements in oncology – An assessment of their methodological quality. *PLoS One, 9*(10), e110469.

Jacobs, P., MacMahon, K., & Quayle, E. (2018). Transition from school to adult services for young people with severe or profound intellectual disability: A systematic review utilizing framework synthesis. *Journal of Applied Research on Intellectual Disabilities, 31*, 962982. https://doi.org/10.1111/jar.12466

James, D., & Warren-Forward, H. (2015). Research methods for formal consensus development. *Nurse Researcher, 22*(3), 35–40.

Johnson, C. B., Pomeranz, J. L., & Stetten, N. E. (2018). Consensus and majority statements derived from life care planning summits held in 2000, 2002, 2004, 2006, 2008, 2010, 2012, 2015, and 2017 and updated via Delphi study in 2018. *Journal of Life Care Planning, 16*(4), 15–18.

Jokela, M., Airaksinen, J., Virtanen, M., Batty, G. D., Kivimaki, M., & Hakulinen, C. (2020). Personality, disability-free life years, and life expectancy: Individual participant meta-analysis of 131,195 individuals in 10 cohort studies. *Journal of Personality, 8*(3), 596–605. https://doi.org/10.1111/jopy.12513

King, G., Curran, C. J., & McPherson, A. (2013). A four-part ecological model of community-focused therapeutic recreation and life skills services for children and youth with disabilities. *Child: Care, Health, and Development, 39*(3), 325–336.

Landon, T., McKnight-Lizotte, M., Connor, A., & Peña, J. (2019). Rehabilitation counseling in rural settings: A phenomenological study on barriers and supports. *Journal of Rehabilitation, 85*(2), 47–57.

Macy, M., & Rusch, F. R. (2010). *Life care planning evaluation.* In E. Mpofu, & Oakland, T. (Eds.), *Rehabilitation and health assessment applying ICF guidelines* (pp. 297–312). Springer Publishing Company. https://bojidarivkov.files.wordpress.com/2012/08/rehabilitation-and-health-assessment.pdf

Mann, S. (2017). What life are planners need to know about the professional discipline of physician physiatrist. *Journal of Life Care Planning, 17*(1), 19–21.

Mauk, K. L. (2017). Revisiting the concept of transdisciplinary life care planning. *Journal of Life Care Planning, 17*(1), 5–6.

McCollom, P. (1998, May 15). Dialogue for tomorrow. *Academy Letter, 1*(1), 3–5.

McLinden, M., Douglas, G., Hewett, R., Cobb, R., & Lynch, P. (2017). Facilitating participation in education: The distinctive role of the specialist teacher in supporting learners with vision impairment in combination with severe and profound and multiple learning disabilities. *Journal of Blindness Innovation and Research, 7*(2). https://nfb.org/images/nfb/publications/jbir/jbir17/jbir070203.html

Melchiorre, M. G., Di Rosa, M., Lamura, G., Torres-Gonzalez, F., Lindert, J., Stankunas, M., Ioannidi-Kapolou, E., Barros, H., Macassa, G., & Soares, J. J. F. (2016). Abuse of older men in seven European countries: A multilevel approach in the framework of an ecological model. *PLoS ONE, 11*(1), e0146425. https://doi.org/10.1371/journal.pone.0146425

Merriam-Webster. (n.d.-a). Foundation. In *Merriam-Webster.* https://www.merriam-webster.com/dictionary/foundation

Merriam-Webster. (n.d.-b). Method. In *Merriam-Webster.* https://www.merriam-webster.com/dictionary/method

Merriam-Webster. (n.d.-c). Standard. In *Merriam-Webster.* https://www.merriam-webster.com/dictionary/standard

Mertes, A. (2018). Content analysis of the research priorities in the *Journal of Life Care Planning* 2004–2017. *Journal of Life Care Planning, 16*(2), 3–9.

Mertes, A., & Harden, T. (2017). What life are planners need to know about the professional discipline of rehabilitation counselors. *Journal of Life Care Planning, 17*(1), 39–44.

Metekingi, J. P. (2013). An introduction to evidence-based practice for the nurse life care planner. *Journal of Nurse Life Care Planning, 13*(3), 88–92.

Neulicht, A. (2006). The life care plan RACE: Review, analysis, critique, and evaluation? *Journal of Life Care Planning, 5*(3), 91–98.

O'Leary, L., Cooper, S. A., & Hughes-McCormack, L. (2018). Early death and causes of death of people with intellectual disabilities: A systematic review. *Journal of Applied Research in Intellectual Disabilities*, *31*(3), 325–342. https://doi.org/10.1111/jar.12417

Online Library of Liberty. (2022). *Novum organum by Sir Francis Bacon*. https://oll.libertyfund.org/title/bacon-novum-organum

Owen, T. R. (2012). Organizational viewpoints on research in life care planning. *Journal of Life Care Planning*, *11*(3), 39–51.

Paul M. Deutsch & Associates, P. A. (n.d.). *Publications*. www.paulmdeutsch.com/LCP-introduction.htm#tbolcp

Pedrinelli, V. J., Rodrigues, G. M., Campos, C., de Almeida, F. R., Polito, L. F. T., & Brandão, M. R. F. (2018). A bioecological perspective of human development on autonomy of an athlete with intellectual disabilities. *Revista de Psicologia del Deporte/Journal of Sport Psychology*, *27*(Suppl 1), 9–14.

Polinder, S., Haagsma, J. A., Stein, C., & Havelaar, A. H. (2012). Systematic review of general burden of disease studies using disability-adjusted life years. *Population Health Metrics*, *10*, 21–35. https://doi.org/10.1186/1478-7954-10-21

Pomeranz, J. L., & Shaw, L. R. (2007). International Classification of Functioning, Disability, and Health: A model for life care planners. *Journal of Life Care Planning*, *6*(1&2), 15–24.

Preston, K. (2019). Guest editorial. *Journal of Life Care Planning*, *17*(1), 3.

Ravindran, N., & Myers, B. (2012). Cultural influences on perceptions of health, illness, and disability: A review and focus on autism. *Journal of Child & Family Studies*, *21*(2), 311–319.

Riddick-Grisham, S. (2006). 2006 life care planning summit proceedings. *Journal of Life Care Planning*, *5*(3), 57–90.

Riddick-Grisham, S. & Deming, L.M. (Eds.). (2011). *Pediatric life care planning and case management* (2nd ed.). CRC Press.

Roseen, E. J., Rajendran, I., Stein, P., Fredman, L., Fink, H. A., LaValley, M. P., & Saper, R. B. (2021). Association of back pain with mortality: A systematic review and meta-analysis of cohort studies. *Journal of General Internal Medicine*, *36*, 3148–3158. https://doi.org/10.1007/s11606-021-06732-6

Rutherford-Owen. T. M., & Wilkins, M. J. (2019). Practice challenges identified by life care planners in the United States. *Journal of Life Care Planning*, *17*(2), 33–39.

Rutherford-Owen, T. M., Thomas, L. B., & Dunlap, K. (2021). Evolution of life care planning with technology. *Journal of Life Care Planning*, *19*(1), 65–80.

Rutherford-Owen, T. M. (2022). *Life care plan peer review* [PowerPoint slides]. Capital University Law School, Life Care Planning Program.

Schewcik, A. Y. (2017). *The impact of the environmental factors in poverty settings on children's participation: A systematic literature review from 2012 to 2017*. Jönköing University, School of Education and Communication. www.diva-portal.org/smash/get/diva2:1106604/FULLTEXT01.pdf

ScienceDirect. (2008a). Mesosystem. In *Science Direct*. www.sciencedirect.com/topics/psychology/mesosystem#:~:text=The%20mesosystem%20is%20a%20combination,part%20of%20a%20child's%20exosystem.

ScienceDirect. (2008b). Macrosystem. In *Science Direct*. www.sciencedirect.com/topics/psychology/macrosystem#:~:text=The%20macrosystem%20refers%20to%20the,and%20relationships%20among%20the%20systems.

ScienceDirect. (2018). Exosystem. In *Science Direct*. https://www.sciencedirect.com/topics/psychology/exosystem#:~:text=An%20exosystem%20refers%20to%20one,setting%20containing%20the%20developing%20person.

ScienceDirect. (2019). Microsystem. In *Science Direct*. https://www.sciencedirect.com/topics/psychology/microsystem

Seid, A. A., Woday, T. A., & Hasen, A. A. (2022). Severity and mortality of COVID-19 among people with disabilities: Protocol for a systematic review and meta-analysis. *BMJ Open*, *12*(6), e061438.

Simeonsson R. J., Sauer-Lee, A., Granlund, M., & Björck-Åkesson, E. (2010). *Developmental and health assessment in rehabilitation with the ICF for children and youth*. In E. Mpofu, & Oakland, T. (Eds.), *Rehabilitation and Health assessment applying ICF guidelines* (pp. 27–46). Springer Publishing Company. https://bojidarivkov.files.wordpress.com/2012/08/rehabilitation-and-health-assessment.pdf

Skarbek, D., Hahn, K., & Parrish, P. (2009). Stop sexual abuse in special education: An ecological model of prevention and intervention strategies for sexual abuse in special education. *Sexuality and Disability, 27*, 155–164. https://doi.org/10.1007/s11195-009-9127-y

Smit, S., Preston, L. D., & Hay, J. (2020). The development of education for learners with diverse learning needs in the South African context: A bio-ecological systems analysis. *South African Journal of Disability*, 1–9.

Sorenson, J. (1995, July-August). …Beyond the Courtroom . *Inside case management, 1*(1), p. 3.

Stetten, M. E., Pomeranz, J., Moorhouse, M., Yuresk, A., Blue, A. V., & Yu, N. S. (2022). An exploratory study of medical marijuana's impact on patients with chronic pain beyond an individual's level of function: Implications for life care planning. *Journal of Life Care Planning, 20*(1), 43–68.

Suarez-Balcazar, Y., Viquez, F., Miranda, D., & Early, A. R. (2020). Barriers to and facilitators of community participation among Latinx migrants with disabilities in the United and Latinx migrant workers in Canada: An ecological analysis. *Journal of Community Psychology, 48*, 2773–2788.

The Kahn Academy. (2022). *The scientific method*. www.khanacademy.org/science/biology/intro-to-biology/science-of-biology/a/the-science-of-biology

Tyrer, F., Kiani, R., & Rutheford, M. (2021). Mortality, predictors and causes among people with intellectual disabilities: A systematic narrative review supplemented by machine learning. *Journal of Intellectual & Developmental Disability, 46*(2), 102–114.

Úbeda-Colomer, J, Fís, M. A., Pieró-Velert, C., & Devís-Devís, J. (2018). Validación de una version reducida en español del instrument *Barriers to Physical Activity Questionnaire for People with Mobility Impairments. Salúd Pública de México, 60*(5), 539–548/

Weed, R. (2003, June 6–7). Life care planning topics, tenets, process, procedures and ethics (Module 1). Intelicus, San Antonio, TX.

Weed, R. O. (2018). Life care planning: Past, present, and future. In R. O. Weed & D. E. Berens, *Life care planning and case management handbook* (4th ed., pp. 3–20). Routledge.

Weed, R., & Berens, D. (Eds.) (2000, April 12). *Life care planning summit 2000 proceedings* [Paper presentation]. Intelicus, International Academy of Life Care Planners, International Association of Rehabilitation Professionals, and the Commission on Disability Examiner Certification, Dallas, Texas.

Weed, R. O., & Berens, D. E. (2018). *Life care planning and case management handbook* (3rd ed.). CRC Press.

Weed, R. O., & Field, T. F. (2012). *Rehabilitation consultant's handbook*. Elliott & Fitzpatrick, Inc.

Weed, R. O., & Owen, T. R. (2018*). Life care planning: a step-by-step guide* (2nd ed.). Elliott & Fitzpatrick, Inc.

World Health Organization. (2001). *International classification of functioning, disability, and health*: Author.

World Health Organization. (2017a). *Comprehensive and brief ICF core sets for spinal cord injury – chronic situation.* www.icf-research-branch.org/images/ICF%20Core%20Sets%20Download/ICF_Core_Sets_for_SCI_longterm.pdf

World Health Organization. (2017b). *Comprehensive and brief ICF core sets for spinal cord injury – early post-acute situation.* www.icf-research-branch.org/images/ICF%20Core%20Sets%20Download/ICF_Core_Sets_for_SCI_early_post_acute.pdf

Yin, R. K. (2018). *Case study research and applications: design and methods* (6th ed.). SAGE Publications, Inc.

Appendix A: IALCP *Standards of Practice for Life Care Planners* (4th ed.)

STANDARDS OF PERFORMANCE

Standards of performance are intended to describe a competent level of skills and behaviors that may be expected of a life care planner. The professional discipline (e.g., counselor, physician, registered nurse, therapist) of a life care planner determines whether a life care planner is permitted to practice in that profession. However, professional disciplines do not typically exercise authority over specialty practice roles. Life care planning represents such a specialty practice. Life care planners are expected to be aware of, and follow, standards of performance that have been determined by the community of life care planners.

The practice competencies provide ways that the life care planner demonstrates compliance with the standards. The competencies listed may not be exhaustive and may change as the specialty practice and the needs of those who use life care plans evolve.

1. STANDARD: The life care planner has an educational background and professional preparation suitable for life care planning.

    PRACTICE COMPETENCIES:

    a. Possesses the appropriate educational requirements in a rehabilitation or healthcare field as defined by their professional discipline
    b. Maintains the current professional licensure, provincial registration, or national board certification that is required to practice their professional rehabilitation or healthcare discipline
    c. Demonstrates that the professional discipline provides sufficient education and training to assure that the life care planner has an understanding of human anatomy and physiology, pathophysiology, psychosocial and family dynamics, the healthcare delivery system, the role and function of various healthcare professionals, and clinical practice guidelines and standards of care. Within their profession's scope of practice, the education and training allow practitioners in the discipline to independently perform assessments, analyze and interpret data, make judgments and decisions on goals and interventions, and evaluate responses and outcomes
    d. Participates in specific continuing education as required to maintain the individual practitioner's licensure, registration, or certification within their profession
    e. Obtains continuing education and/or training to remain current in the knowledge and skills relevant to life care planning

2. STANDARD: The life care planner practices within their professional scope of practice.

    PRACTICE COMPETENCIES:

    a. Remains within the scope of practice for their profession as determined by state, provincial, or national credentialing bodies
    b. Independently makes recommendations for care items/services that are within the scope of practice of their own professional discipline

3. STANDARD: The life care planner must have skill and knowledge to understand the healthcare needs addressed in a life care plan.

    PRACTICE COMPETENCIES:

    a. Consults with others and obtains education when the life care planner must address healthcare needs that are new or unfamiliar

b. Locates appropriate resources when necessary
   c. Uses a consistent, objective, and thorough methodology to construct the life care plan
   d. Relies on appropriate medical and other health related information, resources, and professional expertise for developing the content of the life care plan
   e. Uses specialized skills such as the ability to research, critically analyze data, manage and interpret large volumes of information, attend to details, demonstrate clear and thorough written and verbal communication skills, develop positive relationships, create and use networks to gather information, and work autonomously

4. STANDARD: The life care planner shall practice in an ethical manner and follow the Code of Ethics of their respective professions, roles, certifications, and credentials.

   PRACTICE COMPETENCIES:

   a. Follows the Code of Ethics for their profession
   b. Follows the Code of Ethics for their professional roles, certifications, and credentials

5. STANDARD: The life care planner uses the scientific principles of medicine, rehabilitation, and healthcare as a basis for life care planning.

   PRACTICE COMPETENCIES:

   a. Uses and, when possible, participates, in research relevant to life care planning practice
   b. Evaluates literature for application to life care planning
   c. Uses appropriate clinical practice guidelines and research findings in the development of life care plans

6. STANDARD: The life care planner considers cultural and linguistic factors that may influence the assessment, development, and implementation of the plan.

   PRACTICE COMPETENCIES:

   a. Recommends care that is culturally appropriate
   b. Considers multiple evaluee/client/patient-centered factors such as age, sex, race, ethnicity, religion, gender identity, sexual orientation, disability, and geographic location
   c. Uses qualified interpreters

STANDARDS OF PRACTICE

Standards of practice describe the authoritative process that is followed in life care planning. All the disciplines that engage in life care planning follow a planning process. Standards of practice are organized by the steps that life care planners are expected to follow to perform competently. Steps may be followed sequentially, however, this is a fluid process.

During the complete process, the life care planner may find it beneficial to return to earlier steps or perform some steps simultaneously. Some standards and practice competencies may be applicable to more than one step. It is incumbent upon all life care planners to adhere to the standards of practice, regardless of their primary professional background, professional affiliation, referral source, and/or nature of the case.

The practice competencies provide ways that the life care planner demonstrates compliance with the standards. The competencies listed may not be exhaustive and may change as the specialty practice and the needs of those who use life care plans evolves.

Case initiation

This step refers to the activities performed in the process of responding to requests for life care planning services and determining the appropriateness and parameters for accepting cases.

7. STANDARD: The life care planner facilitates understanding of the life care planning process.

    PRACTICE COMPETENCIES:

    a. Provides information about the life care planning process
    b. Requests the information necessary to start the life care planning process

8. STANDARD: The life care planner establishes working expectations with the referring party.

    PRACTICE COMPETENCIES:

    a. Seeks mutual acknowledgment of the scope of services requested
    b. Seeks clarity regarding jurisdictional requirements that may affect work product
    c. Identifies conflicts or potential conflicts of interest

Assessment and evaluation of an evaluee

This step refers to the activities performed in gathering the information necessary for preparation of a life care plan.

9. STANDARD: The life care planner performs comprehensive assessment through the process of data collection involving multiple elements and sources.

    PRACTICE COMPETENCIES:

    a. Uses a consistent, valid, and reliable approach to data collection
    b. Collects data in a systematic, comprehensive, and accurate manner
    c. Collects data about health, biopsychosocial, medical, financial, educational, and vocational history and current needs
    d. Obtains information from records, evaluee/family (when available or appropriate), and relevant treating or consulting healthcare professionals and others
    e. If access to any source of information is not possible (e.g., denied permission to interview the evaluee), this should be noted
    f. Assesses need for further evaluations or expert opinions

Analysis and Synthesis to Identify Functioning, Disability, and Health

This step refers to organizing collected data into an empirically derived and conceptually coherent format that incorporates case-salient factors.

10. STANDARD: The life care planner analyzes data using a consistent, valid, and reliable process.

    PRACTICE COMPETENCIES:

    a. Analyzes data to determine evaluee needs
    b. Follows a consistent method for organizing and interpreting data
    c. Synthesizes data to identify current functioning, disability, and health, and to provide structure for care recommendations
    d. Identifies current standards of care, clinical practice guidelines, services, and products from reliable sources to evaluate potential functioning, disability, and health
    e. Uses knowledge of human growth and development, including the impact of aging on disability and function
    f. Considers factors such as age, sex, race, ethnicity, religion, gender identity, sexual orientation, disability, and geographic location

Delineating Future Care Recommendations

This step involves the identification of services and products that will be needed with appropriate foundation or rationale.

11. STANDARD: The life care planner uses a consistent, valid, and reliable approach to determining evaluee's needs.

    PRACTICE COMPETENCIES:

    a. Ensures appropriate foundation or rationale for each recommendation
    b. Uses, relies upon, and identifies relevant research and references in the development of the life care plan
    c. Uses current standards of care, clinical practice guidelines, services and products from reliable sources, such as current literature or other published sources, collaboration with other professionals, education programs, and personal clinical practice to make recommendations
    d. Determines consistency of care recommendations with standards of care
    e. Considers person-centered care criteria such as settings, admission criteria, treatment indications or contraindications, program goals and outcomes, consistency of services relative to standards of care, duration and frequency of services, ability of the evaluee to effectively benefit from services and products, responsiveness of services to changing evaluee needs, whether care is the least restrictive relative to the needs of the individual, and availability

f. Considers factors such as age, sex, race, ethnicity, religion, gender identity, sexual orientation, disability, and geographic location
g. Considers recommendations that are age-appropriate, using knowledge of human growth and development, including the impact of aging on disability and function
h. Considers the rationale/reason for inclusion or exclusion of recommendations
i. Considers factors such as pre-existing conditions and causally related needs in forensic cases
j. Considers the likely benefit of recommendations and how a recommendation may affect other recommendations (i.e., multidimensional influences throughout the life care plan)
k. Considers the probability versus possibility of need
l. Researches appropriate options for recommendations, using sources that are reasonably available to the evaluee
m. Uses a consistent method to determine available choices

12. STANDARD: The life care planner seeks collaboration.

    PRACTICE COMPETENCIES:

    a. Seeks recommendations from other qualified professionals and/or relevant sources for inclusion of items and services outside the life care planner's scope of practice
    b. Shares relevant information to aid in formulating recommendations and opinions

13. STANDARD: The life care planner facilitates understanding of the life care planning process.

    PRACTICE COMPETENCIES:

    a. Provides information about the life care planning process to involved parties to elicit participation
    b. Maintains objectivity while collaborating with others in determining appropriate content for the life care plan

Delineating Costs

This step includes methodology for determining the costs of future care recommendations.

14. STANDARD: The life care planner uses a consistent, valid, and reliable approach to costs.

    PRACTICE COMPETENCIES:

    a. Uses a consistent method to determine costs for various categories of available/needed services
    b. Uses geographically relevant and representative costs
    c. Identifies services and products from reliable sources
    d. Follows a consistent method for organizing and interpreting data for projecting costs
    e. Explains the life care planning process to involved parties to obtain needed information
    f. Cites verifiable cost data

Work Product Creation

This step addresses communication about future care recommendations and costs.

15. STANDARD: The life care planner communicates their opinions.

    PRACTICE COMPETENCIES:

    a. Follows a consistent method for creating the narrative component of the life care plan report
    b. Develops and uses documentation tools for reports and cost projections
    c. Considers classification systems (e.g., International Classification of Diseases [ICD], Current Procedural Terminology [CPT], Healthcare Common Procedure Coding System [HCPCS], International Classification of Functioning, Disability, and Health [ICF]) to provide clarity regarding care recommendations and costs
    d. Records lack of access to pertinent information

Evaluation for Consistency Within the Life Care Plan and Adherence to Standards of Practice

This step describes the use of the published standards of practice for the evaluation of the quality of the work practices and work product.

16. STANDARD: The life care planner ensures that opinions and work product are congruent, consistent, and follow accepted methodological practices.

    PRACTICE COMPETENCIES:

    a. Reviews and revises the life care plan to seek internal consistency and completeness
    b. Reviews the life care plan for consistency with standards of care and standards of practice, and seeks resolution of inconsistencies

Education of Consumers/Users of Life Care Plans

This step identifies activities to ensure that the life care plan, and the process by which it is created, is understood.

17. STANDARD: The life care planner, as an educator, facilitates understanding of the life care planning process, the life care plan, and work product.

    PRACTICE COMPETENCIES:

    a. Maintains objectivity and assists others in understanding the content of the life care plan
    b. Provides information about the life care planning process to involved parties
    c. Provides follow-up consultation as appropriate and permitted to facilitate understanding and interpretation of the life care plan

Forensic Application

This step provides guidance for life care planners who are involved in life care planning for litigation purposes.

18. STANDARD: The life care planner may engage in forensic applications.

    PRACTICE COMPETENCIES: If the life care planner engages in practice that includes participation in legal matters, the life care planner:

    a. May act as a consultant to legal proceedings related to determining care needs and costs
    b. May provide expert sworn testimony regarding work process and product
    c. Maintains records generated for the development of the life care plan for a period of time consistent with applicable requirements
    d. Seeks clarity regarding jurisdictional requirements that may affect work product

Source: International Association of Rehabilitation Professionals, International Academy of Life Care Planners. (2022). Standards of practice for life care planners (4th ed.). *Journal of Life Care Planning*, 20(3), 7–23. [Printed by permission]

Appendix B: Consensus and Majority Statements, 2018 Update and Revision

1. Life care planners may come from a variety of disciplines, provided they have qualifications including five years' experience in a primary discipline, complete supervised time under a qualified life care planner and belong to a life care planning professional association
2. Life care planners shall seek out mentor relationships, educating students and unaffiliated professionals about life care planning training, education, experience, special knowledge and required credentials
3. Life care planners shall disseminate information regarding their area of practice through electronic collaboration, web sites, peer-reviewed journals, books, conferences and symposia, and professional associations
4. Life care planning research shall be reviewed by peers through an objective and "blind" process that addresses methodology
5. Life care planners shall understand the definition of reliability and consistently practice in such a manner
6. Life care planners shall have knowledge of relevant laws and regulations as well as local and national care standards
7. Life care planners shall understand optimal outcomes achievable for particular injuries
8. Revised: Life care planners shall promote and participate in a national organization for life care planners that serves as a collective voice for the specialty practice and as a repository for resources
9. Life care planners shall complete 120 hours of training including courses that focus on disability issues and is specific to life care planning
10. Life care planning programs shall be based on the latest knowledge and practices
11. Life care planning programs shall cover certification preparation as well as advanced topics and complex issues

12. Life care planning programs shall be offered in accessible geographic locations and electronically
13. Life care planning continuing education units shall be available at an increasing number of forums
14. Life care planning continuing education units shall be available at forums that may not focus solely on life care planning
15. Life care planners shall keep up to date on best practices in life care planning by completing and encouraging others to participate in continuing education
16. Life care planner certification shall render its holder a qualified life care planner, provided that certification is maintained
17. Life care planner certification shall be renewed every five years with the accumulation of 60 continuing education units
18. Life care planners shall be licensed and/or certified in their professional discipline before being certified as a life care planner
19. The International Commission on Health Care Certification shall apply for National Commission for Certifying Agencies accreditation
20. Life care planners shall hold a certification that has mechanism for complaints and resolution
21. Life care planning certification shall flow from a practitioner-created core curriculum
22. The life care planning certifying body shall not be proprietary
23. The life care planning certifying body shall manage and disclose ethical complaints and violations
24. Life care planning certification exams shall be developed and maintained by an advisory group
25. Life care planning certification exams shall be administered by an autonomous entity independent of any organization that provides life care planning training and/or education
26. Standards of practice terminology shall be reviewed
27. Standards of practice terminology shall be defined
28. Standards of practice shall delineate educational requirements for entry into the practice of life care planning
29. Standards of practice shall assert the role and accountability of life care planners
30. Standards of practice shall be based on a study defining the role and accountability of life care planners
31. Standards of practice shall allow for individual judgment and expertise
32. Standards of practice shall be utilized in the development of the practice of life care planning
33. Standards of practice shall be applicable to current practices
34. Life care planners shall accept referrals only in their area of expertise
35. Life care planners shall maintain objectivity
36. Life care planners shall maintain strict adherence to confidentiality practices
37. Life care planners shall renounce inappropriate, distorted, or untrue comments about peers
38. Life care planners shall renounce inappropriate processes and training
39. Life care planners shall disclose and differentiate between the roles in which they may be called upon to act
40. Life care planners shall avoid dual relationships when objectivity may be challenged
41. Life care planners shall establish themselves within their primary field of practice
42. Life care planners shall objectively place their client's interests before any personal or professional consideration
43. Life care planners shall adhere to relevant codes of ethics
44. Life care planners shall have access to recourse/corrective action process for ethical violations
45. Life care plans shall be individualized

46. Life care plans shall be objective and consistent
47. Life care plans shall be lifelong and flexible
48. Life care plans shall be clear, concise, and user friendly documents
49. Life care plans shall be comprehensive and based on multidisciplinary data
50. Revised: Life care planners shall utilize research (including identifying relevant literature to provide a foundation for recommendations, costing for equipment and services, etc.) in life care plan that is reasonable, relevant, and appropriate
51. Life care planners shall consider the integrity of data
52. Life care planning shall depend on data collection, analysis, and synthesis
53. Life care planners may request additional data, testing, and evaluation if required
54. Life care planners shall research condition, resources, services, and costs
55. Life care plans shall utilize established procedures
56. Revised: Life care planning methods shall be peer reviewed (formally or informally reviewed by other experts in the field) at national organization meetings and summits
57. Revised: Life care plans shall be developed in the client's/evaluee's best interest
58. Life care plans shall include a basis for recommendations
59. Life care planners shall utilize a reliable, consistent method for reaching conclusions
60. Life care planners shall utilize adequate medical and other data for opinions
61. Life care plans shall include an annotated list of requested and reviewed data/sources
62. Revised: Life care planners shall utilize standardized procedures and tools for gathering and reporting information and feature standardized forms and formats
63. Revised: Life care planners will use consistent methodologies to evaluate similar cases
64. Life care plans shall rely on medical/allied health professional opinions
65. Life care planners shall methodically handle divergent opinions
66. Revised: Life care planners shall properly inject professional expertise
67. Life care planners shall utilize credible, evidence-based guidelines
68. Life care planners shall conduct an in-person interview whenever permitted
69. Life care planners shall utilize protocols for cost research
70. Life care planners shall gather geographically relevant and representative prices
71. Life care planners shall utilize protocols for using local versus national resources
72. Life care planners shall follow generally accepted methodology
73. Differences in clinical judgment can result in different recommendations
74. Life care planning databases, templates, and software shall have appropriate foundation
75. Life care planning products and processes shall be transparent and consistent
76. Revised: Life care planners as a whole/or part of the specialty practice of life care planning through ethical practice will contribute to the reliability, validity, and accuracy of life care plans
77. Revised: Life care planners, as a whole and/or part of the specialty practice of life care planning will encourage and participate, if able, in longitudinal studies on life care planning
78. Life care planners shall study the impact of life care plans upon quality-of-life
79. Life care planners shall understand and explain research used in a life care plan
80. Life care planners may independently make recommendations for care items/services that are within their scope of practice
81. Life care planners seek recommendations from other qualified professionals and/or relevant sources for inclusion of care items/services outside the individual life care planner's professional scope(s) of practice
82. The cost of private-hire home care includes care giver compensation and associated expenses
83. Life care planners shall consider the impact of aging

84. Review of evidence-based research, review of clinical practice guidelines, medical records, medical and multidisciplinary consultation, and evaluation/assessment of evaluee/family are recognized as best practice sources that provide foundation in life care plans
85. Best practices for identifying costs in life care plans include:
    a. Verifiable data from appropriately referenced sources
    b. Costs identified are geographically specific when appropriate and available
    c. Non-discounted/market rate prices
    d. More than one cost estimate, when appropriate
86. Life care planners will define terminology of our work product(s)
87. Life care planners have the option to use support staff under their direction and guidance in completing life care plans
88. Life care planners shall identify conflicts of interest
89. Life care planners shall identify the sources of their recommendations
90. *Life care planners shall explore markets for life care planning outside litigation
91. *Life care planner certification standards shall be augmented
92. *Life care planners shall draft life care plans under supervision for one year
93. *Life care planners shall better define dual relationships
94. *Life care plans shall be limited to the planner's expertise and scope of practice
95. *Life care planners shall be involved in research
96. *When the life care planner includes home care, both private-hire and agency-procured services are options to be considered

*Those statements with an asterisk (*) did not receive a consensus to maintain, delete, or revise.

Source: Johnson, C. B., Pomeranz, J. L., & Stetten, N. E. (2018). Consensus and majority statements derived from life care planning summits held in 2000, 2002, 2004, 2006, 2008, 2010, 2012, 2015, and 2017 and updated via Delphi study in 2018. *Journal of Life Care Planning, 16*(4), 15–18. [Printed by permission]

Appendix C: An Evaluation Framework for Life Care Plans

CRITERION 1: COMPREHENSIVE DATA COLLECTION (CASE RECORDS, DEPOSITIONS, MEDICAL RECORDS, AND OTHER TEXT MATERIALS)

DEFINITION OF ATTRIBUTE	TASKS PERFORMED AND PROCESS	CONSEQUENCES OF DEFICITS IN THIS AREA	REPRESENTATIVE REVIEW QUESTIONS	SUMMARY CRITIQUE OF TEXT-BASED DATA GATHERING
Collect and review all relevant information: medical history, current strengths, deficits, capabilities, and needs.	Thorough review. Determine that they are complete and up to date for all treaters, with no gaps in service. Request missing information as needed. Complete records may include the following: • Pre- and postmorbid medical records. • Up to date records of all current treaters. • Rehab, vocational, and outpatient service records including assistive technology needs. • Additional tests and assessment requested by the planner. • Drug and supply records. • Employment records. • Records from SSI (Social Security Insurance), Medicaid, Medicare, or other objective public sources of payment.	• Insufficient information about the client's needs and circumstances. • Will under- or overestimate needs for particular resources. • Inadequate foundation. • Will be subject to challenge. • Inadequate foundation for testimony.	1. Was the information reviewed by the planner current? 2. How much of the available text material did the planner review? 100%? 50%? 20%? 10%? 3. Did the planner review material describing current community functioning? 4. Did the planner request additional information if the information received was not current? 5. Did the planner review pre-incident services? 6. Did the planner actively gather information from a variety of public and private sources to obtain a balanced perspective on the client's needs? 7. Was the planner restricted from reviewing or requesting more current materials? 8. Did the planner provide, in an objective form, the precise scope and range of needs for which the person requires support?	• Summarize total amount of material available. • Identify type and percent of total materials actually reviewed. • Summarize planner's attempts to request updated or additional records, (e.g., educational records on school age children, daily nursing care records for children with severe developmental delay, records of annual school planning meetings, records from school consultants) required to assess educational progress, records from public vocational rehabilitation services or records from Medicaid, Adult Services, or Social Security Disability Income) to objectively validate planner's portrayals of client functioning. • What current problems does the planner identify? How does this list compare to problems identified by current treating team? • Summarize the factual and conjectural inaccuracies in planner's characterization of client problems when balanced against client functioning reported by providers with no vested interest in case outcome. • Identify all current providers available to be interviewed as documented in the current case records.

(Continued)

CRITERION 2: COMPREHENSIVE AND INDIVIDUALIZED DATA COLLECTION (CLIENT-BASED)				
DEFINITION OF ATTRIBUTE	TASKS PERFORMED AND PROCESS	CONSEQUENCES OF DEFICITS IN THIS AREA	REPRESENTATIVE REVIEW QUESTIONS	SUMMARY CRITIQUE OF COMPREHENSIVE CLIENT-BASED DATA-GATHERING EFFORTS
An effective life care plan must reflect the specific obstacles, circumstances, and needs of the individual. All recommendations must be unique to this person. The plan should reflect extensive research into the details of this individual's life. The plan should be rich in information that relates solely to this person.	Data collection can only be accomplished through onsite and direct contact. Specifically, the planner should conduct the following interviews: 1. The in ed and how to access.	A plan completed without direct consumer contact will lack detail and specificity. Recommendations will necessarily be general. Crucial areas of need will be overlooked or under allocated. Without the data collected through these interviews, the plan will lack the necessary foundation required for testimony.	1. Did the planner complete a home visit? 2. If not completed, was a good faith effort made by the planner to have access to the client in their home surroundings? 3. If a home visit was completed, did the planner collect sufficient information about size to the home, equipment used, consumer access barriers, space, equipment storage, to render specific advice. 4. Did the planner know the proximity to, community access of, or other types of restrictions regarding needed services? 5. Can the planner provide an accurate depiction of architectural barriers present in all settings that affect the consumer?	To document evidence of the standard not being met: 1. Describe all factual inaccuracies in planner's descriptions of client functioning. 2. Describe inconsistencies between known aspects of client functioning and resources recommended by planner. 3. List untested assumptions, conjecture and speculative conclusions held by planner after planning process. 4. List every resource historically relied upon by client but not included in plan recommendations. 5. List every plan resource recommended by planner which is inappropriate or for which client would not meet eligibility criteria.

(Continued)

CRITERION 2: COMPREHENSIVE AND INDIVIDUALIZED DATA COLLECTION (CLIENT-BASED)				
DEFINITION OF ATTRIBUTE	TASKS PERFORMED AND PROCESS	CONSEQUENCES OF DEFICITS IN THIS AREA	REPRESENTATIVE REVIEW QUESTIONS	SUMMARY CRITIQUE OF COMPREHENSIVE CLIENT-BASED DATA-GATHERING EFFORTS
A comprehensive plan that reflects the specific needs of one individual can only be achieved through direct interaction with the consumer, family, care providers, and other individuals with whom this individual has frequent contact.			6. Can the planner enumerate detailed information about the age, use, appropriateness of equipment used, and issues regarding current technology, adaptive equipment, adapted transport, medical services, and home services and training needs for family members and care staff who will operate equipment? 7. Did the planner identify client and family members' likelihood to self-advocate for all services needed, skills in self-advocacy, additional training needed over time to determine scope, range, and intensity of case management supports needed? 8. Did the planner assess need for further tests and baseline data gathering to provide additional factual basis for recommendations made, e.g., neurological functioning, custom wheelchair and seating needs, auditory processing evaluations, neuroophthalmology evaluations, nutritional evaluations, occupational or physical therapy evaluations, technology evaluations, or evaluations for architectural access?	

(Continued)

Methodology, Scope of Practice, Standards of Practice, & Consensus ■ 71

		CRITERION 3: COLLABORATIVE PLANNING PROCESSES		
DEFINITION OF ATTRIBUTE	TASKS PERFORMED AND PROCESS	CONSEQUENCES OF DEFICITS IN THIS AREA	REPRESENTATIVE REVIEW QUESTIONS	SUMMARY CRITIQUE OF COLLABORATIVE EFFORTS
The planner should consult with other professionals involved with the consumer for their opinions to reinforce the foundation of the life care plan and to provide detail and inside into the needs of the consumer. Each provider will have details of the individual's functioning otherwise unavailable to the planner because of the history this provider shares with the individual.	The life care planning process requires soliciting the involvement and concurrence of providers currently involved with the person. Specifically, these professionals should be interviewed to obtain the following information: 1. What guidance do they have for resources for this consumer now and in the future? 2. If this individual is not currently providing these services, why not? Do services need to be reinitiated? 3. For what period of time is it likely that the services will be required? 4. What is the expected outcome from the provision of the services and why is this important? 5. What is the cost of these services?	Recommendations developed in isolation from current treating providers of service will necessarily be subjective. These recommendations will not demonstrate a sufficient knowledge base from which to draw conclusions. It is also likely that these recommendations will not match the perspectives of treating professionals and will not have their concurrence. Without the concurrence of treating professionals the plan may lack legal foundation even if the planner has expertise in the particular area in question.	1. Is the planner able to name all currently active providers? 2. Did the planner request all documentation on services provided, and course of treatment or intervention with providers? 3. Can the planner document problems in services provided, deficiencies in scope, and range of services offered? 4. Were providers across all necessary life domains interviewed to understand their attitudes toward the consumer? Were problems with provider attitudes known? 5. Were efforts were made to solicit the active involvement of current providers? Were efforts made to solicit adequate time with providers, direct observation of the consumer interacting with their providers, or a face-to-face visit with providers?	To critique this aspect of plan development, document evidence of inadequate collaboration in the following ways: 1. Identify all current providers available to be interviewed as documented in the current case records. 2. Identify planner attempts to involve relevant treating providers in plan development processes. 3. Identify if planner completed consultation with relevant treating providers in plan development processes. 4. If interviews were conducted, compare planner's deposition testimony to provider involvement and guidance from available treater documentation. 5. Compare provider recommendations to planner's for congruity. 6. Identify each instance in which the planner exceeded background, training, and expertise in prescribing a resource for the client. 7. Identify each instance in which the planner had no factual or experiential basis from which to prescribe a resource.

(Continued)

		CRITERION 3: COLLABORATIVE PLANNING PROCESSES		
DEFINITION OF ATTRIBUTE	TASKS PERFORMED AND PROCESS	CONSEQUENCES OF DEFICITS IN THIS AREA	REPRESENTATIVE REVIEW QUESTIONS	SUMMARY CRITIQUE OF COLLABORATIVE EFFORTS
	6. Are there additional services available from another provider that would enhance the services recommended by this provider? 7. If these services were included in a life care plan, is there documentation that the provider supports the planner's conclusions about services needed or changes?		6. Did the planner involve providers from planning. If no, how was this choice was made? 7. Did the planner seek recommendations for services across all affected life domains, or only focus on one aspect of service? 8. Did the planner identify provider problems or attitudes that would restrict services? 9. Did the planner provide solutions to service delivery problems?	

(Continued)

Methodology, Scope of Practice, Standards of Practice, & Consensus

CRITERION 4: REPRODUCIBLE PLANNING METHODS

DEFINITION OF ATTRIBUTE	TASKS PERFORMED AND PROCESS	CONSEQUENCES OF DEFICITS IN THIS AREA	REPRESENTATIVE REVIEW QUESTIONS	SUMMARY CRITIQUE OF REPPRODUCIBILITY
Another person should be able to duplicate and reproduce data collected, planner methods, and plan formation. A reproducible plan development process defines each method used logically and clearly. The process is standardized and consistent throughout.	The planner provides a clear and logical rationale for each step. The planner defines all text data collected and summary conclusions drawn. The planner identifies all information from the client and family members and relates data collected to conclusions. The planner describes provider information on the individual and shows how it confirms needs. The planner can identify how data collection and planning efforts provide a base for each resource recommended.	No logical rationale for plan development or conclusions regarding client need. Defines source of conclusions as "background, training, and experience," not a database or logical thought processes. Another person seeking to replicate these cannot determine methods or thought processes underlying recommendations. Methods are undependable and do not conform to widely used and accepted data-gathering methods. Little to no information on databases relied upon, cannot state the relevant characteristics of each, their reliability, or how they support the conclusions.	1. Does the planner demonstrate a knowledge of the key steps in long-term plan development? 2. Did planner use generally accepted analytic methods? 3. Did the planner use multiple analytic methods to support conclusions identify eccentric facts? 4. Did the planner reconcile alternatives in the final conclusions? 5. Did the planner disclose analytic assumptions and important variables affecting future treatment and assumptions about the person and circumstances? 6. Could another person obtain the same results by duplicating the planner's steps?	How well can planner's methods be reproduced and/or duplicated. How the planner specifies all actions and provides the data collected. Steps to perform critique: 1. Summarize and define each step of plan development. 2. Compare steps with generally accepted methods for long-term plan development. 3. Summarize deviations and how they affect reproducibility. 4. Identify each method, approach, or technique for which the planner has no identifiable training, skills, or educational background. 5. Document appropriate use of primary and secondary databases and research studies. 6. Identify implications for conclusion reliability. 7. Summarize every database or resource identified by the planner that cannot be located and verified.

(Continued)

DEFINITION OF ATTRIBUTE	TASKS PERFORMED AND PROCESS	CRITERION 4: REPRODUCIBLE PLANNING METHODS		
		CONSEQUENCES OF DEFICITS IN THIS AREA	REPRESENTATIVE REVIEW QUESTIONS	SUMMARY CRITIQUE OF REPPRODUCIBILITY
		The planner will not be able to explain the data on which they relied, and the conclusions they drew.	7. Did the planner critically evaluate information for logical consistency, reliability, and relevance? 8. Is the evidence quoted consistent with evidence identified in records and other appraisals? 9. Can each research, database, or literature source cited be identified and located? 10. Can the planner show how research cited was applicable? 11. Does the planner confirm findings from a database through independent verification, e.g., labor market analyses? 12. Is each resource cited accurate for duration and cost? 13. Does the plan include recommendations or conclusions by which the planner exceeds licensed scope of practice? 14. Can this plan be implemented? 15. Does the planner evidence familiarity with the databases they relied upon?	8. Summarize deficiencies that would arise with plan implementation.

(Continued)

Methodology, Scope of Practice, Standards of Practice, & Consensus ■ 75

CRITERION 5: INFORMED PLANNING—GENERAL KNOWLEDGE, SKILLS, AND EXPERIENCE BASE

DEFINITION OF ATTRIBUTE	TASKS PERFORMED AND PROCESS	CONSEQUENCES OF DEFICITS IN THIS AREA	REPRESENTATIVE REVIEW QUESTIONS	SUMMARY CRITIQUE OF GENERAL PLANNING KNOWLEDGE, SKILLS, AND EXPERIENCE
A life care planner must have a significant degree of specialized knowledge, including current trends regarding disability policy, funding and living options, current technological advances, emerging rights of persons with disabilities, current funding policies and options offered by state agencies doing programming with persons with disabilities, architecture, disability rights, economics, law, medicine, social work, physical and occupational therapy, and assistive technology.	The planner: 1. Knows professional standards for analysis, professional literature. 2. Can assess appropriate theories, standards, and techniques. 3. Knows relevant professional organizations and standards. 4. Describes previous knowledge as part of the basis for recommendations. 5. Shows how large-scale research applies. 6. Knows about current research, technological advances, services, programs, and outcomes.	A series of clichés on general resources, not specific enough to support later resource purchase. Lack of informed perspective, out-of-date standards of care, and outmoded forms of assistive technology will result in inaccurate recommendations.	1. Do proposed resources restrict the person to one setting? 2. Does the plan unnecessarily limit the person to living and working only with other persons with disabilities? 3. Does the planner rely on stereotypical, offensive language, e.g., "a bad baby case", " this Super-Quad case?" 4. Did the planner define the person only in terms of disability, e.g., "C3-4 quad", "the blind", "a TBI", instead of a person with (specific condition). 5. Does the plan expose the person to unnecessary health and safety risks, or does the plan recognize and incorporate a strategy to reduce them? 6. Does the plan address potential vulnerability to abuse, neglect, and exploitation, and incorporate legal, medical, or advocacy resources to offset these risks, if needed?	1. Identify significant cross-disciplinary planning and recommendations. 2. Outline specific examples of sensitivity or insensitivity toward individuals with disabilities. 3. Detail resources and recommendations that do not represent current standards of care. 4. Identify all resource recommendations that rely on outmoded technologies, pharmacological guidelines, or present health and safety risks.

(Continued)

CRITERION 5: INFORMED PLANNING—GENERAL KNOWLEDGE, SKILLS, AND EXPERIENCE BASE				
DEFINITION OF ATTRIBUTE	TASKS PERFORMED AND PROCESS	CONSEQUENCES OF DEFICITS IN THIS AREA	REPRESENTATIVE REVIEW QUESTIONS	SUMMARY CRITIQUE OF GENERAL PLANNING KNOWLEDGE, SKILLS, AND EXPERIENCE
A planner refreshes this body of knowledge with continuous study and training.			7. Were all resources' duration, replacement, start/end dates, diagnostic codes, and substantiated cost fully described? 8. Did the plan provide realistic normalizing experiences, e.g., integrating school experiences, emancipation, some degree of work identity during adult years, community-based recreational activities? 9. Do resources reflect current devices, methods, and standards of care? 10. Does the plan use material from a variety of sources?	

(Continued)

Methodology, Scope of Practice, Standards of Practice, & Consensus ■ 77

CRITERION 6: OUTCOMES-BASED PLANNING PROCESSES TARGETING THE SERVICE DELIVERY SYSTEM

DEFINITION OF ATTRIBUTE	TASKS PERFORMED AND PROCESS	CONSEQUENCES OF DEFICITS IN THIS AREA	REPRESENTATIVE REVIEW QUESTIONS	SUMMARY CRITIQUE OF PLANNER'S SERVICE DELIVERY ANALYSIS
People who have catastrophic disability require an array of unfamiliar current and future services. Connecting with these often requires a bewildering set of restrictions, forms, expectations, and rules. For many, limited access is associated with functional declines, worsening health, and abrupt facility placement. Life care planning must identify all relevant service related problems for a consumer, and then assess how each inter-related part of the service delivery system can be coordinated to function for their benefit.	The life care planner: 1. Appraises resources and provider responses to requests for service. 2. Assesses consumer and family members' ability to identify needs and self-advocate. 3. Identifies existing relationships between client and resource network. 4. Assesses how well the service system is accountable to and representative of the consumer's interests. If there are barriers to getting or maintaining services, case management must be included, specifying why, when, and how a case manager will intervene to assure continuity and access to services. The plan must specify why and how resources are recommended and desired outcomes.	• A plan is naive, invalid, and insufficient if it fails to incorporate strategies to support implementation. • No assurance that services will be accessed, secured, and kept. • No information the family can use in seeking services. • The plan is an artifact of litigation and has no "real-world" application. • **The client will not be able to execute the plan.** No provision for updating the plan, assisting the client in identifying when resources will need to be changed, or introducing the client to newer technologies.	1. Service Assessment: Does the planner know the kind of problems the person has had with service providers in the past? What documents this awareness in the record review and interviews with providers or family? 2. Service Comprehensiveness: Can the planner confirm all services now used by the client, both public and private, understand needs? 3. Service Accountability: If the person experiences a problem with service delivery, does the planner define who will locate and fix it, and how? 4. Service Access: Does the planner confirm that needed services are geographically located, or, is the plan designed so that services are reached only at cost and inconvenience? 5. Service Availability: Does the plan have a strategy to remedy fixed or inflexible provider operating schedules?	1. Ascertain whether the planner documents reported service delivery problems, or recognizes the range of typical problems associated with this disability. 2. Review records and note problems in service delivery not identified or reported by the planner. 3. Identify if the planner had any direct contact with the client, or, made requests to interview and observe the client to collect information on problems in service delivery. 4. Identify planner's direct contact with providers in to assess problems, or analyzed provider records documenting problems. 5. Identify whether the planner assessed the information needs and skills in self-advocacy of the client or their family members. 6. Identify if the planner can cite case management specific tasks, contacts, and activities, and short- and long-term CM (case management) objectives. 7. If case management intervention is recommended, identify if the amount proposed is enough to secure and keep necessary services.

(Continued)

CRITERION 6: OUTCOMES-BASED PLANNING PROCESSES TARGETING THE SERVICE DELIVERY SYSTEM			
DEFINITION OF ATTRIBUTE	TASKS PERFORMED AND PROCESS	CONSEQUENCES OF DEFICITS IN THIS AREA	REPRESENTATIVE REVIEW QUESTIONS	SUMMARY CRITIQUE OF PLANNER'S SERVICE DELIVERY ANALYSIS
The desired outcome is a stable, orderly plan that identifies how to locate and keep needed services. Their purposes are defined, rationales for introduction and stopping are clearly identified, and recommendations is documented. Relationships between and among all services and resources are spelled out. Recommendations for case management are appropriate when the consumer needs: a single point of accountability in the service system; a means to establish responsibility within the current delivery system for services; strengthening the consumer's support system to assure service consistency, continuity, and coordination and facilitate links to additional sources if needed.	Timing and introduction for new resources and the discontinuation of those no longer needed must be clearly explained. The life care plan must identify all resources required, define the purpose of each, and give strategies for arranging and timing for receipt. If links between client and resources are lacking, there should be provision for a coordinating case manager and how this will overcome deficiencies.	No reference to difficulties the client has experienced in the past when seeking to obtain resources from medically sophisticated providers. The plan will list a range of resources without noting how to secure or coordinate them.	6. Service Evaluation: Does the plan say how to monitor and follow-up with providers and clients to learn how well services are working? 7. Service Advocacy: Does the plan provide how to correct problems with public agencies, schools, technology, vendors, contractors, adapted transport, durable medical goods, etc.? 8. Service Identification: Does the plan provide a means to periodically re-assess and update the client on newer resources? 9. Service Integration: Does the plan have a person designated to coordinate and help secure other needed services? 10. Service Continuity: Does the plan have a person designated to prevent abrupt, unexplained interruptions in service delivery? 11. Service Responsiveness: Does the plan have a way to assure that service delivery will be adapted to accommodate changes in need?	

(Continued)

CRITERION 7: FACTUAL PLANNING PROCESS—RESOURCE AND COST VERIFICATION					
DEFINITION OF ATTRIBUTE	TASKS PERFORMED AND PROCESS	CONSEQUENCES OF DEFICITS IN THIS AREA	REPRESENTATIVE REVIEW QUESTIONS	SUMMARY CRITIQUE OF PLANNER'S SERVICE RESEARCH
This section shows how to review recommendations and proposed costs for accuracy, reliability, and validity. It also shows how to review evidence-based research on resource safety and benefit. Errors in costs, contact names, services, and recommendations for obsolete goods undermine credibility. Review processes must rely on current and well-researched information. Services should be related to problems. The planner should document current peer-reviewed research for service outcomes and potential risks, benefits, and negative side-effects.	Use a data collection instrument that summarizes resources and costs, a "cost chart". Substantiation data for each plan item should include: • name and location. • source of information. • three representative vendors if available. • start and end dates for use cost. • replacement cycle. • Procedure Code if applicable. This information can be collected throughout the planning process. Cost charts must be accurate, current, and agree with the record or formal recommendation.	Factual inaccuracies, even simple arithmetical errors, reduce credibility. Cumulative errors further diminish plan credibility and value. Common errors include: 1. Simple arithmetic errors. 2. Complex errors as calculations propagate. 3. Omitting a supported resource. 4. Including unsupported resources. 5. Starting/stopping a resource too soon/late. 6. Providing for a resource for an unsupported time frame. 7. Citing a vendor who does not provide the item or service recommended. 8. Incorrect pricing. 9. Items or services that overlap without supported need. 10. Resources may present unanticipated risks or harm. 11. Resources result in little to no benefit after use. 12. Resources result in unexpected progressive complications.	1. Are these charts supported by records and research? 2. Is every resource outside of the planner's field of licensure or expertise supported by a qualified professional in the field? 3. Are resources, start dates, end dates, and exact costs accurate? 4. How are dates/durations supported? 5. How were costs obtained? 6. Are costs verifiable? Can you obtain the same vendor cost quote for the same parameters?	Steps to perform critique: 1. Identify all unsupported or unverified recommendations. 2. Describe all omitted recommendations that are supported in the record, research, or interview. 3. Detail all inaccuracies regarding period of service, starting too early/late or insufficient duration. 4. Ascertain goods/service availability from vendor referenced. 5. List recommendations priced differently than given. 6. Identify calculation errors.

Source: Caragonne, P., Sofka, K., & Howland, W. (2019, October 9). *Frameworks for Evaluating Life Care Plans*. www.americanbar.org/groups/health_law/publications/health_lawyer_home/2019-october/life-care/ [Printed by permission].

Chapter 3

Research in Life Care Planning

Aaron Mertes and Christine Reid

Fundamentals of Research in Life Care Planning

Types of Research

The term "research" is used in various ways in life care planning, depending on the context. Practitioners may research how much a medical service will cost by scanning the internet, using a database service that gathers data about actual charges and organizes costs by region, consulting a published book, or surveying local providers of that service. They may search an individual's medical record to find a diagnosis from a past provider or call an electric wheelchair manufacturer to learn about the recommended replacement schedule on the battery for a given chair. They may review clinical practice guidelines for various professions, or the standards of practice (SOP) for life care planners. In other words, they use the word "research" colloquially to learn things that enhance their personal knowledge.

On the other hand, research is a term used not only to advance individual knowledge or focus on an individual case (n=1), but also to advance knowledge for the entire profession through carefully planned and organized efforts of data collection and manipulation. The distinction between individual information gathering and systemic research to contribute to general knowledge is important, because it relates to the quality of evidence. Even within formal research, there are distinctions between levels of the quality of evidence. The more a piece of research evidence results from a methodology that systematically controls for various sources of potential error, the greater the quality of that evidence. The pyramid diagram in Figure 3.1 illustrates different levels of the quality of evidence, showing the most plentiful (but least methodologically rigorous) types of publications at the base of the pyramid, and rigor improving (but with less published material available) at each subsequent level.

At the peak of the pyramid are meta-analyses, which are the relatively rare systematic statistical integrations of the results of many studies of a specific research question. Among publications at the lowest level of evidence are articles that provide a verbal review of what others have studied,

DOI: 10.4324/9781003388456-4

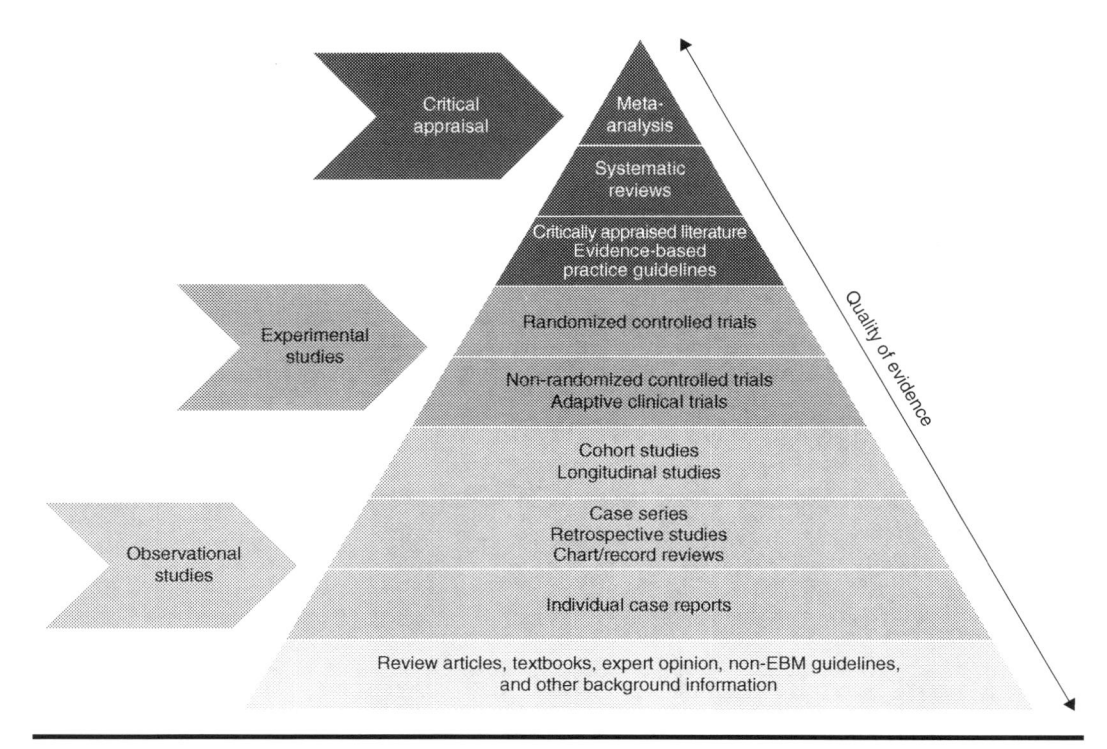

Figure 3.1 Hierarchy of Evidence Pyramid

textbooks, opinions by people considered to have expertise in an area (but not necessarily supported by formal research), or guidelines that are not derived from an evidence-based methodology.

The next three levels in the pyramid are types of observational studies. They involve gathering data through observation, and because they do not manipulate conditions to test hypotheses, they do not reach the next level, experimental studies. The key distinction between observational studies and experimental studies is that in experimental studies, the researchers can assign subjects to specific conditions to systematically test their research hypotheses. Looking within the three levels of observational studies, the lowest level of evidence quality is individual case reports; the next level expands beyond a single case, examining series of cases, retrospective studies, and record or chart reviews. The highest level of evidence quality within the three observational studies' categories is the level of cohort studies or longitudinal studies. At the cohort or longitudinal study level, you not only look beyond just one individual case; but you also look at more than one point in time for all of the individuals studied.

The next two levels in the pyramid are types of experimental studies, in which the researchers can assign subjects to conditions, to test research hypotheses. The lower level of these two includes non-randomized controlled trials, and adaptive clinical trials. A non-randomized controlled trial is best understood by contrasting it to a randomized controlled trial. In a randomized controlled trial, subjects (or research participants) are randomly assigned to one condition (or treatment) or another. They have no choice in the matter. In a non-randomized controlled trial, the researcher might do something like examine data from people receiving services at three hospitals that are implementing a new protocol, versus data from people receiving services at three other similar hospitals that are continuing with treatment as usual. In such a design, there is a chance that other factors related to the various hospitals might affect treatment and obscure the effect of the new protocol. Another type of experimental study that is at the lower of the two levels of rigor is the category of adaptive clinical trials. In such trials, the methodology can be adapted along the way as new information is gathered. The rigor is less than for a non-adaptive randomized controlled trial (the next level on the quality of evidence pyramid), but there can be important ethical considerations that balance the need for rigor. For example, if we conduct a trial to test the efficacy of a vaccine that prevents a serious illness and discover part-way through the trial that the vaccine prevents serious illness in 100% of the group receiving it, yet a large percentage of the group receiving a placebo becomes hospitalized or dies, should we continue withholding the real vaccine from those receiving the placebo?

Moving beyond the experimental studies' levels on the quality of evidence pyramid are three levels of critical appraisal. These involve integrating and critically evaluating multiple studies of the same problem or experience. The first of these three levels includes critically appraised literature, and evidence-based practice guidelines. The critical appraisal should involve more than just an expert giving an opinion about the quality of various studies; it should involve a systematic process of assessing the rigor of those studies, and the degree to which they control for various types of error. Chan et al. (2016) addressed this within the context of applying an evidence-based process to clinical practice. That five step process involves: 1) developing the kinds of well-defined, answerable questions that are clinically relevant to the problem; 2) seeking the best evidence you can find to answer those questions (using systematic search approaches); 3) applying logic to judiciously appraise the evidence (keeping in mind both the levels of quality of the evidence and the direct applicability to the situation); 4) integrating that evidence with your clinical expertise, to apply it to the clinical situation; and 5) evaluating the effectiveness and efficiency of your process to identify and apply evidence-based practices.

Evidence-based clinical practice guidelines integrate the best available research evidence with clinical expertise and a focus on the needs of patients (DePalma, 2002; Sacket et al., 2000). They are developed through a rigorous process of systematically reviewing existing research and integrating it with expert evaluation of how that research applies to clinical practice. Criteria for developing clinical practice guidelines were described by the Agency for Healthcare Research and Quality (2021), which maintained a collection of clinical practice guidelines until funding for this endeavor was cut in 2018. Hopefully, funding for such a repository of vetted clinical practice guidelines will become available again in the future.

At the next level among the critical appraisal categories in the pyramid of evidence is the category of systematic reviews. Cook et al. (1997) explained that a systematic review "involves the application of scientific strategies, in ways that limit bias, to the assembly, critical appraisal, and synthesis of all relevant studies that address a specific clinical question" (p. 376). A very helpful database for identifying healthcare-related systematic reviews is the Cochrane collection. Information about these reviews and their protocols is available through www.cochranelibrary.com/cdsr/about-cdsr

At the peak of the quality of evidence pyramid is the category of meta-analyses. Haidich (2010) described meta-analysis as a "quantitative, formal, epidemiological study used to systematically assess previous research studies to derive conclusions about that body of research" (p. 29). The "quantitative" part of that description refers to the statistical techniques used to combine data from multiple studies in a way that both integrates findings from diverse studies and more precisely and reliably assesses the extent of the observed effects, across many participants in multiple studies. Even if a life care planner is not an expert researcher, Umesh et al. (2016) reminds us that "critical appraisal of scientific literature is an important skill to be mastered not only by academic medical professionals but also by those involved in clinical practice" (p. 670) Those authors provide guidance for evaluating the robustness of study methodologies, which should be understood by practitioners, as well as researchers and scientists. Examples of appraisal items include: ethics and funding; design methodology; randomization; sample size and statistics; reliability; generalizability of results; and limitations. These are among the elements evaluated to make sure the science is solid before trusting the results. Meta-analyses are generally conducted by those who have mastered the skill of evaluating these elements, so that each individual study that is included in a meta-analysis meets scientific standards. Without appraisal of the science, there is room for logical fallacies like "appeal to authority" in which people trust the findings of well-known scientists from well-known universities even if the methodology is not scientifically sound. In a perfect world, people would earn their reputations by producing methodologically sound work, but it is incumbent on consumers of science to have the skills to evaluate evidence themselves.

Applying Research to Life Care Planning

In addition to standards of practice being a direct application of higher levels of evidence, there are other ways a life care planner can use these charts to discuss the level of evidence a life care plan incorporates. An individual life care plan, the result of a systematic process of gathering, analyzing, and applying relevant information, can be considered an observational study or an individual case report. However, the information the life care planner gathers in the process of developing that plan should be collected in a defensibly systematic manner, informed by understanding (and citation) of relevant published research and clinical practice guidelines. Life care planners should be able to articulate the process they use for systematically gathering information needed for life care plans, using processes designed to minimize error, such as the Attendant Care Survey Methodology described by Barros-Bailey et al. (2022).

Part of the process of gathering relevant information for a life care plan should involve reviewing relevant published research, using evidence-based literature to inform the development of life care plans. Life care planners should be familiar with available literature that addresses functional limitations and appropriate accommodations for the disabilities involved, how the disabilities interact with the aging process over time, efficacy of various treatments and rehabilitation approaches related to the disabilities, etc. Although there may have been a time in the past when life care planners who did not have an affiliation with a university or medical center were unable access to such publications, that is no longer the case. Most public libraries now provide access to databases such as EBSCO, CINAHL, etc. to assist people in searching for relevant literature, and can provide access to most of the needed publications free of charge. Often, electronic access to those publications is immediate and for publications not immediately available electronically, librarians may use interlibrary loan (ILL) services to assist their patrons with finding articles not otherwise available in their collection. Life care planners can use the Boolean search functions within the databases (such as EBSCO) to appropriately expand or narrow their searches for relevant literature. For a quick tutorial on how to use Boolean functionality in a search, just run an internet search on terms such as "using Boolean operators," and you will find guidance about how to effectively use those "AND," "OR," "NOT," and "AND NOT" operators to expand or focus the results of a search. Integrating an understanding of the levels of evidence quality into a search for relevant literature, it would be wise for life care planners to run literature searches using the disabilities or rehabilitation approaches involved in conjunction with search terms such as "meta-analysis," "evidence-based," "practice guidelines," "systematic review," "longitudinal study," and "clinical trial."

Another way of categorizing types of research was described by Bellini and Rumrill (2018), who distinguished between primary, secondary, and tertiary research. Primary research refers to "efforts that generate new knowledge and relate directly to the status/participation of people with disabilities in society" (p. 279), or applied to life care planning, studies relating to subjects of a life care plan. Secondary research "measures competencies, attitudes, and dispositions of pre-service or practicing rehabilitation counselors" (p. 279), or the professionals developing life care plans. Tertiary research, then, focuses on "professional issues that are relevant to counselors and educators, but they do not center directly on experiences, perspectives, and concerns of rehabilitation consumers and professionals" (p. 279). These are important distinctions because not only can any of these types of research have a varying quality of evidence, but also, they provide the field with different kinds of information.

The terms primary, secondary, and tertiary are used in different ways by Yin (2008, 2011, 2013, 2017) in an Evidence Source Model (ESM). Barros-Bailey (2018) adapted this for clinical forensic practice, which addresses data collection during an assessment, asking the question, "What evidence can I consider in an assessment?" (Barros-Bailey, 2018, p. 117). The ESM model Barros-Bailey describes includes data collection from evaluee interviews, record review, and from research, with a focus on relevance to forensic report development. Bellini and Rumrill (2018) focus on the terms primary, secondary, and tertiary in terms of research evidence.

Mertes (2018) performed a content analysis of all available articles in the *Journal of Life Care Planning* from 2004 to 2017 to assess several different variables relating to the type and quality of life care planning research. First, he found that of the 214 articles, 73% fell into the tertiary category, meaning more research is being published about the profession itself than about the subjects of life care plans or their authors. Also, the overwhelming majority (86%) were conceptual in nature, meaning they were written to describe a certain condition from a particular professional perspective, not using statistical data or advanced statistical procedures. While these seem like potentially unreliable forms of evidence, Mertes emphasized that life care planning is a relatively new practice and is in the stages of building its foundations. Using the hierarchy of evidence pyramid, one can see how a foundation must be established before the upper parts can be created. The findings revealed a need for more primary research about the outcomes of subjects of life care plans as well as more statistical information gathered across the geographical scope of where life care plans are written, and across time.

In the same article, Mertes (2018) performed a comparison between what the field desired to research and what was actually being researched in the *Journal of Life Care Planning*. He noted that the field is self-reflective and assesses the need for more research of various types. Deutsch and Allison (2004) discussed areas of need in the field and Mertes (2018) compared that to what had been published following that article to identify gaps in research. The greatest area of need identified was efficacy and implementation studies, i.e., research on how accurate and valid life care plans are for those who are using them as a guide to future care. The topic of validity will be discussed below, but the big questions related to "Do life care plans accurately do what they set out to do?" are a great area of interest to life care planners, attorney clients, life care planning evaluees, and their families.

While understanding what types of research are needed will help us later on in the chapter when we discuss future directions, we should also look at what foundational documents and research have laid the groundwork for the practice thus far.

Foundational Documentation and Research

Two of the fundamental questions asked about any professional practice are: What is the practice of life care planning? and does it work? In this case, life care planners have been working to further identify and strengthen understanding of what life care planning is and how it is done well. By defining who life care planners are and what they do, trust in the life care planning process can be built. In other words, if a life care plan is valid, or measures what it says it is measuring, then we can trust that the contents of it accurately outline future disability-related needs and costs. Below are some of the foundational documents that help us answer these questions. Each of these various research efforts provides something unique to the field, even though there may be apparent overlap in the purpose of those research efforts. Not only will the research efforts involved be described, but also, we will try to explain how and why they are important.

Role and Function Studies

Role and function studies define what the role of a life care planner is and what essential functions are necessary to complete a life care plan. There have been three main studies to identify the roles and functions of life care planners (May & Moradi Rekabdarkolaee, 2020; Pomeranz et al., 2010; Turner et al., 2000). Each of these studies is slightly different and has provided the field with new information.

In the initial study, Turner et al. (2000) used an expert panel to determine the frequency of job tasks. In other words, they asked how often certain tasks were performed by life care planners to determine what life care planners actually do in the development of a life care plan. A factor analysis is a statistical tool that allows researchers to categorize a wide variety of information into groups based on similarity of items. In this case, of the 56 job tasks that life care planners were asked to rate for frequency of performance, three factors were identified: need and cost of medical services; assessing the need for vocational services; and serving as an expert witness.

In a subsequent study, Pomeranz et al. (2010) surveyed life care planners in several phases to establish validity for an instrument to be used. The resulting survey was then given to life care planners to rate the level of frequency and importance of a job task. In this case, 21 separate themes were identified, which helped expand understanding of specific skills used in life care plan development.

Most recently, May and Moradi Rekabdarkolaee, (2020) used factor analysis to identify job tasks, and asked several additional questions relating to differences among life care planners. This study identified 16 factors, with 24 subfactors. Despite apparent differences in the number of factors and subfactors between these three studies, May and Moradi Rekabdarkolaee discussed the similarities among all three studies and attributed some of the differences in factors to the growth of the field and maturity of understanding of the process of life care planning.

Of the four additional research questions that May and Moradi Rekabdarkolaee, (2020) asked, there were some interesting outcomes. First, there were differences in the way nurse life care planners and non-nurse life care planners view their roles in the life care planning process. Second, there were no differences between doctoral and non-doctoral-level practitioners. Third, there were differences among those who spent more or less time on developing life care plans. Fourth, there were significant differences in perceptions of the roles and functions based on degree level. While there was apparently no difference between doctoral and non-doctoral-level participants, the specific knowledge domains were emphasized differently among the varying degree levels. As their discussion proposed, the differences were less attributed to level and more attributed to the underlying philosophy of the specific degree, meaning various professions may emphasize the importance of certain tasks more than others based on their prior training. As an example, nurse life care planners place more importance on reviewing records, whereas rehabilitation counselors emphasize knowledge of the psychosocial and cultural impact of disability. This finding makes sense, given the training background and skill sets of these two groups.

Overall, the role and function studies provide an important foundation both for training new life care planners and preparing them for practice, as well as setting and maintaining standards to help provide a more reliable practice. As May and Moradi Rekabdarkolaee (2020) pointed out, varying professions have slightly different views about what the most important parts of a life care plan are, but these studies help standardize the practice so that all life care planners can agree on a complete picture of the process of life care plan development. In other words, this research is essential for understanding the transdisciplinary process of life care planning across professional disciplines.

Consensus and Majority Statements

Consensus statements are a list of statements about what life care planning is and what it should be. While the above description of role and function studies identifies job tasks, the consensus statements identify a broader degree of what life care planning is and should be. While there is overlap in what the consensus statements say and what the roles and functions say about plan development, the consensus statements address other areas regarding the organization of the field in addition to what life care planners do.

The development of these statements started in 2000 when a group of life care planners began meeting to standardize the process of life care planning at a summit. Since then there have been 11 summits, the last one being in 2022. The last time consensus statements were addressed and changed was in 2017; between 2000 and 2017, participants added to the list of statements that further clarify what the practice is and how it should be conducted. "The goal [has been] to *develop* ethics, *standards of practice*, standard of care, etc., specifically using the power of the group of attendees (grass roots)" (Johnson, 2019). The important point to know about the consensus statements is that they were developed by a rigorous democratic process (Delbecq et al., 1975) that invites the voice of all life care planners, not just a select body of experts. For a full description of the methodology, see Johnson (2019). The consensus statements now contain 97 statements that guide life care planners in their practice and plan development.

Standards of Practice

The International Academy of Life Care Planners (IALCP) publishes practice standards for life care planning (IALCP, 2022). If the role and function (R&F) studies are a scientific approach to understanding what life care planners do, then the *Standards of Practice* (SOP) are the formalized result of that research. Similarly, if the consensus statements are the results of collective brainstorming about practice, then the SOP are a formalized place to use the R&F research and consensus statements to establish practice guidelines. It can be confusing to people what the differences are because there is redundancy, but the consensus statements include a wider range of topics from ethics to establishment of a professional journal for publication of research. One could imagine a working committee gathering research on a topic (R&F studies) and deciding how to report the information using that research and all other available information (consensus statements) to others. The resulting report (*Standards of Practice*) that committee generates would be the refined result of their work. The actual methodology used for creating and periodically revising the *Standards of Practice for Life Care Planners* was detailed by Preston and Reid (2015).

It is worth mentioning that although the IALCP practice standards are written to be all inclusive, other organizations publish their own practice standards as they apply to their differing philosophies. The American Association of Nurse Life Care Planners (AANLCP) and the American

Association of Physician Life Care Planners have written their own standards as they apply to their unique vision of practice.

Definitions of what life care planning is can be found in many places, but the SOP should be the formal authoritative place to reference. Also included is an important note about the philosophical perspective of the field regarding what kind of professionals life care planners are. Given the litigious pressure to establish credibility of life care planners, it should be no surprise that discussions of who is *credible* are a result. However, the SOP establishes that life care planning is a transdisciplinary practice (Mauk, 2019), meaning that healthcare professionals of various primary backgrounds with the appropriate training and experience can learn the requisite skills to develop life care plans. It is the individual skill of the life care planner that establishes credibility, not the primary discipline from which they emerge. In addition to these definitions and the philosophical context, there are additional sections related to standards of performance and standards of practice. The reader can refer to the SOP document for specifics on what those are (IALCP, 2022).

Professional Guidelines of Life Care Planning Practitioners

Life care planning is a specialty practice that is performed by various professionals (see prior discussion about the transdisciplinary practice above). This means that a life care planner must follow the professional standards and ethics of their primary discipline. It also means that they are qualified to include recommendations in a life care plan if it is part of their professional training and experience. For example, counselors are able to make recommendations about counseling needs of evaluees, if applicable, because they are trained to assess those needs and provide effective treatments. Counselors are not trained to assess the need for and to provide surgical interventions for evaluees, if applicable, so counselors must rely on the recommendations of qualified surgeons for that. Each life care planner must understand the scopes of practice of not only their own profession, but the professions of other members of the rehabilitation team contributing recommendations to life care plans. When critiquing life care plans developed by others, life care planners should consider whether the recommendations made independently by those life care planners are within the scopes of practice for those individuals. In part, a critique of a plan assesses whether other professionals are qualified to make authoritative recommendations in a plan within their training or experience or whether they need to refer to the recommendations of other professionals trained in other aspects of rehabilitation. A critique will also assess appropriateness of the methodology used by a life care planner, reliability, and applicability of the information used to make decisions about recommendations, etc. As another example, a physiatrist is not trained or experienced in the long-term career outcomes of evaluees, just like the vocational counselor is not trained in the diagnosis of physical disorders or medical treatment necessary to restore or maintain physical functioning after injury. In any collaborative environment, various practitioners are charged to know their roles, as well as the limitations, i.e., when to make a referral. Life care planning requires that same understanding and various professional guidelines are used to ensure that those boundaries are maintained.

In 2019, the *Journal of Life Care Planning* published a special edition of various professionals explaining their foundational professions to provide insight for others into the scope of their work (IARP, 2019). In this issue, professionals described the training and educational requirements, licensing requirements, professional development common beyond formal education, and other information to help readers understand professions commonly seen in life care planning including nursing, occupational therapy, physiatry, speech therapy, and other professional disciplines.

Reliability and Validity of Life Care Plans

There is a clear and acknowledged need to know whether life care plans actually identify real needs and accurate costs (validity), and whether they continue to be accurate over time and across life care planners (reliability) (Countiss & Deutsch, 2002; Sutton et al., 2018). Basically, all research studies are like pieces of a puzzle, providing information about one part of the phenomenon studied, but not addressing all aspects of it. Each type of study has its strengths and limitations. Both strengths and limitations will be discussed below.

In prior editions of this text, Sutton et al. (2018) discussed foundational research regarding the reliability of life care plans. McCollom and Crane (2001) reviewed 130 life care plans from 65 evaluees in cases where two separate life care plans were written. Their goal was to see whether there were statistically significant differences between those plans over time in some key areas of a life care plan. While they acknowledged some limitations, their results gave some evidence that changes were not statistically significant following chi-square tests. In other words, in the case of each evaluee where two plans were written, they were similar enough to be reliable.

In another study (Kendall & Casuto, 2005), participants were interviewed about the type and frequency of medical care they had been receiving following development of a life care plan. Those were compared with the life care plan itself via qualitative coding, then analyzed to determine which recommendations were being followed. In this study, they found that physical therapy, occupational therapy, speech therapy, and attendant care were being followed in a way that was consistent with the life care plan, but counseling services were not. They did not discuss potential reasons for this, but it is some evidence of life care plan accuracy.

Aside from studies previously mentioned in prior editions of this text, Casuto and Gumpel (2003) also conducted a study to understand accuracy of life care plans. In that study, 22 plaintiff families who received life care plans were contacted to discuss the outcomes and potential causes for discrepancy. Some of those outcomes included: consistent emergency room visit expectations; specialist visits were lower than expected, but the volume of primary care visits were as expected, indicating that people were preferring their primary providers; families were hesitant to use recreational programs or sought out their own programs; under-utilization of psychological counseling; and, although it is not necessarily expected that the family assume primary caregiving duties, some mothers exited the workforce to care for their children. The highlight of this research is not only providing information on the accuracy (validity) of life care plans, but it also provides an understanding of what evaluees are doing differently than what is recommended in a life care plan and why. For example, parents were accessing some therapies through the public education system, which may or may not be appropriate, but it is understandable that they would rely on expertise accessed there for support. These outcomes highlight the need for evaluee and parent education on what therapies are appropriate.

Aside from these early studies, little else has been documented in recent history regarding evidence of validity and reliability of entire life care plans. There are studies that address the accuracy or necessity (validity) of certain parts of a life care plan. For example, Marini et al. (2009) asked several research questions to understand if recommendations are based on patient need and "what their patients would really benefit from, or whether their therapy opinion and recommendations are constrained by what they are aware of regarding what the insurance benefits of the patient are" (p. 116). In other words, would that recommendation in the life care plan be genuinely, validly based on patient need if it was limited to what the provider knew could be easily reimbursed? How can life care planners ensure that life care plan recommendations are based on real patient needs, not on financial incentives for providers?

In another study, Rutherford-Owen and Marini (2012) asked questions about implementations of life care plans, or whether people followed the recommendations within. By asking questions regarding demographics, disability type, and funding status, they were able to identify some patterns related to which parts of the life care plan were used, and why they were implemented. There were clear trends that patients who had life care plans implemented the recommendations within, particularly those who were awarded funding. This is evidence of validity because recommended items and services were used.

With only these two studies in mind, we can see that the validity of the life care plan may not only be an issue of whether the life care planner "got it right." There are reasons based on provider incentives and patient circumstances, like funding accessibility, which affect the assessment of life care plan validity and the recommendations therein. This points to the complexity of validity and reliability research and the need for more of it.

Johnson (2019) noted that the need for research assessing the reliability and validity of life care planning has been identified consistently over the years, but barriers exist to incentivizing people to engage in research. First, most life care planners are clinicians with limitations in both time and expertise to design, conduct, and report on research findings. There is a recognized need for academic scholarship, but most life care planners are not academics. Second, for scholars to access life care plans for research purposes, they need life care planners to volunteer access to life care plans, and contact information for following up with the life care plan evaluees. However, in many cases life care planners are not willing or able to do that. It may be unclear whether the protected health information used in a life care plan belongs to the evaluee, the attorney who paid for the life care plan to be written, or the life care planner who wrote it. Understandably, there is reservation on behalf of life care planners to share information with researchers without consent of someone, but even when the approval of ethics boards like the Institutional Review Board (IRB) require stringent data privacy and consent practices, life care planners are generally still reluctant to participate. Even if it would be clear from whom that consent would come, and likely evaluees would need to be part of that, life care planners do not always have access to evaluee contact information or it is not current enough to be useful for research purposes. Note: Some life care planners are now including in their fee agreement a statement that they will be following up with the evaluee at a future point in time, in part to gather information needed to assess reliability and validity of the life care planning process. That may be an approach that will be helpful into the future.

Third, much of the current reliability and validity research has been conducted by life care planners using only their own life care plans. While this should not be considered unvaluable, it does create limitations for generalizability of results to the practices of other life care planners. In other words, it might hint that one life care planner may be reliable in their development of life care plans, but not that the process of life care planning in general is reliable. For a study to properly generalize beyond the practice of one individual, multiple life care planners would need to participate in a research effort to assess reliability of the life care planning process. Some life care planners are reluctant to share life care plans with other fellow planners (including those who are conducting research about life care planning) because of concern that information provided in those plans could be used against them in court later. Even if life care planners have appropriate consent to share life care plans, they are not necessarily incentivized by the legal process to do so. What is important to reiterate to practitioners is that good scientific research takes measures to "blind" the researcher from knowing details that would bias the outcomes AND that steps are taken through IRB ethics boards to ensure ethical practice.

Much of this section has been focused on reliability—the dependability and consistency of the life care planning results, across individuals and over time. Specific types of reliability that should be assessed related to life care planning are consistency of the processes used and results obtained over time (similar to test-retest reliability), consistency between different life care planners in their processes and recommendations (similar to inter-rater reliability), and consistency between processes and recommendations made in similar situations by the same life care planner, regardless of who retained the life care planner (similar to intra-rater reliability). Reliability (dependability, consistency, and minimizing the effect of potential errors) is a prerequisite for validity. If a life care planner's process and outcomes are unreliable, how can they be valid? How can the life care plan accurately predict future disability-related needs and associated costs if the results are prone to error? If a practitioner's life care planning process satisfies the requirement of reliability, we can then look at validity in its various forms.

Face validity refers to whether a life care plan "looks like" the recommendations and conclusions made (content) in the life care plan and related to the evaluee's actual needs. Other ways people talk about face validity are "on the surface…" or "at first glance…." The life care plan is considered to have evidence of face validity if it helps the individual and family understand the plan and the importance of following it, as well as effectively conveying to others (such as judges and juries) the impression that the recommendations are valid. The perception of face validity can be enhanced by clearly tying recommendations to specific needs identified through the evaluation process and explaining how those recommendations are expected to address the identified needs. Technically, face validity is not "true" validity, in the sense of whether the recommendations made really ARE what the evaluee genuinely needs. However, face validity is still an important construct because it relates to whether people THINK recommendations are valid by bringing clarity and understanding. If a life care plan is developed with attention to "real" validity but neglects consideration of face validity, it may never be understood, implemented, or trusted as an accurate roadmap outlining the disability-related services that the person will need to maximize remaining function and quality of life, while minimizing complications. That lack of face validity interfering with effective plan implementation could then negatively affect actual outcomes.

Content validity goes beyond whether recommendations "look like" they are directly related to an evaluee's needs. It asks, are the recommendations and cost estimates (content) within the life care plan tables actually related to the assessed needs of the evaluee? To assess content validity in life care planning, it is important to look at the foundation for each of the recommendations made. Are recommendations logically tied to deficits identified in the medical records, to findings from the life care plan evaluation, etc.? For example, if a recommendation for visual therapy is made for a person who has experienced a brain injury, is there evidence of a visual problem presented in the medical summary or the evaluation interview summary? If that recommendation for visual therapy is not tied to evidence of a visual problem, the recommendation lacks content validity.

Criterion-related validity assesses whether a process is valid by comparing its outcomes to some external criterion. It could be either concurrent (with the criterion to which the outcome is compared occurring at the same time) or predictive (with the criterion for comparison happening later, at some time in the future). An example of concurrent criterion-related validity applied to an individual life care plan would be examining whether a healthcare provider's recommendation for a particular therapeutic regimen is consistent with published clinical practice guidelines for individuals with similar injuries. In that situation, the relevant clinical practice guideline would be the criterion against which the clinician's recommendation is compared. If there is a discrepancy, it would be wise for the life care planner to follow up with that clinician, to seek clarification. It could be that the clinician was not aware of the relevant clinical practice guideline and may recommend a different approach based on information provided in that guideline. Alternately, the clinician may be able to explain why that guideline is not applicable, because the evaluee's situation is different from that of those for whom the guideline was designed, because newer research supports a different approach, etc. Ideally, we should have researchers look at such concurrent validity beyond the individual plan level, and examine the extent to which, across life care planners and across evaluees (with similar injuries), life care plan elements are consistent with clinical practice guidelines. We should expect some exceptions due to individual circumstances in some cases, but hopefully we would find a significant percentage of life care plan recommendations relating well to recommendations published in relevant clinical practice guidelines.

Predictive validity assesses whether a process is valid by comparing its outcomes to a criterion that occurs in the future. For example, if a life care planner includes a recommendation for wheelchair replacement for a given individual every four years, and we follow up with that individual 20 years later, how many times was that wheelchair actually replaced during those 20 years? It is important to recognize that predictive validity is more complex than simply reporting whether recommendations were followed, and how much they actually ended up costing. For example, what happens if insufficient funding is available to carry out the life care planning recommendations? Given that life care plans are designed to maximize remaining function and quality of life while minimizing complications, if the recommendations are not followed, we would predict increased complications, decreased quality of life, and perhaps even decreased life expectancy (Rutherford-Owen & Marini, 2012). Looking at the predictive validity of life care plan recommendations requires not only assessing whether the recommendations were followed, but also why any of them were not followed, and what consequences occurred if they were not followed.

Both concurrent and predictive criterion-related validity can also be categorized as either convergent or divergent. Convergent evidence of validity is found when we expect two things to be related (such as degree of implementation of life care plan recommendations and later measures of quality of life), and then they actually are statistically related in a study. That would be an example of evidence of predictive, concurrent, criterion-related validity. In contrast, divergent evidence of validity is evidenced when we expect two things to NOT be related, and they are in fact NOT related. A lifecare planning example would be examining whether the total dollar amount estimates for comparable case situations are related to whether that life care planner was hired by plaintiff or defense. If life care planners are using consistent methodologies regardless of whether they were hired by plaintiff or defense sides, we would expect there to NOT be a difference in the total dollar estimates for similar cases when their plans were developed for plaintiff, versus for defense sides; there should be no relationship between hiring party and dollar estimates for similar cases. If we found that there was NOT such a relationship (as expected), that would be evidence of concurrent, divergent criterion-related validity. However, if we found that a life care planner's cases (for comparable cases in otherwise similar circumstances) DID differ based on whether that planner was hired by defense or plaintiff sides, we would find that there WAS a relationship between type of hiring party and costs detailed in the life care plan, and we would fail to find evidence of concurrent, divergent criterion-related validity.

Discriminant validity is evidenced when a process accurately differentiates between those who are and those who are not in a particular group. For example, if we hypothesize that people with spinal cord injuries who are able to implement fully funded and appropriately developed life care plans will live longer than those with similar injuries who do not have such services, will the implementation of such plans differentiate between survivors and those who are deceased 20 years later?

Fundamental Principles for Research in Life Care Planning
Scientific Method and Process

As mentioned previously, there are two ways in which we can understand research. There is the kind that practitioners use in practice to find information to include in the life care plan; then there is research of the primary, secondary, and tertiary kind that addresses the practice and advances the knowledge of the entirety of the field. While some of those will certainly involve sample groups, statistical error rates, statistical significance based on p values (the probability of finding such a "significant" result by chance alone when there is not actually a difference or relationship in reality), and other quantitative data analysis tools, there is a large part of the practice that involves less formal data collection and analysis processes. That does not mean that it is not scientific in nature. The following steps of the scientific process can guide life care planning practice processes.

According to the Global Learning and Observations to Benefit the Environment (GLOBE) (2022) program website (www.globe.gov/do-globe/research-resources/student-resources/be-a-scientist/steps-in-the-scientific-process) that is sponsored by the National Aeronautics and Space Administration and supported by the National Science Foundation and the United States Government, there are nine steps to the scientific process. Below, these are applied in the development of the life care plan.

Step 1: Observe Nature

Early in the life care plan process is interviewing evaluees or reading background medical records to establish an understanding of what the disabling conditions might be. The life care planner must understand the etiology of the condition, the prognosis and developmental history, and the recommendations of providers who have cared for the evaluee. This process is merely observing the condition of the evaluee and the nature of their treatment.

Step 2: Pose Questions

After the life care planner acquires an understanding of the condition and development of the evaluee's care to the current point in time, they must ask many questions. This is not an exhaustive list, but some questions include:

- What recommendations for services or products are founded on documented diagnoses?
- What are the expected costs associated with recommendations for future services or products?
- Do the elements of a life care plan have foundation in medical record and research literature?
- Are recommendations made from qualified providers and within their respective scopes of practice?
- Are the costs associated with recommendations relevant to the evaluee's geographical area?
- Are the numbers being used usual, customary, and reasonable (UCR) according to standard practice?

Step 3: Develop Hypotheses

Since a hypothesis is an "educated guess" about something that can be tested using systematic processes, life care planners rely on their training and experience, combined with the strongest level of evidence available, to determine appropriate recommendations and costs in a life care plan. Because medical treatment is reliant on collaborative treatment teams of multiple trained individuals, the life care planner is also reliant on the sufficient training of fellow providers to develop some of the hypotheses that lead to life care planning recommendations. Just as a researcher might re-evaluate the hypothesis questions of other researchers, there are times when life care planners might question the recommendations of providers, and then seek additional evidence to either confirm or disconfirm their hypotheses.

Step 4: Plan Investigation

To test the hypotheses about individual items that could be included in a life care plan, the life care planner may examine the medical records to find foundation for an item. As a very simplistic example, if a provider recommends a wheelchair for a patient, the life care planner may investigate medical records to find a written diagnosis that justifies that expense. This is the basis for some of the foundation for a life care plan. In another example, the life care planner might report a particular recommended medical procedure, but not know how much it costs. That planner may investigate the cost by calling the recommended provider and other area providers, research the costs using a database of procedure costs applied to the geographic area, etc. If they determine that the cost seems low or high compared to what they know from their education, training, and experience, they may test that hypothesis by calling more providers, checking larger databases for healthcare costs, or discussing with other professionals. In any case, they are investigating individual elements and testing them for appropriateness and accuracy.

Step 5: Assemble Data

As individual elements are investigated and tested for appropriateness, they begin to be collected in a cohesive format to be used for later presentation. Sometimes this involves special software programs, spreadsheets, word processing document templates, or whatever individual conventions each life care planner uses to systematically record information.

Step 6: Analyze Data

Data analysis is an ongoing part of life care plan development. When a life care planner establishes a hypothesis about a recommendation or cost, they then investigate through their resources to test the hypothesis. Data are gathered from different relevant sources (medical records, interview with and observations of the evaluee, discussions with treating providers, review of relevant published literature about the needs of individuals with such disabilities, review of relevant clinical practice guidelines), compared, and integrated, with a view toward confirming or disconfirming hypotheses generated. Logical, clear assembly of the data happens during this process; once conclusions are reached with appropriate foundation, data are assembled and documented.

Additional analysis may also occur after conclusions are documented (step 7). Once the life care plan is documented and ready for presentation, it is either presented to the evaluee/evaluee's family to discuss the elements of the plan, or it is exposed to deposition or examination through the litigation process. This process is an analysis done by another party to further assess the data for appropriate foundation, appropriateness of costs, etc. Similar to the way that a researcher analyzes their own data and presents data and findings to others for continued analysis, this happens with a life care plan through the litigation process as well.

Step 7: Document Conclusions

As foreshadowed in the previous step, documentation is the final formatting of the life care plan for consistency. Since many life care planners are writing into the life care plan as they research individual elements, this could be seen as a final review and formalizing of the life care plan. Attention should be paid not only to consistency, but also to sufficient foundation for each recommendation, and for the costs associated with those recommendations.

Step 8: Present Findings

Presenting findings could be seen in two ways. As life care plans are often paid for by attorneys who represent someone who has a vested interest in a legal case, presentation might be offered to the attorney or their client. One could also see the presentation of findings as offering the information to judges or juries to determine the appropriateness of the plan. Life care planners should recognize that there may be many different audiences for a life care plan. They may or may not be used in litigation but should always be written in a manner that is understandable by the people who need to implement those plans.

Step 9: Pose New Questions

This final step depends in part on the specifics of a situation. Sometimes attorneys or evaluees have new information about a case and offer it to the life care planner, which requires new hypotheses to be developed, and then further analysis to be undertaken. Other times, when challenges arise through the litigation process, they might pose new questions to the life care planner to re-evaluate their plan. It is important to mention here that this does not refer only to rectifying errors in an individual's life care plan. The legal process also challenges life care planners to pose new questions about the process of life care planning as a whole. When legal interpretation of law evolves, life care plans must pose new questions. For example, when a precedent is set in an individual state regarding collateral sources of costs and whether they should be considered by the life care planner or not, the life care planner may need to adjust their plans. This does not invalidate the plan, but means that it needs revision to be useful, given the specific legal environment in which they are working.

Rules of Evidence

It is worth making a specific mention of how the above research process relates to federal rules of evidence. There are several cases that famously contribute to the evidentiary standard of expert witness testimony (*Daubert v. Merrell Dow Pharmaceuticals, Inc.*, 1993; *Frye v. United States*, 1923; *General Electric Co. v. Joiner*, 1997; *Kumho Tire Co. v. Carmichael*, 1999). Other resources outline these in great detail (Field, 2011; Field & Choppa, 2005; Robinson, 2013; Stein, 2006; Weed & Field, 1994), but suffice to say that the issue addressed in these cases is whether the evidence is trustworthy enough to be considered fact and, thus, admissible in court. In other words, is the expert presenting information that is vetted by an established method, i.e., the scientific method and established standards accepted by life care planners? The process described above affirms this and the following section will discuss this in more detail. For further reading on this topic, see chapter Forensic Issues in Life Care Planning in this text.

Practical Statistics for the Life Care Planner

The ability to understand and interpret research is an important skill in rehabilitation. More complete resources exist that outline research interpretation skills with research design, but for the practicing life care planner, there are some important concepts that become crucial to decision-making in life care plan development. For example, this section will discuss the concept of usual, customary, and reasonable (UCR) medical costs and the percentile forms in which they are typically presented. For more information on operational definitions of UCR, see the following resources, (Alison et al., 2022; Busch, 2017; Maniha, 2020). Then we will discuss, the term "error rate" which is a statistical tool used in quantitative analysis and is used as an admissibility test according to *Daubert* (*Daubert v. Merrell Dow Pharmaceuticals, Inc.*, 1993). We will discuss what error rates are and how they relate to life care planning. Finally, validity and reliability are an important part of any scientific pursuit, so we will discuss those concepts as they relate to life care planning.

Usual, Customary, and Reasonable (UCR) and Percentile Costs

Before examining exactly what a percentile is, applied to costs, it may be helpful to gain an understanding of what it means to be average, in statistical terms. In simple form, when a large amount of data referring to the varying charge amounts of multiple providers are collected, one of the first things done is to find the mean, or arithmetic average of those costs. If these quantitative data are "normal" they can be represented on a curve where the greatest proportion of the observations is at or around the center of the distribution (the "peak" of the normal curve), with fewer and fewer observations moving out toward the extremes at the higher and lower ends. In a normal distribution, the pattern of decreasing numbers of observations as you move farther in either direction from the middle point is symmetrical; there is not a "bump" of more observations at one end or another, or an asymmetrical skew leaning more toward one extreme or another. The mean is the average of all of the prices available for a given medical service, if we add up all the costs and divide that sum by the number of observations.

We can also look at the median, which is the center value if we line up all of the costs from lowest to highest, meaning half of all providers are charging more and about half of all providers are charging less than that median value. A normal distribution will have the same value for the mean and the median, although a skewed distribution (one that "leans" in one direction or another or has a "bump" of extra observations at one end) will have slightly different values for the mean and median. An example of a skewed distribution, for which the mean is not the best representation of "average" and the median makes more sense, is level of income in the United States. If you include billionaires in the data you are collecting to estimate "average" income level, the mean will seriously overestimate the amount of salary that an average person in the United States earns. For that reason, people often report income averages using median values, instead of mean values. A valuable case for why life care planners should use the median value can be found in Allison et al. (2022).

A third measure to report "averageness" is the mode, which it the most common value in a distribution, or in the case of costs, the most frequently reported cost. In a normal distribution, the mean, median, and mode will all be the same value, right at the midpoint of the distribution. In that normal, symmetrical distribution, we can also know that half (50%) of the observations will be below the mean/median/mode center point, and half (50%) will be above it. That middle value is at the 50th percentile rank level.

A percentile rank level (often just called a "percentile") is the level at which that percentage of the observations fall below it. For example, the 50th percentile is the level where half of the observations (or costs, in this case) fall below it. The 75th percentile is the value below which 75% of the observations lie (75% of the costs are lower than this level). If a life care plan lists the cost of a procedure at $100 dollars because that cost is at the 75th percentile, that means the evaluee should be able to afford 75% of the providers used in the sample. Various forensic experts have proposed which percentile should be used, but as of this writing no consensus has been established (Allison et al., 2022; Research and Planning Consultants, 2021).

One example of how percentiles are used in practice is by looking at one provider of cost benchmarks for medical services, such as FAIRHealth (2022). If a life care planner is relying on cost evidence, it is incumbent on them to know how the costs were derived, using a specific methodology. In the case of FAIRHealth, they collect cost information from 493 geographical areas via zip code. Extremely low or high outliers are removed to avoid distortions of data that could inappropriately skew means, then costs are arrayed from lowest to highest to determine percentiles. "A percentile is a position in a distribution of values below which a specified percentage of values fall" (FAIRHealth, 2022, para 4). With an understanding of the methodology published by FAIRHealth, a life care planner can choose what percentile is appropriate (with an understanding that there must be a defensible rationale for that choice) and find the corresponding value. In situations where too little information is available to accurately represent the range of costs and associated percentiles, FAIRHealth reports "normalizing" data to consider relative values of other codes. It would be like trying to purchase a car from a friend and not knowing if he is giving you a good deal. You would go online to look at other cars of similar year and condition, then compare the average price of those cars to the one your friend is offering. You would also consider the median value in case there are any cars that are skewing the costs based on outrageously high or low prices. Once you know where your friend's charge falls on the range relative to other cars, then you can understand if their price is UCR based on the percentile level you consider is fair. It is important to mention that whatever costing resources a life care planner uses, they should understand and be able to describe the methods used to derive those costs. This does not mean the methods have to be memorized, but they should be understood and available to report as needed.

This begs the question regarding which percentile to use when including costs in a life care plan. Would the fair thing be to just add up all of the costs in an area and use the average? This is where the conversation gets a bit more complicated and a little history is warranted. First, when we are talking about the percentile of a cost, we are essentially saying that whatever a life care planner determines a specific product or service will cost, we are talking about whether that number is similar enough to what others charge, and not outrageously high or low. Second, what is important to know is that the percentile that is most commonly considered UCR by many is the 75th or 80th percentile (Johnson & Woodard, 2022). This is where a little history comes in.

The question about why to use 75th or 80th percentile has to do with two stakeholders that have much to lose or gain by a change in the number: providers (doctors or other healthcare providers) and insurers. It seems like the goal from a fee-for-service perspective has always been to establish some conformity of fees. If everyone simply charged the same for a particular service, then insurers could reimburse at that rate. However, because services can be different in different places, because no two patients are the same, and because there is no regulation regarding what providers can charge, providers are continually challenging the idea that a reimbursement rate should be uniform. In struggling to figure out what to do about this, what we now know as UCR was being worked out as early as 1945 (Teall, 1969). Some insurers were experimenting with different pricing structures based on average fees (Teall, 1969) and by 1979 "most UCR policies define the prevailing fee as the 90th percentile fee in the area" (Korcok, 1979, p. 380). As time went on and decades of negotiation between providers and insurers were influenced by market trends, the industry standard landed somewhere between the 70th and 80th percentile (Riner, 2016). As you can see by the example above, insurance companies would advocate to reimburse at a lower percentile because that would allow them to pay less. They argue that it keeps premiums down, higher percentile numbers incentivize predatory providers from charging exorbitant fees, outlier fees distort UCR charge databases, and it incentivizes patients to use in-network providers (Riner, 2016). On the other hand, many physicians want to be reimbursed at a higher percentile for various reasons (i.e., cost of living is different, cost of education is different, talent differences, standard of care might be higher, some patients just require more time, etc.).

With an understanding of percentiles and why the 75th or 80th percentile is commonly chosen, life care planners can prepare life care plans with an understanding that those numbers are often considered within the UCR definition that has evolved as industry standard. In addition to having a basic understanding about what constitutes statistical "averageness" (measures of central tendency—mean, median, and mode), life care planners should also understand basic principles of statistical variability and relationship, to be informed consumers of relevant research literature.

Measures of variability statistically describe how "different" observations tend to be from each other, in a standardized way. One way of looking at how different an observation is from average would be to look at how far away that observation is from the mean. What is the difference between that observation and the average? Subtracting the average value (mean) from that observation will give us the "deviation from the mean" for that observation. If the observation is above average, the deviation from the mean will be a positive value; if it is below average, the deviation from the mean will be a negative value. An observation right at the average, mean level will have a value of zero for its deviation from the mean. The greater a deviation from the mean is above zero, the more that observation is above average. Similarly, the farther a deviation from the mean is below zero, the more that observation is below average.

What if we wanted to describe the average amount of variation in a distribution? In other words, on average, how far do observations tend to deviate from the mean? Why not just add up all of the deviations from the mean for all of the observations, and divide by the number of those observations? That should give us the average deviation from the mean, right? The problem is that around half of the deviations from the mean will be positive, and half will be negative, so adding them all up will always give us exactly zero. So, statisticians found a way to eliminate those negative values, in a manner that can be mathematically reversed—squaring each deviation from the mean. A positive number squared is positive, and a negative number squared is also positive. So, we can take the average of the squared deviations from the mean for all of the observations in a group. That average of squared deviations from the mean is the variance—a measure of variability. However, it is a little difficult to interpret something in terms of a squared value. For example, what is a squared dollar? We understand what a dollar is, but it is difficult to think of what something means in dollars squared. So, statisticians have a solution—take the square root of the variance, to get rid of the problem of interpreting values as squares. The square root of the average squared deviation from the mean is called the standard deviation (often abbreviated as s.d. or SD in research articles). The standard deviation is basically a standardized measure of the average amount that observations vary around the mean for a group. Thinking back to the normal curve distribution we described when looking at the concept of averageness, for a normally distributed population of observations, we would find about 68% of the observations clustered around the mean, within the range of plus or minus one standard deviation. For example, if an IQ test has a mean of 100 and a standard deviation of 15, around 68% of the IQ scores would tend to fall within the range of 85–115. Around 95% of the IQ scores will fall within two standard deviations from the mean, in the range of 70–130. If we extend the range out to three standard deviations below or above the mean, in the range of 55–145, more than 99% of the observations will fall within that range. Interpreting these differences into functional implications, someone with an IQ more than two standard deviations below the mean (below 70) would meet criteria for diagnosis with intellectual disability (if they also have a corresponding documented measure of adaptive functioning). Similarly, someone with an IQ above 130 is as far above average in intelligence score as somebody with an intellectual disability has a below average intelligence score.

Another measure of variability in a group of observations is the range—the distance between the lowest and the highest observation. A variation on this is the interquartile range, in which the range is divided up into four chunks, and we look at the distance between the observation at the lower end of the second chunk and the upper end of the third chunk.

Occasionally, we need to compare the results of tests or other measurements that are not using the same scale. For example, if someone has an IQ score of 85 on a test with a mean of 100 and standard deviation of 15, but a score 60 on a reading test with a mean of 50 and a standard deviation of 5, how does the IQ of 85 compare to the reading score of 60? A standardized way of comparing scores on measurements with different scales (different means and standard deviations) is to convert them into standardized scores. An example is a Z-score, which is obtained by subtracting the mean from that person's score, and then dividing that difference by the standard deviation. Basically, it is how far away that person is from average, compared to the average amount that people tend to vary. In our example, the Z-score for intelligence would be (85–100)/15, yielding a Z-score of –1.0. The Z-score for reading would be (60–50)/5 = +2.0. So, that person measured one standard deviation below the mean in intelligence, but two standard deviations above the mean in reading. That person is a MUCH better reader than we might have predicted from their intelligence test score.

In addition to Z-scores, other standardized score systems can be used to compare the results of tests or rating using different scales. For example, T-scores are similar to Z-scores, but they have a mean of 50 and a standard deviation of 10 (in part to get around having to explain what a negative Z-score means). Someone with an IQ of 70 on a test with a mean of 100 and standard deviation of 15 would have a T-score of 30. Looking at the higher end of T-scores, someone with a T-score above 80 on a measure of depression should immediately get follow-up assessment of suicide risk, because that score is higher than three standard deviations above the mean, which is higher than the scores of more than 99% of the population. A commonly used standardized score is conversion to percentile ranks, which are more easily understood by the general population than are other types of scores. As discussed earlier in this chapter, the percentile rank is the level where the person (or cost, etc.) is above that percentage of the population.

In statistics, it is important to look not only at measures of averageness (central tendency) and variability, but also measures of relationship. How can we assess whether as one thing goes up, something related to it goes up? Conversely, what if when one thing goes up, the other thing goes down? One way of looking at this is to examine two variables (such as age and income, for example) in the context of each observation's relationship to the mean for that variable and compare them. If one person is above average in age, is that person also above average in income? If another is below average in age, is that person's income also below average? If we multiply the deviation from the mean (that person's score the mean score) for each person's age by the deviation from the mean for that person's income, we could start looking at how age and income go together. If a person is very high above average in age and very high above average in income, but a person who is very far below average in age is very far below average in income, that would suggest a relationship between age and income, right? Conversely, if a person above average in age has a below average income, that would suggest less of a relationship between age and income. A way to pull together all of these observations to describe how the variables tend to go together (co-vary) is the covariance. Covariance is calculated by multiplying the deviation from the mean for one variable by the deviation from the mean for the other variable (for each person), adding those products of deviations from the mean for the two variables, and dividing by the number of people. Basically, the covariance is the average of how the two variables tend to go in the same direction together.

Much like Z-scores and other standardized scores can help us to better compare the results of tests or measurements with different means and standard deviations, covariances can be standardized to something that can be more universally interpreted—correlations. As a Z-score divides the distance between the mean by the standard deviation to standardize a score, the covariance can be standardized by dividing it by the standard deviations of the two variables. Specifically, to convert a covariance to a correlation, you divide it by the product of the standard deviations for the two covarying variables. Keep in mind that the first step in getting the covariance was to multiply the deviation from the mean for one variable by the deviation from the mean for the other variable, so it makes sense that we would need to multiply the two standard deviations together to get a standardized measure. The resulting standardized measure of relationship is the correlation, which has values ranging from −1 to +1, with zero in the center. A correlation value of −1 is a perfect negative correlation; as one variable goes up, the other goes down (such as number of days lived and number of days left to live in the rest of one's life). A correlation value of +1 is a perfect positive correlation; as one variable goes up, the other goes up (such as a person's height in feet and in centimeters). A correlation of zero means that there is no measured relationship between the variables. The closer the correlation is to zero, the weaker it is. The farther it is from zero, the stronger it is.

Correlations can be conceptualized as the group's average product of Z-scores for the two variables. Keep in mind that there are different formulas for calculating the standard deviations, correlations, etc. for an entire population, versus calculating them on data from just a sample to estimate population values. The explanations here consider the sets of observations available to constitute the entire population of interest; if we were using those figures to estimate values for a greater population than our sample, we would include an additional degree of freedom (n-1, instead of just n) in the denominator of our calculations.

Correlations can be used to assess the strength of statistical relationships that we would like to see, such as high inter-rater reliability between life care plan recommendation costs developed by different planners. They can also assess relationships that we hope not to see, such as a relationship between type of referral source and resulting costs outlined in life care plans. Correlations can also be used to identify patterns of variables that tend to vary together, in techniques such as factor analysis, which have been used in some studies related to identifying roles and functions of life care planners.

Most statistical analyses are based on combinations of these basic building blocks: measures of central tendency (averageness), measures of variability, and measures of relationship. For example, t-tests compare two means and divide that difference by the standard deviation. Regression analyses assess the relative contributions of different variables in predicting an outcome/criterion variable through analysis of the strengths of the correlations between those predictors and the criterion. Complex techniques such as MANCOVA (multivariate analysis of covariance) look at differences between multiple independent and dependent variables, as well as their interactions, after first pulling out the effect of a control variable which could otherwise get in the way of assessing the effects of the variables of interest; that technique relies on measures of central tendency, variability, and relationship in a complex manner.

Error Rates

Error should be important to the expert witness because if an expert's testimony includes too many (or too significant) errors, that expert could be disqualified from testifying. However, making errors in a life care plan is not the same as a statistical error rate, as it is outlined in the *Daubert* standards (*Daubert v. Merrell Dow Pharmaceuticals, Inc.*, 1993). When *Daubert* was decided in 1993, life care planners initially claimed that life care planning was not a "bench science" and *Daubert* did not apply. However, subsequent decisions (including *Kumho Tire co. v. Carmichael*, 1999) required all expert witnesses to address the scientific evidentiary standards more seriously, which includes error rates of scientific evidence. So, what are error rates, and what do they have to do with life care planning expert testimony?

The short explanation is that error rates refer to statistical testing, specifically Type I and Type II errors in analysis. There may be thousands of explanations on the internet about what statistical error is, but this chapter is focused on the language applicable to life care planning. Type I error refers to false positives, or some element looking like it is correct when it is not. Type II error refers to false negatives, or some element that is said to be false when it is not. For example, a positive pregnancy test result from the urine of a biological male would be a false positive. A negative pregnancy test from the urine of a biological female who is in her third trimester of pregnancy would be a false negative. It is relatively easy to determine the error rate of a pregnancy test, by administering the test to many people and then comparing the test results with objective outside evidence of whether or not each person taking the test is actually pregnant. The calculated error rate would be inclusive of both Type I and Type II errors. However, in the practice of life care planning, to calculate similar error rates for each and every item within a life care plan, we would need (for each item): 1) a sufficiently large sample size of nearly identical evaluees in nearly identical situations; 2) a way of gathering data after the plan is actually implemented; and 3) consistent criteria for determining whether the data collected support the validity of the recommendations, or are evidence of error. If we had sufficient follow-up data and found that a particular recommendation was commonly made but not necessary in reality, that would be evidence of Type I error. In contrast, if follow-up data showed that a particular recommendation was NOT commonly made, but was necessary in reality, that would be evidence of Type II error. Unfortunately, due to logistical and financial barriers, these kinds of follow-up data are not yet commonly collected, although they would be of great value.

Because life care plans involve predictions of future needs, the "error rate" for a single life care plan cannot be known at the time of plan development. No statistical analyses can be conducted on the accuracy of projections within a single life care plan without knowing what the future holds when that plan is implemented. However, we do know that if life care planners use inconsistent and unsupported methodologies, they decrease the reliability and validity of their life care plans, increasing the likely error rate. Life care planners should be able to demonstrate that their methods for gathering data, making recommendations, and providing cost estimates are evidence-based, reliable, and appropriately applied. Minimizing the potential error rate depends on each life care planner consistently and appropriately following the same process for evaluees in the same situations, regardless of whether the party hiring the planner is from a plaintiff, defense, or other perspective.

A significant danger when developing a life care plan is presenting costs for services that are not needed, or significantly overestimating the costs of needed services; those errors could be false positives. Another danger is not including the costs for services that are needed, or significantly underestimating the costs of needed services; those errors could be false negatives. False positives inaccurately inflate the total costs of goods and services in a life care plan; false negatives inaccurately underestimate the total costs of those goods and services.

Since there are no mathematical tests that determine the "correctness" of a cost in a life care plan, what life care planners do is establish standard systematic methods to arrive at an individual cost. That way, two people given the same information and using the same methods should arrive at similar end costs. This is why standardization of the methodology is so important to the life care planner. So, when someone asks about error rates to determine the admissibility of life care plans or individual items, what the life care planner should be prepared to do is talk about the process by which they arrived at the item (method) and the quality of the resources they used (foundation). The more inconsistent that the methods are to standard practices and the less valid and reliable the resources, the more error there will likely be in the life care plan.

Practitioners also have a vested interest in supporting the conduct of research examining the reliability and validity of life care planning processes, in general. Although we can address questions about reliability and error rate through a focus on the consistency and solid foundation for our own methodology, it would be helpful to point to studies examining aspects like inter-rater reliability (degree of agreement in recommendations about costs between different life care planners using the same methodology with the same evaluees) to address error rate of life care planning methodology in general. Keep in mind that error rate is related to unreliability. The more reliable, dependable, and consistent a process is shown to be, the lower the error rate is likely to be for that process.

Probability vs. Possibility

A final statistical concept that comes up in life care planning is the concept of probability. Somewhere between impossible and absolutely certain is every forensic opinion about a medical recommendation, meaning we all want to know how likely something is going to happen. There are many ways in which we can linguistically describe the ways we try to understand these concepts: absolute diagnostic certainty, reasonable degree of medical certainty, and possibility. The concept that seems to come up more often is probability, perhaps because it can be quantified. When we speak of probability, we might use a number like 5% or 95% probability. To use an example, if one throws a dart at a dartboard 100 times and hit the bull's eye five times, we could say that there is a 5% chance (probability) that one would get a bull's eye. If one throws a dart 200 times and hits the middle ten times, the probability is still 5%. In other words, with any event, including prognostic outcomes of medical procedures, the probability of success is somewhere between 0 and 100 percent.

There are a few terms related to these probabilities that could use some clarification. When we say something is "possible" in life care planning, what we are saying is there a probability greater than zero. There might be a one in one trillion chance that it will happen, but it is still possible. When we say that there is a reasonable degree of medical *probability*, that is typically referred to as "having a probability greater, but not significantly higher, than 50%" (Guileyardo, 2015, p. 248). That is slightly different than when we say there is reasonable degree of medical *certainty*, which is "generally considered as *significantly exceeding* 50% likelihood" (Guileyardo, 2015, p. 248).

Generally, in life care planning, we use the standard of "more likely than not" (reasonable degree of medical or rehabilitative probability) for including an item in the recommendations of a life care plan. Items that are considered "possible" but not "probable" are included in a list of potential complications (for educational purposes), but costs for those items are not included in the life care plan totals.

As this is a section on statistics, we would be remiss if we did not mention p values. P values refer to statistical probabilities, namely that when finding statistical significance of a hypothesis, the p value of .05 refers to the probability of Type I error. In plain terms, it is the probability of getting significant results by chance alone, when there really is not an actual difference or relationship going on. This is an incredibly important concept to the quantitative researcher comparing differences between or relationships among groups of data. However, because the life care planner is working with a single evaluee (n = 1), p values do not apply because there is no statistical analysis that can be done at the time of plan development.

Future Directions in Research

Now that the foundations of research in life care planning have been identified, and concepts discussed to promote understanding of research in life care planning, we can comment on the future directions. It should be clear that research is important for the progression of the practice of life care planning. Not only is it a daily practice to consume research in life care plan development, but also the development of research is an inherent value of life care planners, as evidenced by their continued discussion of the need for it. However, there is much work to be done.

There is still need for validity and reliability research. The Foundation for Life Care Planning Research was developed in 2002 (Marcinko, 2019) to encourage and incentivize research and development of the field. Its mission continues today and has recently been renamed (as the Foundation for Life Care Planning and Rehabilitation Research) and revitalized to encourage more opportunities for people to participate. Despite the barriers discussed above regarding difficulty in conducting reliability and validity research in the field, it is primary-type research that is the most challenging, but also the most needed. To know whether life care plans achieve the desired outcome, to accurately predict the long-term care needs of people with disabilities, is paramount to the practice.

References

Agency for Healthcare Research and Quality. (2021). *Clinical guidelines and recommendations.* www.ahrq.gov/prevention/guidelines/index.html

Alison, A., Corwin, A., Albers, M. J., White, H., & Taylor, R. H. (2022). An analysis of usual, customary, and reasonable charges in life care planning, *Journal of Life Care Planning, 20*(2), 5–20.

Barros-Bailey, M. (2018). An evidence source model for clinical and forensic practice. *Rehabilitation Professional, 26*(3).

Barros-Bailey., Brown, S., Maxwell, A., Malloy, S., Latham, S., Thompson, A., & Donohoe, E. (2022). Attendant care survey methodology (ACSM): Introducing a costing model. *Journal of Life Care Planning, 20*(1), 5–26.

Bellini, J. L., & Rumrill, P. D. (2018). *Research in rehabilitation counseling: A guide to design, methodology, and utilization.* (3rd ed.). Charles C. Thomas Publisher.

Busch, R. M. S. (2017). Managing the notion of UCR in a life care plan. *Journal of Life Care Planning, 15*(3).

Casuto, D., & Gumpel, L. (2003). A retrospective study of pediatric life care plan outcomes: One life care planner's experience. *Journal of Life Care Planning, 2*(1), 13–20.

Chan, F., Keegan, J., Muller, V., Kaya, C., Flowers, S., & Iwanaga, K. (2016). Evidence-based practice and research in rehabilitation counseling. In I. Marini & M. A. Stebnicki (Eds.), *The professional counselor's desk reference* (pp. 605–610). Springer Publishing Company.

Cook, D. J., Mulrow, C. D., & Haynes, R. B. (1997). Systematic reviews: Synthesis of best evidence for clinical decisions. *Annals of Internal Medicine, 126*(5), 376–380. https://doi.org/10.7326/0003-4819-126-5-199703010-00006

Countiss, R. N., & Deutsch, P. M. (2002). The life care planner, the judge, and Mr. Daubert. *Journal of Life Care Planning, 1*, 35–43.

Daubert v. Merrell Dow Pharmaceuticals, Inc., 509 U.S. 579, 113 S. Ct. 2786, 125 L. Ed. 2d 469 (1993).

Delbecq, A. L., Van de Ven, A. H., & Gustafson, D. H. (1975). *Group techniques for program planning: A guide to nominal and Delphi processes*. Scott Foresman and Company.

DePalma, J. A. (2002). Proposing an evidence-based policy process. *Nursing Administration Quarterly, 26*(4), 55–61.

Deutsch, P. M., & Allison, L., (2004). Proceedings of the Life Care Planning Summit 2004 Atlanta, GA, April 24–25, 2004. *Journal of Life Care Planning, 3*(3), 193–202.

FAIRHealth. (2022). *FH charge benchmarks methodology*. www.fairhealth.org/methodologies

Field, T. F. (2011). *Federal Rule 702: In light of the Daubert, Kumho and Joiner rulings on the admissibility of expert testimony*. Elliott & Fitzpatrick, Inc.

Field, T. F., & Choppa, A. J. (2005). *Admissible testimony: A content analysis of selected cases involving vocational experts with a revised clinical model for developing opinion*. Elliott & Fitzpatrick, Inc.

Frye v. United States, 293 F. 1013 (D.C. Cir. 1923)

General Electric Co. v. Joiner, 522 U.S. 136, 118 S. Ct. 512, 139 L. Ed. 2d 508 (1997).

Global Learning and Observations to Benefit the Environment (GLOBE). (2022). www.globe.gov/do-globe/research-resources/student-resources/be-a-scientist/steps-in-the-scientific-process

Guileyardo J. M. (2015). Probability and uncertainty in clinical and forensic medicine. *Proceedings (Baylor University. Medical Center), 28*(2), 247–249.

Haidich, A. B. (2010). Meta-analysis in medical research. *Hippokratia, 14*(Suppl 1), 29–37.

International Academy of Life Care Planners. (2022). *Standards of practice for life care planners* (4th ed). https://rehabpro.org/general/custom.asp?page=ialcp-standards-of-practice

International Association of Rehabilitation Professionals (IARP). (2019). *Journal of Life Care Planning (17)*1, 1–74.

Johnson, C. B., & Woodard, L. (2022). Life care planning cost techniques: History, methodology, and literature review. *Journal of Life Care Planning, 20*(2), 37–55.

Johnson, C. B. (2019). A historical review of life care planning summits since 2000. *Journal of Life Care Planning, 17*(3), 37–51.

Kendall, S. L., & Casuto, D. (2005). A quantitative reappraisal of a qualitative survey to assess reliability & validity of the life care planning process. *Journal of Life Care Planning, 4*(2–3), 75–84.

Korcok, M. I. L. A. N. (1979). US physicians' earnings. Part II: Usual, customary and reasonable. *Canadian Medical Association Journal, 120*(3), 378–384.

Kumho Tire Co. v. Carmichael, 526 U.S. 137, 119 S. Ct. 1167, 143 L. Ed. 2d 238 (1999).

Maniha, A. (2020). Components of a cost/charge scenario as utilized in the life care plan. *Journal of Life Care Planning, 18*(4), 13–35.

Marcinko, D. A. (2019). International Academy of Life Care Planners: Yesterday and today. *Journal of Life Care Planning, 17*(3), 31–35.

Marini, I.. Luckett, K., Miller, E., & Blanco, E.L. (2009). A survey of physical therapists: Long term therapy needs for persons with severe disabilities. *Journal of Life Care Planning, 8*(3), 107–123.

Mauk, K. L. (2019). Revisiting the concept of transdisciplinary life care planning. *Journal of Life Care Planning, 17*(1), 5–6

May III, V. R., & Moradi Rekabdarkolaee, H. (2020). The International Commission on Health Care Certification Life Care Planner Role and Function Investigation. *Journal of Life Care Planning, 18*(2). 3–34.

McCollom, P., & Crane, R. (2001). Life care plans: Accuracy over time. *The Case Manager, 12*, 85–87.

Mertes, A. (2018). Content analysis of the research priorities in the Journal of Life Care Planning from 2004–2017. *Journal of Life Care Planning, 16*(2), 3–9.

Pomeranz, J. L., Yu, N. S., & Reid, C. (2010). Role and function study of life care planners. *Journal of Life Care Planning*, *9*(3), 57–118.

Preston, K., & Reid, C. (2015). Revision process for the *Standards of Practice* for Life Care Planners. *Journal of Life Care Planning*, *13*(3), 21–30.

Research and Planning Consultants. (2021). Determining usual, customary, and reasonable charges for healthcare services [Accessed: 2022-03-01]. www.rpcconsulting.com

Riner, R. M. (2016). Are usual and customary charges reasonable? *Western Journal of Emergency Medicine*, *17*(6), 684–685.

Robinson, R. (Ed.). (2013). *Foundations of forensic vocational rehabilitation*. Springer Publishing Company.

Rutherford-Owen, T., & Marini, I. (2012). Life care plan implementation among adults with spinal cord injuries. *Journal of Life Care Planning*, *10*(4).

Sackett, D. L., Straus, S. E., Richardson, W. S., Rosenberg, W., & Haynes, R. B. (2000). Evidence-based medicine: How to practice and teach EBM (2nd ed.). Churchill Livingstone.

Stein, D. B. (2006). *Rules, civil procedure, and evidence*. Elliott & Fitzpatrick, Inc.

Sutton, A. M., Deutsch, P. M., Weed, R. O., & Berens, D. E. (2018). Reliability of life care plans: A comparison of original and updated Plans, In R. O. Weed & D. E. Berens (Eds.), *Life care planning and case management handbook* (4th ed., pp. 703–709). Routledge.

Teall, R. C. (1969). Usual—customary—reasonable. A California perspective. *California Medicine*, *110*(4), 337–341.

Turner, T., Taylor, D., Rubin, S., & May, R. (2000). Job functions associated with the development of life care plans. *Journal of Legal Nurse Consulting*, *11*(3), 3–7.

Umesh, G., Karippacheril, J. G., & Magazine, R. (2016). Critical appraisal of published literature. *Indian Journal of Anaesthesia*, *60*(9), 670–673. https://doi.org/10.4103/0019-5049.190624

Weed, R. O., & Field, T. F. (1994). *Rehabilitation consultant's handbook*. Elliot & Fitzpatrick.

Yin, R. K. (2008). Case study research: Design and methods (4th ed.). SAGE.

Yin, R. K. (2011). Applications of case study research (3rd ed.). SAGE.

Yin, R. K. (2013). Case study research: Design and methods (5th ed.). SAGE.

Yin, R. K. (2017). Case study research: Design and methods (6th ed.). SAGE.

Chapter 4

Credentialing in Life Care Planning

Sherry A. Latham

Editor's Note

Following completion of this chapter, the Certified Nurse Life Care Planner Certification Board became the Certified Licensed Life Care Planner Certification Board and now issues the Certified Licensed Life Care Planner (CLLCP) as well as the Certified Nurse Life Care Planner (CNLCP) professional designations. The reader is referred to their website at cllcpcb.org for updated information relevant to these credentials.

Credentialing in Life Care Planning

Life care planning has always been a transdisciplinary practice (International Academy of Life Care Planners [IALCP], 2019; Mauk, 2019; May & Moradi Rekabdarkolaee, 2020), meaning that it is comprised of healthcare professionals from multiple disciplines. These individuals come from various primary disciplines, specialize in the field of rehabilitation, and project future medical needs following catastrophic injuries and/or chronic health conditions. Even though life care planning has existed for 40 years, no licensure in life care planning has emerged. Rather, individuals who practice life care planning must demonstrate knowledge, skill, and experience in their primary profession and then acquire skills in life care planning.

In credentialing language, a general scope of practice is based upon educational standards that everyone in the profession is trained into. In contrast is the individual scope of practice, a subset of the general scope of practice that provides an additional expertise in a particular subject area to qualify the professional in a subspecialty. In life care planning, one's individual scope of practice of life care planning starts with the life care planner's general scope of practice and then specializes with a cross-section of knowledge, skills, and abilities across a variety of healthcare and allied health professions (rather than of a single profession). Therefore, the life care planning individual scope of practice derives from cross-sectional skills that allow the life care planner to go beyond their general scope of practice into a specialty that is shared by other professionals from other disciplines who, similarly, have the same training and experience in life care planning.

Since the term "life care plan" was published in *Damages in Tort Actions* (Deutsch & Raffa, 1982) and *A Guide to Rehabilitation* (Deutsch & Sawyer, 1985, Rev. 2002), the scope and practice of life care planning has developed and grown (Neulicht et al., 2001, 2010). Role and function studies are evidence-based studies of the knowledge, skills, and activities performed by individuals in a profession or a specialty practice, and requirements (Leahy et al., 2003; Pomeranz et al., 2010). Role and function studies serve to understand the level of practice upon which the educational standards for training programs are developed and credentialing assessment with their particular evaluative process. Life care planning role and function studies have been completed at the University of Florida and published by Pomeranz et al. (2010) in the *Journal of Life Care Planning*. The most recent updated role and function study was completed by the International Commission on Healthcare Certification (ICHCC™) and published by May and Moradi Rekabdarkolaee (2020). The heterogeneity of skills in life care planning was reflected in the most recent role and function study where life care planners reported 15 different academic degrees including diploma nurses, medical providers, and doctoral level rehabilitation providers (May & Moradi Rekabdarkolaee, 2020). In life care planning, practicing life care planners are determined to be "qualified healthcare providers" (May & Moradi Rekabdarkolee, 2020).

Qualified Healthcare Provider

Gunn (2018) identified two levels of qualification that are required for life care planning experts to present their opinions in a life care plan in court. First, the individual must be qualified generally in the area of life care planning. Second, the expert must be qualified to "substantiate each element of the plan to the degree required under the particular jurisdiction's substantive law" (p. 656). To be qualified generally in life care planning, the individual should have the requisite education and training to demonstrate specialized knowledge in life care planning that can assist the trier of fact, and their opinions should be derived from reliable principles and methods with sufficient data or facts.

To gain knowledge in life care planning, most individuals complete post-graduate training in life care planning. Such programs incorporate subjects including pediatric and adult disabilities (e.g., spinal cord injury, brachial plexus injury, chronic pain), pricing, and forensic principles. Upon completion of the training program, individuals may be granted a certificate of completion, indicating that the student of the life care planning program has successfully met those standards of completion of the educational curriculum including the methodology of life care planning. Life care planning educational programs available in the United States in 2022 include those listed below. Links to each program can be found in the resources section of this chapter.

- AAACEU
- Capital University Law School (CULS) Life Care Planning Program
- FIG Services
- Institute on Rehabilitation Education and Training (IRET)
- Kelynco
- Thomas Jefferson University

Educational programs involved in the preparation for those life care planners who practice in Canada are the following:

- AAACEU
- IRET

For more details on life care planning educational programs, the reader is referred to Chapter 1 of this text.

Licensure

Licensure, which is typically issued by governmental entities, grants an individual legal authority to practice a profession within a scope of practice. To date, there is no specialty license or *licensure* in life care planning (Berens & Weed, 2018). Rather, life care planners rely upon their primary healthcare licensure or related credentialing. In the most recent life care planning role and function study conducted, life care planners reported various professional licensures including registered nurse, occupational therapy, licensed professional counselor, physical therapy, etc. (May & Moradi Rekabdarkolaee, 2020). According to Tracy Raffles Gunn:

> In the absence of separate licensure, life care planners must be mindful of the limitations that are imposed by related and existing state licensure laws. The long-term solution is the creation of a national standards organization that becomes recognized by the states and lobbies for enactment of statutory licensing.
>
> (Gunn, 2018, p. 664)

Dependent upon the primary healthcare profession, some licenses are now available as compact licenses. Compact licensure essentially affords the holder of a professional license in one state the permission by another (compact) state(s) to practice in their location by recognizing the license as a multistate license. The result, therefore, is that a nurse licensed in one state may cross state lines and work in another state if that state has an agreement (compact) with the first state to allow this practice. This may be important to healthcare professionals who specialize in life care planning and work on a national level who provide a hands-on assessment or evaluation of the evaluee, as they would in their primary healthcare licensure. Examples of those would include, but are limited to physicians, physician assistants, chiropractors, nurses, physical therapists, occupational therapists, and speech therapists. A sample of some of the relevant compact agreements for professionals involved in life care planning include:

Audiologists and Speech Language Pathologists: Audiology and speech language pathology interstate compact (ASLP-IC) is a licensure compact that allows these practitioners to practice in multiple states without having to obtain additional state licenses with 23 participating states as of August 2022 (American Speech Language Hearing Association, 1997–2002).

Counselors: The Counseling Compact was funded and created by the American Counseling Association. It was finalized in 2020 and has been introduced in 21 states and passed in nine states (American Counseling Association, 2022).

Nurses: The Nursing Licensure Compact was developed in 2000 as a result of the national nursing shortage. The compact licensure agreement between states allows nurses to practice in other states in addition to their primary licensure. This was streamlined to the Enhanced Nurse

Licensure Compact (eNLC), which requires applicants to undergo state and federal fingerprint-based background checks. As of April 18, 2022, there were 39 states participating in the eNLC (Gaines, 2022).

Occupational Therapists: The Occupational Therapy Licensure Compact (OT compact) is a joint initiative of the American Occupational Therapy Association (AOTA) and the National Board for Certification in Occupational Therapy (NBCOT®). The OT compact is an interstate professional licensing compact for occupational therapy which will address licensure portability. This is a multi-year initiative which requires legislation to be passed in each state where the OT compact will apply. As of July 8, 2022, there are 21 states that are actively allowing compact licensure (American Occupational Therapy Association & National Board for Certification in Occupational Therapy, 2022).

Physical Therapists: The Physical Therapy Compact is an agreement between member states to improve access to physical therapy services for the public by increasing the mobility of eligible physical therapy providers to work in multiple states. As of July 8, 2022, there were 22 states that accept compact privileges (PT Compact, 2022).

Physicians: The Interstate Medical Licensure Compact offers physicians an expedited pathway to licensure for qualified medical professionals to practice in multiple states. As of July 8, 2022, according to the Interstate Medical Licensure Compact (2022), there were 39 members of the compact, including 37 states and two territories.

Historically, from the rehabilitation and case management roles, the life care planner did not conduct a physical evaluation or assessment, but as life care planning has evolved as a specialty, many of the qualified healthcare providers of a clinical nature, evaluate the evaluee as they would in a clinical setting, assessing the evaluee's physical status. For clarification purposes, they do not provide ongoing care, and this should be well documented by the life care planner to the evaluee prior to the evaluation/assessment both in the form of a disclosure statement as well as verbally and astutely documented in the life care plan. Licensure, when performing these tasks can be important.

Certification

Whereas licenses are typically state or federal government issued with the purpose of protecting the health and welfare of citizens (Matkin,1995 as cited in Berens & Weed, 2018), certifications are issued in recognition of an individual having met certain professional qualifications (Berens & Weed, 2018). Certification has been available to life care planners since 1996 (May, n.d.). Having met the standards associated with a certification in life care planning represents that the applicant has met the threshold of minimum standards of training specific to the methodology utilized in life care planning. It is an independent professional entity that provides a certification when the candidate has successfully passed the certification exam. The intent of the development of a separate entity providing the certification was for the protection of the community in which the life care planners develop life care plans as well as those they reach through service provision.

More than one certification exists in life care planning. Some life care planners choose to hold more than one life care planning certification, as they have achieved the requirements of more than one of the certifying bodies. However, there are also life care planners who practice without certification in life care planning. Even without certification, these life care planners are held to the same standards of practice (IALCP, 2022a) and expectations of conformity to the consensus and majority statements (Johnson, 2015; Johnson, 2018; Johnson & Preston, 2012; Johnson et al., 2018). In 2022, multiple certifications in life care planning exist, the details of which will be outlined below.

Certified Life Care Planner (CLCP™)

One of the credentialing organizations in life care planning is the International Commission on Healthcare Certification (ICHCC™). The ICHCC™ issues the certifications of the Certified Life Care Planner (CLCP™) and the Certified Canadian Life Care Planner (CCLCP™). As of June 6, 2022, ICHCC™ had issued CLCP™ certificate #1658, with 1240 active certifications (K. May, personal communication, June 6, 2022).

CLCP™ History

According to Bullins and Reid (2019, p. 23), "The path to developing certification in life care planning was driven by the need for accountability and protection." The International Commission on Health Care Certification (ICHCC, 2021) was the first governing body of the certification of life care planners, originally founded in 1994 as the Commission on Disability Examiner Certification (CDEC) (ICHCC, 2020). The ICHCC™ developed the certification in life care planning as a response to the rapid growth in the field and it eventually led to certification for those who practice in Canada as the CCLCP™. The ICHCC™ notes that the CLCP™ credential was "to measure the CLCP™ applicant's working knowledge of medical systems, associated disabilities, and treatment/maintenance protocol required for a catastrophically disabled individual to sustain life within an acceptable comfort level." (ICHCC, 2023, para. 4). Certification in life care planning is important, according to the ICHCC™, because of the "litigious nature of this specialized health delivery service and the need to protect the consumer of services" (Bullins & Reid, 2019, p. 5). Validity and reliability research of the CLCP™ credential was completed through Southern Illinois University and was based specifically on the roles and function of case managers and rehabilitation nurses who provided this service.

CLCP™ Eligibility

According to the ICHCC™ *Candidate Handbook*, qualifying for the CLCP™ credential is based upon the following:

> Each candidate must have a minimum of 120 hours of post-graduate or post-specialty degree training in life care planning or in areas that can be applied to the development of a life care plan or pertain to the service delivery applied to life care planning. There must be 16 hours of training specific to a basic orientation, methodology, and standards of practice in life care planning within the required 120 hours. The 120 hours may be obtained through online training/educational programs as well as onsite presentations and conferences.
>
> (ICHCC, 2020, p. 6)

Applicants should have a minimum of three years field experience within the five years preceding application for certification. Final approval of any application with ambiguity regarding experience will be left to the discretion of the administration following a thorough review of the respective applications. The opinion of the ICHCC™ is final (ICHCC, 2021, p. 10). Training hours acquired over a time frame of five years from the date of application are counted as valid for consideration. Documentation of such coursework and participation verification is required in the form of attendance verification forms and/or curriculum documentation from the training agency. Each candidate must:

> Meet the minimum academic requirements for their designated health care related profession (or hold a master's degree in a health-related field).
> Be certified, licensed, or meet the legal mandates of the candidate's respective state that allow him or her to practice service delivery within the definition of his or her designated healthcare related profession.
>
> (ICHCC, 2021, p. 11)

As of 2022, the ICHCC™ has four pre-approved educational programs to provide the educational components necessary to sit for the CLCP™ exam:

- AAACEU
- Capital University Law School (CULS) Life Care Planning Program
- Institute on Rehabilitation Education and Training, (IRET)
- Thomas Jefferson University

CLCP™ Exam

The CLCP examination consists of 100 questions in multiple-choice format, which the examinee has three hours to complete. The examination undergoes online scoring with a pass/fail status immediately provided to the examinee (ICHCC, 2020, p. 8). Examination content knowledge domains can be found on the ICHCC™ website at https://ichcc.org/images/PDFs/CLCP_Candidate_Handbook_10-21-2020_Repaired.pdf.

CLCP™ Fees

The fee associated with the certification exam is $445. If the exam candidate has not previously had one of their life care plans peer-reviewed, an additional fee of $350 should be submitted for life care plan peer review by ICHCC™ Commissioners (ICHCC, 2020, p. 19).

CLCP™ Recertification

The CLCP™ and CCLCP™ certifications are renewable every five years, requiring 80 continuing education units (CEUs), eight of which are specific to ethics. For pre-approved CEUs, a renewal fee of $350 is applicable; $400 for non-pre-approved CEUs.

CLCP™ Accreditation

The ICHCC™ is working toward accreditation by the ANSI National Accreditation Board (ANAB). This is a non-governmental organization which provides accreditation services to public- and-private-sector organizations, with more than 2,500 organizations accredited in approximately 80 countries (ANSI National Accreditation Board, 2022). According to the ANAB, certification demonstrates the conformity to the requirements of a standards, whereas accreditation is the procedure by which an authoritative body gives formal recognition that a body or person is competent to carry out specific tasks. Their accredited bodies operate within the international guidelines and have been verified by government and peer review assessments (ANSI, 2022).

Canadian Certified Life Care Planner (CCLCP™)

Beginning in October 2005, (K. May, personal communication October 19, 2021), the ICHCC™ began issuing the CCLCP™ in response to the growth of life care planning in Canada. The CCLCP™ has issued #215 certification and have approximately 176 active CCLCP™ (K. May, personal communication, June 6, 2022). The knowledge domains, fees, and renewal requirements for the CCLCP™ are the same as the CLCP™ outlined above. The Canadian Certified Life Care Planning training is available through two pre-approved programs, AAACEUs and IRET.

Certified Nurse Life Care Planner (CNLCP®)

CNLCP® History

The CNLCP Certification Board, incorporated in 2009 as a non-profit entity, collaborates with the American Association of Nurse Life Care Planners (AANLCP®) Executive Board (CNLCP Certification Board, 2022a). The CNLCP® is currently offered as a certification in life care planning. The CNLCP® has similar qualifications to the CLCP™ but the CNLCP® is available only to nurses and has an emphasis on the nursing process and nursing diagnosis. As of 2021, there were 268 CNLCP® certificate holders (CNLCP Certification Board, 2022b). The CNLCP® credential is as follows:

> Certification…is a formal recognition that validates knowledge, experience, skills and clinical judgement within a specific nursing specialty; and, as such, is reflective of a more stringent professional practice standard. It reflects achievement of proficiency beyond basic licensure.
> (CNLCP Certification Board, 2022c, para 2)

CNLCP® Eligibility

Candidates for the CNLCP® must meet the following eligibility criteria at the time of original application:

Licensure. Proof of valid, active, without restriction, Registered Nurse licensure or its equivalent in other countries, for at least the prior three years immediately preceding application.

Experience. Verification of a minimum of 2,000 hours paid or "billable" professional experience in a role (e.g., life care planning, community based case management, medical cost projections, Medicare set-aside allocations, lifetime nurse care planning, community based rehabilitation nursing, public health nursing, community based legal nurse consulting) that uses the nursing process in assessing and determining an individual's long-term/lifetime treatment needs and costs, across the continuum of care.

Education/Skills. Completion of 120 CEUs relating to life care planning or equivalent areas that can be applied to the development of a life care plan or pertain to the service delivery applicable to life care planning, within the five years immediately preceding application.

There must be a minimum of ten hours specific to a basic orientation, methodology, and standards of practice relevant to the nurse life care planning process contained within the continuing education curriculum OR verification of two years life care planning experience, or a variant thereof (e.g., lifetime nurse care planner [LNCP-C], CLCP™), that incorporates the nursing process and skill set inherent to the assessment and determination of treatment needs and their respective costs, across the continuum of care, within the past five years immediately preceding the application (CNLCP Certification Board, 2022d, para. 3).

The core topics include life care planning, spinal cord injuries, burns and amputations, acquired and traumatic brain injury, neonatal and pediatric injuries/illnesses, chronic pain, and life care plan construction (CNLCP Certification Board, 1998–2022). Of the education programs to qualify for the CNLCP®, there must be a minimum of ten hours specific to basic orientation, methodology and standards of practice relevant to the nurse life care planning process contained within the continuing education curriculum (CNLCP Certification Board, 2022d, para. 3). Life care planning training programs are offered through Capital University Law School, FIG, IRET and Kelynco (CNLCP Certification Board, 2022d). While the (CNLCP®) does not endorse any one program, FIG and Kelynco offer programs using the nursing process.

CNLCP® Exam

The CNLCP® uses on demand testing with the Professional Testing Corporation (PTC). The PTC provides testing Monday through Saturdays with the exception of nationally recognized holidays within the United States and Canada. The fees associated with the CNLCP® Exam are:

- AANLCP® Association Member, $450; Exam, Non-Member, $550
- Re-Schedule of Exam (Transferring to a new three-month window), $235
- Exam Re-Testing (Failure less than or equal to 80%), $235 (CNLCP, 2022e)

CNLCP® Recertification

Nurse life care planning recertification is recognized for five years at which time recertification is required either through CEUs or through retaking the Certification Examination for Nurse Life Care Planners (CNLCP, 2022f). Continuing education credits can be met by the following categories:

60 CEUs

Verification of the 12 academic semester credits of nursing coursework related to nurse life care planning.

Presentations: Five points of credit for a maximum of ten within the five-year renewal period for each presentation, for which national or state approved CEUs have been granted to participants.

Publications or research related to nurse life care planning should be submitted to the CNLCP Certification Board for review/approval of points of credit 90 days prior to the application for renewal deadline. Five points of credit will be awarded for one article published in a peer-reviewed journal related to nurse life care planning. Certificant must be the author or co-author. Ten points of credit will be awarded for one chapter published in a peer-reviewed book related to nurse life care planning. Certificant must be the author, co-author, editor, co-editor, or reviewer. Forty points of credit will be awarded for an institutional review board (IRB) research project, a completed dissertation, thesis, or graduate-level scholarly project related to nurse life care planning completed during the five-year certification period, for which the certificant is clearly identified as one of the primary researchers/authors.

Item Writing/Test Questions: One point of credit, for a maximum of ten points of credit, within the five-year renewal period for every five questions submitted that are supported by evidence-based nursing practice/medical references. Questions with reference supported answers should be submitted to the CNLCP Certification Board for review/approval of points of credit 90 days prior to the application renewal deadline.

Participation on the AANLCP® Executive Board, the CNLCP Certification Board, or an AANLCP® Committee: Ten points of credit per year will be granted, up to a maximum of 20 points within the five-year renewal period. Additional points of credit may be granted, by and at the discretion of the CNLCP Certification Board, for non-board member participation on specialty CNLCP Certification Board committees (CNLCP Certification Board, 2022f, p. 2–4).

CNLCP® Fees

Fees for recertification of CNLCP® every five years (by continuing education):

- AANLCP® Association Member, $375 Recertification of CNLCP® every five years (by continuing education) Non-Member, $475
- Recertification of CNLCP® every five years (by exam), AANLCP® Association Member, $425
- Recertification of CNLCP® every five years (by exam), Non-Member, $525
- Late Recertification, AANLCP® Association Member (within 30 days of expiration), $575
- Late Recertification, Non-Member (within 30 days of expiration), $675

Examination fees include a non-refundable $50 administrative fee. A flat fee of $20.00 will be added to all credit/debit card payments (CNLCP Certification Board, 2022e).

CNLCP® Accreditation

The CNLCP® board has filed for accreditation and is in the process of working with the Accreditation Board for Specialty Certification (ABSNC) toward a portfolio pathway. The ABSNC accreditation was established in 1991 as the ABNS Accreditation Council (ABSNC, 2022a). Since 2009, the ABSNC has been a separate and autonomous accreditation board that serves as the only accrediting body specifically dedicated to evaluating nursing certification programs, with more than 61% of nursing certification programs being accredited through them (ABSNC, 2022b).

Participation in either organization's certification process is voluntary. Obtaining ABSNC accreditation requires a specialty certification board policy to document compliance with specific standards to demonstrate that it has a mechanism in place to respond to issues of discrimination, test security, confidentiality, appeals, and non-compliance. The ABSNC also requires documentation that the candidate certification examination construction, evaluation, and passing score criteria are developed using psychometrically sound and fair methods (ABSNC, 2022b).

Certified Physician Life Care Planner (CPLCP™)

CPLCP™ History

The CPLCP™ certification recognizes life care planners who "adhere to specific, highest-level medical and rehabilitative methodological standards" (CPLCP Certification Board, 2016a, para. 3). The CPLCP™ Certification Board is an independent, non-profit entity that collaborates with the American Academy of Physician Life Care Planners for the purpose of advancing the discipline of life care planning through the certification of qualified physicians (CPLCP Certification

Board, 2016a, para 1). The board consists of both physician and non-physician members (CPLCP Certification Board, 2016e). No additional historical content was provided.

CPLCP™ Eligibility

Requirements for the Certified Physician Life Care Planner (CPCLP™) are as follows:

- Be a licensed Medical Doctor (MD) or Doctor of Osteopathic Medicine (DO) in the United States or equivalent in other countries for at least three years following the completion of residency (unrestricted, active licensure)
- Be board certified in Physical Medicine and Rehabilitation (Physiatry) as designated by the American Board of Physical Medicine and Rehabilitation or by the American Osteopathic Board of Physical Medicine and Rehabilitation
- Be a CLCP™ (CPLCP Certification Board, 2016a)

CPLCP™ Exam

In 2022, the CPLCP™ examination was scheduled at the PTC with time periods that were the entire months of April and October. The examination consists of a maximum of 120 questions, in multiple-choice format with a total testing time of three hours. The exam material consists of basic concepts (10%), tenets and methods (45%), and best practices (45%) (Certified Physician Life Care Planner Certification Board, 2021, p. 12).

CPLCP™ Recertification

The CPLCP™ certification is recognized for five years and can be renewed by taking and passing the most recent CPLCP™ Certification Examination or recertified through 60 CEUs, 15 of which can be continuing medical education (CME) credits applicable to physician life care planning (CPLCP Certification Board, 2016b). Credit hours for recertification can be earned through:

Continuing Education Hours: One hour of approved life care planning education, or medical education applicable to life care planning = 1 credit hour. Examples of courses that would be approved: 1) Physiatric education regarding spinal cord injury, traumatic or acquired brain injury, amputations, burns, orthopedic injuries, chronic pain, etc.; 2) life care planning education approved/accepted by ICHCC, etc. Course outlines should be submitted to the CPLCP™ Certification Board for review/approval of points of credit hours 90 days prior to the application for renewal.

Presentations: five points of credit for each presentation, for which national or state approved continuing education has been granted to participants, for a maximum of ten points per five-year renewal period. Presentation outlines should be submitted to the CPLCP™ Certification Board for review/approval of points of credit hours 90 days prior to the application for renewal.

Research and Publication: Publications or research related to a life care planning article, or clinical articles applicable to the practice of life care planning, should be submitted to the CPLCP™ Certification Board for review/approval of points of credit 90 days prior to the application for renewal. Five points for each publication/research project will be awarded, with a maximum of ten credits per five-year period.

Item Writing/Test Questions: one point of credit for every five questions submitted that are supported by evidence-based medical references for a maximum of ten points of credit per five-year renewal period. Questions with reference supported answers should be submitted directly to the CPLCP™ Certification Board, which will, at its sole discretion, accept/reject questions for credits.

American Academy of Physician Life Care Planners (AAPLCP™) or CPLCP™ Certification Board membership or committee participation: five points of credit per year with documented or verified annual participation will be awarded. Participation is defined as 85% attendance/participation on the applicable boards/committees. The maximum points of credit that can be earned are 20 points in a five-year period (CPLCP Certification Board, 2016b, para. 2-6).

CPLCP™ Fees

The fees associated with the CPLCP™ are follows:

- Examination (AAPLCP Members): $325.00
- Examination (AAPLCP Non-Members): $475.00
- Transfer Fee: $295.00
- Rescheduling of examination: $200.00
- Recertification (AAPLCP Member): $295.00
- Recertification (AAPLCP Non-Member): $195.00
- Late Recertification: $200.00 (CPCLP Certification Board, 2016d)

CPLCP™ Accreditation

At this time, the CPLCP™ is not accredited (W. Davenport, personal communication September 21, 2022).

FIG's Life Care Planning—Certified (LCP-C)

LCP-C History

FIG Education added a certification for all qualified healthcare and rehabilitation professionals in 2021. According to FIG's website, "FIG's Life Care Planning Certification Class is taught from the perspective that the rehabilitation/case management and nursing model is the foundation of Life Care Planning" (FIG Services, Inc., 2022, para. 4).

LCP-C Eligibility

FIG's LPC-C criteria include:
　　Minimum of bachelor's degree in the medical, healthcare, or rehabilitation field.
　　Current, active, and unrestricted licensure or certification in the candidate's primary practice within the medical, healthcare, or rehabilitation field.
　　Minimum of two years of full-time paid employment within the primary practice of medical, healthcare, or rehabilitation field.
　　Completion of FIG's 120-hour Life Care Planning Certification Class, which includes submission or a redacted case study life care plan to be peer-reviewed by the FIG Advisory Board with a passing score.

FIG's 120-hour Life Care Planning Certification Class is divided into 24, five-hour lessons consisting of an independent study with recorded presentations, reading assignments, and a homework assignment consisting of multiple-choice questions and short essays. This program is asynchronous, in that each individual may advance at their own pace. A life care plan case study is presented toward the end of the 120-hour online class. The life care plan case study report will then be peer-reviewed by the FIG Advisory Board. The course work should be completed in 6–12 months. Upon completion of FIG's 120-hour online class and peer-reviewed life care plan case study report, the individual receives a certificate of completion and can then apply for LCP-C Certification. FIG's LCP-C Certification is open to individuals who have successfully completed FIG's LCP Certification Class.

LCP-C Exam

FIG's LCP-C Certification exam is included within FIG's 120-hour Life Care Planning Certification Class at the end of each lesson. A passing score of 70% is required in all 24 lessons

LCP-C Recertification

FIG's LCP-C renewal period is every five years. Recertification criteria include a current, active, and unrestricted licensure/certification in the LCP-C's primary practice and specialty practice of life care planning; and there is a requirement of 60 CEUs related to the primary practice and specialty practice of life care planning.

LCP-C Fees

The cost of FIG's LCP-C credential is included in the class tuition. There is no additional charge for FIG's LCP-C credential. There is a $199 fee for processing at the time of each LCP-C renewal period.

LCP-C Accreditation

FIG's LCP-C credential is not accredited at this time.

Fellow Designation

In addition to certification, involvement in life care planning related professional organizations became important as the specialty practice of life care planning grew (Latham, 2021). Currently, there are three life care planning related professional organizations, each of which holds annual conferences with presentations related to life care planning. The organizations include The International Academy of Life Care Planners (IALCP), now under the formal umbrella of the IARP, AANLCP and the AAPLCP. One of these organizations, the IALCP, offers the opportunity for life care planners to apply for the designation of Fellow of the International Academy of Life Care Planners, a designation which has existed since 1996 (Albee, 2019; Shahnasarian, 2015). This designation is awarded to those individuals who "have achieved a high level of skill and who use their skills and knowledge to promote the advancement of life care planning" (IARP, 2022a, para 2). To apply for consideration for Fellow designation, the professional must submit two redacted life care plans for blind review that the applicant has completed within the last 12 months. The application fee is $350 with renewal occurring every five years (with a renewal fee of $175). The application is scored based upon the following criteria:

- Applicant maintains license and certifications to practice in his/her healthcare discipline
- Applicant contributes to the development of the field through providing education, conducting research, publishing in professional journals/texts, and/or providing mentoring for other life care planners
- Applicant demonstrates satisfactory acceptance of the life care plan product by obtaining at least two letters of recommendation from referring sources (i.e., the sources requesting the life care plan) within the past five years
- Applicant has completed a minimum of 50 life care plans and a minimum working five years as a life care planner
- Applicant demonstrates systematic, comprehensive data collections (consistent method of collecting data from appropriate, relevant, and authoritative sources)
- Applicant demonstrates analysis of data that reflects whether evaluee's needs are being met, comparison to expected norms, and comparison to expected standards of care
- Applicant demonstrates a consistent planning process that includes methods for organizing data, consistent documentation tools, a process of validating inclusion/exclusion of content, and use of expert resources in formulating opinions
- Applicant demonstrates evaluation of the life care plan for completeness and internal consistency; all information is detailed completely or marked as not applicable; there are properly sourced references with supporting foundation; and there is a method for the recipient of the life care plan to contact the life care planner
- Applicant who acts as an expert witness or consultant in legal matters demonstrates accuracy of record keeping for participation in sworn testimony and can describe his/her activity
- Applicant maintains professional knowledge and skills through continuing education
- Applicant provides a one-paragraph blinded-biography summarizing, at a minimum, their credentials, their years of life care planning experience, and a brief history of the industry segments in which they have worked (IARP, 2022c).

Life Care Planning in Litigation

In the medicolegal context, the judge determines if the life care planner is qualified as an expert witness under court, state, or federal rules, to testify and provide opinions. The *Federal Rules of Evidence* are used by the "gatekeeper" or judge, as to whether the life care planner can be of assistance to the trier of fact. The judge determines if the life care planning expert is qualified to give opinion if the testimony is relevant and reliable.

Federal Rule of Evidence 702 is the rule concerning the qualifications of an expert to give an opinion. An expert witness qualifies as such based on his/her knowledge, skills, experience, training, or education. The expert is permitted to testify if:

- The expert's scientific, technical, or other specialized knowledge will help the trier of fact (e.g., jury) to understand the evidence or determine a fact in issue
- The testimony is based on sufficient facts or data
- The testimony is the product of reliable principles and methods
- The expert has reliably applied the principles and methods to the facts of the case (Brown-Henry, 2018, p. 650)

Brown-Henry (2018) notes that challenges to a life care planner's qualification may be predicated on the professional's education and training (or lack thereof) and concludes, "Certifications in life care planning help obviate these types of challenges" (p. 51). Additionally, Gunn (2018) notes that a lack of completion of certification can be a deficit in a professional's qualification as an expert.

Conclusion

With four decades of life care planning materials now accumulated and thousands of individuals who have or are practicing in the specialty practice of life care planning, the evidence base for life care planning as a discipline has grown. As life care planning evolved, codification of the methods for developing a life care plan as well as the requirements necessary for individuals to serve as life care planners have emerged.

As life care planning is transdisciplinary in nature, there exists no licensure specifically available in life care planning. Without licensure, certification in life care planning is often relied upon as evidence that the individual preparing the life care plan has the requisite skills and knowledge to do so. By 2022, there are various training programs as well as professional certifications available to life care planners. Certification in life care planning, like life care planning itself, continues to evolve and will remain a topic for discussion in life care planning. It is anticipated that as life care planning continues to become identified as an evidence-based practice with an accepted standard methodology, established standards of practice, consensus statements, dedicated ethics with disciplinary actions, those practicing life care planning will be held to higher standards. This may result in the necessity for certification bodies to meet the criteria for accreditation for their certifications. To date, none of the available certifications have achieved a form of national or international accreditation, despite this being of high importance to the profession, a priority listed among the consensus statements, and particularly important for life care planners who testify as experts to meet the thresholds required by courts. A necessary vision and commitment of the field of life care planning has trudged through the movements of the certifications CLCP™, CCLCP™, and the CNLCP® toward accreditation to provide the recognition and status of competency of high standards and quality control. The CLCP™, CCLCP™, and CNLCP® governed respectively by the ICHCC™ and the Certified Nurse Life Care Planner Board (CNLCP® board) are pursuing forms of accreditation.

Resources

AAACEU: www.aaaceus.com/CLCP-Certified-Life-Care-Planners.asp
Capital University Law School (CULS) Life Care Planning Program: www.capital.edu/academics/graduate-programs/law-school/life-care-planner-program/
FIG Services: www.figeducation.com
Institute on Rehabilitation Education and Training (IRET): https://iretprograms.com/
Kelynco: https://kelynco.com/
Thomas Jefferson University: www.jefferson.edu/academics/colleges-schools-institutes/rehabilitation-sciences/departments/outcomes-measurement/education/life-care-planning-graduate-certificate.html

References

Accreditation Board for Specialty Nursing Certification. (2022a). *About*. https://absnc.org/about
Accreditation Board for Specialty Nursing Certification. (2022b). *Frequently asked questions*. https://absnc.org/frequently-asked-questions
Albee, T. (2019). A historical look at the fellow of the International Association of Life Care Planning (FIALCP) designation. *Journal of Life Care Planning, 17*(3), 53–56.
American Counseling Association. (2022). *Florida and Kentucky become eighth and ninth states to sign interstate Counseling Compact into law*. www.counseling.org/news/updates/news-detail/2022/04/12/florida-and-kentucky-becomes-eighth-and-ninth-states-to-sign-interstate-counseling-compact-into-law#:~:text=Currently%2C%20the%20Counseling%20Compact%20has,to%20recognize%20another%20state's%20license
American Occupational Therapy Association & National Board for Certification in Occupational Therapy. (2022). *Occupational therapy licensure compact*. https://otcompact.org/compact-map/
American Speech Language Hearing Association. (1997–2002). Audiology and speech-language pathology interstate compact (ASLP-IC). www.asha.org/advocacy/state/audiology-and-speech-language-pathology-interstate-compact
ANSI National Accreditation Board (2022). *About ANAB*. https://anab.ansi.org/about-anab
Berens, D. & Weed, R. (2018). Credentialing and other issues in life care planning. In R. O. Weed & D. E. Berens (Eds.), *Life care planning and case management handbook*, (4th ed., pp. 813–818), Routledge.
Brown-Henry, K. (2018). A plaintiff's attorney's perspective on life care planning. In R. O. Weed & D. E. Berens (Eds.), *Life care planning and case management handbook*, (4th ed., pp. 641–654), Routledge.
Bullins, S. M., & Reid, C. A. (2019). Certification in life care planning practice. *Journal of Life Care Planning, 17*(3), 23–29.
Certified Nurse Life Care Planner (CNLCP®) Certification Board. (1998–2022). Certification examination for nurse life care planners Handbook for candidates. https://ptcny.com/pdf/cnlcp.pdf
Certified Nurse Life Care Planner (CNLCP®) Certification Board. (2022a). https://cnlcp.org/
Certified Nurse Life Care Planner (CNLCP®) Certification Board. (2022b). *Certification*. https://cnlcp.org/certification/
Certified Nurse Life Care Planner (CNLCP®) Certification Board. (2022c). *Our certification*. https://cnlcp.org/certification/#:~:text=Certification%20is%20a%20formal%20recognition,of%20proficiency%20beyond%20basic%20licensure
Certified Nurse Life Care Planner (CNLCP®) Certification Board. (2022d). *Education resources*. https://cnlcp.org/education-resources/
Certified Nurse Life Care Planner (CNLCP®). (2022e). CNLCP certification and recertification fees. https://cnlcp.org/cnlcp-certification-re-certification-fees/
Certified Nurse Life Care Planner (CNLCP®). (2022f). Recertification. https://cnlcp.org/recertification/
Certified Physician Life Care Planner Certification Board. (2021). Certification examination for physician life care planners. https://ptcny.com/pdf/CPLCP.pdf
CNLCP Certification Board. (2022f). 2022 CNLCP® Recertification guidelines. https://ptcny.com/pdf/CNLCP_RecertGuidelinesAndApplication.pdf
CPLCP™ Certification Board. (2016a). CPLCP™ Examination. https://cplcp.org/Certification.aspx
CPLCP™ Certification Board. (2016b). Recertification. https://cplcp.org/Recertification.aspx
CPLCP™ Certification Board. (2016c). Fees. https://cplcp.org/Fees.aspx
CPLCP™ Certification Board. (2016d). *Recertification guidelines*. https://ptcny.com/pdf/CNLCP_RecertGuidelinesAndApplication.pdf
CPLCP™ Certification Board. (2016e). Our board. https://cplcp.org/Board.aspx
Deutsch, P. M., & Sawyer, H. W. (1985, Rev. 2002). *A guide to rehabilitation*. AHAB Press.
Deutsch, P., & Raffa, F. (1982). *Damages in tort action* (Vols. 8 & 9). Matthew Bender.
FIG Services, Inc. (2022). www.figeducation.com/life-care-planning/
Gaines, K. (2022, April 19.) What are compact nursing states? https://nurse.org/articles/enhanced-compact-multi-state-license-eNLC/
Gunn, T. R. (2018). *A defense attorney's perspective on life care planning*. In R. Weed & D. Berens (Eds.), *Life care planning and case management handbook*, (4th ed., pp. 655–668). Routledge.

International Academy of Life Care Planners. (2019). Transdisciplinary practice position paper. *Journal of Life Care Planning*, *17*(2), 3–4.
International Academy of Life Care Planners. (2022). Standards of practice for life care planners, 4th edition. *Journal of Life Care Planning*, *20*(3), 5–20.
International Association of Rehabilitation Professionals. (2022a). Fellow program. https://connect.rehabpro.org/lcp/fellow/fellow-program
International Association of Rehabilitation Professionals. (2022b). *Current fellows*. https://connect.rehabpro.org/lcp/fellow/current-fellows
International Association of Rehabilitation Professionals. (2022c). IARP IALCP Fellow Designation Program Application. https://higherlogicdownload.s3.amazonaws.com/REHABPRO/c6d14bd5-fe3a-4d20-855c-14bd56ffa0a4/UploadedFiles/k4I5ZfHRomQ7AGpBHq4p_Application_for_Fellow_2019_.pdf
International Commission for Health Care Certification. (2022). *Certification programs*. www.ichcc.org/certifications.html
International Commission on Health Care Certification. (2020). *Candidate handbook*. https://ICHCC™.org/images/PDFs/CLCP_Candidate_Handbook_10-21-2020_Repaired.pdf
International Commission on Health Care Certification. (2021). *Practice standards and guidelines*. https://www.ichcc.org/images/PDFs/Standards_and_Guidelines.pdf
International Commission on Health Care Certification. (2023). Certified life care planner. https://www.ichcc.org/certified-life-care-planner-clcp.html
Interstate Medical Licensure Compact. (2022, July 8). www.imlcc.org/wp-content/uploads/2022/07/Information-Release-Rhode-Island-becomes-39th-member.pdf
Johnson, C., & Preston, K. (2012). Consensus and majority statements derived from life care planning summits held in 2000, 2002, 2004, 2006, 2010 and 2012. *Journal of Life Care Planning*, *11*(2), 9–14.
Johnson, C. (2018). A historical review of life care planning summits since 2000. *Journal of Life Care Planning*, *17*(3), 37–51.
Johnson, C. (2015). Consensus and majority statements derived from life care planning summits, held in 2000, 2002, 2004, 2006, 2008, 2010, 2012, 2015. *Life Care Planning Journal*, *13*(4), 35–38.
Johnson, C., Pomeranz, J., & Stetton, N. (2018). Life care planning consensus and majority statements, 2000–2018: Are they still relevant and reliable? A Delphi study. *Journal of Life Care Planning*, *16*(4), 5–14.
Kelynco. (2022). https://kelynco.com/
Latham, S. (2021, August). The history and evolution of life care planning. *Oklahoma Bar Journal*, *92*(6), 20–24.
Leahy, M., Chan, F., & Saunders, J. (2003). A work behavior analysis of contemporary rehabilitation counseling practices. *Rehabilitation Counseling Bulletin*, *46*, 66-81.
Mauk, K. L. (2019). Revisiting the concept of transdisciplinary life care planning. *Journal of Life Care Planning*, *17*(1), 5–6.
May, V. R. (n.d.). Commission reports on first five months of certifying life care planners. *Inside Life Care Planning*, *1*(6), 5,12.
May, V. R., & Moradi Rekabdarkolaee, H. (2020). The International Commission on Health Care Certification Life care planner role and function investigation. *Journal of Life Care Planning*, *18*(12), 3–68.
Neulicht, A. T., Riddick-Grisham, S., & Goodrich, W. R. (2010). Life care plan survey 2009: Process, methods, and protocols [Special issue]. *Journal of Life Care Planning*, *9*(4), 131–200.
Neulicht. A. T., Riddick-Grisham, S., Hinton, L., Costantini, P. A., Thomas, R., & Goodrich, B. (2001). Life care planning survey 2001: Process, methods and protocols. *Journal of Life Care Planning*, *1*(2), 97–148.
Pomeranz, J., Yu, N., & Reid, C., (2010), Role and function study of life care planners. *Journal of Life Care Planning*, *17*(3), 57–106.
PT Compact. (2022). https://ptcompact.org/ptc-states
Shahnasarian, M. (2015). Insights into the International Association of Life Care Planning Fellow Program: Questions and answers from program developers. *Journal of Life Care Planning*, *13*(4), 21–25.

Chapter 5

Ethics in Life Care Planning

Mary Barros-Bailey

How we practice as professionals in any context—clinical, forensic, academic, research, or other—tells the world about who we are as individuals or groups that share common practices. Ethics can shape not only our professional behavior, but also our professional thoughts and expressions. The purpose of this chapter is to explore the realm of professional ethics, and its application to the specialty of life care planning.

The earliest literature found on ethics in life care planning started with a two-page reflection by a rehabilitation ethicist briefly outlining life care planner responsibilities, integrity, objectivity and independence, and professional care and competence (Blackwell, 1995). As life care planning glimpses the threshold of the fifth decade of its formation as a specialty, dialogues about professional behavior are now more ample and present in our textbooks (Berens & Weed, 2018; Savage, 2011) and professional journals. Review of archives from the *Journal of Life Care Planning* and the *Journal of Nurse Life Care Planning* as well as comprehensive searches on academic databases,[1] found that ethics in life care planning are captured or woven in some way in the following literature:

- *Professional Community Consensus and Standards Development*
- Forums on professional discourse involving consensus building in practice (Albee et al., 2018; Berens 2018a, 2018b, 2018c; Deutsch et al., 2018; Gamez & Johnson, 2017; International Association of Rehabilitation Professionals, 2018; Johnson, 2012; Johnson, 2015a, 2015b; Johnson et al., 2011; Johnson et al., 2018a, 2018b; Preston et al., 2018; Riddick-Grisham, 2003, 2018)
- General issues in life care planning for credentialed practitioners (Pettengill, 2013)
- Research content reviews (Mertes, 2018)
- Standards development (Preston & Reid, 2015)
- *Specialized Topical Advice and Guidance*

- Business issues such as general practice (Preston, 2006), payments (Howland, 2014a) or fees (Howland, 2014b)
- Evaluee/client/patient relationships (Barros-Bailey et al., 2008, 2009; Cimino-Ferguson, 2005; Manzetti & Howland, 2013; Schofield & Huntington-Frazier, 2015)
- Evidence-based practice (Howland, 2014c; Metekingi, 2013)
- Life care planner roles (Gonzales & Zotovas, 2014)
- Multicultural issues (Barros-Bailey, 2017, 2018)
- Professional responsibility including conflict of interest (Howland, 2013a) and invalid credentials (Howland, 2013b)
- Report writing (Barros-Bailey, 2020)
- Special issues such as underestimating life expectancy (Reid, 2013), special populations like individuals with spinal cord injuries (Priebe et al., 2007), or the ethics of other damages team members (Gibbs et al., 2013)

Evaluees in Life Care Planning

Who is considered the client in life care planning, the person evaluated, the one who sent the referral, or the one paying the bill? For many years, this question was a hot and controversial topic in professional conversations, literature, and online discussion boards in forensic rehabilitation, including life care planning. The issue was put to rest in 2008 when a group of professionals, including several life care planners, converged to deliberate the definition (Barros-Bailey et al., 2008, 2009). We stripped away semantics and examined the intent of relationships in clinical and forensic contexts. The vital difference in these relationships is that in forensics a life care planner or other professional does not develop a client–counselor, patient–physician, or other such relationship where primary care is expected; however, in a normal course of clinical treatment, primary care services are expected. As a result of the evaluee definition published in a white paper, it was broadly disseminated in the rehabilitation literature and unanimously adopted by the boards of the American Board of Vocational Experts, the Commission on Rehabilitation Counselor Certification, and the International Association of Rehabilitation Professionals. Consequently, the *evaluee* definition entered the life care planning lexicon as a clear and distinct term to describe the person who is the subject of a forensic evaluation where there is no clinical relationship beyond that of an evaluative one. The person who requested that the life care planner provide such evaluative services is the *referral source*, who may or may not be the same as the *payor* (Barros-Bailey et al., 2008, 2009). If a life care planner is hired to perform services in a forensic or clinical case, it is vital to distinguish such differences to an evaluee because of the resulting standard of care expectations.

Standards of Care in Life Care Planning

Standards of care are not standards of practice. While standards of practice are developed by a discipline to provide guidelines for best practices, a *standard of care* is a legal concept that is defined as the "degree of care a prudent and reasonable person will exercise under the circumstances" (The Law Dictionary, n.d., para. 2). Life care planners delivering services in a medical malpractice case, for example, may read discovery in the liability side of the case (see chapter in this text titled A Defense Attorney's Perspective on Life Care Planning) where the breach of the standard of care may be the issue at hand. That is, the question a liability side of a malpractice case needs to answer is: Did the adverse outcome from the act/failure to act breach the duty of care that would be expected by a reasonable provider within the same profession? Even if life care planning does not have formally defined standards of care or a life care planner holds no formal credentialing in the field, if a life care planner is sued for negligence, the guidelines that will be used by defense and plaintiff sides to make their case will include the main documents in life care planning such as standards of practice, codes of ethics, consensus statements, etc. Typically, duty is established when the life care planner develops the relationship with the evaluee to provide life care planning services. The relationship could start at the time of a signed retainer agreement, when the disclosure and informed consent process is performed at the start of a data collection interview, or at the time of any other defined event that could mark the start of the relationship.

Moral vs. Ethics vs. Legal

Before exploring ethical dilemmas in the life care planning literature, we will explore basic theoretical foundations of ethics. Morals refer to the behavioral tenets we hold as individuals, while ethics are tenets held by society. For example, I may not believe it is okay to ingest any mind-altering substances (moral), although societally, this behavior may be acceptable (ethics). Different from individual morals and society ethics, legal rules provide a measure of behavior and its societal acceptance. Individuals in societies can hold different morals. I may have a different opinion of what is morally acceptable to charge for services based on someone's ability to pay compared to my colleagues. Similarly, groups within a population may have differing opinions as to appropriate behaviors. One professional discipline may have defined guidelines of appropriate pricing for services while another discipline may not. Legal behavior, on the other hand, goes beyond a discipline's guideline and may use government mechanisms to establish and enforce fee schedules. Reverting to the above substance use example, while drinking alcohol may be acceptable ethical behavior in a culture or population or by individuals, the legal level of ingested alcohol could be regulated by the laws of different jurisdictions.

Professional Ethics

The study and practice of professional ethics comes in many forms. Such study could be about "moral thought and moral language," or what is called metaethics (Wilson, 2016), rather than practice. Providing processes or guidelines for individual actions and behaviors for practice is called normative ethics (Cavalier, 2002). Applied ethics is what we are most familiar with in the disciplines that feed into the life care planning specialty as it deals with "specific realms of human action and [crafting] criteria for discussing issues that might arise" (Cavalier, 2002, para. 3); it is the category of ethical discourse under which medical or bioethics falls.

Principle Ethics

For over four decades in bioethics and beyond, Beauchamp and Childress's principle ethics framework has influenced codes of ethics, ethical decision-making, and the lexicon used when discussing ethical dilemmas and their resolution in medicine and related allied health professions (Shea,

2020). The initial four principles introduced in 1979 were: autonomy, nonmaleficence, beneficence, and justice.

Autonomy concerns individuals making their own choice. To make a choice, however, the individual needs to be informed about the scope of that choice and potential impacts. One of the ways this concept is manifested in healthcare is in the disclosure and informed consent form and process: Life care planners disclose the scope of their services and any limitations of their role and the informed evaluee elects to proceed—or not—with the described services.

Nonmaleficence is the essence of the Hippocratic oath—to do no harm—and covers omissions or commissions of behaviors. An example of this principle is a life care planner voiding basic needs for an evaluee in an opposing expert's plan although there is probable evidence for the needed services; or, on the other extreme, a life care planner vastly overstating needed services for the evaluee beyond probability, thus risking the admission of the plan into testimony before the trier of fact and precluding the evaluee's ability to present the plan as a measure of damages.

While nonmaleficense is avoiding harm, the principle that embraces proactive action is *beneficence*. This principle focuses the behavior on appropriate and good acts to safeguard an individual, group, or population. An example during a home evaluation would be for the life care planner to identify an area of services the evaluee desperately needs and providing the evaluee, the family, and the referral source with information about the recommended resources so they could access the services immediately and receive better care. Because a life care planner acts benevolently does not mean the professional is advocating for the evaluee, just taking the right and ethical action.

The last of the four original ethical principles is *justice*, which is the concept of the impartial distribution of benefits or burdens. In life care planning, this principle is illustrated in the expectation of unbiased and objective opinions regardless of the referral source or evaluee. That is, regardless of who is paying the life care planner's invoice, given the same set of facts, the results of a life care plan for the same evaluee would be the same.

Since Beauchamp and Childress (2001) introduced principle ethics, an additional principle—*fidelity*—was proposed by Welfel and Kitchiner (1992). They described fidelity as "promise keeping, trustworthiness, and loyalty" (p. 180). Whereas a related principle—*veracity*—meaning being honest, is used by the ethical codes of some helping professions (Commission on Rehabilitation Counselor Certification, 2017), honesty could be construed as inherent to the principle of fidelity. An example for this last principle of fidelity is demonstrated in life care planning as providing the services for which the life care planner was retained.

Values' Clarification

Savage (2011) explored the clarification of values in life care planning ethical decision-making. Values' clarification is defined by Kulich and Chi (2014) as:

> … reflexive, personal, sociocultural, and intercultural processes whereby one seeks to identify the undergirding or influential value priorities that guide one's interests, choices, actions, and reactions in a variety of interpersonal and social contexts. By helping an individual to better understand what one considers most important related to the complex makeup, diverse contexts, and variable roles of the society in which one is situated, this process of guided, cognizant self-reflection can facilitate a more realistic understanding of oneself in relation to social norms, expectations, and options (para. 1).

A variety of values clarification exercises, assessments, worksheets, quizzes, and tests exist online to assist the professional to become more self-aware of their reaction when presented with simple or complex ethical dilemmas.

Elements of Professional Ethics for Life Care Planners

Professional Discipline Codes

Practitioners of life care planning come into the specialty from varied professions, each of which have established ethical codes, and congregate in professional or credentialing groups ascribing to ethical guidelines. The fourth edition of the *Standards of Practice for Life Care Planners* (International Academy of Life Care Planning, 2022) formalizes the expectation that the first stop is the life care planner's professional code of ethics or those guiding their professional activities:

4. STANDARD: The life care planner shall practice in an ethical manner and follow the Code of Ethics of their respective professions, roles, certifications, and credentials.

   a. Follows the Code of Ethics of their profession.
   b. Follows the Code of Ethics for their professional roles, certifications, and credentials (p. 8).

Beyond main professional codes of ethics for the discipline each life care planner derives, there are currently four organizations with established codes of ethics providing guidance to their members or certificants: American Academic of Nurse Life Care Planners (AANLCP, 2015), American Academy of Physician Life Care Planners (AAPLCP, 2014); International Association of Rehabilitation Professionals, International Academy of Life Care Planning (IALCP, 2022); and International Commission of Health Care Certification (ICHCC, 2015). Each of these codes presents a threshold of behavior starting with what is expected in the law. Therefore, it is important for life care planners to understand what they can legally do in a particular jurisdiction as well as based on their professional and respective life care planning code of ethics.

The Service Role and Relationship: Clinical v. Forensic

Because life care planning was born out of the need for an organizational framework to present the current and future needs of an individual with physical, mental, or cognitive conditions (see chapter in this text titled Life Care Planning: Past, Present, and Future) to the trier of fact, there is the assumption that life care planning is performed within a forensic setting. However, services may also be clinical (e.g., case management for special needs trusts, elder care), so it is wise to address ethics from both clinical and forensic perspectives. Ethical dilemmas in the life care planning literature provide guidance in both arenas.

Ethical Decision-Making

Life care planners facing ethical dilemmas are often best served through guidance, such as that of an ethical decision-making model. Many disciplines offer professionals in their fields models geared toward resolving ethical dilemmas based on specialized consideration. More recently, Barnao et al. (2022) proposed a model for ethical decision-making in forensic practice. Foundational to their decision-making model is the concept of ethical blindness, or when professionals overlook matters in practice that are not within the practitioner's view. They state that:

> Ethical dilemmas, conflicts, gaps and so on are simply not identified because the ethical framework relied on by clinicians does not contain the general theoretical resources, or specific standards, that flag them as issues to be noted and responded to.
> (Barnao et al., 2022, p. 83)

Instead of providing a model that is based on a step-by-step process that goes from one phase to the next or organically between considerations, Barnao et al. (2022) proposed an Ethical Evaluation Guide based on a cluster of heuristic questions designed to have forensic practitioners look beyond guidance in ethical codes of ethics. The questions have been adapted below for life care planning:

What ethical issues are present for the life care planner and their role within forensic practice and what kind of harm or benefit could arise? CONSIDERATION: Any problems detected as a result of this question should be viewed from the perspective of human rights and dignity of the individual.

- What implications result when considering outcomes of dignity from the dilemma?
- Are all stakeholders affected by the issue considered? Is the evaluee receiving equal attention compared to other parties involved with the issue?
- Is the response to the ethical dilemma generalizable to other evaluees? That is, if the evaluee were different but the circumstances and issues similar, would the life care planner arrive at the same conclusions and responses?

These questions are helpful to tie into traditional models that recommend consultation with peers, mentors, or others who can provide objective input to a proposed action before such action is taken and the practitioner can document their ethical decision-making process.

Ethics Guidance in Life Care Planning

The most extensive collection of ethical dilemmas and advisory opinions for life care planners comes from the Ethics Interface Panel appearing in nearly every issue of the *Journal of Life Care Planning* since 2006. From the inception of the panel, Nancy Mitchell has chaired the team of professionals including practitioners in nursing, occupational therapy, psychology, and rehabilitation counseling to address and research various ethical dilemmas or issues cited by life care planners, and provide advisory opinions based on researched codes of ethics or the literature from life care planning, medical, and allied health disciplines. Before each Ethics Interface is published, it undergoes a secondary review by a small group of individuals from legal and life care planning specialties. The following series of tables summarize and categorize the advisory opinions by the panel published through to 2022 by theme. Note that some of the ethical dilemmas can be classified into one or more ethical categories, but have been placed in the theme found to be predominant.

Relationships with Evaluees

Codes of ethics in the helping professions typically lead with standards surrounding person-centered services. The evaluation by a life care planner is primarily for the benefit of the evaluee, no one else, although the referral may have been received from a number of different sources and the invoice could be paid by the same or other individuals or institutions. Therefore, within the domain of relationship with the evaluee, there typically exist themes associated with professional behaviors resulting in the individual's welfare, dual or multiple roles by the life care planner, understanding and adhering to evaluee rights, respecting culture, and avoiding imposing the evaluator's values upon the process that could bias it, termination of services, and similar topics. Of no surprise, this domain of ethics garners the most questions from the life care planning community.

Dual or Multiple Roles

Predominant are questions about playing two roles with the same evaluee or, namely, switching between case manager and life care planner, friend/family member to life care planner, etc.

Table 5.1 Dual or Multiple Roles

ETHICAL DILEMMA	*ADVISORY OPINION*
Dual Relationships	
Can a longstanding case manager provide an objective and defensible life care plan in a forensic setting for the same client/evaluee? (Mitchell et al., 2013a)	Generally, codes of ethics discourage dual relationships especially during the course of case management service. However, there may be circumstances when the needs of the evaluee are best met by the existing case manager in developing the life care plan. If switching roles on the same case (clinical–forensic, forensic–clinical, etc.), it is important that full disclosure and informed consent be provided to the evaluee about the new role and the implications of the role change.
I have provided case management services to an individual with disabilities who is now in need of a life care plan and have been requested to develop it by her legal counsel. I have become close to the family and know I could write an objective plan. Is it ethical for me to accept this assignment and prepare the life care plan? (Mitchell et al., 2008a)	It is clear that the original intent for the avoidance of dual relationships was the potential of the loss of objectivity and the prevention of exploitation for personal gain. It is now suggested that evaluee benefit versus harm to the evaluee be the guiding principle in determining the ethics of dual relationships.
I recently completed a life care plan for a child who needs case management services. The case has settled and my work on the case is completed. The family has indicated they want to contract with me to work as the case manager. Would this be considered a dual relationship? (Mitchell et al., 2011b)	Life care planners should avoid dual relationships as it is best practice to avoid a potential line of questioning for opposing counsel if it appears the life care planner is conflicted, such as making case management recommendations and then providing such services.
One of my close relatives was seriously hurt in a motor vehicle accident. A life care plan is needed. Can I offer to do the life care plan at no cost? (Mitchell et al., 2009c)	If you are questioning yourself, then you probably know the answer: Suggest the attorney refer the life care plan elsewhere. The basis for the decision is found in our ethics codes governing impartiality, dual relationships, and conflict of interest.

Traditionally, the advice in those circumstances was to avoid dual or multiple relationships. While this is still by far the predominant recommendation, depending on the details of the case, that avoidance may actually be harmful to the evaluee. The dual role ethical dilemmas described by life care planners involve the principles of nonmaleficence, beneficence, and autonomy. One example is a case manager with a very specialized skillset that is unique to a particular case where there may not be access to a colleague with equal credentials to develop the life care plan fairly and accurately. The decision to mindfully engage in a dual role should not be made in a void or taken lightly, but be part of a documented ethical decision-making process where the potential benefits (beneficence) to the evaluee far outweigh harms (nonmaleficense), such as the appearance of a conflict of interest, bias, or objectivity before the trier of fact. As part of the decision-making process, the evaluee and the referral source must be fully aware of the potential hazards of the life care planner playing both roles. After the disclosure of potential harms that may arise in the dual relationship are discussed, if the evaluee elects to move forward (autonomy), a specialized informed consent form outlining potential positive and negative consequences of switching roles should be signed by the individual and the professionals.

Welfare of Those Served

By the nature of the scope of our work as life care planners and through our historical clinical practice, we have access to many sources and resources across a large spectrum of conditions, care, and geographies that provide us with opportunities to advance the quality of lives for those we evaluate or for their families. The role of an objective and unbiased evaluator does not negate the ethical responsibility to do no harm or to be beneficent. Because the life care planner in a forensic setting is an evaluator and does not deliver primary care, the referral source or payor should be informed of the professional's observations and the life care planner's recommendations.

Regarding transportation and independent living or housing recommendations, the principles of nonmaleficense and justice counterbalance in the ethical dilemma posed to the Ethics Interface Panel. The question the life care planner must weigh is whether the housing situation is one that is sustainable over the evaluee's life expectancy given the person's care needs and stability of their caregiver staffing over the lifespan: Just because someone rented at the time of an incident, does not necessarily indicate they would rent for the rest of their lives. Having control over their housing environment may be a short- and long-term critical care issue. Because life care planning requires individualized assessment, the customized issues in each case must be weighed. If rental properties do not allow for needed renovations and may create a hazardous and unsafe situation for the evaluee that might be neutralized by more stable, owned housing, that may be the clear and ethical option. Offsets by forensic economists or earning capacity evaluations could introduce the principle of justice into the final damages figures but are typically within the scope of practice of other members of a transdisciplinary team, rather than the life care planner.

Also relevant to professional responsibility is the need for life care planners to understand that the purpose of life care planning is to return the evaluee to the maximal functional state possible held at the time of an incident, exposure, or event. The life care planner is an educator to all parties, including the evaluee, about the importance of recommendations. If the evaluee does not have the functional ability or will to make adequate financial decisions in their behalf, potentially causing self-harm, it is ethically incumbent upon the life care planner to help prevent such harm by providing awareness of these issues to the referral source.

Table 5.2 Welfare of Those Served

ETHICAL DILEMMA	ADVISORY OPINION
Evaluee Welfare	
I just completed an in-home evaluation for a new case. The evaluee and her family are wonderful but unsophisticated people. It is clear this person has been provided inadequate care by her treatment team who continues to be involved in her care. Where can I share my opinions to make sure this evaluee gets the care she needs before the life care plan is implemented? (Mitchell et al., 2015c)	Share your opinions with the appropriate people, particularly the referral source. Our standards and professional ethics direct us to assist the evaluee in achieving optimal outcomes. Be prepared to offer suggestions for alternative medical professionals who can evaluate the person to obtain needed care.
I am developing a life care plan for an injured individual whose family has always rented their housing, as have previous generations of family members. Is it ethical to include architectural renovation costs if rental housing for people with disabilities is available in their home community? (Mitchell et al., 2020a)	If the evaluee is living in accessible rental housing that meets that person's needs and has no intention to move, renting can be advantageous because home maintenance, lawn care, and snow removal may not be the responsibility of the person with a disability or the caregivers. Still, the average person living in the United States moves 11.7 times in their lifetime,[2] so, the life care planner must consider the evaluee's needs over that lifetime. Depending on the age of the person, it may be important to consider a move to another community where the accessible rental housing is limited or not available. Consider inclusion of home modifications in the typical section with the comment "as needed" or list these in the "potential complications" section of the report.
During the process of performing a life care plan evaluation, I described to the evaluee many items that would be of obvious benefit who declared he would never use these but would prefer to use funds for vacations and other items unrelated to the disability. Do I include the items? How should I proceed? (Mitchell et al., 2016a)	It is important to contact the referring attorney to discuss this issue who may wish to recommend that any funds received be put in a trust. People with (or without) disabilities may change their mind over time as to what they need as circumstances change. It is your role to educate the evaluee about current and future needs and the reason for the inclusion of items in the life care plan. If the person understands the reasons for items but still does not want them, the standards support the person's right to their point of view. However, if the person is unable to understand the reason for certain items, it would be prudent to document the evaluee's rejection of any items as well as your reasons for including them in the plan.

[2] www.census.gov/topics/population/migration/guidance/calculating-migration-expectancy.html#:~:text=Using%202007%20ACS%20data%2C%20it,one%20move%20per%20single%20year.

Respecting Diversity

Culture does not pertain alone to evaluees who are from ethnic or linguistic groups that are different from the mainstream society. Multicultural issues involve evaluees from any minority group who share same or similar "race, color, religion, sex (including pregnancy, sexual orientation, or gender identity), national origin, age (40 or older), disability, and genetic information (including family medical history)" (U.S. Equal Employment Opportunity Commission, 2022, para. 1). By the very fact that life care planners are evaluating someone who has a physical, mental, or cognitive disability, the life care planner must be sensitive to cultural issues as the evaluee falls into a protected group—individuals with disabilities. There is no heterogeneity in the group of people with disabilities served by life care planners. Instead, much variability exists within the disability culture

Table 5.3 Respecting Diversity

ETHICAL DILEMMA	ADVISORY OPINION
Cultural Issues	
The retaining law firm hired an interpreter for my life care plan evaluation for a non-English speaking evaluee and family. I worry about accuracy of the information I collected during my interview when I have not understood something "first hand." (Mitchell et al., 2015b)	Various codes emphasize the life care plan must provide accurate information. Language that is clear and understandable to all parties must be used. A life care planner should avoid using a friend or family member to interpret in a professional setting. It may be prudent to only agree to work on a case when a professional interpreter is provided. Accuracy and lack of bias are the critical ethical issues governing the interview process. A friend or family member used as an interpreter may have a bias or be embarrassed by a question and not present the information accurately to either the evaluee or the life care planner. Obtaining a list of approved court interpreters, who often contract for work outside the court system, may be an option when seeking a qualified interpreter and other professional interpreters.
My evaluee's functional medicine physician comes from the same refugee ethnic community as her and provides medical recommendations that are very different from those of the consulting rehabilitation physician. The consulting physician's recommendations are more consistent with what we learned in our life care planning training from mainstream medical practitioners. How can I be culturally sensitive to the needs of the evaluee and her functional medicine physician as well as the recommendations of the consulting rehabilitation physician? How do I address cultural issues in my life care plan? (Mitchell et al., 2017c)	Our standards of practice direct us to recognize and embrace cultural differences. This is easy for most of us when our cultural practices align. The challenge comes when the other person's cultural beliefs and practices are not in tandem with our personal and professional way of thinking. The most prudent way to handle this is to provide both options in the life care plan. It will be important to fully disclose this approach to the injured person, the family, and your retaining attorney as appropriate to your role in the case.

that may itself have smaller subgroups from any of the other cultural demographic groups that could impact everything from collecting the primary data because of linguistic, religious, or other differences or norms to the final recommendations and contents of the life care plan. Obviously, addressing culture is a complex issue.

Where the cultural dilemma involves linguistic differences, written language is referred to as translation and oral language (including sign) is called interpretation. The key in this situation is verifying the accuracy of cross-cultural communication between the life care planner and the evaluee or other stakeholders.

Some evaluees may come from individualistic societies like Australia, Canada, United Kingdom, United States, or South Africa and others may come from collectivistic societies such as Brazil, India, Italy, Spain, or Taiwan. Linguistic and cultural differences may dictate who provides information and how many people are part of a life care interview or home visit. These added cultural differences could add greater complexity to the communication. Because accuracy of information is vital in the life care planning process, it is incumbent upon the life care planner to have a professional interpreter as part of the interview process to minimize the introduction of undue bias (fidelity). Having an evaluee paraphrase back to the life care planner through an interpreter their understanding of vital information, such as the content of disclosure and informed consent or care needs, facilitates the principle of autonomy.

A second communication-related dilemma involves conflict between two physician opinions—that of the functional medicine physician and that of the consulting physician. A consensus statement (#65) that provides help in this scenario states that life care planners "shall methodically handle divergent opinions" (Johnson et al., 2018a, p. 17), which could result in presenting both sets of opinions and leaving it to the trier of fact which one to select or choosing another method to systematically handle the differing opinions.

Termination and Referral

Although rare, sometimes issues arise in a case that necessitate termination of services by the life care planner. Unless completely unavoidable (e.g., impairment or death of the life care planner), the practitioner should try to resolve any issues or misunderstandings (e.g., fees, communication) within a reasonable timeline to comply with their retained role (fidelity). If termination appears to be the only option (autonomy), providing referral options to the referral source to colleague life care planners is advisable (justice).

Table 5.4 Termination and Referral

ETHICAL DILEMMA	ADVISORY OPINION
In reviewing a copy of the life care plan I developed, the evaluee became very upset by some of the reported information about her challenges, which was subsequently removed. Should I withdraw myself from the case because the evaluee is angry? (Mitchell et al., 2018a)	Discuss this issue with your referral source. In very rare circumstances, it may be necessary to terminate involvement should issues arise that cannot be resolved, and the life care planner cannot or wishes not to continue to provide services. Some codes of ethics and standards of practice provide guidance for a specific method to terminate services. It will be important to review the areas of concern and see if they are a critical part of the life care plan or if the objectionable parts can be stated differently without losing information that is critical to the plan while adhering to life care planning methodology.

Professional Responsibility

Life care planners have a responsibility, not only to their primary profession that supplies them the general scope of practice to enter life care planning, but also to their individual scope of practice as life care planners, which includes competency and advertised qualifications.

Competency

In a forensic capacity, who is competent to provide life care planning services falls to the courts to determine, not to colleagues from other disciplines. There is not a single discipline that is trained or qualified to address all aspects of life care planning needs for the heterological population served by life care planners. Making absolutist comments about any professional discipline suggests accusation and is a matter of opinion, not reality, given the breadth of trained, credentialed, and qualified disciplines who have individual scopes of practice in life care planning. For more information, please see the chapter 'Life Care Planning: Past, Present, and Future'.

What a life care planner has done to obtain and maintain competency is important and an ethical area covered in most professional codes of ethics. Competency in life care planning requires understanding that in forensic practice, the primary ethical responsibility is to be objective and unbiased, which can be challenging in environments that are dynamic, such as life care planning. It is up to the life care planner to establish professional boundaries, adhere to methodological precepts, and navigate systematic road bumps competing with that ethical responsibility to adhere to nonmaleficence and fidelity principles. Because an environment is dynamic does not mean that changes will result in opinions that do not rise to probability and life care planning certainty. Emergent factors in a case require the life care planner to adhere to competency ethical standards calling for attaining and maintaining their competency at the highest level possible and avoiding harming the evaluee (nonmaleficence), who is the person to whom the life care planner is ultimately ethically responsible.

Qualifications

The ethical dilemmas in this section concern the principles of integrity, nonmaleficence, and autonomy. There is substantial overlap among the ethical standards in codes of ethics of the disciplines feeding into the specialty of life care planning. The life care planner must be aware of any differences in the codes pertaining to their practice and transparency in retainer letters or other documents where the life care planner clearly identifies which standards predominate where there may be a conflict. An example of an ethics statement in a retainer letter could read:

> Ethics Statement: In forensic practice, ABC, Inc. abides by the DEF *Code of Ethics* (GHI Commission, 2022), those of the JKL and MNO professional organizations. Should there be any discrepancy between the codes, the provisions of the DEF code predominate.

Concurrent with awareness of the professional ethical codes of practice, the principle of integrity dictates not only those actions a life care planner takes within a case, but also how the professional presents their qualifications and credentials to the public. Only the highest-held degree associated in life care planning is advertised. For example, if a life care planner has a doctoral in the

Table 5.5 Competency

ETHICAL DILEMMA	ADVISORY OPINION
What do you do when a physician colleague testifies that in their opinion only nurses and physicians are qualified to author life care plans, as they have the appropriate medical background? (Mitchell et al., 2012c)	The specialty practice of life care planning is recognized as a transdisciplinary practice for a number of professionals. Each person's educational background and work experience provides a unique set of skills and experiences that they bring to their life care planning practice. The life care planning process follows a methodology that can be broadly applied across disabilities and conditions. Life care planners often lack awareness of the full scope of the education and experience of other life care planners when the primary profession is different from their own. It is important for life care planners to inform themselves about the education of their peers and demonstrate respect for all disciplines who do the work.
Often, I am on the opposing side of a local life care planner who I believe does extremely poor work. She is certified as a life care planner but her reports do not reflect the basic tenets taught in life care planning training programs or of the credential. It is unclear if the work product reflects incompetence or the intention to inflate costs to satisfy referral sources. At what point should I report a peer? (Mitchell et al., 2008d)	The standards of practice for our varied professions do not offer recommendations on when a life care planner should report the work product of a peer if it is considered to be of poor quality. The work product needs to be the focus of your concerns. It is important to inform your referral source of the pertinent standards of practice of life care planning. This, along with your critique of the work product, can illuminate the poor work quality of the opposing life care planner.
I have worked on cases where I think the opposing life care planner develops a plan that is largely biased by the referral source. I have seen many exaggerated recommendations on plaintiff plans and significant omissions and cost cutting on defense plans. At what point is it just a bad life care plan and when does it breach ethical standards? (Mitchell et al., 2020a, 2021a)	Life care planners come from different educational and clinical backgrounds, which can impact not only their individual scope of practice and work experiences, but also ultimately the items they include in their life care plans. Share your concerns with the referral source. The opposing attorney working with an expert witness, like a life care planner, also has ethical responsibility to assure that all relevant facts are provided to the life care planner and no misrepresentations are made. Standards of practice are clear that life care planners must maintain objectivity. Life care planners should be mindful that it is not their job to please their referral source, but rather to develop a life care plan that is safe and reasonable. Recommendations that breach standards of care or present harm to the evaluee deserve a different consideration. You should consider the report of another life care planner when the recommendations are dangerous or egregious; this should not be done to air a grievance with or disparage another life care planner. Unless the situation presents imminent harm to the evaluee, confidentiality and/or other issues may require waiting until the case is settled to submit or discuss details regarding a potential ethical violation.

(Continued)

Table 5.5 (Continued)   Competency

ETHICAL DILEMMA	ADVISORY OPINION
The night before my deposition, I read in the testimony transcript of another damages team member reference to a neuropsychology evaluation that was not a part of the records I received. In my call to the retaining counsel on my way to the deposition, he stated, "You did not have it because I did not want you to have it." I believe the neuropsychology report as represented in the other witness's testimony would have definitely changed my life care plan. How do I handle this situation? (Mitchell et al., 2018c)	If the opposing attorney notes the missing report in the questions asked, and depending on the questions during the deposition, you must be forthright about the fact that you were not provided this report and that it is possible your review of this record could change your opinion. You should not state that it will change your opinion, as you cannot draw any conclusion without reviewing the evaluation. Prior to changing your opinion however, you must carefully review the referenced neuropsychology report outside of the deposition setting. It is important to reserve the right to read and analyze new information in an unpressured environment. Our standards provide clear guidelines that our work should be accurate and unbiased. It is your professional obligation to provide a valid and reliable life care plan. As noted, it is prudent to have a standard part of your narrative report state that you reserve the right to change your opinions if other information becomes available.
The retaining plaintiff attorney asked that I not consult with the evaluee's treating doctor as this is not required in that jurisdiction. Is not consulting with the treating physician an ethical violation? (Mitchell et al., 2012b)	It is important for your competency as a life care planner to have adequate foundation for items included in the life care plan. You must also understand the rules governing the jurisdiction in which you practice. The input of other health professionals is needed for foundation beyond your scope of practice. Treating physicians and therapists are often the ideal consultants to the process. The attorney who retained you may have valid reasons for this request as there are times when the input of members of the treatment team is inappropriate. If for whatever reason, the treating physician cannot be used, medical foundation for the plan is still needed for items beyond your scope of practice.
I continue to practice in my clinical field as I grow my life care planning business. For my formation in the specialty, I obtained the requisite certification and continue to participate in continuing education specific to my clinical work. Is there a concern if I choose not to attend educational programs focused on forensics or life care planning? (Mitchell & Barros-Bailey, 2010)	It is important for life care planners to remain current in life care planning. Competence in our primary profession contributes to the foundation of our life care plans but does not necessarily assure competence in life care planning. While it may not be a serious breach of ethics, non-attendance at continuing education specific to life care planning or forensic work is training poor business practice.

(Continued)

Table 5.6 Qualifications

ETHICAL DILEMMA	ADVISORY OPINION
I received my certification as both a CLCP™ (Certified Life Care Planner) and a CNLCP® (Certified Nurse Life Care Planner) years ago, but I never renewed them. Is it okay that I continue to use those acronyms after my name? I did everything to apply for and earn those credentials. (Mitchell et al., 2019a)	An awarded credential may only be used during the valid time period of the certification/license. If you fail to recertify or renew your certification you must immediately stop using the credential designation. The misuse of credentials is a clear violation of our standards of performance and ethical standards. Individuals who continue to use a credential beyond its expiration should be reported to the certifying board. The fraudulent use of credentials will likely have a negative impact on one's professional reputation.
As a nurse, I hold two certifications in life care planning: Certified Life Care Planner and Certified Nurse Life Care Planner. I maintain active memberships with the International Academy of Life Care Planners and the American Association of Nurse Life Care Planners. Both organizations/certifications have their own standards of practice and ethical guidelines. If there are differences between these standards and guidelines, how do I provide the best service and protect myself from potential ethical infractions? (Mitchell et al., 2016c)	It is the responsibility of life care planners to understand all applicable scope and standards of practice as well as ethical guidelines pertinent to their practice. Examples of conflicts in the standards could include the life care planner providing dual roles such as case management, legal nurse consulting, vocational rehabilitation training, or placement for the evaluee for whom a life care plan is developed. It is prudent for the life care planner to address such conflicts in the standards openly and directly as a part of the business practice. If conflicts exist and these present an ethical dilemma, it may be best to use an ethical decision-making process. Ultimately, it will be important to document your personal resolution to the conflict of standards in your case acceptance letter, fee agreement, or case file should this become fodder for questions at deposition or trial.

history of music, but a master's in occupation therapy, they would not use the title "Dr." in their life care planning practice as history of music is not a closely related field to the disciplines qualified to enter and form independent scopes of practice in life care planning, although occupational therapy is such a discipline.

Relationships with Other Professionals

Because life care planners work in transdisciplinary teams in clinical or forensic practice, sometimes issues arise with their peers, colleagues, or with adjunct professionals who are members of the treatment or damages team that might call into question boundaries, competencies, confidentiality, and research and publication.

Respecting Colleagues

Although each of these ethical dilemmas are very different, the underlying value in each scenario is one of respect—for the other professional and to the process.

A competent, ethical, and secure life care planner does not have to advance in their practice by disparaging a colleague. It can be uncomfortable to be on the receiving end of disparaging remarks and work product critiques. Barros-Bailey and Neulicht (2006) explained the difference between the terms disparaging and critique. Disparaging remarks are personal attacks on the person's character, immutable characteristics, or other such factors that have little to do with what the person did in their life care plan analysis and conclusions. In other words, these remarks tend to be portrayed in the vernacular as "cheap shots," are unprofessional, and can be fodder for an ethical complaint. A critique, on the other hand, does not focus on the person per se, but the work product; it is a written response to a body of work that made its way into the forensic and professional arena from academia where such debate is expected for the advancement of scholarship and advancing critical and creative thought. The four ethical dilemmas in this section illustrate different sides of these two concepts.

The third ethical dilemma where the life care planner received a review of their life care plan most concretely addresses where a critique ends, and a disparaging remark begins and embodies the principle of fidelity. If the life care planner has used sound methodological practices and feels certain about their assessment outcome, although the critique might be uncomfortable and feel like a vicious attack, if the focus is on the work product and not an on the life care planner, it is not necessarily unethical but a role and function of the life care planner practicing in an adversarial forensic arena. The fine line between the two definitions not only marks whereby a response from an opposing life care planner is measured, but is also a guideline for the authoring life care planner providing a peer review of a plan or while assisting a referral source to query the planner's bases and methodological approaches to the assessments, findings, conclusions, and opinions as in the fourth dilemma.

In the first ethical dilemma where there is an overt attempt to wrestle a case from a colleague who has already been retained and with whom the vocational life care planner consults is not only potentially unethical based on the professional's code of ethics, but can also be a poor business decision as the planner's actions could be interpreted by the retaining and retained party as unprofessional, conniving, and desperate. Whatever the expert may say in the process of trying to detour the case can be interpreted as disparaging if it is a personal attack. It is always easier to establish a reputation than to turn a negative one around; thus, misdirected short-term "marketing" efforts could blow back and result in long-term impacts on the expert's reputation and ability to work with other colleagues on future cases. Respect for professional boundaries in the life care planning context is advisable.

Lastly, in the second scenario where the life care planner is hired as a testifying consultant whose reputation will be affected by the contents of the plan who bears the planner's name, the contracting party must respect the professional boundaries inherent in that relationship. Safeguarding one's work product against changes but allowing for comments for later discussion between the life care planning professionals equalizes the power differential as well as the level of authorship and content responsibility. Contracting agreements should clearly identify the level of final review editing before a life care plan is published to the referral source to protect both parties and avoid the introduction of bias by either contracting entity.

Table 5.7 Respecting Colleagues

ETHICAL DILEMMA	ADVISORY OPINION
I frequently provide referrals to vocational experts (VEs) for those aspects of the case outside of my scope of practice. I learned that one individual has tried to persuade referral sources to use him instead of me on cases, although I have already been retained. Is this behavior an ethical breach by the VE, or just poor business practice? (Mitchell et al., 2018b)	Our standards of practice consistently promote positive relationships, professionalism, and integrity. This act by the vocational expert, is an exploitation of your professional relationship.
In subcontracting life care planning work with a local case management/life care planning company, my work product was edited and submitted before I received the final copy. The editing went beyond typographical errors to foundational content such as replacement frequencies that amplified plan costs. My name is on the report but it does not accurately represent my research or opinions. What should I do? (Mitchell et al., 2008c)	You will have a record of the foundation of the plan in your file. This must agree with your plan. It is clear that changing your work product in terms of pricing and replacement schedules is unethical; this must be addressed promptly with the company for whom you subcontract. The report must be changed to accurately reflect your research and opinions. To guard against changes in your work product, it is highly advised that you learn to password protect your report before sending anything electronically.
I just received a report written by the defense life care planner viciously attacking my plan. This has happened many times with the same life care planner. When does the criticism of another person's work cross the line? At what point is this unprofessional or unethical? (Mitchell et al., 2017b)	It can be painful and even embarrassing to have our work critiqued in a written and public forum. However, a boundary is crossed when the life care planner is attacked rather than the work or methodology. Such statements can be considered disparaging remarks. Life care planners can minimize criticism by using well-established and accepted methodology, staying within their scope of practice, and using consistency as they develop life care plans. A life care planner retained to review another's life care plan must be mindful that critiques should be focused on the work, the methodology, and conclusions of the opposing life care planner rather than a personal attack about the value of the person.
Is there an ethical problem when a life care planner assists an attorney with deposition questions for the opposing life care planner? Does this make the life care planner an advocate? How far should we go to "rip apart" the opposing life care plan/life care planner? (Mitchell et al., 2011a)	To educate and assist the retaining attorney in preparing deposition and/or trial questions, it is common practice in litigation for life care planners, consultants, and others to review the plans and opinions of the opposing attorney's expert witnesses. It is important, however, to be professional and objective when providing this service. The critique should be a review of the life care planner's education and training as well as the methodology and contents of the life care plan. The review should be based on

(Continued)

Table 5.7 (Continued)   Respecting Colleagues

ETHICAL DILEMMA	ADVISORY OPINION
	clinical practice guidelines, published protocols and tenets, and standards of practice; analysis should never be personal or mean-spirited. It is imperative for life care planners to be clear on the distinction between the role of a consultant in a case versus the role of a retained expert witness. Fellow life care planners should be treated with respect and not critiqued in a disparaging manner.
I was hired to develop a life care plan by a defense attorney. When I arrived at the evaluee's home the plaintiff life care planner was present to monitor the evaluation. I had no previous knowledge this would occur. The opposing expert introduced me as "the enemy." Is this an ethical violation? (Mitchell et al., 2019b)	While the plaintiff's introduction may have been an attempt to lighten the mood, it may have had unintended negative consequences for you and your work on the case. Even if it was meant in jest, the statement is not objective, and can be seen as harassing and disparaging because it characterizes you based on who hired you, not your work product. This can be a violation of our ethical standards. It is important to try to determine the intent in the moment. It may be important to have a private conversation with the other expert to clarify your roles and expectations. Inform your retaining attorney of the incident. Should this happen again, it may be necessary to terminate the evaluation, then follow through with the retaining attorney and certifying body.

Confidentiality

Keeping something private or secret comes along a continuum from that which is protected under the law—called privilege—and that which is required by codes of ethics in helping professions except in circumstances that could provide harm, which is called confidentiality. Life care planners practice in both clinical and forensic settings where the interplay of different parties in a case may result in different expectations for the life care planner along this continuum. Because confidentiality is typically one of the areas of greatest publication in the helping professions, it is not surprising that the Ethics Interface Panel has addressed it in several dilemmas presented by life care planners.

Confidentiality, Privilege, and Privacy

Privilege communication is a legal concept and does not exist for life care planners in forensic cases. Consequently, life care planners should be aware that the information they obtain during their primary data collection, such as interviews with the evaluee, their family, or providers, can be queried under oath. If the life care planner is part of the damages team, any information obtained during the evaluation process relevant to other parts of the case—such as liability or damages—is fair game, so the life care planner needs to determine why that or any other kind of information is

Table 5.8 Confidentiality, Privilege, and Privacy

ETHICAL DILEMMA	ADVISORY OPINION
I was retained in my first defense case to peer review a life care plan and possibly develop my own plan. In an unrelated social situation, I was introduced to plaintiff's counsel on the same case and mentioned we were on opposing sides. When I mentioned the interaction to my retaining attorney, she was furious. What did I do wrong and why? Who is it okay to talk to and who is off limits in these cases? (Mitchell et al., 2006, 2008b)	When working on a case, it is important to know if you are retained as a consultant or as an expert. If you are retained as a consultant, the attorney has the right to not reveal your involvement in the case. If you are retained as an expert, your name is still considered confidential until such time as discovery dictates when your retention is disclosed. Confidentiality covers all aspects of the case, including your retention. Do not disclose the name of the patient/client to any party, without a release by the evaluee. If the opposing attorney attempts to retain your services on a case you already are engaged with, but your name is not disclosed, it is not necessary to explain the nature of the conflict or the reasons for the conflict when you do not take a case.
I continue to work clinically in a rehabilitation hospital in my profession. A defense attorney asked for my services on a case. His client had been injured in an accident and had been a patient at my facility. I received permission from the administration at the hospital to work on the case. However, I overheard a conversation between two nurses regarding the manner in which the accident of this evaluee occurred—information that would be very valuable to the defense retaining counsel. Do I have a conflict in this case? (Mitchell et al., 2007)	Information about a patient that is obtained from any source in the health care workplace is protected by the Health Insurance Portability and Accountability Act of 1996 (HIPAA). Not only are you under no obligation to share the information with your retaining attorney; you cannot breach the confidentiality of your hospital work setting. It is important to understand the difference in your role as a life care planner and as a consultant to the case. As a life care planner, you have been retained and brought into the case to address the issue of damages, not liability. Liability concerns do not have a place in your role as a life care planner unless you feel the conversation you heard will compromise your ability to provide an unbiased life care plan. In that instance, do not take the case.
I frequently have other experts on the same damage team assigned to a case contact me by e-mail. I am uncomfortable with the informality and content of some of these communications. What should go in an e-mail and what is off limits? What are the ethics of e-mail communications for the life care planner? (Mitchell et al., 2008b)	Information received and remitted online is the same as a hard copy. A question sometimes arises about the privacy and security of e-mails. If a subpoena or court order requests copies of those e-mails, they could be obtained without too much effort from various servers if they no longer reside on the life care planner's inbox or trash bin. The next question that arises is whether the work product is protected. It is best to assume that e-mail is not protected, although this may vary per jurisdiction.

(Continued)

Table 5.8 (Continued) Confidentiality, Privilege, and Privacy

ETHICAL DILEMMA	ADVISORY OPINION
I just completed a plaintiff interview where I learned that the plaintiff is selling his opioid medications. How should I proceed? (Mitchell et al., 2015d)	This is a serious claim, so you must first assess the credibility of the information you obtained and how you obtained it prior to determining how to proceed. Did you properly inform the plaintiff that any of the information provided you might not be confidential? The retaining attorney may elect to have you refrain from writing a report and discontinue your services, but it is you, and not the retaining attorney, who must determine if the information is relevant to your life care plan. It is your responsibility to draft an unbiased report that includes any credible information you have that affects the plaintiff's life care plan.
Who are the parties I can talk to when working on a forensic life care planning case? (Mitchell et al., 2009b)	In the United States, the Health Insurance Portability and Accountability Act (HIPAA) Privacy Rule provides guidance regarding records and documents.
I was retained to develop a life care plan for a teenager with a spinal cord injury. During the interview, the evaluee disclosed they believed they were transgender and contemplated transition. This information has been shared with friends, however, the medical and legal communities, as well as the parents were apparently unaware of the circumstance. While this may or may not impact the contents of the life care plan, I want to be respectful in my report with the use of correct pronouns. How should I proceed? (Mitchell et al., 2017d)	Unless life care planners are very new to their primary professions, it is unlikely their educational backgrounds have prepared them to appropriately address the transgender population, as the mainstream public and professional discourse on this topic is relatively new. Beyond the use of the correct pronoun, there are many issues to consider when developing a life care plan for someone who presents as transgender. Provisions within our standards prohibit any type of discrimination toward an evaluee, including gender and sexual orientation. Lack of knowledge may be considered a type of discrimination in that it may not be possible to provide correct and/or adequate provisions for the life care plan. During the disclosure and informed consent process, at the time of the formal evaluation with the teen, the life care planner should cover the confidentiality rules under which the assessment is taking place, including the limits of such confidentiality. With this new information, it will be important to disclose to the evaluee your role in the assessment and the need for disclosure of the information to the retaining attorney who is the advocate for this young individual.

relevant. Disclosure of those limits into the content of an interview can easily be addressed during the disclosure and informed consent process (autonomy), so the evaluee understands topics that might be on or off the table to discuss.

Confidentiality, however, does exist for the life care planner, regardless of clinical or forensic practice setting. Not only is it likely covered in the professional code of ethics for the planner's clinical code, but also it is an expectation within forensic practice. For those in clinical practice, their respective professional codes will provide guidance. For those in forensic settings, members of the Section of Litigation of the American Bar Association (ABA) adopted the *Guidelines for Retention of Experts by Lawyers* (ABA, 2011). Although the standards did not pass the ABA general assembly, the document's approval by the Section provides a glimpse into how attorneys view confidentiality in litigated cases with the following standard:

> The lawyer must assure that the expert treats any information received or work product produced by the expert during an engagement as confidential, and secure an understanding from the expert that he or she shall not disclose any such information except as required by law, as retaining counsel shall determine and advise, or with the consent of the client.
>
> (ABA, 2011, p. 4)

Therefore, the extent of confidentiality to maintain in a case is one that is delineated by the retaining source and the life care planner's professional organizations. In some cases, the retained expert may need to sign a confidentiality or gag agreement about anything associated with the case that might have a higher level of protection beyond basic confidentiality. Confidentiality has its limits, however, in circumstances where the individual can cause harm to themselves or others. Indeed, if the life care planner observes issues of neglect and eminent or egregious harm to the evaluee, under *Tarasoff* case law (1974), adopted by most—if not all—professional codes of ethics in the helping professions, in most jurisdictions it is the life care planner's duty to warn the appropriate authorities or parties of such neglect (Ewing, 2005).

Records

Hard copy or digital records are how life care planners review, record, document, and report their process, observations, findings, conclusions, and opinions. Guidelines of how to ethically perform this process including maintaining or disposing of relevant documents, could come from internal policy guidelines, your retainer agreement, the referral source, the jurisdiction, professional or credentialing organizations, or regional or national laws or statutes. Therefore, to manage these documents ethically and legally, the life care planner must be aware of each guideline that controls the maintenance and transfer of the records upon case termination, or the incapacity or death of the life care planner. Ultimately, the safeguard and disposal of these records is associated with autonomy and nonmaleficence ethical principles.

Remote Assessment

Post COVID-19, the acceptance of remote mechanisms for life care planning assessment has increased. Barros-Bailey et al. (2022) performed a survey of remote life care planning practice and found that, while convenient, in more complex or complicated matters, if there is a choice between performing the assessment remotely or on-site and it is practical, the latter would be

Table 5.9 Records

ETHICAL DILEMMA	ADVISORY OPINION
My concern is the proper and ethical way to dispose of medical records provided with the referral. Is it adequate to remove the person's name from the records and dispose of the rest in a recycling bin? (Mitchell et al., 2010a, 2011c)	When a person files a lawsuit, they waive their right to medical privilege. However, depending on the jurisdiction, medical records in civil cases may still be protected by HIPAA. Privacy laws are likely to continue and become even more restrictive. It seems clear from various guidelines that life care planners need to responsibly destroy medical records to maintain the confidentiality of their evaluees.
Recently, one of my life care planning single-practice colleagues with a vibrant practice passed away. Neither the referral sources reaching out to me to take over the development of life care plans nor I know how to obtain copies of the working records of my deceased colleague. What is my responsibility as a life care planner and single practitioner regarding record maintenance and retention should I become impaired to practice or pass on? (Barros-Bailey, 2010)	This whole topic calls attention to how records are kept and maintained and the notification of the parties as well as an In Case of Emergency (ICE) policy and provision that could be included in disclosure to clients/evaluees as well as referral sources.
I was advised that the case I worked on settled and I was directed to "shred the records." Does this pertain to my own working file? If I keep these, is this a violation of our standards? (Mitchell et al., 2022b).	Official guidelines will vary by the jurisdiction relative to a specific case. Often, there are professional conduct rules for attorneys. "Specific rules may also apply to other professions. For those who are covered under the Health Insurance Portability and Accountability Act (HIPAA Journal, 2021), records retention is for a minimum of six (6) years from the time the record was created (CFR §164.316(b)(1))" (Mitchell et al., 2022b, p. 53). Follow the direction of your retaining attorney and shred the records that were provided to you. It is likely a wise business decision to keep a copy of your report as it is your personal work product, or any documents you may want to use in the future to defend a potential malpractice claim or to explain a particular decision. Check the law of your state to determine the limitation period for malpractice actions, and retain the records beyond that time to assure they are available in the event a claim is filed. It is, of course, critical that any records are destroyed in a manner that assures confidentiality.

Table 5.10 Remote Assessment

ETHICAL DILEMMA	ADVISORY OPINION
I am a life care planner with a medical condition that currently makes it difficult for me to travel. I would like to develop a life care plan and do my evaluation with the use of technology rather than visit the person in their home. As a part of the assessment I typically do my own testing, some of which must be done face-to-face. Do our standards of practice address our ability to perform remote assessments? (Mitchell et al., 2020b)	Life care planners are required to perform a comprehensive evaluation, preferably face-to-face. Life care planning consensus statement number 73 says, "Life Care Planners shall conduct an in-person interview whenever permitted." It is likely an evaluation will be less complete if not done in the person's home; the physical accessibility and condition of a person's home as well as family interactions can provide the life care planner valuable information that may be lost using a telephone or video format. The life care planner's ability to administer tests typically performed during an in-person assessment may be greatly limited, if not impossible. While there may be some remote options for testing, validity and proctoring issues must be addressed; reliable testing results are critical. If available, life care planners should be aware of guidelines for remote testing as provided by their primary profession. The impact of reduced or absent testing should be disclosed in the report. There are a variety of reasons why it may be difficult to perform an in-person assessment at a given time, e.g., there may be a very significant inconvenience to the evaluee or the life care planner. At other times, critical health concerns for either party may be an issue or an opposing attorney may not allow the assessment. Most recently, physical distancing constraints have challenged all life care planner's typical methodologies. Discuss with your referral source the reason you are unable to conduct an in-person assessment and suggest solutions. Make every effort to ascertain confidentiality and security in your chosen method of technology. The use of various technology platforms may challenge not only the evaluee but also the life care planner; those with less technology knowledge and experience are likely to find this arrangement more frustrating. Plan extra time for technology adjustments and be mindful of potential equipment limitations of the evaluee. Obtain a phone number at the beginning of the session in the event of technology failure. Be sensitive to potential cultural groups that may distrust technology or possibly fear being recorded. The need for an interpreter may necessitate programming that allows for three parties. It will be important to be transparent in your report about the reasons an assessment was conducted remotely and how that may have limited/impacted the evaluation. If feasible, conduct a face-to-face assessment at a later date.

preferrable to avert omissions in observations. Many professional organizations have provided guidelines to practitioners to safeguard the ethical delivery of services through digital means. Absent the ability to perform an on-site assessment, best practices dictate that the life care planner become aware of these guidelines for ethical remote assessment while also learning techniques to gather relevant data needed for the assessment (e.g., having evaluee/family member walk the house to demonstrate the home's condition and allowing the life care planner to record that part of the session).

Legal Issues in Forensic Ethics

Life care planning is highly specialized, as are the environments in which life care planners practice, especially in forensics. These environments sometimes place life care planners in ethical situations that are thorny to navigate from a legal perspective and could create demands that result in the life care planner acting illegally. The following ethical dilemmas are illustrative of two such circumstances encountered by life care planners.

Someone's legal responsibility is the gold standard guideline in ethical behavior. Perjury violates the ethical principles of integrity and fidelity, and could result in criminal charges. If the attorney's request is inappropriate, it places the life care planner in a compromising legal position, and should be rejected.

Similarly, except for most government documents that are in the public domain, most publications protect intellectual property through copyright. That means that the life care planner cannot make copies of the documents and provide them to another party without the permission of the copyright holder or risk violating copyright law. If parties are interested in getting copies of copyrighted materials relied upon by a life care planner, that planner can provide a list of references whereby the soliciting party can obtain them on their own.

Whether in reports or in publications, any use of another life care planner's intellectual property, such as copying sections of an article, chapter, book, software, or a report in another case and adopting the same exact terminology as your own without giving credit or attribution to the author for each and every citation infringes upon the author's intellectual property and is an ethical conflict of fidelity.

Research and Publications

Research and publications advance practice and innovation, keep a discipline vibrant, and apprise professionals of changes in medical, rehabilitation, and life care planning practice. Although this area of ethical dilemmas may be distant for some life care planners, for others who may be emerging or engaging in their interest in research and writing, the dilemma presented covers important points in protecting intellectual property.

Life care planners typically come into the specialty from clinical rather than research or academic disciplines where these kinds of ethical issues may arise. Yet, contributing to the field through publication helps advance the specialty and a life care planner's practice.

Attention to the order of authorship arose out of the publish-or-perish stressors of academics who need to demonstrate scholarship through research, publications, and professional engagement to rise through the tenure ladder. The pressures of achieving tenure might cause some academics to place their names as first authors on publications where their students or mentees did the majority of the work, therefore, violating issues of integrity and nonmaleficence as it appropriates the student's intellectual property for the sake of status and financial gain of the academic or mentor. In practice, names on publications are normally listed in the order of greatest contribution to least while those who do not contribute to the publication are not listed. Having the idea of the research or publication, having greater experience or professional status, or some other hierarchal factor is insufficient reason to have a name listed first in a publication, presentation, or similar activity. Similarly, those who are listed as senior authors should not expect those who are listed as subsequent authors to do more work than them; to do so could result in issues of maleficence to those given inadequate credit for their contribution.

Ethics in Life Care Planning ■ 147

Table 5.11 Legal Issues in Forensic Ethics

ETHICAL DILEMMA	ADVISORY OPINION
I was referred a case in which I was the second life care planner retained. The first planner did an extensive report that the attorney decided not to use due to scope of practice concerns—she had learned the life care planner had been found to lack credibility in other cases and wanted a fresh report. The first life care planner's report was within the referral documents, but I was requested to not disclose that I had seen the prior plan if asked while under oath. Is this an ethical request? (Mitchell et al., 2021b).	The attorney is asking you to perjure yourself; willfully telling an untruth when under oath is quite simply wrong.
Today I received a subpoena duces tecum requesting I bring to my deposition a variety of materials I relied upon that are protected by copyright including articles, books, software, and psychometric instruments. How do I legally and ethically handle copyrighted materials but also comply with the subpoena? (Mitchell et al., 2016b)	The codes of ethics for life care planners require obeying the law and copyright laws are no exception. Unless the materials requested are in the public domain or permission from the copyright holder has been obtained, peer-reviewed research articles, books, theses/dissertations, and other such materials contain intellectual property that is typically covered by copyright law. Sharing these materials is illegal and against any code of ethics that is central to a life care planner's practice. Life care planners can share these materials with the permission of the copyright holder or with a court order demanding distribution of the requested resources. Those items not covered by copyright, within the public domain (e.g., government data), or allow for partial dissemination under Creative Commons or open source publications, as well as the internet link to the sources, can be shared in a bibliography. A life care planner may be requested to provide copyrighted materials as part of a subpoena duces tecum (subpoena which requests documents) in a court action. A subpoena is a court order but issued only by an attorney. Court rules generally provide an opportunity for an objection when the subpoena requires disclosure of "privileged or other protected material" (Federal Rule of Civil Procedure 45(d)(2)(B) — state rules may vary.) Because copyrighted material is protected under the law, the life care planner should not produce copyrighted material until after an objection is entered and a court overrules the objection. At that point, the life care planner should provide the materials to the court for copying, without making copies themselves. This protects both the life care planner from an unethical act of breaching the copyright, and provides the copyright holder with some protection by assuring the material is copied only for use in court proceedings.

Table 5.12 Research and Publications

ETHICAL DILEMMA	ADVISORY OPINION
I recently participated in a research project with several people, and we want to publish the findings in our professional journal. One of the senior members of the group thinks the authors should be listed alphabetically, but individual efforts varied greatly. I invested a lot of time in the project and my name falls at the end of the alphabet. Are there ethical standards that address this issue? (Mitchell et al., 2022a)	Journals vary in their approach and publication protocol, so one needs to know the procedures of the particular journal. Certain journals may mandate an author's CRedIT (Contributor Roles Taxonomy), which allows for detailed information on each author's contributions. It is expected that all contributors will have reviewed and approved the submission for accuracy. Other journals require written confirmation that all authors take responsibility for the contents of the submitted work. Within codes relevant to professions typically feeding into life care planning, the stance is that the issue should be dealt with in advance and principal contributors should be listed first.

Business Practices

Business practices are those that the life care planner engages in to run a business operation and contains such components as fee setting to determine income and finances to cover business operations, marketing operations, accounting, and other business systems. One of the fundamental areas of decision-making is that associated with fees, which is the area of business practices where life care planners—particularly those new to the specialty—have a lot of questions.

Fees

Compensation in life care planning, particularly when performed in a medico-legal setting, can present potential ethical dilemmas, to the point that this it is not only addressed in ethical codes from professional organizations, but also from legal codes of ethics. The ABA has the *Model Rules of Professional Conduct* (2019) that directly address this issue in Rule 3.4 (b) which prohibits counsel from assisting "a witness to testify falsely, or offer an inducement to a witness that is prohibited by law" (para. 2). The ABA's Section of Litigation *Guidelines for Retention of Experts by Lawyers* (ABA, 2011) is even more explicit: "Contingent Compensation of Experts in Litigated Matters: No lawyer may offer compensation that is contingent on the outcome of litigation" (p. 8). Many state bar associations either use the ABA Rule or have similar provisions in their codes of ethics. Therefore, neither should a referral source offer a bonus for the positive outcome of a case or be requesting that the life care planner take a reduction in their invoice for the negative outcome of a case, nor should colleagues offer or accept kickbacks for referrals. In each instance, the potential tarnish to the life care planner's reputation for implied or explicit financial conflicts of interest overriding the main tenet of objectivity could have enduring problematic consequences.

Reporting Ethical Violations

The question of whether to file an ethical complaint against a colleague can be anxiety-provoking. Many of the recommendations in ethical decision-making models of how to resolve an ethical

Table 5.13 Fees

ETHICAL DILEMMA	ADVISORY OPINION
I am a life care planner who works mostly in the state/province of my residence. I recently was in court in another state and testified on the same day as another member of the damages team who provided expert testimony on the injured person's earnings losses. He offered to potentially refer me more cases for a percentage of my fees on the referred work. (Mitchell et al., 2012a)	Some decisions are related to ethics and others are primarily business in nature. It is critical to the standards of our field that the opinion of the life care planner field not be compromised by the referral source. Paying money or a "kick back" to a referral source may present an appearance of impropriety. Any appearance of impropriety could result in reduced credibility of the life care plan and ultimately harm the person who is the subject of the life care plan. Whether to accept work from this source is a business decision as well as an ethical one. It is crucial that a life care planner analyze how a "kick back" would appear if this had to be defended in testimony. There should be no influence or appearance of influence by a referral source.
After a successful settlement, the retaining plaintiff attorney wanted me to issue him an additional bill for "file consultation services" because the settlement exceeded what he anticipated and he wanted to show his appreciation. Am I wrong to accept this type of "bonus?" (Mitchell et al., 2015a)	The ethical standards are clear: It is wrong to accept this bonus as it can be perceived as affecting our ability to provide unbiased, objective opinions depending on the outcome of a case.
I was recently asked by an attorney to take a reduction on my bill because the case was lost at trial. The law firm is an important referral source and I want to stay in their good graces. Is there an ethical problem with me providing a discount? (Mitchell et al., 2009a)	Life care planners should not enter into financial commitments that may compromise the quality of their services or raise questions as to their credibility. Payment should never be contingent on outcome or awards.
Please address ethical pricing and billing practices for life care planners. (Mitchell et al., 2013b)	The fee structure for life care planning services can vary greatly between individuals and even between regions of the country. This in itself is not a problem but it is important to have a fee agreement that clearly spells out fees and payment arrangements, preferably signed by the referral source. Life care planners should also not enter into financial commitments that may compromise the quality of their services or otherwise raise questions as to their credibility. A life care planner must consider how the appearance of a specific practice may be viewed by the opposing attorney, the judge, or jury.

dilemma can likewise be used when a life care planner attempts to determine if an ethical threshold has been surpassed by another practitioner and what to do about it.

In ethical proceedings, a life care planner who is defending an ethical complaint will usually have the complaint adjudicated by a group of peers. Therefore, a life care planner who suspects

Table 5.14 Reporting Ethical Violations

ETHICAL DILEMMA	ADVISORY OPINION
I am certified as a life care planner working on the opposing side of another life care planner with the same credential. During the course of the opposing life care planner's work on a case, I believe an ethical standard was breached. What is my responsibly to report this alleged ethical breach to the certifying agency? Should the legal case be resolved prior to such reporting? Should I just ignore this behavior? (Mitchell et al., 2017a)	The issue should be discussed with the retaining attorney. While standards of our various professions vary greatly in the amount of detail addressing this issue, almost universally there is an obligation to report an ethical breach. The timing of reporting potential ethical violations is a more complex issue that may vary depending on the severity of the issue and potential harm that may occur as a result of the breach. Engage in a decision-making process using a model that includes consultation with others as appropriate to the situation. Document the decision-making process and ultimate decision you choose, and avoid the appearance or intent to influence the outcome of the case.

an ethical breech by a colleague may consult with peers while maintaining the privacy and confidentiality of the case specifics and the offending colleague as well as consult with the retaining source. The peer consultation should not only be with colleagues who they believe would be sympathetic to their point of view, but those who could help them see other perspectives and traverse the issues.

Some adjudicating boards want to verify that the professional filing the complaint has followed a due process procedure. The first step of this procedure involves the life care planner contacting the colleague to make them aware of the ethical issue with attempts to resolve it at that level before submitting a formal complaint to the professional or credentialing board. If a case is active and prolonged, it may be some time before that due process conversation could take place. Should the behavior be egregious, it may be necessary to file the ethical complaint directly and usurp the normal due process procedure. Because there are always two sides to an ethical complaint, it is normal that about 50% of complaints are discontinued once both sides of a situation are examined by an ethics committee.

Summary and Conclusion

No life care planner is free of ethical dilemmas in practice. This chapter provides a comprehensive review of the known literature in life care planning, including pivotal definitions used in the specialty that might be different than terminology a life care planner may use in their predominant profession. It further attempts to clarify the difference between standards of care that are anchored in legal tenets and standards of practice that are affixed to best practices in the specialty. Similarly, an attempt to bridge theoretical concepts of professional ethics, particularly principle and virtue ethics, and how these apply to life care planning is made through actual ethical dilemmas presented in the literature and made practice through advisory opinions offered by a panel of experienced life care planners from various disciplines.

Note

1 *Keywords*: "life care plan*", "ethic*"
   Databases: Academic OneFile; ACM Digital Library; Business Insights: Global; Cabell's Directory of Published Opportunities; Child Welfare Information Gateway; Choice Reviews; Chronicle of Higher Education Online; Consumer Health Complete; CQ Researcher; Dissertations & Theses Full Index; EBSCO; Educator's Reference Complete; Europeana; Gale; JSTOR; OSTI.GOV; Oxford Reference Online; PubMed (Medicine); PubMed Central Archive of Life Science Journals; Sage Journals; Sage Knowledge; SAGE Research Methods; Science Direct; UNData; US Government Documents Catalog of US Government Publications; Web of Science; World Bank Open Data

References

Albee, T., Gamez, J. N., & Johnson, C. B. (2018). 2017 life care planning summit proceedings. *Journal of Life Care Planning*, *16*(4), 201–211.

American Academy of Nurse Life Care Planners. (2015). *Ethics in nurse life care planning: The AANLCP code of ethics and conduct*. www.aanlcp.org/ethics-in-nurse-life-care-planning-the-aanlcp-code-of-ethics-and-conduct/

American Academy of Physician Life Care Planners. (2014). *Ethics and professional conduct*. https://aaplcp.org/About/Ethics.aspx

American Bar Association, Section of Litigation. (2011). *Guidelines for retention of experts by lawyers*. https://nysba.org/NYSBA/Sections/Commercial%20Federal%20Litigation/Com%20Fed%20PDFs/ABA%20proposal%20on%20experts%20011412.pdf

American Bar Association. (2019). *Rule 3.4: Fairness to opposing party & counsel*. www.americanbar.org/groups/professional_responsibility/publications/model_rules_of_professional_conduct/rule_3_4_fairness_to_opposing_party_counsel/

Barnao, M., Robertson, P., & Ward, T. (2022). Ethical decision making and forensic practice. *The British Journal of Forensic Practice*, *14*(2), 81–91. https://doi.org/0.1108/14636641211223648

Barros-Bailey, M. (2010). Ethics interface. *Journal of Life Care Planning*, *9*(3), 119–122.

Barros-Bailey, M. (2017). Cultural experience and international practices of life care planners: Results of an exploratory research study. *Journal of Life Care Planning*, *15*(2), 7–12.

Barros-Bailey, M. (2018). Cultural considerations for life care planning. In R. O. Weed & D. E. Berens (Eds.), *Life care planning and case management handbook* (4th ed., pp. 833–841). Routledge. https://doi.org/10.4324/9781315157283-36

Barros-Bailey, M. (2020). Life care planning report writing foundations, standards, methods, and ethics: Development of a checklist. *Journal of Life Care Planning*, *18*(2), 69–79.

Barros-Bailey, M., & Neulicht, A. (2006). Understanding disparaging remarks in ethics. In *Commission in Rehabilitation Counselor Certification. Ethics for Rehabilitation Counselors, Program II* (pp. 7–9). CRCC.

Barros-Bailey, M., Carlisle, J., Graham, M., Neulicht, A. T., Taylor, R., & Wallace, A. (2008, 2009). Who is the client in forensics? [White paper]. Published in: *Estimating Earning Capacity*, *1*(2), 132–138; *Journal of Forensic Vocational Analysis*, *12*(1), 31–33; *Journal of Life Care Planning*, *7*(3), 125–132; *Journal of Rehabilitation Administration*, *33*(1), 59–64; *The Rehabilitation Professional*, *16*(4), 253–256; *Rehabilitation Counselors & Educators Journal*, *2*(2), 2–6; *Vocational Evaluation and Career Assessment Professionals Journal*, *5*(1), 8–14.

Barros-Bailey, M., Knott, M., Neulicht, A. T., Mitchell, N., Albee, T., Robinson, R., Riddick-Grisham, S., & Marcinko, D. (2022). *Results of the 2021 survey of remote life care planning practice: Pandemic edition*. [Manuscript submitted to publication.]

Beauchamp, T. L., & Childress, J. F. (2001). *Principles of biomedical ethics* (5th ed.). Oxford University Press.

Berens, D. E. (2018a). 2006 life care planning summit/town hall meeting: A celebration of life care planning … 10 years later. *Journal of Life Care Planning*, *16*(4), 95–96.

Berens, D. E. (2018b). Life care planning summit 2004: The progress continues. *Journal of Life Care Planning*, *16*(4), 81–84.

Berens, D. E. (2018c). Summary of the life care planning summit 2002. *Journal of Life Care Planning*, *16*(4), 47–50.

Berens, D. E., & Weed, R. O. (2018). *Ethical issues for the life care planner.* In R. O. Weed, & D. E. Berens (Eds.), *Life care planning and case management handbook* (4th ed., pp. 691–700). Routledge.

Blackwell, T. L. (1995). Ethical principles for life care planners. *Inside Life Care Planning*, *1*(2), 1, 9.

Cavalier, R. (2002). *Online guide to ethics and moral philosophy.* Carnegie Mellon University. http://caae.phil.cmu.edu/cavalier/80130/part2/II_preface.html

Cimino-Ferguson, S. (2005). Multiple relationships in the field of life care planning. *Journal of Life Care Planning*, *4*(1), 11–16.

Commission on Rehabilitation Counselor Certification. (2017). *Code of professional ethics for rehabilitation counselors.* Author. https://crccertification.com/wp-content/uploads/2023/01/2023-Code-of-Ethics-1.pdf

Deutsch, P. M., Allision, L., Berens, D., Corcoran, J. R., Gisclair, B., McKinley, L., Neulicht, A. T., Preston, K., Shaw, L., Sutton, A., Wirt, S., & Yuhas, S. (2018). Proceedings of the life care planning summit 2004, Atlanta, GA, April 24–25, 2004. *Journal of Life Care Planning*, *16*(4), 85–94.

Ewing, C. P. (2005). Tarasoff reconsidered. *Judicial Notebook*, *36*(7). www.apa.org/monitor/julaug05/jn#:~:text=In%201985%2C%20the%20California%20legislature,injury%20upon%20a%20reasonably%20identifiable

Gamez, J. N., & Johnson, C. B. (2017). Why should you attend the 2017 life care planning summit? *Journal of Life Care Planning*, *15*(1), 41–43.

Gibbs, R. L., Rosen, B. S., & Lacerte, M. (2013). Published research and physiatric opinion in life care planning. *Physical Medicine and Rehabilitation Clinics of North America*, *24*, 553–566. https://doi.org/10.1016/j.pmr.2013.03.002

Gonzales, J. G., & Zotovas, A. (2014). Life care planning: A natural domain of physiatry. *PM&R*, *6*, 184–187. https://doi.org/10.1016/j.pmrj.2014.01.011

Howland, W. (2013a). Conflict of interest. *Journal of Nurse Life Care Planning*, *13*(2), 61–62.

Howland, W. (2013b). Possible invalid credential. *Journal of Nurse Life Care Planning*, *13*(4), 137.

Howland, W. (2014a). An issue with a vendor. *Journal of Nurse Life Care Planning*, *14*(1), 8–9.

Howland, W. (2014b). Fixed-rate life care plans, a conflict? *Journal of Nurse Life Care Planning*, *14*(3), 591–592.

Howland, W. (2014c). Rush job, iffy documents? *Journal of Nurse Life Care Planning*, *14*(4), 725–726.

International Academy of Life Care Planning. (2022). *Standards of practice for life care planners* (4th ed.). International Association of Rehabilitation Professionals.

International Association of Rehabilitation Professionals. (2018). Life care planning summit 2000. *Journal of Life Care Planning*, *16*(4), 19–45.

International Commission on Health Care Certification. (2015). *Code of professional ethics.* www.ichcc.org/images/PDFs/ICHCC_StandardsandGuidelines_2018.pdf

Johnson, C. B. (2012). The 2012 life care planning summit: Third time is a charm. *Journal of Life Care Planning*, *16*(4), 187–192.

Johnson, C. B. (2015a). 2015 life care planning summit: Moving forward and looking ahead. *Journal of Life Care Planning*, *16*(4), 193–199.

Johnson, C. B. (2015b). Consensus and majority statements derived from life care planning summits held in 2000, 2002, 2004, 2006, 2008, 2010, 2012, and 2015. *Journal of Life Care Planning*, *13*(4), 35–38.

Johnson, C. B., Lacerte, M., & Weed, R. (2011). Canadian life care planning summit 2011 proceedings. *Journal of Life Care Planning*, *10*(3), 3–24.

Johnson, C. B., Pomeranz, J. L., & Stetten, N. E. (2018a). Consensus and majority statements derived from life care planning summits held in 2000, 2002, 2004, 2006, 2008, 2010, 2012, 2015, and 2017 and updated via Delphi study in 2018. *Journal of Life Care Planning*, *16*(4), 15–18.

Johnson, C. B., Pomeranz, J. L., & Stetten, N. E. (2018b). Life care planning consensus and majority statements, 2000–2018: Are they still relevant and reliable? A Delphi study. *Journal of Life Care Planning*, *16*(4), 5–13.

Kulich, S. J., & Chi, R. (2014). Values clarification. In A. C. Michalos (Ed.), *Encyclopedia of quality of life and well-being research.* Springer. https://doi,org/10.1007/978-94-007-0753-5_3563 https://link.springer.com/referenceworkentry/10.1007/978-94-007-0753-5_3563#citeas

Manzetti, C., & Howland, W. (2013). Patient, client, or? *Journal of Nurse Life Care Planning, 13*(2), 58–60.

Mertes, A. (2018). Content analysis of the research priorities in the *Journal of Life Care Planning* 2004–2017. *Journal of Life Care Planning, 16*(2), 3–9.

Metekingi, J. P. (2013). An introduction to evidence-based practice for the nurse life care planner. *Journal of Nurse Life Care Planning, 13*(3), 88–92.

Mitchell, N., & Barros-Bailey, M. (2010). Ethics interface. *Journal of Life Care Planning, 9*(1), 53–54.

Mitchell, N., Apuna, D., Barros-Bailey, M., & Simmons-Grab, D. (2015a). Ethics interface. *Journal of Life Care Planning, 13*(1), 33–35.

Mitchell, N., Apuna, D., Barros-Bailey, M., & Simmons-Grab, D. (2015b). Ethics interface. *Journal of Life Care Planning, 13*(2), 33–38.

Mitchell, N., Barros-Bailey, M., & Simmons-Grab, D. (2015c). Ethics interface. *Journal of Life Care Planning, 13*(3), 65–69.

Mitchell, N., Apuna, D., Barros-Bailey, M., & Simmons-Grab, D. (2013a). Ethics interface. *Journal of Life Care Planning, 12*(1), 75–76.

Mitchell, N., Apuna, D., Barros-Bailey, M., & Simmons-Grab, D. (2013b). Ethics interface. *Journal of Life Care Planning, 12*(2), 91–92.

Mitchell, N., Apuna, D., Barros-Bailey, M., & Simmons-Grab, D. (2012a). Ethics interface. *Journal of Life Care Planning, 11*(2), 43–44.

Mitchell, N., Apuna, D., Barros-Bailey, M., & Simmons-Grab, D. (2012b). Ethics interface. *Journal of Life Care Planning, 11*(4), 33–34.

Mitchell, N., Apuna, D., Barros-Bailey, M., & Simmons-Grab, D. (2012c). Ethics interface. *Journal of Life Care Planning, 10*(4), 49–53.

Mitchell, N., Apuna, D., Barros-Bailey, M., & Simmons-Grab, D. (2011a). Ethics interface. *Journal of Life Care Planning, 10*(3), 57–60.

Mitchell, N., Apuna, D., Barros-Bailey, M., & Simmons-Grab, D. (2011b). Ethics interface. *Journal of Life Care Planning, 10*(2), 21–24.

Mitchell, N., Apuna, D., Barros-Bailey, M., & Simmons-Grab, D. (2011c). Ethics interface. *Journal of Life Care Planning, 10*(1), 47–49.

Mitchell, N., Apuna, D., Barros-Bailey, M., & Wallace, A. (2006). Ethics interface. *Journal of Life Care Planning, 5*(4), 203–204.

Mitchell, N., Apuna, D., Barros-Bailey, M., & Wallace, A. (2007). Ethics interface. *Journal of Life Care Planning, 6*(1&2), 61–62.

Mitchell, N., Apuna, D., Barros-Bailey, M., & Wallace, A. (2008a). Ethics interface. *Journal of Life Care Planning, 7*(1), 27–29.

Mitchell, N., Apuna, D., Barros-Bailey, M., & Wallace, A. (2008b). Ethics interface. *Journal of Life Care Planning, 7*(2), 85–87.

Mitchell, N., Apuna, D., Barros-Bailey, M., & Wallace, A. (2008c). Ethics interface. *Journal of Life Care Planning, 7*(3), 153–155.

Mitchell, N., Apuna, D., Barros-Bailey, M., & Wallace, A. (2008d). Ethics interface. *Journal of Life Care Planning, 7*(4), 203–206.

Mitchell, N., Apuna, D., Barros-Bailey, M., & Wallace, A. (2009a). Ethics interface. *Journal of Life Care Planning, 8*(1), 57–59.

Mitchell, N., Apuna, D., Barros-Bailey, M., & Wallace, A. (2009b). Ethics interface. *Journal of Life Care Planning, 8*(3), 135–138.

Mitchell, N., Apuna, D., Barros-Bailey, M., & Wallace, A. (2009c). Ethics interface. *Journal of Life Care Planning, 8*(4), 207–208.

Mitchell, N., Apuna, D., Barros-Bailey, M., & Simmons-Grab, D. (2015a). Ethics interface. *Journal of Life Care Planning, 13*(1), 33–35.

Mitchell, N., Apuna, D., Barros-Bailey, M., & Simmons-Grab, D. (2015b). Ethics interface. *Journal of Life Care Planning, 13*(2), 33–38.

Mitchell, N., Barros-Bailey, M., & Simmons-Grab, D. (2015c). Ethics interface. *Journal of Life Care Planning, 13*(3), 65–69.

Mitchell, N., Barros-Bailey, M., & Latham, S. (2015d). Ethics interface. *Journal of Life Care Planning, 13*(4), 55–57.

Mitchell, N., Barros-Bailey, M., & Latham, S. (2016a). Ethics interface. *Journal of Life Care Planning, 14*(1), 97–100.
Mitchell, N., Barros-Bailey, M., & Latham, S. (2016b). Ethics interface. *Journal of Life Care Planning, 14*(2), 47–48.
Mitchell, N., Barros-Bailey, M., & Latham, S. (2016c). Ethics interface. *Journal of Life Care Planning, 14*(3), 59–62.
Mitchell, N., Barros-Bailey, M., & Latham, S. (2017a). Ethics interface. *Journal of Life Care Planning, 15*(1), 37–40.
Mitchell, N., Barros-Bailey, M., & Latham, S. (2017b). Ethics interface. *Journal of Life Care Planning, 15*(2), 49–51.
Mitchell, N., Barros-Bailey, M., & Latham, S. (2017c). Ethics interface. *Journal of Life Care Planning, 15*(3), 45–53.
Mitchell, N., Barros-Bailey, M., & Latham, S. (2017d). Ethics interface. *Journal of Life Care Planning, 15*(4), 27–31.
Mitchell, N., Barros-Bailey, M., & Latham, S. (2018a). Ethics interface. *Journal of Life Care Planning, 16*(1), 65–69.
Mitchell, N., Barros-Bailey, M., & Latham, S. (2018b). Ethics interface. *Journal of Life Care Planning, 16*(2), 47–50.
Mitchell, N., Barros-Bailey, M., & Latham, S. (2018c). Ethics interface. *Journal of Life Care Planning, 16*(3), 41–45.
Mitchell, N., Barros-Bailey, M., & Latham, S. (2019a). Ethics interface. *Journal of Life Care Planning, 17*(1), 75–79.
Mitchell, N., Barros-Bailey, M., & Latham, S. (2019b). Ethics interface. *Journal of Life Care Planning, 17*(4), 39–41.
Mitchell, N., Barros-Bailey, M., & Latham, S. (2020a). Ethics interface. *Journal of Life Care Planning, 18*(1), 65–68.
Mitchell, N., Barros-Bailey, M., & Latham, S. (2020b). Ethics interface. *Journal of Life Care Planning, 18*(2), 107–112.
Mitchell, N., Barros-Bailey, M., & Latham, S. (2021a). Ethics interface. *Journal of Life Care Planning, 19*(1), 81–91.
Mitchell, N., Barros-Bailey, M., & Latham, S. (2021b). Ethics interface. *Journal of Life Care Planning, 19*(3), 39–43.
Mitchell, N., Barros-Bailey, M., & Latham, S. (2022a). Ethics interface. *Journal of Life Care Planning, 20*(1), 69–72.
Mitchell, N., Barros-Bailey, M., & Latham, S. (2022b). Ethics interface. *Journal of Life Care Planning, 20*(3), 53–55.
Mitchell, N., Barros-Bailey, M., & Simmons-Grab, D. (2015c). Ethics interface. *Journal of Life Care Planning, 13*(3), 65–69.
Mitchell, N., Barros-Bailey, M., Apuna, D., & Simmons-Grab, D. (2010). Ethics interface. *Journal of Life Care Planning, 9*(2), 47–49.
Pettengill, A. (2013). Ethical issues and the Certified Nurse Life Care Planning™ Certification Board. *Journal of Nurse Life Care Planning, 13*(2), 63–65.
Preston, K. (2006). Tools for creating an ethical practice. *Journal of Life Care Planning, 5*(3), 109–114.
Preston, K., & Reid, C. (2015). Revision process for the *Standards of Practice for Life Care Planners*. *Journal of Life Care Planning, 13*(3), 21–30.
Preston, K., Pomeranz, J., & Walker, C. (2018). Life care planning summit 2008 proceedings. *Journal of Life Care Planning, 16*(4), 131–142.
Priebe, M. M., Chiodo, A. E., Scelza, W. M., Kirshblum, S. C., Wuermser, L. A., & Ho, C. H. (2007). Spinal cord injury medicine: Economic and societal issues in spinal cord injury. *Archives of Physical Medicine and Rehabilitation, 88*(Supp. 1), S84–S88.
Reid, C. (2013). Ethical risks of underestimating life expectancy in life care planning practice. *Journal of Life Care Planning, 11*(1), 61–73.
Riddick-Grisham, S. (2003). Life care planning summit 2002. *Journal of Life Care Planning, 2*(2), 57–140.

Riddick-Grisham, S. (2018). 2006 life care planning summit proceedings. *Journal of Life Care Planning*, *16*(4), 97–130.

Savage, T. A. (2011). Ethical and moral issues in caring for children with special needs. In S. Riddick-Grisham, & Deming, L. M. (Eds.), *Pediatric life care planning and case management* (2nd ed., pp. 959–973). Routledge.

Schofield, S., & Huntington-Frazier, M. (2015). Advocacy on trial: Are the nurse life care planner's roles on advocate and expert witness in conflict? *Journal of Nurse Life Care Planning*, *15*(4), 928–932.

Shea, M. (2020). Forty years of the four principles: Enduring themes from Beauchamp and Childress. *Journal of Medicine and Philosophy*, *45*, 387–395.

Tarasoff v. Regents of University of California, 13 Cal. 2d 177, 118 Cal. Rptr. 129, 529. www.lexisnexis.com/community/casebrief/p/casebrief-tarasoff-v-regents-of-univ-of-cal

The Law Dictionary. (n.d.). Standard of care. In *TheLawDictionary.com dictionary*. Black's Law Dictionary. https://thelawdictionary.org/?s=standard+of+care

U.S. Equal Employment Opportunity Commission. (2022). *Who is protected from employment discrimination?* www.eeoc.gov/employers/small-business/3-who-protected-employment-discrimination

Welfel, E. R., & Kitchener, K. S. (1992). Introduction to the special issue: Ethics education – An agenda for the '90s. *Professional Psychology: Research and Practice*, *23*(3), 179–181. https://doi.org/10.1037/0735-7028.23.3.179

Wilson, C. (2016, February 9). *What is metaethics?* https://doi.org/10.11647/OBP.0173.0022

Chapter 6

Multicultural and Cross-Cultural Considerations for Life Care Planning

Mary Barros-Bailey

Culture \ˈkəl-chər\ is a noun and is defined as:

> the beliefs, customs, arts, etc. of a particular society, group, place, or time; a particular society that has its own beliefs, ways of life, art, etc.; a way of thinking, behaving, or working that exists in a place or organization.
> (Merriam-Webster, 2022b, para. 1)

Sometimes, culture can be limited by ethnicity, country, or area of origin, or other descriptive variables. In general terms, however, ethnicity or geography are only two of the potential delimiters of culture. Any unit of people in any society or region that share common beliefs, lifestyles, ethnicity, or customs can be a cultural group.

Culture is the root term for two other important related definitions that carry the underlying structure of this chapter: multicultural and cross-cultural. Using Merriam-Webster (2022c), multicultural is defined as, "relating to or including many different cultures" (para. 1) within a society no matter regional or national boundaries such as the culture of people with disabilities, the culture of allied health professionals in any country, the culture of First Peoples, or the culture of ex-patriots living abroad. The concept of multiculturalism is that the multitude of cultures is contained *within* a single society. The more cultures contained in such a society, the more heterogeneous that society is in its beliefs, customs, arts, or other variables. Cross-culturalism, on the other hand, involves the interaction of people *between* more than one society instead of a single society or country. Using the Merriam-Webster (2022a) source again, cross-culturalism is defined as, "relating to and involving two or more different cultures or countries" (para. 1). Cross-cultural relationships may be when a person or group from one country interacts with an individual or group located in another country. As it involves life care planning, the terms used in this chapter are as follows:

Multicultural: the life care planner provides services nationally within the country of residence and the evaluee/client/patient/family comes from a different culture than the planner's (e.g., a life care planner in Canada develops a life care plan for a refugee residing in Canada).

Cross-cultural: the life care planner provides services for the evaluee/client/patient in another society than their own main country of practice (e.g., a life care planner in the United States [U.S.] develops a life care plan for a South Korean national in the evaluee/client/patient's country of residence).

Therefore, if the life care planner and the evaluee/client/patient are within the same dominant culture, like a country, and the services are to be delivered within that dominant society, but the life care planner and the evaluee/client/patient come from two different cultures, it is multicultural life care planning. However, if the life care planner is to develop and/or deliver services across societies, regardless of whether the life care planner and the evaluee/client/patient come from the same or different culture, the fact that the life care planner will be interacting with individuals in other societies makes the relationship a cross-cultural one. Sometimes, in the latter example, this is called international life care planning.

Foundations of Multicultural and Cross-Cultural Issues in Life Care Planning

The body of the life care planning literature that directly addresses issues of culture in practice is nascent and emerging (Caragonne, 2016; Cosby, 2016; Phillips, 2016). It is explored along with calls for the consideration of cultural issues in practice within the seminal literature in the field.

There are some foundational documents and studies that allude to the knowledge of culture in practice. First, Pomeranz et al. (2010) performed a role and function study of life care planners to "help define a profession and provide an empirical basis for establishment of educational standards and certification requirements" (p. 57). As part of their study, they included the knowledge of multicultural issues within a composite question that also involved knowledge of family dynamics and geographical issues. This area was included in the needed knowledges required in Counseling and Services—or, the domain that included those "items that represent the process of helping individual and/or family/caregivers adjust to the psychological and/or behavioral impact of disability" (p. 113). The International Commission on Health Care Certification (ICHCC™), in their most recent role and function study, had a similar question about the application of "knowledge of family dynamics, gender, multicultural, and geographical issues" (May & Moradi Rekabdarkolaee, 2020, p. 44).

Second, there are practice and ethical standards that include the consideration of cultural issues. For a discussion of ethics involving cultural issues, see the Ethics in Life Care Planning chapter. One of the six standards of performance outlined in the *Standards of Practice for Life Care Planners* (Preston, 2022) is that the life care planner "… considers cultural and linguistic factors that may influence assessment, development, and implementation of the plan" (p. 14), with a practice competency being that the life care planner "recommends care that is culturally appropriate" (p. 14). Specific to the broader professions from where life care planners may come, respective credentialing and professional bodies contain provisions for cultural considerations in practice. For nurse life care planners, for example, the standards of practice of the professional organization for all nurses, the American Nurses Association, addresses consideration of "cultural preferences, beliefs, and spiritual and health practices in plans of care" (Cosby, 2016, p. 13). In credentialing, the ICHCC™ for those in the US and Canada notes in its *Practice Standards and Guidelines* (2015) the adoption of a code of ethics that rests upon other codes, such as that of Commission on Rehabilitation Counselor Certification (2023), that clearly outline the consideration of cultural issues in clinical and forensic practice.

Missing from the collection of professional consensus statements in life care planning is culture. The summits for life care planners from 2000 to 2018 (Johnson, 2015; Johnson et al., 2018; Preston & Johnson, 2012) identified consensus on a variety of majority statements dealing with qualifications, professional and ethical standards, and methodological principles and procedures, with contributions from the American Association of Nurse Life Care Planners (AANLCP®); American Association of Legal Nurse Consultants; Care Planner Network; Commission on Disability Examiner Certification (now ICHCC); Commission on Health Care Certification (now, ICHCC™); Case Management Society of America; Foundation of Life Care Planning Research; Georgia State University; Intelicus; International Academy of Life Care Planners (IALCP); International Association of Rehabilitation Professionals (IARP); IARP-Canada; University of Florida; and, Vocational Rehabilitation Association of Canada (VRA). None of the 96 statements directly addresses cultural issues in life care planning.

Regardless of the scant treatment of the topic within the role and function studies, in standards of practice, or in consensus statements, it is a fact that life care planners face multicultural and cross-cultural issues in life care planning. In their survey of life care planners and their processes and methods, Neulicht et al. (2010) asked respondents if they had provided services in the international arena in the preceding five years. A total of 25 (11.26%) respondents indicated providing life care planning in such a setting. The 2022 updated decennial practice survey data for this area of practice are not available at the publishing of this text. However, given the ever increasing movement of people across borders, results may show that there is a strong likelihood that life care planners who choose to do international life care planning will have more opportunity to perform life care planning in various countries.

Barros-Bailey (2017) performed exploratory research on multicultural and cross-cultural issues in life care planning by collecting data from life care planners who are members of AANLCP®, IALCP, IARP, and the Life Care Planner Network. The results of the study suggested that in the multicultural area, the most significant issues encountered by life care planners were in communication; family; access/use of medical, mental health, or related care; housing; and advocacy. In cross-cultural life care planning, the most significant issues identified were in the access/use of medical, mental health, or related care; providers; legal services; cost resources; communication; society; and referral source education. Therefore, it appears that from a multicultural framework, life care planners are more concerned with relational and contextual factors whereas from a cross-cultural perspective life care planners are more concerned with resources for the life care plan development and only secondarily with the relational and contextual issues.

Multicultural and Cross-Cultural Issues in Life Care Planning

When considering the fundamental concepts in life care planning involving culture, it is important to explore definitions about cultures and adaptation to cultural values and tenets.

Individualistic and Collectivistic Cultures

Conceptually, if the life care planner understands the difference between the two types of societal structures, it may greatly assist in the approach, understanding, development, and delivery of services across all types of cultures over the lifespan. The concept of life care planning, or what has been known in Canada as a Cost of Future Care Plan (Phillips, 2016), was developed in cultures that are considered individualistic, namely, the US. The definition of an individualistic culture is one where "the culture focuses on the individual's needs and looks for happiness on an individual level before looking to the group" (Reference*, 2016b, para. 1). In contrast, collectivistic cultures are those that "emphasize family and work group above individual needs or desires" (Reference*, 2016a, para. 1). Individualistic cultures are found in countries including Australia, Belgium, Canada, Ireland, Israel, New Zealand, Poland, Slovakia, South Africa, Sweden, the US, and the United Kingdom. Collectivistic cultures are found in countries including Argentina, Brazil, Egypt, Ethiopia, Ghana, India, Japan, Korea, Mexico, Portugal, Russia, and Saudi Arabia.

How people cooperate (Boles et al., 2010; Marcus & Le, 2013; Nguyen et al., 2010), practice professionally (Shilo & Kelly, 1997), are treated over the lifespan (North & Fiske, 2015), and even their ethical behavior (Ralston et al., 2014), can be correlated with the type of society (i.e., collectivistic or individualistic) from which they come. If life care planners can comprehend the socially constructed views of their evaluees/clients/patients and how those differ from their own, it becomes the first step in bolstering potential areas of agreement or understanding conflict in life care planning.

Acculturation and Enculturation

At least in the US, which has been described as an individualistic country that has one of the most diverse societies on the planet, the merging of individualistic and collectivistic cultures over time has been studied. Results suggested that long term, there were no differences among the immigrant cultures in cultural assimilation (Vargas & Kemmelmeier, 2013). The adjustment process is dynamic and can happen in the short term or over generations. This process is often referred to as acculturation.

Formally, acculturation is "the process of adopting the cultural traits and social patterns of another group" (Dictionary.com, 2022, para. 1). This definition assumes that an individual started off in one culture, is being exposed to another culture, and is adopting some of the traits of the second culture. The distinction is different than when someone is born into a culture and undergoes the process of learning about their own culture, which is called enculturation. Various acculturation models exist, but they generally involve how well someone is integrated or assimilated into the dominant culture or retains remnants of their own culture, and may also suggest whether the individual is segregated or marginalized by their own or dominant culture or society.

The level of someone's acculturation can affect how the individual communicates with those within the culture, or with other cultures. Members of a family can have various levels or rates of acculturation. Where someone lives, the kind of housing they choose, or the members within the household itself can be affected by the level of acculturation. Further, how diverse members of a culture advocate for themselves or their loved ones can also be affected by acculturation. Important to life care planning is what health, mental health, other care or related services someone considers, participates in, or administers. This, too, can be substantially impacted by the level of acculturation of the evaluee/client/patient, caregiver, partner, or the family.

Consequently, in multicultural matters, understanding the level of acculturation of the evaluee/client/patient, as well as understanding one's own level of acculturation to the specific subculture, is a good second step to assessing the dynamic context in which the practitioner operates. Assessing someone's level of acculturation could be done informally first through the review of the secondary data in the records that might provide evidence as to these issues, and more directly through primary data collection as a part of the life care planning diagnostic interview and observation. If more formal assessment measures are necessary to determine someone's level of acculturation, a variety of instruments exist. Celenk and Van de Vijver (2011) for example, summarize approximately 50 such tools that could be used with different populations.

Life Care Planner Cultural Competence

Beyond understanding the level of acculturation of the evaluee/client/patient and their immediate support system, it is also important that the life care planner understand their own level of cultural competency. The competency standards for professional practice are outlined by a variety of organizations including those in counseling and psychology (Yoon et al., 2011), nursing (American Association of Colleges of Nursing, 2011; Beard et al., 2015), and social work (National Association of Social Workers, 2001) to name a few. Like tools to measure someone's level of acculturation, there are also a number of instruments that could be useful for a life care planner to test their level of cultural competency. One resource that may be helpful is the National Institutes of Health's (NIH) *Tools for Assessing Cultural Competence* (NIH, National Library of Medicine, 2014). This resource includes direct access to tools including the *Self-Assessment Checklist for Personnel Providing Services and Supports to Children and Youth With Special Health Needs and Their Families* and the *Multicultural Competent Service System Assessment Guide*. However, a query on an online search engine provides a multitude of cultural competency checklists and guidelines specific to the many cultural groups the life care planner may encounter in an individualized assessment.

To enhance cultural competence with regards to recommendations in life care plans, there is an emerging body of critical appraisal literature on cultural issues in treatment approaches, such as psychosocial interventions for burn patients and caregivers (Williams et al., 2020). To find additional literature and resources, please refer to the Life Care Planning, Costing, Literature, and Summary of Resources chapter in this text.

Multicultural and Cross-Cultural Communication

Given that communication was the greatest concern for life care planners identified in the Barros-Bailey (2017) study, specific discussion of communication—whether oral, bodily, or written—becomes important when addressing multiculturalism. In its simplest form, communication comes down to information that is expressed and received. How the information or thought is encoded by one individual and decoded by another individual becomes increasingly complex when both people come from different cultures. The complexity is due to how the context, words, or actions affect how the life care planner and evaluee/client/patient or caregiver intend to communicate and how that intent is interpreted.

MindTools (2016) describes the 7Cs of communication that may be helpful to the life care planner to ensure expression and reception of information not only with evaluee/client/patients and caregivers, but also with service providers, care team members, or others involved in the process. The 7Cs are: 1) Clarity of message; 2) Conciseness by sticking to the message and keeping it simple and brief; 3) Concreteness of the message by giving a clear picture and presenting vivid facts; 4) Correctness of the message and keeping it free of errors; 5) Coherent messages are those that are logical and points are connected together; 6) Complete messages that include what the evaluee/client/patient or caregiver needs to be informed about in order to make decisions; and, 7) Courteousness of the message so that it is honest and friendly.

Communication would be incomplete if the provision of translation and interpretation within the life care planning process were not addressed. Both words are used almost as synonyms, but they are different based on the medium used. In translation, it is text that is being transferred from one form of communication to another while interpretation is the oral transfer. Taking a medical record from one language to another is a translation. However, the individual in a medical appointment who takes the medical information from the physician and provides it in sign or other language to the patient is an interpreter. Typically, in life care planning, most practitioners will more frequently use interpreters rather than translators. Under the cultural and linguistic Standards of Performance of the fourth edition of the *Standards of Practice for Life Care Planners*, a practice competency states that life care planners should "use qualified interpreters" (Preston, 2022, p. 14). Best practices in using an interpreter (Refugee Health Technical Assistance Center, 2016) as adapted to life care planning include:

- Introducing self to interpreter
- Acknowledge interpreter as the professional communicator
- Speak to the evaluee/client/patient, not the interpreter
- Slow down the rate of speech so the interpreter can catch the totality and intent of what is being communicated
- Speech should be broken up into short segments and be at an even pace
- Assume everything being said is being interpreted
- Do not hold the interpreter responsible for what the evaluee/client/patient says or does not say

Understand that some concepts in one language have imprecise or nonexistent equivalents in another language; therefore, describing a concept in more than one way or asking for clarification from the evaluee/client/patient to ascertain understanding may be necessary

Give the Interpreter Time to Relate Information from Both Parties

What may be personal or sensitive in one culture may not be so in another; therefore, be aware of the potential sensitive issues that might be important to explore through an interpreter in a variety of different modes of communication to obtain the information that is needed for the life care plan:

- Avoid complex language or concepts; keep the communication clear and simple
- Encourage the evaluee/client/patient, caregiver, or interpreter to ask questions
- Avoid patronizing or minimizing the evaluee/client/patient
- Paraphrase, paraphrase, paraphrase to ensure you understand what the evaluee/client/patient is expressing and that the evaluee/client/patient interprets your communication correctly
- Allow extra time for the communication process, including a session with the interpreter beforehand that might provide insights about the communication

Professional interpreters are advised where there are linguistic differences. In situations where there may not be a professional interpreter and others may be used (e.g., friend, family member, community advocate), professional ethics should be the cautionary filter. This helps to verify that the evaluee/client/patient or caregiver understands the intent, purpose, or question and, in return, to confirm the life care planner's understanding of the information being expressed and collected.

With tools to effectively understand, measure, and interpret multicultural issues, the life care planner can best navigate the specific factors that may be present in the development of a plan. They may be better able to address social issues in the family and their relationship to the development and delivery of the life care plan, access and use of medical, mental health, or other care, advocacy or lack thereof, adequate housing or transportation, or any number of factors that may be present in the delivery of services.

Communication between cultures within a society may not be materially different than those in a cross-cultural setting. The difference may be that multiculturally, the life care planner and evaluee/client/patient may be speaking the same language and the concepts being communicated may be the same or similar. The life care planner and evaluee/client/patient may have been born in the same society, speak the same language, and have similar understandings of personal, geographical, societal, and other constructs, procedures, programs, or other factors although attitudes, beliefs, values, and customs may be different. In cross-cultural communication, the life care planner may be attempting to communicate in a society they have no or limited information about, even if the life care planner has lived in that society. Not only the language and ethnic or social culture may be different, but also everything associated with the life care planner's culture that impacts the development or management of the life care plan may also be different. Therefore, the issues of communication cross-culturally may be more complex than they are multiculturally. The level of life care planner cultural competency, therefore, becomes more important in a cross-cultural setting. The 7Cs of communication and the best practices identified previously are just as relevant in a cross-cultural environment. The life care planners must have greater awareness of the customs, attitudes, beliefs, and values of the society in which they develop the life care plan.

Methodological Framework for Cross-Cultural/International Life Care Planning

No methodological frameworks were found specific to developing multicultural life care plans. The first and only methodological framework found in the literature considering any kind of culture is for the development of life care plans in the cross-cultural or international context. In describing life care planning in such a setting, Caragonne (2016) states, "to be valid and truly useful post litigation, a plan must exactly fit the cultural and healthcare infrastructure of the country where it will be used" (p. 18). Dr. Caragonne goes on to detail a useful nine-stage process for developing a cross-cultural life care plan including:

Stage 1: Initial request for work: Determinations to be made
Stage 2: Plan translations
Stage 3: Planner and subject safety
Stage 4: Plan research
Stage 5: Skills and familiarity in equipment and services for disability
Stage 6: Plan documentation and transparency
Stage 7: Physician, nursing, and paraprofessional validation
Stage 8: Researching quantitative databases
Stage 9: Representing services available through federal health systems

Not only does Dr. Caragonne provide an important framework for the development of a life care plan cross-culturally, but also a multi-stage process that could be modified to the development of a life care plan in a multicultural context. With its introduction into the literature, it throws open the door to the discussion of guidelines, procedures, and methods in the development and delivery of life care planning services multiculturally and cross-culturally. Forefront in this process are emerging critical appraisal resources that life care planners use. For example, clinical practice guidelines have been developed with cultural and international comparison approaches, such as for cryptogenic stroke (Bray et al., 2019) or pediatric gastroesophageal reflux disease (Harris et al., 2022), while recent research demonstrates a movement toward international clinical practice guidelines for the treatment of some populations such as children or youth with cerebral palsy (Jackman et al., 2022; Morgan et al., 2021) or post-traumatic stress disorder (Ennis et al., 2020).

Conclusion

Perhaps because the specialty of life care planning is relatively new, just now entering its fifth decade, and has been preoccupied with activities relevant to the establishment of the specialty practice across a host of different rehabilitation and allied health professionals, cultural factors in life care planning have not enjoyed much attention, deliberation, and discussion in the professional literature until 2016. Mertes (2018) performed a content analysis of the *Journal of Life Care Planning* from 2004–2017 and identified the following as part of the research priorities:

- Topics related to the creation of plans, legal proceedings, and expert witnessing: … Impact/importance of family wishes (and cultural beliefs) on life care planning.
- Topics of the efficacy of plans, including reliability studies, meaning assessing the outcomes of the plans or planning process: … Explore the relationship between geographic location and cultural diversity of life care planners and clients (p. 5).

Yet, no further research on multicultural or cross-cultural issues was found since the 2019 publication of this chapter, although it is evident that such matters are facing life care planners on a regular basis. It is time to begin this discussion and to delve deeply into those elements life care planners should be aware of in practice, whether these be within multicultural or cross-cultural contexts.

Much of the literature in the field focuses on the medical/mental/cognitive, functional, development, resource, or other immediate issues for the dominant culture. However, if someone is not a member of that culture, this presents the life care planner with a host of quandaries of how to develop a life care plan or manage one that is individualized to the evaluee/client/patient. This updated chapter starts at a very high level by introducing concepts and definitions into the life care planning literature that may help life care planners understand the underlying dynamics that may be at play when two cultures meet—what kind of society one comes from or ascribes to (individualistic vs. collectivistic), the level of acculturation or enculturation, modes of communication and the use of interpreters in that process, and a methodological framework for the development of a life care plan cross-culturally.

There are more thematic topics that need to be tackled. For example, from a practical standpoint, what resources exist that can be used for the development of plans in these contexts? How are providers and costs located? How does a life care planner effectively educate a referral source about the issues in a case, particularly if these vary from what is common in life care planning where the same cultural questions do not exist? Those who provide life care plans in these contexts have anecdotal and practical experience that can benefit the entire specialty practice of life care planning. A proposed starting point may be to compare how life care plans have been developed within the dominant culture to those developed in multicultural or cross-cultural contexts (e.g., Phillips,

2016). Such an exercise would focus the discussion not only on philosophical or theoretical topics, but also on practice considerations in various life care planning settings. Let the discussion begin.

References

American Association of Colleges of Nursing. (2011). *Tool kit for cultural competence in master's and doctoral nursing education.* www.aacnnursing.org/Portals/42/AcademicNursing/CurriculumGuidelines/Cultural-Competency-Grad-Tool-Kit.pdf

Barros-Bailey, M. (2017). Cultural experience and international practices of life care planners: Results of an exploratory research study. *Journal of Life Care Planning, 15*(2), 7–12.

Beard, K. V., Gwanmesia, E., & Miranda-Diaz, G. (2015). Culturally competent care: Using the ESFT model in nursing. *American Journal of Nursing, 115*(6), 58–62.

Boles, T. L., Le, H., & Nguyen, H. D. (2010). Person, organizations, and societies: The effects of collectivism and individualism on cooperation. In R. M. Kramer, A. E. Tenbrunsel, & M. H. Bazerman (Eds.), *Social decision making: Social dilemmas, social values, and ethical judgments* (pp. 171–200). Psychology Press.

Bray, E. P., McMahon, N. E., Bangee, M., Al-Khalidi, A. H., Benedetto, V., Chauhan, U., Clegg, A. J., Georgiou, R. F., Gibson, J., Lane, D. A., Lip, G. Y. H., Lightbody, E., Sekhar, Al, Chatterjee, K., & Watkins, C. L. (2019). Etiologic workup in cases of cryptogenic stroke: Protocol for a systematic review and comparison of international clinical practice guidelines. *Systematic Reviews, 8*(1), 1–5. https://doi.org/10.1186/s13643-019-1247-6

Caragonne, P. (2016). Life care planning in Mexico and Latin America. *Journal of Nurse Life Care Planning, 16*(3), 18–23.

Celenk, O., & Van de Vijver, F. (2011). Assessment of acculturation: Issues and overview of measures. *Unit 8 Migration and Acculturation, Subunit 1 Acculturation and Adapting to Other Cultures.* http://scholarworks.gvsu.edu/cgi/viewcontent.cgi?article=1105&context=orpc

Commission on Rehabilitation Counselor Certification. (2023). *Code of professional ethics for certified rehabilitation counselors.* https://crccertification.com/wp-content/uploads/2022/10/2023-Code-of-Ethics.pdf

Cosby, M. F. (2016). Cultural considerations for life care planners: Religious traditions and health benefits. *Journal of Nurse Life Care Planning, 16*(3), 13–17.

Dictionary.com (2022). Acculturation. In *Dictionary.com.* www.dictionary.com/browse/acculturation

Ennis, N., Shorer, S., Shoval-Zuckerman, Y., Feedman, S., Monson, C. M., & Dekel, R. (2020). Treating posttraumatic stress disorder across cultures: A systematic review of cultural adaptations of trauma-focused cognitive behavioural therapies. *Journal of Clinical Psychology, 76*(4), 587–611. https://doi.org/10.1002/jclp.22909

Harris, J., Chorath, K., Balar, E., Xu, K., Naik, A., Moreira, A., & Rajasekaran, K. (2022). Clinical practice guidelines on pediatric gastroesophageal reflux disease: A systematic quality appraisal of international guidelines. *Pediatric Gastroenterology, Hepatology, and Nutrition,* (2), 109–120. https://doi.org/10.5223/pghn.2022.25.2.109

International Commission on Health Care Certification™. (2015). *Practice standards and guidelines.* www.ichcc.org/images/PDFs/ICHCC_StandardsandGuidelines_2018.pdf

Jackman, M., Sakzewski, L., Morgan, C., Boyd, R. N., Brennan, S. E., Langdon, K., Toovey, R. A. M., Greaves, S., Thorley, M., & Novak, I. (2022). Interventions to improve physical function for children and young people with cerebral palsy: International clinical practice guideline. *Developmental Medicine & Child Neurology, 64*(5), 536–549.

Johnson, C. B. (2015). Life care planning summit: Moving forward and looking ahead. *Journal of Life Care Planning, 11*(2), 27–33.

Johnson, C. B., Pomeranz, J. L., & Stetten, N. E. (2018). Consensus and majority statements derived from life care planning summits held in 2000, 2002, 2004, 2006, 2008, 2010, 2012, 2015, and 2017 and updated via Delphi study in 2018. *Journal of Life Care Planning, 16*(4), 15–18.

Marcus, J., & Le, A. H. (2013). Interactive effects of levels of individualism-collectivism on cooperation: A meta-analysis. *Journal of Organizational Behavior, 34*, 813–834.

May, V. R., & Moradi Rekabdarkolaee, H. (2020). The International Commission on Health Care Certification life care planner role and function investigation. *Journal of Life Care Planning, 18*(2), 3–67.

Merriam-Webster. (2022a). Cross-cultural. In *Merriam-Webster.* www.merriam-webster.com/dictionary/cross-cultural

Merriam-Webster. (2022b). Culture. In *Merriam-Webster.* www.merriam-webster.com/dictionary/culture

Merriam-Webster. (2022c). Multicultural In *Merriam-Webster.* www.merriam-webster.com/dictionary/multicultural

Mertes, A. (2018). Content analysis of the research priorities in the *Journal of Life Care Planning* 2004–2017. *Journal of Life Care Planning, 16*(2), 3–9.

MindTools. (2016). *The 7Cs of communication.* www.mindtools.com/pages/article/newCS_85.htm

Morgan, C., Fetters, L., Adde, L., Badawi, N., Bancale, A., Boyd, R. N., Chorna, O., Cioni, G., Damiano, D. L., Darrah, J., de Vries, L. S., Dusing, S., Einspieler, C., Eliasson, A. C., Ferriero, D., Fehlings, D., Forssberg, H., Gordon, A. M., Greaves, S., Guzzetta, A., … Novak, I. (2021). Early intervention for children aged 0 to 2 years with or at high risk of cerebral palsy: International clinical practice guidelines based on systematic reviews. *JAMA Pediatrics, 175*(8), 846–858. https://doi.org/10.1001/jamapediatrics.2021.0878

National Association of Social Workers. (2001). *NASW standards for cultural competence in social work practice.* Author. https://www.socialworkers.org/LinkClick.aspx?fileticket=7dVckZAYUmk%3D&portalid=0

National Institutes of Health, National Library of Medicine, National Center for Biotechnology Information. (2014). *Improving cultural competence: Tools for assessing cultural competence.* www.ncbi.nlm.nih.gov/books/NBK248429/

Neulicht, A. T., Riddick-Grisham, S., & Goodrich, W. R. (2010). Life care plan survey 2009: Process, methods[,] and protocols. *Journal of Life Care Planning, 9*(4), 129–214.

Nguyen, H. D., Le, H., & Boles, T. (2010). Individualism-collectivism and co-operation: A cross-society and cross-level examination. *International Association of Conflict Management and Wiley Periodicals, Inc., 3*(3), 179–204.

North, M. S., & Fiske, S. T. (2015). Modern attitudes toward older adults in the aging world: A cross-cultural meta-analysis. *American Psychological Association, 141*(5), 993–1021.

Phillips, K. (2016). A comparison of Canadian and US life care planning. *Journal of Nurse Life Care Planning, 16*(3), 23–28.

Pomeranz, J. L., Yu, N. S., & Reid, C. (2010). Role and function study of life care planners. *Journal of Life Care Planning, 9*(3), 57–118.

Preston, K. (2022). Standards of practice for life care planners (4th ed.). *Journal of Life Care Planning, 20*(3), 7–23.

Preston, K., & Johnson, C. (2012). Consensus and majority statements derived from life care planning summits held in 2000, 2002, 2004, 2006, 2008, 2010[,] and 2012). *Journal of Life Care Planning, 11*(2), 9–14.

Ralston, D. A., Egri, C. P., Furrer, O., Kuo, M. H., Li, J., Wangenhelm, F., Dabic, M., Naoumova, I., Shimizu, K., Carranza, M. T. G., Fu, P. P., Potocan, M. V., Pekerti, A., Lenartowicz, T., Srinivasan, N., Casado, T., Rossi, A. M., Szabo, E., Butt, A., Palmer, I., Ramburth, P., … Weber, M. (2014). Societal-level versus individual-level predictions of ethical behavior: A 48-society study of collectivism and individualism. *Journal of Business Ethics, 122*, 283–306.

Reference*. (2016a). Collectivist culture. In *Reference*.* www.reference.com/world-view/examples-collectivist-cultures-ac597798cdac77fe

Reference*. (2016b). Individualistic culture. In *Reference*.* www.reference.com/education/individualistic-culture-12e6b48e73cf5fd7

Refugee Health Technical Assistance Center. (2016). *Best practices for communicating through an interpreter.* http://refugeehealthta.org/access-to-care/language-access/best-practices-communicating-through-an-interpreter/

Shilo, A. M., & Kelly, E. W. (1997). Individualistic and collective approaches to counseling: Preference, personal orientation, gender, and age. *Counseling and Values, 41*(3), 253–264.

Vargas, J. H., & Kemmelmeier, M. (2013). Ethnicity and contemporary American culture: A meta-analytic investigation of horizontal-vertical individualism-collectivism. *Journal of Cross-Cultural Psychology, 44*(2), 195–222.

Williams, H. M., Hunter, K., Clapham, K., Ryder, C., Kimble, R., & Griffin, B. (2020). Efficacy and cultural appropriateness of psychosocial interventions for paediatric burn patients and caregivers: A systematic review. *BMC Public Health, 20*(1), 1–16. https://doi.org/10.1186/s12889-020-8366-9

Yoon, E., Langrehr, K., & Ong, L. A. (2011). Content analysis of acculturation research in counseling and counseling psychology: A 22-year review. *American Psychological Association, 58*(1), 83–96. https://doi.org/10.1037/a0021128

LIFE CARE PLANNING ACROSS THE LIFESPAN 2

Chapter 7

Pediatric Care Management in Life Care Planning[1]

Kristi B. Bagnell and Elizabeth Moberg-Wolff

This chapter is adapted from Riddick-Grisham, S. & Deming, L. (Eds.) (2011). *Pediatric life care planning and case management handbook*. Routledge.

Unique Considerations in Pediatric Life Care Planning

According to the U.S. Department of Health and Human Services, Health Resources & Services Administration (HRSA, 2020), children and youth with special healthcare needs (CYSHCN) are defined as those "who have or are at increased risk for chronic physical, developmental, behavioral, or emotional conditions" (p. 1). These individuals are identified as "requiring health and related services of a type or amount beyond that required by children generally" (HRSA, 2020). The most recently available data published by the HRSA in the National Survey of Children's Health reflected that in 2017–2018, approximately 13.6 million children in the United States had a special healthcare need (HRSA, 2020). A wide range of severity and thus specific needs are encountered based upon the child's level of function and medical condition. Survey data from 2017–2018 revealed that functional limitations were evident in 26.6% of these children and 19.9% were documented to consistently and/or significantly be impacted by their health condition(s) (HRSA, 2020). There was also a higher prevalence of children with special healthcare needs diagnosed with mental health conditions. For example, anxiety was nine times greater, and depression was 16 times greater among children with special healthcare needs. Additionally, rates of emergency department (ED) use were nearly 2–3 times higher among children and youth with special healthcare needs in the survey, with 30.8% having at least one ED visit in the past year, and 10.9% with two or more visits (HRSA, 2020).

Since the passage of the Americans with Disabilities Act (ADA) in 1990, further legislation has been implemented in support of persons with disabilities. In the last decade, the Achieving a Better Life Experience Act (ABLE) of 2014 improved the financial stability and employment options for individuals with disabilities by authorizing tax-advantaged savings accounts for youth and adults with disabilities (Achieving a Better Life Experience Act of 2014, 2014). In 2015, the Every Student Succeeds Act (ESSA) reauthorized the Elementary and Secondary Education Act of 1965 and replaced the No Child Left Behind Act of 2001. This legislation has empowered state and local decision-makers to develop their own strong systems for school improvement. It ensures accountability and guarantees that when students fall behind, steps are taken to help them, and their school to improve (U.S. Department of Education, 2015). The ADA has undergone several revisions. In 2016, this included updated guidelines for electronic and information technology, telecommunications products and services, as well as amended regulations for transportation and equal employment opportunity (U. S. Department of Justice Civil Rights Division, 2022).

There is emerging evidence that several factors have led to an increase in life expectancy for individuals with disabilities and thus, the number of these persons within our population. Clearly, respiratory status, gross motor functioning, presence of epilepsy, and cognitive factors, especially as related to neurological injury, are extremely important (Day & Reynolds, 2018). Historically, the quality of care has not properly been accounted for in models of life expectancy. For instance, care for individuals diagnosed with cerebral palsy has been shown in studies to be affected by where they live, the provider that they see, and how their care is financed (Novak, 2014). Furthermore, medical innovations are leading to longer lives in cerebral palsy patients as well as those with other neurocognitive and neuromotor disorders (Lichtblau, 2021).

Children with chronic healthcare needs are diverse, and comprised of all racial, ethnic, gender, and socio-economic backgrounds. Their families are faced with managing an increasingly complex healthcare system and are likely to encounter multiple treating physicians as well as a vast array of allied health professionals. The life care planner must recognize that the parents of these children are responsible for constant organization of physician visits, therapy sessions, recommended treatments, equipment purchases, medication administration, and interface with the educational system, all while providing hands-on care in the home. As the child ages, the parents must make important decisions about guardianship, transition out of the school environment, and establishment of medical care with a whole new set of physician providers. This transition into adulthood can be daunting for families and may include selection of long-term living options due to the aging, disability, or death of the primary caregiver (Riddick-Grisham, 2011).

Because advances in medicine have resulted in more children surviving conditions that were once life-threatening, there has been an increased demand for all levels of care for children who have experienced catastrophic injury or have chronic healthcare needs, that the life care planner must consider. This spans from the primary care provider to community and educational services, to the specialty healthcare services required by these children. The provision of care includes multiple entities, often with different missions, consisting of independent healthcare professionals, third-party payers, private organizations, and public agencies funded by a variety of sources. Care coordination can become quite complicated but is critical in life care plan development to prevent duplication of services and ensure the efficient use of resources and funding (Riddick-Grisham, 2011).

Common Diagnoses in Pediatric Life Care Planning

Individuals in the pediatric age group for whom life care plans are developed present with a wide variety of diagnoses. As with their adult counterparts, life care plans for children and adolescents are requested for those who have experienced traumatic brain injury, spinal cord injury, catastrophic burns, amputation, or other musculoskeletal injuries, including brachial plexus injury or developmental dysplasia of the hip. Other conditions encountered are organ failure requiring transplantation, cancers, or genetically inherited disorders like Down syndrome, cystic fibrosis, or hemoglobinopathies. The evaluee may have met the diagnostic criteria for autism spectrum disorder, cerebral palsy, intellectual disability, or other neurodevelopmental disorders. Complications from medical errors or toxic exposures are other potential issues faced by the individual. Vision and hearing impairment are common findings. Those with cerebral palsy secondary to a hypoxic ischemic encephalopathic event and/or acquired brain injury, as well as those with a spinal cord injury may experience similar sequelae, such as spasticity, weakness, pulmonary compromise, bowel and bladder dysfunction, seizures, osteopenia, and skin disruption, all of which the life care planner must identify or anticipate.

Typical Versus Atypical Development

Distinguishing typical versus atypical development is critical in identifying children with disabilities. The term *development* refers to the characteristic and predictable ways that human behavior changes through time, which can be described in terms of specific functional domains (Pellegrino & Myers, 2019). These domains are comprised of motor development (gross motor and fine motor skills as well as oral motor function), cognitive development (receptive and expressive language abilities, non-verbal problem-solving, perceptual reasoning), and neurobehavioral development (social and emotional behavior, self-regulation, mental status) (Pellegrino & Myers, 2019). The term *typical* is preferred to *normal* when defining developmental change as experienced by most children. *Atypical* development is characterized by delays from expected trajectories, either in some domains more than others (dissociated development) or across all domains of function (globally impaired development). *Developmental delay* is apparent when milestones in one or more areas of development are attained in the typical sequence but at a slower rate. Delays of 22.5–25% or greater, or performance that is 1.5–2 standard deviations or more below the norm are considered significant (Pellegrino & Myers, 2019).

Developmental Surveillance in Children with Atypical Development

Developmental surveillance is the process of reviewing developmental progress over time. Primary care providers (i.e., pediatricians, family practitioners, nurse practitioners, physician assistants) are uniquely positioned to provide such surveillance due to the frequent contact with young children throughout the critical early stages of their development. However, clinicians vary considerably in their level of experience and expertise in identifying developmental differences. Consequently, studies have indicated that many children with potentially significant developmental concerns may not be recognized for early intervention services (Thomas et al., 2012). Therefore, surveillance is considered necessary, but not a sufficient practice to identify delayed development.

In 2006, the American Academy of Pediatrics (AAP) published guidelines recommending that all children routinely undergo developmental screening using a standardized screening tool at 9, 18, and 24, or 30 months of age. The screening tool should also be utilized at any visit when surveillance suggests a developmental problem (Council on Children with Disabilities, 2006). Commonly used developmental screening tests include the Ages & Stages Questionnaire, third Edition (ASQ-3) (Squires et al., 2009), and the Parents' Evaluation of Developmental Status

(PEDS) (Brothers et al., 2008). Due to increasing concerns about identifying children with autism spectrum disorder, the AAP has additionally recommended screening with the Modified Checklist for Autism in Toddlers – Revised ([M-CHAT – R], Robins et al., 2014) to be administered at 18 and 24 months of age (Zwaigenbaum et al., 2015). These screening tests have been designed to be easily completed by parents or caregivers and have been shown in research as effective in identifying children with developmental delays (favorable sensitivity) and children who do not exhibit developmental delays (favorable specificity).

The purpose of developmental surveillance and screening is to distinguish those children who will benefit from early intervention services. The importance of providing early intervention has been well documented in many studies to optimize developmental outcomes in children at risk for or already manifesting delayed milestones (Wallander et al., 2014). Although developmental surveillance and screening have become important for recognizing atypical development in children, diagnostic testing is necessary for proper identification and assessment of their condition and functional status.

Neuropsychological Evaluation of Children with Neurological Impairments

The National Academy of Neuropsychology (NAN) defines a neuropsychologist as a professional within the field of psychology with special expertise in the applied science of brain-behavior relationships (NAN, 2001). These clinicians have a doctoral degree and use psychological, neurological, cognitive, behavioral, and physiologic tests to evaluate a client's function and potential capabilities.

A pediatric neuropsychologist specializes in the assessment of children and adolescents. They assess the neurocognitive, behavioral, sensory, psychomotor, and emotional strengths and weaknesses of children with a variety of challenges or disabilities (Fluss & Lidzba, 2020). They have expertise in the areas of pediatric and adolescent behavior, psychosocial adjustment, learning disorders, mental illness, and cognitive disability. This training and experience allows them to identify cognitive deficits that impact daily function, learning disabilities such as Attention Deficit Hyperactivity Disorder (ADHD), dysgraphia, dyslexia, non-verbal learning disabilities, post-traumatic stress syndrome and other behavioral disorders, and developmental disorders such as autism that may benefit from intensive treatment.

Neuropsychologists have typically earned a PhD in clinical neuropsychology, but also complete additional internships, practice, and examination requirements to obtain their subspecialty certification. The focus and depth of their training and evaluations differs significantly from that of a psychologist, who is often the individual initially seeing a child who is having difficulty. The pediatric neuropsychologists' assessment and opinions help guide educators and families in how to best assist a child with behavioral or learning challenges and make recommendations that extend beyond the educational environment into adulthood.

Children's hospitals often employ pediatric neuropsychologists, as the presence of psychiatric, trauma, oncology, and epilepsy units, and complex care teams, often requires their expertise. Evaluations are often conducted prior to seizure surgery or cancer treatments (such as chemotherapy and radiation) that may impact cognition. They assess children post-injury or post-surgery to help formulate educational and medical treatment plans. Many also work in non-academic and private practice settings doing individualized testing and evaluations and serve as consultants to schools or legal firms.

Neuropsychology evaluations are ongoing in children, as their cognitive and skill development allows different types of testing as time goes on. Typically, testing is recommended every 2–4 years in a child with developmental or cognitive difficulties, through to completion of high school. Testing may be initiated after an injury, when delays are noted, when genetic or developmental disorders are diagnosed, or when a large disparity in a child's areas of abilities are noted (Limond et al., 2014).

A review of medical, academic, vocational, social, and psychological histories is part of every pediatric neuropsychology assessment. They also perform and interpret a variety of neuropsychological tests and evaluations, which are far more in depth that what a typical educational setting would provide. They interview the family/caregivers and evaluate the child's behavior and demeanor both with and without family present (Silver, 2014).

A child's current function, as well as their future needs and capabilities are incorporated into neuropsychology recommendations and treatment plans. It is important that not only are a child's weaknesses identified, but also their strengths. This can be essential to guiding a family and child to successful vocational or avocational opportunities, and providing hope, not frustration. In summary, a pediatric neuropsychologist may:

- Evaluate cognitive, sensory, psychomotor, and emotional function
- Assess coping and psychosocial skills
- Identify special educational or other services a child is eligible for
- Identify mental health issues that may need medical referral
- Recommend when pharmacologic intervention might be beneficial
- Prognosticate about cognitive and academic function
- Identify helpful educational interventions and compensatory learning strategies
- Assess cognitive remediation treatment and its impact over time
- Recommend counseling for an individual or family
- Prognosticate individual's independent living skills
- Assist with guardianship decisions
- Recommend physical, occupational, or speech therapy
- Suggest appropriate vocational training or vocational accommodations

The neuropsychologist's expertise not only assists the life care planner in providing a foundation for care recommendations, but also assists the physicians seeing the patient—including psychiatrists, physiatrists (physical medicine and rehabilitation [PM&R]), and neurologists in understanding their cognitive and behavioral needs.

Seizure Activity in Children with Neurological Injury

Seizures are transient disturbances of brain function resulting from an abnormally excessive excitation of cortical neurons. A seizure is classified as generalized when it involves both hemispheres at onset, or focal when it starts in one hemisphere with or without subsequent spread to the other hemisphere (Zelleke et al., 2019). It is well established that children with developmental disabilities are at an increased risk for having epilepsy. For instance, a child with cerebral palsy has five times the risk of developing epilepsy than a typically developing child (Hundozi-Hysenaj & Boshnjaku-Dallku, 2008). For children with intellectual disability, the epilepsy risk is 15–20% in their lifetime (Besag, 2002). Comorbid conditions also increase the risk for epilepsy. As an example, individuals with autism spectrum disorder (ASD) are at risk for developing epilepsy. If the child has intellectual disability associated with ASD, this risk increases to 35% at five years and 67% by ten years of age (Holmes, 2002).

Epilepsy control in children with developmental disabilities has historically been more difficult to achieve, and medically refractory epilepsy is more common (Airaksinen et al., 2000). Additionally, both epilepsy and anti-seizure medications may contribute to learning difficulties and disruptive behavior. Children with epilepsy are more likely to exhibit cognitive impairment, attention deficit/hyperactivity disorder, anxiety disorder, and depression (Zelleke et al., 2019).

Treating Seizure Activity in Children

Once the diagnosis of epilepsy is made, the initiation of an anti-epileptic medication is typically the first line of treatment. These medications can be categorized as narrow spectrum, which are effective for focal or secondarily generalized epilepsies, or broad-spectrum medications that have efficacy in both focal and generalized epilepsies (Asconapé, 2010). Carbamazepine, oxcarbazepine, levetiracetam, and lamotrigine are considered first-line drugs for focal seizures with or without secondary generalization, while valproate, lamotrigine, topiramate, and levetiracetam are used to treat generalized epilepsies (Shih et al., 2017).

Lennox-Gastaut syndrome is a disorder defined by a mixture of seizure types including atypical absence, tonic, drop or atonic, myoclonic, tonic-clonic, and focal seizures with an impairment of awareness. Children diagnosed with Lennox-Gastaut syndrome have an increased risk for frequent falls and injury. Seizure control and resolution of the EEG abnormalities are thought to be necessary for improved cognitive and behavioral outcomes in these children. Their seizures have proven to be difficult to control, and most children with Lennox-Gastaut syndrome exhibit intellectual disability. Rufinamide, clobazam, and felbamate are commonly used for anti-epileptic treatment (Zelleke et al., 2019).

In 2018, cannabidiol was approved by the Food and Drug Administration (FDA) as an add-on anti-epileptic drug in children with Dravet syndrome and Lennox-Gastaut syndrome. A purified preparation of cannabidiol, Epidiolex, has now become commercially available. Stockings et al. (2018) found, in a systemic review on 17 observational studies, that Epidiolex was efficacious in reducing seizure frequency and improving quality of life in childhood epilepsy scores. In addition, four clinical trials in children with Dravet and Lennox-Gastaut syndromes have demonstrated a reduction in seizure frequency in cannabidiol treated patients (Lattanzi et al., 2019). A study by Pietrafusa et al. (2019) also suggested that Epidiolex may have beneficial effects in patients with developmental and epileptic encephalopathy with an acceptable safety profile.

The goal of treatment with anti-seizure medication is to prevent seizures with no or minimal side effects and an acceptable quality of life. If two or more appropriate anti-seizure medications at reasonable doses have failed in the treatment of focal epilepsy, other treatment modalities should be considered (Zelleke et al., 2019). For children with epilepsy who do not respond to one or two first-line anti-seizure medications, evaluation by an epileptologist is recommended. This neurology specialist will review the child's seizure history, as well as the EEG and brain MRI findings. For children who continue to demonstrate seizures despite two or more appropriate anti-epileptic medications, the chance of success of an additional one is low. The epileptologist will consider other treatment options to include dietary treatment, surgery, and neuromodulatory therapies. At this point, the child is often admitted for inpatient video EEG monitoring to characterize the typical seizure activity (Zelleke et al., 2019).

A ketogenic diet is the treatment of choice for glucose transporter deficiency, which is associated with epileptic encephalopathy due to impaired glucose transport to the brain (Klepper, 2008). Children who are treated for a wide variety of seizure types and epilepsy refractory to anti-seizure medications can benefit from a ketogenic diet (Freeman et al., 2007). These patients must be monitored with urine and blood ketone levels to ensure adequate ketosis. Early side effects can include lethargy, gastrointestinal disturbance, hypoglycemia, and metabolic acidosis. Over the long term, renal stones, dyslipidemia, and failure to thrive have occurred (Freeman et al., 2007).

When there are multiple seizure foci, palliative epilepsy surgery may reduce seizure frequency or severity in children with refractory seizures. Although these procedures rarely result in a resolution of seizures, they can improve quality of life. A corpus callosotomy is a treatment option for refractory epilepsy, including atonic (drop) seizures and secondarily generalized epilepsy (Rosenfeld & Roberts, 2009).

Neuromodulatory therapies has been found effective in the management of medication resistant epilepsy in children. Vagal nerve stimulation has been proven as an effective option for this group, with a statistically significant reduction in number of seizures, a decreased morbidity of the seizures, and decreased number of days in inpatient care (Terra et al., 2014). According to 14 published studies of vagal nerve stimulation in children with Lennex-Gastaut syndrome, 55% were responders (Starnes et al., 2019). The vagal nerve stimulator must be surgically implanted, requires regular physician programming, as well as ongoing replacement of batteries, all of which must be anticipated by the life care planner. A systematic review of deep brain stimulation for the treatment of drug-resistant epilepsy in childhood was published in 2018 by Yan et al. It was concluded that deep brain stimulation should be considered as an alternative or adjuvant treatment for these children, as favorable outcomes were reported. Future clinical trials were recommended to identify the optimal deep brain stimulation target in pediatric patients.

Mortality in children with epilepsy is most attributed to an accident (especially swimming related), the underlying cause of the epilepsy (for example, a brain tumor), and sudden unexpected death in epilepsy (SUDEP) (Zelleke et al., 2019). Sudden unexpected death in epilepsy is thought to be related to post-ictal alterations in respiratory and cardiac function. A meta-analysis of studies showed an incidence of 0.22 per 1,000 patient-years in childhood, making it a very rare occurrence (Harden et al., 2017). Generalized tonic-clonic seizures and nocturnal seizures are risk factors for SUDEP, as well as early childhood onset of epilepsy, developmental delay, and refractoriness to multiple anti-seizure medication. However, for children with epilepsy associated with multiple disabilities, the prognosis is more related to the disabilities and underlying causes than to the epilepsy itself (Morse & Kothare, 2016).

Oral Health Concerns Children with Neurological Impairment

Children with developmental disabilities are considered at higher risk for developing oral disease and more likely to have unmet dental needs than typically developing children (Norwood et al., 2013). Those with intellectual developmental disabilities are more likely than the general population to exhibit poor hygiene and an increase in decay and periodontal disease (Binkley et al., 2014). This increased risk is attributed to cariogenic diets, medications that are high in sugar or have the detrimental side effect of gingival overgrowth, the inability to clear foods from the oral cavity, an increased incidence of malocclusion, physical or cognitive limitations preventing proper oral hygiene, and dependence on a caregiver for their oral healthcare. In addition, children with disabilities are now more likely to survive into adulthood which poses a long-term risk for dental problems (Norwood et al., 2013).

Dental decay in those with moderate to profound neurocognitive and neuromotor deficits is often associated with regurgitation or pouching/pocketing of food within the mouth. Altered salivary function, either reduced due to medications or increased (sialorrhea), can also lead to decay. Fractured and avulsed teeth can occur secondary to falls, trauma during seizure activity, pica, and self-injurious behavior. Gingival overgrowth due to seizure medication can lead to the delayed loss or eruption of primary teeth as well as the delayed eruption of permanent teeth leading to periodontal disease. Bruxism is commonly found in children with neurological injury. The continued grinding erodes the structure of the teeth which can cause sensitivity and need for restoration. Temporomandibular joint disorders can present long-term difficulties for these adults (Scheifele et al., 2019). When a non-verbal child is irritable, occult dental issues must be considered in the differential diagnosis.

Sialorrhea

Excessive drooling (sialorrhea) is also a significant social, dental, and medical issue that many pediatric patients with disabilities, including about 30–40% of cerebral palsy patients have (Dias et al., 2016; Speyer et al., 2019). Drooling can be related to head position, inattention, poor oral motor control, lack of sensory awareness or all of the above. It is not typically related to excessive production of saliva, but can be exacerbated by medications, seizures, reflux, or movement disorders. The risk of aspiration, skin chafing, excessive laundry, electronic equipment breakdowns, and social rejection that can result from excess salivation are troubling (Dias et al., 2016).

Speech therapy can help address some of the positional and oral motor issues. Medications such as glycopyrrolate, a scopolamine patch or atropine drops can dry up secretions but titrating them to the most effective level can be a challenge. Overly thick secretions and constipation can be side effects.

Intraoral appliances, such as a Bluegrass appliance, are typically used to reduce anterior tongue thrusting and thumb sucking (Chhabra & Chhabra, 2020). They can help localize tongue movements in those with oral motor dystonia to reduce anterior spillage of saliva. These devices must be placed under sedation by an experienced dentist or orthodontist.

Botulinum toxin injections to the salivary glands can also be effective in reducing salivation but are not FDA approved for pediatric patients. These injections typically last 4–6 months (Porte et al., 2014; Ture et al., 2021) and are often performed by a PM&R physician or an otolaryngologist (ENT) in clinic or with sedation. The procedure should be coordinated with any other botulinum toxin use in the patient so risk of overdose or tolerance to the medication is reduced.

Surgical ductal ligation or rerouting of the ducts is a last resort when conservative measures have failed. If aspiration and respiratory complications are occurring frequently, treatment of sialorrhea should be anticipated. The American Academy of Cerebral Palsy and Developmental Medicine (AACPDM) care pathway provides a possible algorithm for treatment options.

Maintaining Oral Health in Children with Atypical Development

Tools for preventative dentistry include brushing, flossing, fluoride application, and dental sealants for permanent teeth exist within the dental home (American Academy of Pediatric Dentistry, 2021). According to McKinney et al. (2014), not having a medical home is the strongest predictor of having dental problems. The need for specialized dentistry must be considered for children with disabilities, as well as an understanding of how associated medical conditions will affect their oral health. Their cooperation and tolerance for dental procedures, abrupt or uncontrolled movements, presence of seizures, diminished protective reflexes, and need for prolonged dental interventions often require the need for sedation or general anesthesia, which should be considered by the life care planner.

As oral health is an important part of general health and well-being, preventative and regular visits should be provided for these children through a dental home. Oral healthcare for children with developmental disabilities requires specialized knowledge, and the providers must demonstrate methods of accommodation and an increased awareness beyond what are considered routine (American Academy of Pediatric Dentistry, 2021).

Nutritional Guidelines for Children with Atypical Development

Children with disabling conditions such as acquired or traumatic brain injury, cerebral palsy, or spinal cord injury often have a variety of gastrointestinal complications. Some may feed safely from birth, but have reflux, gastric retention, or constipation. Others will have dysphagia and aspiration, and never master oral feeding. Still others may tolerate feeds for enjoyment but are not able to consume enough calories in a timely manner to sustain their weight. Specialty formulas may, therefore, be a lifelong need, either as primary nutrition or to supplement oral feeds (Arvedson, 2013).

It is the role of the gastroenterology (GI) physician and the pediatric dietitian, to determine the type and volume of feedings needed. Fortunately, there are many more nutritional choices on the market, including organic, gluten free, dairy free, and blended "real food" options (Oral Cancer Foundation, 2022).

Each varies in its nutritional makeup, and supplementation of Vitamin D, B vitamins, etc. may be necessary. Laboratory studies to check nutritional status should be included in a life care plan. The life care planner needs to be aware that some home care companies may only carry certain formula brands, so that multiple formula changes are not necessary. Additionally, caloric needs increase with age, and this must be anticipated when determining future formula volumes (Bell & Samson-Fang, 2013).

The speech pathologist helps determine feeding safety with the aid of radiographic swallow studies. They help determine the type of food or liquid that is currently tolerable, and repeated studies over time, as abilities progress, may be needed. Some children can improve their oral intake through outpatient speech therapy. Others, often with a sensory or behavioral component, require an inpatient intensive feeding program in which a psychologist is an important team member (Arvedson, 2013).

Gastrostomy or jejunostomy placement and/or Nissen fundoplication may be indicated for some patients and can be a lifetime need. Gastrostomy tubes are surgically placed and after the tract heals, are typically replaced quarterly. This can be done either in the clinic or by a trained caregiver. Extra tubes should be provided, as they can pull out unexpectedly and need to be replaced quickly. Jejunostomy tubes must be placed under radiologic guidance by interventional radiology and require replacement less frequently (Villela et al., 2014).

The pediatric dietitian should use specialty growth charts for diagnoses such as cerebral palsy, as they differ significantly from normal developmental curves (Brooks et al., 2011) This avoids the parental guilt associated with poor weight gain, and also avoids overfeeding a child. Either situation can lead to skin integrity issues, ill-fitting equipment, or difficulty with mobility. Dietitian costs are typically included in a GI clinic visit charge.

Attention to specialty diets needed for children with diabetes, seizures, short gut syndrome, burns, or other medical conditions is essential. Some children with sensory issues or oral motor coordination problems require specific food textures or flavors. Many require stool softeners and bowel stimulants to avoid chronic constipation issues (Vande Velde et al., 2018). In rare cases, total parenteral nutrition (TPN) may be initiated, or become an ongoing need. In these instances, long-term venous access, frequent laboratory studies, and social worker involvement should be anticipated (Dibb et al., 2013).

Musculoskeletal Considerations in Children with Atypical Development

Injuries to the brain and spinal cord impact both musculoskeletal function and growth. Factors such as immobility, the presence of spasticity, hypotonia, and dystonia or other movement disorders, nutritional challenges, and sensory impairments also impact bone and muscle function.

Surveillance for typical problems (e.g., scoliosis, hip dysplasia, osteopenia) associated with brain or spinal injury that can rapidly progress is essential. Pediatricians, PM&R physicians, and developmental pediatricians are often the ones who identify and make referrals for surgical or other interventions when function is impaired. The interventions chosen will depend on factors such as the child's age, disability, severity of deformity, presence of pain, and/or the rapidity of progression. They might include the use of orthotics/splints, equipment (standers, walkers), physical or occupational therapy, oral or injectable medications, intrathecal baclofen pumps for spasticity management, or orthopedic or neurosurgical procedures.

Spasticity and Other Movement Disorders

Spasticity, dystonia, and hypotonia are common muscle tone and movement difficulties that result from injury to the brain or spinal cord. Their presence can affect respiratory effort, sleep, comfort, caloric needs, caregiver needs, and general functional abilities such as rolling, sitting, crawling, walking, feeding, and talking. Spasticity can be advantageous functionally, however, when substituting for strength, such as when doing stand pivot transfers. Thus, choosing an appropriate treatment that enhances function and prevents long-term injurious consequences can be a challenge in a growing child. Spasticity and dystonia can also be focal or generalized, and multiple patterns (e.g., hemiplegia, diplegia, quadriplegia) result, depending on the type of brain or spinal cord injury.

Treatment options vary according to not only the problematic muscle groups, but also are adapted to how much of the movement needs to be diminished. Treatment interventions are often done in tandem and vary at different developmental stages or with growth. For example, in a toddler, therapy is more likely to be recommended, while in a teenager, surgery might be more likely (Novak, 2014) Treatment generally falls in four categories:

- Therapeutic options
- Oral medications
- Injectable medications
- Orthopedic or neurosurgery

Physical and occupational therapists commonly use positioning devices such as standers, walkers, and splints to improve joint position, and work on muscle strength and motor planning to overcome abnormal movement patterns. They may use electric stimulation, casting, or kinesiotaping to align the body correctly. Splints are typically replaced annually due to growth and wear and tear. The use of a qualified orthotist to fabricate devices is essential.

Common oral medications for spasticity and dystonia include baclofen, dantrolene, benzodiazepines, trihexyphenidyl, and levodopa while seizure medications, gabapentin, and cannabinoids are less common options. Consideration of G tube compatibility, frequency of dosing, sedating or other side effects, and interactions with other medications impact choice (American Academy for Cerebral Palsy and Developmental Medicine, 2022a; Gormely & Deshpande, 2021). Dose ranges generally change with weight.

Injectable medications include botulinum toxins (BoNT) for muscle relaxation, and phenol or alcohol for nerve block. Botulinum toxins are costly, last about three months, and can be repeated for functional benefits for years, but can also be done primarily during growth spurts. Multiple toxin brands exist, with good evidence for efficacy. Alcohol and phenol last longer and are less costly, but most pediatric patients require sedation for these e-stim or EMG guided injections (Gormely & Deshpande, 2021).

Orthopedic procedures for the spine, hip, and lower extremities due to contractures that impair function, comfort, or caregiving are common and fairly predictable. As these fix a mechanical problem, but not the underlying spasticity, repeat procedures are not uncommon (Koman et al., 2003).

Selective dorsal rhizotomy is a permanent neurosurgical procedure that requires lengthy and intense physical therapy post-procedure and is appropriate for only a select group of generally higher functioning children. A reversible intrathecal baclofen pump is an alternative to this, with wider patient selection, but a need for routine refill appointments and battery replacements over time. Dosing is not weight based (Gormely & Deshpande, 2021).

The frequency of medications, clinic visits, adaptive devices, splints, and surgical procedures can often be anticipated by a PM&R physician or pediatric neurologist, and consultation with the treating physician can be helpful in predicting outcomes. The life care plan should plan for ongoing treatment until growth is complete.

Neuromuscular Scoliosis

Neuromuscular scoliosis is a common consequence of an injury to the brain or spinal cord, and its incidence is especially high in those who are wheelchair dependent. It is more severe and more progressive and is associated with greater morbidity. Curves over 50 degrees that are not corrected can lead to problems such as cardiopulmonary compromise, difficulty with seating due to pelvic obliquity, pressure sores, pain, and gait and balance difficulties. Self-image and social interactions can also be affected (Allam & Schwabe, 2013; Wishart & Kivlehan 2021).

Typically, screening x-rays are done at least annually, with initiation varying with the particular disability. If a curve is progressing quickly, frequency of x-rays increases. Use of custom seating, thoracolumbar sacral orthosis (TLSOs), and spinal technology that "grows" with the child (VEPTR – vertical expandable prosthetic titanium rib, MAGEC rods – MAGnetic expansion control) can delay the time to final spinal fusion. These technologies involve a series of surgical interventions prior to final fusion, which must be anticipated by the life care planner (Brooks & Sponseler, 2016).

Hip Dysplasia

Hip dysplasia is another common problem, with one in three children with cerebral palsy developing this (Murphy et al., 2021). Interventions include physical therapy, splinting, serial casting, BoNT injections, and surgery. Common surgical procedures needed are varus derotational osteotomies and adductor muscle lengthenings. Hamstring contractures and Achilles tendon contractures are also common consequences of spasticity (Vargus-Adams et al., 2021). In many cases, the earlier a surgery is performed, the higher the likelihood repeat surgeries will be needed (Chang et al., 2018; Joo et al., 2011). The American Academy of Cerebral Palsy and Developmental Medicine ([AACPDM], 2022b) website has a helpful care pathway for surveillance of hip problems which can be found at www.aacpdm.org/publications/care-pathways/hip-surveillance-in-cerebral-palsy.

Osteoporosis

Osteoporosis is an often-overlooked consequence of immobility, tube feedings, lack of exposure to outdoor activities, seizures medications, and spasticity. Fragility fractures are not uncommon in children with severe cerebral palsy, and can be difficult to quickly diagnosis in young, dependent, non-verbal children. Poor bone density also impacts orthopedic surgical outcomes. Monitoring calcium and Vitamin D intake, increasing weight bearing, and getting DEXA scans (bone densitometry) can help in the prevention of osteoporosis. As this is a lifelong concern, routine monitoring is needed, and treatment can be initiated far earlier than in a non-disabled individual. Calcium and Vitamin D supplementation, as well as the use of bisphosphonates is often initiated by an endocrinologist, PM&R physician, or a nephrologist, in at risk children (Boyce et al., 2014). The AACPDM has a care pathway for monitoring and treatment of osteoporosis in children at www.aacpdm.org/publications/care-pathways/osteoporosis-in-cerebral-palsy

Essential Concepts in Pediatric Medical Equipment and Assistive Technology

As anyone anticipating the birth of a child knows, the "equipment" needed to keep them safe, comfortable, and entertained can be formidable. Add to that the additional needs of medical equipment for a child with disabilities, who will grow in size, but might never change in terms of need. Additionally, "special needs" items are often exorbitantly priced, are difficult to obtain, require frequent repairs, and can become outdated quickly.

As most equipment for children is custom, not off-the-shelf, equipment acquisition is a team sport involving at least four members—the physician, the therapists, the family, and the assistive technology professional (ATP). Multidisciplinary clinics or coordination with a PM&R physician who has expertise in this area is most common, as the majority of primary care physicians do not feel comfortable or have the training to determine what equipment is needed (Sneed et al., 2001). The physician plays an integral part in determining and anticipating the medical needs (current and future), and the ability of the child and family to utilize a device.

The physical, occupational, or speech therapists (medical and/or school based) also know the family's capabilities, and frequently trial devices to see how the child responds. The family must prioritize what they can practically use, what they have room for, what they can transport if needed, what their child might cooperate with, and then can determine the features of devices that are most beneficial to them.

The ATP is someone who can assist in analyzing the needs of a client in the selection of equipment and training them how to use it. They are most often employed by a durable medical equipment (DME) company and are typically paid on commission. Their certification requires varying hours of work experience based on background, a required number of required AT education courses, and a written exam (Rehabilitation Engineering and Assistive Technology Society of North America [RESNA], 2022). Thus, expertise can vary dramatically. Their ability to recommend and obtain appropriate equipment may depend on their experience, their ability to code equipment and understand funding sources, and their technical ability to modify equipment, anticipate growth, and understand the unique medical needs of the child.

Factors Considered for DME Use

Issues that must be considered when evaluating for and recommending equipment include medical diagnosis; growth potential of the child; cognitive, sensory, and behavioral characteristics of the child; space and home environment; replacement needs; transport needs; and overall practicality and functional benefits.

Medical Diagnosis

A child's medical diagnosis helps inform the equipment they will need. Some patient diagnoses are progressive, while others are static. Some children are physically active, while others are not. Some have significant cognitive deficits, while others self-direct their care. Some have significant movement disorders or skin integrity issues that must be accommodated. Some need a long-term fitness plan and compete in adapted sports, while others need only comfortable and safe positioning.

Functional classification scales designed for use in cerebral palsy help classify the abilities of many pediatric patients. The Gross Motor Functional Classification Scale (GMFCS), Manual Ability Classification System (MACS), and Communication Function Classification System (CFCS) can be used as guides for potential equipment needs (Eliasson et al., 2006; Hidecker et al., 2011; Palisano et al., 1997). The reader is referred to www.macs.nu for more information.

Children grow and their bones and muscles need proper positioning to do so. Their vision, cognitive and emotional skills depend on access to their environment. While the needs of a child with paraplegia who has intact cognitive and verbal skills, and a child with quadriplegia who is non-verbal with cognitive deficits will vary dramatically, basic principles and goals apply. Equipment should facilitate and address the medical purposes of the following factors (Ward et al., 2021):

- Maintenance of appropriate boney alignment to prevent orthopedic issues
- Weight bearing to facilitate stand pivot transfers and/or bone density
- Stretching to promote functional range of motion
- Head and body positioning to promote visual integration and communication
- Maintenance of hygiene and skin integrity
- Safe mobility with as much independence as possible

Growth and Aging

It is important to anticipate a child's growth, which may be impacted by endocrine issues, nutrition, genetics, and their injury or diagnosis. Equipment must be replaced to accommodate these changes. Some wheelchair frames have "growth kits" included in their initial pricing. The chair seating needs replacement each time the chair is grown, but also intermittently due to use. Standers, gait trainers, special needs car seats, activity chairs, and walkers also have weight and height limits, and vary in their weight and durability, which impacts what the child can most easily and safely use.

Weight gain must also be considered, and patient lifts are recommended by the National Institute for Occupational Safety and Health when transferring a patient over 35 lbs., as back protection for the caregiver is important. A variety of types exist, and consideration of anticipated growth, as well as planning around potential spine, hip, or leg surgeries that alter positioning is important (Ward et al., 2021).

Physical/Psychological Needs

A child's physical, cognitive, sensory, behavioral, and psychological needs for activity must be considered. Questions to ponder:

As they grow, are they likely to become more independent and able to use different equipment on their own, or are their caregivers going to be utilizing the equipment to keep them safe and comfortable?

Will they become mobile or likely remain dependent on others?

- Do they have the cardiorespiratory capacity, and orthopedic and skin integrity to continue to use equipment as they age?
- Would they benefit from adapted sports equipment to maintain fitness as they grow?
- Do they have sensory issues that make certain devices more tolerable than others?
- Will they be utilizing adapted technology devices (speech generating systems, special computers, etc.) that require mounting or special accessibility?
- Will the device be socially acceptable to the patient, so they will utilize it in functional settings outside the home?

Additional Concerns

The home environment has to accommodate needed equipment, so adequate storage space, flooring that will allow equipment to move easily, widened doorways, at least ramped entrances for egress in emergency, and outdoor accessibility for recreational or fitness equipment (adapted bicycles, swings, etc.) must be considered. If the equipment is kept outside, rain, snow, and heat can affect its use, and certain climates may necessitate canopies, covers, or electric components compatible with the weather.

Items may need to be transported to school, therapy, family events, on vacations, or between the homes of divorced parents. Consideration of their size, caregiver vehicles, and ease of breaking items down into transportable components should be addressed. If the client is being transported in the device, which avoids lifting transfers, transit tie downs must be present. "Valet chairs" that rotate and lift a client into the car can provide another practical option to avoid lifting.

Maintenance and eventual replacement of equipment due to wear and tear needs to be considered, as well as upgrading due to size, additional components related to anticipated decline or improvement in physical or cognitive abilities, or transfer to a group home where equipment may or may not be provided. Some devices (respiratory vests) provide lifelong replacement vests free of charge after initial purchase, and wheelchairs may include growth kits, so replacement cost should not be included in a life care plan. Prosthesis and orthosis typically require more frequent replacement due to growth than DME products.

Utilizing equipment also takes a lot of time, effort, and compliance on the part of the child and caregiver. Assessing whether the caregiver is physically capable and willing to help the client in and out of a device should be discussed. The need for multiple devices if there are two caregiver homes versus transporting devices should also be considered. If power is needed to maintain equipment (ventilator), a generator must be provided.

Major Equipment Categories

Medical Strollers

A lightweight medical stroller with minimal seating is a practical alternative when transport in the wheelchair is not possible (vehicle or caregiver issues.) They are able to tie down in a vehicle, but durability and customization are less. They visually also infantilize a child and limit independence, as they are not self-propelled (Ward et al., 2021).

Manual Wheelchairs

The physical abilities of the client and caregiver need consideration. Some clients can walk, but not for long distances. Others can push independently, but only for brief periods. Others are athletic and risk overuse injuries. Caregivers who push dependent children vary in height, strength, and ability to break down equipment for transport. Manual frames are either foldable, rigid, or tilt, and materials can be lightweight or ultralight. Their durability, growth potential, and weight all vary, and must match their users (Ward et al., 2021).

Wheelchairs can be propelled with two arms, with a one-arm drive, or can have power assist wheels or a clip-on power device to reduce energy expenditure and stress on joints. Tire and wheel configurations depend on the weight, height, and physical environment the child will be pushing or pushed in. No-flat inserts can save families much time and effort. Dynamic components added to footrest hangers or chair backs can minimize wear and tear for children with spasticity or rocking behaviors. The "amount" of seating varies by the child's ability to maintain a midline position, but more is generally heavier and more costly. The frame and seating systems need to be considered separately in both growth and replacement. Modifications such as a "Smart Drive" or power assist wheels might be needed if a child's endurance no longer matches ability based on changes in their weight, or to reduce the potential for commonly seen shoulder overuse injuries (Walford et al., 2019).

Power Wheelchairs

Power wheelchairs provide independence to users with limited physical capabilities, via a joystick, body switch, or head mount. Power chairs are also routinely provided to young pediatric users who have the cognitive, motor, and attentional skills to use them safely, but environment of use, and ability to transport the chair must be considered (Mockler et al., 2017).

The need for tilt, recline, or standing, or all of the above, impact the complexity and cost of the electronics needed, and the cognitive needs for the client to use them independently. Batteries typically require more frequent replacement than the wheelchair itself (Ward et al., 2021).

Seating and Accessories

Wheelchair seat backs and cushions come in a variety of materials and need replacement every time the chair is "grown," or often after orthopedic procedures such as hip or scoliosis surgery. Custom molded systems better accommodate pressure areas and orthopedic deformities but are more costly and are not as modifiable. Warranties vary. Most cushions are replaced every 2–3 years due to either growth or wear and tear. Headrests, armrests, trays, and seat/chest belts are also accessories that add additional cost to a chair but are medically necessary for most patients.

Standers

Standers promote proper alignment and weight bearing, which facilitates transfer training, contracture reduction, bowel evacuation, circulation, and bone density. Prone, supine, and rolling standers exist, but the ability of the caregiver to singlehandedly position the child in the device can be difficult. Standers that go from sitting to standing with a crank, are easiest. Accessories to maintain head, knee, and trunk position are not included in the baseline cost. Mobile standers that can be self-propelled are available but are not typically covered as they can be considered a mobility device, duplicative of a wheelchair (Ward et al., 2021).

Bath Equipment Considerations

Lifting and carrying a wet, wiggly child out of the tub is difficult enough, but when they have spasticity, paralysis, or are heavy and dependent, it can be dangerous. Bath and shower chairs, which may include a toileting system for positional support during bowel programs or toilet training, are essential for safety. However, they often need to be moved for others to use the facilities, so wheels are essential. Most bathrooms are not modified well to accommodate equipment, so size matters. Lifts that lower and raise a child onto bath equipment or into a toilet chair provide back protection and safety. An adapted bathroom that allows the child to be bathed, dried, and dressed in the same environment is also helpful for temperature stability.

Recreational Equipment

The need for fitness continues despite disability, and lifelong recreational activities such as bike riding or adapted sports can promote both physical and psychological benefits. Adaptive equipment is typically customized to the child's specific orthopedic or neurologic needs, is not easily rentable, and typically costs more than traditional sports equipment. Sport specific wheelchairs differ in wheel position and weight, to reduce risk of injury and improve competitiveness, so the client's regular chair usually would not suffice (Miller & Meilhan, 2021).

Assistive Technology

Communication

Fortunately, with Alexa, Siri, Voice to Text, and the many Bluetooth-enabled devices available today, environmental controls (lights, temperature, music, computers, etc.) are achievable for many people with physical disabilities. However, for those with speech that is unintelligible or who are non-verbal, augmentative and alternative communication (AAC) devices are needed. As a speech therapist's scope is vast, one that specializes in augmentative technology is necessary. They often practice in a hospital clinic or outpatient practice with this special focus, but sometimes can be found in a school system. Appropriate devices may range from an iPad with inexpensive applications, to an eye gaze-controlled Tobii Dynavox. An appropriate device must account for the child's visual abilities, positional abilities, and manual dexterity. Sign language or picture exchange cards do not engage many children with disabilities, as like their peers, they are more interested in cell phone applications and computer games. Using this interest is important and often does not require a high level of manual dexterity. If using a wheelchair, an appropriate tray or mount is needed for the device to be accessible. This highly specialized equipment is also likely to be updated as technologies advance, and frequent re-evaluations may be needed (Light et al., 2019).

Activities of Daily Living

An occupational therapist provides input about devices that enable independence in activities of daily living. Many items are available on the internet, as they are also utilized by aging or disabled adults. Kitchen equipment, adapted shoes that do not require ties, looped socks, magnetic buttons and zipper closures and "tear away" clothing, make life easier. An allowance for the difference in cost, is appropriate to include in a life care plan.

Sleep

Sleep is often complicated in children with special needs due to continuous feeding needs, seizures, sleep apnea, or disrupted sleep. While semi electric or fully electric hospital beds provide some measure of safety and height adjustment for transfers, mesh or wooden enclosed beds may be needed for children with agitation or ability to wander unsafely (Ward et al., 2021).

Driving

As adolescents transition into adulthood, many are cognitively and visually able to drive, but require an adaptive equipment evaluation and specialty driving lessons. The equipment and driver's training needed to use it must be anticipated, as it can enhance access to vocational activities and independent living (Ward et al., 2021).

Orthoses

Physiatrists and orthopedists often recommend either soft or hard orthoses for ankles, knees, hips, and spine to provide stability and improve function for children with spasticity, hypotonia, or orthopedic deformities. They may be custom or prefabricated. Most require annual replacement through the growth years. Ability to independently don and doff orthotics is a goal some may not be able to achieve due to limitations of range or motion, cognition, or hand function. Due to coding differences, orthosis that are soft and have no rigid components, are often not covered by insurance. An experienced orthotist is vital to obtaining a wearable, functional splint, or brace, as the materials and styles utilized for braces are quite variable (Ward et al., 2021).

E-stimulation devices (e.g., Walk-Aide, Bioness, Smart Glove) can provide not only biofeedback for therapeutic reasons, but also replace heavy or hot orthoses with something that may be more functional or cosmetically acceptable to the patient. These devices are costly, however, and as regular orthoses might provide the same functional benefit, are not typically covered by insurance (El-Shamy et al., 2016).

Overall, most medical equipment for children and teens with disabilities is customized, obtained through a DME provider for warranty and repair purposes, and will require upsizing and replacement over time.

Therapy Needs for Children with Neurocognitive and Neuromotor Deficits

Children with brain and spinal injuries, for whom life care plans are commonly requested, frequently have a multitude of neurologic issues. These include sensory, visual, auditory, motor, emotional, behavioral, and cognitive impairments. These are addressed by different strategies, by different professionals, at multiple different times in the lifespan, and require different levels of intervention (Novak, 2014; Vargus-Adams et al., 2021)

Therapeutic goals are typically to improve functional skills and promote independence. However, they can also prevent regression, reduce pain, and ameliorate the impact of aging or other inherent problems related to the disability. Thus, therapy can be a lifelong need, as goals, abilities, environment, medical status, and needs for adaptive equipment will change over a lifetime. Therapy evaluations can be scheduled on a routine basis, so that the need for renewed therapy intervention can be identified quickly. Determining how and when to intervene, and the appropriate frequency and intensity of the intervention can be challenging. Factors that may impact this include:

- Medical issues and stability of the child
- Motivation and historical progress of the child
- Functional needs and age of the child
- Procedures or surgeries that require therapy intervention to regain or improve function
- Goals of the family
- Goals of the child/adolescent
- Expertise and availability of local therapists
- Availability of specific types of therapies (robotics, aquatics, hippotherapy)
- Ability of the family to transport the child to therapy
- Ability of the family to follow through with therapy strategies at home
- Opportunities for adapted sports, therapeutic recreational activities which may augment therapeutic goals

Adapted sports and recreational physical activities such as yoga, martial arts, etc. provide physical as well psychological benefits. Strength, balance, endurance, and aerobic /anaerobic capacity can be improved. These activities can augment the goals set in a skilled medically based therapy session, but as all children are not able to participate in adapted or recreational sports, they cannot replace skilled therapy needs (Miller & Meilahn, 2021). Therapy in a different environment such as a pool or on a horse (hippotherapy), when provided by a licensed therapist, can also be very motivating and effective for a child (Muñoz -Blanco et al., 2020; Park et al., 2014).

Growth, and the anticipation of a surgery or medical procedure, such as botulinum toxin injections, hip surgery, or selective dorsal rhizotomy, will also frequently necessitate more intensive therapy, to either regain skills, maximize skills prior to a temporary loss, or to take advantage of a time period where medication is most actively working (Josenby et al., 2012).

The intensity of therapy may vary with the child's tolerance, the scheduling capacity of agencies involved, and the availability of the child (summers vs. school year). Much like practicing the piano daily, versus once weekly, the repetition provided by intensive therapy can be more effective to achieving a goal, than would weekly therapy for months. Specific therapy interventions (constraint-induced therapy for hemiplegia, robotics for gait) may require this greater intensity over a specific time frame to be effective (Christy et al., 2012; Meyer-Heim & van Hedel, 2013; Sakzewski et al., 2014; Vargus-Adams et al., 2021).

Complementary and alternative therapies (CAM) are often requested by parents of children with disabilities because they are seeking anything that might help their child. These therapies might include massage, hyperbaric oxygen, conductive education, Adeli suite therapy, Doman-Delacato patterning therapy, and craniosacral therapy. Complementary and alternative medicine includes practices that have not yet met standards of safety and efficacy through clinical trials or through consensus of the medical community. While the potential benefit/risk in terms of function, health, cost, and time of these interventions vary, the vulnerability of the families is a commonality (Vargus-Adams et al., 2021). The inclusion of CAM interventions in a life care plan must be carefully weighed.

The public educational system under PL 108-446, the Individuals with Disability Education Improvement Act (IDEA, 2004) and Every Student Succeeds Act (ESSA, 2015) only provide what is educationally relevant for a disabled child to learn in the current environment of their individualized education program (IEP). Therapy services provided by school districts are typically limited to those services needed to meet educational goals and access to instruction in the classroom and other school environments to comply with requirements for a free and appropriate public education (FAPE). In many school districts, therapists serve in a consultative role to develop plans to be carried out by teachers or teacher's aides, with periodic re-evaluations performed within the IEP. This contrasts sharply with the work of therapists in a clinical setting who provide therapeutic encounters as treatment to enhance physical status through range of motion and strengthening modalities as well as application of orthoses to mitigate the influence of spasticity, as possible, and prevent deformity. Dysfunctional swallowing is another example of an issue that therapists address in the medical model that are not addressed in school-based services, due to concerns for possible aspiration. Therefore, functional restoration and general habilitation of children with cerebral palsy and other conditions resulting in neurocognitive and neuromotor disabilities is generally considered beyond the school's mandate or scope of service requirements that are limited to therapeutic services to meet the child's educational goals and objectives. For more discussion regarding special education for children with disabilities, please refer to the special education chapter in this text.

To be effective, therapy must be individualized, engaging, and interesting to the patient if they have the cognitive ability to participate, be reinforced by the family and school caregivers, and be provided at an intensity, frequency, and duration that matches the child's current needs. All of these issues must be taken into consideration when forming a lifelong therapy plan. Weekly therapy throughout the lifetime is rarely the most appropriate model . A pediatric PM&R physician can be a valuable resource in identifying therapy needs, as well as equipment and medical needs specific to disability, given their training and expertise.

Life Expectancy

Undoubtedly, the costliest part of many life care plans is the long-term home care or facility care needs of the client. The intensity and length of time for which this care is needed is often hotly debated. The patient's life expectancy can be defined as the age at which they will likely pass away, although some define it as the additional years, from the current age, the patient will live. To avoid confusion, the physician determining life expectancy, the attorney, and the life care planner need to agree as to how they will reference life expectancy.

There are numerous articles, websites, and actuarial models that attempt to predict life expectancy for varying disabilities. Mortality tables may be used, with the economist projecting cost in some adult cases, depending on the state where litigation is occurring. However, for pediatric patients in particular, the individual must be considered. Statistics do not consider or account for the quality, access, or level of care that the patient receives, their individual health history, their family situation, or educational level, socio-economic status, or so many other factors which can have a great impact. The implementation of the life care plan, which provides for the type of care that can affect health and longevity, is also not accounted for in these models. The treating physician and physician experts will consider the medical records, client's health history, and the many elements of their past, present, and future care, as delineated in the life care plan, to opine on life expectancy.

The Role of the Medical Home

Medical home implementation in pediatric care has been shown to improve the quality and efficiency of care, and there have been demonstrated benefits in relation to preventative care outcomes and specific conditions. Provision of coordinated services through an effective medical home has resulted in reduced hospitalizations and emergency visits for children with several chronic conditions (Kuo & Houtrow, 2016).

The medical home is defined as a model of primary healthcare that is accessible, family-centered, continuous, comprehensive, coordinated, compassionate, and culturally effective (HRSA, 2020). Six components have been identified for an effective system of care for CYSHCN:

- Children are screened early and continuously for special healthcare needs
- Families of CYSHCN are partners in decision-making
- Community-based services are organized so families can use them easily
- CYSHCN receive care in a medical home
- There is adequate insurance and funding to cover services
- CYSHCN receive services necessary to make the transition to adult healthcare

Children with medical complexity (CMC) are further defined as those who have multiple significant chronic health problems that affect multiple organ systems and result in functional limitations, high healthcare need or utilization, and often the need for or use of medical technology (Cohen et al., 2011). Approximately 1% of children, most of whom are children with medical complexity, account for up to one-third of overall healthcare spending for children, an increasing percentage of pediatric hospitalizations, and recurrent hospital admissions (Cohen et al., 2011). Evidence suggests that these children have among the highest risk of all children for adverse medical, developmental, psychosocial, and family outcomes. Care coordination through a primary care physician or comanaged with a complex care service (ideally including a physician specializing in PM&R

within a hospital or clinic setting can reduce the number of visits necessary to the tertiary care center, increase adherence to the care plan, raise satisfaction for families, and decrease costs through reduced hospital utilization (Cohen et al., 2011). Regardless of the setting, a child with complex medical needs should have periodic scheduled contact with their medical home as part of the care plan to address growth and nutrition, health maintenance and preventative care (including dental care), developmental and psychosocial needs, family functioning, medical management of underlying chronic conditions, long-term planning, and timely intervention in the case of an adverse event. The health maintenance visit is additionally one of the best times for review of home health services, if applicable.

Unfortunately, the most recent National Survey of Children's Health revealed that less than half (42.7%) of CSYHCN had a medical home (HRSA, 2020). This provides the pediatric life care planner an opportunity to guide families regarding the importance of obtaining a medical home to ensure optimal healthcare for the child. Utilizing a family-centered approach, life care planning facilitates collaborative relationships. This, in turn, results in an integrated continuum enabling shared communication and expectations among the patient, the family, and all care providers (Riddick-Grisham, 2011).

Transition Medical and Legal Services for Adolescents with Special Needs

Transition to adolescence is another significant stage that requires decision-making. Many young females will naturally experience the onset of menstruation, but the effects of a disease or disability can sometimes complicate normal hygiene. Consultation with a specialist in gynecology with experience in treating individuals with disabilities is helpful to families in consideration of options for birth control and menstrual flow. Seizures can change and/or increase in frequency with the hormonal fluctuations of adolescence. Social interactions can sometimes be limited to the school environment, so it is important that the life care planner consider recreational opportunities that allow for appropriate and stimulating social contact. Many clinical centers are now including transition centers or teams specializing in the identification and management of issues related to transition. Due to the expansion in pediatric subspecialty care, adolescents and young adults now often transfer to an adult subspecialty counterpart, for instance in the fields of PM&R, neurology, urology, gastroenterology, pulmonology, and orthopedic surgery. There has been more focus to ensure a patient-centered medical home in the adult healthcare system, and life care planners have a unique opportunity to encourage families to always pursue this team approach to caring for their loved one.

Guardianship and Supported Decision-Making

As many children and adolescents needing a life care plan have catastrophic injuries that lead to lifelong cognitive impairments, guardianship is often necessary. This must be done prior to their eighteenth birthday, and entails at minimum, a psychological evaluation of the child, filing an application in court, and participating in a hearing. Guardians must meet requirements set by each state, as laws vary. If this process is not completed until after their eighteenth birthday, the child is appointed a guardian-ad-litem and the process is a bit more complicated. Guardianships can be temporary or can be reversed if the client's medical problems are likely to improve to a point where guardianship is not needed. Guardianships are also able to finesse the different abilities of the client, to allow decision-making for some things, but not others (e.g., placement decision, but not finances).

For individuals who need assistance making decisions about things like healthcare, finances, relationships, and living arrangement, "supported decision-making" is an alternative to guardianship. It allows individuals with disabilities to make their own choices with the support of a team of people they select. The structure and process for choosing this option varies state to state, but the individual and supporters execute a Supported Decision-Making agreement.

Educating families about these options and processes is a role the life care plan's case manager can play, as well as a licensed state attorney or guardianship clinic. By working with a case manager or life care planner, families can help design a plan to facilitate continued health and well-being with access to the least restrictive living environment in a setting that provides for the individual's daily care needs, socialization, recreation, and, when appropriate, work. More information can be found through the Center for Public Representation (2022).

Long-Term Living Options

One of the major challenges faced by life care planners and families is the availability of long-term living options for the child, adolescent, or young adult with disabling conditions. When young, the child most often remains in the family home with the necessary supports in place. Full- or part-time skilled nursing or home health attendant care must be considered as well as respite care. Unfortunately, the ongoing nursing shortage makes the reliability and sustainability of these options difficult. It is not news that nurses are leaving the healthcare profession in droves, and many blame the COVID-19 pandemic. Since the start of the pandemic in March 2020, it is estimated that almost 500,000 employees have left healthcare (U.S. Department of Labor, 2022). It has been suggested that the pandemic only served to shine a light and exacerbate issues that have long been present in healthcare.

An additional concern is that nurses who care for children with disabilities need specialized pediatric training to provide appropriate care. To assume a nurse who has worked with adults is competent to care for a medically fragile child in a family home is ill-advised. Even experienced nurses need training to deal with the issues of the child and family. Those who care for children with disabilities need to understand that they live within complex family systems that will change over time. Healthcare providers must have a special awareness of how to maximize life outcomes as the child matures within this changing dynamic (Riddick-Grisham, 2011).

Depending on the medical needs of the child, the life care planner will assess if full- or part-time care can be rendered by skilled nursing or home healthcare attendants. Some families may choose to independently hire a private healthcare worker to reside in the home. Families who pursue this course must be cognizant of the requirement to provide the live-in employee a private room and benefits, such as health and workers' compensation insurance coverage. If a caregiver is to be hired directly, it is important to have a written agreement setting out the terms of the employment as well as the defined duties to be performed. The Family Caregiver Alliance (caregiver.org) suggests that the following areas be considered:

- Personal care: bathing, eating, dressing, toileting
- Household care: cooking, cleaning, laundry, shopping
- Healthcare: medication management, physician's appointments, physical therapy
- Emotional care: companionship, meaningful activities, conversation

While these general services are to be included in the design of the private-hire home care plan, there are many other considerations to be addressed by the family, such as:

Prescreening Activities

Bonding
Check auto general liability policy regarding "household employee" coverage
Check homeowners' insurance for injury coverage
Credit check
Criminal check
Do Not Hire checklist
Driving record
Drug and alcohol screen
Medical examination
Reference checks

Contract for Services

Attorney fees (for contracts, employment agreements)
Clearly stated outline of services to be provided
Employment schedule, need for pool of providers
House rules
Overtime pay
Payroll schedule
Performance reviews
Repeat drug and alcohol screen
Termination policy
Vacation/leave policy
Accounting fees if not utilizing payroll software
Bank fees
Federal
Payroll taxes
Social Security/Medicare
State
Unemployment insurance
Workers' compensation

Attention must be given to food and utility costs, parking restrictions, and emergency contact systems. Additional hours for case management coordination to assist with identification, screening, and scheduling will be required, if the case manager agrees to this responsibility.

Providing respite care either in or outside of the home is essential to avoid caregiver burnout. The day-to-day requirements of caring for a child with special health needs often becomes overwhelming and can cause severe stress and the potential of family breakdown. Camps can be considered as an option for respite care. Some programs require a family member, nurse, or other healthcare provider to accompany the child during the camp experience.

If the young adult with special health needs continues to reside in the family home, it is important that the family create a plan that will address the time when the aging parent(s) will no longer be available to provide medical care or care supervision. It is essential that the family and caregivers look for ways to promote socialization, stimulating recreation, and, if appropriate, employment for their young person.

If necessary, residential placement options for children, adolescents, and young adults with significant disability are very limited and may be some distance from the family home. As their child ages, families should begin looking at all options for long-term living. Unfortunately, even group homes for individuals with neurocognitive and/or neuromotor disabilities have extensive wait lists for placement. Some young adults who can live in a community setting often require full- or part-time help from lay persons or home healthcare providers. To ensure their continued independence and safety, all transportation, socialization, financial, and legal issues must be addressed.

Assisted living programs may be another option for families. If a placement is being considered, it is important to select a program that allows for socialization and recreation for the young person with disabilities through interaction with age-related peers. In addition, the decision-makers should be mindful of the medical care and daily assistance the facility will provide. In certain situations, it is also important to confirm that the program can support access to community events and work, if appropriate (Riddick-Grisham, 2011).

The Pediatric Life Care Planner

As a transdisciplinary specialty practice, life care plans are developed by a variety of professionals. It is the responsibility of the life care planner to abide by the scope and standards of practice within their own profession as well as the standards of life care planning according to industry standards and organizational governance (International Academy of Life Care Planners, 2022; Preston & Reid, 2015; Weed & Berens, 2018). The specific professional education, training, and experience of each life care planner has likely included interactions with pediatric and adolescent age groups, and these should be relied upon when developing a pediatric life care plan. As part of an established methodology, the planner must consider not only the evaluee and the family, but also the process of aging with disability. The treatment team's recommendations should be discussed based upon "needs-driven" considerations and the most current research on the disability. Because life care plans are designed to cover a lifetime of needs, the process must be structured to allow for updating and revision as changes occur over time (Riddick-Grisham, 2011).

To begin work, the life care planner will request several different items, as described in Riddick-Grisham & Deming (2011).

Case Referral

Request all medical records, medical and therapeutic consults, early intervention records, school records (including IEP documents), medical and pharmaceutical billing records, photographs, and videos. Request that the referral source notify the family and any experts of life care plan involvement, as well as the clinical treatment team, school, and home care personnel if appropriate. Obtain a signed contract and retainer. Request time to meet with the child and family. Confirm a requested date of report completion and other important time frames (e.g., trial and discovery dates). Recommend a vocational consultant to the referral source, as appropriate. Determine who will be addressing life expectancy.

Medical Records Review

Review primary and secondary diagnoses; problem lists; current providers and specialized consultants; frequency, duration, and treatment of complications, including hospitalizations and surgeries as well as invasive procedures; medication usage and response. Chart developmental surveillance. Note standardized assessments (e.g., Apgar scores, developmental screenings). Document significant laboratory studies, radiological and diagnostic findings, as well as immunization status. Outline rehabilitation outcomes.

Supporting Information

Determine if additional evaluations are required (neuropsychological evaluation, current therapy assessments, IEP evaluation). Obtain information from case management/social work or other sources as indicated. If available, obtain additional information from the family (e.g., personal logbooks). Review depositions of the child, family, treatment team, or other experts, as well as videos as indicated and available. When appropriate, obtain pre- and post-injury school records, including test scores. Academic, vocational, and employment history of immediate family members as available and appropriate.

Initial Interview

Perhaps the most important step in the life care planning process is the family interview. When possible, conduct interviews in the family home or other living environment. Prepare family by requesting that they have equipment and medications available for inspection. If home-based therapy is being administered, try to meet with the therapist if possible while in the home. Observe child at school or at outpatient therapy as appropriate. Use a structured interview form. Request that the responsible party sign a HIPAA-compliant medical release form. Photograph the child and their equipment, supplies, and home. Observe the child for social interaction, physical function, behavior, complications (seizure frequency, suctioning requirements), and play.

Multiple family visits may occur over the course of developing a life care plan, but none is more important than the first. The reality of having a child that will require a significant amount of healthcare has a profound effect on both the child's and the family's future. Many such families are caring sometimes for a very young child who, in some ways, may seem to be typically appearing, but whose developmental delay will become increasingly evident as the child grows and matures. Reaction to this life crisis varies widely because of cultural, religious, individual beliefs, family structure, and support systems. The challenge for the life care planner and the child's treatment team is to be culturally aware and knowledgeable about different cultural values, beliefs, and practices because they can greatly influence all aspects of healthcare. Parents experience intense stress during the grieving process that accompanies an atypical birth or a disability diagnosis, particularly because most parents are poorly prepared for anything but a "normal" child and often have had little or no exposure to the specific disability (Riddick-Grisham, 2011).

Building a relationship involves taking the time to listen to family members as they describe the day-to-day challenge of managing care requirements for their child and the emotional and psychosocial impact on the family unit. It is important that the life care planner develop an intimate understanding of the child's daily schedule, including hygiene, feeding, therapy, school, medication, and outside appointments. When dealing with a family with limited English proficiency, qualified professional interpreters must be used to gather information, provide instructions, or obtain consent.

The planner can sometimes ascertain subtle information that can give a great deal of insight into the understanding of the family dynamics. For example, in many instances when families are asked where the child sleeps, they will report that the child sleeps in the parental bed, although the child is well beyond the age when they typically would sleep in a separate room. When this information is presented to the life care planner, it can result in the exploration of issues impacting the decision to keep the child in the parental bedroom. One would want to consider the need for counseling support to help ease the anxiety of this normal transition, or an understanding of what types of interventions that the parents are providing through the night.

During the interview process, the family will be asked to provide an overview of the child's medical history. Asking the family to review the child's medical history allows the life care planner to evaluate the family's understanding of the disability, relationship with service providers, and insight into the future course of the disability. It also reveals relevant information pertaining to the family's level of empowerment and how its members will approach the decision-making process.

In each individual instance, the life care planner must address specific challenges and bring them to the attention of the family. As an example, families caring for children in wheelchairs need to consider the accessibility issues that will allow for care, hygiene, therapy, transportation, and recreation. Frequently, the use of photographs can document accessibility and the condition of equipment and can be a useful tool if the life care planner requests additional evaluations done by an architect or contractor skilled in understanding home modification needs. In addition, many families with very young children will likely have spent a limited amount time thinking about a future in which they may be unable to adequately care for their child. In the face of daily challenges, this essential issue can get lost, giving the life care planner an opportunity to address this important consideration. These types of interactions give the life care planner insight into the fears as well as the maladjustment issues that exist within the family (Riddick-Grisham, 2011).

To gather such information, most life care planners rely on a comprehensive interview form that documents:

- Medical history: History of treatment since birth and/or onset of the disability
- Growth and development: Charting the achievement or delay in developmental milestones
- Treatment team: Identification by name, location, and specialty of each medical provider
- Therapy team: Identification by name, location, and specialty of each therapy provider
- School/education: Identification by name and location of early intervention program, schools, teachers, school-based therapists, and a description of the IEP that includes a list of the child's achievements
- Medications: Detailed listing of all medications, including dosages and administration schedules
- Supplies: Detailed listing of supplies, including their purchase, use, and replacement patterns
- Equipment: Detailed listing of equipment including purchase dates and use, maintenance, and replacement schedules
- Family configuration: Age and health of both parents and each sibling, location of the family residence, the parents' (and in some instances the siblings') acquired educational and training levels, work experience, and work schedules
- Family adjustment: Identification of the primary care giver, back-up and respite support systems, family or individual counseling resources, family recreation needs, and sibling support resources

- Activities of daily living: Detailed analysis of the child's mobility, communication skills, and ability to perform hygiene, dressing, toileting, and medication administration
- Daily schedule: Detailed description of the child's daily schedule
- Home accessibility: A review of the accessibility issues that limit the child's access to and within the home environment
- Transportation: Description of the family vehicle and any modifications necessary to ensure the child's safe transport
- Future thoughts: An important overview of the family's thoughts, concerns, and fears regarding their child's future

Understand Daily Care Requirements

Document time, equipment, and level of assistance required for daily hygiene, dressing, grooming, feeding, toileting, behavior management, medication administration, transport to school, and outside appointments. Identify primary caregivers, respite care, and home health providers. Recognize other family demands including sibling care, work, and school.

Team Collaboration

When possible and/or indicated, consult with the current clinical team (i.e., physicians and therapists), school personnel, community providers, home healthcare providers, DME sources, and pharmacies. Use researched literature, standards of care, and clinical guidelines as needed. If access to an entity is denied, consult with the expert evaluators and document all attempts to secure information. Using a team approach, analyze needs through the developmental process; always consider aging and quality of life. Create the medical foundation for medically related items.

Because the next step in the completion of the life care plan may include collaboration with the clinical, therapy, and school teams, the life care planner should ask the family to sign a Health Insurance Portability and Accountability Act (HIPAA)-compliant medical release form (Health Insurance Portability and Accountability Act of 1996 [HIPAA], updated in 2020 in response to the COVID-19 pandemic). The life care planner can consult, either in writing or in person, with members of the clinical team to gather their opinions regarding the child's future needs (see Figure 7.1). Soliciting input from team members and drawing from their unique training and experience allow for development of a care plan that is based on medical and habilitative or rehabilitative probability and focuses on achievement of successful long-term outcomes in the least restrictive environment; at the same time, it considers issues of safety, well-being, and quality of life. It is important that the life care planner create the medical foundation or rationale for medically related items contained in the life care plan. For instance, during collaboration with the life care planner, the treating or consulting pediatric neurologist will base medical recommendations on clinical protocols and practice guidelines that the life care planner should appropriately incorporate to provide a valid foundation for the application of the specific recommendations.

The life care planner should not only rely on the experience and input from the clinical team, but also address issues surrounding equipment and supplies, therapeutic recreation, case management, home modifications, and transportation. Because case management is foundational to life care planning and long-term living is traditionally an area that, when implemented, uses case

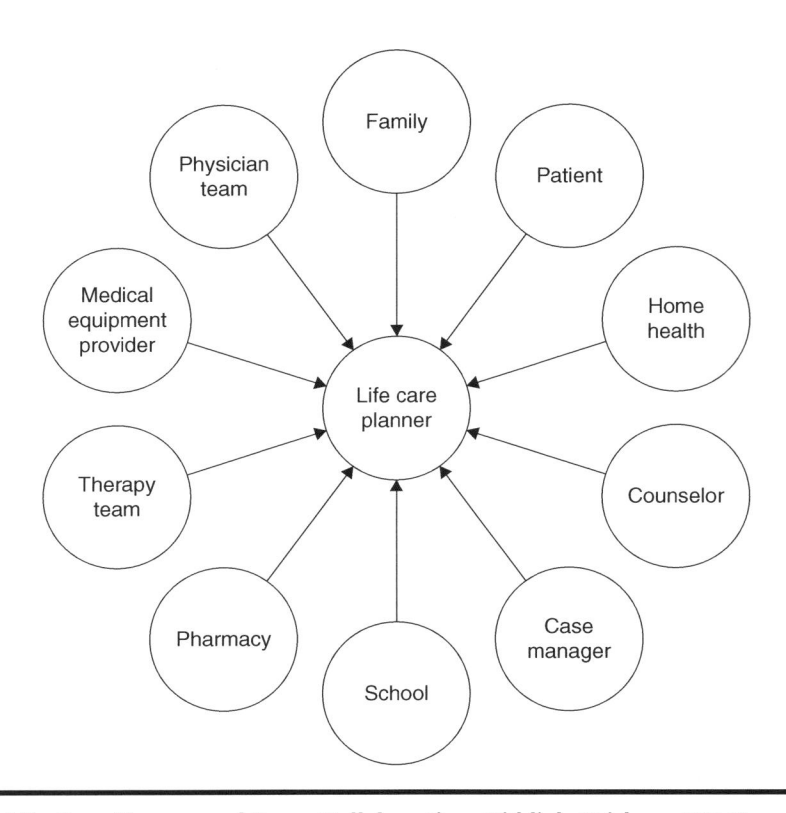

Figure 7.1 Life Care Planner and Team Collaboration (Riddick-Grisham, 2011)

management services, the life care planner is often more aware than other team members of the variety of living options available to the child and family. Additionally, the life care planner may be more familiar with the rules of state and federal regulatory agencies as they apply to home healthcare and the role and function of home healthcare providers. As an example, currently in many states, administration of nutrition via a gastrostomy tube is considered a skilled nursing activity as defined by the Nurse Practice Act, and home health agencies must send in a licensed practical nurse (LPN) or registered nurse (RN) in those states for the management of tube feeding. If the life care plan includes a home health aide to provide this service rather than a skilled nurse, it can be a costly error that could have been avoided if the principles of case management were applied (Riddick-Grisham, 2011).

An integral component of life care planning and case management involves the child's access to educational opportunity and services available through the public school system. As part of the information-gathering process, the life care planner may wish to interview the child's early intervention and special education team members to review the services for which the child is eligible. Section 504 of the Rehabilitation Act of 1973, the ADA of 1990, and the Individuals with Disabilities Education Act ([IDEA], 2004) are the legislative efforts that established the framework for provision of special education and related services for children. As previously noted, IDEA requires that all children with disabilities who meet eligibility criteria for special education services have a free, appropriate public education available to them. This education must include the related services designed to meet their unique needs and to prepare them for employment and independent living (IDEA, 2004).

Research Costs

Determine usual and customary costs utilizing statically valid and reliable data sources and methodology. Use vendors and manufacturers to determine costs as well as replacement and maintenance schedules. Use geographically relevant vendors as indicated.

Finalizing the Life Care Plan

Review the plan to confirm that it is individualized, family-centered, reasonable, appropriately lifelong, and based upon a sound foundation of medical research data and experience. Check for overlaps, computation, or other errors. A major part of life care planning methodology involves the use of a reliable system for information accumulation and documentation. The categories outlined in Table 7.1 are considered in the development of each life care plan. Even though each category

Table 7.1 Pediatric Life Care Plan Checklist

Projected evaluations: Have you planned for different types of nonphysician evaluations (e.g., physical therapy, speech therapy, recreational therapy, occupational therapy, music therapy, dietary assessments, audiology, vision screening, swallow studies)?
Projected therapeutic modalities: What therapies will be needed based upon the evaluations? Is behavior management with psychological counseling warranted?
Diagnostic testing/educational assessment: What testing is necessary for the child and at what ages? Vocational evaluation? Neuropsychological evaluation?
Wheelchair needs: What types and configuration of wheelchair(s) will the child require? Power? Shower? Manual? Specialty? Ventilator, reclining, quad pegs features?
Wheelchair accessories and maintenance: Has each chair been listed separately for maintenance and accessories if indicated (e.g., bags, cushions, trays)? Have you considered the child's activity level?
Aids for independent functioning: What items can this individual use for assistance? Environmental controls? Adaptive devices?
Orthoses/prostheses: Will the child require orthoses or prostheses? Have you planned for replacement and maintenance?
Home furnishings and accessories: Will the child need a specialty bed? Portable ramps? Hoyer or other lift?
Drug/supply needs: Have prescription and non-prescription drugs been listed, including size, quantity, and dose? All supplies such as bladder and bowel program, skin care, etc.?
Home care/facility care: Is it possible for the child to live at home? How about specialty programs such as yearly camps? What level of care will the child require? Eventual facility care?
Future medical care routine: Which medical specialties? Specialty dentistry? Additional primary care physician visits? Laboratory or radiological studies?
Transportation: Is a specialty van needed? Vehicle modifications, such as hand controls, etc.?

(Continued)

Table 7.1 (Continued) Pediatric Life Care Plan Checklist

Health and strength maintenance: What specialty recreation is needed? Adaptive exercise equipment? (Specialty wheelchairs should be placed on wheelchair page)
Architectural renovations: Have you considered ramps, hallways, kitchen, fire protection, alternative heating/cooling, floor coverings, bath, attendant room, equipment storage, etc.?
Future medical care/surgical intervention or interventional treatment: Are interventional treatments planned? Or additional surgeries, such as reconstruction, contracture releases, hip procedures, scoliosis surgery?
Orthopedic equipment needs: Is a gait trainer, stander, or body support equipment needed?
Vocational/educational plan: What are the costs of vocational counseling, job coach/life skills training, tuition, fees, books, supplies, technology, etc.?
Potential complications: Have you considered a list of potential (possible rather than probable) complications that can occur?

Source: Adapted from Weed, R., 2001.

should be evaluated, not all will apply in each case, nor will they all be necessary for the formulation of an effective pediatric life care plan.

The life care planner must assess the frequency and duration of each need within all applicable categories. Although report formats vary among life care planners, they should clearly document the need for and the usual and customary cost of each given item, the expected duration of that need, and the projected frequency and cost of the item's replacement. For example, when the life care planner addresses the future needs of a child with a seizure disorder, creating an individualized life care plan requires close examination of the unique characteristics of the case. Future medical care and therapeutic interventions vary dramatically based on the type of seizure disorder and associated complications, the standards and protocols implemented by the clinical management team, as well as other considerations. Furthermore, the interrelationships among all the child's needs must be anticipated by the life care planner.

Life care plans are dynamic documents and will require periodic updating and revision to accommodate changes in family structure, new diagnoses, medical complications, or any change in the child's functional status. Life care plans are often used in civil litigation to outline the future needs of a child with subsequent trust fund establishment. Once the case is completed and the funds are in place in the form of a trust, the life care plan can be implemented according to the provisions of the trust in consultation with a case manager or life care planner. In other situations, a life care plan is implemented using the funds and resources available to the family (Riddick-Grisham, 2011).

Summary

Life care planning for children, adolescents, and young adults with significant disabling conditions is both challenging and rewarding. Life expectancy for these individuals has improved, resulting in an increase in demand for all levels of care, from the primary care provider to community and educational services, to required specialty healthcare services. Medical home implementation in pediatric care has been shown to improve quality and efficiency of care and should be ensured by the life care planner. Additionally, there are many unique considerations for children with special healthcare needs. The planner should understand the child's individual delays and how they were diagnosed. For children with neurocognitive and neuromotor deficits, a seizure disorder may need to be included in projected care. This group is also at higher risk for developing oral health disease and sialorrhea that must be addressed. Nutritional guidelines for children and adolescents with disabilities require special attention and may include feedings via gastrostomy tube. These children may require orthopedic surveillance, often due to immobility, and they may face issues with osteopenia. During the years of growth and development, individual therapy needs are important, and close attention should be given to pediatric medical equipment and assistive technology, including the appropriate replacement cycles. Specific home modifications and travel accessibility may need to be included. The interview and evaluation process are critical for building a relationship with the family to understand their challenges and the child's care requirements. The life care planner must then create the medical foundation for the medically related items from the clinical team, treatment protocols, and practice guidelines, as well as their own training and experience within their individual scope of practice. The life care plan is meant to establish an integrated continuum to improve outcomes and reduce complications throughout the child's entire lifespan.

Key Points for Life Care Planners

Pediatric life care planning is unique, as it involves multiple medical specialists over time, the educational system, specialized equipment, guardianship, and transition needs, and as well as an extended impact of aging with a disability.

- Neuropsychology testing is often repeated as children develop cognitively, verbally, and emotionally.
- Seizure interventions require modification as the child ages, and inpatient monitoring, special diets, medication dosing adjustments, and surgical interventions can occur.
- Dental problems are common due to cariogenic diets, difficulty with oral hygiene, and dependence on caregivers, and can be missed in non-verbal patients. Sedation is often needed for treatment.
- Dietary requirements must be updated, as swallowing and feeding skills as well as caloric needs change over the lifetime. Special growth charts and formulas are available to assist the dietitian and pediatric provider.
- Spasticity treatments involve therapies, orthoses, oral and injectable medications (which are not necessarily weight based), orthopedic and neurosurgical procedures. Interventions increase in intensity during the periods of growth and development and occur in tandem.
- The treatment of scoliosis involves an interplay between seating systems, orthoses, and possible surgery, which can be multi-step over time to allow for growth.
- Osteoporosis and related fragility fractures are common and can affect the child's comfort level, the outcome of orthopedic surgical procedures, and their equipment needs. Proactive versus reactive treatment should be highly considered.
- Adapted mobility equipment has physical and psychological benefits for the growing child and their needs will change over time. Reduction of lifting the child and adolescent will also protect the caregivers.
- Alternative communication systems and other assistive technologies should be introduced as early as possible, to encourage independence and autonomy.

- Adapted recreational equipment can improve cardiovascular and musculoskeletal fitness and provides social opportunities that might otherwise be impossible.
- Therapy, both medically and educationally based, is valuable, and variable in timing, frequency, and duration, and provides habilitative, not just rehabilitative benefits.
- Consideration of the family's, and the adolescent's (if appropriate) wishes should be incorporated in long-term care planning.
- The interview and evaluation process are critical for building a relationship with the family to understand their challenges and the child's care requirements.
- Medical home implementation in pediatric care has been shown to improve quality and efficiency of care and should be ensured by the life care planner.
- The life care plan is meant to establish an integrated continuum to improve

Note

1 This chapter is adapted from Riddick-Grisham, S. & Deming, L. (Eds.) (2011). *Pediatric life care planning and case management handbook.* Routledge.

References

Airaksinen, E. M., Matilainen, R., Mononen, T., Mustonen, K., Partanen, J., Jokela, V., & Halonen, P. (2000). A population-based study on epilepsy in mentally retarded children. *Epilepsia*, *41*(9), 1214–1220.

Allam, A. M., & Schwabe, A. L. (2013). Neuromuscular scoliosis. *PM&R: The Journal of Injury, Function, and Rehabilitation*, *5*(11), 957–963. https://doi.org/10.1016/j.pmrj.2013.05.015

American Academy of Cerebral Palsy and Developmental Medicine (2022a). Sialorrhea in cerebral palsy. www.aacpdm.org/publications/care-pathways/sialorrhea-in-cerebral-palsy

American Academy for Cerebral Palsy and Developmental Medicine. (2022b). *Dystonia in cerebral palsy.* www.aacpdm.org/publications/care-pathways/dystonia-in-cerebral-palsy

American Academy of Pediatric Dentistry. (2021). Policy on oral health care programs for infants, children, adolescents, and individuals with special health care needs. *The Reference Manual of Pediatric Dentistry. American Academy of Pediatric Dentistry*, 9–42.

Arvedson J. C. (2013). Feeding children with cerebral palsy and swallowing difficulties. *European Journal of Clinical Nutrition*, *67*(Suppl 2), S9–S12. https:doi.org/10.1038/ejcn.2013.224

Asconapé, J. J. (2010). The selection of antiepileptic drugs for the treatment of epilepsy in children and adults. *Neurologic Clinics*, *28*(4), 843–852.

Bell, K. L., & Samson-Fang, L. (2013). Nutritional management of children with cerebral palsy. *European Journal of Clinical Nutrition*, *67*(Suppl 2), S13–S16. https://doi.org/10.1038/ejcn.2013.225

Besag, F. M. (2002). Childhood epilepsy in relation to mental handicap and behavioural disorders. *Journal of Child Psychology and Psychiatry*, *43*(1), 103–131.

Binkley, C. J., Johnson, K. W., Abdi, M., Thompson, K., Shamblen, S. R., Young, L., & Zaksek, B. (2014). Improving the oral health of residents with intellectual and developmental disabilities: An oral health strategy and pilot study. *Evaluation and Program Planning*, *47*, 54–63. https://doi.org/10.1016/j.evalprogplan.2014.07.003

Boyce, A. M., Tosi, L. L., & Paul, S. M. (2014). Bisphosphonate treatment for children with disabling conditions. *PM&R: The Journal of Injury, Function, and Rehabilitation*, *6*(5), 427–436. https://doi.org/10.1016/j.pmrj.2013.10.009

Brooks, J., Day, S., Shavelle, R., & Strauss, D. (2011). Low weight, morbidity, and mortality in children with cerebral palsy: New clinical growth charts. *Pediatrics*, *128*(2), e299–e307. https://doi.org/10.1542/peds.2010-2801

Brooks, J. T., & Sponseller, P. D. (2016). What's new in the management of neuromuscular scoliosis. *Journal of Pediatric Orthopaedics*, *36*(6), 627–633.

Brothers, K. B., Glascoe, F. P., & Robertshaw, N. S. (2008). PEDS: developmental milestones—An accurate brief tool for surveillance and screening. *Clinical Pediatrics*, *47*(3), 271–279.

Center for Public Representation. (2022). About supported decision making. https://supporteddecisions.org/about-supported-decision-making/

Chang, F. M., May, A., Faulk, L. W., Flynn, K., Miller, N. H., Rhodes, J. T., Zhaoxing, P., & Novais, E. N. (2018). Outcomes of isolated varus derotational osteotomy in children with cerebral palsy hip dysplasia and predictors of resubluxation. *Journal of Pediatric Orthopedics*, *38*(5), p. 274–278. https://doi.org/10.1097/BPO.0000000000000809

Chhabra, N., & Chhabra, A. (2020). Evaluation of the efficacy of the modified Bluegrass appliance in cessation of thumb-sucking habit: An in vivo study with 12 months follow-up. *Medicine and Pharmacy Reports*, *93*(2), 190–194. https://doi.org/10.15386/mpr-1329

Christy, J. B., Chapman, C. G., & Murphy, P. (2012). The effect of intense physical therapy for children with cerebral palsy. *Journal of Pediatric Rehabilitation Medicine*, *5*(3), 159–170. https://doi.org/10.3233/PRM-2012-0208

Cohen, E., Kuo, D. Z., Agrawal, R., Berry, J. G., Bhagat, S. K., Simon, T. D., & Srivastava, R. (2011). Children with medical complexity: An emerging population for clinical and research initiatives. *Pediatrics*, *127*(3), 529–538.

Council on Children with Disabilities, Section on Developmental Behavioral Pediatrics, Bright Futures Steering Committee, & Medical Home Initiatives for Children with Special Needs Project Advisory Committee. (2006). Identifying infants and young children with developmental disorders in the medical home: An algorithm for developmental surveillance and screening. *Pediatrics*, *118*(1), 405–420.

Day, S. M., & Reynolds, R. J. (2018). Survival, mortality, and life expectancy. In Al-Zwaini IJ (ed.), *Cerebral palsy – Clinical and therapeutic aspects* (pp. 45–64). http://dx.doi.org/10.5772/intechopen.80293

Dias, B. L., Fernandes, A. R., & Maia Filho, H. S. (2016). Sialorrhea in children with cerebral palsy. *Journal de Pediatría*, *92*(6), 549–558. https://doi.org/ 10.1016/j.jped.2016.03.006

Dibb, M., Teubner, A., Theis, V., Shaffer, J., & Lal, S. (2013). Review article: The management of long-term parenteral nutrition. *Alimentary Pharmacology & Therapeutics*, *37*(6), 587–603. https://doi.org/10.1111/apt.12209

Eliasson, A. C., Krumlinde-Sundholm, L., Rösblad, B., Beckung, E., Arner, M., Öhrvall, A. M., & Rosenbaum, P. (2006). The Manual Ability Classification System (MACS) for children with cerebral palsy: Scale development and evidence of validity and reliability. *Developmental Medicine & Child Neurology*, *48*, 549–554.

El-Shamy, S. M., & Abdelaal, A. A. (2016). WalkAide efficacy on gait and energy expenditure in children with hemiplegic cerebral palsy: A randomized controlled trial. *American Journal of Physical Medicine & Rehabilitation*, *95*(9), 629–638. https://doi.org/10.1097/PHM.0000000000000514

Fluss, J., & Lidzba, K. (2020). Cognitive and academic profiles in children with cerebral palsy: A narrative review. *Annals of Physical and Rehabilitation Medicine*, *63*(5), 447–456. https://doi.org/10.1016/j.rehab.2020.01.005

Freeman, J. M., Kossoff, E. H., & Hartman, A. L. (2007). The ketogenic diet: One decade later. *Pediatrics*, *119*(3), 535–543.

Gormely M., & Deshpande S. (2021). Hypertonia. In K. P. Murphy, M. A. McMahon, & A. J. Houtrow (Eds.), *Pediatric rehabilitation principles and practice* (6th ed., pp. 100–124). Springer Publishing.

H.R. 647–113th Congress (2013-2014): Achieving a Better Life Experience Act of 2014. (2014, December 3). www.congress.gov/bill/113th-congress/house-bill/647

Harden, C., Tomson, T., Gloss, D., Buchhalter, J., Cross, J. H., Donner, E., French, J. A., Gil-Nagel, A., Hesdorffer, D. C., Smithson, H., Spitz, M. C., Walczak, T. S., Sander, J. W., & Ryvlin, P. (2017). Practice guideline summary: Sudden unexpected death in epilepsy incidence rates and risk factors: Report of the guideline development, dissemination, and implementation subcommittee of the American Academy of Neurology and the American Epilepsy Society. *Epilepsy Currents*, *17*(3), 180–187.

Hidecker, M. J., Paneth, N., Rosenbaum, P. L., Kent, R. D., Lillie, J., Eulenberg, J. B., Chester, K., Jr., Johnson, B., Michalsen, L., Evatt, M., & Taylor, K. (2011). Developing and validating the Communication Function Classification System for individuals with cerebral palsy. *Developmental Medicine and Child Neurology*, *53*(8), 704–710. https://doi.org/10.1111/j.1469-8749.2011.03996.x

Holmes, G. L. (2002) Childhood-specific epilepsies accompanied by developmental disabilities causes and effects. In O. Devinsky & L. E. Westbrook (Eds.), *Epilepsy and developmental disabilities* (pp. 23–40). Butterworth-Heinemann. www.hhs.gov/hipaa/for-professionals/index.html

Hundozi-Hysenaj H., & Boshnjaku-Dallku I. (2008). Epilepsy in children with cerebral palsy. *Journal of Pediatric Neurology*, *6*, p. 43–46.

International Academy of Life Care Planners. (2022). *Standards of practice for life care planners* (4th ed). https://rehabpro.org/general/custom.asp?page=ialcp-standards-of-practice

Joo, S. Y., Knowtharapu, D. N., Rogers, K. J., Holmes, L., Jr, & Miller, F. (2011). Recurrence after surgery for equinus foot deformity in children with cerebral palsy: Assessment of predisposing factors for recurrence in a long-term follow-up study. *Journal of Children's Orthopaedics*, *5*(4), 289–296. https://doi.org/10.1007/s11832-011-0352-4

Josenby, A. L., Wagner, P., Jarnlo, G. B., Westbom, L., & Nordmark, E. (2012). Motor function after selective dorsal rhizotomy: A 10-year practice-based follow-up study. *Developmental Medicine and Child Neurology*, *54*(5), 429–435. https://doi.org/10.1111/j.1469-8749.2012.04258.x

Klepper, J. (2008). Glucose transporter deficiency syndrome (GLUT1DS) and the ketogenic diet. *Epilepsia*, *49*, 46–49.

Koman, L. A., Smith, B. P., & Barron, R. (2003). Recurrence of equinus foot deformity in cerebral palsy patients following surgery: A review. *Journal of the Southern Orthopaedic Association*, *12*(3), 125–134.

Kuo, D. Z., & Houtrow, A. J. (2016). Council on Children with Disabilities. Recognition and management of medical complexity. *Pediatrics*, *138*(6), e20163021.

Lattanzi S. M., Trinka E., Russo E., Striano P., Citraro R., Silvestrini M., & Brigo, F. (2019). Cannabidiol as adjunctive treatment of seizures associated with Lennox-Gastaut syndrome and Dravet syndrome. *Drugs Today*, *55*, 177–196.

Lichtblau, C. H. (2021). Cerebral palsy life expectancy: Discrepancies between literature and community data. *International Journal of Physical Medicine and Rehabilitation*, *9*(4), 1–5.

Light, J., McNaughton, D., Beukelman, D., Fager, S. K., Fried-Oken, M., Jakobs, T., & Jakobs, E. (2019). Challenges and opportunities in augmentative and alternative communication: Research and technology development to enhance communication and participation for individuals with complex communication needs. *Augmentative and Alternative Communication*, *35*(1), 1–12. https://doi.org/10.1080/07434618.2018.1556732

Limond, J., Adlam, A. L., & Cormack, M. (2014). A model for pediatric neurocognitive interventions: Considering the role of development and maturation in rehabilitation planning. *The Clinical Neuropsychologist*, *28*(2), 181–198. https://doi.org/10.1080/13854046.2013.873083

McKinney, C. M., Nelson, T., Scott, J. M., Heaton, L. J., Vaughn, M. G., & Lewis, C. W. (2014). Predictors of unmet dental need in children with autism spectrum disorder: Results from a national sample. *Academic Pediatrics*, *14*(6), 624–631.

Meyer-Heim, A., & van Hedel, H. J. (2013, June). Robot-assisted and computer-enhanced therapies for children with cerebral palsy: Current state and clinical implementation. *Seminars in Pediatric Neurology*, *20* (2), 139–145.

Miller M., & Meilahn, J. (2021). Adaptive sports and recreation. In K. P. Murphy, M. A. McMahon, & A. J. Houtrow (Eds.), *Pediatric rehabilitation principles and practice* (6th ed., pp. 243–259). Springer Publishing.

Mockler, S. R., McEwen, I. R., & Jones, M. A. (2017). Retrospective analysis of predictors of proficient power mobility in young children with severe motor impairments. *Archives of Physical Medicine and Rehabilitation*, *98*(10), 2034–2041. https://doi.org/10.1016/j.apmr.2017.05.028

Morse, A. M., & Kothare, S. V. (2016). Pediatric sudden unexpected death in epilepsy. *Pediatric Neurology*, *57*, 7–16.

Muñoz-Blanco, E., Merino-Andrés, J., Aguilar-Soto, B., García, Y. C., Puente-Villalba, M., Pérez-Corrales, J., & Güeita-Rodríguez, J. (2020). Influence of aquatic therapy in children and youth with cerebral palsy: A qualitative case study in a special education school. *International Journal of Environmental Research and Public Health, 17*(10), 3690. https://doi.org/10.3390/ijerph17103690

Murphy K., Sobus K., Moberg-Wolff, E., Dubon M., & Pico E. (2021). Musculoskeletal conditions. In K. P. Murphy, M. A. McMahon, & A. J. Houtrow (Eds.), *Pediatric rehabilitation principles and practice* (6th ed., pp. 371–409). Springer Publishing.

National Academy of Neuropsychology. (2001). NAN definition of clinical neuropsychologist. www.nanonline.org/docs/paic/pdfs/nanpositiondefneuro.pdf

Norwood, K. W., Slayton, R. L., Liptak, G. S., Murphy, N. A., Adams, R. C., Burke, R. T., Friedman, S. L., Houtrow, A. J., Kalichman, M. A., Kuo, D. Z., Levy, S. E., Turchi, R. M., Wiley, S. E., Bridgemohan, C., Peacock, G., Strickland, B., Wells, N., Wiznitzer, M., Mucha, S., Segura, A., Boulter, S., Clark, M., Gereiger, R., Krol, D., Mouradian, W., … & Keels, M. A. (2013). Oral health care for children with developmental disabilities. *Pediatrics, 131*(3), 614–619.

Novak, I. (2014). Evidence-based diagnosis, health care, and rehabilitation for children with cerebral palsy. *Journal of Child Neurology, 29*(8), 1141–1156.

Oral Cancer Foundation. (2022). Commercial formulas for the feeding tube. https://oralcancerfoundation.org/nutrition/commercial-formulas-feeding-tube/

Palisano, R., Rosenbaum, P., Walter, S., Russell, D., Wood, E., & Galuppi, B. (1997). Development and reliability of a system to classify gross motor function in children with cerebral palsy. *Developmental Medicine and Child Neurology, 39*(4), 214–223. https://doi.org/10.1111/j.1469-8749.1997.tb07414.x.

Park, E. S., Rha, D. W., Shin, J. S., Kim, S., & Jung, S. (2014). Effects of hippotherapy on gross motor function and functional performance of children with cerebral palsy. *Yonsei Medical Journal, 55*(6), 1736–1742. https://doi.org/ 10.3349/ymj.2014.55.6.1736

Pellegrino L., & Myers, S. M. (2019) Developmental assessment. In M. L. Batshaw, N. J. Roizen, & L. Pellegrino (Eds.), *Children with disabilities* (8th ed., pp. 194–198). Paul H. Brookes Publishing Co.

Pietrafusa, N., Ferretti, A., Trivisano, M., De Palma, L., Calabrese, C., Carfi Pavia, G., Tondo, I., Cappelletti, S., Vigevano, F., & Specchio, N. (2019). Purified cannabidiol for treatment of refractory epilepsies in pediatric patients with developmental and epileptic encephalopathy. *Pediatric Drugs, 21*(4), 283–290.

Porte, M., Chaléat-Valayer, E., Patte, K., D'Anjou, M. C., Boulay, C., & Laffont, I. (2014). Relevance of intraglandular injections of botulinum toxin for the treatment of sialorrhea in children with cerebral palsy: A review. *European Journal of Paediatric Neurology, 18*(6), 649–657. https://doi.org/10.1016/j.ejpn.2014.05.007

Preston, K., & Reid, C. (2015). Revision process for the standards of practice for life care planners. *Journal of Life Care Planning, 13*(3), 21–30.

Rehabilitation Engineering and Assistive Technology Society of North America. (2022). Assistive technology professional (ATP) certification. www.resna.org/Certification/Assistive-Technology-Professional-ATP

Riddick-Grisham, S., & Deming, L. (Eds.). (2011). *Pediatric life care planning and case management handbook*. Routledge.

Riddick-Grisham, S. (2011). The role of the life care planner in pediatric life care planning. In S. Riddick-Grisham & L. M. Deming, *Pediatric life care planning and case management* (2nd. ed., pp. 49–89). Routledge.

Robins, D. L., Casagrande, K., Barton, M., Chen, C. M. A., Dumont-Mathieu, T., & Fein, D. (2014). Validation of the modified checklist for autism in toddlers, revised with follow-up (M-CHAT-R/F). *Pediatrics, 133*(1), 37–45.

Rosenfeld, W. E., & Roberts, D. W. (2009). Tonic and atonic seizures: What's next—VNS or callosotomy? *Epilepsia, 50*, 25–30.

Sakzewski, L., Gordon, A., & Eliasson, A. C. (2014). The state of the evidence for intensive upper limb therapy approaches for children with unilateral cerebral palsy. *Journal of Child Neurology, 29*(8), 1077–1090. https://doi.org/10.1177/0883073814533150

Scheifele E., Patel, M. Y., Tate, A. R., & Waldman, H. B. (2019). Oral health. In M. L. Batshaw, N. J. Roizen, & L. Pellegrino (Eds.), *Children with disabilities* (8th ed., pp. 708–709). Paul H. Brookes Publishing Co.

Shih, J. J., Whitlock, J. B., Chimato, N., Vargas, E., Karceski, S. C., & Frank, R. D. (2017). Epilepsy treatment in adults and adolescents: Expert opinion, 2016. *Epilepsy & Behavior*, *69*, 186–222.

Silver, C. H. (2014). Sources of data about children's executive functioning: Review and commentary. *Child Neuropsychology: A Journal on Normal and Abnormal Development in Childhood and Adolescence*, *20*(1), 1–13. https://doi.org/10.1080/09297049.2012.727793

Sneed, R. C., May, W. L., & Stencel, C. (2001). Physicians' reliance on specialists, therapists, and vendors when prescribing therapies and durable medical equipment for children with special health care needs. *Pediatrics*, *107*(6), 1283–1290. https://doi.org/10.1542/peds.107.6.1283

Speyer, R., Cordier, R., Kim, J. H., Cocks, N., Michou, E., & Wilkes-Gillan, S. (2019). Prevalence of drooling, swallowing, and feeding problems in cerebral palsy across the lifespan: A systematic review and meta-analyses. *Developmental Medicine and Child Neurology*, *61*(11), 1249–1258. https://doi.org/10.1111/dmcn.14316

Squires, J., Bricker, D. D., & Twombly, E. (2009). *Ages & stages questionnaires* (pp. 257–182). Paul H. Brookes.

Starnes, K., Miller, K., Wong-Kisiel, L., & Lundstrom, B. N. (2019). A review of neurostimulation for epilepsy in pediatrics. *Brain Sciences*, *9*(10), 283.

Stockings, E., Zagic, D., Campbell, G., Weier, M., Hall, W. D., Nielsen, S., Herkes, G. K., Farrell, M., & Degenhardt, L. (2018). Evidence for cannabis and cannabinoids for epilepsy: A systematic review of controlled and observational evidence. *Journal of Neurology, Neurosurgery & Psychiatry*, *89*(7), 741–753.

Terra, V. C., Furlanetti, L. L., Nunes, A. A., Thomé, U., Nisyiama, M. A., Sakamoto, A. C., & Machado, H. R. (2014). Vagus nerve stimulation in pediatric patients: Is it really worthwhile? *Epilepsy & Behavior*, *31*, 329–333.

Thomas, S. A., Cotton, W., Pan, X., & Ratliff-Schaub, K. (2012). Comparison of systematic developmental surveillance with standardized developmental screening in primary care. *Clinical Pediatrics*, *51*(2), 154–159.

Ture, E., Yazar, A., Dundar, M. A., Bakdik, S., Akin, F., & Pekcan, S. (2021). Treatment of sialorrhea with botulinum toxin A injection in children. *Nigerian Journal of Clinical Practice*, *24*(6), 847–852. https://doi.org/10.4103/njcp.njcp_85_20

U. S. Department of Justice Civil Rights Division. (2022). Information and technical assistance on the Americans with Disabilities Act. www.ada.gov/2010_regs.htm

U.S. Congress. (2004, December 7). Individuals with Disabilities Education Improvement Act, Sec 300.34 Related services. www.congress.gov/bill/108th-congress/house-bill/1350

U.S. Department of Education. (2015). Every Student Succeeds Act (ESSA) www.ed.gov/essa?src%3Drn

U.S. Department of Health and Human Services, Health Resources & Services Administration. (2020, July). Children with special health care needs. *NSCH Data Brief*.

U.S. Department of Labor. (2022, January 7). The employment situation—December 2021. *News Release—Bureau of Labor Statistics*. www.bls.gov/news.release/empsit.toc.htm

Vande Velde, S., Van Renterghem, K., Van Winkel, M., De Bruyne, R., & Van Biervliet, S. (2018). Constipation and fecal incontinence in children with cerebral palsy. Overview of literature and flowchart for a stepwise approach. *Acta Gastro-enterologica Belgica*, *81*(3), 415–418.

Vargus-Adams J., Collins A., & Paulson A. (2021). *Cerebral palsy pediatric rehabilitation principles and practice*. (6th ed., pp. 320–347). Springer.

Villela, E. L., Sakai, P., Almeida, M. R., Moura, E. G., & Faintuch, J. (2014). Endoscopic gastrostomy replacement tubes: Long-term randomized trial with five silicone commercial models. *Clinical Nutrition (Edinburgh, Scotland)*, *33*(2), 221–225. https://doi.org/10.1016/j.clnu.2013.04.015

Walford, S. L., Requejo, P. S., Mulroy, S. J., & Neptune, R. R. (2019). Predictors of shoulder pain in manual wheelchair users. *Clinical Biomechanics* (Bristol, Avon), *65*, 1–12. https://doi.org/10.1016/j.clinbiomech.2019.03.003

Wallander, J. L., Biasini, F. J., Thorsten, V., Dhaded, S. M., de Jong, D. M., Chomba, E., Omrana, P., Goudar, S., Wallade, D., Chakraborty, H., Wright, L. L., McClure, E., & Carlo, W. A. (2014). Dose of early intervention treatment during children's first 36 months of life is associated with developmental outcomes: An observational cohort study in three low/low-middle income countries. *BMC Pediatrics*, *14*(1), 1–11.

Ward, M., Johnson, C., Klein, J. Farber, J., Nolm, W., & Peterson, M. (2021). Orthotics and assistive devices. In K. P. Murphy, M. A. McMahon, & A. J. Houtrow (Eds.), *Pediatric rehabilitation principles and practice* (6th ed., pp.196–229). Springer Publishing.

Weed, R. (2001). Contemporary life care planning for persons with amputation. *Orthotics and Prosthetics Business News*, *10*(23), 20–30.

Weed, R. O., & Berens, D. E. (Eds.) (2018). *Life care planning and case management handbook* (4th ed.). Routledge.

Wishart, B. D., & Kivlehan, E. (2021). Neuromuscular scoliosis: When, who, why and outcomes. *Physical Medicine and Rehabilitation Clinics of North America*, *32*(3), 547–556. https://doi.org/10.1016/j.pmr.2021.02.007

Yan, H., Toyota, E., Anderson, M., Abel, T. J., Donner, E., Kalia, S. K., Drake, J., Rutka, J. T., & Ibrahim, G. M. (2018). A systematic review of deep brain stimulation for the treatment of drug-resistant epilepsy in childhood. *Journal of Neurosurgery: Pediatrics*, *23*(3), 274–284.

Zelleke, T. G., Depositario-Cabacar, D. F., & Gaillard, W. D. (2019). *Epilepsy*. In M. L. Batshaw, N. J. Roizen, & L. Pellegrino (Eds.), *Children with disabilities* (8th ed., pp. 457–479). Paul H. Brookes Publishing Co.

Zwaigenbaum, L., Bauman, M. L., Fein, D., Pierce, K., Buie, T., Davis, P. A., ... & Wagner, S. (2015). Early screening of autism spectrum disorder: Recommendations for practice and research. *Pediatrics*, *136*(Supplement_1), S41-S59.

Resources

Tube feeding basics: www.feedingtubeawareness.org/g-tube/
Feeding tube formulas: https://oralcancerfoundation.org/nutrition/commercial-formulas-feeding-tube/
Sialorrhea treatment algorithms: www.aacpdm.org/publications/care-pathways/sialorrhea-in-cerebral-palsy

Chapter 8

Elder Care Management in Life Care Planning

Jennifer Crowley and Shanna Huber

The aging population has helped increase demand for services, including life care management. Eighty percent of individuals aged 65 years and over have at least one chronic health condition and 68 percent have two or more chronic health conditions (National Council on Aging [NCOA], 2021). With the exponential rise in the number of adults living into old age, precipitated by the baby boom generation, there is an anticipated rise in the number of older Americans living with multiple comorbidities and potential frailty due to declining health. By 2030, one in six people in the world will be aged 60 years and older (World Health Organization [WHO], 2021). Recommendations to address the challenges of the baby boom generation, including structured long-term care savings plans, improving health in aging populations, and changing societal behaviors and perceptions around aging often take decades for any measurable impact (Knickman & Snell, 2002).

Healthcare systems have enhanced their own services using multidisciplinary professionals who are assigned to work more closely with individuals who may be considered high risk or have more complicated healthcare needs. This may be referred to as the patient-centered medical home model of care, designed to provide greater access to care and improved communications to patients and their families with more robust social services, care coordination, and discharge planning (National Conference of State Legislators [NCSL], 2012). Despite this, healthcare is still complex for most consumers, being overwhelming to navigate. Consumers may have poor information and lack access to resources, leading to confusion and a failure to effectively manage their health conditions. Additional barriers for effective self-management and engagement of consumers in their own healthcare include low healthcare literacy, lack of experience navigating healthcare in general, and a failure of providers to utilize a person-centered approach for informed decision-making (Lewis & Pignone, 2009). Consumers may not have any experience caring for themselves or others in the context of normal aging, with any sudden shift causing significant disruption.

Increasingly, insurers and other stakeholders mention "value-based care," which means that payment or reimbursement depends upon the measurable outcomes in certain populations or disease cohorts. Providers are tasked with demonstrating positive outcomes but are limited in their ability to spend the time necessary to completely understand the breadth of the situation or focus on more than one area. There may be limitations in the ability to provide the necessary education for the consumer to effectively self-manage and follow through with recommendations. Information sharing among different providers, such as primary care and specialists, may be fragmented and unreliable if the electronic documentation system lacks sophistication.

The electronic health record (EHR) can support other care-related activities that interface with the role of the life care manager, including measurement of quality and outcomes, and evidence-based decision support (Centers for Medicare & Medicaid Services [CMS], 2021). Healthcare systems have made tremendous progress expanding their networks and capabilities for communication and sharing of EHRs. Electronic health records have been widely adopted since 2009 following implementation of the Health Information Technology for Economic and Clinical Health Act (Yan et al., 2021). Electronic health records help provide transparency, efficiency, and accountability. However, Yan et al. (2021), found that EHRs contribute to more problems, including health information technology (HIT)-related stress, which has been associated with burnout among providers. The systems designed to improve lives may create more barriers for those more commonly tasked with helping individuals and families through the myriad of situations more likely to occur during older adulthood. Electronic health records help providers see other data relevant to their patient depending on the application and network, so this has helped improve information sharing, data collection, and billing practices. However, there are still gaps and silo-effects in healthcare, where provider offices, such as specialists and other non-conventional provider practices—as well as community partner organizations—are left out of the loop.

Healthcare systems and stakeholders need capable, competent professionals who are adept at reducing burden and meeting measurable outcomes in the population they serve. Increasingly, healthcare needs a powerful liaison who can help connect the team players and maintain the client/patient as the center of focus, working collaboratively to improve outcomes. Individuals and families need knowledgeable professionals who are proficient at performing assessments, creating care plans with recommendations, communicating with the entire healthcare team, and assisting with ongoing management.

The care management model emerged to help manage the health of populations, providing a collaborative, person-centered approach to improve patient outcomes (Farrell et al., 2018). Today, care management has grown into a promising discipline of practice for healthcare professionals to help others across the continuum of care and play an important role in reducing healthcare burden. Life care planners have attributes, skills, and experience that make them ideal candidates for adding care management to their portfolio of services.

Although additional research is needed to determine how best to engage consumers with their healthcare and how to evaluate consumer experiences working with professional care managers, research has shown that consumers value having a care manager who listened to them, provided education on their health conditions in terms they can understand, helped them navigate community supports and services, connected them to vital resources, and helped monitor their chronic health conditions, especially following a hospitalization (O'Malley et al., 2017).

The Role of the Life Care Manager

Without prior exposure and experience working with a professional care manager, the most common question for aging professionals and healthcare providers may be "what is a life care manager?" Professional care managers may also be referred to as geriatric care managers, life care managers, or elder care managers. The National Institute on Aging (NIA, 2017) recognizes the geriatric care manager as often being a licensed nurse or social worker who acts as a professional relative and specializes in geriatrics, helping individuals and families identify needs, and make recommendations to help meet those needs. The role may include tasks that improve well-being and are highly individualized according to the identified needs, including making home visits, coordinating medical services, discussing difficult issues, and providing alternative living options (NIA, 2017).

The care manager often works in the community, helping to resolve elder issues, plan for care, and perform tasks related to chronic disease management. The care manager may also identify as a patient advocate, care coordinator, care navigator, aging life care professional, or care planner.

Crowley and Huber define life care management as:

> … a field of practice, utilizing educated and experienced professionals specializing in the assessment and care planning, connecting to vital services and resources, coordinating care through collaboration, managing care and providing professional oversight, and helping to resolve issues to achieve optimal health regardless of age or ability.
> (Crowley & Huber, 2021, p. 3)

Historically, the first known terminology associated with the advancement of the profession known as geriatric care management came from a group of social workers, psychologists, and nurses located in the state of New York who eventually formed the National Association of Geriatric Care Managers (NAPGCM), now known as the Aging Life Care Association® (ALCA®), a professional organization with over 2,000 members (Davis, 2012).

Life care managers may work in private practice or as an employee or contracted professional within a larger organization, with opportunities to play a pivotal role using a multidisciplinary, holistic approach to care. Increasingly, life care managers find avenues for helping others through their various relationships with aging industry partners within their own community, including financial advisors, home health agencies, and other stakeholders, such as insurers and attorneys (Crowley & Huber, 2021).

Benefits of Care Management

Life care managers are valuable assets, who help improve the lives of others, resolve some of the biggest challenges in healthcare, and help to navigate complex situations. The Agency for Healthcare Research and Quality ([AHRQ], 2018) recognizes care management as an effective mechanism for managing the health of populations, especially those with modifiable risks.

Sometimes interchanged with the nomenclature of case management, the benefits of care management delivered by competent professionals include improved coordination of care, reduced healthcare utilization, and enhancement of the interdisciplinary, person-centered approach (Giardino & De Jesus, 2021). Care managers can provide support to other professionals who are limited in their scope of practice and allotted time by discussing important and often complex topics with individuals and their families based upon the individual's values and wishes. Care managers can provide expertise and support to stakeholders, such as insurers, attorneys, fiduciaries, and physicians, to facilitate understanding of situations using a holistic perspective and perform tasks outside the traditional medical home model of care.

Increasingly, the healthcare industry is recognizing the need to deliver care that is aligned with the individual's needs. Care managers are trained in utilizing a holistic approach to care which encompasses a person-centered approach. This approach is based on key principles of practice which recognize the individual as central to the plan of care, focusing on the individual's defined priorities and capacity for achieving goals and taking into consideration the individual's education level, socioeconomic status, family dynamics, and level of understanding about their own health and how to manage their conditions.

The life care manager can perform tasks that are typically outside the time allotted for primary care providers to visit with their patients. Care managers often have greater time allowance and insights to the living environment which is helpful to guide other professionals with treatment planning. A meta-analysis of 24 studies showed interventions that included self-management, telephone follow-up, and medication reconciliation activities were most likely to be effective in reducing re-hospitalization (Tomlinson et al., 2020). These are tasks familiar and customary to the care manager.

Care managers can elevate the consumer healthcare experience by providing support which underscores the interconnectedness of mental and physical health and focuses on the individual's health goals and other attributes that help to achieve the intended outcomes. Care managers develop an understanding of the unique individual characteristics that impact the care plan. They are skilled in navigating complex situations and have good communication skills.

Kinds of Patients and Problems Usually Seen and Addressed

Life care managers obtain referrals from professionals, individuals, and concerned family or friends, who recognize a need for assistance. Typically, the individual for whom the assistance is being requested is experiencing a setback in their health or has acquired a new health condition resulting in a temporary or permanent functional loss. Many clients are aging clients who have a sudden or progressive change in mental or physical status. Considering the common occurrence of chronic health conditions in the aging population, the arrival of a more complex, progressive health condition or disability has the capability of causing significant disruption to well-being. Chronic health conditions may aggravate normal aging-related changes, increasing burden and risk. Individuals with chronic illness are at higher risk for more severe illness, which became more apparent during the coronavirus pandemic as public health measures raised awareness of those more vulnerable to complications or increased mortality (Roberts et al., 2021). Although the aging population makes up most cases, care managers also work with individuals with special behavioral or physical challenges as well as those with progressive diagnoses such as Multiple Sclerosis and Parkinson's disease.

Many life care managers work with individuals with diverse needs. Even if the life care manager specializes in a specific area of practice, the interplay of other health conditions and aging-related changes influence their recommendations. Many of the common chronic health conditions care managers help manage include those which are more complex or progressive in nature. The most common chronic health conditions in the 65 years and older population include hypertension, hypercholesterolemia, arthritis, heart disease and heart failure, diabetes, chronic kidney disease, depression, dementia, and chronic obstructive pulmonary disease (NCOA, 2021). Some of these health conditions may seem minor in comparison to more complicated disease states. However, when considering normal aging-related changes that may be aggravated by a health condition, there can exist a significant number of challenges for individuals. There may be difficulty with self-management, occurrences of complications such as falls or other accidents, a lack of education, and a mindset which is disruptive to being proactively engaged in their own health.

Additionally, the public may not fully understand the expected changes related to normal aging. Individuals may get caught up in the anti-aging, youth-oriented mindset that keeps them from accepting their current and future healthcare needs and focusing on effectively managing their health. There may be a personal belief in a lack of control over the future, a fatalistic view which is disruptive to focusing on health and engaging in strategic care planning.

Many clients and clients' families pay out of pocket for services. For this reason, the length of time and scope of involvement is often dictated by the available funds and financial resources of each individual. Some individuals may have family pooling together funds for an assessment and recommendations and therefore, implement the plan of care themselves. Others give full rein to the care manager to implement every recommendation in the plan of care and follow-up with ongoing care needs, communicating with all parties involved. The bulk of cases are somewhere in-between, where families may take on some tasks themselves while asking the care manager to complete the more advanced and skilled recommendations such as attending physician visits, communicating with providers, coordinating skilled care professionals, and ensuring smooth transitions of care. For these reasons, life care managers may be involved in a case for a couple of weeks while at other times, care managers may be involved for years until the end of life. It is the goal of the care manager to put services and items in place for optimal independence and quality of life. Oftentimes, care managers work with clients to get them on a stable course, but as their disease or condition progresses and circumstances change, the care manager will become re-involved in the same case over time.

It is important for life care professionals to help communicate the potential physiologic changes and educate clients on what to expect and how to manage their health. Table 8.1 provides a basic review of normal aging-related changes to help professionals educate their clients on realistic expectations for resolving certain symptoms and developing an acceptance for what they can or cannot control.

Methodology: Learn-Create-Manage

Using a consistent method helps streamline an otherwise complex process. The ALCA® recognizes several domains of expertise of the care manager, which demonstrates the vast areas of understanding the care manager must obtain when working with individuals. These include health and disability, financial, advocacy, legal, housing, crisis intervention, family, advocacy, and resources (ALCA®, n.d.).

The methodology for a life care manager is similar to that of a life care planner, especially in the initial phases of working with an individual. The life care manager receives the referral and is provided a brief introduction to the case and develops an understanding of what is needed and the potential urgency or other priorities. Once any potential conflicts are removed, the life care manager then executes a service or contract agreement with the responsible party, ensuring authorizations are obtained for the sharing of protected health information. Once the formalities are established, the life care manager makes initial contact with the individual to schedule an in-person visit. The agreed upon financial arrangements when getting hired or retained for services will vary depending on the individual professional or the agency organization of the care manager. Some care managers charge a retainer fee whereas others do not. Most care managers charge an hourly professional rate of service and have detailed fee schedules to include billable rates for mileage, travel time, and special rates for evenings, weekends, and holidays.

Table 8.1 Age-Related Changes

Normal age-related changes	Expected change	Disease/illness	Functional consequences
Vision	Farsightedness, sensitivity to glare	Common eye-related conditions include glaucoma, cataracts, macular degeneration, and diabetic retinopathy	Falls, difficulty reading/learning, safety issues
Hearing	Age-related hearing loss (or presbycusis) is the gradual loss of hearing in both ears. One in three adults over the age of 65 years has hearing loss (John Hopkins Medicine, 2020). Speech of others sounds muffled or slurred. High-pitched sounds such as "s" or "th" are hard to distinguish. Conversations are difficult to understand, especially with background noise. Some sounds are overly loud and annoying	Tinnitus, deafness	Social isolation, loneliness, cognitive decline
Sleep disturbance	Delayed sleep onset, fragmented sleep, decreased stages 3 and 4 sleep (which are the more profound REM sleep stages) (Neubauer, 1999)	Pain causing sleep disturbance	Depression, falls
Pain/discomfort	The most common types of pain in elderly adults are low back or neck pain (65%), musculoskeletal pain (40%), peripheral neuropathic pain (40%), and chronic joint pain (20%) (Jones et al., 2016)	Arthritis	People with osteoarthritis have a 30% increase in falls with a 20% greater risk of fractures than those without osteoarthritis (Arthritis Foundation, 2020)
Decreased appetite	Low appetite, slower metabolism, decreased saliva production	Medication side effects, hormonal changes, gastrointestinal changes, chronic disease states, cancer	Dehydration, poor nutrition, weight loss
Cardiovascular	Cardiovascular system changes include stiffening of the blood vessels and arteries, causing the heart to work harder to pump blood (Mayo Clinic, 2020)	Hypertension, congestive heart failure, myocardial infarction	Fatigue, shortness of breath, decreased endurance

(Continued)

Table 8.1 (Continued) Age-Related Changes

Normal age-related changes	Expected change	Disease/illness	Functional consequences
Bones/joints/muscles	Bones shrink in size and density (Mayo Clinic, 2020), muscles lose strength and flexibility	Degenerative disk disease, atrophy	Decreased coordination, balance issues, higher risk for falls
Gastrointestinal	Constipation	C-diff	Nutritional deficit, irritability, social withdrawal, urinary incontinence
Genitourinary	More frequent urination, difficulty emptying bladder, enlarged prostate	Urinary tract infections, bladder prolapse	Increased risk for falls, increased confusion (delirium), behavior issues, social self-isolation
Reproductive organs and sexuality	Vaginal wall shortening and wall becoming thinner and stiffer, erectile dysfunction becomes more common	Vaginal prolapse	Reduced sexual pleasure and drive, isolation
Neurological	The hippocampus in the brain, which is responsible for memory, progressively atrophies, and may have inflammation and reduced plasticity (Dause & Kirby, 2019). Reduced neurotransmitters which will cause difficulty with concentration and handling multiple tasks at once	Alzheimer's disease, Lewy Body, Parkinson's, Sundowners syndrome	Social isolation, social withdrawal, falls, decreased executive function
Dental	Gums recede from the teeth making them looser and creating pathways for bacteria	Tooth decay	Difficulty eating, pain
Integumentary	Fatty tissue below the skin decreases, making skin less elastic, thinner, and fragile, bruises more easily, dry skin due to decreased production of natural oils, wrinkles, age spots, and skin tags are more common	Infection of the skin, skin cancer, bedsores, non-healing wounds	Sepsis, skin breakdown, decreased resistance to infection, decreased flexibility, and mobility
Endocrine	Increased insulin sensitivity	Diabetes, hypoglycemia	Increase risk for falls, nutritional deficits, dehydration

Learn About the Situation, the Case Details, and the Needs

The life care manager gets to know the case through learning about the background and the status. The life care manager is adept at collecting data quickly, especially involving cases which may have a more urgent need for professional assistance. These might include cases in which there is a sudden shift in health, an accident, or other crises necessitating swift attention. Using a comprehensive assessment tool and other helpful resources, the life care manager develops a thorough understanding of the situation. The methodology for collecting information and learning about the client should be consistent, ensuring a workflow is established helping to capture the numerous data in a time-efficient manner (Crowley & Huber, 2021). The areas of the assessment are provided in Table 8.2. The assessment may be referred to as an evaluation or an interview. Several areas of discovery help to provide the most suitable recommendations, which need to be highly individualized according to education level, social structure, and financial means.

The life care manager seeks to maximize resources, always identifying collateral sources available such as public assistance, insurance benefits, aging services, and other community-level support which may be available to the client. Once litigation ends, if the individual receives funds, those funds can be set aside in a formal arrangement such as a special needs trust. The goal of a special needs trust is to ensure the financial security of an individual with a disability or complex chronic health condition. A trust can be managed by an individual such as a parent or loved one, or professionally managed by a trust officer in a bank or financial entity. Care managers are often called upon to implement the life care plan, or if time has passed, to provide a new assessment and recommendations. The current care plan helps guide the distribution of funds to improve quality of life and provide sustainability of finances.

Payor sources in elder care management are very important, creating either opportunity or limited choices, depending on the situation. One's financial portfolio and financial stability are often the most determining factors for choices and options for long-term care (Crowley, 2017). The most well-known payor sources for long-term care include long-term care insurance, veteran's benefits, and Medicaid. Other possible payor sources include grants for programs dedicated to specific disease cohorts and disabilities, state initiatives, philanthropic or charitable donations, and non-profit organizations. The reliability of public benefits may be uncertain. It is the responsibility of everyone to be prepared for their future care needs. The life care manager will need to fine-tune their skills for learning about the familial, cultural, and geographic circumstances which make it difficult for individuals to engage in their own healthcare. They build trust and rapport by taking the time to learn about what makes the client unique to develop solutions for optimizing well-being (Davison et al., 1992).

The assessment may be cumbersome, depending on the number of individuals and family members involved, societal and situational factors, whether the individual is able to participate, and the effective recall of relevant health information. Developing a good understanding of who is involved in decision-making, providing care or other support, or depending upon the client for financial or other support is very important. Some individuals will have a designated, legally authorized person who provides support in decision-making, defined as the proxy or power of attorney. The power of attorney may also make decisions independently of the client in cases involving diminished capacity, such as with cognitive impairment. In some situations, there may be a court-appointed guardian who the care manager will work with to understand the situation. Other cases may involve an individual who has not identified a primary contact person to assist with such matters or perhaps they have no next of kin, commonly referred to as a solo ager. Many individuals have not yet completed any advance care planning which identifies who will assist in the event they cannot make their own decisions, either because they did not understand the need

Table 8.2 Areas of the Assessment

Demographics	Address
	Relatives/emergency contacts
	Education level
Support Services	Home health
	Community programs
	Therapist/counselor
Medical/Health Status	Diagnosis
	Hospitalization(s)
	Medications
	Pharmacy
	Medical providers
	Pain & daily symptoms
	Vision & hearing
	Allied health providers/other team members
Daily Habits & Routines	Daily routines
	Exercise
	Nutrition
	Sleep habits
Function	Activities of daily living
	Instrumental activities of daily living
Cognitive	Memory & decision-making
Safety	Driving
	Fall risk
	Home safety
	Pressure sore risk scale
Financial	Medical insurance
	Income/other assets
	Debt/liability
	Contracts-banking/retirement accounts
	Long-term care insurance
	Veterans Administration
	Legal documents
	Signs of financial abuse/fraud
Legal	Healthcare power of attorney
	Financial power of attorney
	Advance directives
	Funeral arrangements
Psychosocial	Social support: Caregiver(s)/family/friends
	Emotional & spiritual support Faith community
	Alcohol/substance use
	Smoking history

Reprinted with permission, The Life Care Management Institute.

to complete such designations or for other reasons, such as no identifiable, capable person in their life who is willing or able to take on the responsibility. It is during this initial phase the life care manager starts creating the needs list, which often includes completion of the appropriate legal documents. This may require additional visits and a coordination of meetings between the client and their family member or friend who is involved.

Various tools are available to help the life care manager assess the individual and collect the comprehensive data. These include standardized forms, protocols, and templates which help guide the conversation and provide a framework for handling the vast amount of information. Some tools are specific to the needs of the situation or case, such as the memory screening tests, which are available in cases involving memory loss or suspected cognitive decline. The life care planner working in the field of care management will find it necessary to become familiar with the various resources available to them when performing an assessment or evaluation. Many of the tools available help to create the story but are not necessarily diagnostic in nature. The results of screening and other assessment data can be shared with the medical provider to develop a greater understanding of the individual, perhaps helping better define a new medical diagnosis or identify recurring or new problem areas, which then helps to create the most effective treatment plan.

There are several resources available online through reputable organizations. For example, the Hartford Institute for Geriatric Nursing (www.consultgeri.org) offers a comprehensive selection of assessment tools for the best practices in the care of older adults as well as guidelines for the care of older adults with chronic disease. Their "Try This" series includes topics such as alcohol use, assessing nutrition, assessment of the fear of falling, and evaluating caregiver strain. Assessment tools which provide an opening for more targeted discussion and focus on specific concerns can be valuable when working with clients who need longer development time to understand and come to terms with their own situation and to move toward greater acceptance. The care manager may strengthen their own recommendations by relying upon the evidence-based tools to support findings which suggest a particular need.

The care manager may move back and forth between the learning phase and the creation of the care plan, similar to future discovery in life care planning. Working with older adults and their health conditions is a dynamic process, evolving as health or situations change. The care manager establishes a needs list early on, identifying the problem areas or areas of concern. This needs list will change as goals are achieved, with changes in the treatment plan, or as new information becomes available. The areas of concern become addressed through implementation of the care plan.

Create the Care Plan

Once enough information is gathered and the assessment is complete, the life care manager creates the care plan. This is based on the primary concerns of the individual and family, provider and other input, and the observations and recommendations of the life care manager. Goals are established, along with identification of barriers to achieving those goals. Life care managers rely upon their assessment data and needs list to clearly define the area(s) of concern. The area of concern is the problem or issue which needs attention. The primary concern(s) is sometimes clearly stated by the individual or family member, and other times overwhelming for them to clearly understand. The life care manager can assist with navigating the conversation to define the areas of concern more clearly. Once the concerns are understood, the care plan moves into the area of goal setting or defining what needs to be achieved. Sometimes this is easier than knowing what the problem is. Individuals may be more likely to be able to state what it is they want, rather than what the problem is. Additionally, the barrier to achieving what they want may be difficult to

Table 8.3 Sample Basic Care Plan

Area of concern	Mr. Rich needs help with bathing
Goal	*Mr. Rich will have a meeting with his financial advisor to determine the best approach for freeing up funds to pay for care*
	Mr. Rich will review options for obtaining in-home support
	Mr. Rich will decide on the home health provider to hire and execute service agreements
	Mr. Rich will have in-home personal care assistance within 2–4 weeks to assist on a weekly basis with bathing
Barrier	*Finances*
	Home health in his area is limited
Recommendation	*Schedule meeting with financial advisor*
	Review list of home health and personal care options in the community
	Hire non-medical home health provider
	Schedule initial visit with caregiver

identify. Barriers include anything that might be a challenge or something that needs to be overcome to achieve the goal. Table 8.3 provides a sample basic care plan to help with understanding the areas of focus for the care plan that is completed by the life care manager. Recommendations are actions needed to fulfill the primary objective, or goal, and help resolve the primary concern(s). These could be simple steps listed as tasks or action items. As the care plan is implemented, the recommendations will be updated to reflect any changes or completion of the tasks. Life care managers will often utilize the care plan as an ongoing tool for providing recommendations in written format, having the understanding that working with individuals and their families is often a dynamic process. This is a process that is expected to evolve and may require multiple efforts.

Management of the Care

The management of a case will depend on whether professional assistance is needed to resolve one issue, more often referred to as a task assignment, or if the client requires ongoing or indefinite involvement by a life care manager. Stakeholders sometimes hire care managers to help resolve a single issue. For example, an individual who needs to see a specialist but does not have the support or wherewithal to know where to start. The care manager will still need to utilize their formal process for initiating professional services and accepting a referral and then develop an understanding of the situation. More often, life care managers provide ongoing support and care management of cases for sometimes a prolonged period, possibly several years.

While the life care planner may stop at the completion of a life care plan, the life care manager can be a valuable resource to ensure appropriate follow through with education and support. The life care manager can be an extension of the life care planner, working in the community to help implement the life care plan. Once a life care plan has been completed and the case is settled, the life care manager can be the professional who implements the life care plan, following up and making appropriate modifications to the plan of care.

The role of the life care manager in the management phase will depend on several factors. These may include whether there is a capable support person, such as an adult child, if there are other in-home services, if the individual resides in assisted living or another support community, and the number of tasks needing accomplished. For example, the life care manager may assist an older adult with chronic disease who needs to relocate, and the family has requested help identifying options in the community. The task was helping find the family a suitable location and once that is achieved the care manager may not be involved. Some care managers may obtain a referral fee from residential care communities in their area if the client moves into their facility. In other situations, the care manager will stay on indefinitely, to be somewhat of a proxy for adult children or other loved ones who live at a distance. Perhaps there are several family members who just feel incapable, for whatever reason, of providing the level of support required by the situation. Short-term versus long-term tasks will depend on each case and the presenting problems, such as a family who is concerned about their loved one's ability to drive and requests help to persuade their loved one to give up the car keys; or the family is looking ahead at potential needs because their loved one has dementia.

Some of the long-term tasks the life care manager can assist with include professional oversight of the home health or residential care team; coordination of care needs; accompanying to medical appointments; performing routine check-ins either in person or telephonically; or education and support of the medical treatment plan. The care plan with the recommendations helps guide the ongoing management of a case.

Life Care Planner and Care Manager Interface

Life care managers are the care coordinators for not only seniors, but also serve individuals with special needs and chronic health conditions. The life care manager can implement the life care plan and have continuity of services to follow-up and make any changes as the individual's needs change. To find a local life care manager, the life care planner can visit the ALCA® at https://www.aginglifecare.org/. The professional organization for life care managers is the ALCA®. The ALCA® has *Standards of Practice and a Code of Ethics*. Members of the ALCA® have specialized degrees and experience in human services, such as social work, psychology, gerontology, or nursing, and are expected to adhere to ALCA's® *Standards of Practice and Code of Ethics* (ALCA®, 2021). The life care planner can seek the professional background that fits the specific evaluee's needs.

Life care managers may also write reports for family members, trust officers, payor sources, the courts, attorneys, and other stakeholders. There may be a need to assist guardians and conservators with the ongoing effective management of their case, helping to prevent or resolve problems to improve the well-being of the individual.

Referral Sources for the Life Care Manager

Life care managers are most successful when they have created their network of possible referral sources. Life care planners often work with litigation professionals. Life care managers typically work outside of the litigation arena. Although some life care managers may contribute to a case involving legal matters, such as with guardianship proceedings or in special situations where the professional becomes a court-appointed care manager. The most common referral sources for life care managers include elder law attorneys, trust officers, financial advisors, and other professionals that serve seniors.

Elder Law Attorneys

Elder law attorneys are the most common referral source for care managers. Seniors, as well as children and loved ones of seniors, often seek counsel to help them plan for the future, or more often, reach out to elder law attorneys in times of crisis. Elder law attorneys make excellent referral sources as they come across the clients that need help with guidance, advocacy, options for aging in place versus facility placement, and help with families in crisis. A good way to find a local elder law attorney is by going to the National Academy of Elder Law Attorneys found at www.naela.org

Elder law attorneys are typically in local estate planning councils. Local estate planning councils are common in most populated areas and are composed of the very target audience the life care manager markets to, including estate planning attorneys, elder law attorneys, trust officers, financial advisors, and other professionals who work in the aging profession. It is typically well worth it to join a local estate planning group for networking or ask to present to the group. Other ways to find elder law attorneys is through the local and state bar association. Providing a presentation on a relevant topic, or sponsoring lunch at local meetings, can be beneficial.

Trust Officers

A trust officer is a professional, usually within a bank, who is responsible for administering and managing assets within a trust for an individual or family. Trust officers do not typically have the knowledge or background to know the special needs of seniors, individuals with special needs, or those with chronic health conditions. The trust officer appreciates guidance on how to preserve wealth while optimizing quality of life for their beneficiary. Not all banks have trusts or trust officers. Primary referral sources are mid-size regional banks that are larger than small local banks, but smaller than large national chains that often have trust officers who work from a distance but are not as hands-on. Trust officers can be difficult to find unless the care planner attends networking groups, such as estate planning groups or a personal introduction is made. Most elder law attorneys have good relationships with local trust officers and can make an introduction once a relationship is established.

Financial Advisors

As individuals grow older and begin to decline or have difficulty, families often reach out to a financial planner to seek help in crisis. Financial advisors also have local network meetings. Sometimes the care manager can join or ask to speak at a meeting. The financial advisor can work with the life care manager to help determine the next steps. The financial advisor is often involved with helping families determine what is feasible in the long term with recommendations from the life care manager. Different options can be given to determine which option is best for the individual and fits within their means. Once the recommendations are made, the proper allocations can be made to help sustain the financial arrangements or set aside funds for future care.

Aging Services Professionals

The life care manager makes many recommendations for connecting clients to the most appropriate services and professionals in the community. The life care manager should attend any local networking groups for aging professionals to become familiar with the available services and build relationships. The life care manager may find it rewarding to assist other professionals in helping provide value to clients in their community by working collaboratively to resolve issues and improve outcomes. This may include situations involving end-of-life care, integrative care in mental health, and promotion of healthy aging. The life care manager may also work alongside community partners to volunteer or organize charitable events aimed at a specific cause or public health improvement effort. These types of activities in the community help the life care manager to be recognized and build relationships that are likely to result in referrals. The life care professional should network with their peers and colleagues, similar to any other business that provides a service or product. Handing out business cards and educating community partners on the role of the life care manager helps to get referrals.

Standards of Practice, Professional Guidelines, and Code of Ethics for Care Managers

The National Academy of Certified Care Managers (NACCM) is the accrediting organization that administers the formal certification program for professionals to become Certified Care Managers (CMC). An individual is not required to be certified to practice as a life care manager.

NACCM (2020) published the *Standards of Practice and a Code of Ethics* in 2020. The NACCM code helps define standards of practice supporting ethical principles. These principles include:

- Integrity: the care manager always acts in a manner consistent with the professional values
- Loyal and responsible: the care manager maintains confidentiality, avoids conflict of interest, and always pursues the best interest of the clients
- Promoting benefit and avoiding harm: the care manager strikes to ensure that clients' individual choices are maximized and is aware of potential conflicts that may arise
- Respect: the care manager exercises care and compassion in planning for care and respects the client as an individual with their own history, narrative, and unique cultural identity
- Justice: the care manager acts justly and fairly with no form of discrimination

Guidelines for practice are also available through the International Association of Rehabilitation Professionals (IARP) (IARP, n.d.). The IARP guidelines address professional standards for medical case management, which include working within the professional's qualifications and formal background, understanding conditions and rehabilitation principles, and developing and implementing a plan of care that integrates the client in the decision-making process

Challenges exist in this field of care management, mostly due to a lack of uniform language, general awareness and acceptance, limited studies on outcomes, and the varying nomenclature used when referring to the professional role. The AHRQ published a guide on implementation of care management for primary care practices, noting the many names for the type of role including health coach, nurse educator, health navigator, care coordinator, case manager, and care manager (AHRQ, n.d.).

Care managers help to optimize well-being and recovery from exacerbation of health, injury or new onset of illness, advocate for the client while providing professional oversight to ensure quality of care, helping with goal attainment, and promotion of self-management skills.

Despite the many reputable sources for obtaining practice guidelines, there is limited research that correlates with the overall benefits to the consumer and whether care management helps to both improve quality of care and reduce healthcare expenditure. The Center for Healthcare Research and Transformation reviewed two models, the Eric Coleman Care Transitions Intervention and Mary Naylor's Transitional Care Model, aimed at targeting high risk, high-cost elderly patients following discharge from the acute care setting. Both demonstrated at least a 30% reduction in readmissions and costs, both underscoring that the most successful programs provide face-to-face interactions between individuals and care managers, education in self-management, use of EHRs, and integration and collaboration with primary care practices (Center for Healthcare Research and Transformation, 2014).

Case Study

Common case of adult children deciding if a parent is safe at home alone

Kelly is a 60-year-old female who has five siblings who live in various states. Her mother, Opal, is a widow who is 80 years old and currently lives independently at home. Opal has fallen three times in the past few months and has a diagnosis of mild cognitive impairment. Opal has a small poodle that she adores but she gets more confused at night and is afraid to open the door and let the dog out, so the dog is defecating on her carpeted lanai each evening. Opal often calls her children afraid in the evening and seems confused. She is driving short distances to the store during the day but does not go out at night.

Kelly reached out to a local care manager, Lisa, to help determine what to do with Opal. Kelly and her five siblings have been discussing what to do with Opal for almost a year. They all want what is best for their mother, but an agreement cannot be made between the children. One child thinks Opal would do best in an assisted living facility, one child believes she would be best in a dementia care unit, one believes she would do best in her home and is happiest there, although it may not be safe, and one child believes all the children should take turns checking in regularly.

The care manager, Lisa, is retained to help the family determine the next steps and provide guidance in the best interests of Opal. The children are paying for Lisa's services by splitting the bill between them. Lisa begins the assessment (learning) phase by interviewing the family on concerns, medical history, functionality, emergency contacts, and what help Opal is currently receiving. Lisa then meets Opal in person, describes her services, lets Opal know she is working on behalf of Opal, and wants to do what is in her best interest. A full assessment is completed with Opal (learning) and a Health Insurance Portability and Accountability Act (HIPAA) release is obtained to gather more information on specific diagnoses and medications Opal is taking.

After completing the assessment, key areas of concern identified were:

- Medications are being taken incorrectly (specifically blood pressure and blood sugar medications)
- The lanai smells of dog urine and feces are found on the carpet
- Rotting food is found in the refrigerator
- Opal has difficulty remembering to eat at times and cannot recall what she had the prior day to eat
- Although in Opal's chart it states she has "mild cognitive impairment," no definitive diagnosis was made, and she has never been seen by a neurologist
- Falls happen more in the evening

The goal is to have a plan in place where Opal will have optimal independence while remaining safe. The barrier is that Opal wants to remain in her home and is refusing to consider any other living facility options. She is not willing to even tour a facility.

Recommendations Included:

- Organizing medications in a medication reminder system to ensure proper administration of medications that may be contributing to falls and confusion
- Having a home care aide come in the morning and then again at night to have a set schedule, cook healthy meals for breakfast and dinner and set out a lunch, light housekeeping duties, run errands, help provide socialization, and put her to bed at night
- That the life care manager make an appointment with the primary care physician and attend the visit to discuss a definitive diagnosis and explore Alzheimer's vs vascular dementia or other medical reasons for her cognitive decline
- Scheduling weekly visits and keep in communication with the home care aide to determine if providing a regular schedule, regular meals, taking medications correctly, and socialization in the evening helps improve cognition
- Asking provider for orders to check blood sugar daily to determine if this could be the cause of the falls and order physical therapy to improve strength and gait to decrease chance of falls.

Lisa went on to meet with Opal weekly, then monthly. She communicated with all the children to keep them updated on her progress and communication with the physician (with appropriate releases from Opal). Opal did improve and went on to live in her home with assistance for another ten years until she declined cognitively. Eventually her cognitive impairment worsened, and she no longer recognized her own home. Her quality of life was at risk due to safety concerns as well as self-neglect, and she was more fearful in her own home, with her care needs exceeding the help that could be provided in the home cost effectively. It was determined that facility placement was the best option.

Following this course, the life care manager can provide assistance with planning for the relocation, making the appropriate referral once the family is able to choose the preferred location, and providing ongoing management as appropriate.

A formal care management report includes a combination of a narrative report with subjective and objective data collected at the time of the assessment, similar to the narrative portion in a life care plan. The care plan is provided in a grid as shown in Table 8.3 and reviews the areas of concern, barriers, goals, and recommendations.

Resources

7 Steps to Long-Term Planning www.sevenstepplanning.com
AAA Foundation for Traffic Safety: Vulnerable Adults https://aaafoundation.org/category/vulnerable-road-users/
AARP® (American Association of Retired Persons) www.aarp.org/

(Continued)

Accessible Home Modifications Page: Find home modification specialists https://homemods.org/
ADA (Americans with Disabilities Act) www.ada.gov/ https://adata.org/
Administration on Aging https://acl.gov/about-acl/administration-aging
Age Safe America www.agesafeamerica.com
Aging Life Care Association® www.aginglifecare.org/
AHRQ (Agency for Healthcare Research and Quality www.ahrq.gov/
AGS (American Geriatrics Society) www.americangeriatrics.org/
AGS (American Geriatrics Society) Health and Aging Foundation www.healthinaging.org/
Alzheimer's Association www.alz.org
Alzheimer's Disease Education and Referral Center at the National Institute of Aging www.nia.nih.gov/health/alzheimers
American Association for Geriatric Psychiatry www.aagponline.org/
American Association for Homecare www.aahomecare.org/
American Geriatric Society 2019 Beers Criteria ® http://files.hgsitebuilder.com/hostgator257222/file/ags_2019_beers_pocket_printable_rh.pdf
American Society of Clinical Oncology (Older adult resources) www.cancer.net/navigating-cancer-care/older-adults/resources-older-adults
American Society on Aging www.asaging.org/
ARCH National Respite Network and Resource Center https://archrespite.org/
Arthritis Foundation www.arthritis.org/
Benefits Check Up: National Council on Aging www.benefitscheckup.org/
Brookdale Center for Healthy Aging https://brookdale.org/
Campaign to End Loneliness www.campaigntoendloneliness.org
Care.com (Personal caregiver search) www.care.com

(Continued)

Certified Aging in Place Specialist (CAPS) through National Association of Home Builders www.nahb.org/education-and-events/education/Designations/Certified-Aging-in-Place-Specialist-CAPS	
Centers for Disease Control and Prevention: Promoting Health for Older Adults www.cdc.gov/chronicdisease/resources/publications/factsheets/promoting-health-for-older-adults.htm	
Centers for Medicare & Medicaid Services www.cms.gov/	
Dementia Society of America www.dementiasociety.org	
Diverse Elders Coalition www.diverseelders.org	
Elder Care Directory www.eldercaredirectory.org/	
Eldercare Locator https://eldercare.acl.gov/Public/Index.aspx	
Eldercare Workforce Alliance https://eldercareworkforce.org/	
Fisher Center for Alzheimer's Research Foundation www.alzinfo.org/	
Hartford Institute for Geriatric Nursing www.HIGN.org	
Health and Age https://healthandage.com/index.html	
Hospice Foundation of America https://hospicefoundation.org/	
Lewy Body Dementia Association (LBDA) www.lbda.org	
Life Care Management Institute www.LCMexpert.com	
Life Care Planning Law Firm Association https://www.lcplfa.org/	
Living in Place Institute www.livinginplace.institute	
Medicare Nursing Home Reviews www.medicare.gov/nursinghomecompare	
National Academies Press https://nap.nationalacademies.org/	
National Academy of Certified Care Managers www.naccm.net	
National Academy of Elder Law Attorneys www.naela.org	
National Academy of Social Insurance www.nasi.org/	

(Continued)

National Adult Protective Services Association (NAPSA) www.napsa-now.org
National Asian Pacific Center on Aging www.napca.org/
National Center for Caregiving www.caregiver.org/support-groups
National Center on Elder Abuse https://ncea.acl.gov
National Council of Certified Dementia Practitioners (NCCDP) www.nccdp.org
National Council on Aging: Evidence-Based Health Promotion and Disease Prevention Programs www.ncoa.org/resources/ebpchart/
National Council of Certified Dementia Practitioners www.nccdp.org/about.htm
National Elder Law Foundation www.nelf.org
National Hispanic Council on Aging https://nhcoa.org/
National Institute on Aging Alzheimer's Disease Research Center www.nia.nih.gov/health/alzheimers-disease-research-centers
National Association of State Units on Aging https://nasua.org/
National Caregivers Library www.caregiverslibrary.org/
National Center on Elder Abuse https://ncea.acl.gov/
State Elder Abuse Hotlines https://elderprotectioncenter.com/state-elder-abuse-hotlines/
National Committee to Preserve Social Security and Medicare www.ncpssm.org/
National Council on Aging www.ncoa.org/
National Hospice and Palliative Care Organization www.nhpco.org/
National Institutes of Health www.nih.gov/
National Institute on Aging www.nia.nih.gov/
National Senior Games Association https://nsga.com/
Nutrition and Aging Resource Center (Administration for Community Living) https://acl.gov/senior-nutrition
Research Institute for Aging https://the-ria.ca/

(Continued)

Senior Helpers (Find senior in-home care) www.seniorhelpers.com/	
Social Security Administration www.ssa.gov	
The Association for Frontotemporal Degeneration www.theaftd.org	
The Gerontological Society of America www.geron.org/	
The Hartford Institute for Geriatric Nursing www.consultgeri.org	
The Life Care Management Institute www.lcmexpert.com	
US Aging www.usaging.org/	

References

Agency for Healthcare Research and Quality. (2018). *Care management: Implications for medical practice, health policy, and health services research.* www.ahrq.gov/ncepcr/care/coordination/mgmt.html

Aging Life Care Association (ALCA). (2021.). *Standards of practice and code of ethics.* www.aginglifecare.org/ALCAWEB/About%20Us/Code_of_Ethics_and_Standards_of_Practice/ALCAWEB/About_Us/Code_of_Ethics_and_Standards_of_Practice.apx

Aging Life Care Association (ALCA). (n.d.). *What you need to know: What is aging life care™?* www.aginglifecare.org/ALCAWEB/What_is_Aging_Life_Care/What_you_Need_to_Know/ALCAWEB/What_is_Aging_Life_Care/What_you_need_to_know.aspx

Arthritis Foundation. (2020). *Osteoarthritis.* www.arthritis.org/diseases/osteoarthritis

Center for Healthcare Research & Transformation. (2014, April). *Best practice in care management for senior populations.* https://chrt.sites.uofmhosting.net/wp-content/uploads/2014/04/CHRT-Best-Practices-in-Care-Management-for-Senior-Populations-.pdf?_ga=2.110823429.1049327284.1678824605-1983749630.1678824605

Centers for Medicare & Medicaid Services. (2021). *Electronic health records.* www.cms.gov/Medicare/E-Health/EHealthRecords

Crowley, J. & Huber, S. (2021). *The life care management handbook.* Author Academy Elite.

Crowley, J. (2017). Determining financials. *7 Steps to Long-Term Care Planning, 7*(1), 40–47.

Dause, T. J., & Kirby, E. D. (2019). Aging gracefully: Social engagement joins exercise and enrichment as key lifestyle factors in resistance to age-related cognitive decline. *Neural Regeneration Research, 14*(1), 39–42. https://doi.org/10.4103/1673-5374.243698

Davis, J. (2012, Spring). Our national association history. Inside GCM, *23*(1), 7–8.

Davison, C., Frankel, S., & Smith, G. D. (1992). The limits of lifestyle: Re-assessing 'fatalism' in the popular culture of illness prevention. *Social Science & Medicine, 34*(6), 675–685. https://doi.org/10.1016/0277-9536(92)90195-v

Farrell, T., Tomoaia-Cotisel, A., Scammon, D., Day, J., Day, R., & Magill, M. (2018). *Care management: Implications for medical practice, health policy, and health services research.* Agency for Healthcare Research and Quality. www.ahrq.gov/ncepcr/care/coordination/mgmt.html

Giardino, A. P., & De Jesus, O. (2021). *Case management.* StatPearls Publishing. www.ncbi.nlm.nih.gov/books/NBK562214/

Holtrop, J. S., Fitzpatrick, L., Jortberg, B. T., Staton, E. W., Clark, R., Sue Voss, & Saffer, K. (n.d.). Care management an implementation guide for primary care practices. https://www.ahrq.gov/sites/default/files/wysiwyg/evidencenow/tools-and-materials/care-management-implementation-guide.pdf

International Association of Rehabilitation Professionals (IARP). (n.d.). *Standards of practice and competencies*. https://rehabpro.org/page/standards

John Hopkins Medicine. (2020). Age-related hearing loss (presbycusis). www.hopkinsmedicine.org/health/conditions-and-diseases/presbycusis.

Jones, M. R., Ehrhardt, K. P., Ripoll, J. G., Sharma, B., Padnos, I. W., Kaye, R. J., & Kaye, A. D. (2016). Pain in the elderly. *Current Pain and Headache Reports*, *20*(4), 23. https://doi.org/10.1007/s11916-016-0551-2

Knickman, J. R., & Snell, E. K. (2002). The 2030 problem: Caring for aging baby boomers. *Health Services Research*, *37*(4), 849–884. https://doi.org/10.1034/j.1600-0560.2002.56.x

Lewis, C. L., & Pignone, M. P. (2009). Promoting informed decision-making in a primary care practice by implementing decision aids. *North Carolina Medical Journal*, *70*(2), 136–139.

Mayo Clinic. (2020). *Healthy lifestyle, healthy aging*. www.mayoclinic.org/healthy-lifestyle/healthy-aging/in-depth/aging/art-20046070

National Academy of Certified Care Managers (NACCM). (2020, July). *Code of ethics and standards of practice*. www.naccm.net/about/code-of-ethics/

National Conference of State Legislators. (2012). *The medical home model of care*. www.ncsl.org/research/health/the-medical-home-model-of-care.aspx

National Council on Aging. (2021, April). *The top 10 most common chronic health conditions in older adults*. www.ncoa.org/article/the-top-10-most-common-chronic-conditions-in-older-adults

National Institute on Aging. (2017, May). *What is a geriatric care manager?* www.nia.nih.gov/health/what-geriatric-care-manager

Neubauer, D. N. (1999). Sleep problems in the elderly. *American Family Physician*, *59*(9), 2551–2560.

O'Malley, A. S., Peikes, D., Wilson, C., Gaddes, R., Peebles, V., Day, T. J., & Jin, J. (2017). Patients' perspectives of care management: A qualitative study. *The American Journal of Managed Care*, *23*(11), 684–689.

Roberts, M. K., Ehde, D. M., Herring, T. E., & Alschuler, K. N. (2021). Public health adherence and information-seeking for people with chronic conditions during the early phase of the COVID-19 pandemic. *PM & R: The Journal of Injury, Function, and Rehabilitation*, *13*(11), 1249–1260. https://doi.org/10.1002/pmrj.12668

Tomlinson, J., Cheong, V. L., Fylan, B., Silcock, J., Smith, H., Karban, K., & Blenkinsopp, A. (2020). Successful care transitions for older people: A systematic review and meta-analysis of the effects of interventions that support medication continuity. *Age and Ageing*, *49*(4), 558–569. https://doi.org/10.1093/ageing/afaa002

World Health Organization (WHO). (2021). *Ageing and health*. www.who.int/news-room/fact-sheets/detail/ageing-and-health

Yan, Q., Jiang, Z., Harbin, Z., Tolbert, P. H., & Davies, M. G. (2021). Exploring the relationship between electronic health records and provider burnout: A systematic review. *Journal of the American Medical Informatics Association*, *28*(5), 1009–1021. https://doi.org/10.1093/jamia/ocab009

3

THE TRANSDISCIPLINARY TEAM

Chapter 9

The Role of the Physiatrist in Life Care Planning

Richard Paul Bonfiglio and Debbe Marcinko

The American Academy of Physical Medicine and Rehabilitation (AAPM&R, 2022a) states that physical medicine and rehabilitation (PM&R), also known as physiatry or rehabilitation medicine, aims to enhance and restore functional ability and quality of life. Physiatrists strive to restore maximum function lost through injury, illness, or disabling diagnoses, treating the whole person, often leading a team of professionals. Physiatrists are experts in designing comprehensive, patient-centered treatment plans, and are integral members of the care team, their patients ranging in age from infants to octogenarians (AAPM&R, 2022a). Physiatrists and life care planners share similar goals on patient/evaluee assessment and care planning, making collaboration a seamless partnership. "The team approach that is essential to life care planning development and implementation is also key to rehabilitation physicians' approach to patient care" (Bonfiglio, 2018, p. 22). Similar to physiatry goals, life care planning goals include enhancing functional capabilities, reducing suffering, preventing secondary complications, increasing independence with activities of daily living, improving cognitive and linguistic capabilities, and enhancing psychological adjustment to impairments (Weed & Owen, 2018).

Physiatry and Life Care Planning Collaboration

According to Paul Deutsch Ph.D. (1992), widely considered to be the founder of life care planning, no single physician or rehabilitation professional completing a life care plan can do so in a vacuum. Each must reach out to establish a medical, case management, rehabilitation, and psychological foundation for the plan. Physiatry has played an integral role in life care planning evolution. In the fall 1992, five rehabilitation professionals, including physiatrist Richard Bonfiglio, MD; Paul Deutsch, Ph.D.; Julie Kitchen, CDMS; Susan Riddick, BS, RN; and Roger Weed, Ph.D., met to discuss the apparent problems associated with life care planning practices (Weed, 2018a). They developed the first training modules and the foundation for the training programs today.

At the 2010 Life Care Planning Summit, life care planners debated establishing the necessary foundation for life care plan recommendations (Preston, 2019). The following two consensus and majority statements were created:

- Life care planners may independently make recommendations for care items/services that are within their scope(s) of practice.
- Life care planners seek recommendations from other qualified professionals and/or relevant sources for inclusion of care items/services outside the individual life care planner's professional scope(s) of practice (Johnson, 2018, p. 878).

The International Academy of Life Care Planners (IALCP) has published peer-reviewed *Standards of Practice for Life Care Planners*, developed in 2000 with revisions in 2006, 2015, and 2022. These state the life care plan reflects a collaborative effort among the various parties, when possible, and goals that are preventive, habilitative, palliative, and rehabilitative in nature and should optimize outcomes (IALCP, 2022).

The *Life Care Planning and Case Management Handbook* (Weed & Berens, 2018), and the *Pediatric Life Care Planning and Case Management* (Riddick-Grisham & Deming, 2011) publications, represent two of the most comprehensive texts on the topics of life care planning and case management currently on the market (Deutsch, 2018). In both publications, the value of consulting with physiatry is referenced in the chapters addressing chronic conditions and selected disabilities. Both have included chapters on the role of the physiatrist in life care planning.

Dr. Roger Weed, the editor of the *Life Care Planning and Case Management Handbook*, opined that it is reasonable to retain the services of a physician or other individuals as appropriate when treatment team members are not available to discuss the case or the caregivers are not specialized. Dr. Weed noted that some treating physicians may not be experts in the particular disability or may be reluctant to provide recommendations, in which case it may be appropriate to arrange for specialty evaluations by other qualified medical professionals (Weed, 2018a). While there are many ways to obtain a medical foundation for certain items included in a life care plan, one way is through collaboration with a qualified physician (or several if differing specialties are required) (Weed, 2018b).

A medical foundation is required for any recommendation that is exclusively medical in nature. Treating physicians including primary care physicians, orthopedists, neurosurgeons, neurologists, and other medical specialists can provide a medical foundation within their scope of practice. Physicians specializing in PM&R contribute to the development of life care plans by providing a medical foundation addressing an individual's medical condition, premorbid medical issues, patient and family input, and desired functional outcomes. The physiatrist's understanding of the holistic needs of the patient/evaluee assists the life care planner, contributing to a comprehensive plan. Gibbs et al. (2013) noted that rehabilitation physicians are uniquely qualified to provide expert opinions for a life care plan by nature of their medical specialty. Additional foundation from other medical specialists or allied healthcare providers is required for all items that fall outside of the physiatrist's area of expertise.

History of Physical Medicine and Rehabilitation

The origins of rehabilitation therapy, an essential component of the physiatry treatment approach, began thousands of years ago with the ancient Chinese, Greek physician Herodicus' (5th century BC), Roman physician Galen (2nd century CE), and others (Atanelov et al., 2015)

The development of physiatry in the United States has its origins in rehabilitation programs for persons following polio, tuberculosis, and returning veterans. Franklin Delano Roosevelt became an avid proponent of rehabilitation following contracting polio with resulting lower limb paralysis in 1921. Philadelphia physician Dr. Frank Krusen contracted tuberculosis during medical school at Jefferson Medical College. After his recovery, Dr. Krusen pursued research in the uses of physical medicine, establishing a program in physical therapy, and an inpatient rehabilitation unit at Temple University in 1929 before moving to the Mayo Clinic in 1936, where he developed a department of physical medicine and the field's first United States residency training program (AAPM&R, 2022a).

Dr. Krusen published *Physical Medicine and Rehabilitation for the Clinician* in 1951 (AAPM&R, 2022b), the first comprehensive textbook, and is credited with coining the term "physiatrist" to identify a physician specializing in physical medicine. Although rehabilitation medicine treatments were established before World War I, rehabilitation medicine used physical medicine approaches, multidisciplinary interventions, and medications for soldiers returning from World War II. The Army Air Forces Convalescent Training Program established in 1942 under the direction of Dr. Howard Rusk, focused on comprehensive rehabilitation services including physical, neuropsychological, and occupational therapies (Atanelov et al., 2015). Dr. Rusk, recognized as "the father of comprehensive rehabilitation," founded the first university-affiliated comprehensive rehabilitation center at New York University (later renamed Howard A. Rusk Institute of Rehabilitation Medicine) in 1951. Dr. Gabriella E. Molnar is the recognized founder of the field of Pediatric Rehabilitation Medicine. Her guiding principle was always that children are not miniature adults, but individuals with changing physical, intellectual, and emotional abilities and needs (Murphy et al., 2021, p. 3).

In 1938, The American Society of Physical Therapy Physicians, the organization that later became the American Academy of Physical Medicine and Rehabilitation (AAPM&R, 2022b) was founded. The American Medical Association (AMA) established the section on PM&R in 1945 (AAPM&R, 2022b). By 1946, 25 hospitals had residency and fellowship training programs in physiatry (AAPM&R, 202b), and the first board examinations were administered in 1947 (ABPM&R, 2022a). Additional notable dates in the history of PM&R can be found at www.aapmr.org/about-physiatry/history-of-the-specialty and www.abpmr.org/About

In 2019, Esquenazi and Frontera reported that the United States had the largest contingent of trained physiatrists with 11,800 trained physiatrists, nearly 9,000 board certified, and 2,500 in academic practices. Physiatrists in the United States are represented by three organizations; the American Board of Physical Medicine and Rehabilitation (ABPMR), a certification and training body; the American Academy of Physical Medicine and Rehabilitation (AAPM&R), a national specialty organization; and the Association of Academic Physiatrists (AAP).

The Americas are composed of North America (i.e., United States, Canada, Mexico, and Caribbean nations) and 24 Latin American countries representing Central and South America. Canada has an estimated 500 physiatrists served by the Canadian Association of Physical Medicine and Rehabilitation. According to Esquenazi and Frontera, Mexico has 1,300 practicing physiatrists represented by two major organizations: The Mexican Society of Physical Medicine and Rehabilitation for academic and scientific development and the Mexican Board of Rehabilitation Medicine for certification. Not every physiatrist has to be certified or recognized by the accrediting body, the Academia Mexicana de Medicina Física y Rehabilitación (Esquenazi & Frontera, 2019). Organized in 1961, the Latin American Medical Association of Rehabilitation (AMLAR), represents the growth and development of physiatry in Central America, South America, and some countries in the Caribbean regions. As of 2019, there were 24 official member countries of AMLAR, with biannual meetings, subregional organizations, and three scientific journals (Esquenazi & Frontera, 2019).

For those who may be seeking physiatric collaboration outside of the United States, information can be found at the International Society of Physical and Rehabilitation Medicine (ISPMR, 2022), a global non-governmental organization with the World Health Organization, an international umbrella organization of PM&R physicians.

Physiatry Education and Training

Through training, experience, and ongoing education, physiatrists provide lifelong care to individuals who have sustained an injury or illness that has resulted in permanent impairment(s) and subsequent disabilities. Physiatrists are medical doctors who have completed training in the specialty of PM&R. Training involves close collaboration with other medical specialists such as orthopedic surgeons, neurologists, and neurosurgeons, as well as physical therapists, occupational therapists, vision therapists, speech and language therapists, rehabilitation nurses, psychologists, and neuropsychologists. The physiatrist develops a thorough understanding of the physical, cognitive, emotional, and social impact of chronic disabling illnesses (Law & Matthews, 2011).

Physical medicine and rehabilitation is one of 24 medical specialties board certified by the American Board of Medical Specialties. The American Board of Physical Medicine & Rehabilitation (ABPM&R) offers this primary certification and subspecialty certifications in the following areas (ABPM&R, 2022d):

- Brain injury medicine
- Neuromuscular medicine
- Pain medicine
- Pediatric rehabilitation medicine
- Spinal cord injury medicine
- Sports medicine

To become board certified in PM&R in the United States, physiatrists must complete a postgraduate degree in medicine (medical doctor or doctor of osteopathy), four years of postdoctoral residency training, and pass both a written (Part I) and oral (Part II) examination administered by the American Board of Physical Medicine and Rehabilitation (ABPM&R, 2022c). Once board certified in physiatry and meeting the eligibility requirements (typically after completing a fellowship) they can sit for a subspecialty examination. The continuing certification process varies based on the year certified or recertified. Certifications issued after 2020 are on a five-year cycle requiring 150 continuing medical education (CME) credits (ABPM&R, 2022b).

Physiatrists may seek additional certification as a Certified Life Care Planner (CLCP™) through the International Commission on Health Care Certification (ICHCC™, 2022). The reader is referred to Chapter 4 in this text for the criteria to obtain this certification.

Scope of Practice

The physiatrist diagnoses, develops treatment plans, and leads comprehensive rehabilitation teams in delivering individualized treatment programs. They provide lifelong care coordination for children through developmental transitions into adulthood, providing anticipatory guidance on life issues such as reproduction, function, aging, adjustment, work, and recreation. The physiatrist overlaps and collaborates with other medical specialists such as physical therapists, occupational therapists, speech and language therapists, nutritionists, nurse practitioners, nursing, social workers, case managers, neurologists, neurosurgeons, orthopedic surgeons, and others.

Pediatric Rehabilitation Medicine Subspecialty

Pediatric rehabilitation medicine is the subspecialty of physiatry whose role is to understand the natural history of the primary disorder and to anticipate the primary and secondary medical and physical complications that often accompany the disorder. Pediatric physiatrists are physicians who specialize in the rehabilitation care and medical management of children with brain injuries, spinal cord injuries, neuromuscular disorders, and an array of musculoskeletal conditions (University of Pittsburgh Medical Center, Children's Hospital of Pittsburgh, 2022). Accomplishments of developmental milestones help to clarify deficits by comparing the child's function with expected standards for their age. Rehabilitation management of children with physical impairments requires the identification of functional capabilities and the selection of the best rehabilitation intervention strategies, with an understanding of the natural history, the usual course of the disability, and the effect of treatment in a continuum of care (Association of Academic Physiatrists [AAP, 2022a; Law & Matthews, 2011).

The process of growing up with a disability has an impact on the individual and how the family functions in society (Matthews & Wilson, 1999). Children with disabilities not only struggle with physical and cognitive impairments but also the lifelong social implications of their disability. Pediatric physiatrists fill a unique niche in the care of medically complex children resulting in improved continuity of care, improved coordination across multiple providers, more efficient use of therapeutic and technological interventions, and better patient and family satisfaction (Vova & Sholas, 2016).

The ability of the pediatric physiatrist to predict the future needs of a child with a disability is extremely valuable in the development of a life care plan. Their training, experience, and knowledge of disabilities enable them to assist the life care planner in developing an accurate projection of future needs. This collaboration can make the life care plan a more valuable guide to families, providers, and legal professionals (Law & Matthews, 2011)

Physician Physiatrist Contributions to Life Care Plan Recommendations

Each profession brings to the process of life care planning their practice standards. Each professional works within the specific standards of practice for their discipline to assure accountability, provide direction, and mandate responsibility for the standards for which they are accountable. Katz et al. (2015) noted that medical opinions "must be limited to the physiatrist's areas of expertise and be based on a solid medical foundation resulting from the physician's clinical experience and review of applicable medical literature" (p. 74).

In 2019, the *Journal of Life Care Planning* (International Association of Rehabilitation Professionals [IARP]) explored the scope of practice of the most common professions engaged in life care planning (i.e., occupational therapy, physical therapy, physiatry, psychologist/neuropsychologist, registered nurse, rehabilitation counselor, and speech/language pathologist) and included detailed articles and tables for each profession (see Table 2.2 in Chapter 2). This compilation is a valuable resource for practicing life care planners to identify the various professional's scope of practice, and how each profession can provide additional foundation to the life care plan. Mann (2019) provided an overview of physiatry and its contribution to life care planning recommendations.

Table 9.1 JLCP Vol 17 No1 (2019) Appendix B Table 3

Care category	Can physician physiatrist make recommendation?
Physician (MD, DO, DC, DDS) referral to evaluate/consult	Within scope of practice
Physician (MD, DO) ongoing visits	Within scope of practice
Chiropractic visits	Collaborative
Dentist ongoing visits and sedation	Within scope of practice
Ancillary (non-physician professionals) referrals	Within scope of practice
Ancillary ongoing visits	Collaborative
Diagnostic testing	Within scope of practice
Surgery	Within scope of practice to identify need; may be collaborative to determine some details
Aggressive interventions (e.g., invasive procedures, specialty programs)	Within scope of practice or collaborative depending on intervention
Wheelchairs, including features and accessories	Within scope of practice to identify need; may be collaborative to determine some details
Other mobility equipment	Within scope of practice to identify need; may be collaborative to determine some details
Orthotics	Within scope of practice or collaborative
Prosthetics	Collaborative
Other medical equipment	Within scope of practice or collaborative depending on equipment
Adaptive aids for independent function	Within scope of practice to identify need; may be collaborative to determine some details
Drugs requiring prescription	Within scope of practice
Over-the-counter drugs	Within scope of practice
Disposable supplies	Within scope of practice to identify need; collaborative to determine details
Home care skill level (to attend to person) (i.e., unlicensed aide, licensed nurse)	Collaborative
Home care hours	Collaborative

(Continued)

Table 9.1 (Continued)   JLCP Vol 17 No1 (2019) Appendix B Table 3

Care category	Can physician physiatrist make recommendation?
Household (housekeeping, yard care, house repairs) services and hours	Collaborative
Adapted transportation (evaluation, training, equipment)	Within scope of practice to identify need; collaborative or outside of scope of practice to determine equipment details
Alternative transportation	Collaborative
Architectural modification	Within scope of practice to identify need; collaborative or outside of scope of practice to determine details
Home furnishings	Outside of scope of practice
Health maintenance	Within scope of practice
Adaptive or therapeutic recreation	Collaborative
Potential complications	Within scope of practice

Common Problems Seen by the Physiatrist

Physiatrists provide treatment and interventions to a diverse group of adult and pediatric patients, practicing in outpatient settings, rehabilitation hospitals, rehabilitation units within hospitals, and private practice, often providing consultations in acute care and trauma, long-term care, and skilled nursing facilities. Virtual visits with physiatrists have become much more common during the COVID-19 pandemic benefiting individuals with limited mobility and stamina.

Physiatrists take a patient-centered approach, considering the biopsychosocial and ecological factors that affect function and quality of life (Sandel, 2019). Physiatrists consider the impact of the diagnosis and related impairments (pain, weakness, other symptoms or conditions) on the patient's day-to-day activities, maximizing the patient's function and quality of life (Sandel, 2019). They incorporate many evaluation scales in their practice to communicate with other health providers, plan appropriate interventions, allow accurate functional prognostication, and demonstrate progress (Vova & Sholas, 2016). According to AAPM&R (2022c), physiatrists undertake the following:

- Determine and lead a treatment/prevention plan
- Diagnose and treat pain as a result of an injury, illness, or disabling condition
- Focus treatment on function
- Have broad medical expertise that allows them to treat disabling conditions throughout a person's lifetime
- Lead a team of medical professionals, which may include physical therapists, occupational therapists, and physician extenders to optimize patient care
- Treat patients of all ages
- Treat the whole person, not just the problem area
- Work with other physicians, which may include primary care physicians, neurologists, orthopedic surgeons, and many others

Depending on the injury, illness, or disabling condition, physiatrists may evaluate and treat their patients using the following procedures/services (AAPM&R, 2022c):

- Complementary-alternative medicine (acupuncture, etc.)
- Disability/impairment assessment
- Discography, disc decompression, and vertebroplasty/kyphoplasty
- Electromyography (EMG)/nerve conduction studies (NCS)
- Fluoroscopy guided procedures
- Injections of joints
- Injections of spine
- Manual medicine/osteopathic treatment
- Medicolegal consulting
- Nerve and muscle biopsy
- Nerve stimulators, blocks, and ablation procedures—peripheral and spinal
- Prescription of physical, occupational, speech, vision, and recreational therapies
- Prolotherapy
- Prosthetics and orthotics
- Referrals to other healthcare providers including medical specialists and subspecialists, nurse case managers, psychologists, and neuropsychologists
- Spasticity treatment (Phenol and botulinum toxin injections, intrathecal baclofen pump trial, and implants)
- Topical, oral, and injected medications
- Ultrasound-guided procedures

According to the AAPM&R (2022a), the practice of physiatry aims to enhance and restore functional ability and quality of life to those with physical impairments or disabilities affecting the brain, spinal cord, nerves, bones, joints, ligaments, muscles, and tendons. Common health problems and populations seen by physiatrists include neurological conditions (e.g., acquired and traumatic brain injury, spinal cord injury, stroke), musculoskeletal injury and conditions, amputation, chronic pain, and neuromuscular disorders (e.g., amyotrophic lateral sclerosis (ALS), burn care, multiple sclerosis, muscular dystrophy, myopathic disorders, neuropathy, osteoarthritis, and Parkinson's disease). Pediatric care may include acquired and traumatic brain injury, brachial plexus palsy, cerebral palsy, gait abnormalities, limb deficiencies, musculoskeletal conditions, neuromuscular disorders, spina bifida, and spinal cord injury.

Some conditions commonly treated by physiatrists will be explored below. Additionally, the reader is referred to the chapters about each condition.

Amputation

Recognizing the extent of impairments and medical conditions caused by amputation is within the experience of many physiatrists. The impact of an amputation goes beyond the loss of the affected limb causing increased energy demands with mobility and daily activities, chronic phantom and stump pain, psychological issues due to loss of body image, and increased mechanical stress on adjacent joints. Physiatry recommendations can be further detailed by collaboration with the orthotist, prosthetist, psychologists, and therapists.

The prosthetist is an integral part of the assessment and provision of a prosthesis and evaluee education. According to American Board for Certification in Orthotics, Prosthetics, and Pedorthics

(2022), the prosthetist provides assessment and analysis, determines the prosthetic requirements, evaluates for environmental barriers, and need for physical and occupational therapy. They formulate the prescription with rationale and functional goals. They select the material, oversee fabrication and assembly, perform the diagnostic fitting, and develop functional exercises and training. The prosthetist performs needed modifications and develops a long-term treatment plan.

Orthoses are used to improve function, prevent further deformity, and/or maintain positioning gained with other interventions, and are intended to produce a more typical gait pattern and improve balance and stability (Ward et al., 2021). In children, orthotic management is guided by growth and development which often requires regular reevaluations and adjustments. While the physiatrist will prescribe, the orthotist or therapist will formulate, fit, align, deliver, and review the orthosis as part of a multidisciplinary, patient-centric approach involving the orthotist, therapist, caregivers, and patient.

Brain Injury

Brain injury can be traumatic (TBI) or non-traumatic ([NTBI], often referenced as an acquired brain injury). According to the Brain Injury Association of America ([BIAUSA], 2020), a non-traumatic brain injury causes damage to the brain by internal factors, such as a lack of oxygen, exposure to toxins, and pressure from a tumor. A traumatic brain injury is defined as an alteration in brain function, or other evidence of brain pathology, caused by an external force. Traumatic impact injuries can be defined as closed (or non-penetrating) or open (penetrating).

The Rancho Los Amigos Scale, used in traumatic brain injury, categorizes patients from level I (most impaired) to level X (least impaired) (Vova & Sholas, 2016). It allows providers to move beyond the binary notion of injured or intact and give more indication of the degree of function. Using such a scale can be useful information for future expectations and challenges. It also allows interventions to be structured in a manner most appropriate for the patient's cognitive and functional impairment, as well as in measuring progress in the patient's recovery. In addition to disorder-specific scales, there are more global scales like WeeFIM, the adaptation for children of the Functional Independence Measure (FIM), helpful in classifying functional skills by developmental/age expectation (Vova & Sholas, 2016).

A person with a mild to moderate traumatic brain injury may experience a significant disruption of daily activities and may be unable to function as usual at home, school, or work. Neuropsychological testing may be helpful to the physiatrist in determining the nature and extent of ongoing impairments and strengths. Some individuals, especially after recurrent concussions, experience long-term symptoms and medical issues including post-traumatic headaches, impaired cognition, and seizures. Ongoing assistance with daily activities, medications, therapies, physician visits, and psychological counseling may be needed. A physiatrist can help to translate functional limitations and collaborative evaluations into life care planning components.

Brain injury can cause profound disorders of consciousness ranging from the minimally conscious state to a persistent vegetative state/unresponsive. Accurate diagnosis requires a multidisciplinary rehabilitation team, providing the information needed to optimize prognosis and treatment decisions. A person in a persistent vegetative state is completely detached from the environment and unable to appreciate pleasure, pain, and suffering. In contrast, an individual in a minimally conscious state has some awareness of the environment with limited ability to make thoughts, desires, and preferences known. According to the American Academy of Neurology practice guidelines (Giacino et al., 2018), clinicians should identify and treat confounding conditions, optimize arousal, and perform serial standardized assessments to improve diagnostic accuracy in adults and children with prolonged disorders of consciousness. Patients with prolonged disorders of consciousness frequently experience significant medical complications that can slow recovery and interfere with treatment interventions. An accurate diagnosis of the level of consciousness has implications for prognosis and management. Frequent neurobehavioral reevaluations/serial evaluations aid in diagnosis and prognosis. Patients with prolonged disorders of consciousness may have a prolonged recovery over months to years, and many will remain severely disabled. Lifelong coordination of medical and rehabilitative care is required. A physiatrist can collaborate with various disciplines to establish and coordinate long-term care planning, monitoring, and management of concomitant medical needs and complications.

In the absence of pediatric-specific evidence for disorders of consciousness, it is reasonable to apply the diagnostic recommendations for adult populations. No tests have been shown to improve prognostic accuracy in children (Giacino et al., 2018).

Brain injuries in children, especially birth-related hypoxic-ischemic injuries, can necessitate extensive, lifelong daily, medical, and rehabilitative care. Life care planning is further complicated by the impact of brain injury on developmental and growth processes, new learning, and socialization. Designing a lifelong plan to meet the needs of these children is bolstered by a physiatrist who has experience taking care of children and adults with childhood-onset impairments and functional limitations.

Cerebral Palsy (CP)

All non-progressive permanent disorders of movement and posture attributed to disturbances that occurred in the developing fetal and infant brain can be described as CP (Vargus-Adams et al., 2021). A 2019 international multidisciplinary consensus statement clarified that CP is a neurodevelopmental disorder diagnosed on clinical signs, not etiology. Cerebral palsy (CP) is the most common motor disability in children with an estimated prevalence of 2.6–2.9 per 1000 births in the United States between 2011–2013 (Yi et al., 2019).

Cerebral palsy itself is not progressive, but secondary complications or conditions can develop and may worsen over time. Concomitant communication disorders are common. In addition to disorders of movement and posture, other neurologic impairments are not uncommon. These include sensory deficits (e.g., vision and hearing), intellectual disability, emotional and behavioral concerns, and seizures (Vargus-Adams et al., 2021).

Children with complex needs require a multidisciplinary treatment team, typically led by the physiatrist, to coordinate educational and transition support, home and nursing care, ongoing diagnostics, therapy, medications, equipment and supplies, home modifications, transportation, and case management. Team members vary but may include the physiatrist, developmental pediatrician, orthopedist, neurologist, physical therapist, occupational therapist, pediatrician, speech and language pathologist, therapeutic recreational specialist, orthotist, neuropsychologist, psychologist, social worker, and nutritionist. Treatment goals should address neuromuscular concerns (maintaining range of motion, tone control), general health nutrition, fitness, and functional goals (self-care skills, mobility, communication).

Scales used to assess the functioning of children with neuromotor disabilities are very helpful in guiding interventions as well as gauging the benefits of interventions and progress. Children with CP are classified by gross motor function. The Gross Motor Function Classification System (GMFCS, Levels I–V) is one of the common classification systems used (Vova & Sholas, 2016). The levels are further defined by age to show the developmental progression of a child at a given level over time, predict what functional tasks are within the future ability of a given patient, and to plan for appropriate mobility support over the lifetime of the child (Vova & Sholas, 2016).

Adults with CP will need continued monitoring and management along with the increased rate of chronic health conditions and eventual decline in strength and functional reserve, decrease in physical activity, increased musculoskeletal complications, and gradual change in swallowing ability (Yi et al., 2019).

A physiatrist with experience in both pediatric and adult management of CP will be an asset in collaborating with the various healthcare team members to make recommendations from childhood, transitioning into adulthood, and throughout the lifespan.

Chronic Pain

Objectively determining the etiology and pathophysiology of chronic pain for an individual can be difficult. Pain cannot be objectively measured, compared, or validated. The impact of pain physically, cognitively, and psychologically is variable. Pain for all of us becomes a common occurrence with the aging process. Some individuals are profoundly affected due to the nature and extent of the pain, previous pain experiences, and the presence of contributing medical conditions such as depression, anxiety, post-traumatic stress disorder, sleep disorder, peripheral neuropathy, and traumatic brain injury. Physiatry input can help design a life care plan by looking at the functional implications.

For musculoskeletal pain and inflammation, injection of local anesthetics along with or in place of steroids is efficacious. Bursal injections, joint space injections, and trigger point injections (or dry needling) are done by pediatric physiatrists, especially for older teens. Finally, EMG and NCS are diagnostic extensions of the physical exam that clarify pathologies of the peripheral nervous system and muscles (Vova & Sholas, 2016).

Lymphedema

Lymphedema is a chronic progressive condition with physical and psychosocial consequences. The physiatrist, along with a multidisciplinary team, sets up strategies for the management and rehabilitation that require constant monitoring. Pressure garments need to be renewed at 6–9 month intervals. Imaging may include lymphoscintigraphy, ultrasonographic evaluation, low-flow color Doppler ultrasound, lymphofluoroscopy, and near-infrared imaging of the lymphatic system. Therapies include complete decongestive therapy, multilayer short stretch bandages, lymphedema exercises, manual lymphatic drainage, compression garments, and pneumatic pressure pumps. Physical therapy modalities can include low-level laser therapy, far-infrared radiation (fir), and extracorporeal shock wave therapy (EsWt) (Borman, 2018).

Spasticity

Spasticity is an abnormal increase in muscle tone or stiffness of muscle, which might interfere with movement and speech, or be associated with discomfort or pain. Spasticity is usually caused by damage to nerve pathways within the brain or spinal cord that control muscle movement. It may occur in association with ALS, brain or head trauma, CP, hereditary spastic paraplegias, multiple sclerosis, spinal cord injury, stroke, and metabolic diseases such as adrenoleukodystrophy, phenylketonuria, and Krabbe disease. Symptoms may include hypertonicity (increased muscle tone), clonus (a series of rapid muscle contractions), exaggerated muscle stretch reflexes, muscle spasms, scissoring (involuntary crossing of the legs), and fixed joints (contractures). The degree of spasticity varies from mild muscle stiffness to severe, painful, and uncontrollable muscle spasms. Spasticity can interfere with rehabilitation in patients with certain disorders, and often interferes with daily activities (National Institute of Neurologic Disorders and Stroke, 2022).

Spasticity requires treatment if this abnormal tone interferes with function or ability to provide care. According to Law and Matthews (2011), physiatrists are experts in the management of spasticity. The physiatrist understands the hierarchical approach to effective management and can prescribe medications and perform botulinum toxin and phenol blocks to reduce or control this abnormal tone. Using a team approach, complex spasticity management can include interventions such as intrathecal baclofen or selective dorsal rhizotomy. These treatment options are recommended only as part of a total rehabilitation program for the specific goal of improving function, easing care, or preventing suffering.

Spinal Cord Injury

For those persons with complete or nearly complete spinal cord injuries, especially cervical-level injuries, virtually every organ system is affected. A physiatrist's comprehensive training and holistic philosophy provides valuable insight.

The American Spinal Injury Association created a consensus classification system across medical and surgical specialties with input from therapists. It classifies a spinal cord injury based on motor and sensory function. In addition to being descriptive of the child's level and extent of paralysis, there are accepted functional abilities for each level and clear associated prognoses of recovery (Vova & Sholas, 2016).

Alterations in physiology after a spinal cord injury may cause constipation, impaired sweating, and thermal regulation. Secondary complications include bowel, bladder, kidney dysfunction, cardiovascular problems, chronic pain, contractures, heterotopic ossification, osteoporosis, overuse syndrome, pressure injury, psychological needs, respiratory limitations, sexual/fertility issues, spasticity, urinary tract infections, and stones. Designing a life care plan that addresses the altered physiology, functional limitations, and potential secondary complications necessitates medical input by experienced professionals caring for persons with similar issues. Children and adolescents with spinal cord injury must deal with multisystem involvement imposed by an injury, compounded by physical and psychological growth and development, which cause complications not seen in adults.

Postural hypotension can be especially problematic during the acute hospitalization and rehabilitation process but may become a chronic issue. Persons following spinal cord injury, especially with injuries above the T6 level, may develop autonomic dysreflexia (AD) or hyperreflexia. In AD, sensory stimulation below the level of injury caused by bladder overdistention, excessive and prolonged skin pressure, and constipation trigger dysreflexia with hypertension, facial flushing, sweating, and headache. Untreated, this condition can cause life-threatening hypertension and cardiac arrhythmias.

The rehabilitation of spinal cord injury is a lifelong process. Goals of rehabilitation should include maintenance or attainment of good health along with prevention of secondary complications while promoting maximal and age-appropriate functional independence. This can range from primarily family education in higher level injuries, to facilitating complete functional independence in lower level injuries. The involvement of a team of experts in the management of children and adolescents with spinal cord injury is recommended into adulthood (Hornyak & Wernimont, 2021).

According to a Turkish study of PM&R specialists on the management of neurogenic bladder due to spinal cord injury, differences were found in current surveillance and management, with no definitive guidelines (Akkoç et al., 2021). Per the Paralyzed Veterans of America (PVA) Consortium for Spinal Cord Medicine (2006), a urologic evaluation is done every year, although there is no consensus among doctors on the frequency of this type of exam or the range of tests that should be included. According to the PVA Clinical Practice Guideline, history, level of injury, and signs and symptoms alone are not enough to determine if a person is experiencing high intravesical pressures, which may cause renal complications over time. The goal of bladder management is to gain continence, promote independence, minimize infections, and protect the kidneys.

Bladder management will depend on the residual function and other variables. Options may include medications, clean intermittent catheterization, indwelling catheters, suprapubic cystostomy, transurethral sphincterotomy, electrical stimulation, and posterior sacral rhizotomy, bladder augmentation, urinary diversion, and cutaneous iliovesicostomy. According to Kreydin et al. (2018) at a minimum, patients should undergo an annual history and physical examination, renal functional testing (e.g., serum creatinine), and upper tract imaging (e.g., renal ultrasonography). The existing evidence does not support the use of other modalities, such as cystoscopy or urodynamics, for routine surveillance.

Functional Considerations

Functional independence involves performing daily living tasks without anyone's direct support and ensures individuals' full participation in life situations that are meaningful and purposeful (Guess et al., 2015). This includes activities of daily living (i.e., bathing, grooming, dressing, eating, and toileting), mobility (i.e., ambulation, bed mobility, driving, transfers), communication, home management, school, work, and leisure skills. The physiatrist's focus on restoring or acquiring functional skills may require the use of durable medical equipment, orthotics, and technology. The physiatrist, collaborating with the rehabilitation team, can identify equipment options, including the advantages and disadvantages, to create an individualized plan. Ambulation aids include canes, walkers, crutches, and standing devices that are individually selected and sized by physical, occupational therapy, and equipment vendors based on the individual's functional requirements. Mobility or standing devices allow play or work in an erect or semi-reclining position maintaining joint range of motion through a functional stretch with or without orthotics. Wheelchairs, specialized strollers, and scooters can provide children the opportunity to explore their environment providing stability, optimal body alignment, head control, trunk balance, and upper extremity use for interaction with the environment. In addition to input from the physical and occupational therapists, the durable medical equipment vendor knowledgeable in current equipment and trends, and seating specialists or rehabilitation engineers are valuable resources. While the physiatrist will provide the medical rationale for these devices, the rehabilitation team provides the specifications needed to meet the needs of the evaluee that will ultimately affect maintenance, replacement, and cost.

Augmentative and alternative communication (AAC) involves the use of signs, gestures, communication books, speech generating devices, or electronic tablets with communication applications to enhance communication function whenever speech does not meet the functional needs of an individual's either acute or chronic condition (Ward et al., 2021). While recommended by the physiatrist, AAC evaluation and device-specific recommendation should be provided by a speech and language pathologist, and if a more comprehensive assessment is needed, an occupational therapist to aid in the ability to use the device, and rehabilitation engineer for custom solutions.

Driving allows access to the community, work, medical and rehabilitation appointments, and social events. A certified driving evaluator will assess vision, reaction time, and cognitive skills. If appropriate, a behind-the-wheel assessment will determine safe driving practices and the need for adaptive driving technology. The physiatrist can provide the medical rationale and incorporate these specifications into their recommendations.

Input by occupational or recreational therapists provides additional detailed recommendations for accomplishing activities of daily living, community reintegration, exercise, and leisure activities.

Shorter hospital stays have resulted in increased use of outpatient settings for comprehensive rehabilitation services and procedures. Earlier discharge of persons with complex care needs can greatly increase their daily care needs at home or in extended care facilities. Individuals with functional limitations often require additional assistance with daily activities later in life. The need for supportive services can vary from a few hours per day of attendant care to 24 hours per day of nursing care. The physiatrist explains the physiologic changes, medical conditions, and impairments caused by the injury or illness including the physical, cognitive, and psychological implications, and the impact on the family. The physical and psychological stress of caring for a family member with complex needs impacts family dynamics.

Technology and Future Rehabilitation

The field of PM&R is being propelled by new and innovative technologies including myoelectric prostheses and orthoses that provide more precise prehension and function than standard devices. Robotic exoskeletons provide wearable powered hip and knee motion to facilitate individuals with spinal cord injuries to be able to ambulate. Therapy-assisted robotics facilitate functional movements in stroke rehabilitation and assist with gait, posture, and trunk control. Smart homes and environmental control systems enhance daily activities for individuals with severe mobility limitations, increase their independence, and reduce energy demand. Virtual and augmented reality systems stimulate cognition and allow individuals with profound physical and/or cognitive impairments to experience life more fully.

Environmental control can be accomplished through touch (sip and puff, head pointing, pointers), adaptive equipment, eye gaze, or voice activation. With many technologies available, it is important to integrate systems. Some have built-in capability through Bluetooth or other technology. Referral to an occupational therapist or technology specialist is helpful, ideally with the provider going to the home for assessment, setup, and training. Smart homes allow control of doors, lights, security systems, music, computer, television, thermostat, and more.

The most current technological advancements should be reflected in the life care plan.

Ambulation and stair climbing for persons with paraplegia are possible with computerized and powered bionic external support systems like ReWalk. Improvements with prostheses include computerized control of key components like the knee joint for above-the-knee amputees; these sophisticated joints allow amputees to ambulate with a variable cadence and enhanced stability and safety. Lower limb orthoses utilizing functional electrical stimulation allow persons with hemiplegia following strokes to ambulate with more normal gait patterns with reduced energy demands. Advances in wheelchair technology, environmental control systems, and augmentative communication devices advance independent functioning. Forward-looking life care plans that provide the most up-to-date equipment can greatly improve function and quality of life.

Life Expectancy Opinions

The Centers for Disease Control (CDC) and Prevention provide United States life expectancy data via the National Center for Health Statistics annual *Life Tables* (CDC, 2022). Life tables are used to measure mortality, survivorship, and the life expectancy of a population at varying ages. These tables provide data for populations reflecting age, gender, race, and state of residence. These population studies include all individuals regardless of their underlying medical conditions.

To accurately project lifetime daily, medical, and rehabilitative care in a life care plan, an accurate prediction of life expectancy is needed. There is no medical literature for individuals with catastrophic injuries or illnesses that projects life expectancy based on the level of care that is typically outlined in a life care plan. Medical literature limitations include the use of statistical projections without a medical foundation and lack of current healthcare provision or technological advances. Additionally, population studies do not address the unique medical and personal situations of individual persons. Therefore, in these authors' opinion, an opinion provided by an experienced physiatrist can help predict the life expectancy of a specific individual for whom a life care plan is being developed. Such determinations require a thorough review of available medical records to recognize underlying medical conditions, catastrophic injury or illness impact, and potential complications. A comprehensive evaluation including a physical examination provides a further basis for life expectancy projections.

Qualification for opinions predicting life expectancy should be based on education, training, medical literature, and clinical experience. A physiatrist's opinions should not be based merely on anecdotal experience, but on available medical and biostatistical data, coupled with clinical experience. Having a consulting physiatrist with a relevant clinical practice, combined with board certification is ideal, ensuring the consultant has the basic medical foundation and experience to provide opinions to a life care planner (Rosen et al., 2013).

Questions Life Care Planners Should Ask the Physiatrist When Developing a Life Care Plan

A physiatrist can provide a medical foundation addressing areas medical in nature. Their goal is to restore and maximize functional ability and quality of life using a comprehensive, whole-person approach. They have broad medical expertise working in various settings with diverse populations and patients of all ages. The physiatrist should match the needs of the evaluee, and limit opinions to his or her scope(s) of practice.

General Questions to Consider

Qualification—does the physician's education, experience, and qualifications match the evaluee's needs? Is there additional subspecialty experience or certifications concomitant with the disability? Experience with the age group? Training in additional procedures and services (EMG, injections, etc.). Are there areas where additional medical specialization will be needed to supplement the medical foundation (durable medical equipment (DME), surgery, medical specialty, prosthetics/orthotics, psychology, complementary-alternative medicine, etc.)?

Life expectancy—is this physician qualified, experienced, and comfortable providing a life expectancy estimate? Should this information be sought elsewhere?

To be thorough, it is helpful to consider the categories outlined in the Life Care Plan Checklist (Weed & Berens, 2018) as a guide, individualizing each category to the evaluee. The physiatrist may or may not need to collaborate with other healthcare providers depending on the evaluee needs, the expertise of the physiatrist, and recommendations made. Depending on circumstance (condition, age, specialized needs), consideration should be made for growth and development, life transitions, and aging in each category. The impact of pre-existing conditions on current needs should be considered; have they been exacerbated by the injury of disease and if so, to what extent?

Medical Basis and Foundation Questions to Consider

The following is not meant to be all-inclusive. Medical foundation and collaboration needs will be specific to the evaluee and recommendation.

- **Projected evaluations (non-physician)—within PM&R scope of practice**
  - Is there a need for non-physician evaluations now and over the evaluee's lifetime in the areas of: audiology, educational, driving, neuropsychological, optometry, physical therapy (PT), psychology/counseling, occupational therapy (OT), recreational therapy, respiratory, speech/language, and others.
  - If so, how often? Will frequency change over time? With aging?
- **Projected therapeutic modalities—within the scope of practice to identify needs, collaboration may be indicated**.
  - These recommendations are often an extension or follow-up to the above-identified evaluations. Will therapies (specify) be needed over the evaluee's lifetime? Routine or intermittent? Lifelong or during periods of transition?
  - If so, how often (frequency) and for how long (duration)?
- **Collaboration consideration**
  - Adaptive devices and equipment recommendations, specifications, and replacement.
  - Audiology specifics for hearing aid recommendations, interventions, and appropriate follow-up and monitoring.
  - Driving evaluation and training, ability to drive safely, vehicle modifications, and replacements. Educational specialists to identify the need for tutors, home, and other learning supports.
  - Neuropsychology for specific cognitive, behavioral, and treatment recommendations, identification of strengths and weakness, additional testing, and follow-up.
  - Nutritionist for special dietary needs, parenteral or supplemental nutrition, failure to thrive needs, monitoring.
  - Orthotist/prosthetist to identify evaluee specific needs, follow-up, replacements.
  - PT, OT, psychologist, etc. providing further insight or specialized recommendations related to frequency and duration of treatment and follow-up. PT or OT may have specific modalities to be included (splinting, e-stimulation, compensatory strategies), need for home exercise program updates, seating re-evaluations.
  - Psychology to identify specific testing, counseling needs, and treatment for issues such as adjustment, addiction, pain, post-traumatic stress disorder, related family/marriage dysfunction, exacerbation of underlying conditions, etc.
  - Cognitive therapy recommendations and follow-up.
  - Recreational therapy for community reintegration planning, functional activities, and leisure activity.
  - Respiratory therapy for specific requirements for management of the tracheostomy or ventilator-dependent evaluee, bilevel positive airway pressure (BiPAP)/CPCP management.
- **Seating and wheelchair specialist for specifications**.
  - Speech and language therapist for augmentative communication recommendations, device choice, training, and monitoring. Additional studies or modalities for the evaluee with swallowing deficits. Vocational counseling, testing for capacity and transferable skills, work reintegration and accommodation, transition planning from school or to work, vocational potential, career guidance, and exploration, placement, coaching, training, supported employment, and work-life expectancy.
- **Diagnostics**—within the scope of practice to identify needs, collaboration may be indicated. Will routine or periodic lab, radiology, or other testing be needed?

- Educational testing, vocational evaluations, other?
- If so, how often (frequency) and for how long (duration)?
■ **Wheelchair needs/accessories**—within the scope of practice to identify needs, collaboration may be indicated.
  - Will the evaluee require a wheelchair for mobility? Manual or power? Scooter? Recreational? Standing or power assist?
  - If the evaluee uses a manual wheelchair, or a child is currently dependent for propulsion, will there be a transition to power? When?
  - If the evaluee is power chair dependent, is there need for a manual as backup?
  - How often would each chair be replaced, considering usage, activity level, and aging?
  - Is there a need for accessories (oxygen or ventilator carrier, activity/work/feeding tray)? (these specifics are typically recommended by OT).
  - Collaboration consideration: PT, OT, technician, and vendor input would be needed for specifications of specialized or customized wheelchairs, seating systems (tilt/recline, positioning), pressure relief options, accessories, etc.
■ **Aids for independent function**—within the scope of practice to identify needs, collaboration may be indicated.
  - Will the evaluee need adaptive equipment or devices to facilitate activities of daily living, work, and recreation?
  - Does the evaluee require aids and software for environmental control?
  - Need for adaptive clothing?
  - Learning devices or software for children? Adapted toys?
  - Collaboration considerations: OT can define customized adaptive equipment and rationale. OT, rehabilitation engineer, or technology specialist can identify environmental control devices to meet the functional ability and need of the evaluee.
■ **Orthotics**—within the scope of practice to identify needs, collaboration IS indicated. Will the evaluee require an orthotic? Please specify (AFO, resting hand splint, heel protectors, etc.).
  - How often should these be replaced? More frequently during growth years, transitions? Collaboration considerations: PT, OT, and orthotist (or all) to choose and fit the orthotic, determine replacement frequencies, and need for training and monitoring.
■ **Prosthetics**—within the scope of practice to identify needs, collaboration IS indicated. Will a prosthetic be needed? Cosmetic, functional, specialized?
  - Collaboration considerations: Prosthetist to define the prosthetic(s), components and supplies, fitting, training, replacement frequencies, and monitoring.
■ **Equipment/home furnishing**—within the scope of practice to identify needs, collaboration IS indicated.
  - Questions would depend on the needs of the evaluee but may include: Will the evaluee need crutches, cane, walker, standing frame, or gait trainer? Continuous positive airway pressure (CPAP), BiPAP, nebulizer, oxygen concentrator, equipment to monitor vital signs? Ventilator (portable and/or stationary), suction machine, other? Backup generator? Hospital or specialty bed, specialty mattress for pressure relief, turning, etc.? Mechanical or overhead lift for transfers?
  - Shower chair/tub bench? Portable commode? Elevated toilet seat?
  - Collaboration considerations: Appropriate therapists and vendors will provide the specifications and rationale for recommended equipment.
■ **Medications (prescription and non-prescription)**—within the scope of practice to identify needs, collaboration may be indicated.

- What medications are required? Dosage, frequency, route of administration? Short-term, intermittent, or lifetime? Changes with aging?
- Collaboration considerations: Neurology collaboration may be needed for difficult neurological conditions or seizure management, adjustments with growth, and aging. Specialty collaboration for management of medications such as Gattex, growth hormone, fertility/erectile dysfunction, hormones, mood and psychiatric management, etc. Other difficult or unstable conditions outside of the scope of the physiatrist.

- **Supplies**—within the scope of practice to identify needs, collaboration may be indicated. The physiatrist can support the need for various supplies based on the condition or treatment. Does the evaluee require supplies for feeding, bowel management, bladder management, incontinence, skin protection or wound care, etc.?
  - Collaboration consideration: Usually, items and usage frequencies are obtained from the family/evaluee and vendor. In the case of the amputee, the prosthetist.

- **Home care/facility care**—within the scope of practice to identify needs, collaboration IS indicated. Is the evaluee able to remain independently at home, or with support? Explain.
  - Alternative residential recommendation?
  - Parent/family/caregiver respite?
  - Does the evaluee require household and homemaking support? Home maintenance assistance?
  - Would the evaluee benefit from participation in camp, summer programming, adult day care?
  - Do you anticipate the need to transition to a higher level of support or care (group home, assisted living, skilled nursing facility)? Timeline?
  - Collaboration consideration: OT, case management, and/or nursing are knowledgeable in state regulations related to the level of care guidelines and are typically consulted to assess and define the level of care and number of hours needed.

Summary

Life care plan recommendations should remain within each practitioner's scope of practice, with an appropriate foundation or rationale providing for reasonable and necessary items to meet daily, medical, and rehabilitative care needs. Physicians can provide medical foundation within their scope of practice. The physiatrist is a logical partner for the life care planner by combining the traditional medical model with a functional approach. Unlike other medical practices that are disease or system-specific, physiatrists have a broad scope of practice, trained to provide holistic lifelong care for multiple conditions, illnesses, and injuries to persons of all ages with the goal of restoring function and improving quality of life. They are comfortable collaborating with a variety of healthcare professionals, frequently participating as members of a multidisciplinary team. While the physiatrist can provide the basis or rationale for medical recommendations, collaboration for individualized and specialized details from other healthcare practitioners may be needed. By nature of their origin in rehabilitation and holistic philosophy, the physiatrist is a valuable resource and contributor to the life care planner and the life care planning process.

References

Akkoç, Y., Ersöz, M., Çınar, E., & Gök, H. (2021). Evaluation and management of neurogenic bladder after spinal cord injury: Current practice among physical medicine and rehabilitation specialists in Turkey. *Turkish Journal of Physical Medicine and Rehabilitation*, 67(2), 225.

American Academy of Physical Medicine and Rehabilitation. (2022a). *About physical medicine & rehabilitation.* www.aapmr.org/about-physiatry

American Academy of Physical Medicine and Rehabilitation. (2022b). *History of the specialty.* www.aapmr.org/about-physiatry/history-of-the-specialty

American Academy of Physical Medicine and Rehabilitation. (2022c). *What is a physiatrist?* www.aapmr.org/about-physiatry/about-physical-medicine-rehabilitation/what-is-physiatry

American Board of Physical Medicine & Rehabilitation. (2022a). *About ABPMR: ABPMR's history.* https://www.abpmr.org/About

American Board for Certification in Orthotics, Prosthetics, and Pedorthics. (2022). *Scope of practice.* www.abcop.org/publication/scope-of-practice

American Board of Physical Medicine & Rehabilitation. (2022b). *Continuing certification program.* www.abpmr.org/CC/About/Overview

American Board of Physical Medicine & Rehabilitation. (2022c). *Getting board certified.* www.abpmr.org/Primary

American Board of Physical Medicine & Rehabilitation. (2022d). *Subspecialty certification.* www.abpmr.org/Subspecialties

Association of Academic Physiatrists. (2022a). *Pediatric rehabilitation medicine.* www.physiatry.org/page/Peds_fellowships

Association of Academic Physiatrists. (2022b). *What is physiatry.* https://www.physiatry.org/page/WhatIsPhysiatry

Atanelov, L., Steins, S. A., & Young, M. A. (2015). History of physical medicine and rehabilitation and its ethical dimensions. *American Medical Association Journal of Ethics, 17*(4), 568–574.

Bonfiglio, R. P. (2018). The role of the physiatrist in life care planning. In R. O. Weed & D. E. Berens (Eds.), *Life care planning and case management handbook* (4th ed., pp. 21–28). Routledge.

Borman, P. (2018). Lymphedema diagnosis, treatment, and follow-up from the view of physical medicine and rehabilitation specialists. *Turkish Journal of Physical Medicine Rehabilitation, 64*(3), 179–197

Brain Injury Association of America. (2020). *What is the difference between an acquired brain injury and traumatic brain injury.* www.biausa.org/brain-injury/about-brain-injury/nbiic/what-is-the-difference-between-an-acquired-brain-injury-and-a-traumatic-brain-injury

Centers for Disease Control, National Center for Health Statistics. (2022). *Life tables.* www.cdc.gov/nchs/products/life_tables.htm

Consortium for Spinal Cord Medicine Clinical Practice Guidelines. (2006). Bladder management for adults with spinal cord injury: A clinical practice guideline for health-care providers. *Paralyzed Veterans of America.* https://pva.org/wp-content/uploads/2021/09/cpgbladdermanageme_1ac7b4.pdf

Deutsch, P. M. (1992). Profile. *The Case Manager* (Jan/Feb/Mar).

Deutsch, P. M. (2018). Forward. *Life care planning and case management handbook* (4th ed., pp. 21–28). Routledge.

Esquenazi, A., & Frontera, W. (2019). 7.3 The organizations of physical and rehabilitation medicine in the world: Physical and rehabilitation medicine in the Americas. *The Journal of the International Society of Physical and Rehabilitation Medicine, 2*(5), 139.

Gibbs, R. L., Rosen, B. S., & Lacerte, M. (2013). Published research and physiatric opinion in life care planning. *Physical Medicine and Rehabilitation Clinics, 24*(3), 553–566.

Giacino, J. T., Katz, D. I., Schiff, N. D., Whyte, J., Ashman, E. J., Ashwal, S., Barbano, R., Hammond, F. M., Laureys, S., Ling, G. S., Nakase-Richardson, R., Seel, R. T., Yablon, S., Getchius, T. S, Gronseth, G. S., & Armstrong, M. J. (2018). Practice guideline update recommendations summary: Disorders of consciousness. *Archives of Physical Medicine and Rehabilitation, 99,* 1699–1709.

Guess, E., Paul, D., & Lane, A. E. (2015). *Achieving functional independence.* https://clinicalgate.com/achieving-functional independence/#:~:text=The%20achievement%20of%20functional%20independence,to%20health%20and%20well%2Dbeing.

Hornyak, J. E., & Wernimont, C. W. (2021). Spinal cord injury. In K. R. Murphy, M. A. McMahon, & A. J. Houtrow (Eds.) *Pediatric rehabilitation principles and practice.* (6th ed., pp. 7676–701). Springer Publication Company.

International Academy of Life Care Planners. (2022). Standards of practice for life care planners, (4th ed.). *Journal of Life Care Planning, 20*(3), 5–20.

International Association of Rehabilitation Professionals. (2019). *Journal of Life Care Planning, 17*(1), 1–88.

International Commission on Health Care Certification. (2022). *Certification programs*. www.ichcc.org/certified-life-care-planner-clcp.html
International Society of Physical and Rehabilitation Medicine. (2022). https://isprm.org/
Johnson, C. B. (2018). Appendix II: Consensus and majority statements derived from life care planning summits held in 2000, 2002, 2004, 2006,2008, 2010, 2012, and 2015. In R. O. Weed & D. E. Berens (Eds.), *Life care planning and case management handbook* (4th ed., pp. 875–878). Routledge.
Katz, R. T., Bonfiglio, R. P., Zorowitz, R. D., & Kirschner, K. L. (2015). Expert testimony: Implications for life care planning. *PM & R: The Journal of Injury, Function, and Rehabilitation*, *7*(1), 68–78.
Kreydin, E., Welk, B., Chung, D., Clemens, Q., Yang, C., Danforth, T., Gousse, A., Kielb, S., Kraus, S., Mangera, A., Reid, S., Szell, N., Cruz, F., Chartier-Kastler, E., & Ginsberg, D. A. (2018). Surveillance and management of urologic complications after spinal cord injury. *World Journal of Urology*, *36*(10), 1545–1553.
Law, C. R., & Matthews, D. J. (2011). The role of the pediatric physiatrist in life care planning. In S. Grisham & L. M. Deming (Eds.) *Pediatric life care planning and case management* (2nd ed., pp. 91–95). CRC Press.
Mann, S. (2019). What life care planners need to know about the professional discipline of physician physiatrist. *Journal of Life Care Planning*, *17*(1), 19–21.
Matthews, D. J., & Wilson, P. (1999). Cerebral palsy. In G. E. Molnar & M. A. Alexander (Eds.), *Pediatric rehabilitation*. Hanley & Belfus.
Murphy, K. P., McMahon, M. A., & Houtrou, A. J. (Eds.) (2021). Dedication. *Pediatric rehabilitation principles and practice*. (6th ed., p. 3). Springer Publishing Company.
National Institute of Neurologic Disorders and Stroke. (2022). *Spasticity definition*. www.ninds.nih.gov/health-information/disorders/spasticity
Preston, K. (2019). Guest editorial. *Journal of Life Care Planning*, *17*(1), 3.
Riddick-Grisham, S., & Deming, L. M. (Eds.). (2011). *Pediatric life care planning and case management* (2nd ed.). CRC Press.
Rosen, B. S., Gibbs, R. L., & Crtalic, A. K. (2013). Estimating life expectancy: A physiatric perspective. *Journal of Life Care Planning*, *12*(1), 3–11.
Sandel, E. M. (2019). *The philosophical foundations of physical medicine and rehabilitation*. https://now.aapmr.org/the-philosophical-foundations-of-physical-medicine-and-rehabilitation/
University of Pittsburgh Medical Center, Children's Hospital of Pittsburgh. (2022). *Pediatric rehabilitation medicine*. www.chp.edu/our-services/rehab-medicine
Vargus-Adams, J., Collins, A., & Paulson, A. (2021). Cerebral palsy. In K. R. Murphy, M. A. McMahon, & A. J. Houtrow (Eds.) *Pediatric rehabilitation principles and practice* (6th ed., pp. 440–461). Springer Publication Company.
Vova, J., & Sholas, M. G. (2016). Pediatric aspects of physiatry and function. In I. L. Rubin, J. Merrick, D. E. Greydanus, & D. R. Patel (Eds.), (pp.1017–1025). *Health care for people with intellectual and developmental disabilities across the lifespan*. Springer International.
Ward, M., Johnson, C., Klein, J., Farber, J. M., Nolin, W., & Peterson, M. J. (2021). Orthotics and assistive devices. In K. R. Murphy, M. A. McMahon, & A. J. Houtrow (Eds.), *Pediatric rehabilitation principles and practice* (6th ed, pp. 269–304). Springer Publication Company.
Weed, R. O., & Berens, D. E. (Eds.). (2018). *Life care planning and case management handbook* (4th ed.). Routledge.
Weed, R. O. (2018a). Life care planning: Past, present, and future. In R. O. Weed & D. E. Berens (Eds.), *Life care planning and case management handbook* (4th ed., pp. 3–20). Routledge.
Weed, R. O. (2018b). Forensic issues for life care planners. In R. O. Weed & D. E. Berens (Eds.), *Life care planning and case management handbook* (4th ed., pp. 609–630). Routledge.
Weed, R., & Owen, T. (2018). *Life care planning: A step-by-step guide* (2nd Ed.). Elliott & Fitzpatrick.
Yi, Y. G., Jung, S. H., & Bang, M. S. (2019). Emerging issues in cerebral palsy associated with aging: A physiatrist perspective. *Annals of Rehabilitation Medicine*, *43*(3), 241–249.

Resources

A searchable database to locate a practicing physiatrist by name, specialty, practice area, and city/state can be found at https://members.aapmr.org/AAPMR/AAPMR_FINDER.aspx

Chapter 10

The Role of the Rehabilitation Nurse in Life Care Planning

Amy M. Sutton

Qualified life care planners present with a variety of backgrounds and experiences, as well as various medical, psychological, and nursing licensures and certifications. These professionals include, but are not limited to nurses, physiatrists, psychologists, rehabilitation counselors, and physical, occupational, and speech therapists. The life care planning training programs and certification processes were designed to train specialists to practice in the field of life care planning, utilizing standards of practice to guide the life care planning process and set expectations regarding methodology and an ethical approach (Weed, 2018). This chapter will outline the training, licensing, and scope of the professional nurse as well as the advantages and expected roles of involving the rehabilitation nurse in consultation and/or the development of a life care plan. Many areas covered in this chapter will be discussed in further detail in subsequent chapters of this text, as some of these issues apply to life care planners from all rehabilitation backgrounds.

The Educational and Licensure Requirements for the Professional Registered Nurse & Nursing Subspecialties

The nursing profession has continuously evolved since the nineteenth century when nurses first began formal educational training. In the United States, the Civil War and the World Wars created a demand for nurses that was satisfied by universities and colleges initiating training programs for nurses. In the 1960s, the American Nurses Association suggested three tracts for nursing students including a baccalaureate degree, an associate degree, and a vocational program (Carey & Marcinko, 2019). Both the baccalaureate and the associate degree students are eligible for becoming a registered or professional nurse (RN). The associate degree requires two to three years of study including clinical training. The baccalaureate degree is generally a four-year program with both general academic education as well as practical nursing training in a variety of clinical settings (i.e., medical-surgical, pediatrics, operating room, emergency care, obstetrics, home health). Once coursework is complete, the graduate nurse must take the licensure exam known as the National Council Licensure Examination for Registered Nurses (NCLEX-RN°) to obtain a license to practice as a RN. More than 50% of the states require continuing education units (CEUs) for the RN to maintain licensure throughout their career. Graduate degrees in nursing are also available including the Master of Science in Nursing (MSN) and a Doctorate in Nursing (PhD or DPN). An Advance Practice RN (APRN) is a graduate-prepared nurse who has completed the required education and licensing and is permitted to diagnose, order tests, and prescribe medication. Each state has specific regulations outlining the parameters of APRN practice (American Nurses Association, 2015).

One of the specialty areas in nursing is rehabilitation. The rehabilitation nurse is a nurse who has procured special expertise in maximizing and maintaining function and quality of life in patients with various disabilities or chronic illnesses that have limited their ability to function in their daily lives (Association of Rehabilitation Nurses, 2007). A rehabilitation nurse may decide to obtain special certification by the Association of Rehabilitation Nurses (ARN) which results in the credentials CRRN (Certified Rehabilitation Registered Nurse). Certification as a CRRN requires an RN licensure, 1–2 years of rehabilitation nursing experience, and successful completion of a proctored examination (Association of Rehabilitation Nurses, 2022). Continuing education units are required to maintain certification. Certainly not all competent rehabilitation nurses are CRRNs. It is an optional credential available and is becoming more popular as rehabilitation facilities encourage their nursing staff to obtain this certification. More information about certification is included at the end of this chapter.

Practice Settings for Rehabilitation Nurses

Rehabilitation nurses are employed in inpatient and outpatient rehabilitation hospitals, as well as in the home health industry. They are frequently used by insurance companies or work in private practice as case managers to manage long-term care and associated costs for patients with lifelong disabilities or illnesses. The roles of the rehabilitation nurse include:

1 *Educator*: The rehabilitation nurse educates the patient, family, and caregivers about the disability or disease. They train the self-care skills necessary to achieve independence, if possible, such as managing bowel and bladder function, monitoring skin condition, safety with mobility, etc. When a family member or caregiver is involved, they train those individuals to provide the necessary care, assistance, and reminders. The rehabilitation nurse also educates the family regarding expectations for the future regarding possible future equipment needs, potential complications, and changing needs over time due to the aging process. For example, a child with a spinal cord injury may require the caregiver to catheterize them while they are too young but with maturity, the child may learn to catheterize themselves, thereby achieving increased independence. In contrast, an individual with a disability who has been independent most of their lives may require more assistance than the average person in the later years of their life.
2 *Caregiver*: The rehabilitation nurse, depending on their type of employment, may provide ongoing assessment of the patient, develop and implement a nursing care plan, and evaluate and adjust the care plan as needed (see description of the nursing process).
3 *Collaborator*: The rehabilitation nurse, as with all nurses, works with other specialists to develop goals and facilitate communication between all healthcare professionals involved with the patient's care. Often, the rehabilitation nurse is working with a large interdisciplinary

team given the nature of long-term disability and chronic illness. For example, individuals with spinal cord injury or traumatic brain injury may have multiple therapists (physical, occupational, speech, psychological, vocational, etc.), as well as multiple physicians (physiatrist, neurologist, orthopedist, neurosurgeon, psychiatrist, etc.). The collaboration process in these complex cases often requires team conferences or frequent interdisciplinary communication. The rehabilitation nurse or nurse case manager may be the point of convergence where all these disciplines are informed about the current plan of care.

4 *Client Advocate*: Depending on the role, the rehabilitation nurse advocates for services and equipment that will promote quality of life for the patient and assist the patient to achieve their maximum potential. When appropriate, they may refer the patient to resources in the community to provide additional services at low to no cost to the patient or family. They may assist patients and families in the process of finding and obtaining appropriate and affordable equipment, supplies, and services, and negotiating with insurance case managers to fund items and/or services (Association of Rehabilitation Nurses, n.d.).

5 *Consultant*: The nurse may be retained by insurance companies, lawyers, families, trusts, and others to provide expertise and suggestions for management of long-term care needs, referrals to appropriate medical specialists for further evaluation, and other similar functions. In some situations, these consultants are not disclosed but rather work behind the scenes to achieve a variety of goals.

The Nursing Process and Care Plan Development

Nurses from every field of healthcare delivery share the basic tenets of the nursing process (Wilkerson, 2012). They are the foundation for patient-focused care, and this includes:

Assessment: This step involves physical assessment of the patient, as well as psychological, sociological, economic, lifestyle, past and current health history, and past and present stressors, and coping strategies assessment.

Nursing Diagnoses: While nurses do not make medical diagnoses, they are expected to diagnose the patient's response to a current or potential diagnosis. These diagnoses are broken down into physical and psychological components including diagnoses such as "at risk for falls," "impaired skin integrity," "adjustment difficulties," "nutritional deficits," "ineffective airway clearance," "anxiety," etc.

Outcomes/Planning: Following assessment and after the resulting nursing diagnoses are determined, the nurse sets goals, both short and long term, to address and ultimately resolve/treat the identified diagnoses. The result of this process is called the nursing care plan which is typically documented so that other nurses and healthcare professionals can participate in the process and provide continuity of care. The nursing care plan and the process of its development are quite similar to the development and implementation of a life care plan.

Implementation: Once the care plan is developed, it is implemented to facilitate progress toward the identified goals.

Evaluation: The care plan is continually evaluated, updated, and modified as it is a living document, just as a life care plan is a dynamic document which is adjusted based on the needs of the patient.

The nursing care plan, resulting from *Outcomes/Planning*, is an organized list of nursing diagnoses and goals for each patient based on their unique medical and psychosocial diagnoses, the patient's own expectations and family expectations, and considers both the potential of the patient and their limitations. These documents are a means of communication between nurses and other healthcare professionals and are educational tools for patients, families, and caregivers. Nursing care plans are often used as a guide for duration of hospitalization, home health services, and reimbursement by third-party payers. The nursing care plans are updated based on changes in the patient's condition on an as-needed basis. Similarly, the life care plan identifies the needs and goals of a patient, incorporates the services and equipment to achieve these goals, and is updated and re-evaluated based on the changing needs of the patient over time (Weed, 2018).

The Contributions of the Rehabilitation Nurse in Life Care Planning

In life care planning, nurses have two options for certification: Certified Life Care Planner (CLCP™) which is open to all eligible licensed healthcare professionals (or Canadian Certified Life Care Planner [CCLCP™] for Canadian practitioners) or Certified Nurse Life Care Planner (CNLCP®) which is open only to nurses. Each of these certifications have requirements that the candidate be licensed as a nurse, receive life care planning training from a specialized training program, and on-the-job training experience (Carey & Marcinko, 2019). As the specialty practice of life care planning expands, there is an emerging emphasis on having a baccalaureate degree as a minimum to practice as a life care planner. The RN also has the option of obtaining certification as a CRRN. The steps to certification include having a current license as a RN, demonstrating two years of rehabilitation nursing experience or one year of experience and one year of advanced study (post-baccalaureate), and passing the formal CRRN examination (Association of Rehabilitation Nurses, 2022).

As previously noted, the nursing care plan is a tool very similar to the life care plan. Rehabilitation nurses are trained to develop and implement the nursing care plan early in their nursing career. There are significant advantages to involving a rehabilitation nurse with life care planning training in the development or evaluation of life care plans.

As part of nursing education, student nurses are educated in almost all areas of nursing specialties. There are classes in pediatrics, obstetrics, gerontology, intensive care, cardiology, psychiatry, home health, rehabilitation, and much more. Students are required to participate in practicum experiences in these various areas to learn hands-on care for patients with a variety of conditions. Following graduation, nurses often work in a variety of settings before landing in a specialty area. Clinical nurses in a hospital are frequently required to work in many different areas of the hospital depending on staffing needs and therefore must be proficient in most specialties. This background is especially beneficial in the field of life care planning due to the range of illnesses and disabilities presented to the life care planner during his or her career.

Rehabilitation nurse life care planners who have worked as clinical nurses have hands-on experience with procedures, supplies, equipment, post-operative needs, etc. For example, a rehabilitation nurse who has catheterized or taught a patient to self-catheterize has first-hand knowledge about the types of supplies necessary, the difference between catheter types, and the amount of training time required to learn this skill. They have used a hydraulic lift, a pulse oximeter, a ventilator, and so on. They have dressed, bathed, and transferred a completely dependent patient, and they understand the burden on caregivers and the equipment that can ease that burden. This practical knowledge is an advantage when developing a life care plan and when educating an attorney or a jury about why something should or should not be included in a future care plan.

Scope of Practice

The life care planning process is collaborative and interdisciplinary, requiring the input from multiple specialists via direct contact or through medical records (International Academy of Life Care Planners, 2015). Nurses in every field have extensive experience collaborating with a variety of specialists. Rehabilitation nurses have regular contact with speech, physical, and occupational therapists, neuropsychologists, physicians, respiratory therapists, etc., and have at least some training in most of these areas. The development of a life care plan is an extension of this collaborative process. However, the broad experiences and training of the rehabilitation nurse does not allow them to make recommendations in every category of the life care plan. The nurse life care planner must stay within their scope of practice. It is essential for the nurse to establish a foundation for recommendations outside of their scope. For example, medications, frequency and type of physician visits, surgeries/hospitalizations, and diagnostic testing require input from a medical doctor. If the nurse life care planner has additional expertise in other areas, such as being a physical therapist or psychologist, they may include independent recommendations in those areas as well (International Academy of Life Care Planners, 2015).

In many life care plans, the most important and most expensive category of the plan is home/facility care (Sutton et al., 2002). This area of the life care plan is within the scope of a rehabilitation nurse if they rely upon the medical experts' or treating physicians' assessment of the patient's abilities and limitations. When needed, the recommendations may include a companion, a nursing assistant (or home health aide), a nurse, a case manager, a nursing home, a group home, an assisted living facility, or some combination of any of these services. Following hospital discharge, the amount and level of care needed is typically determined by a home health or rehabilitation nurse during an initial evaluation based on the medical skills necessary and the level of independence demonstrated by the patient. During the development of a life care plan, the rehabilitation nurse life care planner discusses these issues with the physicians, therapists, and neuropsychologist (depending on the specialists involved) to determine the patients' abilities and limitations. They can then use their background and training to determine the appropriate amount and level of care indicated. Each state has a Nurse State Practice Act which lays out the roles and responsibilities of the professional nurse which can be a tool to guide the nurse life care planner in recommendations for home care services. The life care planner may also need to consult with published Attorney General statements and Welfare & Institution Codes for the appropriate state of residency to establish the rules and regulations for in-home caregivers and their scopes of practice.

Overall, the rehabilitation nurse, in the role of a life care planner, is expected to have the background, education, and experience to fulfill the aforementioned expectations. The care planner is often in situations that are complex, stressful, and require critical thinking skills and a great deal of patience. See Table 10.1 for additional desirable traits for the rehabilitation nurse life care planner.

Research Issues for the Rehabilitation Nurse in Life Care Planning

The issue of research in the field of life care planning is applicable to all life care planners, not just the nurse life care planner. Some nurse life care planners are conducting or participating in current life care planning research. While others may not be actively involved in research, all life care planners should be familiar with the past and present research in the field and understand the research process. This is especially relevant considering the *Daubert* challenges, which highlight

Table 10.1 Desirable Traits for Rehabilitation Nurse Life Care Planners

1. Know inpatient medical-surgical or acute rehabilitation services
2. Have emergency medical experience
3. Possess verbal and analytical reasoning skills
4. Have the ability to communicate with a variety of cultural, educational, and experiential backgrounds
5. Possess problem-solving, negotiation, and conflict resolution skills
6. Are computer literate for research and communication
7. Have knowledge of professional resources and access to resources
8. Have the ability to critically analyze literature
9. Understand the scope and limitations of medical and allied health fields
10. Have pharmacology knowledge
11. Know normal laboratory values
12. Know drug actions/interactions
13. Know pathophysiology of different disabilities
14. Have basic abnormal psychology knowledge
15. Know the effects of trauma on coping and psychological functioning
16. Deal effectively with stress
17. Pay attention to details
18. Are well organized
19. Document the work in the file
20. Maintain meticulous files
21. See the big picture
22. Have self-confidence
23. Are objective and professional
24. Stay within area of expertise

Source: Riddick-Grisham, S. (2010). Reprinted from the 3rd edition of the *Life care planning and case management handbook*, p. 34.

the importance of scientific and quantifiable life care planning research that can demonstrate the reliability and validity of the life care planning process in forensics (Countiss & Deutsch, 2002). With the availability of the internet, information has become accessible to everyone, including attorneys who would like to discredit a life care planner. The research process assists the nurse life care planner in staying current with standards of practice, expected outcomes of various disabilities and treatment modalities, conducting a market survey of costs, determining replacement frequency of equipment, researching applicable case law depending on where the case is tried, and finding organizations which provide services for various disabilities, cultures, and belief systems.

Although nurse life care planners commonly rely on the input from physicians regarding expected outcomes for medical diagnoses and specific medical interventions, there is a large body of research available to help guide the life care planner with future care recommendations specific to each type of disability. For example, the Consortium for Spinal Cord Medicine (sponsored by the Paralyzed Veterans of America) has published guidelines and expected outcomes for spinal cord injured patients based on the level of injury (Paralyzed Veterans of America, 2002). Medical journals have published outcome studies for various pain management procedures like spinal cord stimulators and baclofen/morphine pumps. These types of publications can be helpful in guiding discussions with experts or treating physicians regarding the needs of a patient following an intervention or specific injury and facilitate an educated discussion with experts, defending a plan during deposition, or testifying at trial.

Collateral Sources

The nurse life care planner should be familiar with the services offered by the state in which the patient resides. Some services are federally funded such as the Individuals with Disabilities Education Act (IDEA) 1990, as amended, which finances a variety of services for school-aged children with disabilities. Some services are privately funded such as Easter Seals, assisting adults and children with disabilities. Each state has programs in place such as Early Intervention for children under age three. Life care planners often practice in multiple states and should research the resources available, as well as the bases for those resources. For example, in California, the Regional Center and California Children's Services are available to assist with therapy needs, parenting needs, medical and equipment needs, respite care, and case management for children (State of California Department of Developmental Services, 2022a). The Regional Center also provides group home services for adults with a qualifying diagnosis and who were disabled prior to age 18 years. The funding for the Regional Center is protected by the Lanterman Act that was passed in 1977 (State of California Department of Developmental Services, 2022b). Researching these types of details specific to each source and each state goes a long way in providing the foundation for including these sources in a life care plan.

Life Care Planning Costing

Researching the costs for the life care plan is a fundamental step in the process of creating a useful tool for future planning, as well as determining the overall cost of funding the life care plan. Life care planning standards of practice (International Association of Rehabilitation Professionals, 2022) provide the basic tenets of cost research and the life care planner chooses their preferred method of determining the reasonable market rate. The Consensus and Majority Statements derived from Life Care Planning Summits (Johnson et al., 2018) also provide guidance for the cost research process. Life care planners are encouraged to use verifiable and geographically specific costs. Cost estimates should be based on more than one source (when possible) and reflect market rates. Some life care planners prefer using databases, while others conduct a market survey by calling, on average, 3–5 local providers for current prices. A 2020 technology survey found that 73% of respondents (n = 81) used costing databases in their practice (Owen et al., 2021). Another more recent survey of practicing life care planners, presented at the May 2022 life care planning summit, identified that more than 90% of the respondents use databases for at least some of the costs in some of their plans. The same study also identified that more than 90% of the respondents use telephonic surveys for at least some of the costs in some of their plans (Pomeranz & Yu, 2022). Service providers often disclose different rates depending on the payer source. When contacting providers for pricing, one must specify whether they are seeking a private-pay rate, a contracted rate, or the amount billed to a third-party payor. They may have a specific rate negotiated with each insurance company, which is likely different than the rate they bill the insurance company, and a private-pay or cash rate for patients who are uninsured or choose to pay out-of-pocket (Busch, 2022). Determining which rate to use will likely depend on the payer source that is expected to fund the life care plan as well as applicable state and federal rulings which specify admissible data. If the life care plan is for litigation and third-party payers are excluded from being named as a collateral source, the cash rate may be appropriate. However, it is not appropriate for the life care planner to negotiate a discounted rate that would not be readily available to the public (International Academy of Life Care Planners, 2015). Each state has case laws that may help guide the life care planner in selecting the applicable rates. Most states have case law specific to past medical care cost recovery and some have case law that either states or implies future care costs and recovery rates. Each state also has case laws that set forth whether collateral sources may be utilized and may depend upon whether the case is medical malpractice or personal injury (Stern & Owen, 2022). The life care planner should research and be familiar with the applicable case law in the state where the case is pending litigation. Finally, when researching the cost of community or medical services, the focus should be on conducting a market analysis rather than determining a list of specific locations where the patient must receive future care. The survey is used to establish the reasonable cost of a service in a particular area, not a list of precise referrals which would be subject to scrutinization by opposing attorneys. For pricing home/facility care options, private *and* agency hire options should be considered (Johnson et al., 2018). If a facility or group home is included, the appropriateness for each specific patient should be considered especially regarding diagnosis, average age of the residents, and the level of care provided. Due to the complexity and high cost associated with attendant care, a costing model (ACSM) has been introduced to specify methodology for life care planners (Barros-Bailey et al., 2022). This is a 12-step model to assist the life care planner in collecting, reporting, and defending the cost research specific to attendant care.

Some nurse life care planners require assistance in collecting data in all these areas and employ a research assistant (Pomeranz & Yu, 2022). These individuals are not expected to provide expert testimony but, instead, may assist the life care planner with researching costs of services and equipment, identifying resources available in the community, conducting a literature search for applicable publications on a particular topic, and researching availability of specialty services and checking ratings of specialty facilities. The research assistant should be familiar with the nursing/medical field and be educated by the life care planner regarding market survey or cost research methodology. Research assistants must be directed and supervised by the life care plan author to assure they follow the process and methodology of the author and to assure that the patient's confidentiality is protected.

Other Roles of the Rehabilitation Nurse in Life Care Planning

Rehabilitation nurse life care planners provide a variety of services during the life care planning process, as well as consulting on cases without developing a life care plan. See Table 10.2 for a description of some of these services and responsibilities. See Table 10.3 for questions for the attorney. See Table 10.4 for questions the nurse life care planner should ask the vocational expert (if one is involved).

Table 10.2 Additional Roles and Expectations of the Rehabilitation Nurse Life Care Planner

Educate attorneys in selecting a life care planner and how to evaluate the background and credentials of the opposing life care planner (see Table 10.3)
Assist attorneys in selecting other specialties that could or should be retained or consulted (i.e., vocational expert, physiatrist, urologist, plastic surgeon, neuropsychologist) depending on the specifics of the case
Assist attorneys in preparing deposition questions for patients, family members, experts, and treating physicians
Review pre- and post-incident medical records to determine services that are unrelated or pre-existing, then confirm with appropriate medical experts
Rely upon nursing diagnoses and life care planning standards of practice to assist other retained experts or treating physicians in identifying future care needs: a. Collaborate with experts and/or treating providers on expected outcomes of treatment that may affect long-term prognoses (i.e., eventual increase or reduction in medications, increase or decrease in attendant care needs, increase or reduction in palliative care needs)   b. Cover all categories of the life care plan with each expert and/or treating provider to promote a thorough future care plan (i.e., an orthopedic expert may recommend follow-up visits and a future surgery only but if asked about future diagnostic testing, post-operative home health, or post-operative physical therapy, he or she may realize that the recommendations exceed just surgery and follow-up visits)   c. Educate experts and/or treating providers in the legal standards for including services in the life care plan (greater than 50% probability)   d. Communicate recommendations of all experts and/or treating providers with other involved experts/treating providers to avoid overlap or contradictions in recommendations   e. Develop one's own or use published lists of questions to guide discussions with other retained experts to maintain consistency in methodology. The types of questions will depend on the area of expertise: vocational expert, psychological or neuropsychological expert, physicians (specific to specialty), therapists (specific to specialty), and the economist (source-example of questions for the vocational expert)   f. Evaluate one's own or the opposing life care plan as a whole, not in parts, to determine whether the plan is reasonable and feasible (i.e., number of hours per day in therapy, caregiver services overlapping with school or day treatment programs, including intensive interventions without reasonable expectation of benefiting from those services)   g. Educate attorneys and other experts regarding the standards of practice in life care planning. The standards of practice can protect one life care planner while highlighting the methodological flaws in another (Fick & Preston, 2015)

Related Certifications and Organizations

There are a number of organizations that offer credentials for life care planning, rehabilitation nursing, legal nurse consulting, case management, and related certifications. This is a list of many of the credentials that are related to nursing and life care planning:

- CRRN: Certified Rehabilitation Registered Nurse, offered by the Association of Rehabilitation Nurses (ARN); www.rehabnurse.org

Table 10.3 Questions for the Attorney: Life Care Planner Qualifications and Expertise

Does the life care planner have specific training in this specialized profession and the type of disability involved?
Is the person board certified? (e.g., CLCP™, CNLCP™, or CPLCP™)
Does the life care planner belong to the International Academy of Life Care Planners (IALCP), the International Association of Rehabilitation Professionals (IARP), the American Association of Nurse Life Care Planners (AANLCP), or the American Association of Physician Life Care Planners (AAPLCP)?
Does the life care planner subscribe to the *Journal of Life Care Planning* and/or other relevant journals (i.e., *Rehabilitation Nursing*)?
Do they have publications related to life care planning in their library (i.e., *Guide to Rehabilitation* by Deutsch & Sawyer [out of print], *Life Care Planning and Case Management Handbook* (1st–4th Edition), *Pediatric Life Care Planning and Case Management* (1st & 2nd edition edited by Grisham & Deming), *Life Care Planning and Case Management Across the Lifespan* 5th Edition— an integration of the Weed & Riddick-Grisham texts with a focus on life care planning across the lifespan, other relevant publications)?
Does the life care planner offer vocational and life care planning expertise? If so, do they have the background, training, and credentials to provide both services?
Does the life care planner have the medical foundation for necessary recommendations, or do they collaborate with medical professionals who *can* provide the foundation?
Does the life care planner project *future* needs in addition to current needs (i.e., needs that may increase or decrease over time)?
Is the life care planner familiar with and do they subscribe to the published standards of practice for life care planning, including methodology, omission, or removal of costs for pre-existing conditions, ethical guidelines, etc.?

Source: Adapted from Sutton, A. M., & Weed, R. O. (2004, Winter). Life care planning issues for the attorney. *The ATLA Docket*, 10–22.

Table 10.4 Questions the Nurse Life Care Planner Should Ask the Vocational Expert

First determine if vocational aspects have been considered or are already underway (e.g., already initiated by insurance company or attorney).
What vocational interview information has been obtained from the evaluee (e.g., work skills, leisure activities, education, work, functional abilities based on Department of Labor and/or physician)?
Have you obtained copies of relevant medical records?
Have you obtained work related information (such as tax returns, job evaluations, school and test records, training history, and treating or consulting MD comments)?
Does the evaluee need testing before determining vocational potential (e.g., vocational evaluation, psychological, neuropsychological, or physical capacities testing)? Also, is the evaluation a "reliable" and "valid" appraisal which can stand the scrutiny of talented reviewers/opposing experts?
If there is work potential, is there a need for justifying a plan by performing a Labor Market Survey (LMS)? If LMS, what method is used (e.g., direct contact with employers vs. statistics, computer program and/or publications)?

(Continued)

Table 10.4 (Continued) Questions the Nurse Life Care Planner Should Ask the Vocational Expert

What is the evaluee's expected income including benefits? (If personal injury litigation, then pre- vs. post-injury capacity)
If there is an apparent market for the evaluee's labor, is there a need for a job analysis? (And if an analysis was completed, was it compliant with the Americans with Disabilities Act guidelines?)
What are the estimated costs of the vocational plan? For example:
Counseling, career guidance? When does it start/stop, frequency, and cost
Job placement, job coaching, or supported employment costs?
Tuition or training, books, supplies? Include dates for expected costs
Rehabilitation or assistive technology, accommodations, or aids, costs for work, education and/or training (e.g., computer, printer, workstation, tools, audio recording applications, attendant care, transportation—include costs and replacement schedules)?
What effect, if any, does the injury have on work life expectancy (e.g., delayed entry into workforce, less than full-time, earlier retirement, expected increased turnover, or time off for medical follow-up or treatment)?

Source: © Roger O. Weed, PhD (1997, rev, 2002, 2016), with permission. R. Weed personal communication September 6, 2022).

- CLCP™: Certified Life Care Planner, offered by the International Commission on Health Care Certification (ICHCC™); www.ichcc.org
- CNLCP®: Certified Nurse Life Care Planner, offered by the American Association of Nurse Life Care Planners (AANLCP®); www.aanlcp.org
- CPLCP™: Certified Physician Life Care Planner; www.aaplcp.org
- LNC: Legal Nurse Consultant, offered by the American Association of Legal Nurse Consultants (AALNC); www.aalnc.org
- CCM: Certified Case Manager, offered by the Commission for Case Manager Certification (CCMC); www.ccmcertification.org
- CMCN: Certified Managed Care Nurse, offered by the American Board of Managed Care Nursing (ABMCN); www.abmcn.org
- CMC: Care Manager, Certified, offered by the National Academy of Certified Care Managers (NACCM); www.naccm.net
- COHN: Certified Occupational Health Nurse, offered by the American Board for Occupational Health Nurses (ABOHN); www.abohn.org

Conclusion

The rehabilitation nurse can offer a variety of services in the ongoing treatment, future care planning, and long-term maintenance of patients with catastrophic injuries and chronic health concerns. The combined rehabilitation and nursing expertise with the life care planning training allows nurse life care planners to apply their broad nursing training and experience to future care plan development. The nurse life care planner has extensive clinical experience in collaborating across multiple disciplines to achieve patients' goals and maximum potential. The nursing care plan process is both similar and complementary to the process of developing life care plans and designed to predict needs and prevent complications. When the rehabilitation nurse incorporates the nursing process with standards of practice in life care planning and has the attributes, skill set, and qualifications described in Tables 10.1–10.3, they can be an excellent choice for providing life care planning services in forensics or the private sector.

References

American Nurses Association. (2015). *Nursing: Scope and standards of practice* (3rd ed.). Author.

Association of Rehabilitation Nurses. (n.d.). *Rehabilitation nurses play a variety of roles.* https://rehabnurse.org/about/roles-of-the-rehab-nurse

Association of Rehabilitation Nurses. (2007). *Role of the nurse on the rehabilitation team.* https://rehabnurse.org/about/position-statements/role-of-the-nurse

Association of Rehabilitation Nurses. (2014). *Standards and scope of rehabilitation nursing practice.* Author.

Association of Rehabilitation Nurses. (2022). *Steps to CRRN certification.* https://rehabnurse.org/crrn-certification/earn-your-crrn

Barros-Bailey, M., Brown, S., Maxwell, A., Malloy, S., Latham, S., Thompson, A., & Donohoe, E. (2022). Attendant care survey methodology (ASCM): Introducing a costing model attendant care survey methodology. *Journal of Life Care Planning, 20*(1), 5–26.

Busch, R. M. (2022). Healthcare service costing: Pricing perspectives and case studies for life care planners. *Journal of Life Care Planning, 20*(2), 21–35.

Carey, E. M., & Marcinko, D. A. (2019). What life care planners need to know about the professional discipline of registered nurse. *Journal of Life Care Planning, 17*(1), 31–38.

Countiss, R. N., & Deutsch, P. M. (2002). The life care planner, the judge and Mr. Daubert. *Journal of Life Care Planning, 1*(1), 35–43.

Fick, N., & Preston, K. (2015). An attorney perspective on standards of practice: A weapon or a shield? *Journal of Life Care Planning, 13*(3). 17–20.

International Academy of Life Care Planners. (2015). Standards of Practice for Life Care Planners (3rd ed.). IARP.

International Association of Rehabilitation Professionals. (2022). Standards of practice for life care planners (4th ed.). *Journal of Life Care Planning, 20*(3), 5–20.

Johnson, C. B., Pomeranz, J. L., & Stetten, N. E. (2018). Consensus and majority statements derived from life care planning summits held in 2000, 2002, 2004, 2006, 2008, 2010, 2012, 2015, and 2017 and updated via Delphi study in 2018. *Journal of Life Care Planning, 16*(4), 15–18.

Owen, T. R., Thomas, L. B., & Dunlap, K. (2021). Evolution of life care planning with technology. *Journal of Life Care Planning, 19*(1), 65–80.

Paralyzed Veterans of America. (2002). *Expected outcomes: What you should know—A guide for people with C4 spinal cord injury.* Consortium for Spinal Cord Injury Medicine.

Pomeranz, J. L., & Yu, N. S. (2022, May 13–14). *Explanation of life care planning costing survey and presentation of results* [Conference presentation]. 2022 Life Care Planning Summit, Dallas, TX.

Riddick-Grisham, S. (2010). The role of the nurse case manager in life care planning. In S. Riddick-Grisham (Ed.). *Pediatric life care planning and case management* (1st ed., pp. 25–34). CRC Press.

State of California, Department of Developmental Services. (2022a). Services. www.dds.ca.gov/services/

State of California, Department of Developmental Services. (2022b). *Lanterman developmental disabilities services act and related laws.* www.dds.ca.gov/wp-content/uploads/2022/02/Revised_LantermanAct_February2022.pdf

Stern, B., & Owen, T. R. (2022). Collateral source rule approaches and its implications for usual, customary and reasonable pricing. *Journal of Life Care Planning, 20*(1), 27–41.

Sutton, A. M., & Weed, R. O. (2004, Winter). Life care planning issues for the attorney. *The ATLA Docket,* 10–22.

Sutton, A. M., Deutsch, P. M., Weed, R. O., & Berens, D. E. (2002). Reliability of life care plans: A comparison of original and updated plans. *Journal of Life Care Planning, 1*(3), 187–194.

Weed, R. O. (2018). Life care planning: Past, present, and future. In R. O. Weed & D. E. Berens (Eds.), *Life care planning and case management handbook* (4th ed., pp. 3–20). Routledge.

Wilkerson, J. M. (2012). *Nursing process and critical thinking*. Pearson.

Chapter 11

The Role of the Rehabilitation Counselor in Life Care Planning

Debra E. Berens and Ann T. Neulicht

This chapter answers the question of what role the rehabilitation counselor (RC) plays in life care planning. Recognizing that RCs have been part of the healthcare landscape for over 100 years (originally known as vocational rehabilitation counselor), the profession has evolved through the years and the role of the contemporary RC covers the lifespan of individuals with a disability and/or chronic health condition. A summary of the various roles that RCs have within the specialty practice of life care planning is detailed in this chapter and includes RC as vocational expert (VE) and life care planner (dually qualified as both VE and life care planner), RC as case manager to implement the life care plan (dually qualified as both life care planner and case manager), RC as VE only to collaborate with non-RC life care planners to provide vocational recommendations for the life care plan and/or to provide wage loss/loss of earnings capacity opinions, or any combination of the above roles.

Historical Roots of the Profession of Rehabilitation Counselor

A review of the literature shows that the profession of RC is not new (Berens & Weed, 2018; Mertes & Harden, 2019; Rubin & Roessler, 2007). During Colonial America, the first general hospital was established in Philadelphia in 1751 and by 1769, Dr. Benjamin Rush, a general surgeon, is considered to have implemented the beginning of what we know today as the rehabilitation team concept. Medical practices during early colonial times included restorative surgery, exercise, massage, and the use of heat, water, and bracing. Additionally, an emphasis was placed on the importance of pleasant surroundings, talking and listening, and consideration of the child as an individual with needs separate from adults (Neulicht & Berens, 2011). Although limited, this description might be considered somewhat analogous to being a RC across the lifespan today.

An historical look at the definition of RC finds that the occupation of "Vocational Advisor" (code 0-39.84), with an alternate title of "Vocational Counselor," first appeared in 1939 in the inaugural edition of the *Dictionary of Occupational Titles* (*DOT*), defined as one who:

> … advises students or others relative to the occupations for which they are best suited; confers with students to determine their aptitudes and plans for the future; studies occupations to keep in touch with employment trends; [and] advises students as to formal training needed (p. 997).

In contrast, the entry for "Counselor" in the 1939 edition of the *DOT* refers to "Lawyer." It is not until the 1965 revision of the *DOT* that there is an entry for "Counselor II" (code 045.108) with alternate titles of guidance counselor; vocational advisor; vocational counselor; counselor, college; and counselor, school, with definitions similar to various types of psychologists. While "Counsellor, Rehabilitation" (2399-114) and "Rehabilitation Specialist" (2399-110) are listed in the 1971 *Canadian Classification and Dictionary of Occupations* (Volume 2), the actual title of "Vocational Rehabilitation Counselor" does not appear in the *DOT* until 1977 (J. Truthan, personal communication, April 9, 2022).

The last (and most recent) definition of (code 045.107-042) "Vocational Rehabilitation Counselor" was updated in the *DOT* in 1981 and included:

> …counsels handicapped [sic] individuals to provide vocational rehabilitation services; interviewing and evaluating clients, conferring with medical and professional personnel and analyzing records to determine type and degree of disability, developing and assisting clients throughout the rehabilitation plan (or program), and aiding clients in outlining and obtaining appropriate medical and social services; may specialize in a particular type of disability (e.g., mental illness, alcohol abuse, hearing and visual impairment).
>
> (U.S. Department of Labor, 1991a, p. 52)

Although the *DOT* itself, as a foundational source for occupational information, has not been updated since 1991 (with no plans for future updates), the categorization and definition of RC has continued to evolve. It is noteworthy that the 1981 definition described above is overall consistent with the role of the RC in life care planning and is consistent with the general steps to develop a life care plan detailed later in this chapter. Indeed, it is perhaps meaningful to note that life care planning was first published in the literature approximately one year after the latest definition of RC was published in the *DOT* (Deutsch & Raffa, 1982).

Evolution of Rehabilitation Counselor

In an attempt to replace the *DOT* as well as expand and update available occupational information using an electronic database, the Occupational Information Network (O*NET, n.d.) was launched in 1998 under sponsorship of the U.S. Department of Labor/Employment and Training Administration (USDOL/ETA) through a grant to the North Carolina Employment Security Commission (Tippins & Hilton, 2010). The Bureau of Labor Statistics National Compensation Survey, funded by the Social Security Administration, is collecting new occupational data as part of its effort to develop an Occupational Information System to replace the *DOT* for disability purposes. The new Occupational Requirement System (ORS) data include cognitive/mental requirements, education/training/experience, environmental conditions, and physical demands (U.S. Bureau of Labor Statistics, 2022a). For the ORS *Handbook of Methods*, which is equivalent to the *Revised Handbook for Analyzing Jobs* (U.S. Department of Labor, 1991b) for the *DOT*, the reader is referred to www.bls.gov/opub/hom/ors/concepts.htm

As defined in the O*NET and ORS (using the Standard Occupational Classification/SOC) (U.S. Bureau of Labor Statistics, 2022b), RCs are those who:

> …counsel individuals to maximize the independence and employability of persons coping with personal, social, and vocational difficulties that result from birth defects, illness, disease, accidents, or the stress of daily life; coordinate activities for residents of care and treatment facilities; assess client needs and design and implement rehabilitation programs that may include personal and vocational counseling, training, and job placement.
>
> (https://www.onetonline.org/link/summary/21-1015.00)

Thus, the role of the RC has continued to evolve and expand, and RCs in today's workforce practice in varied settings that serve a wide range of individuals with disabilities and/or chronic medical conditions, as well as provide diverse types of service delivery. Such settings include, but are not limited to, private rehabilitation companies, government agencies including the Department of Veterans Affairs and Veterans Administration, self-employed practitioners, personal injury, health or disability insurance/managed care, hospitals, mental health centers, hospice or end of life care, litigation, rehabilitation centers (e.g., specialty centers of excellence such as the Shepherd Center in Atlanta, Georgia and Craig Hospital in Denver, Colorado), disability services at postsecondary education programs, and other educational institutions/schools. Specifically, the area of transition services for students with special needs to facilitate their transition from the K-12 school setting into adult activity (postsecondary education, integrated employment/supported employment, adult services, independent living, and/or community participation) has grown as an active area of employment for RCs due to the passage of the Workforce Innovation and Opportunity Act (WIOA) that was signed into law on July 22, 2014 (U.S. Bureau of Labor Statistics, 2014). While the topic of transition services is beyond the scope of this chapter, the reader is referred to Chapter 31 in this text for more information.

Contemporary Role of the Rehabilitation Counselor

Today, RCs are, once again, being called to expand what might be considered one of the initial roles of RCs in the early 1900s, to help veterans receive effective rehabilitation services and to facilitate their reintegration into society. According to Berens (2023), combat soldiers/veterans with physical or psychological war wounds who have returned from recent wars are seeking counseling services in greater numbers, and RCs are specially trained to provide the needed services. The goal of receiving effective treatment, reintegration into society, and productivity is still a valid outcome for today's veterans who are strongly motivated to be as independent as possible (Nichols & Martindale-Adams, 2020). These same goals are true today regarding long-term outcomes for veterans who received service-connected injuries, the greatest numbers being traumatic brain injuries resulting from blast injuries from bombs, grenades, land mines, missiles, and mortar/artillery shells (Traumatic Brain Injury Center of Excellence, 2022). The incidence of TBIs from recent wars has caused TBI/ABI to be commonly referred to as "the signature wound" of modern wars (Okie, 2006). A meta-analysis published by the U.S. Department of Defense (2021), which discusses evidence-based TBI mitigation efforts that have demonstrated the best clinical evidence in treatment of individuals with TBI, shows that rehabilitation as a "treatment" reflects the highest number of studies included in the meta-analysis, with pharmacology as the second highest, and behavioral health as the third highest (U.S. Department of Defense, 2021). Rehabilitation counselors are trained in at least two of these treatment areas, namely rehabilitation practices and behavioral health.

Rehabilitation Counselor Across the Lifespan

The Centers for Disease Control and Prevention (CDC) estimate that there are more than 61 million adults (26% of the total U.S. population) living in the United States with a disability (CDC, 2020), while the estimate of children with a disability living in the United States is 4.3% (U.S. Census Bureau, 2021). Given these numbers, it is clear to see that disability occurs across the lifespan and touches people of all ages. In responding to this reality, RCs are uniquely trained to work with evaluees (the individual with a disability or chronic medical condition), young and old, who have a disability and/or chronic health condition across the lifespan (Berens, 2023). As part of the continuum of care across the lifespan from childhood to adulthood, RCs provide a valuable service to children, adolescents, young adults, adults, and senior adults with disabilities in planning for their lifetime needs. Over the lifespan of individuals with disabilities, RCs are also working with senior adults, or those adults who choose to work past the normal age of retirement (age 67 years), or who establish "encore" careers. Given improvements in medicine, science, and technology, there has also been a corresponding improvement in the life expectancy of adults living in the United States such that adults are now living and working longer into old age (Berens, 2023). Medina, Sabo, and Vespa (2020) document that over the last four decades (approximately 1980–2020), life expectancy in the United States has generally risen among most, though not all, groups and by 2060 life expectancy for the total U.S. population is projected to increase to 85.6 years old. Although increases in life expectancy are projected to be larger for men than women, all racial and ethnic groups are projected to have longer life expectancies by 2060 (Medina et al., 2020). This trend parallels worldwide estimates by the World Health Organization (WHO) Global Health Observatory data that confirm the trend for longevity and verify that lifespans are getting longer (WHO, 2019). The WHO confirms that, globally, life expectancy has increased by more than six years between the years 2000 and 2019 (from 66.8 years in 2000 to 73.4 years in 2019). Based on these trends, adults are living longer than at any other point in history and, with that, older adults have distinct psychological and physical issues associated with aging of which the RC must be aware. Current estimates are that 85% of individuals over age 65 years have at least one chronic health condition and 60% have at least two chronic conditions (National Institute on Aging, 2017). With regard to older adults working longer, the CDC recognizes that workers who are older actually tend to experience fewer workplace injuries than their younger colleagues and that younger workers (19–34-year-olds) with chronic medical conditions have significantly higher medical costs than medical costs for older workers aged 65–74 years (CDC, 2015).

By examining the role of the RC in life care planning over the lifespan, the benefits of providing rehabilitation counseling services not only to the evaluee (the individual with a disability or chronic medical condition), but also to the individual's family and/or those persons significant to the individual are important components to the role of the RC. Additionally, prevocational and vocational recommendations, including applicable avocational and non-remunerative recommendations, fall within the role of the RC. Further, the development and implementation of transition plans or habilitation/rehabilitation plans are also within the scope of the RC as are opinions regarding wage loss and earnings capacity, all of which fall within the role of a qualified RC in life care planning.

What is a Rehabilitation Counselor?

From an historical perspective, Szymanski (1985) defines rehabilitation counseling as "a profession that assists individuals with disabilities in adapting to the environment, assists the environments in accommodating the needs of the individual, and works toward full participation of persons with disabilities in all aspects of society, especially work" (p. 3). Maki (1986) further defines rehabilitation counseling as an individualized holistic process that is comprehensive in scope and prescriptive in nature and serves to develop or restore one's capacities with a goal of attaining functional independence. Mertes and Harden (2019) state that RCs are uniquely trained "to understand how disabilities affect an individual's vocational and psychosocial life" (p. 41). The above definitions are consistent with the Commission on Rehabilitation Counselor Certification (CRCC) definition of RC as:

> …the only professional counselors educated and trained at the graduate-level who possess the specialized knowledge, skills, and attitudes to work collaboratively with individuals with disabilities. Through a comprehensive unique counseling process, rehabilitation counselors help individuals with disabilities achieve their personal, social, psychological, career, and independent living goals. Rehabilitation counselors are the bridge between the individual and self-sufficiency, helping their clients live fully integrated lives.
>
> (CRCC, 2022a, para 2)

Further, the CRCC defines the practice of rehabilitation counseling as:

> …a systematic process that assists persons with physical, mental, developmental, cognitive, and emotional disabilities to achieve their personal, career, and independent living goals in the most integrated setting possible through the application of the counseling process. The counseling process involves communication, goal setting, and beneficial growth or change through self-advocacy, psychological, vocational, social, and behavioral interventions.
>
> (CRCC, 2022c, para 1)

Philosophical tenets that form the foundation for rehabilitation counseling include a fundamental belief in the worth and dignity of each individual (Maki et al., 1978), consumer choice, empowerment, informed consent, integration, as well as the right of an individual to contribute to society in a citizen capacity. Inherent in these rights is the assessment of risk and the need for ethical decision-making on the part of the RC that is consistent with the rights and best interests of the individual with a disability being served.

Scope of Practice of Rehabilitation Counselor

The qualified RC is a professional trained to engage in a systematic process when evaluating individuals with disabilities and providing services (Neulicht & Costantini, 2002). Such services include assessing evaluee needs, developing a plan to meet identified needs, and coordinating not only vocational and avocational, but medical and rehabilitative services over an evaluee's lifespan that facilitate achievement of the evaluee's optimal level of independence and/or productivity in an effort to restore them to as close to pre-injury/incident status as possible. As Mertes and Harden explain:

> …just like 'doctor' is a general term for a specific type of doctor, such as a physiatrist, a rehabilitation counselor may be named based on a specialty area with titles such as vocational expert, vocational consultant, rehabilitation case manager, forensic vocational counselor, rehabilitation specialist and/or vocational placement specialist.
> (Mertes & Harden, 2019, p. 40)

The Scope of Practice Statement for RCs, as defined by the CRCC, outlines specific activities in which RCs are trained and for which they can make recommendations for the life care plan:

- Assessment and appraisal
- Diagnosis and treatment planning
- Career (vocational) counseling
- Individual and group counseling; treatment interventions focused on facilitating adjustments to the medical and psychological impact of disability
- Case management, referral, and service coordination (Author note: Life care planning falls under this activity)
- Program evaluation and research
- Interventions to remove environmental, employment, and attitudinal barriers
- Consultation services among multiple parties and regulatory systems
- Job analysis, job development, and placement services, including assistance with employment and job accommodations
- Consultation about and access to rehabilitation technology

(CRCC, 2022d, para 2).

The scope of practice for RCs can be compared to the core competencies of VEs, as defined by the American Board of Vocational Experts (ABVE), which include life care planning and life care planning related competencies:

- Vocational assessment (forensic vocational reporting, medical/functional aspects of disability, forensic vocational rehabilitation tools, psychometric evaluation)
- Forensic vocational practice venues and systems (disability systems, legal system, civil litigation, life care planning)
- Professional standards/practice (clinical judgment, research and statistics, professional standards and ethical issues)

(ABVE, 2022a, paras 1–3).

A section on the scope of practice for RCs would also be relevant to include standards related to the education of RCs that outline specialty educational and competency requirements of RC training programs. In 2019, the Council for the Accreditation of Counseling and Related Educational Programs (CACREP), the accreditation body for RC education programs, appointed a standards revision committee to examine the existing 2016 CACREP standards with the potential for revision. The committee was charged with, among other tasks, examining how to infuse disability concepts into the eight core curricular areas established by CACREP (CACREP, 2022, para 4). The CACREP Board adopted the 2024 CACREP Standards at its February 2023 meeting and the new Standards go into effect July 1, 2024.

Credentialing for Rehabilitation Counselors

Rehabilitation counselors can be credentialed in a number of areas, most notably Certified Rehabilitation Counselor (CRC) and its Canadian equivalent, Canadian Certified Rehabilitation Counselor, Certified Vocational Evaluation Specialist, College of Vocational Rehabilitation Professionals (CVRP), and ABVE. The authors note that although the Canadian CRC credential was discontinued in 2007, Canadian CRCs who were certified prior to 2007 and who desire to maintain their credential can continue to renew it through obtaining the requisite continuing education credits (CRCC, 2022b, para 16).

While this section will provide a brief overview of the above RC credentials with corresponding websites to view for more information, the reader is strongly encouraged to thoroughly research the history and requirements of any credential, confirm the credential is founded upon published role and function research studies, and scrutinize the validity of any credential in which they are interested.

Certified Rehabilitation Counselor (CRC)

The CRCC established the first credentialing process in the U.S. in 1974 with the mission to certify RCs in the United States (and later Canada) (CRCC, 2022b, para 4, 10). To become certified, RCs must demonstrate knowledge by passing a board certification examination in 12 knowledge domains areas (CRCC, 2022e, para 1). Recognizing that the functions of a RC overlap with the functions of a life care planner in multiple areas, one of the 12 knowledge domains requires that RCs "understand and facilitate life care planning and life care planning services" as a knowledge domain that underlies rehabilitation counseling (CRCC, 2022e, para 12). The reader is referred to the CRCC website for more information, https://crccertification.com/about-crcc/

Certified Vocational Evaluation Specialist

The CRCC also provides a national board certification examination to certify vocational evaluators (CVEs). Similar to other specialty practice areas, CVEs possess "unique, comprehensive, and holistic proficiencies, education, and insights in rehabilitation counseling, evaluation, and career assessment services … and serve individuals in need of rehabilitation services addressing personal, social, and vocational goals" (CRCC, 2022f, para 1). Additionally, the Code of Professional Ethics for Vocational Evaluation Specialists, Work Adjustment Specialists, and Career Assessment Associates (CRCC, 2009) emphasizes that CVEs use a holistic approach to assist individuals in the identification of vocational goals and recommendations as well as the transition to and attainment of vocational goals. CVEs provide, utilize, and/or incorporate vocational information and services in order to measure, observe, and document an individual's interests, values, temperaments, work-related behaviors, aptitudes, skills, physical capacities, learning style, training needs, and employment needs (CRCC, 2009). The reader is referred to the CRCC website for more information on the CVE credential, https://crccertification.com/cve-get-certified/

College of Vocational Rehabilitation Professionals (CVRP)

The CVRP was developed by and for Canadian rehabilitation practitioners and is headquartered in Ontario, Canada; however, the credential is available to practitioners internationally. The CVRP defines a VR professional as one who assesses, evaluates, and identifies persons who are experiencing, or are at risk of experiencing, a vocational disability or disadvantage, and who seek to develop and execute vocational rehabilitation and return to work (RTW) plans designed to achieve or restore optimum vocational and avocational outcomes through the application of knowledge, skills, interventions, and strategies that are unique to the discipline and the vocational rehabilitation (VR) profession (CVRP, 2022a, para 4). According to the CVRP Scope of Practice statement, CVRPs assist individuals to access, maintain, or return to vocational and/or avocational activities, and to determine and facilitate access to any vocational rehabilitation and/or support services needed to achieve the individual's desired goals (CVRP, 2022b, para 1). The reader is referred to the CVRP website for more information, https://cvrp.net/about-us/?lang=usa

American Board of Vocational Experts (ABVE)

Many RCs also are certified through the ABVE. The ABVE promotes competence in forensic vocational evaluation, testimony and psychometric assessments and requires specific knowledge or (sic) vocational assessment, functional capacity measures, psychological tests and measurement, job analysis, job placement, and job surveys (ABVE, 2022a, para 1). As defined by the ABVE *Code of Ethics* (2020), VEs are primarily committed to determining the vocational capacities of individuals taking into consideration the age, education, previous work experience, earnings record, mental and physical status of the person with the disability as well as test data and the expert's own vocational experience in order to provide a vocational opinion. Further, VEs may be called upon to provide psychological, vocational, and rehabilitation testimony that may include information concerning vocational testing, vocational exploration, job placement, and job development in addition to evaluation of social, medical, vocational, and psychological data, as well as economic information (ABVE, 2020). The reader is referred to the ABVE website for more information, https://abve.net/

While other certifications exist (e.g., certified disability management specialist/CDMS), a certificant's background (e.g., registered nurse, certified case manager) does not necessarily provide someone with the specialized training, education, knowledge, or experience to be qualified as a RC. Qualified RCs usually belong to several professional associations (e.g., International Association of Rehabilitation Professionals, National Rehabilitation Counseling Association, and American Rehabilitation Counseling Association) and many also belong to organizations that focus on specific disabilities (e.g., National Spinal Cord Injury Association, the Brain Injury Association, American Burn Association) or organizations specific to life care planning (e.g., International Academy of Life Care Planners).

In addition to the RC and VE credentials described in this chapter, some workers' compensation laws or policies provide guidelines as to the qualification of rehabilitation providers working within the workers' compensation jurisdiction of the particular state. These guidelines generally address education, work experience, licensure, and certification requirements for RCs and other rehabilitation providers in order to provide rehabilitation services in the particular state. Additionally, many RCs, trained as professional counselors with specialized knowledge in rehabilitation and disability practices seek licensure as a mental health counselor with designations such as Licensed Professional Counselor (LPC), Licensed Clinical Mental Health Counselor (LCMHC), Licensed Clinical Professional Counselor (LCPC), and Licensed Mental Health Counselor (LMHC). Counseling licensure is now available in all U.S. states, and at least four states have rehabilitation counseling specific licensing aside from the state's licensure for professional counselors (e.g., Licensed Rehabilitation Counselor/LRC in the State of Louisiana). Given that requirements for licensure are regulated at the state level, the reader is referred to www.counseling.org/knowledge-center/licensure-requirements and https://crccertification.com/advocacy-and-legislation/state-licensure-boards for state-by-state counseling licensure requirements.

Rehabilitation Counselors in Life Care Planning

As described above, RCs who work within the life care planning arena generally hold one or more national certifications in the field of rehabilitation, are professionals who have a minimum of a master's degree in rehabilitation counseling or a related discipline, and have extensive training and experience in the areas of evaluation and assessment, catastrophic case management, transferable work skills, earnings capacity analysis, and job placement (Weed & Field, 2012). Related to life care planning, RCs may perform one or more roles within the life care planning context depending on the referral request and/or the RC's individual scope of practice. These roles commonly include:

- Vocational expert (VE): Specific vocationally-focused assessment, analysis of wage loss, loss of earnings capacity opinion (with consideration of non-remunerative work, and lifespan issues/encore careers as appropriate).
- Life care planner: Rehabilitation counseling expertise used for comprehensive needs assessment, independent living options, adaptive devices/assistive technology, disability accommodations, case management needs, vocational/educational assessment, and overall long-term care planning.
- Vocational expert and life care planner (if dually qualified): Uses skills within both areas. See above for descriptions.
- Clinician/Case Manager: Implements life care plan (if dually qualified).
- Other aspects of rehabilitation counseling/service delivery that are within an individual's scope of practice based on the individual's education, training, and experience. Also see below for CRC scope of practice.

The roles and specialization of RCs in life care planning have evolved since the early 1980s (Deutsch & Sawyer, 1985, 2003), and employment opportunities in forensic rehabilitation is perhaps the fastest growing area for RCs in the current labor market. As cited in Peterson (2022), there is an increasing need for RCs to provide forensic vocational rehabilitation services in workers' compensation cases, personal injury cases, and Social Security Administration disability determination appeal hearings (Robinson, 2014). While the importance of using evidence-based practices is applicable for RCs who provide services in public or private rehabilitation settings, Barros-Bailey (2018) emphasizes that RCs in private forensic rehabilitation settings must use evidence-based practices especially with regard to opinions and testimony concerning assessment of vocational losses, future vocational capacities, and potential interventions for individuals who have acquired disability conditions throughout their lifespan and that the evidence is either primary (what the RC collects) or secondary (what someone else collected or exists, which they review). It is important to recognize that recommendations for vocational rehabilitation (VR) services (e.g., evaluation and ongoing service delivery) are included in several clinical practice guidelines as part of the care recommendations related to specific medical diagnoses or conditions. For example guidelines, the reader is referred to the list of Clinical Practice Guidelines by Select Diagnostic Groups that Contain VR Recommendations at the end of the chapter. Additionally, a checklist for selecting a RC in life care planning is provided in Table 11.1.

Rehabilitation Counseling Worldwide

Establishing the International Classification of Functioning (ICF) Core for Vocational Rehabilitation

In an effort to provide a universal or worldwide description of functioning for individuals who participate in VR services, as well as to standardize the provision of rehabilitation services globally, the WHO collaborated with other partners on a project to develop an ICF-based Core Set (2017) to describe the functioning and health of individuals who participate in multidisciplinary VR (ICF, 2017; Momsen et al., 2019). The outcome of the project resulted in development of 90 ICF categories identified as "core considerations" for conducting a comprehensive, multidisciplinary assessment of individuals participating in multidisciplinary VR (ICF, 2017). Of the 90 core categories, 13 ICF categories were selected to comprise the Brief ICF Core for VR (ICF, 2017). The intent of the ICF Core Sets is to serve as a worldwide guide on measures to help clinicians and researchers implement optimal rehabilitation programs for individuals of working age with limited or restricted work participation due to disease, injury, or health-related events. In addition, the core sets are intended to cover a broad spectrum of health conditions and types of job (ICF, 2017). For more information on what comprises the comprehensive categories and brief core categories for VR services, the reader is referred to www.icf-research-branch.org/icf-core-sets-projects2/diverse-situations/icf-core-sets-for-vocational-rehabilitation

Rehabilitation Counselor as a Team Member

As emphasized by Mertes and Harden (2019), RCs serve as instrumental members of the rehabilitation team to coordinate assessments to measure a person's aptitude, achievement levels, transferable work skills, as well as potential for independent living. Rehabilitation counselors must be knowledgeable and stay within their scope of practice as well as accepted standards and guidelines of the particular jurisdiction for which they are preparing the life care plan (e.g., workers' compensation, long-term disability, personal injury). For example, within the personal injury arena, a RC's role is to determine if the evaluee has the potential to work/live independently and to what degree. The RC's role is to also provide information on the cost of expected future needs to identify damages associated with the injury or disability. Regardless of the specific jurisdiction, RCs in life care planning must be able to determine first if an evaluee can work and, if so, what work (remunerative and/or non-remunerative) is viable. This determination would include providing information on not only the types of vocational activity an evaluee can be expected to perform, but also the cost, frequency, and duration or replacement of any training or assistance (such as job coach, vocational counseling, rehabilitation technology, modified or custom-designed workstation, supported employment, tuition/books, or other specialized education programs) that may be required to

Table 11.1 Checklist for Selecting a Rehabilitation Counselor in Life Care Planning

Qualifications
Education, including degrees and continuing education, from accredited universities
Certifications or licenses (e.g., CLCP™, CRC, CVE, ABVE, CVRP, LPC, LRC, other)
Experience: work, life care planning, research
Industry experience
Specialization in working with individuals within a particular disability or age group (e.g., pediatrics)
Special education and/or early intervention experience (if pediatric evaluee)
Case management experience (e.g., care coordination, transition planning)
Vocational rehabilitation experience (e.g., state VR program, Workers' Compensation or Federal Office of Workers' Compensation programs, Jones Act, Federal Employees Liability Act (FELA), short- and long-term disability)
Testimony experience (e.g., Social Security, personal injury)
Commitment to the profession
Active membership in professional and/or disability specific organizations
Participation in professional development activities
Contribution of time and effort by volunteering, speaking, holding office in professional organizations, writing articles, chapters, or books
Recipient of awards, honors, or other forms of peer recognition
Standard procedures and methodology for life care planning
Awareness of and familiarity with life care planning across the lifespan, including procedures, processes, resources, references, and specific training
Follows peer-reviewed methodologies and standards of practice
Uses peer-reviewed and published checklists and forms
Foundation for opinions established (e.g., medical/treatment provider opinions, consulting specialist opinions, clinical practice guidelines, medical records)
Consultation with healthcare team to obtain information and identify needs (e.g., physician, physical therapist, occupational therapist, speech-language pathologist, audiologist, neuropsychologist, school personnel)
Other considerations
Possesses effective communication skills
Experience preparing life care plans
Current résumé or CV
No ethics complaints or arrests
Billing for services (e.g., different rates for deposition and/or trial testimony?)
Forensic experience testifying in the past 4 years; defense/plaintiff referral ratio
Knowledge of guidelines pertaining to experts (e.g., hearsay rules, collateral source rules)

Adapted from Weed, R. O. (2018). Checklist for selecting a life care planner. In *Life care planning and case management handbook* (4th ed.). Weed, R. O. & Berens, D. E. (Eds.). Routledge.

reach the goal (Weed & Riddick, 1992). Depending on the type of disability, the RC works with a variety of medical and allied health professionals in determining an individual's potential and providing information for the life care plan. Table 11.2 outlines primary life care planning questions regarding vocational needs that the qualified RC should be able to answer.

As with other disciplines that develop life care plans, a RC must rely on an evaluee's treatment team for recommendations outside their professional scope of practice. Professionals such as physicians and medical specialists, physical therapists, occupational therapists, speech/language pathologists,

Table 11.2 Life Care Planning Questions Regarding Vocational Needs

Are all applicable records available for review? Medical/treatment records? Depositions of the evaluee, family, consulting experts, and/or treatment team? School records including standardized test scores (if applicable)? Vocational and employment records (if applicable)? Job/Performance evaluations? Union records (if applicable)? Training history? Tax returns?
Have vocational aspects been considered or already underway (e.g., already initiated by family, referral source, other)?
Do the records indicate (and does the RC address) whether the evaluee is at his or her optimum level of functioning (e.g., maximum medical improvement)?
Is documentation of physical, psychological, and/or cognitive restrictions or limitations, especially relevant to determining vocational options, available? Are other members of the evaluee's team (e.g., physicians, therapeutic team members, school personnel) involved? If applicable, have pre-injury schoolteachers and/or employers been contacted? Have objective and relevant questions been asked to obtain the necessary information regarding function, prognosis, and limitations/restrictions (e.g., functional capacity evaluation/FCE)?
Has a personal interview been conducted with the evaluee/family, when allowed? Has one been requested? If not allowed, has the request (and denial) been documented?
Does the interview follow a standardized format? Does the interview address essential areas to be considered in evaluating vocational potential (e.g., medical history, treatment providers, medication intake, sleeping patterns, self-reported physical tolerances, interests, values, educational and employment background/history, specific vocational preparation, work skills, social, cultural, environmental, economic and psychosocial factors, functional capacity, functional abilities based on *DOT*, O*NET, ORS and/or Department of Labor definitions)?
What hobbies, avocational, and/or leisure/recreational activities did the evaluee participate in prior to the incident/injury (typically does not apply to birth-related injuries or conditions)? School sports? Organized sports (e.g., Little League baseball, travel or club sports, soccer, basketball, karate, tennis, swimming, gymnastics, football, other sports activities)? Music-related activities (e.g., piano, drums, guitar, school chorus, church choir)? Dance? Robotics? Coding? Other?
Are appropriate referral recommendations made to solicit additional information as needed (e.g., neuropsychological/psychological assessment, vocational evaluation/situational assessment, functional capacity evaluation/FCE)?
Does the evaluee need testing before determining vocational potential (e.g., vocational evaluation, psychological, neuropsychological, or functional capacity evaluation/FCE)? If testing is performed, is the evaluator credentialed and qualified in the area of testing? Are appropriate tests utilized to provide the needed information? In what manner does the RC integrate test results into assessment opinions? (For example, are results of interest tests appropriately used to indicate the evaluee's ability to perform in the area of interest?) Is the evaluation a quality and valid appraisal?

(Continued)

Table 11.2 (Continued) Life Care Planning Questions Regarding Vocational Needs

Are test modifications/deviations from standardized testing protocols utilized when necessary, and results appropriately interpreted? Are the test results meaningful?
If work or vocational potential is relevant, should the vocational plan be justified by performing labor market research? If so, what method is to be used (e.g., employer sampling/direct contact with employers, statistics/databases, computer program, industry publications)?
If a market appears to exist for the evaluee's labor, is there a need for a job analysis to provide objective data? If a job analysis was completed, was it done according to the Americans with Disabilities Amendments Act of 2008?
What is the evaluee's expected income including benefits? In cases of personal injury litigation, is pre- vs. post-injury capacity included?
Are there expenses or estimated costs for the vocational plan? *See Note below.
Therapeutic modalities (e.g., speech, physical, occupational, recreational, visual, other)?
Vocational counseling/career guidance? If so, are the initiation/suspension dates included? Frequency/cost? (e.g., 30 hrs. over 6 months at $100 to $150/hr)
If job placement assistance, job coaching, and/or supported employment is required, what are the expected costs?
If training or education is required, what are the expected costs for tuition or training, books, supplies? Include dates for expected costs (e.g., career technical education, 2 years @ $8,000/yr. for 2023–2025)
If rehabilitation or assistive technology, accommodations, or aides are required, what are the costs for work, education, and/or training (e.g., specialized computer/printer, adapted workstation, tools, specialized software, attendant care, transportation), include initial charges and replacement schedules as applicable)
*Note: If the evaluee does not have vocational potential or the expected ability to work for pay or remuneration, the RC's role is to make appropriate recommendations and costs for services to enhance the evaluee's avocational participation, including recommendations for their community integration and involvement, as applicable.
What effect, if any, does the injury have on work life expectancy (e.g., delayed entry into workforce, less than full-time work, earlier retirement, expected increased turnover or time off work for medical follow-up or treatment, consideration of lifespan with pre- and post-productive activity past the traditional "retirement age")?

Sources: Adapted from R. O. Weed, Ph.D. (Berens & Weed, 2018; Neulicht & Berens, 2004, 2011; Riddick-Grisham, 2011); Berens, D. E., & Weed, R. O., Life care planning questions regarding vocational needs. In Weed, R. O. & Berens, D. E. (Eds.). (2018). Life care planning and case management handbook (4th ed), 57. Routledge; Neulicht, A. T., & Berens, D. E. (2004, 2011). The role of the vocational consultant. In S. Riddick-Grisham (Ed.). (2004). Pediatric life care planning and case management. CRC Press. With permission.

recreation therapists, nurses, psychologists, neuropsychologists, audiologists, counselors or other mental health professionals, and, in the case of school-age evaluees, school personnel, all have a potential role in working with the RC to provide information for the life care plan. For evaluees for whom a nurse or other professional may be the primary author of the life care plan, the RC must work in conjunction with them to gather and disseminate vocationally-relevant information. It is the responsibility of the RC to collaborate with the team to establish a medical or psychological foundation to support an evaluee's work and independent living opinions.

Rehabilitation Counselor Involvement Across the Lifespan

The needs of a child with a disability are not a smaller or scaled-down version of the needs of an adult with a disability who has sustained impairments that impact work and/or activities of daily living (ADLs). Instead, factors unique to working with children with a disability must be considered. Factors that address pediatric emotional, social, familial, educational, and prevocational needs require qualified professionals and programs that are appropriate and responsive to ages and stages of development. Traditional rehabilitation models historically have not placed much emphasis on rehabilitating children with disabilities; rather, that was left up to the healthcare providers involved in the child's care. These providers typically followed a medical model of treating acute illnesses/complications as they presented rather than preventing complications from occurring or providing services to ameliorate or lessen the impact of the disability, especially in the long term (Neulicht & Berens, 2011).

As recent as the 1960s and 1970s, children with disabilities were either cared for at home with little support and services or were placed in institutional settings with little expectation for improvement in either medical status or functional abilities, not to mention community integration. In the 1980s, with the advent of life care planning as a case management tool and the continuing deinstitutionalization/independent living movement, the value of pediatric case management and life care planning became more apparent. Furthermore, advances in medical technology as well as better prenatal and neonatal healthcare created the opportunity for infants and children who previously did not survive disabling medical conditions, illnesses, or injury to be effectively treated and often discharged home to the community under the care of their parents, family, or other caregivers. Through assessment, collaboration, planning with the family and other members of the healthcare team, teaching, counseling, supportive interventions, ongoing evaluation of care, and identification of costs associated with recommended care, pediatric case managers and life care planners provide a valuable service to children with disabilities (Deutsch & Sawyer, 2005; Hillis et al., 2016; Neulicht & Berens, 2011).

Beyond certifications, the qualified RC providing pediatric life care planning services must have a firm foundation and specific knowledge of service delivery and coordination issues pertinent to each developmental stage (i.e., from birth to young adulthood). In assessing evaluees and forming opinions, the RC follows a standard methodology for life care plan development and/or earnings capacity assessment that begins with the information-gathering process. This process includes a review of medical and related records, an initial interview with and observation of the child and family or caregiver, and consultation with the pediatric healthcare team (e.g., physicians and allied health professionals, including pediatric neuropsychologist, if applicable), as well as school service providers (e.g., early intervention providers, special education coordinator/teacher, therapists, guidance counselors, school administrators). The technical aspects of VR and life care planning for children vary from the planning used for adults such that pediatric planning is based on the unique needs of the child (as opposed to those of an adult) and the setting in which services are provided. However, the essential elements of rehabilitation counseling are constant and consistent with the RC scope of practice that includes conducting a needs assessment, assisting the evaluee/family in developing goals, developing a plan to achieve the goals, and coordinating therapeutic and medical services and/or interventions to meet those needs, including recommended follow-up services throughout the evaluee's lifetime (CRCC, 2022c).

The role of the RC in pediatric life care planning is unique and differs from that of a medical or nurse consultant in that the RC is specially trained to identify and address disability related as well as vocational issues relevant to the child's future. Obviously, due to age factors, the RC may not be able to rely on a child's past work history or, in cases of a very young child, delineation of aptitudes or academic achievement. While issues related to loss of employment options, loss of choice in selecting a job, wage loss, and earnings capacity analysis for pediatric cases must be adapted from a traditional transferable skills analysis approach that is used for adult evaluations, the RC must still follow a standard methodology.

When conducting a pediatric rehabilitation evaluation, the RC obtains standard interview data and will want to focus particularly on the following information as related to the child evaluee:

- Child's level of education, including attainment of developmental milestones (for the toddler or young child), preschool or nursery school records, church school records, elementary school records, etc.
- Family characteristics and trends/patterns (including parents, siblings, grandparents, aunts, and uncles, and/or whomever the child defines as being "family" as well as those that provide the most influential impact on the child's development)
- Family attitudes toward and emphasis on learning, education, and work
- Environmental influences
- Psychosocial and socioeconomic factors
- Standardized test data of the child (and parents and siblings, if appropriate)
- Statistical information (e.g., compiled by the U.S. Census Bureau, U.S. Bureau of Labor Statistics, U.S., state departments of labor, and other sources for data on educational attainment/labor force participation)

Using these and other relevant data, the RC is then able to determine the child's educational and vocational development options. Appropriate vocational and avocational alternatives are based upon interview information and labor market data with consideration of issues such as:

- Which of the child's pre-injury developmental options remains feasible?
- Impact of the disability in performance of job-specific tasks?
- Residual functional limitations and vocational handicaps as a result of injury/illness?
- Like or similar occupational groups appropriate to the child's capabilities?
- Range of specific job alternatives appropriate to the child's capabilities?

Rehabilitation Counselor and Pediatric Life Care Planning

Pediatric case management, as with adult case management, is most effective when it begins soon after a child acquires a disability (Weed & Field, 2012). In instances of prenatal injury to the child or expected neurodevelopmental disease, case management may begin antepartum (prior to birth) in an effort to prepare the family and the treatment providers and to provide the best possible intervention not only from time of delivery forward but also *in vitro*, where possible. In pediatric life care planning, the RC must determine first if the child has the expected capacity to work when they reach working age and, if so, what work the child will likely be capable of performing. This determination includes providing information not only on the types of vocational or avocational activity a child can be expected to perform as an adult but also the cost, frequency, and duration, or replacement of any training or assistance (e.g., job coaching, vocational counseling, rehabilitation technology, modified or custom-designed workstation, supported employment, tuition and books, or other specialized education programs) that may be required to reach the child's goals (Weed & Riddick, 1992).

The pediatric life care planner with expertise as a RC must account for services and recommendations appropriate to the child's needs to properly manage the child's disability, reduce or prevent potential problems, and plan for a vocation or independent living as an adult. The following list is an adaptation from one contained in *A Guide to Rehabilitation* (pp. 7C-52–7C-53) and includes some of the more critical factors to consider when evaluating a child or adolescent (Deutsch & Sawyer, 2005). Although originally written for children with acquired brain injury, the authors have adapted the list to apply to children with other catastrophic and permanently disabling conditions:

- Degree of interaction with the environment and with family and caregivers
- Ability to grow in relation to chronological age and reach developmental milestones
- Ability to take food/nourishment by mouth vs. reliance on tube feedings
- Ability to move one's body voluntarily and purposefully to crawl, walk, reach, etc.
- Occurrence of uncontrolled or unmanageable seizures
- Other factors, such as existence of cardiac problems, upper respiratory or pulmonary problems, aspiration or choking, swallowing difficulties, contractures, or spasticity
- Ability for education and potential for learning, allowing for necessary modifications and accommodations

The following list, also adapted from *A Guide to Rehabilitation*, includes discussion of preventive services designed to effectively prevent and/or reduce complications considered in the development of life care planning recommendations for children with disabilities (Deutsch & Sawyer, 2005):

- Utilization of educational and behavioral support programs to work with the child as well as provide family education, support, and resource
- Provision of appropriate medical care and support to provide intervention and prevention services
- Integration of physical, occupational, and speech therapy to provide ongoing therapeutic intervention as part of the child's daily routine
- Application of stimulating environments and interaction with other children to provide peer and social interaction, appropriate behavior modeling, and support to encourage the child or young adult to reach the highest level of cognitive, social, behavioral, emotional, motoric, and vocational development

For the RC working with a child with a disability, it is important to recognize the demands required of typical stages of development for a child. Hamilton and Vessey (1992) suggest five distinct developmental stages within childhood that have an influence on the delivery of case management and life care planning services:

- *Newborn and early childhood stages* (*first two stages*): Parents or guardians are the primary caregivers and decision-makers. Focus of planning for infants is caregiver education directed toward management of the infant's condition
- *Preschool stage*: Planning is affected by developmental themes of affective, cognitive, and physical growth in areas such as toilet training, safety and injury prevention, sibling rivalry, caregiver separation, and developmental delay
- *School age*: Planning is focused on the child's needs as they become more active in self-care and medical planning (to the extent possible)
- *Adolescence*: Continuation of school-age stage with goal of assisting the teenager in greater independence and self-care in preparation for adulthood. The extent of an adolescent's participation can be affected by the person's maturity level, family emotional responses, and severity of diagnosis, among others

Table 11.3 Three Stages in the Occupational Choice Process

Period	Age	Characteristics
Fantasy	Childhood (before 11 years)	Play gradually becomes work oriented
Tentative	Early adolescence (11–17 years)	Transition to recognition of work requirements/rewards, awareness of interests, abilities, values, and responsibilities accompanying a career choice
Realistic	Middle adolescence (17 years to young adult)	Further values development, integration of interests and abilities, identification of specific occupational choices, commitment to a specific career

Source: Adapted from Zunker, V. G. (2006). Theories of career development, In Career counseling: A holistic approach (7th ed). Thomson Brooks/Cole. With permission.

In addition, Super (1972) focused on the development of self-concept and formalized vocational development stages:

Table 11.4 Development of Self-Concept and Formalized Vocational Development Stages

Period	Age	Characteristics
Growth	Birth to 14 or 15 years	Development of capacity, attitudes, interest, and needs
Exploratory	15–24 years	Tentative phase in which choices are narrowed but not finalized
Establishment	25–44 years	Trial and stabilization through work experiences
Maintenance	45–64 years	Continual adjustment process to improve working position and situation
Decline	65+ years	Pre-retirement considerations and eventual retirement

As discussed in Zunker (2006), occupational choice may also be viewed from a developmental standpoint. Ginzberg et al. (1951) describe three stages in the occupational choice process shown in Table 11.3.

Further, as cited in Zunker (2006), Super (1972) also outlines career patterns for men and women as well as the cycling/recycling of developmental tasks through the lifespan. By using a life-stage model, Super illustrates a "life rainbow" and "archway" that highlights the various roles and the interdependency/interactions of roles for a "full" life. Vocational considerations over the lifespan also include issues such as image norms (Giannantonio & Hurley-Hanson, 2006), age and work-related motives (Kooig et. al, 2011), work values (Jin & Rounds, 2012), stereotypes (Ng & Feldman, 2012), personality (Woods et al. 2013), and career commitment (Katz et al., 2019).

While a disability may impact the rate at which a child moves through their developmental stages (and delays or prevents attainment of certain tasks), the facilitation of typical developmental tasks and roles must be encouraged. Failure on the part of the RC to acknowledge the child's developmental stages and appropriately plan for necessary services at each stage will have consequences that could negatively impact the child's ability to achieve their optimal level of

Super et al. (1963) also identify developmental tasks associated with each stage. For example, *during the growth and exploratory stages, tasks include*:

Table 11.5 Developmental Tasks

Task	Ages	General Characteristics
Crystallization	14–18 years	Cognitive process of developing vocational goals through exposure to resources, contingencies, interests, values, and planning
Specification	18–21 years	Progression from a tentative vocational preference to a specific goal
Implementation	21–24 years	Period in which training toward a vocational goal is completed and employment begins

Source: Adapted from Zunker, V. G. (2006). Theories of career development, In Career counseling: A holistic approach (7th ed.). Thomson Brooks/Cole. With permission.

independence and productivity as well as fail to prevent or reduce future complications from occurring. The reader is referred to Taveira et al. (2016) for a literature review using an ecological perspective as a framework for children's career development, Schiariti et al. (2021) for an intervention framework of child-environment interactions to optimize function, Bronfenbrenner (1977) as a foundational source of the experimental ecology of human development, and Curry and Milsom (2022) for in-depth coverage of career and college readiness counseling (e.g., assessment, diversity/cultural considerations, legal/ethical/collaboration issues as well as developmental/theoretical overview, curriculum, targeted interventions, developmental tasks, sample activities and case studies by grade/developmental levels). Using visual models such as a career genogram may also be helpful for detailing family educational/occupational history and career influences. One example of a genogram that can be used by RCs and focuses on an evaluee's family's education, career choices, and values is developed by the University of Chicago's Network for College Success (n.d.), https://ncs.uchicago.edu/sites/ncs.uchicago.edu/files/uploads/tools/NCS_PS_Toolkit_ESF_Set_A_GenogramLessonPlan.pdf. The genogram can help evaluees (and RCs) understand the influence that the evaluee's family's education, career choices, and values can have on their postsecondary and career decisions. To be most effective, career genograms used for purposes of vocational rehabilitation counseling should focus on those individuals that are closest (emotionally, physically, familially, socially) and/or serve as a role model to the evaluee as opposed to distant relatives or relatives that do not live with, near, or have a connection with the evaluee.

Tasks of the Rehabilitation Counselor in Life Care Planning

Interview Process

At the time of referral for services, the RC must obtain information from the referral source as to how the RC can gain access to the child, parents, and/or guardian to conduct the interview and obtain necessary information. The intake interview for pediatric evaluees is typically conducted in the child's home or place of residence, with their parents or guardians serving as primary historians.

As part of lifespan considerations, depending on the child's age and capabilities, the RC will want to spend time during the interview observing the child (for children too young or too impaired to actively participate in the interview), and/or interact with the child to obtain their view of things, interact and engage with them, and to encourage them to take as active a role in their future care planning as appropriate. For older adolescents and young adults, the RC will want to assess the evaluee's ability to perform their ADLs and instrumental activities of daily living to gain an appreciation of how functional the evaluee is at home and how independent they are with their personal needs and daily activities. The RC also will want to inquire about additional activities appropriate for the evaluee's age, including the ability to drive (pre- and post-injury), transition from school to independent living, vocational and/or avocational or productive activity as an adult. For adult evaluees, the RC will obtain information regarding the evaluee's past education and work history, including identification of their transferable skills, with a goal of determining their post-incident vocational and avocational goals as well as their loss of earnings capacity, if any.

An important factor in pediatric life care planning is the inclusion and involvement of the child's parent or guardian from case referral and throughout each step of the process of life care planning. As a first step, the RC must first assess the parents' or guardians' level of understanding of the child's disability and their ability to participate in the care planning physically, emotionally, and intellectually. If, in the professional judgment of the RC and in consultation with the child's treatment team, the parents/guardian are not yet ready to participate with the team in making effective decisions and determining the child's future needs, the RC must provide appropriate support, patience, and education to facilitate their active participation (assuming there are no time constraints for the RC's involvement in the case). Regardless of any time constraints that may exist with the case, creating an atmosphere of reciprocal trust, care, and communication will go a long way toward enhancing the parent or guardian's sense of involvement in the child's future and restore some control over the child's life that often is lost (or perceived as being lost) as a result of the child's life-long disability or medical condition. A second step is providing information or access to resources to the child's parents/guardian to offer education and support for the child's current and expected future care needs. Deutsch and Sawyer (2005) assert that "the life care plan is designed with primarily two objectives in mind ... [the second of which is] to provide a format for the families of the disabled individual [sic]" (pp. 7A-3). The authors emphasize that the only way for parents or guardians to obtain the knowledge they need to support their child with a disability or chronic illness is to be active participants of the child's healthcare team, including the life care planning process. One study that supports the parent's/guardian's involvement in their child's care found that a survey of parents' satisfaction and dissatisfaction with pediatric rehabilitation and care planning services revealed that highly satisfied parents most often mentioned respectful and supportive care, such as feeling listened to and having a sense of rapport with service providers. Conversely, dissatisfied parents most often mentioned lack of access to existing services and lack of continuity and coordination of care (King et al., 2001). The life care plan is an ideal mechanism to address the parents or caregivers' concerns regarding lack of continuity and coordination of care and to ensure that services are coordinated across all disciplines, needs, and developmental stages over the child's lifetime.

Identification of Vocationally-Related Needs

If the life care planner is not a RC and qualified to complete a vocational assessment to address the evaluee's vocationally-related needs, the life care planner must collaborate with and/or recommend consultation with a qualified RC, as appropriate, to address vocational needs and services. In addition to a standardized approach to creating a life care plan (see Chapter 2 in this text), below is a list of vocationally-related issues to consider when preparing life care plans for pediatric evaluees and for evaluees across the lifespan:

- Identify and obtain relevant medical, educational, vocational/employment, and other vocationally-related records (e.g., school records, tax returns, evaluee's résumé/curriculum vita, work performance evaluations, Union membership records, if applicable), depositions, interrogatories, etc.
- Use a consistent methodology to organize the information so that the foundation for opinions is readily available. This is consistent with the *Standards of Practice for Life Care Planners* (2022) that require life care planners follow a consistent method for organizing data; provide a consistent, objective, and thorough methodology for constructing the life care plan; and demonstrate the ability to research, critically analyze data, manage and interpret large volumes of information, [and] attend to details (IARP, 2022).
- Present the appropriate health privacy act compliant consent form for evaluee/guardian signature.
- Obtain pre- and post-injury school records of evaluee (including standardized test scores), including early intervention, daycare or preschool records for the young, preschool age evaluee.
- Obtain school records of immediate family members (if applicable and available).
- In addition to obtaining an evaluee's vocational and employment history, obtain the vocational and employment history of parents and immediate family members (e.g., siblings, maternal and paternal grandparents, aunts/uncles, etc.).
- Request and schedule a personal interview with the evaluee/family. If not allowed, document that the request was made (and ultimately denied).
- Follow a standardized format for interviews; include vocational as well as avocational issues.
- Determine if vocational issues have already been considered or are underway; consider formal/informal testing needs, as well as assessment modifications, to determine vocational potential.
- Establish adequate medical and vocational foundation for opinions from qualified physician(s), evaluee records/consultations, published and peer-reviewed literature, and/or clinical practice guidelines; clarify whether the evaluee is at optimum level of functioning (e.g., clinical practice guidelines for many conditions include referral to and use of VR services in their criteria).
- Obtain recommendations from appropriate team members (e.g., therapeutic team members, school personnel, pre- and post-injury providers if applicable).
- Document date of consultation and source(s) of information.
- Appropriately address services that might be covered in part through the school system under the Individuals with Disabilities Education Act (IDEA) and Amendments as opposed to medically (but not educationally) necessary services (Individuals with Disabilities Education Act, 2004).
- Determine work potential, expected income; projected vocational plan costs, work life expectancy; conduct labor market research as necessary.
- Consider programs and/or accommodations to address avocational tasks that would provide productive activity for the evaluee.
- Ensure congruency and consistency of vocational recommendations in life care plan, so that there is no overlap or duplication of services (Neulicht, 2006; Weed, 2007).

A thorough interview is a crucial step in the life care planning process and gives the RC relevant information needed to continue future vocational and/or avocational planning over the evaluee's lifespan. By understanding the evaluee's abilities obtained and observed through the interview, the RC can make appropriate recommendations for adaptive equipment and devices and evaluations or services that can assist the evaluee in overcoming some of the barriers associated with the disability and can lead to a productive and fulfilling life. Additionally, the RC contributes important vocationally-related recommendations to the life care plan that might otherwise be overlooked or remain unidentified by a non-RC (e.g., summer jobs, volunteer activities/community participation, internships or co-ops, extracurricular activities).

Rehabilitation Counselor as Part of the Healthcare Team

The RC is frequently called upon to make recommendations for evaluees to reach their optimal level of functioning. Examples of possible recommendations include: (1) additional medical or rehabilitation evaluations to assess the need for related services; (2) modifications to the school or work environment; or (3) accommodations to facilitate a safe and productive entry into the labor market. Determination of growth rates and present value issues typically are beyond the scope of practice of a vocational rehabilitation consultant and generally are determined by an economist. For more information on this topic, see publications by Dillman (1987), Stephenson and Macpherson (2021), or Chapter 18 in this text. The RC's written report must include the details and data upon which recommendations and opinions are based. A report typically includes information such as the referral source, purpose of the evaluation, demographic data, records reviewed, other sources of information (e.g., interviews, observations, telephone consultations), medical history and status, educational and vocational history (if appropriate, including military history or previously developed vocational plans), hobbies and leisure activities, residual functional capacity profile, and conclusions and recommendations.

Depending on the evaluee's disability, the RC will interact with a variety of medical and allied health professionals in determining the evaluee's optimal functional capacities. In pediatric life care planning, it is common for the RC to rely on the child's primary physician (typically a pediatrician, developmental pediatrician, or pediatric physiatrist) in determining recommendations for future care, expected functional educational and/or vocational potential, and services required to reach their potential (Weed, 1998; Mertes & Harden, 2019). Although RCs rely on medical and other appropriate providers involved in the child's care to obtain relevant information about the child's functional abilities and anticipated future needs, RCs are uniquely qualified to use the information to determine the child's likely or expected future vocational needs and recommendations to be implemented to reach their expected outcomes. As such, a RC serves as an instrumental member of the pediatric healthcare rehabilitation team to coordinate age-appropriate assessments to measure the child's physical capabilities, aptitudes, achievement levels, temperament, and other factors that might affect future vocational skills. These assessments help determine the child's potential for future productive activity when the child reaches working age, i.e., competitive employment, employment in a supported employment environment, or avocational activity (Weed & Berens, 2018).

If work or productive activity is an appropriate goal for the evaluee, then the RC must include recommendations for the needs and steps to achieve that goal in the life care plan. When working with an adolescent or young adult with a disability for whom work activity is not a realistic goal, the RC is instrumental in designing a plan to help the individual achieve their highest level of productivity and/or independent living, with an understanding that their plan may include volunteer/

non-remunerative work and/or avocational activities. For adults, including older adults, vocational planning may also involve remunerative and/or non-remunerative activities depending on the evaluee's abilities and vocational or productive activity goals. Additional texts such as Fong et al. (2019) and Strauser (2020) may be useful to review with regard to assessment of vocationally-related needs.

Special Considerations Across the Lifespan

Collaborating with Early Interventionists and School Personnel as Part of the Team

Consultation with the child's early intervention providers (for children birth to age 3) and, later, their school personnel, is critical to provide a foundation for educational and vocational recommendations for the evaluee later in their life. Federal regulations require states to provide a statewide early intervention program for children from birth to three years of age who have a disability and for those services to be provided in a natural environment (usually in the child's home or wherever the child resides). Furthermore, IDEA regulations require that all school-age children with a disability be provided special education and receive educationally necessary support services (e.g., PT, OT, Speech, adapted physical education, adapted transportation) if the child is determined qualified and eligible to receive these services. Special education is specially designed instruction to meet the needs of the child with a disability, at no cost to the parents (Smith et al., 2001), and includes career development or transition services when the child reaches adolescence (Curry & Milsom, 2022). An important distinction to make is that educationally necessary support services are not synonymous with the same or similar services that may be medically necessary for a child to reach their full potential. The reader is referred Chapter 31 in this text for a discussion of federally mandated services for children with disabilities and IDEA provisions and parameters.

As part of the information-gathering process as well as collaborating with providers involved in the child's care, it is recommended that the RC establish contact with the child's early intervention and special education team members to review early intervention and school-based services that the child is receiving or for which they are eligible. The provision (or lack thereof in some cases) of school-based services could impact the child's treatment and care needs such that it is incumbent on the RC to know what is offered from an educational perspective and, for older children, what is expected for the child as they transition from high school to adulthood. Life skills and later, vocational needs, are a common thread throughout the child's school years and must be kept at the forefront to prepare for the child's future adequately and effectively beyond school. The RC is uniquely trained to facilitate vocational exploration within the school system and ensure that issues of vocational relevance are addressed. By knowing what services are provided by the school system, the RC can better determine what additional services the child needs outside the school environment to achieve the short- and long-term goals and enhance the child's optimal functioning.

Transition Planning for the Adolescent/Young Adult

The next step of the life care plan process involves transitioning students with a disability out of the school system (generally between ages 18 and 22 years) and into employment, independent living, or community support. Transitions are a natural occurrence in life for all individuals. For children with a disability, the period of transition from childhood to adulthood may occur differently, as the adolescent or young adult is usually not able to be fully independent and may have difficulty assuming the role of an adult in society. The goals for transition planning may include performing ADLs without assistance or with minimal assistance, living in an independent or unsupervised setting, working in a competitive employment setting, and/or integration into the community with non-disabled peers (Turnbull et al., 2014; Turnbull et al., 2022). While transition plans are required in Individualized Education Plans (IEPs) for students between ages 14 and 22 years (U.S. Department of Education, n.d.), once a child turns age 16, transition plans must include measurable goals as well as transition services needed for the student to meet their goals in employment, education, training and, if appropriate, independent living skills. By collaborating with school personnel, healthcare team members, parents, and the child, the RC is an integral part of the transition planning team to ensure that services are identified, and to describe a means for the services to be provided during the student's transition from school to work. In this way, the life care plan is a tool that can be used to identify the following:

- The support and services necessary to optimize the child's capabilities and to enhance their capacity for employment.
- Activities that will help the child achieve their optimal level of productivity, prevent complications, and provide for services to achieve and maintain a reasonable quality of life, including work and/or avocational activities.

For the life care planner who is not trained as a RC, identification and inclusion of transition services is best outsourced to a qualified RC. Through collaboration, the RC involved in transition planning can decrease the fragmentation of education, healthcare services, and other types of intervention that young adults with disabilities often experience when moving from school-based services to work or related activities. According to Kirby et al. (2019), an analysis of the National Longitudinal Transition Study (NLTS) reveals that youth expectations may play a stronger predictive role than parent expectations for postsecondary education and independent living. The NLTS also emphasizes the importance of involving the evaluee, parents, and school team to develop collaborative expectations and support for adult independence (Kirby et al., 2019). The reader is referred to additional resources such as Shogren and Plotner (2012) and Chen (2019) for an analysis of transition issues related to school/parent perspectives, curriculum, employment, legislation, accountability, individualized programs, and transition planning. More detail is also found in Chapter 31 of this text.

For the adolescent or young adult with a disability, mastery of prevocational skills is a necessary building block in achieving mastery of job skills and is one goal of transition planning. In the educational setting, the focus of service delivery is on the development or rehabilitation of skills that are educationally driven. These skills include self-care tasks such as taking off and putting on a jacket, snapping fasteners, pulling pants up or down for toileting purposes, handling a spoon or fork for feeding, drinking from a cup, toileting, and manipulating tools for drawing, coloring, painting, cutting, and writing. Prevocational skills are also frequently emphasized at the school level as many students with disabilities often do not attend postsecondary education and generally are placed directly out of high school into a job setting suitable to their capabilities (McCaigue, 2004).

Working with Adult Evaluees

As a RC developing a life care plan for an evaluee who is expected to enter the workforce, activities and services that will enhance the evaluee's ability to successfully be placed in a job should be addressed, including services to develop:

- Appropriate job skills and work behaviors
- Effective social support network
- Self-confidence and competence
- Understanding of and motivation for the world of work

Further, the RC must carefully consider issues relevant for the life care plan by asking questions such as these:

- What is the ultimate goal for the evaluee (employment or highest level of productivity)?
- What are the vocational services to achieve the identified goal?
- What services are included to ensure continuation of programming and services?
- What is the level of spousal/partner/significant other/family involvement, if applicable?
- What counseling and support services are needed to assist the evaluee (and family or significant other, if applicable) with coping and adjustment issues?
- What amount of support is needed (e.g., 24-hour supervision, periodic check-in, onsite staff availability as needed)?
- What type of living arrangement is most appropriate? Include preferences (if evaluee is able to communicate them), family preferences, physical/cognitive abilities, availability of services/programs, geographical limitations, etc.
- What is the evaluee's ability to drive? For young adults who were able to drive before the onset of their disability or chronic medical condition, what is their ability to resume safe driving? Clearly, the ability to drive has implications for independence and employment across the lifespan.
- What is the evaluee's style of learning (hands-on, visual, didactic, multimodal, simulated tasks, etc.)?
- What are the evaluee's short-term needs (1–5 years) as well as expected long-term needs across their lifespan?

Vocational Contributions to the Life Care Plan

For non-RC life care planners, consultation with a qualified RC is important to answer vocationally-related questions and identify recommendations (items or services) for the evaluee's life care plan that may be outside of the non-RC life care planner's scope of practice (but are within the RC's scope of practice). Specific examples of how a qualified RC evaluates and makes recommendations for an evaluee's life care plan across their lifespan include recommendations for:

Vocational Testing, Assessment, and/or Evaluation

- Clarification of physical/functional capacities (physical/functional capacity evaluation)
- Vocational counseling (to include career and/or guidance counseling)

- Additional education or training (e.g., postsecondary education, career technical programs, short-term certificate programs, on-the-job training programs, other)
- Job-seeking skills training (e.g., résumé writing, online or in-person job lead identification, application techniques, interviewing, and employer communication)
- Labor market search to include labor market research and employer sampling/census data
- Job analysis of potential jobs
- Work adjustment training
- Job coaching/supported employment
- Selective job placement
- Post-placement services to monitor employment (typically provided for 90 days post placement to assure success)
- For evaluees without vocational potential, recommendations regarding avocational or non-remunerative activities are made (e.g., volunteer activities, adult day programs)

A brief definition of the above vocational services that may be recommended for the life care plan follows:

Vocational testing: An objective assessment of an individual's aptitudes, interests, skills, abilities, and temperaments as they relate to the workforce (Weed & Field, 2012).

Vocational assessment: A comprehensive informal process that takes place over a period of time, usually involving a multidisciplinary team. The purpose of vocational assessment is to identify individual characteristics (e.g., functional capacities, limitations, and preferences), rehabilitation, education, training, and placement needs. Vocational assessment forms the basis for planning rehabilitation, employment, career development, education, and/or transition programs as well as provides an individual with insight into their own vocational and career potential (Dowd, 1993 modified from McCray, 1982; Whiston, 2016). Note that vocational assessment and vocational evaluation (see next bullet) are terms that sometimes are used interchangeably (CRCC, 2023).

Vocational evaluation: A comprehensive process that systematically uses work, either real or simulated, as the focal point for assessment and vocational exploration to assist individuals in vocational development. Vocational evaluation incorporates medical, psychological, social, vocational, educational, cultural, and economic data into the process to attain the goal of evaluation (Dowd, 1993; Tenth Institute on Rehabilitation Services, 1972).

Physical/functional capacity evaluation: An objective evaluation of physical and functional capabilities and limitations as they relate to work, recreation, and ADLs that describes the optimum and maximal capabilities of an individual's strength, endurance, fine and gross motor coordination, limiting factors, and methods of functional and task performance (Weed & Berens, 2018). Capacities testing generally includes strength, flexibility, balance, coordination, cardiovascular condition, and body mechanics, all in relation to performing work tasks.

Vocational counseling: The process of helping evaluees analyze and synthesize vocational evaluation results, assisting the evaluees to understand the relationship of evaluation data to real jobs in the labor market, and aiding evaluees with identifying and clarifying feelings about personal vocational strengths and weaknesses as they relate to the goal of vocational independence (Weed & Field, 2012).

Job-seeking skills training: Training to help educate and prepare evaluees in effective job search techniques, including where to find information about job openings, how to complete applications/take pre-employment tests, develop a résumé, and make a positive impression before, during, and after the interview (e.g., role play interviews, wear appropriate interview attire). Training can be provided individually or in a job club arrangement with other individuals seeking employment.

Labor market search (*LMS*): A methodological process of determining the pattern of employment in a specific geographic area with corresponding earnings capacity. Composed of *Labor Market Research* and *Employer Sampling* approaches:

– *Labor market research*: An investigation and vocational analysis of the buyers and sellers of labor services (e.g., employers, job seekers, workers) using a variety of resources. Information may be gathered and interpreted on specifically defined labor markets (international, national, state, local) to examine trends, analyze policy issues, or provide a context/benchmark to focus a search on specific industries, occupations, and geographical areas. Labor market research includes personal contact and/or use of printed/internet resources and data. Personal contact is most often made with an employer, State Employment Security Commission, or via a professional network. With regard to published/printed information, VEs most often rely on the U.S. Bureau of Labor Statistics, online job openings, and classified ads (Neulicht et al., 2007).

– *Employer sampling*: Involves direct contact/communication with a select set of employers in a designated locale to collect information about the labor market in which specific occupations, skill sets, and/or education/training is required or can be supplied, as well as to determine a pattern of employer variables. In a forensic setting, information most often provided is work experience, education and skills, strengths, and abilities. Information most often obtained includes jobs currently available, job description, and minimum qualifications (Neulicht et al., 2007). The reader is referred to Barros-Bailey (2012) for labor market survey methodology that includes the use of survey research to design labor market surveys, collect the data through samples or censuses, data analysis using qualitative or quantitative methods that may include descriptive statistics (e.g., measures of central tendency or variability, error rates), and reporting on the results of the collected data of labor market research in the overall labor market search process.

Job analysis: A detailed analysis of a particular job (e.g., a position in a single establishment) that identifies and describes, in a systematic and comprehensive manner, what the worker does in terms of activities or functions (essential and non-essential functions); how the work is done (methods, techniques, or processes involved and work devices used); results of the work (goods produced, services rendered, or materials used); and worker characteristics (skills, knowledge, abilities, and adaptations) required to accomplish the tasks. Also includes identification of the context of the work in terms of environmental and organizational factors and the nature of the worker's discretion, responsibility, or accountability (U.S. Bureau of Labor Statistics, 2022c; U.S. Department of Labor, 1982).

Work adjustment training: Services to enable evaluees prepare to RTW, including cleanliness and personal hygiene, social skills, appropriate work behaviors, adjustment to work, need for internal and external support, etc.

Job coach/supported employment: Training of evaluees in real work environments by a job coach; designed to assist evaluees in obtaining and maintaining employment in real jobs by providing individualized one-on-one assistance in job placement, travel training, skill training at the job site, and ongoing assessment and follow-up (Wehman & Melia, 1985). As cited by the Rehabilitation Act Amendments of 1986 and 1992, PL 99-506 and PL 102-569, supported employment is competitive employment in an integrated setting with ongoing support services for individuals with the most severe disabilities.

Selective job placement: A placement process which, because of the nature or severity of an individual's limitations, involves close attention and matching of both the demands of the job and the individual's skills. In some cases, job or work site modification may be necessary to accomplish the goal of placement. Further, the number of possible work sites that represent a match between job requirements and the evaluee's skill may be quite limited (Rusch et al., 1982).

Post-placement services: Follow-up contact with evaluee and employer after placement has been achieved to ensure both are satisfied with the job placement and to identify services, if any, to promote job maintenance. From the first day of employment, the RC should work with the evaluee, employer, family, and other integral members of the team to plan for support and services to ensure a successful employment tenure as well as plan for career advancement.

Local rehabilitation programs in the evaluee's geographic area can often provide current rate/data and current statistics may be available from local rehabilitation programs and/or a state VR agency (e.g., average hours for assessment, planning, job search/job development, training, fading, ongoing support, average cost for purchased services, average total months in service, average hours worked the week, average weekly earnings, average hourly earnings at closure). Excerpted items from a life care plan by one of the authors are included in Table 11.6 as an illustration of vocationally-relevant services.

Table 11.6   Example Excerpts for Vocationally-Related Recommendations from a Life Care Plan

Vocational Plan			
Recommendation (by Whom)	*Year Initiated*	*Purpose*	*Expected Cost*
Vocational evaluation, to include testing, analysis, exploration of vocational choices, and review of results (RC*)	2023–25 (age 16–18) for 1 X evaluation	Assess and identify vocational interests, aptitudes, work behaviors, skills, temperaments, target vocational goals, etc.	$1,000–1,500 (avg.) for 1 X only evaluation to include report and recommendations
Career technical education (RC)	2025–29 (age 18–22)	Higher education to enhance employment within capabilities	Approximately $2,500–$3,400 for application fee, tuition, mandatory fees, and books for 2–3-quarter program (depends on specific program)
Vocational rehabilitation counseling/guidance, job placement services, and post-placement activities (RC)	2028–29 (completion of career technical education) to work life expectancy	Job-seeking skills training, labor market research employer sampling, job analysis, and selective job placement assistance	$3,000–$6,000 for 20–40 hrs. (average) for RC services @ $150/hour (avg.).
	2029–2030 or whenever evaluee obtains employment	Post-placement or placement retention services to maintain employment over work life expectancy	$1,500–$3,000 for 10–20 hrs. (average) for placement monitoring and follow-up and $1,500 – $3,000 at time of two expected job changes over work life expectancy
Specialized computer software (RC)	2023–2030 (age 16-23)	Develop language skills and/or compensate for communication disorder	Software: $300 per year (average) over and above general population to 2030 or whenever obtain employment

* *RC = Rehabilitation Counselor* recommendations for the Life Care Plan.

When employment is not a realistic option for the evaluee, possible alternate life care planning goals include referral and linkages with adult community services such as independent living centers and long-term residential community participation. When appropriate, volunteer, recreation, and non-remunerative activities should be recommended as part of the evaluee's overall life care plan with the cost of support services and interventions that would facilitate the evaluee's independence and enhance their self-esteem. Once recommendations for future care services are identified, determination of growth rates and present value issues over the evaluee's lifespan typically are beyond the RC's scope of practice and are determined by an economist. For more information on the economist's role in the life care plan, see publications by Dillman (1987) and Stephenson & Macpherson (2021), as well as Chapter 18 in this text.

Note regarding the above vocationally-related services: The evaluee may be eligible for vocational rehabilitation (VR) services through their state division of vocational rehabilitation; however, any cost-sharing and/or private pay charges required by the state cannot be determined until the evaluee is evaluated by the state VR program and found eligible to receive services. State VR services are often considered a collateral source and the reader is referred to Chapter 27 of this text for more information on the collateral source rule.

Loss of Earnings Capacity (LOEC)

In addition to contributing vocationally-related recommendations for a life care plan, the qualified RC can also provide an analysis of the evaluee's LOEC due to the disability and/or chronic medical condition that may prevent the evaluee from working or from working full-time. History shows that forensic vocational rehabilitation began shortly after the beginning of private and public rehabilitation programs with rehabilitation counselors testifying in workers' compensation cases regarding earnings capacity of injured workers as early as the 1920s (Barros-Bailey, 2014). Although an in-depth discussion of earnings capacity (EC) is beyond the scope of this chapter, a basic definition of EC may be helpful. According to Horner and Slesnick (1999), EC is defined as what an evaluee is able to earn over their entire work life (as opposed to the terms "actual earnings" and "expected earnings" which have different though related meanings), and is considered the most common standard for [vocational] loss in personal injury cases (Horner & Slesnick, 1999). Horner and Slesnick (1999) further delineate the role that RCs play in determining "vocational capacity" and the role that economists play in determining EC. Specifically, the authors suggest that, in determining the vocational capacity/ies of an evaluee, the qualified RC examines "many complex questions involving medical and psychological issues" (p. 29), and identifies specific jobs or classes of jobs that describe the evaluee's vocational capacity, i.e., jobs that the evaluee would be able to perform. From the list of jobs or classes of jobs prepared by the RC, the economist then "reduces" the list to a number or a range of numbers that represent the evaluee's EC (Horner & Slesnick, 1999).

Historically, in cases where employment in the competitive labor force has been determined by the RC as an unrealistic goal, many evaluees who previously were determined to be unemployable in the competitive labor market were recommended to be "placed" in sheltered employment settings (Berens & Weed, 2018; Weed & Field, 2012). Sheltered employment generally means performing "work-like" activities in a setting alongside other workers with disabilities, and is not considered part of the "competitive" labor force. Historically, sheltered employment "workers" typically receive wages for their work-like activities that are below the federal minimum wage (Berens & Weed, 2018; Weed & Field, 2012). However, the Association of People Supporting

Employment First (APSE) published a recent white paper that shows a declining trend in payment of "subminimum wages" (US Department of Labor, Wage and Hour Division, 2022) to individuals with disabilities who are "working" under active 14(c) certificates held by community rehabilitation providers. The declining trend represents a 46% decrease since 2018 with a corresponding increase in preference for competitive, integrated employment, largely due to students with disabilities transitioning out of high school and into adult services and community support (APSE, 2021). The 14(c) certificates referenced above refer to Section 14(c) of the Fair Labor Standards Act (1986) that authorizes employers, after applying for and receiving a certificate from the U.S. Department of Labor Wage and Hour Division, to pay wages less than the federal minimum wage to workers who have disabilities for the work that they perform (U.S. Department of Labor, 2022, para 2).

For evaluees who are not able to enter the competitive workforce due to their catastrophic disability or chronic medical condition, their loss of access to the labor market and subsequent LOEC can be substantial. In such cases, it becomes the role of the qualified RC to determine the loss. As the evolution of VR progresses over time, and as the trend to place individuals in the Least Restrictive Environment continues, it is important for the RC to include or contribute recommendations to the life care plan for avocational activities that would allow the evaluee who does not have employment potential with an opportunity to perform productive and meaningful activity, even if it is volunteer and/or non-remunerative activity.

The qualified RC can serve a vital role in determining the evaluee's EC and potential LOEC as related to their disability or chronic medical condition. For evaluees who have an established work history, the qualified RC can assess and determine the evaluee's transferable skills (based on the evaluee's past training, education, and vocational and avocational history), determine pre- and post-injury occupational profiles, research the labor market and occupational statistics/databases, and provide an opinion of the evaluee's expected or likely capacity to work, with a corresponding wage analysis (e.g., Bast et al., 2002; Berens & Weed, 2018; Blackwell, 1991; Boyd & Toppino, 1995; Cohen & Yanklowski, 1997; Dunn & Growick, 2000; Field, 1999; Field & Field, 2004; Weed, 2002; Weed & Field, 2012; Weed & Taylor, 1990). The reader is referred to Robinson (2014) for a summary of over 20 models that RCs can use to facilitate an EC opinion. In addition, Barros-Bailey (2012) describes a five phase process that uses the 12 steps of the labor market survey process that the RC can follow in formulating an EC opinion. Once the RC determines the evaluee's vocational potential, the need for future vocational and/or educational training as well as job modifications or specialized assistance (e.g., vocational counseling, supported employment, assistive technology) that is recommended by the RC to facilitate the evaluee's potential is detailed in the life care plan (Berens & Weed, 2018; Deutsch & Sawyer, 2005; Field, 2002; Mertes & Harden, 2019). It is important to note that if an intervention is recommended and the costs are included in the life care plan/rehabilitation plan (e.g., vocational counseling, cost of education/training), then the likely consequences or results of that intervention also need to be accounted for in the evaluee's LOEC assessment.

Impact of Education and Other Demographic Factors on Earnings Capacity

Although intelligence has a clear impact on schooling, occupational opportunities, and job success, the most important determinants of EC are educational level and occupation (Brody, 1997; Ceci & Williams, 1997; Sternberg et al., 2003). Data from the U.S. Census Bureau consistently reveal that annual and lifetime earnings are positively correlated with education. Generally, as a person's educational attainment and specific skill level increases, so does their EC. Educational attainment and occupational selection are strongly influenced by aptitude, academic performance, college entrance examination scores, curriculum content (college preparatory courses, advanced placement classes), parental educational level, socioeconomic status of the parents, and gender (Woodside et al., 1991). Occupations vary by gender and, according to data published by the U.S. Department of Labor, the overall ratio of women's earnings to men's earnings is still lower (although increased to 82%) despite higher educational attainment (Evers & Sieverding, 2013; U.S. Bureau of Labor Statistics, 2022d). Earnings also vary by age group, race, and educational level (U.S. Census Bureau, 2022a). One's college major also contributes to earnings differences as "science, technology, engineering and mathematics majors earn much more than teaching and serving majors, which include education, psychology, and social work" (Carnevale et al., 2015, p.8). Studies further indicate that family influence (e.g., social modeling and observation) has a significant effect on males, as most will engage in the same or similar occupations as their father (Hout, 1984), although the impact of mentors, role models, and extended family/community support can make a difference (Wilson et al., 2016). Sapp et al. (2020) found significant positive relationships between caregiver and child educational attainment and occupation, which supports the foundation for PEEDS-RAPEL© described later in this chapter.

The potential negative effects of a one-parent family must also be considered by the RC when developing an EC opinion (e.g., higher incidence of school drop-out, less likely to complete college, more likely to get into trouble with the law), as well as the tendency of children of parents at the extremes of the educational status to regress toward the mean (Weed, 2000). Wilson et al. (2016) assert that a strong relationship with mothers, awareness of father's absence, interaction with mentors and role models, exposure to activities and programs, vision for themselves as fathers, extended family support, religion, not speaking ill of fathers, desire to give back and help others also has an influence on children, especially black children, raised in absent-father homes. Except at high income levels, children tend to do at least as well financially as their parents. A review of multiple studies in the labor economics and sociology literature indicates that parental earnings and educational level are the best predictors of a child's premorbid earning potential (Isom et al., 2001; Schonbrun & Kampfe, 2008), and the probabilities of completing various levels of educational attainment can be computed (Gill & Foley, 1996; Kane et al., 2013; Kane & Spizman, 2001; Mare, 2000; Spizman & Kane, 1992, 2020). For example, children of college-educated parents are more likely to attend college than children whose parents did not attend college (Anderson et al., 1972; Clearinghouse for Military Family Readiness at Penn State, 2020; National Center for Educational Statistics, 2001). In the scenario of attending college, two considerations are apparent based on the literature: 1) if parents believe they [the child] are college bound (Ablin, 2015); and 2) if children believe their family can afford it [college] (National Center for Educational Statistics, 2022a).

As education becomes more of a key factor in obtaining employment and the incidence of college degrees/specific skill training increases, training may reduce gender differences at the low end of the spectrum and potentially widen the gap at the top of the wage distribution (Icardi, 2021). Per Current Population Survey data (U.S. Census Bureau, 2022b), between 2010 and 2020, educational attainment rates among 25- to 29-year-olds increased at each attainment level. During this period, the percentage who had completed at least high school increased from 89 to 95 percent, the percentage with an associate's or higher degree increased from 41 to 50 percent, the percentage with a bachelor's or higher degree increased from 32 to 39 percent, and the percentage with a master's or higher degree increased from 7 to 9 percent (National Center for Educational Statistics, 2022b).

Increased educational attainment may also affect career mobility as well as the opportunity to live in metropolitan settings and command higher salaries (Farley, 1996; Martin & Weinstein, 2012; Stephenson & Macpherson, 2021). Other considerations in determining RC include a lowered labor force participation and earnings ratio for persons with disabilities as well as increased rates of disabilities for individuals who perform unskilled labor or are of Hispanic or African American background (U.S. Bureau of Labor Statistics, 2022e; Weed, 2000). Personal appearance has also been shown to have an impact on earnings (e.g., Benzeval et al., 2013; Halstrom, 1995; Hamermesh & Biddle, 1993; Gvozdenodic, 2013; Johnson et al., 1993;). According to the U.S. Bureau of Labor Statistics (2020), job tenure differs by age (generally longer for older workers) and type of job (highest tenure for managers and professionals; lowest for service occupations). It is important to recognize that published statistics and databases do not take into consideration a specific or individualized vocational plan prepared by a RC for an evaluee that may ameliorate or have an impact on the evaluee's ability for employment and EC.

While at least some postsecondary education or training is becoming the entry-level requirement for many jobs, there are 20 million "middle jobs" (which require career technical education) in the United States that pay $35,000 or more on average and do not require a bachelor's degree. Nevertheless, there are positive returns for human capital accumulation in college even when a student does not complete a degree (gains identifiable for as little as a semester's worth of credit), and there is a significant difference in earnings gains according to field of study. Similar to the differences in college major, in general, earnings gains are higher for career technical or occupational programs, whereas in very few cases are the returns high in the humanities, social sciences, or other academic disciplines (Carnevale et al., 2015, 2021).

Establishing a Foundation for Loss of Earnings

The age of the individual at the time of injury will influence the way a RC obtains information and arrives at a LOEC opinion. Issues related to the identification of EC can be divided into four general categories (Berens & Weed, 2018):

- Injury at birth or in the neonatal period
- Injury before school age (no academic grades or standardized test scores)
- Injury before the establishment of a career identity or viable vocational goal
- Injury after an established work history representative of vocational potential (consider stage of work life at the time of injury; e.g., early, middle, or end of work life and beyond).

As indicated in Table 11.7, using multiple sources of information is critical to an accurate assessment of the pre- and post-injury developmental options available to an evaluee (Berens & Weed, 2018). The broader the base of history and documentation, the more likely a RC can establish an accurate foundation for an EC opinion. Triangulation, or the combination of independent yet complementary research methods or data sources, will strengthen the validity of a RC's opinion (Barros-Bailey & Neulicht, 2005). The qualified RC's goal is to obtain data from sources that have different strengths so they can complement each other and allow the RC to expand their source data and to move from uncontrolled to more controlled data.

Table 11.7 Sources of Information by Age Group for Earnings Capacity Opinion

Age	Information Base
0–1 year	Obtain family history. Establish family patterns of educational attainment, work history (occupations and skill levels). Include information from parents, older siblings, aunts/uncles, grandparents, and/or those adults who are likely to provide a role model for the child. Consider vocational or intellectual testing of parents
2–5 years	Obtain family history and review records from early intervention specialists (e.g., Individualized Family Service Plan/IFSP), pediatrician, and/or other medical/allied health providers, daycare providers, church, and sitters or preschool staff. Obtain family videotapes, baby books (if well documented), or other relevant records. Utilize interview and observational data to clarify pre- and post-injury status and prognosis
6–18 years	Obtain family history and review school records, including aptitude and academic performance, grade point average, achievement test scores, college entrance examination scores, curriculum content, honors, disciplinary records, extracurricular activities, pediatric and/or other medical records, neuropsychology and/or vocational evaluations, as well as other relevant records
18+ years	Review school records, neuropsychology and/or vocational evaluations, employment/personnel records, military records, community/civic involvement, personal observations, and other relevant information

Source: Adapted from Weed, R. O. & Berens, D. (Eds.). (2018). Life care planning and case management handbook (4th ed.). Routledge. With permission.

Forming a Vocational Opinion

Using the preceding information, in conjunction with the evaluee's identified or expected restrictions and limitations, a qualified RC must draw conclusions about the earnings potential of the evaluee in terms of the evaluee's probability of attending college, most likely career choices, and income levels/patterns. For pediatric evaluees, older children/adolescents are more likely to have career goals or objectives that may help to narrow the focus of the vocational analysis. In comparison, the younger the child, the more general the vocational opinion will necessarily be (due to young age and no or minimal demonstrated abilities). Loss of EC may reflect overall averages of pre- and post-injury wage paths by levels of education, gender, geographic area, or specific examples of relevant occupations and, typically, the RC delineates categories and examples of occupations representative of the type of jobs that the evaluee could reasonably have been expected to fill pre- and post-injury (Berens & Weed, 2018; Deutsch & Sawyer, 2005; Horner & Slesnick, 1999). Where possible, general worker trait profiles (based on parental and family history or pre-injury capacities) can be developed and computer programs utilized to compare pre- and post-injury profiles or to provide an estimate of labor market access (e.g., https://mccroskeymvqs.com/; https://skilltran.com/).

The pre- and post-injury options also form the basis for a comparison of salaries, using information from a variety of resources. If specific jobs are identified, publications such as the *Occupational Outlook Handbook* (U.S. Department of Labor, 2022) can be used for general information and as a resource for the names of specific associations or unions to contact for information on salary surveys (www.bls.gov/ooh/). Salary and wage data for specific occupations are also available from various websites (see employment-related computer resources listed at the end of chapter), including publications on educational attainment of employed civilians, employment, and earnings (e.g.,

Irwin et al., 2021; National Center for Education Statistics, 2022b, 2022c; U.S. Census Bureau, 2022a), as well as occupational employment statistics by occupation, state, region, and metropolitan statistical area.

The *Digest of Educational Statistics* also provides educational attainment data by state (National Center for Educational Statistics, 2022d). Additionally, the U.S. Bureau of Labor Statistics is a valuable source of information and offers data on topics such as median years of tenure by occupation, characteristics of workers on flexible and shift schedules, and industry-specific trends (www.bls.gov). Data on earnings by education and gender are available from the U.S. Census Bureau as is information on the employment rate of persons with disabilities (www.census.gov/). Salary information can also be accessed through mega-sites (see examples of online mega-sites at end of chapter) that can be used as a supplement to government data (e.g., individual state employment data, state and metropolitan statistical area/MSA wages, and occupational employment and wage statistics/OEWS). However, the astute RC must be cognizant of and familiar with how the salary information is obtained as well as the reliability and validity of the salary data provided by the mega-sites. Best practices recommend that RCs triangulate this information with other reliable sources to provide the foundation for a valid and credible vocational opinion (Barros-Bailey & Neulicht, 2005). Professional organizations/associations can also be a resource for salary information depending on the particular job being researched and, ultimately, a labor market survey can be performed to verify and provide support for the salary estimates obtained from other sources (Barros-Bailey, 2012). In addition to labor market survey research, the RC may use employer sampling to obtain and provide details regarding the demands of specific occupations and/or vocational settings (Neulicht et al., 2007). International as well as local, state, and provincial agencies and organizations can also provide information on vocational services and potential future costs for evaluees within a specific disability group (e.g., United Cerebral Palsy Association).

A RC's skill and experience in analyzing the evaluee's work history, adjusting their worker trait profile based on their disability, and evaluating labor market research and wage data is critical to produce credible results and accurate calculations as to the evaluee's loss of labor market access and wages or EC (Bast et al., 2002). A RC must consistently and objectively follow a standardized model for analysis and be able to define and discuss the decision-making process that was followed. Although several case conceptualization models are available to the RC to provide a framework (Robinson, 2014), the authors describe one of the more salient models to illustrate the role of the RC in life care planning across the lifespan.

PEEDS-RAPEL©

As previously stated, there are over 20 known and published LOEC models available to the RC when determining an evaluee's LOEC. Of the known and published LOEC models, this section and the case study that follows specifically describe and apply the PEEDS-RAPEL© model to an actual case. Based on the RAPEL model, a widely accepted and recognized format for summarizing life care plan and vocational opinions (Weed, 1993, 1995, 1996, 2000; Weed & Field, 2012), PEEDS-RAPEL© was developed to further delineate issues specific to pediatric vocational opinions (Neulicht & Berens, 2004, 2005, 2015). The chart below defines the acronym RAPEL and PEEDS-RAPEL©. Literature that forms the foundation for PEEDS-RAPEL© includes economics (e.g., socioeconomic status/SES, parental characteristics, social modeling, human capital); psychology (e.g., predictive value of intelligence, non-cognitive factors); family (e.g., environmental/cultural expectations, family systems theory, confounding variables); and characteristics of the child/young adult (e.g., assessment results, functional capacity, aptitudes, interests, skills). Since the publication of PEEDS-RAPEL© in the professional literature (Neulicht & Berens, 2004), authors have elaborated on the original tenets of the model terms such as "sphere of influence" (Leslie, 2018). Additionally, the basis for establishing the relationship of parental to child educational attainment and occupational skill level/physical demand level, a key foundation for expert EC opinions in pediatric cases, is supported by Sapp et al. (2020). Further, much has been published on the relationship between parents' educational attainment and child development within the parenting literature (Davis-Kean et al., 2019).

PEEDS-RAPEL© is an acronym defined as follows:

PARENTAL/FAMILY OCCUPATIONS: Obtain family work history (occupations and skill levels). Include information from parents, older siblings, aunts and uncles, grandparents, and adults who are likely to provide a role model for the child. Also include military experience, volunteer or community service, and avocational activities. Consider vocational assessment of parents, as appropriate, to determine a pattern of aptitudes or trait profile.

EDUCATIONAL ATTAINMENT: Establish family patterns of educational attainment including information from the immediate and extended family (as above). Determine not only the academic level and degrees earned, but also the skills obtained through education and training. Administer or coordinate a referral for achievement, and/or intellectual assessment of parents as needed.

EVALUATION RESULTS: Determine the child's functional capacities through interviews and formal assessment of physical, cognitive, emotional, and vocational capacity. Consider academic skills, interests, aptitudes, personality, assessment of independence and ADLs, and family patterns of hobbies and leisure activities. When appropriate, compare to pre-injury status and function.

DEVELOPMENTAL STAGE: Consider the normal developmental tasks of a particular age (e.g., ADLs, career development). Determine the effects of a disability on function and ability to achieve developmental milestones. Provide recommendations for remediation and accommodations to facilitate the optimum level of function for the child.

SYNTHESIS: Integrate results of the interview, parent and family occupations, educational attainment, evaluation results, developmental stage, and opinions regarding functional capacities to determine the impact of the disability and the likely options that are, within reasonable probability, available to the child.

REHABILITATION PLAN: Determine the rehabilitation plan based on the [evaluees's] vocational and functional limitations, vocational strengths, emotional functioning, and cognitive capabilities. This may include testing, counseling, training fees, rehabilitation technology, job analysis, job coaching, placement, and other needs for increasing employment potential. Also, consider reasonable accommodation. A life care plan may be needed for catastrophic injuries.

ACCESS TO THE LABOR MARKET: Determine the [evaluee's] access to the labor market. Methods include use of computer programs for transferability of skills (or worker trait) analysis, disability statistics, and experience. This may also represent the [evaluee's] loss of choice and is particularly relevant if earnings potential is based on very few positions.

PLACEABILITY: This represents the likelihood that the [evaluee] could be successfully placed in a job. This is where the "rubber meets the road." Consider the employment statistics for people with disabilities, employment data for the specific medical condition (if available), economic situation of the community and availability (not just existence) of jobs in chosen occupations. Note that, where appropriate, the [evaluee's] or family's attitude, personality, and other factors will influence the ultimate outcome.

EARNINGS CAPACITY: Based on the above, what is the pre-incident capacity to earn compared to the post-incident capacity to earn? Consider categories and examples of occupations (e.g., unskilled, semi-skilled, or skilled as a result of elementary and middle school, high school, career technical education, or college educational attainment) that are representative of the type of occupations a child could reasonably have been expected to perform pre- and post-injury. Determine the ability to be educated (sometimes useful for people with acquired brain injury). Utilize relevant research data and computer analysis, as appropriate, based on family work patterns and/or [evaluee's] worker traits.

LABOR FORCE PARTICIPATION: This represents the [evaluee's] work life expectancy. Determine the amount of time that is lost, if any, from the labor force as a result of the disability. Issues include additional time to find employment, part-time vs. full-time employment, medical treatment or follow-up, earlier retirement, etc. Display data using specific dates or percentages. For example, an average of 4 hrs. a day may represent a 50% loss.

Source: Neulicht, A. T., & Berens, D. E. (2005). PEEDS-RAPEL©: A case conceptualization model for evaluating pediatric cases, *Journal Life Care Planning*, 4(1), 27–36. With permission.

Case Study: Elias and the Role of the Rehabilitation Counselor in Life Care Planning Across the Lifespan

To illustrate PEEDS-RAPEL©, the authors present the case of Elias, a six-year-old boy with diagnoses of spastic diplegia with an athetotic component, auditory neuropathy, bilateral sensorineural hearing loss requiring cochlear implants, upward gaze palsy, dental enamel hypoplasia, kernicterus, developmental delay, severe communication disorder with elements of dyspraxia (oral, motor, and peripheral), and developmental delays. Note: For further reading on kernicterus, please see the article by Deming (2006).

Birth records indicate that Elias' mother was healthy, experienced no problems during pregnancy or with labor and (vaginal) delivery. A birth weight of 6 lb. 3 oz. is recorded with Apgar scores of 8 (1 min) and 9 (5 min). Newborn screening labs were within normal limits and Elias passed a hearing screen in the nursery. Due to critical aortic stenosis, aortic insufficiency, and subsequent necrotizing enterocolitis, birth hospitalization surgeries included cardiac catheterization, aortovalvuloplasty, exploratory laparotomy with colon resection, peritoneal debridement, ileostomy, enterostomal enterostomy, and aortic valve repair. Neonatal progress notes indicate elevated bilirubin as well as hyperbilirubinemia. Elias also required a Ross procedure, a heart valve replacement operation, to treat severe aortic valve disease.

At the time of the RC's evaluation, Elias was classified by his school system as a child with hearing impairment and had been placed in a mainstream classroom (80% or more of the time) with consistent therapeutic intervention (auditory-verbal therapy; speech therapy, occupational therapy, physical therapy). Classroom accommodations included a Frequency Modulation system and preferential seating. Current IEP goals included activities to improve expressive skills, sound production, balance and stability, fine/visual motor skills, as well as upper body strength, and functional hand use. Per his current teacher, Elias will likely benefit from two years in a first grade class (e.g., being held back to repeat the 1st grade).

Parental/Family Occupations

Based on the RC's interview with Elias and his family, his mother's work history includes jobs as a fast-food worker, screen printer, and assembler. She currently earns $16.75 per hour as a part-time shipping clerk (25-hour work week). The father's work history includes jobs as a fast-food worker and material handler. He currently earns $15.70 per hour as a construction laborer for a 40+ hour workweek (weather permitting). The maternal grandfather and great grandfather were maintenance/machine mechanics (grandfather disabled). Elias is in close contact with his maternal grandmother, who currently works as a home health aide at the level of a certified nursing assistant, with past work history as a fast-food manager and textile machine operator. An aunt is a phlebotomist, a close cousin is a sheriff, and another cousin is an established rap music artist.

Elias' immediate and extended family have held positions that require at least average to above average manual/finger dexterity and motor coordination. Work tasks have involved dealing with people and attaining precise tolerances.

Educational Attainment

Both parents finished the tenth grade but dropped out of school as they were expecting Elias. The mother is currently taking General Education Development classes. The father has completed some welding classes at a local community college. The maternal grandmother participated in an on-the-job certificate program (for certified nurse assistant); an aunt completed phlebotomy training, and a cousin completed basic law enforcement training. The paternal grandmother has an associate's degree but has no contact with Elias; other paternal educational history is unknown.

Evaluation Results

Developmental screening reveals Gesell figures at the five year level, although the figures are extremely tremulous with demonstrated fine-motor delay. Elias is able to write some of his upper-case letters; however, he needs cueing for proper letter formation sequence, sizing, and spacing. He is able to finger feed (e.g., eat a cookie). He is able to dress and undress himself if there are Velcro fasteners or very large buttons. He can pull on his shirt, don/doff elastic waist pants, but is unable to snap pants. Sometimes he can zip a jacket. He can feed himself using a spoon and fork. He has successfully mastered toilet training. Elias can hold his scissors appropriately and can cut simple shapes within 1/2" of a preordained line although he demonstrates difficulty with motor planning to hold, turn, and cut the paper smoothly (requires hand over hand assistance and adaptive scissors).

With bilateral Ankle Foot Orthotics, Elias is able to walk throughout the school environment with only supervision for safety, and able to go up/down curbs as well as small steps without assistance. He continues to need a handrail plus supervision or hand-held assistance for numerous or steep steps. He occasionally loses his balance when running or when he is not paying close attention. He is unable to hop on one foot.

Elias' weakest areas are in language (reading, speaking, and writing). Based on a score of 8 (out of 78 points), Elias qualifies for Title I reading services. Speech is often very difficult, if not impossible to understand. Spontaneous expressive speech is estimated at less than 50 words. Elias is using two to three word phrases and is 25%–40% intelligible, depending on what kind of day he is having. He is very social and will persist in trying to make his needs known (e.g., will physically take someone to what he wants, if necessary). Picture symbol cards are used to facilitate communication when necessary. Other modes of augmentative communication will likely be needed.

On the WPPSI-III, Elias achieved a performance IQ of 86. He displayed average visual attention and reasoning skills. Auditory memory deficits are recorded. On the Test of Nonverbal Intelligence-III, Elias achieved a standard score of 103, an indication that nonverbal intelligence is in the average range of functioning (considered a minimal estimate).

Developmental Stage

Although Elias expresses an intense interest in becoming a rapper and demonstrates play behavior indicative of this, he is in the fantasy stage of career development. He is too young to express a viable vocational goal, and his play behavior will likely change many times before it becomes work oriented.

Synthesis

Elias will require an IEP with special education placement and an extended school year throughout his developmental period. Based on current function, he will likely earn an occupational diploma and require vocational services throughout his career.

Elias' physical deficits are consistent with cerebral palsy which include likely exertional and functional limitations in the areas of lifting, carrying, pushing/pulling, standing, walking, climbing, balancing, crouching, crawling, handling, reaching, fingering, and exposure to moving mechanical parts, unprotected heights, and operating automotive equipment. Due to dexterity deficits and choreoathetosis, he has a greater need for a computer than the normally developing child and will, more likely than not, require an augmentative communication device to facilitate expressive language as well as provide more options for intelligible verbal communication. He will also likely require computer keyboard adaptations due to poor fine-motor dexterity.

As a consequence of his severe sensorineural hearing loss and continued communication deficits, he will have difficulty working in jobs that require extensive talking and/or public contact. He will require information to be presented visually as well as orally. Elias' ability to maintain attention and concentration for long periods of time will be dependent on medication efficacy and neuromaturation over time. Even with medication, he will likely require accommodations for understanding/memory, social interaction, sustained concentration/persistence, and adaptation. The effect of any kernicterus-related adjustment disorders on educational/personal achievement cannot be specifically determined at this time.

Rehabilitation Plan

Ongoing evaluation of medication, attention deficits, psychoeducational status, and psychological issues is needed. Proactive medical, psychological, educational, and rehabilitation services as well as therapeutic modalities are recommended to maximize Elias' function and vocational/independent living success.

As Elias will be restricted in his choice of jobs, situational assessment and structured placement in trial work experiences that will enhance a positive self-concept as well as match his aptitudes, interests, values, and physical ability are recommended. Services of a transition counselor beginning between ages 14 and 16 years are also recommended.

Access to the Labor Market

Due to the combined effect of Elias' hearing, language, and physical deficits, he will not be capable of independently performing the types of positions his parents or extended family have performed. Consistent with current school accommodations, Elias will require a supported employment work environment. Supported employment is work in an integrated work setting for individuals who, because of their handicaps, need ongoing support services such as a job coach, employer support, specialized instructions, and/or other job modifications/technology to facilitate success. Supported employment success is contingent upon the results of proactive case management and a compatible job coach/employer-match, as well as provision of appropriate vocational rehabilitation services.

Placeability

Given the nature of his injury as well as his age, Elias will benefit from a specialized vocational assessment to provide guidance with respect to post high school career planning. Physical capacity should be addressed through a functional capacity evaluation. Elias will require assistance with career skills preparation, problem solving/planning, school/work accommodations, compensatory work strategies, and selective job placement with follow-up during periods of transition/career changes.

Earnings Capacity

Pre-Incident Opinion

Based on parental and family education/work history, it is likely that Elias, absent his injuries, would have, at the least, graduated from high school. The greatest probability of vocational outcome, assuming a high school education and no injury, would have been for Elias to become employed in service, construction, or transportation/material-moving occupations (U.S. Census Bureau, 2022a, Table 2). Per the Bureau of Labor Statistics, career fields that are projected to have the most openings include construction/installation, maintenance/repair, transportation, healthcare and protective services, healthcare/personal care, office/administrative support, production and sales/transportation (U.S. Bureau of Labor Statistics, 2022f). Individuals with a high school education without additional training are most likely employed as janitors and cleaners, food preparation workers, fast-foods workers, food servers, construction laborers, and material-moving workers (U.S. Bureau of Labor Statistics, 2022g; U.S. Census Bureau, 2022a) with entry wages of $8.09 to $10.50 per hour and median wages of $11.18 to $15.24 per hour (North Carolina Department of Commerce, 2022). With on-the-job or career technical education, jobs such as cook, carpenter, electrician, truck driver, and police officer are most prevalent (median wage: $12.36 to $22.39 per hour). Experienced electricians earn $29.91 per hour, police/sheriff's patrol officers, $32.34 per hour and tractor-trailer truck drivers, $32.43 per hour (North Carolina

Department of Commerce, 2022). Per the American Community Survey (Expectancy Data, 2019), the median wage for a male high school graduate (age 18 to 24) is $24,425; for a male with less than one-year college, $25,280; and for an associate degree, $30,044.

Post-Incident Opinion

Elias will likely graduate from high school with an occupational diploma (Note: An occupational diploma follows an Occupational Course of Study (OCS) that is intended to meet the needs of a select and specified group of students with disabilities who need a modified curriculum that focuses on post-school employment and independent living). The focus of an OCS is to prepare students with disabilities to go directly into employment with marketable skills or to attend a postsecondary education program resulting in licensure or credential upon graduation from high school (www.dpsnc.net/Page/265#:~:text=The%20Occupational%20Course%20of%20Study,funded%20Systems%20Change%20Transition%20Project). Supported employment in an integrated work setting utilizing a job coach/natural supports is the most likely placement option for Elias. Activities that develop Elias' personal strengths will be a key element to his success. Post high school, specific skills training is highly recommended as this will be the most significant factor in achieving sustained employment for Elias. For example, a three course series in records management, payroll, and bookkeeping is offered through the Catawba Valley Community College (CCVC) Workforce Development Innovation Center (total cost ranges from $1,395 to $1,795).

Based on 2020–2021 data from the state VR program in Elias' state of residence, for consumers with deafness and cerebral palsy, the average amount in VR service expenditures per intervention (e.g., work adjustment, job coaching, supported employment) to achieve competitive integrated employment was $20,413 per individual. For the time period July 2020–July 2021, the average hourly earnings for VR consumers at case closure was $9.17 per hour, and the consumers worked an average of 19.8 hours per week for an average weekly wage of about $182.

Labor Force Participation

Elias' EC will be diminished due to lowered productivity, endurance, and need for adaptations such as a part-time work schedule. Even with rehabilitation assistance, skill, or specialized training and workplace accommodation/personal assistance, Elias will likely require additional time to find suitable employment. Although he will likely be able to participate in a supported employment work environment on at least a part-time basis, he will require rehabilitation counseling, selective placement, adaptive equipment, and job accommodations to secure and maintain employment.

Due to his physical deficits, Elias' options for competitiveness, lateral mobility, and upward mobility have been restricted. Elias will not enjoy the same pre-injury opportunities for advancement, nor the same age-earning cycle. In addition, as he ages, functional limitations due to cerebral palsy will become more pronounced and may necessitate an earlier exit (retirement) from the labor market than pre-injury. A loss of work life expectancy is expected but cannot reasonably be measured at this time.

Conclusion

This chapter includes a "story within a story" that not only defines and describes what is a RC, but also the role of the RC in life care planning and in providing a LOEC opinion. As an integral part of the life care planning team, the RC is part of the continuum of care that addresses an evaluee's overall health and well-being across their lifespan, with a focus on providing vocationally-related recommendations. The chapter identifies the value added to a life care plan by a RC that includes vocational recommendations related to vocational (work) activities, avocational activities, and/or productive activities as part of life care planning over the lifespan. Similar to the *Standards of Practice for Life Care Planners* (IARP, 2022) that require life care planners to establish a foundation for recommendations included in a life care plan, RCs must also establish a foundation for including vocational recommendations in a life care plan and/or providing a LOEC opinion that supports the evaluee's goals for optimum functioning over their lifetime. The chapter describes two vocational methodologies for determining loss of wages for both adult and pediatric evaluees (RAPEL for adults and PEEDS-RAPEL© for pediatrics). Through a "real world" case example, the role of the RC in life care planning is illustrated. A comprehensive list of relevant resources is also provided.

Example Online Resources

Clinical Practice Guidelines by Select Diagnostic Groups that Contain VR Recommendations

Amputation

U.S. Department of Veterans Affairs, Department of Defense. (2017). VA/DoD clinical practice guideline for rehabilitation of individuals with lower limb amputation. www.healthquality.va.gov/guidelines/Rehab/amp/VADoDLLACPG092817.pdf

U.S. Department of Veterans Affairs, Department of Defense. (2022). VA/DoD clinical practice guideline for the management of upper limb amputation rehabilitation. www.healthquality.va.gov/guidelines/Rehab/ULA/VADoDULACPG_Final_508.pdf

Back Pain

Verbeek, J. H. (2001). Vocational rehabilitation of workers with back pain. *Scandinavian Journal of Work, Environment & Health, 27*(5), 346–352. www.jstor.org/stable/40958861

U.S. Department of Veterans Affairs, Department of Defense. (2022). VA/DoD clinical practice guideline for the diagnosis and treatment of low back pain. www.healthquality.va.gov/guidelines/Pain/lbp/VADoDLBPCPGFinal508.pdf

U.S. Department of Veterans Affairs, Department of Defense. (2022). VA/DoD clinical practice guideline for the use of opioids in the management of chronic pain. www.healthquality.va.gov/guidelines/Pain/cot/VADoDOpioidsCPG.pdf

Mental Health

Au, D. W. H., Tsang, H. W. H., So, W. W. Y., Bell, M. D., Cheung, V., Yiu, M. G. C., Tam, K. L., & Lee, T-H. (2015). Effects of integrated supported employment plus cognitive remediation training for people with schizophrenia and schizoaffective disorders. *Schizophrenia Research, 166*, 297–303.

Carmona, V. R., Gómez-Benito, J., Huedo-Medina, T. B., & Rojo, J. E. (2017). Employment outcomes for people with schizophrenia spectrum disorder: A meta-analysis of randomized trials. *International Journal of Occupational Medicine and Environmental Health, 30*(3), 345–366. https://doi.org/10.13075/ijomeh.1896.01074

Carmona, V. R., Gómez-Benito, J., & Rojo-Rodes, J. E. (2019). Employment support needs of people with schizophrenia: A scoping study. *Journal of Occupational Rehabilitation, 29*, 1–10.

Fischler, I., Riahi, S., Stuckey, M. I., & Klassen, P. E. (2016). Implementation of a clinical practice guideline for schizophrenia in a specialist mental health center: An observational study. *BMC Health Services Research, 16*, 372–83. https://doi.org/10.1186/s12913-016-1618-9

Hanisch, S. E., Wrynne, C., & Weigel, M. (2017). Perceived and actual barriers to work for people with mental illness. *Journal of Vocational Rehabilitation, 46*, 19–30.

Lockett, H., Waghorn, G., & Kydd, R. (2018). A framework for improving the effectiveness of evidence-based practices in vocational rehabilitation. *Journal of Vocational Rehabilitation, 49*(1), 15–31. https://doi.org/10.3233/JVR-180951

Strassnig, M., Cornacchio, D., Harvey, P. D., Kotov, R., Fochtmann, L, & Bromet, E. J. (2017). Health status and mobility limitations are associated with residential and employment status in schizophrenia and bipolar disorder. *Journal of Psychiatric Research, 94*, 180–185.

Strassnig, M., Kotov, R., Fochtmann, L., Kalin, M., Bromet, E. J., & Harvey, P. D. (2018). Associations of independent living and labor force participation with impairment indicators in schizophrenia and bipolar disorder at 20-year follow-up. *Schizophrenia Research, 197*, 150–155.

U.S. Department of Veterans Affairs, Department of Defense. (2017). VA/DoD clinical practice guideline for the management of posttraumatic stress disorder and acute stress disorder. www.healthquality.va.gov/guidelines/MH/ptsd/VADoDPTSDCPGFinal012418.pdf

Spinal Cord Injury

Consortium for Spinal Cord Medicine. (1999). *Outcomes following traumatic spinal cord injury: Clinical practice guidelines for health care professionals*. Paralyzed Veterans of America.

Traumatic Brain Injury

Gerber, L., Deshpande, R., Moosvi, A., Zafonte, R., Bushnik, T., Garfinkel, S.A., & Cai, C. (2021). Narrative review of clinical practice guidelines for treating people with moderate or severe traumatic brain injury. *Neurorehabilitation 48*(4), 1–17. https://doi.org/10.3233/NRE-210024

MacDonald, S., & Shumway, E. (2016). *Practice standards and guidelines for acquired cognitive-communication disorders*. College of Audiologists and Speech-Language Pathologists of Ontario. www.researchgate.net/publication/290395866_Practice_Standards_and_Guidelines_for_Acquired_Cognitive-Communication_Disorders

Marshall, S., Bayley, M., McCullagh, S., Velikonja, D., Berrigan, L., Ouchterlony, D., & Weegar, K. (2015). Updated clinical practice guidelines for concussion/mild traumatic brain injury and persistent symptoms. *Brain Injury, 29*(6), 688–700. www.researchgate.net/publication/280317242_Updated_clinical_practice_guidelines_for_concussionmild_traumatic_brain_injury_and_persistent_symptoms

Ontario Neurotrauma Institute. (2016). *Clinical practice guideline for the rehabilitation of adults with moderate to severe TBI*. https://braininjuryguidelines.org/modtosevere/fileadmin/Guidelines_components/Rec/Section_1_REC_complete_ENG_final.pdf

Stergiou-Kita, M., Dawson, D. R., & Rappolt, S. (2011). Inter-professional clinical practice guideline for vocational evaluation following traumatic brain injury: A systematic and evidence-based approach. *Journal of Occupational Rehabilitation, 22*(2), 166–8. https://doi.org/10.1007/s10926-011-9332-2

U.S. Department of Veterans Affairs, Department of Defense. (2019). VA/DoD clinical practice guidelines for the management of stroke rehabilitation. www.healthquality.va.gov/guidelines/Rehab/stroke/VADoDStrokeRehabCPGPocketCardFinal8292019.pdf

Education Related Websites

https://sites.ed.gov/idea/about-idea/#:~:text=The%20Individuals%20with%20Disabilities%20Education,related%20services%20to%20those%20children (IDEA provisions and other free appropriate education services for eligible school-age children)

https://www.adainfo.org/resources/international-center-disability-information-icdi-disability-tables/ (International Center for Disability Information at the West Virginia University, statistical information regarding individuals with disabilities according to state, national, and worldwide statistics) www2.ed.gov/about/offices/list/osers/index.html (Office of Special Education Programs, programs for children and youth with disabilities in two main areas: special education and vocational rehabilitation)

https://specialednews.com/sitemap/ (special education news)

www.504idea.org/ (The Council of Educators for Students with Disabilities, Inc., Section 504, and IDEA training and resources for educators)

https://ici.umn.edu/ (The National Center on Secondary Education and Transition [NCSET] coordinates national resources, technical assistance, and information related to secondary education and transition for youth with disabilities)

https://vcurrtc.org/ (Virginia Commonwealth University's Rehabilitation Research and Training Center provides information on a variety of programs for individuals with disabilities)

www.vcu.edu/rrtcweb/facts/jan98.html (Virginia Commonwealth University's Rehabilitation Research and Training Center research report: *Analysis of Transition Plans for Students with Significant Disabilities*)

General Interest Websites

www.apse.org/ (Association of People Supporting Employment First, integrated employment and career advancement opportunities for individuals with disabilities)

www.biausa.org (Brain Injury Association of America with list of state and regional chapters)

www.easterseals.com/ (Easter Seals Disability Services providing services, education, outreach, and advocacy for people living with autism and other disabilities)

https://eric.ed.gov/ (Education Resources Information Center, database of education research and information)

www.epmagazine.com/ (Exceptional Parent, resources for the special needs community, including access to the online *Exceptional Parent* magazine)

https://www.caregiveraction.org/?gclid=Cj0KCQjwuNemBhCBARIsADp74QQF-NK4Hd7QYtCzu0QO_GYvOOEEq0HJMg3pzDIO9BlAM9NpnLN7E-caAq5EEALw_wcB (Family Caregiver Alliance provides information on assistive technology and rehabilitation equipment)

www.fcsn.org (Federation for Children with Special Needs providing information, support, and assistance to parents of children with disabilities)

www.integrationscatalog.com (Integrations, products for children with learning and sensory disabilities)

https://emedicine.medscape.com/ (Medscape, information on diseases and other topics regarding disabilities and medical conditions)

www.nacdd.org/ (National Association of Councils on Developmental Disabilities/ NACDD)

www.fhi360.org/projects/national-dissemination-center-children-disabilities-nichcy (National Dissemination Center for Children with Disabilities, including Center for Parent Information and Resources)

www.merckmanuals.com/professional (online *Merck Manual*)

www.schoolspecialty.com (School Specialty, products and brands in the educational resources market including educational technology and career technical products)

www.ucp.org/ (United Cerebral Palsy Association, information on cerebral palsy and advocacy for the rights of people with any disability)

Government-Related Employment Websites

Canadian

www.canada.ca/en/services/jobs/opportunities.html (Find a Job in Canada to include jobs in the federal government and with employers across Canada)

www.jobbank.gc.ca/home (Job Bank, Canada's national employment service and leading source of jobs and labor market information in Canada)

https://resources.workable.com/tutorial/best-job-sites-in-canada (List of the 10 best job sites in Canada including Indeed Canada, Glassdoor, Monster Canada, CareerBuilder Canada, and local job boards)

International

www.ilo.org/global/lang--en/index.htm (International Labour Organization, devoted to promoting social justice and internationally recognized human and labor rights)

United States

www.acinet.org (America's Career InfoNet is transitioning to CareerOneStop sponsored by the U.S. Department of Labor, Employment and Training Administration)

www.Jobbankinfo.org (A part of CareerOneStop, provides individual state job banks, private-sector job banks and portal Web sites related to employment)

www.careeronestop.org/Toolkit/ACINet.aspx (CareerOneStop, database for career exploration, training, and job information)

www.usa.gov/statistics (demographic and economic data, population, maps, and information about the 2020 U.S. Census)

https://askjan.org/ (Job Accommodation Network, workplace productivity enhancements, reasonable accommodation solutions, and Americans with Disabilities Act information)

www.naceweb.org/ (National Association of Colleges and Employers, quantitative research; forecasting hiring trends in the job market; tracking starting salaries of recent college graduates. See Press Room link for releases on college graduate earnings)

http://nces.ed.gov/ (National Center for Educational Statistics)

www.bls.gov/ooh/ (*Occupational Outlook Handbook*, U.S. Bureau of Labor Statistics, information on various occupations in the U.S. economy)

www.bls.gov/ors/ (Occupational Requirements Survey, U.S. Bureau of Labor Statistics, job-related information regarding physical demands; environmental conditions; education, training, experience; cognitive and mental requirements for jobs in the U.S. economy)

www.doleta.gov/programs/onet (*O*NET*, U.S. Department of Labor Occupational Information Network, occupational requirements and worker attributes including knowledge, skills, abilities, tasks, work activities, and other descriptors of various occupations)

www.onetcenter.org/overview.html (O*NET Resource Center contains hundreds of standardized and occupation-specific descriptors on almost 1,000 occupations covering the entire U.S. economy)

www.ssa.gov/ (Social Security Administration Home Page, includes links to information on Social Security Disability Income/SSDI)

www.trninc.com/ (Training Resource Network provides resources on the full inclusion of persons with disabilities in their communities)

www.bls.gov/ (U.S. Bureau of Labor Statistics measures labor market activity, working conditions, price changes, and productivity in the U.S. economy)

www.census.gov/ (U.S. Census Bureau, data on the U.S. and its economy)

www.dol.gov/ (U.S. Department of Labor, data about the U.S. labor trends)

www.dol.gov/odep/ (U.S. Department of Labor Office of Disability Employment Policy, policies and coordination with employers and government to increase workplace success for people with disabilities)

www.uspublishing.net/catalog/ (U.S. Publishing Occupational Statistics publishes occupational statistics by state with analysis by unskilled, semi-skilled, and skilled employment by occupation)

Job Listing and Salary Comparison Websites

Economic Research Institute, www.erieri.com/ (salary surveys and cost-of-living information)
Glassdoor.com, www.glassdoor.com/
Indeed.com, www.indeed.com/
JobStar Guide to Salaries, http://jobstar.org/tools/salary/index.php
LinkedIn, www.linkedin.com/
Monster.com, www.monster.com/
Payscale.com, www.payscale.com/
Salary.com, www.salary.com/

Print Resources Including Evidence-Based Vocational Rehabilitation Articles

Dillman, E. G., Field, T. F., Horner, S., Slesnik, F., & Weed, R. O. (2002). *Approaches to estimating lost earnings: Strategies for the rehabilitation consultant.* Elliott & Fitzpatrick, Inc.

Farr, J. M., & Shatkin, L. (Eds.). (1998). The *O*NET dictionary of occupational titles.* JistWorks.

Field, J. E., & Field, T. F. (2004). *The transitional classification of jobs: A bridge between the Dictionary of Occupational Titles and the O*NET database* (6th ed.). Elliott & Fitzpatrick, Inc.

Havranek, J., Field, T., & Grimes, J. W. (2001). *Vocational assessment: Estimating employment potential.* E & F Vocational Services.

Leahy, M. J., Del Valle, R., Landon, T. J. Iwanaga, K., & Sherman, S. (2018). Promising and evidence-based practices in vocational rehabilitation: Results of a national Delphi study. *Journal of Rehabilitation*, 48, 37–48. https://doi.org/10.3233/JVR-170914

Lockett, H., Waghor, G., & Kydd, R., (2018). A framework for improving the effectiveness of evidence-based practices in vocational rehabilitation. *Journal of Vocational Rehabilitation*, 49, 15–31. https://doi.org/10.3233/JVR-180951

Office of Hearings and Appeals, Social Security Administration. (2003). *Vocational expert handbook* (2nd ed.). Social Security Administration.

Robinson, R. H. (Ed.). (2014). *Foundations of forensic vocational rehabilitation.* Springer. Publishing Company.

Sherman, S., Del Valle, R., Chan, F., Landon, T. J., & Leahy, M. J. (2018). Contemporary perceptions of evidence-based practices in rehabilitation counseling. *Journal of Rehabilitation*, 84(4), 4–12.

U.S. Department of Labor. (1991a). *Dictionary of occupational titles* (4th ed.). U.S. Government Printing Office.

U.S. Department of Labor. (1992). *Revised handbook for analyzing jobs.* U.S. Government Printing Office.

U.S. Department of Labor. (1993). *Guide for occupational exploration.* U.S. Government Printing Office.

U.S. Department of Labor. (1998). *Standard occupational classification.* U.S. Government Printing Office.

U.S. Department of Labor. (2007). *Employment and earnings.* Bureau of Labor Statistics. U.S. Government Printing Office.

U.S. Department of Labor. (2022). *The occupational outlook handbook.* U.S. Government Printing Office.

Weed, R. O., & Berens, D. E. (Eds.). (2018). *Life care planning and case management handbook* (4th ed.). Routledge.

Weed, R., & Field, T. (2012). *The rehabilitation consultant's handbook* (4th ed.). Elliott & Fitzpatrick, Inc.

Vocationally-Related Computer Software Applications *LifeStep© Software* (Version 5.0). (1998), www.datapeoplethings.com/LifeStep.html

McCroskey Vocational Quotient System, 2009 (MVQS2009), Version 9.0 (2009) and other computer products, https://mccroskeymvqs.com/

SkillTran, LLC to include Occubrowse, Job Browser Pro, OASYS© and other information on work decisions, www.skilltran.com

Voc Rehab, Inc. to include WebTSA™, and Career A.I., www.vocrehab.com

References

Albin, A. (2015). *Children more likely to succeed academically if parents believe they're college bound.* www.universityofcalifornia.edu/news/children-more-likely-succeed-academically-if-parents-believe-theyre-college-bound

American Board of Vocational Experts. (2020). *Code of ethics.* https://abve.net/wp-content/uploads/2020/08/ABVE_Code_of_Ethics_2020.pdf

American Board of Vocational Experts. (2022a, September 16). *Core competencies.* https://abve.net/fellow-diplomate-certification/. Paras 1–3.

Anderson, C. A., Bowman, M. J., & Tinto, V. (1972). *Where colleges are and who attends: Effects of accessibility on college attendance.* McGraw-Hill.

Association of People Supporting Employment First. (2021). *Trends and current status of 14(c)*. https://apse.org/wp-content/uploads/2021/10/10_20_21-APSE-14c-Update-REV.pdf

Barros-Bailey, M. (2012). The 12-step labor market survey methodology in practice: A case example. *The Rehabilitation Professional, 20*(1), 1–10.

Barros-Bailey, M. (2014). History of forensic vocational consulting. In R. Robinson (Ed.), *Foundations of forensic vocational rehabilitation* (pp. 13–31). Springer Publications.

Barros-Bailey, M. (2018). An evidence source model for clinical and forensic practice. *The Rehabilitation Professional, 26*(3), 117–128.

Barros-Bailey, M., & Neulicht, A. T. (2005). Opinion Validity©: An integration of quantitative and qualitative data. *The Rehabilitation Professional, 13*(2), 33–42.

Bast, S., Williams, J. M., & Dunn, P. L. (2002). The classic model of transferability of work skills: Issues affecting the accurate assessment of future vocational options in earnings capacity assessment. *Journal of Forensic Vocational Assessment, 51*, 15–28.

Benzeval, M., Green, M. J., & Macintyre, S. (2013). Does perceived physical attractiveness in adolescence predict better socioeconomic position in adulthood? Evidence from 20 years of follow up in a population cohort study. *PLoS ONE, 8*(5), e63975. https://doi.org/10.1371/journal.pone.0063975

Berens, D. E. (2023). Disability, ableism, and ageism. In D. G. Hays & B. T. Erford (Eds.). *Developing multicultural counseling competence* (4th ed., pp. 267–300). Pearson Education, Inc.

Berens, D. E., & Weed, R. O. (2018). The role of the vocational counselor in life care planning. In R. O. Weed & D. E. Berens (Eds.), *Life care planning and case management handbook* (4th ed., pp. 41–61). Routledge.

Blackwell, T. L. (1991). *The vocational expert primer*. Elliott & Fitzpatrick.

Boyd, D., & Toppino, D. (1995). The forensic vocational expert's approach to wage loss analysis. *NARPPS Journal and News, 103*, 95–102.

Brody, N. (1997). Intelligence, schooling and society. *American Psychologist, 52*(10), 1046–1050.

Bronfenbrenner, U. (1977). Toward an experimental ecology of human development. *American Psychologist, 32*(7), 513–531. https://doi.org/10.1037/0003-066X.32.7.513

Carnevale, A. P., Cheah, B., & Hanson, A. R. (2015). *The economic value of college majors*. Georgetown University Center on Education and the Workforce. https://cew.georgetown.edu/wp-content/uploads/The-Economic-Value-of-College-Majors-Full-Report-web-FINAL.pdf

Carnevale, A. P., Cheah, B., & Wenzinger, E. (2021). *The college payoff: More education doesn't always mean more earnings*. Georgetown University Center on Education and the Workforce. https://cew.georgetown.edu/cew-reports/collegepayoff2021/

Ceci, S. J., & Williams, W. M. (1997). Schooling, intelligence, and income. *American Psychologist, 52*(10), 1051–1058.

Centers for Disease Control. (2015). *Productive aging and work*. www.cdc.gov/niosh/topics/productiveaging/safetyandhealth.html

Centers for Disease Control. (2020). *Disability impacts all of us*. www.cdc.gov/ncbddd/disabilityandhealth/infographic-disability-impacts-all.html

Chen, L. J. (2019). Special education transition issues over the past 60 years: Social network analysis on Web of Science exploration. *European Journal of Special Needs Education, 34*(1), 1–19. https://doi.org/10.1080/08856257.2017.1413805

Clearinghouse for Military Family Readiness at Penn State. (2020). *Parents' educational levels influence on child educational outcomes: Rapid literature review*. https://militaryfamilies.psu.edu/wp-content/uploads/2020/01/Parents-Educational-Levels-Influence-on-Child-Educational-Outcomes.20Jan06.final_.pdf

Cohen, M. D., & Yanklowski, T. P. (1997). Methodologies to improve economic and vocational analysis in personal injury litigation. *Litigation Economics Digest, 22*, 126–135.

College of Vocational Rehabilitation Professionals. (2022a, September 16). *History*. https://cvrp.net/wp-content/uploads/105-CVRP-History-2.pdf

College of Vocational Rehabilitation Professionals. (2022b, September 16). *Certified vocational rehabilitation professional (CVRP) scope of practice*. https://cvrp.net/our-credentials/cvrp/?lang=usa

Commission on Rehabilitation Counselor Certification. (2009). *Code of professional ethics for vocational evaluation specialists, work adjustment specialists, and career assessment associates*.

Commission on Rehabilitation Counselor Certification. (2022a, September 16). *About us: What is a rehabilitation counselor?* https://crccertification.com/about-crcc/

Commission on Rehabilitation Counselor Certification. (2022b, September 16). *About us: What is the history of CRC?* https://crccertification.com/about-crcc/

Commission on Rehabilitation Counselor Certification. (2022c, September 16). *Scope of practice statement.* https://crccertification.com/scope-of-practice/

Commission on Rehabilitation Counselor Certification. (2022d, September 16). *Scope of practice statement.* https://crccertification.com/scope-of-practice/

Commission on Rehabilitation Counselor Certification. (2022e, September 16). *Exam overview.* https://crccertification.com/get-certified/crc-exam-overview/

Commission on Rehabilitation Counselor Certification. (2022f, September 16). *Get certified.* https://crccertification.com/cve-get-certified/

Commission on Rehabilitation Counselor Certification. (2023). *Code of ethics for certified rehabilitation counselors.* https://crccertification.com/wp-content/uploads/2023/01/2023-Code-of-Ethics-1.pdf

Council for the Accreditation of Counseling and Related Educational Programs. (2022, September 16). *Standards revision committee news: Committee charge.* www.cacrep.org/SRC-2023/

Council for the Accreditation of Counseling and Related Educational Programs. (2023). https://www.cacrep.org/wp-content/uploads/2023/06/2024-Standards-Combined-Version-6.27.23.pdf

Curry, J. R., & Milsom, A. (2022). *Career and college readiness counseling in P-12 schools* (3rd ed.). Springer Publishing Company.

Davis-Kean, P. E., Tang, S., & Waters, N. E. (2019). Parent education attainment and parenting. In M. H. Bornstein (Ed.), *Handbook of parenting: Biology and ecology of parenting* (pp. 400–420). Routledge/Taylor & Francis Group, https://doi.org/10.4324/9780429401459-12

Deming, L. (2006). Bilirubin encephalopathy/kernicterus and the newborn infant: Implications for life care planning. *Journal of Life Care Planning, 4*(4), 205–218.

Deutsch, P. M., & Sawyer, H. W. (1985 with updates through 1994). *A guide to rehabilitation, Volumes 1 & 2.* Matthew Bender.

Deutsch, P. M., & Sawyer, H. W. (1995 with updates through 2003). *A guide to rehabilitation, Volumes 1, 2 & 3.* AHAB Press.

Deutsch, P. M., & Sawyer, H. W. (2005). *A guide to rehabilitation.* AHAB Press.

Deutsch, P., & Raffa, F. (1982). *Damages in tort actions* (Vol. 8). Matthew Bender.

Dillman, E. (1987). The necessary economic and vocational interface in personal injury cases. *Journal of Private Sector Rehabilitation, 23,* 121–142.

Dowd, L. R. (Ed.). (1993). *Glossary of terminology for vocational assessment, evaluation and work adjustment.* University of Wisconsin–Stout.

Dunn, P. L., & Growick, B. S. (2000). Transferable skills analysis in vocational rehabilitation: Historical foundations, current status and future trends. *Journal of Vocational Rehabilitation, 14,* 79–87.

Evers, A., & Sieverding, M. (2013). Why do highly qualified women (still) earn less? Gender differences in long-term predictors of career success. *Psychology of Women Quarterly, 38*(1), 93–106. https://doi.org/10.1177/0361684313498071

Expectancy Data. (2019). *Full time earnings in the United States: American Community Survey Analysis* (2017 ed.). https://www.expectancydata.com/

Fair Labor Standards Amendments of 1986 (Pub. L. 99-486, 100 Stat. 1229). U.S. Government Printing Office, www.ecfr.gov/current/title-29/subtitle-B/chapter-V/subchapter-A/part-525

Farley, R. (1996). *The American family: Who we are, how we got there, where are we going?* Russell Sage Foundation.

Field, J. E., & Field, T. F. (2004). *The transitional classification of jobs: A bridge between the Dictionary of Occupational Titles and the O*NET database* (6th ed.). Elliott & Fitzpatrick, Inc.

Field, T. F. (1999). *Strategies for the rehabilitation consultant: Transferability, loss of employment, lost earning capacity and damages* (Rev. ed.). Elliott & Fitzpatrick, Inc.

Field, T. F. (2002). The importance of vocational rehabilitation in life care planning. *Journal of Life Care Planning, 1*(3), 195–202.

Fong, F., Strauser, D. R., & Tansey T. N. (2019). *Assessment in rehabilitation and mental health counseling.* Springer Publishing Company.

Giannantonio, C. M., & Hurley-Hanson, A. E. (2006). Applying image norms across Super's career development stages. *The Career Development Quarterly*, *54*(4), 318 – 330.

Gill, A. M., & Foley, J. (1996). Predicting educational attainment for a minor child: Some further evidence. *Journal of Forensic Economics*, *92*, 101–112.

Ginzberg, E., Ginsburg, S. W., Alexrod, S., & Herma, J. L. (1951). *Occupational choice: An approach to general theory*. Columbia University Press.

Gvozdenodic, V. (2013). Beauty and wages: The effect of physical attractiveness on income using longitudinal data. [Honors Thesis, Pforzheimer Honors College, Pace University] https://digitalcommons.pace.edu/cgi/viewcontent.cgi?article=1135&context=honorscollege_theses

Halstrom, F. N. (1995). Proving partial loss of earning capacity. *Trial*, *31*(10), 70–72.

Hamermesh, D. S., & Biddle, J. E. (1993). Beauty and the labor market. *American Economic Review*, *84*, 1174–1194.

Hamilton, B., & Vessey, J. (1992). Pediatric discharge planning. *Pediatric Nursing*, *185*, 475–478.

Hillis, R., Brenner, M, Larkin, P. J. Cawley, D., & Connolly M. (2016). The role of care coordinator for children with complex care needs: A systematic review. *International Journal of Integrated Care*, *16*(2), 1 – 18. http://doi.org/10.5334/ijic.2250

Horner, S. M., & Slesnick, F. (1999). The valuation of earning capacity definition, measurement and evidence. *Journal of Forensic Economics*, *12*(1), 13–32.

Hout, M. (1984). Status, autonomy, and training in occupational mobility. *American Journal of Sociology*, *89*, 1379–1409. https://apse.org/wp-content/uploads/2021/10/10_20_21-APSE-14c-Update-REV.pdf

Icardi, R. (2021). Returns to workplace training for male and female employees and implications for the gender wage gap: A quantile regression analysis. *International Journal for Research in Vocational Education and Training*, *8*(1), 21–45.

Individuals with Disabilities Education Act, Pub. L. No. 101–476 (1990, amended 1997, 2004). U.S. Government Printing Office.

International Association of Rehabilitation Professionals. (2022). *Standards of practice for life care planners* (4th ed.). https://cdn.ymaws.com/rehabpro.org/resource/collection/D5B16132-B4BE-4918-BA5A-1BABE8C2E1A4/SOP4_101122.pdf

International Classification of Function. (2017). *ICF core sets for vocational rehabilitation*. www.icf-research-branch.org/icf-core-sets-projects2/diverse-situations/icf-core-sets-for-vocational-rehabilitation

Irwin, V., Zhang, J., Wang, X., Hein, S., Wang, K., Roberts, A., York, C., Barmer, A., Bullock Mann, F., Dilig, R., & Parker, S. (2021). *Report on the condition of education 2021* (NCES 2021-144). U.S. Department of Education. https://nces.ed.gov/pubs2021/2021144.pdf

Isom, R., Barton, T. R., & Holloway, L. (2001). Pediatric earning capacity: Developing a defensible estimate of pre-morbid earnings. *Journal of Forensic Vocational Analysis*, *4*, 21–28.

Jin, J., & Rounds, J. (2012). Stability and change in work values: A meta-analysis of longitudinal studies. *Journal of Vocational Behavior*, *80*, 326–339.

Johnson, L. E., Ley, R. D., & Benshoof, P. T. (1993). Estimating economic loss for a facially disfigured minor: A case study. *Journal of Legal Economics*, *3*(2), 1–9.

Kane, J., & Spizman, L. (2001). An update of the educational attainment model for a minor child. *Journal of Forensic Economics*, *14*(2), 155–166.

Kane, J., Spizman, L., & Donelson, D. (2013). Educational attainment model for a minor child: The next generation. *Journal of Forensic Economics*, *24*(2), 175–190. http://www.jstor.org/stable/42756168

Katz, I. M., Rudolph, C. W., & Zacher, H. (2019). Age and career commitment: Meta-analytic tests of competing linear versus curvilinear relationships. *Journal of Vocational Behavior*, *112*, 396–416.

King, G., Cathers, T., King, S., & Rosenbaum, P. (2001). Major elements of parents' satisfaction and dissatisfaction with pediatric rehabilitation services. *Children's Health Care*, *303*, 111–125.

Kirby, A. V., Dell'Armo, K. D., & Persch, A. C. (2019). Differences in youth and parent postsecondary expectations for youth with disabilities. *Journal of Vocational Rehabilitation*, *51*, 77–86.

Kooig, D. T. A. M., Del Lange, A. H., Jansen, P. G., Kanfer, R., & Dikkers, J. S. E. (2011). Age and work-related motives: Results of a meta-analysis. *Journal of Organizational Behavior*, *32*, 197–225. https://doi.org/10.1002/job.665

Leslie, T. P. (2018). Determining the loss of earning capacity in pediatric or young adult cases. *Journal of Forensic Vocational Analysis*, *18*(1), 25–31.

Maki, D. R. (1986). Foundations of applied rehabilitation counseling. In T. F. Rigger, D. R. Maki, & A. W. Wolf (Eds.), *Applied rehabilitation counseling*. Springer Publishing Company.

Maki, D. R., McCracken, N., Pape, D. A., & Scofield, M. E. (1978). The theoretical model of vocational rehabilitation. *Journal of Rehabilitation*, *44*(4), 26–28.

Mare, R. D. (2000). *Assortative mating, intergenerational mobility, and educational inequality* (Working Paper CCPR 004–00). http://papers.ccpr.ucla.edu/index.php/pwp/article/view/1015/397

Martin, G., & Weinstein, M. A. (Eds.). (2012). *Determining economic damages*. James Publishing.

McCaigue, I. S. (2004). The role of the occupational therapist in life care planning. In R. O. Weed (Ed.), *Life care planning and case management handbook* (2nd ed., pp. 77–113). CRC Press.

McCray, P. M. (1982). *Vocational evaluation and assessment in school settings*. University of Wisconsin-Stout Materials Development Center.

Medina, L. D., Sabo, S., & Vespa, J. (2020). Living longer: Historical and projected life expectancy in the United States, 1960 to 2060. *Current Population Reports*, P25–1145. www.census.gov/content/dam/Census/library/publications/2020/demo/p25-1145.pdf

Mertes, A., & Harden, T. (2019). What life care planners need to know about the professional discipline of rehabilitation counselors. *Journal of Life Care Planning*, *17*(1), 39–44.

Momsen, A. H., Stapelfeldt, C. M., Rosbjerg, R., Escorpizo, R., Labriola, M., & Bjerrum, M. (2019). International classification of functioning, disability, and health in vocational rehabilitation: A scoping review of the state of the field. *Journal of Occupational Rehabilitation*, *29*(2), 241–273. https://link.springer.com/article/10.1007/s10926-018-9788-4

National Center for Education Statistics. (2022a, January 12). *Students are more likely to attend college if they believe family can afford to pay*. [Press Release] https://nces.ed.gov/whatsnew/press_releases/1_12_2022.asp

National Center for Education Statistics. (2022d. September 16). *Digest of education statistics*. http://nces.ed.gov/programs/digest/

National Center for Educational Statistics. (2001). *Special analysis 2001—Students whose parents did not go to college: Post-secondary access, persistence and attainment*. https://nces.ed.gov/pubs2001/2001126.pdf

National Center for Educational Statistics. (2022b, September 16). *Fast facts: Educational attainment*. https://nces.ed.gov/fastfacts/display.asp?id=27

National Center for Educational Statistics. (2022c, September 16). *Educational attainment of young adults*. https://nces.ed.gov/programs/coe/indicator/caa

National Institute on Aging. (2017). *Supporting older patients with chronic conditions*. www.nia.nih.gov/health/supporting-older-patients-chronic-conditions

Neulicht, A. T. (2006). The life care plan RACE: Review, analysis, critique, evaluation? *Journal of Life Care Planning*, *5*(3), 91–98.

Neulicht, A. T., & Berens, D. E. (2004). The role of vocational consultant. In S. Riddick-Grisham (Ed.), *Pediatric Life Care Planning and Case Management* (pp. 277–324). CRC Press.

Neulicht, A. T., & Berens, D. E. (2005). PEEDS-RAPEL©: A case conceptualization model for evaluating pediatric cases. *Journal of Life Care Planning*, *4*(1), 27–36.

Neulicht, A. T., & Berens, D. E. (2011). The role of vocational rehabilitation consultant in life care planning. In S. Riddick-Grisham & L. M. Deming (Eds.), *Pediatric life care planning and case management* (2nd ed., pp. 275–318). CRC Press.

Neulicht, A. T., & Berens, D. E. (2015). A case conceptualization model for evaluating pediatric cases with acquired brain injury. *Neurorehabilitation*, *36*(3), 275 – 287.

Neulicht, A. T., & Costantini, P. A. (2002). The vocational expert's role in establishing damages. *Journal of Legal Nurse Consulting*, *133*, 3–10.

Neulicht, A. T., Gann, C., Berg, J. F., & Taylor, R. H. (2007). Labor market search: Utilization of labor market research and employer sampling by vocational experts. *The Rehabilitation Professional*, *15*(4), 29–44.

Ng, T. W. H., & Feldman, D. C. (2012). Evaluating six common stereotypes about older workers with meta-analytical data. *Personnel Psychology*, *65*, 821–858.

Nichols, L. O., & Martindale-Adams, J. (2020). *Interventions for parent caregivers of injured military/veteran personnel*. U.S. Department of Defense: Defense Technical Information Center. https://apps.dtic.mil/sti/citations/AD1108429

North Carolina Department of Commerce Demand Driven Data Delivery. (2022, September 16). *Occupational employment and wages in North Carolina* (OEWS). https://d4.nccommerce.com/OESSelection.aspx

O*NET On-line. (n.d.). *Summary report for: 21-1015.00—Rehabilitation counselors*. http://online.onetcenter.org/link/summary/21-1015.00

Okie, S. (2006). Reconstructing lives—A tale of two soldiers. *New England Journal of Medicine*, 355(25), 2609–2615. www.nejm.org/doi/full/10.1056/NEJMp068235

Peterson, S. (2022). CACREP and the rehabilitation counseling profession. *The Rehabilitation Professional*, 30(2), 51–70.

Rehabilitation Act Amendments, Pub. L. No. 102-569 (1992). U.S. Government Printing Office.

Rehabilitation Act Amendments, Pub. L. No. 99-506 (1986). U.S. Government Printing Office.

Riddick-Grisham (Ed.). (2004). *Pediatric life care planning and case management* (pp. 277–324). CRC Press.

Robinson, R. H. (2014). Forensic rehabilitation and vocational earning capacity models. In R. Robinson (Ed.), *Foundations of forensic vocational rehabilitation* (pp. 33–62). Springer

Rubin, S. E., & Roessler, R. T. (2007). *Foundations of the vocational rehabilitation process* (6th ed.). PRO-ED.

Rusch, F. R., Schutz, R. P., & Agran, M. (1982). Validating entry-level survival skills for service occupations. *Journal of the Association for the Severely Disabled, 8,* 32–41.

Sapp, L. H., Remley, T. P., & Range, L.M. (2020). The validity of exploring educational and attainment levels and occupational skill and physical strength demand levels of caregivers when evaluating loss of earning capacity in pediatric cases. *The Rehabilitation Professional*, 28(1), 5 – 14.

Schiariti, V., Simeonsson, R. J., & Hall, K. (2021). Promoting developmental potential in early childhood: A global framework for health and education. *International Journal of Environmental Research and Public Health, 18,* 2007. https://doi.org/10.3390/ijerph18042007

Schonbrun, S. L., & Kampfe, C. M. (2008). Loss of earning capacity in pediatric cases. *Journal of Forensic Vocational Analysis, 11*(2), 7–15.

Shogren, K. A., & Plotner, A. J. (2012). Transition planning for students with intellectual disability, autism, or other disabilities: Data from the National Longitudinal Transition Study-2. *Intellectual and Developmental Disabilities*, 50(1), 16–30.

Smith, M., Togut, T., Wallace, D., & Myles, M. (2001). *Georgia Individuals with Disabilities Education Act*. Lorman Education Services.

Smith-Fess Act, Pub. L. No. 236 (1920). U.S. Government Printing Office.

Smith-Hughes Act. (1917). U.S. Government Printing Office.

Spizman, L. M., & Kane, J. (1992). Loss of future income in the case of personal injury of a child: Parental influence on a child's future earnings. *Journal of Forensic Economics*, 5(2), 159–168.

Spizman, L. M., & Kane, J. (2020). Update of educational attainment model for a minor child: Round 18 of National Longitudinal Survey of Youth/NLSY (1997). *Journal of Forensic Economics*, 29(1), 131–141. https://doi.org/10.5085/JFE-465

Stephenson, S. P., & Macpherson, D. A. (2021). *Determining economic damages*. James Publishing.

Sternberg, R. J., Grigoreno, E. L., & Bundy, D. A. (2003). The predictive value of IQ. *Merrill Palmer Quarterly*, 49(1), 1–41.

Strauser, D. R. (2020). *Career development, employment & disability in rehabilitation*. Springer Publishing Company.

Super, D. E. (1972). Vocational development theory: Persons, positions, and processes. In J. M. Whiteley & A. Resnikoff (Eds.), *Perspectives on vocational development*. American Personnel and Guidance Association.

Super, D. E., Starishesky, R., Matlin, N., & Jorday, J. P. (1963). *Career development: Self-concept therapy*. College Entrance Examination Board.

Szymanski, E. M. (1985). Rehabilitation counseling: A profession with a vision, an identity and a future. *Rehabilitation Counseling Bulletin, 29*, 2–5.

Taveira, M., Oliveira, I. M., & Araujo, A. M. (2016). Ecology of children's career development: A review of the literature. *Psicologica*, 32(4). https://www.scielo.br/j/ptp/a/sR6RShV9DsWYdFb6pHxkyZJ/?lang=pt

Tenth Institute on Rehabilitation Issues. (1972). *Vocational evaluation and work adjustment in vocational rehabilitation* (reprint series No. 8). University of Wisconsin-Stout Materials Development Center.

Tippins, N. T., & Hilton, M. L.(Eds.). (2010). A database for a changing economy: Review of the Occupational Information Network (O*NET). https://nap.nationalacademies.org/download/1281

Traumatic Brain Injury Center of Excellence (formerly called the Defense and Veterans Brain APA Injury Center). (2022, September 16). www.brainline.org/resource/defense-and-veterans-brain-injury-center-0

Turnbull, A., Turnbull, H. R., Francis, G. L., Burke, M. M., Kyzar, K. K., Haines, S., Gershwin, T., Shepherd, K., Holdren, N., & Singer, G. H. S. (2022). *Families and professionals: Trusting partnerships in general and special education* (8th ed.). Pearson Education.

Turnbull, A., Turnbull, H., Erwin, E., Soodak, L., & Shogren, K. (2014). *Families, professionals and exceptionality: Positive outcomes through partnerships and trust* (7th ed.). Pearson Education.

University of Chicago Network for College Success. (n.d.). *Supporting student identity: Genogram lesson plan and sample*. https://ncs.uchicago.edu/sites/ncs.uchicago.edu/files/uploads/tools/NCS_PS_Toolkit_E SF_Set_A_GenogramLessonPlan.pdf

U S. Bureau of Labor Statistics. (2022f, September 16). *Fast-growing occupations that pay well and don't require a college degree*. www.bls.gov/careeroutlook/2022/article/occupations-that-dont-require-a-degree.htm

U. S. Department of Labor. (1939). *Dictionary of occupational titles*. U.S. Government Printing Office.

U. S. Department of Labor. (1982). *A guide to job analysis*. Materials Development Center, University of Wisconsin–Stout. https://files.eric.ed.gov/fulltext/ED273802.pdf

U. S. Department of Labor. (1991a). *Revised handbook for analyzing jobs*. Government Printing Office.

U. S. Department of Labor. (1991b). *Dictionary of occupational titles* (4th ed.). U.S. Government Printing Office. www.dol.gov/agencies/oalj/topics/libraries/LIBDOT

U. S. Department of Labor. (2022). *The occupational outlook handbook*. U. S. Government Printing Office. www.bls.gov/ooh/

U.S. Bureau of Labor Statistics. (2014). *Workforce Innovation and Opportunity Act (WIOA), Pub. L. 113–128*. www.doleta.gov/WIOA/Docs/WIOA_Factsheets.pdf

U.S. Bureau of Labor Statistics. (2020, September 22). *Employee tenure in 2020*. [News Release]. www.bls.gov/news.release/pdf/tenure.pdf

U.S. Bureau of Labor Statistics. (2022a, September 16). *Occupational requirements survey*. www.bls.gov/ors/

U.S. Bureau of Labor Statistics. (2022b, September 16). *Standard occupational classification*. www.bls.gov/soc

U.S. Bureau of Labor Statistics. (2022c, September 16). *Occupational requirements survey: Handbook of methods*. www.bls.gov/opub/hom/ors/concepts.htm

U.S. Bureau of Labor Statistics. (2022d). *Highlights of women's earnings in 2020, Report 1094*. www.bls.gov/opub/reports/womens-earnings/2020/home.htm

U.S. Bureau of Labor Statistics. (2022e, September 16). *Persons with a disability: Labor force characteristics – 2021*. www.bls.gov/news.release/pdf/disabl.pdf

U.S. Bureau of Labor Statistics. (2022g, September 16). *Labor force statistics from the Current Population Survey, Household Data Annual Averages, Table 39*. www.bls.gov/cps/aa2020/cpsaat39.htm/

U.S. Census Bureau. (2021). *Childhood disability in the United States: 2019*. www.census.gov/library/publications/2021/acs/acsbr-006.html

U.S. Census Bureau. (2022a, September 16). *Educational attainment in the United States: 2021*. www.census.gov/data/tables/2021/demo/educational-attainment/cps-detailed-tables.html

U.S. Census Bureau. (2022b, February 24). Census Bureau releases new educational attainment data. [Press Release Number CB22-TPS.02].

U.S. Department of Defense. (2021). *Report to Congress: Study and report on traumatic brain injury mitigation efforts final report*. file:///C:/Users/debra/Downloads/Study%20and%20Report%20on%20Traumatic%20Brain%20Injury%20Mitigation%20Efforts.pdf

U.S. Department of Education. (n.d.). *Section 1414(d) Individualized education programs*, 20 U.S.C. § 1414 D. https://sites.ed.gov/idea/statute-chapter-33/subchapter-ii/1414/d#:~:text=The%20term%20%E2%80%9Cindividualized%20education%20program,achievement%20and%20functional%20performance%2C%20including%E2%80%94

U.S. Department of Labor, Wage and Hour Division. (2022, September 16). *Subminimum wage*. www.dol.gov/agencies/whd/special-employment

Weed, R. O. (1993, April 23). *The RAPEL method: A common sense approach to life care planning and earnings capacity analysis*. Unpublished document. Presented at *NARPPS Annual Conference*, Atlanta, GA.

Weed, R. O. (1995). Forensic rehabilitation. In A. E. Dell Orto & R. P. Marinelle (Eds.), *Encyclopedia of disability and rehabilitation* (pp. 326–330). Macmillan.

Weed, R. O. (1996). Life care planning and earnings capacity analysis for brain injured clients involved in personal injury litigation utilizing the RAPEL method. *NeuroRehabilitation, 7*(2), 119–35. https://doi.org/10.3233/NRE-1996-7204

Weed, R. O. (1998). Aging with a brain injury: The effects on life care plans and vocational opinions. *The Rehabilitation Professional, 6*(5), 30–34.

Weed, R. O. (2000). The worth of a child: Earnings capacity and rehabilitation planning for pediatric personal injury litigation cases. *The Rehabilitation Professional, 81*, 29–43.

Weed, R. O. (2007). *Life care planning: A step-by-step guide*. E&F Vocational Services.

Weed, R. O. (2018). Checklist for selecting a life care planner. In R. O. Weed & D. E. Berens (Eds.), *Life care planning and case management handbook* (4th ed.). Routledge.

Weed, R. O. (Guest Ed.). (2002). Special issue on the assessment of transferable skills in forensic settings. *Journal of Forensic Vocational Analysis, 5*(1), 1–60.

Weed, R. O., & Berens, D. E. (Eds.). (2018). *Life care planning and case management handbook* (4th ed.). Routledge.

Weed, R. O., & Field, T. F. (2001, rev. through 2012). *The rehabilitation consultant's handbook* (4th ed. rev.). Elliott & Fitzpatrick, Inc.

Weed, R. O., & Riddick, S. (1992). Life care plans as a case management tool. *The Individual Case Manager Journal, 31*, 26–35.

Weed, R. O., & Taylor, C. (1990). Labor market surveys: The backbone of the rehabilitation plan. *NARPPS Journal and News, 54*, 27–32.

Wehman, P., & Melia, R. (1985). The job coach: Function in transitional and supported employment. *American Rehabilitation, 112*, 4–8.

Whiston, S. C. (2016). *Principles and applications of assessment in counseling* (5th ed.). Cengage Learning.

Wilson, A. D., Henriksen, R. C., Bustamante, R., & Irby, B. (2016). Successful black men from absent-father homes and their resilient single mothers: A phenomenological study. *Journal of Multicultural Counseling and Development, 44*, 189–208.

Woods, S. A., Lievens, F., De Fruyt, F., & Wille, B. (2013). Personality across working life: The longitudinal and reciprocal influences of personality on work. *Journal of Organizational Behavior, 34*, S7 – S25. https://doi.org/10.1002/job.1863

Woodside, P., Wiggins, C. D., & Venn, J. J. (1991). Assessing lost earning capacity for an injured minor. *Journal of Legal Economics, 1*(3), 95–101.

World Health Organization. (2019). Global health estimates: Life expectancy and healthy life expectancy. www.who.int/data/gho/data/themes/mortality-and-global-health-estimates/ghe-life-expectancy-and-healthy-life-expectancy#:~:text=Globally%2C%20life%20expectancy%20has%20increased,reduced%20years%20lived%20with%20disability

Zunker, V. G. (2006). Theories of career development. In *Career counseling: A holistic approach* (7th ed.). Thomson Brooks/Cole.

Chapter 12

The Role of the Neuropsychologist in Life Care Planning

Carol P. Walker

Neuropsychology has been conceptualized as falling at the intersection of the neurosciences (neurology, neuroanatomy, neurophysiology, neurochemistry, neuroimaging) and the behavior sciences (psychology, linguistics), including cognitive, emotional, and motivational processes (Vallar & Caputi, 2022). While considering the roles of a neuropsychologist across the lifespan does not change the overall characteristics, it does require consideration of how the roles of neuropsychologists are different depending on the age group with whom they primarily work. Testing of infants and preschool children is an area where most generalist/adult neuropsychologists have limited training or experience. The education and training with school-aged children (typically beginning at age six) and adolescents is more robust for generalists, and many neuropsychologists' practices include evaluating and treating children and adolescents in this age group. There are also different needs in older adults; for example, it is this population for which a neuropsychologist with training in geropsychology might be called upon to perform a capacity evaluation for submission to a court (typically probate court) as part of a determination of civil competence. The most common reason for clinical referrals in this older age group are to assess for a neurodegenerative process (dementia), for post-stoke assessment, post-traumatic brain injury (TBI), metabolic conditions, or the effects of multiple comorbidities (which may include medication effects) on cognition. Confirming a differential diagnosis between cognitive changes and depression or other psychological disorder is often requested.

History of Neuropsychology

Neuropsychology emerged as a field in the United States in the 1930s, however, the concept of the relationships between the brain and behaviors predates this concept by many centuries. The

Edwin Smith Papyrus, dated 2500 BCE to 3000 BCE, represents the oldest written record that described different types of brain injuries causing different symptoms. The Edwin Smith Papyrus is the earliest documentation of medical treatment (Fitzhugh-Bell, 1997). Among the cases described Fitzhugh-Bell notes there are references to head and brain injuries. The descriptions suggest the belief that brain functions are localized in specific areas of the brain. In the fifth century BC, Hippocrates of Kos (who is considered the father of modern medicine) postulated that diseases are physiological rather than punishment from the gods (Heilman & Valenstein, 1993). There was also recognition that the brain was the control center of the body and emotions. Hippocrates of Kos was the first to recognize that paralysis occurred on the side of the body contralateral to the side of a head injury. By the time of Galen (129–199 CE), a Greek physician, surgeon, and philosopher in the Roman Empire, trephining was used in treating skull fractures to relieve pressure, and for removing skull fragments that threatened the dura, and in some instances, for drainage. Galen placed mental functions, described by Aristotle as memory, attention, fantasy, and reason, as well as common sense, to locations in the ventricles (Freemon, 1994). Galen's concept of "humors" persisted for 1,000 years. Gall, a neuroanatomist and physiologist, introduced the concept that the brain was comprised of discrete organs, each localized and responsible for a specific psychological trait. Gall's concept, phrenology, correlated mental abilities to specific brain areas which he attributed to measurements of the skull. He opined this might allow the deduction of moral and intellectual characteristics since the shape of the skull is modified by the underlying brain (Heilman & Valenstein, 1993). Based on his observation that his student with good verbal memory had prominent eyes, Gall suggested that word memory was localized in the frontal lobes. In spite of the erroneous conclusions on which phrenology was based, Gall's phrenology represents the beginning of the modern-day localizationist doctrine.

In the late 1800s, Broca, a French physician, anatomist, and anthropologist, described the well-known case of Tan, Broca's patient who suffered the effects of a left hemispheric stroke. While only able to utter the word "tan," he was able to accurately comprehend language. Broca used this case, in conjunction with others, to demonstrate that the expression of language is subserved by the left frontal lobe. This area subsequently became known as "Broca's area" and individuals with damage to Broca's area are referred to as having "Broca's aphasia." Several years after Broca presented his findings regarding aphasia in frontal lobe lesions, Wernicke, a German physician, anatomist, psychiatrist, and neuropathologist, presented cases of patients with lesions in the superior posterior portion of the left hemisphere leading to language comprehension deficits. This finding led to the idea that the component processes of language were localized, and on this basis, the modern doctrine of component process localization and disconnection syndromes was begun. This doctrine states that complex mental functions, such as language, represent the combined processing of a number of subcomponent processes that are represented in widely diverse areas of the brain.

One of the first uses of the term "neuropsychology" was by Dr. William Osler in 1913 (Vallar & Caputi, 2022). In 1949, Donald Hebb, a Canadian psychologist, published *The Organization of Behavior. A Neuropsychological Theory* (Brown & Milner, 2003). Hebb also co-edited a book titled, *The Neuropsychology of Lashley*, which was the selected papers by Lashley (1960). Both Hebb's and Lasley's research were related to the neurophysiological basis of learning and memory.

Ward Halstead was a primary contributor to the development of the field of clinical neuropsychology; he started the first neuropsychology laboratory in the United States in 1935. Halstead worked in collaboration with neurological surgeons to perform research that helped form the scientific basis for neuropsychological testing. Halstead used neuropsychological testing to study the effects of different types of brain lesions on various cognitive domains, as well as sensory and perceptual functioning. During the early stages in the field, neuropsychological test results were used primarily for lesion localization. Prior to employing testing, Halstead observed individuals with brain damage in a variety of real-world settings to determine the types of problems they experienced. He then assembled a battery of ten tests, which were administered to these patients (Sbordone et al., 2007). In collaboration with his student, the late Ralph Reitan, Halstead created the Halstead–Reitan Battery. In one study, the Halstead–Reitan Neuropsychological Battery (HRNB) compared computerized tomography, electroencephalograms, and the HRNB and found that the HRNB interpretation had the highest degree of accuracy in identifying brain damage (Yantz et al., 2006). The Boston Approach, which was developed at the Boston Veterans Affairs (VA) by Harold Goodglass, Edith Kaplan, and Nelson Butters, focused more on a qualitative strategy, relying heavily on behavioral observations during the performance of a task (Libon et al., 2013). The quantitative approach, based on the use of standardized testing to elicit pathognomonic signs, and often administered by a trained psychometrist, and the qualitative strategy were developed relatively independently; presently, most neuropsychologists employ both of these methods during an examination.

Another prominent figure in the field of neuropsychology was Alexander Luria. Luria developed a theory of brain–behavior relationships that postulated complex behavior may be reduced to individual components and the component studied to determine what functional system had been damaged (Luria, 1973).

Neuropsychology was first recognized as a discipline separate from psychology or neurology in the 1960s when Klove used the term "neuropsychology" in the English biomedical literature and with the inception of the International Neuropsychological Society in 1967 (Bilder, 2011). While diagnosis has remained one focus of neuropsychological testing, it has been supplanted as a primary diagnostic tool to a large degree by the advent of advanced neuroimaging techniques (Roalf & Gur, 2017). Neuroimaging has become highly specific in terms of measurement of neural structure; however, neuropsychological testing and evaluation remain the most sensitive measure of brain function.

Neuroimaging

The advent of methods to visualize structures of the brain allow for the opportunity to understand the structural and physiological concomitants of neurocognitive processes and neurological diseases (Bigler, 1996; Damasio & Damasio, 1989). Neuroimaging has gained widespread utility in neuropsychological research and practice over the recent decades. The study of brain function during health or disease requires integration of data from behavioral and neurophysiological findings (Roalf & Gur, 2017). While functional neuroimaging has been rapidly evolving, it is also the case that the well-established knowledge base of clinical and actuarial inferences derived from neuropsychological approaches are likely to remain salient given that implementations of advances in rehabilitation, forensics, and treatment planning remain basic functions of neuropsychologists (Benitez et al., 2014).

One of the most promising areas of neuroimaging is functional neuroimaging techniques (fMRI). The early goal of fMRI studies in neuropsychology was to understand how psychological processes are localized in brain tissue, to understand the normal organization of the elements of processing, and to predict the nature of the deficits that will arise when the brain is damaged (Berman et al., 2006). Initial studies focused on cognition, and subsequent studies examined neural systems involved in emotion processing and found results suggesting separate brain regions are involved in different aspects of emotions including fear and sadness (Gur et al., 2002).

Brain and Cognitive Development

To better elucidate the roles of pediatric neuropsychologists and adult neuropsychologists, it is necessary to place their roles in the context of brain development. When a neuropsychologist works with infants and children, whether in a clinical setting or completing (or consulting on) a life care plan, it is critical that the age of the child and the accompanying developmental stage be considered. It is also crucial that the life care planner be knowledgeable of and consider normal development to assess qualitatively and quantitatively the effects of trauma or abnormal development on a developing child.

Cognitive development in general refers to the development of the ability to think and reason. Psychosocial development refers to the development of personality and social development. A developmental theory describes the changes over time in one or several areas of behavioral or psychological capabilities. These include, but are not limited to, such skills as language, perception, memory, learning, executive functioning, and behavior.

Nature vs. Nurture

Both historically and currently, a primary issue in the scientific debate on development is the relative contributions of nature and nurture. There is nearly uniform agreement that there is an interaction between innate and environmental factors accounting for both the development of a trait or behavior, as well as variations in the trait or behavior. Or, as Hebb (1980) opined, behavior is determined 100 percent by heredity and 100 percent by environment. Heredity is expressed dependent on the specific environment in which the expression occurs; that is, hereditary influence can have different behavioral effects in different environments. This has been documented in studies of intelligence; Kaufman (1999) reports that unrelated children raised together have measured IQs more similar than biological siblings raised apart. While this provides evidence of the effect of environment on this construct, evidence of a genetic component of intelligence can clearly be seen as well. Overall, the evidence in child development research seems to indicate that nature is vulnerable to nurture, and there are bidirectional and interactive effects between parenting and children's characteristics (Kiff et al., 2011).

It is also well-known that chromosomal influences exist that can negatively affect the developing brain, prenatally, as in the cases of Trisomy-21 (Down's syndrome), Trisomy 13 (Patau's syndrome), and Trisomy 18 (Edward's Syndrome) (Stavljenić-Rukavina, 2008). There are also postnatal effects of chromosomal influences, examples include phenylketonuria (PKU) and microcephaly for which an exemplar is MECP2-related disorder (formerly called Rett Syndrome) (Seltzer & Paciorkowski, 2014). While there is a substantial body of research on the influence of nature versus nurture on intellect (Plomin & von Stumm, 2018), this influence of research findings may be seen in areas other than intellect. It is apparent from findings in multiple lines of research, ranging from premature births (Guarini et al., 2021) to traumatic brain injury (Ryan et al., 2016) and autism (Modabbernia et al., 2017), that the influence of the environment can be a powerful factor on outcomes.

Many of the theories that have been advanced regarding the development of emotion and cognition have been revised or replaced as research and technology have advanced scientific knowledge. For example, the psychoanalytic models of development advanced by Sigmund Freud and others are difficult to support with empirical research due to the reliance, in large part, on unconscious processes that do not lend themselves to scientific inquiry (Freud, 1963). Early studies in developmental psychology were based on descriptive data. For example, in the 1930s, Gessell advanced a maturation theory and began to establish normative data for physical, cognitive, and motor development. His theory is based on the premise that behavior is a function of structure and that humans develop in a patterned and predictable manner. His data collection on hundreds of children resulted in a normative base of normal growth in physical, cognitive, and motor development.

Developmental Theories

Various facets must be considered when examining cognitive and psychosocial development. Simeonsson (1983) postulated four dimensions integral to the developmental process: biological, psychological, cultural, and environmental. Each of these dimensions can be affected by another dimension; for example, malnutrition caused by poverty (environmental) may result in amenorrhea (biological). Throughout history, developmental theorists have clearly distinguished themselves from each other by placing varying levels of importance on each of these dimensions.

The influence of environment is particularly salient in the developmental theories that are behaviorist and view the child as being, in large part, what John Locke described as a *tabula rasa* (blank slate). Beginning in the 1700s with the introduction of Locke's concept and continuing through the work of the behaviorists and social learning theorists, the emphasis has been placed on environment. One familiar example, from John Watson, the theorist who laid the groundwork for B.F. Skinner's operant conditioning, who wrote in *Behaviorism* that:

> Give me a dozen healthy infants, well-formed, and my own specified world to bring them up in, and I'll guarantee to take any one at random and train him to become any type of specialist I might select–doctor, lawyer, artist–regardless of his talents, penchants, tendencies, abilities, vocations, and race of his ancestors (n.d., p. 82).

This is consistent with a mechanistic view of human nature, whereby the organism is formed by developmental influences received from the environment and experiences. Organismal theories incorporate both innate and experiential influences on development into their theories and consider the interactions between the two. The ethological theories focus on biological processes and view the organism as following an evolutionary scheme of development.

In contrast to the mechanistic perspective of development, the organismic model views the developing organism as active and spontaneously interacting with, rather than purely reacting to, the environment from birth. One of the primary reasons for developmental models is to have a representation of normal development that provides an explanation of how a child's thinking changes as they develop. Piaget's theory is the most often cited developmental cognitive theory and is used in educational programs (Miller, 1983).

Piaget's Developmental Cognitive Theory

A basic tenet of Piaget's theory is that knowledge is a process rather than a state. The child "constructs" knowledge through active interactions with the environment. According to his theory, the child's knowledge of the world changes as his/her cognitive system develops. Development occurs through the interaction of the processes of assimilation and accommodation.

A detailed description of Piaget's model can be found in Simeonsson (1983).

Table 12.1 Piaget's Stages of Development

Stage of Development	Age Range (years)	Learning and Mastery During Stage
Sensorimotor	0–2	Learning about objects and their relationships Learn Object Permanence
Pre-Operational	2–7	Egocentric view of the world Characterized by language acquisition and other forms of conceptual development
Concrete Operational	7–11	Capable of concrete problem solving Able to engage in logical, organized thought
Formal Operations	11–15	Capable of abstract thought and able to incorporate principles of deductive hypothesizing

Freud's Theory of Development

Next to Piaget, the most well-known and influential of the developmental theorists is Sigmund Freud. Freud's theory is based on the premise that development through psychosocial stages early in life sets the stage for an individual's personality later in life. Freud introduced the novel theory of the crucial nature of early development on personality; he emphasized the first few years of life as being the most important in development of personality. Freud, like Piaget, focuses of stages of development that are qualitative rather than quantitative.

Behavioral Models of Development

The behaviorist models are also representative of the mechanistic view. The child produces responses to the world like a machine. Behavior is learned by imitation, association, conditioning, or observation. The over-riding belief of the learning theorists is that development is dependent on experience. The developing child acquires new behaviors and modifies existing behaviors by interactions with their social and physical world. The beginning of the behaviorist movement can be traced to John Watson's 1913 "declaration of behaviorism," where he asserted that psychology's goal should be the prediction and control of behavior (Miller, 1983).

Anyone who has taken an introductory psychology class is familiar with the terms "reinforcement," "punishment," "behavior modification," the name B. F. Skinner, and his Skinner box. During the 1930s, Skinner performed research using operant conditioning focusing on the effects of shaping behaviors with schedules of reinforcement. Skinner's approach assumes that the same set of learning principles underlie normal and abnormal behavior. The essence of Skinner's model is the employment of reinforcement contingencies that reward desirable behaviors and ignore undesirable behaviors.

The outcome of this experimental work by behaviorists was a body of research providing empirical support that learning is increasingly under the control of cognition during development. As reported by Miller (1983), several important conclusions were derived from this research, first, as Piaget had expected, children are active in their learning. Instead of passively learning stimulus-response bonds, they try to solve problems. The second conclusion, related to the first, is that the primary changes that occur in learning during development are based on the cognitive processes of language, attention, thinking, and social behavior. Learning theory, as well as social learning theory, focuses on processes of change. Social learning theory had its inception in the 1930s with the works of O. H. Mowrer, Neal Miller, John Dollard, Robert Sears, Leonard Doob, and John Whiting, all of whom attempted to combine learning theory with Freudian concepts. For learning theorists, development involves the accumulation of operantly, or classically, conditioned responses established shortly after birth (Miller, 1983).

Social Learning Theory

Probably the most influential learning theorist in recent developmental thinking is Albert Bandura, who developed social learning theory. Bandura's BoBo doll experiments by Bandura et al. (1961) demonstrated the effects of modeled aggression on children's behaviors. In Bandura's model of observational learning, developmental progress occurs as a result of physical maturation, experience with the world, and cognitive development. Motivational processes are related to the child's reproduction of behavior having desirable outcomes that they observe.

In summary, the key concepts of Bandura's social learning theory are as follows:

- Rather than only mimicking another person's behavior, observational learning can be more general. The child constructs new behaviors by listening to another person or reading and developing the behaviors representatively. Even complex new behaviors can be learned in this way. Overall, overt behavior by the model is not a necessary condition for learning to occur.
- The child is self-regulatory. Although reinforcement is not necessary for observational learning to occur, it is beneficial for self-regulation. The child observes behaviors that result in reinforcement and punishment. These observations are then employed as sources of information to facilitate rule learning, evaluating performance's, developing standards of conduct, set goals, and deciding in what situations the observed behavior will be used.
- Three sources of influence determine behavioral change. These influences are the person, their behavior, and the environmental interaction. Unlike previous behaviorist theories, in Bandura's model, the environment does not consistently exert the greatest control (Miller, 1983).

Vygotsky's social cognition learning model views culture as the primary determinant in an individual's development (Miller, 1983). This model views the importance of culture as twofold, first, children acquire much of their knowledge through their culture and second, the culture teaches the process of dialect. Vyogtsky's theory continues to be influential in educational psychology.

Theoretical Models of Neuropsychology

In neuropsychology, the organismic theoretical model is employed and based on the premise that various types of behavior are neurologically based. These behavior classes include sensory functioning, and higher order functioning such as attention, executive functioning, and affective states. The late Ralph Reitan (1988, p. 333) described the theoretical underpinning of neuropsychology as follows:

> The theories of most relevance for clinical neuropsychology have followed a general organizational plan in which sensory input represents the first element, central

processing the second element, and motor responsiveness the third element. Sensory input is related to the primary receptor areas of the cerebral cortex and these areas, which serve to receive incoming information, are related in turn to secondary sensory areas. The secondary sensory areas are customarily assigned a task involved in additional processing or integration of incoming information.

The normal development of the nervous system and neuropsychological functioning is based on interactions between brain development and experiences. Among the developing systems in the child, the motor system is first to reach maturity. The sensory system also develops early. The systems responsible for language and higher level cognitive integrative functioning develop later. These areas continue to develop into later adolescences and adulthood (Spreen et al., 1995).

Alexander Luria, a Russian neuropsychologist, hypothesized that all functional systems of the brain involve components associated with each of three primary "blocks" or functional units (Luria, 1970). He also noted that as much as three quarters of the cerebral cortex is not directly involved in sensory or motor functions and that the role of neuropsychology is to map the brain's function and systems responsible for the higher, more complex behavioral processes.

Luria's first functional unit, the subcortical division, is associated with the brainstem reticular formation and other subcortical structures. A primary component of this system is the reticular system which is considered to be involved in nearly all functions of the nervous system. Luria (1973) argued that this unit, along with the two other units, is involved in all conscious activity. The reticular formation is important for attention and alertness; one specialized functioning is the maintenance and regulation of waking states.

Luria described three types of sources of cerebral activation in the subcortical division: metabolic, environmental, and cortical regulatory. Metabolic processes are responsible for activation of various responses of the autonomic nervous system (e.g., cardiovascular, respiratory, and gastrointestinal function), as well as consummatory behaviors such as feeding and sexuality. These functions are affected by specific cranial nerves and hypothalamic nuclei. Changes in the normal level of environmental stimuli often require an increased level of alertness. If the subcortical division is disrupted, deterioration in wakefulness and alertness and disorganization of memory may result (Luria, 1973). Some theorists assert that the symptoms of childhood learning problems, such as attention deficit hyperactivity disorder (ADHD) may be associated with subcortical division dysfunction.

Luria also postulates units associated with the cerebral cortex (posterior division and anterior division). The posterior division is comprised of the parietal, occipital, and temporal regions and is functionally specialized to receive, analyze, and store information. The anterior division is functionally specialized for formation of plans and programs and for verification of overt and covert behaviors. Luria described the prefrontal regions as having a prominent role in the formation of intentions and programs, and in regulation of the most complex forms of behavior, including motor, speech, intellectual activities, as well as consciousness, affective states, and memory processes (Luria, 1973).

Luria's model, which in general relies on an information processing model of cognition, also allows for the examination of the effects of individual differences on child development. Learning involves filling out the requisite databases and structure upon which a system operates. Luria focused on the increasing role of language as the child develops (Spreen et al., 1995). Luria postulated that at approximately six years of age, language becomes internalized and mediates and regulates behavior. This is generally consistent with the report of internalized verbal mediation of problem solving by age seven years as reported by Kendler and Kendler (1962).

Developmental Disorders

In the case of developmental disorders, the rate of skill acquisition is slower than that of the normally developing child. Further, in some cases, not only is the acquisition of the skill slower but the final skill level may be lower than the level attained in normally developing children (Miller, 1983). In this way, a delay that appears minor at an early age becomes increasingly noticeable as the trajectory for improved skill increases with the child's developmental maturity. For example, expressive language deficits that are not apparent in a toddler-aged child, may be quite noticeable in the school-aged child. Additionally, an interaction among skills can be observed. A skill that fails to emerge at the expected time may negatively affect a later developing skill which depends, for its foundation, on the earlier developing skill. Again, using the example of language development, Majovski (1989) cites research by Pinker in 1984 and Devilliers and Devilliers in 1979, which found that if speech is absent or poorly established by six years of age, significant intellectual and social deficits are likely. Developmental language disorders are common in a number of developmental conditions further complicating outcomes (Aguilar-Mediavilla et al., 2022).

The influence of brain development is important in pediatric neuropsychology, neuropsychology, and life care planning. The effects of abnormal development on intellectual functioning, emotional functioning, language, education, self-care, instrumental activities of daily living and other aspects of a life care plan are important in both development and implementation of a life care plan, as these issues are critical throughout the life span of an individual.

Neurodevelopmental Delays

Most research documents that the effects of a neurological insult at a young age may be mitigated to some degree as the child matures (Kolb & Gibb, 2011). The concept of brain plasticity was explained in Aram and Eisele (1992) as the capacity of the brain for reorganization based on the substitution of one brain area to subsume functions usually served by another area of the brain. These authors opine this would be accounted for by redundancy in the neural networks such that a specific function might have multiple representations or neural repair mechanisms, thus enabling the restoration of function in a previously damaged area. Others have opined that neuronal plasticity may rely on a number of mechanisms including neuronal regeneration/collateral sprouting, including the concepts of synaptic plasticity and neurogenesis, and functional reorganization, which includes equipotentiality, vicariation (where brain areas of different function assume the function of injured areas), and diachisis (dysfunction in a portion of the brain connected to a remote, damaged brain area) (Puderbaugh & Emmady, 2022).

There have been multiple studies assessing the concept of plasticity of the immature brain. While these studies have found fewer residual effects in children in comparison to adults, children continue to exhibit an overall decrement in intellectual functioning compared to controls (Spreen et al., 1995). Thus, in spite of some restitution of function, subtle deficits remain that impair abilities in ways that while not readily notable, impinge upon the child's ability to learn or function as efficiently as would have been the case but for the neurological event that transpired.

If the immature brain is able to reorganize in response to a neurological insult, how might the etiology of developmental delays be explained? Khan and Leventhal (2021) argue that the cause of most developmental delays is unknown. These authors suggest that there are a broad range of potential etiologies which must be examined individually to help determine the cause and mitigate the deficits. They further state that most developmental delays resolve spontaneously. Indicators that may lead to significant developmental deficits are hearing and vision loss, loss of previously achieved developmental skills, persistent hypotonia or hypertonia, asymmetrical movements, no communicative speech at 16 months old, and disproportionate head circumference.

While it is unknown why plasticity does not operate in the domain of developmental delays, Temple (1997a) postulated several reasons why this may be the case. One, plasticity has an inhibitory effect that when exerted prevents the activation of compensatory systems. Another possibility is that the compensatory system is not activated when the basis of the deficit is genetic or related to growth and development of the underlying brain region. Temple (1997a) concludes that she perceives plasticity as a response to injury or disease with its origin in infancy or childhood rather than a response to an abnormal prenatal process. If correct, then although many children have dyslexia, ADHD, intellectual disability, and other learning difficulties, neuronal plasticity fails to engage and provide deficit compensation. Temple's hypotheses appear supported in part by Martin and Huntsman, (2012), who argue that in order for normal development to occur, the organism requires the capacity for appropriate and effective neuronal plasticity. Neuronal plasticity is the ability of a neuron, or network of neurons, to functionally alter in response to changes in input or activity. Within the central nervous system, this process is involved with the development and refinement of connections, as well as with learning, memory, behavior regulation, and cognition. Problems are believed to arise when the plasticity mechanisms operate abnormally, and the ensuing neuronal networks develop abnormally. Martin and Huntsman (2012) state that abnormal neuronal plasticity is the hallmark of many developmental and cognitive disorders.

Prematurity and Birth Weight

There is a demonstrated link between early neural development and both intrinsic and extrinsic factors. Some of these factors, such as malnutrition of the mother, birth asphyxia, and severe brain injury during a child's birth, are obvious causes of abnormal development. However, there are also subtle factors, such as premature birth, that may cause problems that are less readily apparent. Also, there is often an interaction among factors, such as the effects of neglect, substance abuse (Substance Abuse and Mental Health Services Administration, 2016), poor healthcare, and educational issues, that may accompany maternal malnutrition during pregnancy.

The developmental effects of prematurity and low birth weight are well-documented in the research literature. Intraventricular hemorrhage (IVH) is the most common type of preterm brain injury, usually occurring in the first three days of life in up to 31% of very preterm infants (Strahle et al., 2019). Very low birth weight (VLBW) infants and extremely low birth weight infants (ELBW) are highly susceptible to respiratory distress, necrotizing colitis, septicemia. meningitis, hypoglycemia, hypothermia, intraventricular hemorrhage, periventricular leukomalacia, and recirculation of arterial blood to the lungs. As might be expected, VLBW infants who suffer intracranial hemorrhage have greater likelihood of compromised cognitive and psychosocial development. However, it should be noted that there are mediating factors in the environment that may have a potent effect on the ultimate outcome. The quality of home environment is documented in one meta-analysis as the most important factor, citing the effects of this factor on cognitive development at age 22 months (Pascal et al., 2018).

Some studies have found that children born premature have a higher incidence of academic difficulties than their peers. This is attributed to lower levels of intellectual abilities and behavioral difficulties. Studies addressing school-aged children often find more cognitive lag than studies assessing children during their preschool years; however, a 2017 study using a population of subjects in the United Kingdom suggested that advances in obstetrics and neonatal care may have attenuated the negative consequences between 1958 and 1970 birth cohorts and the cohort born in 2001 (Goisis et al., 2017). A 2018 meta-analysis found that the prevalence of cognitive and motor delays, evaluated using developmental tests, was estimated at 16.9% for cognitive delays and 20.6% for motor delays (Pascal et al., 2018). The authors of the Pascal et al. (2018) meta-analysis found that the delays increase as gestational age and birthweight decrease. They concluded that there are still a wide range of negative neurodevelopmental outcomes associated with very preterm (VPT) and VLBW infant births.

Collectively, a child's risk of problems is inversely correlated with birth weight and gestational age at birth. The long-term consequences for VLBW and ELBW infants are more detrimental. Linsell and her colleague (2018) and her colleagues from the United Kingdom found that the mean cognitive scores of extremely preterm individuals were on average 25.2 points (95% CI −27.8 to −22.6) lower than those of their term-born peers. The scores of extremely preterm males were on average 8.8 points lower than those of extremely preterm girls.

Moderate/severe neonatal brain injury and gestational age of less than 25 weeks also had an adverse effect on cognitive function. Linsell et al. (2018) concluded that: "There is no evidence that impaired cognitive function in extremely preterm individual's materially recovers or deteriorates from infancy through to 19 years. Cognitive test scores in infancy and early childhood reflect early adult outcomes" (p. 363).

Acquired Brain Disorders

Acquired disorders are characterized by a period of normal development followed by disruption by either neurological trauma or illness. Examples of acquired disorders include birth injuries, traumatic brain injury, and illnesses such as meningitis, streptococcus B infections, and human immunodeficiency virus (HIV).

Traumatic Brain Injury (TBI)

Another common cause of acquired developmental difficulties is TBI. It is common to see both cognitive and psychosocial sequelae following TBI. The effects may be seen in any or all domains of cognition, including intellectual capacity, attention, memory, visuospatial functioning, sensory functioning, motor function, and executive functioning. In addition, there are often deficits in behavior and adaptive functioning. The neuropsychological and behavioral effects will vary dramatically depending on age at injury, the age when effects are most prominent, severity of injury, and the environmental conditions at home and other settings (Wade et al., 2016).

Birth Injuries

The effects of an anoxic episode during the prenatal, perinatal, or postnatal period range from immediate death to the absence of significant sequelae. Having an anoxic episode in isolation is a poor predictor of later disability. While there is research by Fitzhardinge and colleagues (1981) demonstrating an association between hydrocephalus, spastic hemiplegia, quadriplegia, and diplegia in term infants treated for clinical evidence of post-asphyxial encephalopathy, the inferences are considered tenuous; these children were followed only until they were 18 months of age (Fitzhardinge et al., 1981). A more recent review of neonatal encephalopathy (NE) following perinatal asphyxia by Van Handel and her colleagues (2007), found that children with NE who also have cerebral palsy (CP) at age 12 months are often severely developmentally delayed. With mild NE without CP, the prognosis is good. In this group, intellect, educational achievement, and neuropsychological functions are comparable to healthy peers at least until middle childhood. While the Van Handel et al. (2007) review does not provide data regarding outcomes as development proceeds; a review of outcomes among children from late childhood through adolescence by Lee and Glass (2021) found that normal neurodevelopmental outcomes in early childhood do not rule out subtle deficits in cognitive and behavioral abilities in later childhood and adolescence. In children with severe NE, there are impairments in every cognitive domain. These children have lower levels of intellect, perform worse in academics and on neuropsychological testing than groups of healthy controls and children with mild NE or moderate NE. Marlow et al. (2005) performed an assessment similar to Van Handel et al. (2007) and found that children who had NE have poorer scores on cognitive, neuropsychological, education and behavioral assessments than their classmates. The differences are worse in children with more severe NE. Children with NE commonly have learning difficulties requiring comprehensive school assessment. Overall, Marlow et al. (2005) confirms a high prevalence of subtle impairment in a subgroup of children without severe encephalopathy.

The effects of convulsive disorders on development can best be considered concomitantly with the underlying etiological condition. The most common and important cause of acute symptomatic neonatal seizures is hypoxic-ischemic encephalopathy (HIE). Perinatal stroke is the second most common cause of symptomatic seizures in the newborn. Almost all types of intracranial hemorrhage can be associated with seizures. The long-term neurodevelopmental effects of neonatal seizures are prevalent. Etiology has been determined to be a primary determinant of outcome for long-term sequelae in neonatal seizures. Hypoxic-ischemic encephalopathy, hemorrhage, central nervous system infections, and cerebral malformations are associated with more adverse outcomes. Prolonged seizures in HIE are shown to worsen brain damage (Kang & Kadam, 2015). Neonatal seizures are also found to correlate significantly with moderate to severe TBI. Overall, there is no reliable guidance regarding the long-term effects that may accrue with seizures. Spreen et al. (1995) reported that approximately 50% will recover without deficits and the other 50% will either die or suffer severe neurodevelopmental difficulties. Focal left temporal and grand mal seizures have the strongest association with developmental issues. Epilepsies are slightly more common in males as compared with females. Psychiatric comorbidities are common in epilepsy and estimated to occur in 25% to 35% of patients (Lu et al., 2021). While males more often have epilepsy, women who have seizures have a higher comorbid incidence of both depression and anxiety. Further, research notes that psychiatric comorbidities are associated with poorer outcomes (Josephson et al., 2017) which is a negative indicator for seizure treatment efforts. Research has also found that approximately 25% of individuals with chronic epilepsy have intellectual disability (Akrout-Brizard et al., 2021; Kaaden & Helmstaedter, 2009). The results of the study by Helmstaedter and Elger (2009) described epilepsy as a developmental hindrance and found that patients became increasingly impaired at the approximate endpoint of functional cerebral plasticity. For this reason, the deficits become most evident during the decade after puberty. A recent study by Hermann et al. (2021), assessed a group of epilepsy patients to assess symptoms of psychopathology. Patients with temporal lobe epilepsy as a group exhibited significantly elevated symptoms of emotional distress. The groups classified as mildly or globally impaired showed differential cognitive abnormalities, particularly in the more severe group where there were impacts on intelligence, memory, and executive functioning.

Genetic or Multifactorial Conditions
Attention Deficit Hyperactivity Disorder

One of the most common diagnoses made in children by mental health professionals is ADHD. There is a high comorbidity between ADHD and conduct disorder, oppositional defiant disorder, mood disorders, learning problems, speech and language disorders, and intellectual disability. There are a number of possible etiologies that have been evaluated in this disorder ranging from genetic to environmental factors. Premature birth is an important risk factor for ADHD, the disorder occurs 2.6–4 times more often in babies born with LBW or VLBW (Núñez-Jaramillo et al., 2021). Perinatal hypoxia also increases risk as does lack of proper nutrients.

Sleep disturbances have been associated with ADHD. A recent review (Bijlenga et al., 2019), proposed that chronic sleep disorders are some of the most common symptoms of ADHD. They suggested that patients presenting with ADHD symptoms should undergo a sleep quantification study.

Studies have suggested a genetic influence on development of ADHD. While there may be multiple genes involved, two seem to have received more attention. First is brain derived neurotrophic factor (BDNF). A meta-analysis completed by Zhang et al. (2018) did not fully support BDNF as etiological, instead finding no statistically significant difference in peripheral BDNF between ADHD patient and control groups overall, but BDNF levels were significantly higher in males with ADHD when compared to controls. There are changes in brain morphology; ADHD patients present with a different trajectory in maturational changes in the brain's development in terms of cortical volume (Núñez-Jaramillo et al., 2021).

Genetic disorders may also affect development. In the case of genetic disorders, there is a clear and specific etiology, which may have an effect beginning during the developmental period and be associated with physiological changes that extend throughout the life span. Examples of common genetic disorders are phenylketonuria (PKU), Turner's syndrome, and sickle cell anemia.

Developmental Language and Social Issues in Children

The presence of cognitive dysfunction in childhood appears to be associated with a risk of development of psychological disorders to a greater degree than that associated with physical deficits. It is widely accepted that psychopathology is multiply determined. However, in some cases, cognitive dysfunction plays a role. Schizophrenia is often characterized by a delay in neurodevelopment and generalized cognitive deficits. These deficits are often present prior to onset of the condition. Difficulties in working memory, attention, processing speed, visual and verbal learning, as well as reasoning, planning, abstraction ability, and problem solving have been estimated as being in a range as high as 98% (Tripathi et al., 2018).

Autism Spectrum Disorder

Autism Spectrum Disorder is a common (1 in 44 children in the United States in 2021—as reported by the CDC), highly heritable, heterogeneous neurodevelopmental disorder associated with cognitive features and commonly co-occurring with other conditions (Lord et al., 2020).

In the 1960s the current conceptualization of autism began to develop. In the 1970s there was recognition of the impairments in language, play, and social interactions in those with autism. The

Diagnostic and Statistical Manual of Mental Disorders (5th ed.; DSM–5-Text Revision) (American Psychiatric Association, 2022) requires deficits in social reciprocity, non-verbal communication, and developing, maintaining, and understanding relationships. There must be evidence of restricted, repetitive behaviors and interests, and symptoms must be present in early development even if not fully manifest until later in life. Environmental risk factors that have been associated with autism include advanced parental age and birth trauma, maternal obesity, a short interval between pregnancies, gestational diabetes mellitus, and valproate use during pregnancy (Lord et al., 2020). Having an older sibling with ASD and neonatal hypoxia also increase the relative risk for ASD. Twin and family studies have consistently demonstrated a genetic contribution to the development of ASD. In a meta-analysis completed by Wang et al. (2017), the heritability of ASD was found to be 92.4%. which was the highest obtained among all of the 149 diseases they studied.

Developmental Language Disorder

Language development is key in the development of cognitive and social skills. Developmental language disorder emerges early in childhood and often persists throughout the lifespan. The prevalence has been reported in a meta-analysis from Great Britain by Norbury et al. (2016) as a total prevalence of 9.92%. In this analysis, children with language disorders displayed elevated symptoms of social, emotional, and behavioral problems relative to peers, and 88% did not make expected academic progress.

Critical Periods in Development and Environmental Toxins

There are critical periods of vulnerability for the developing nervous system. These periods during the development of the nervous system are sensitive to environmental insults.

Multiple clinical disorders in humans (e.g., schizophrenia, dyslexia, epilepsy, and autism) may also be the result of interference with normal developmental processes in the nervous system (Dehorter & Del Pino, 2020). There is also concern that developmental exposure to neurotoxicants may result in an acceleration of age-related decline in function. Dehorter and Del Pino (2020) cite evidence regarding the effects of toxic stress in early development that has been linked to behavioral and health problems. For examples, adverse childhood experiences are found to increase the risk for engaging in harmful behaviors such as substance abuse, gambling, gang involvement, and violent crime. Toxic stress has been correlated with alterations in immune function and markers associated with a variety of chronic illnesses, including cardiovascular disease, autoimmune disease, asthma, liver cancer, and depression. Adverse childhood experiences have been linked to a number of cognitive deficits, including difficulties with memory and executive function, and affective deficits such as problems with reward processing and emotion regulation.

Historically, the field of developmental psychology has produced a number of diverse theories. Regardless of whether the child develops according to the Piagetian theory of assimilation and accommodation or social learning theory, wherein the child modifies their environment, virtually all developmental theories incorporate the effects of both innate influences and experience. More recent research on child development, while not attributed to individual theorists, places an emphasis on how the architecture of the brain is influenced by experiences during the prenatal and early postnatal periods. There is also increasing evidence of the interactions of genetics, environments, and experiences, with findings demonstrating the important role that experiences play during sensitive periods in shaping the capacity of the brain. The role of environment has been found to be a salient factor in both development of neural circuits, expression of characteristics of developmental disorders. Family systems (used here as a proxy for environment) have been found to be a primary factor in recovery after pediatric TBI.

When treating a child, one must consider the confluence of factors that interact to create the behavior(s) of interest. In cases where children have a developmental abnormality, a perinatal or postnatal injury, or a childhood or adolescent injury, behavior(s) can be affected. Changes, which may include alterations in motor development or functioning, language development or acquired language disorders, learning abilities, and social development, are of paramount concern when developing a life care plan and by extrapolation, when consulting with a neuropsychologist to obtain information to utilize in a life care plan. Increased understanding of the brain's structure and effects of lesions within the brain as a consequence of injury provide for an understanding of how structural damage affects functional abilities and allows comparison of the child's abilities to those of their same aged peer group. Evaluation of each child's strengths and weaknesses is essential for life care planning, as it allows for the systematic consideration of ramifications of an injury on the developing child and adolescent.

Beyond the development in childhood and adolescence, there is evidence that brain plasticity continues throughout the life span. This allows for some recovery of brain capabilities, even in adults. One line of research looks at brain plasticity in terms of recovery following strokes in older adults and another line of research on the role of structural plasticity in the hippocampus on neurodegenerative diseases, including Alzheimer's disease, Parkinson's disease, Huntington's disease, and multiple sclerosis (Weerasinghe-Mudiyanselage et al., 2022).

Role and Scope of Practice of Neuropsychologists

The American Psychological Association's Commission for the Recognition of Specialties and Proficiencies in Professional Psychology (CRSSSP, n.d.) describes clinical neuropsychology as a specialty that applies principles of assessment and intervention based upon the scientific study of human behavior as it relates to normal and abnormal functioning of the central nervous system. The specialty is dedicated to enhancing the understanding of brain–behavior relationships and the application of such knowledge to human problems. Both adult and pediatric neuropsychologists are trained in both clinical psychology and neuropsychology; the pediatric neuropsychologist has additional specialized training in brain development. Neuropsychologists are expected to meet the educational requirements to meet the standards of the Houston Conference training (Hannay et al., 1998) model. All neuropsychologists are expected to be knowledgeable in both assessment issues and evidence-based clinical interventions. Cultural and language issues are also necessary elements of learning for competently practicing neuropsychologists. Neuropsychologists are interested in observation of changes in thoughts and behaviors known to be related to the structural integrity of the brain; they then develop inferences regarding the structural integrity of the brain based on evaluation and observation of behaviors. In performing the roles in neuropsychology, at times the neuro aspect is dominant and at other times, the psychology aspect is more important.

Both pediatric and generalists are expected to understand all aspects of individual and cultural diversity and how these are to be applied in practice. There is an increased awareness of and need for neuropsychologists to be aware of their personal, individual, and cultural characteristics and how they might affect assessment and treatment issues. All neuropsychologists are governed by the American Psychological Association's *Ethical Principles of Psychologists and Code of Conduct*

(American Psychological Association, 2017). In a number of states, the code is included in licensing laws or regulations governing psychological practice. Psychologists (including the specialty of neuropsychology) are also governed by the state laws and regulations of the areas where they practice. While the ethics code is a national code, the laws and regulations governing practice differ among the states. Most neuropsychologists are licensed as psychologists; an exception is Louisiana, where there is separate licensure for neuropsychologists.

As is always the case when seeking an expert, knowing the areas in which a neuropsychologist may testify is important. For example, testimony regarding causation of brain damage is allowable in some states but not in others. While the courts may allow the testimony, the licensing law and/or regulations may not. It is also the case that the neuropsychologist should not provide opinions that are not within their scope of practice; for example, a neuropsychologist often makes clinical recommendations for evaluations by other allied health professionals and medical specialists. Most trained neuropsychologists understand key concepts related to disciplines such as neurology, physiatry, psychiatry, neuroradiology, rehabilitation, and education and are able to communicate and interact knowledgeably with professionals in these disciplines. There are often communications related to case conceptualization and treatment issues, participation as part of interdisciplinary treatment teams collaborating with other professionals to provide neuropsychological, and often psychological, information in the development and implementation of treatment goals. However, making recommendations for plans of care for treatment to be provided by these specialists is not in the scope of psychological practice, including that of neuropsychologists. Some neuropsychologists include recommendations for medications in their reports; there are a few states that allow psychologists to prescribe. If the neuropsychologist is not a prescribing psychologist, medication recommendations are not within their scope of practice.

Clinical neuropsychologists have specialized knowledge and training in the science of brain–behavior relationships and apply this knowledge performing assessment, diagnosis, treatment, and rehabilitation of patients across the lifespan who have known or suspected developmental conditions, neurological diagnoses, medical conditions, or psychiatric condition.

Pediatric neuropsychologists are often called upon for evaluating and assisting in the management of children with developmental and acquired brain disorders. Their roles in evaluation and treatment are to understand how problems with the brain may be expressed in cognitive or behavior problems in the school setting, at home, or during interactions with peers, to understand how a child learns most efficiently, and to assist with treatment planning or treatment provision.

In addition to meeting educational requirements to be a neuropsychologist, the experiences each brings to a particular disorder may differ substantially based on training and experience. This being the case, it is incumbent when making a referral for a neuropsychological examination to determine the goals of the examination and whether the neuropsychologist is in a position to address the questions to be answered. In the case of children, it is important that the provider is a pediatric neuropsychologist or if not, demonstrates experience in working with children the age of the child to be evaluated. In children, not only the disorder but the developmental stage of the child must be considered. The application of adult brain–behavior relationships is not consistently appropriate. Family and socio-environmental issues are often more complex when evaluating children or adolescents. While it is preferable to utilize a pediatric neuropsychologist with children, there is not always an available pediatric specialist in all parts of the country. The American Board of Clinical Neuropsychology has a subspecialty board certification for pediatric neuropsychologists. If no pediatric specialist is available, it can be useful to determine the number of evaluations performed (for the relevant age group) per year by the neuropsychologist to whom a referral is to be made for a child or adolescent.

Sbordone and his colleagues (2007) also noted that most psychologists are unfamiliar with cognitive rehabilitation techniques and have minimal to no experience training people to use compensatory strategies and techniques to maximize behavioral and cognitive functioning following brain injury. When these neuropsychologists without these experiences perform evaluations or make recommendations, Sbordone et al. (2007) believed the opinions to often be overly pessimistic. These authors noted that rehabilitation neuropsychologists, on the other hand, may be overly optimistic about the potential for improvement. One way to address this potential over optimism or pessimism is to ask the neuropsychologist about the probability of their opinions in terms of the standard utilized in life care planning of more likely than not. In other words, what is their reliance on the body of literature versus experience, training, and expertise. Whiteneck et al. (2018) have published a reference for adults that collates data from the Model System addressing some of the recovery probabilities for one- and five-years post-injury.

Role of Neuropsychologists

Another issue to address in looking at the opinions of a neuropsychologist is that person's role in the case. This may be particularly important in obtaining information as a life care planner. If the neuropsychologist is the treating neuropsychologist, they may have limited background records, especially pre-injury records, and may not perform an evaluation as comprehensive as would be the case if the injured person is referred for a forensic evaluation with the neuropsychologist serving as an expert. On the other hand, the treating neuropsychologist is likely to have had more experience with the behavior of the individual outside of the one-to-one testing environment which may allow more behavioral observations and inferences. There are a number of differences between the roles of a treating psychologist and expert psychologist. It is beyond the scope of this chapter to address all of these differences. However, for interested readers, they are delineated in a paper by Greenberg and Shuman (1997).

Overall, when selecting a neuropsychologist to perform an independent examination, it is important to ensure that the provider is appropriately trained and has the skills necessary to evaluate the individual for whom referral is sought. Client factors to be considered include ethnicity, age, and presenting diagnosis. Important provider factors to consider include the training environment of the neuropsychologist, the experience in clinical neuropsychology (evaluator versus treater), as well as knowledge and experience in the disorder and referral questions, the theoretical orientation of the neuropsychologist, and their forensic experience. Board certification, by either the American Board of Clinical Neuropsychology (ABCN), American Board of Professional Neuropsychology (ABN), or American Academy of Pediatric Neuropsychology (AAPdN) provides external validation that the individual has undergone examination by his or her peers in terms of neuropsychological competence. While not the only competent neuropsychologists, it gives one greater confidence when referring to a neuropsychologist about whom one knows very little. In many cases it is important that the neuropsychologist understand the medicolegal issues involved in the case, as well as the legal constructs and the case law governing the evaluation. For example, some states allow third-party observers during neuropsychological examinations conducted by the defense. Some states limit the degree to which neuropsychologists can testify regarding causation of a neurological condition such as brain injury and instead, limit the opinions to whether the findings are "consistent with" the brain injury. This issue tends to arise most often in the case of mild TBI.

Selecting a Neuropsychologist

How should one go about selecting a neuropsychologist for a specific case? Division 40 of the American Psychological Association (APA) published a definition of a neuropsychologist in *The Clinical Neuropsychologist* (March 22, 1989). This definition was adopted by the Division 40 Executive Committee and reviewed and accepted again and re-approved in 2003. The necessary educational attributes are listed, and a definition of a neuropsychologist is given. This definition stressed that attainment of the diplomate in clinical neuropsychology from the American Board of Clinical Neuropsychology "is the clearest evidence of competence as a clinical neuropsychologist assuring that all of these criteria have been met" (1989, p. 22). A listing of clinical neuropsychologists who have obtained this board certification may be found at https://theaacn.org. The directory provides a search tool for locating both adult and pediatric neuropsychologists.

The American Board of Professional Neuropsychology, another certifying body for neuropsychologists, has a listing of their diplomates in the directory at http://abn-board.com. Both of these certifying bodies require specific education and training for a neuropsychologist to apply for certification; the applicant must then undergo a rigorous peer-review process to become certified. This is not to suggest that there are not many excellent, well-trained, and experienced neuropsychologists who are not board certified. However, if seeking a neuropsychologist in a particular area, those who are board certified by either of the previously described boards have been evaluated by their peers, and their work has been found to meet the established criteria for expertise. This being the case, when no treating neuropsychologist is available, this allows greater assurance of the training and expertise of the neuropsychologist. Additional information regarding the necessary education and training in clinical neuropsychology, as well as the description of the scope of practice is available at the following resources:

- Policy Statement, Houston Conference on Specialty Education and Training in Clinical Neuropsychology (1998), https://www.nanonline.org/docs/paic/pdfs/hc%20policy%20statement.pdf
- National Academy of Neuropsychology (NAN) (2001), *Definition of a Clinical Neuropsychologist*

Neuropsychological Assessment and Treatment Recommendations

Neuropsychological assessment is a normative-based method to assess cognitive and psychological functioning. The standardized testing instruments are employed, along with behavioral observations and interview, to obtain information to make a differential diagnosis, to discriminate psychiatric versus neurological symptoms, to identify possible neurological disorders, and less often, to provide input regarding localization of a lesion related to test findings. A comprehensive neuropsychological evaluation of cognitive abilities and skills, and emotional and behavioral functioning can provide the foundation for not only accurate diagnosis but also useful recommendations for treatment for use clinically. Recommendations may include individual psychotherapy, family psychotherapy, psychiatric intervention, behavioral interventions, cognitive rehabilitation, special education services, and evaluation of specialized needs such as services provided by other physician specialists and allied health professionals (e.g., occupational therapy, neuro-ophthalmology, speech therapy, pain management consultations, neurological consultations, dietary consultations).

Follow-up neuropsychological testing allows for a determination of changes in the neuropsychological status of an individual. It may also be used to determine the effects of treatment and cognitive remediation strategies. In those individuals whose symptoms are being treated with medications, repeat testing might also help determine the effects of the medication on cognitive functioning. For example, their cognitive abilities may improve due to behavioral stability, better sleep patterns, or reduced depression or anxiety or, conversely, cognitive abilities may decline due to adverse side effects of medications. However, there are issues related to serial testing. The position paper from the American Academy of Clinical Neuropsychology (AACN) (Heilbronner et al., 2010) cites the potentially positive effects and negative effects of serial assessment including assisting in differential diagnosis, tracking neuropsychological strengths and weaknesses over time, and managing a variety of neurological and psychological conditions. However, when tests are administered on a repeated basis, there are two test scores to be interpreted, each with separate variance related to ability and procedure, as well as error variance from factors related to the examinee, examiner, environment, and context of the testing session. Practice effect refers to improvement in performance on retesting rather than to a true change in ability and is considered a primary consideration in serial testing. Heilbronner and his colleagues argue that methodological (e.g., statistical regression to the mean and person-specific (e.g., motivation)) factors may also help explain the change, or lack of change, that occurs with repeated testing. Generally, the effects of repeated examinations have shown increases in test scores as a result of the repeated exposure (Heilbronner et al., 2010). While use of alternate forms is helpful, the examinee benefits from acquiring a testing taking response set or strategy or familiarity with the testing procedure. For the severely brain injured, improvements (practice effects or real change) may be minimal.

Provision of information to patients (clinical cases) regarding strengths and deficits is imperative and must consider the patient's response to findings (Rosado et al., 2018). For neuropsychologists who perform only evaluations (consultations), there is often no way to evaluate the examinee's understanding of the findings as there are no additional sessions to obtain feedback. Anosognosia, or poor self-awareness, regarding the presence of deficits, is a common effect in both acute and chronic stages following moderate to severe brain injury (Steward & Kretzmer, 2021). Individuals who lack self-awareness are at risk of acting-out and self-injurious behaviors. Lack of self-awareness is not analogous to psychological denial, although they may co-exist. Denial is a psychological defense where symptoms are not fully acknowledged. This frequently occurs in situations where the person feels overwhelmed by their injury or illness (e.g., the individual with a complete cervical spinal cord injury who expresses the belief they will walk out of the hospital). Anosognosia is more often a function of frontal lobe/executive dysfunction or other brain lesion. These individuals may be at risk of engaging in illegal activities, either due to impulsivity and poor judgment or vulnerability to the influence of others. Because of deficits in executive functioning, they may not recognize when others are taking advantage of them. Many of them have lost relationships with friends (and/or family) with whom they interacted prior to the injury and due to loneliness are vulnerable in multiple environmental contexts. They may also fail to recognize the dangers inherent in their behaviors (for example, a person with post-traumatic seizures who continues to use alcohol in spite of having a seizure after each episode of drinking).

Neuropsychological testing performed in school-aged children and adolescents can assist in educational placement, curriculum planning, and recommendations to maximize learning. The neuropsychologist may be able to serve as a liaison between the school and the family to provide for a smoother return-to-school transition, cognitively and behaviorally. It is also the case that the neuropsychologist, particularly one who has been involved with the individual during post-acute inpatient rehabilitation or outpatient rehabilitation, is likely to be helpful in developing a behavior management program should one be required.

In children, the information documented regarding serial testing does not apply in the same way as in adults. In children, the variability is greatest in young children (before the age of five) and reduces over time (albeit slowly) throughout childhood and adolescence. Children have been shown to have differential rates of variability based on characteristics of the tests and effects of accelerated periods of brain development. Measuring change in children with acquired brain injury may be particularly challenging as the child is not only trying to recover previously learned skills but also learn new age-expected skills (Heilbronner et al., 2010). This is often the conundrum with recovery in children, they may appear to be progressing well in their recovery and later experience what appears to be a decline as they fail to develop skills expected in children at an older age.

Neuropsychological assessment, particularly for adults, can also provide information regarding an individual's ability to participate and, more importantly, benefit from cognitive neurorehabilitation treatment. This is an area where some neuropsychologists are involved in either helping to develop treatment strategies or as service providers. Research by Leon-Carrion et al. (2013) and Kennedy et al. (2008) have documented findings showing that while an individual may benefit from cognitive remediation regardless of the time post-injury, beginning earlier post-injury is associated with greater improvements in mood, cognitive function, quality of life, and better functional outcomes. A committee from the Institute of Medicine found limited evidence regarding the effectiveness of cognitive remediation training (Cicerone et al., 2019; Koehler et al., 2011). An evidence-based systematic review of the literature on cognitive rehabilitation notes that cognitive rehabilitation should be directed toward improving everyday functioning and should have a goal of generalization or directly apply compensatory strategies to functional settings. Evaluation of rehabilitation effectiveness typically occurs at the impairment level, with the expectation that this will translate into changes in daily functioning. However, this expectation is a limiting factor in evaluation of rehabilitation effectiveness. For example, the Institute of Medicine (Koehler et al., 2011) report on cognitive rehabilitation therapy for TBI documented evidence from controlled trials that internal memory strategies are useful for improving recall on decontextualized, standard tests of memory. Unfortunately, they found limited evidence that these benefits translate into meaningful changes in patients' daily memory either for specific tasks/activities or for avoiding memory lapses. They cited a need for increased emphasis on functional patient-centered outcomes to improve patient functioning (Koehler et al., 2011) for development of interventions and outcome measures that focused on functioning in everyday living skills. Neuropsychological assessment can help to direct cognitive rehabilitation through demonstrating strengths that may be used to facilitate recovery in areas of weakness and to assist the determination of strategies that are likely to provide the optimum effect.

Many patients are referred for clinical neuropsychological evaluation to assess cognitive strengths and weaknesses and to obtain information about behavioral changes and emotional characteristics. Assisting with adjustment to an individual's disability for the patient, their family, and/or their caregiver is also within the purview of neuropsychologists. Primarily, this role consists of educating the family, caregiver, and patient regarding the effects of the neurological condition on the individual's behavior. However, a neuropsychologist's recommendations can address modifications to the environment (to address behavior and cognition); these might include the interactions between over-stimulation, fatigue, sleep disruption, and behavior. Another recommendation might be developing a structured plan for task completion, which might include the model used in some holistic rehabilitation programs (Ben-Yishay & Diller, 2011) of identifying a problem with the potential solutions, and then developing a strategy to meet the desired outcome. Treatment recommendations might also include assisting others in appropriate behavior management techniques; families/caregivers often give mixed messages to the individual leading to high levels of conflict. Additionally, pediatric neuropsychologists may perform a role in the school system developing behavior management programs and making recommendations for

Individualized Education Plan (IEPs). Education of family and other stakeholders through providing a full description of the patient's abilities, deficits, prognosis, and need for rehabilitation services and needed environmental modifications are crucial for the best adjustment of the individual and their entire family. Without this information, it is difficult for families and others involved in the person's care and education to make plans for future care, including the need for and degree of supervision, and other management issues for a patient with acquired brain injury or another neurological dysfunction. The neuropsychologist may answer questions regarding an individual's cognitive capacity in terms of self-care, the ability to follow a therapeutic regimen independently, the cognitive capacity to operate a motor vehicle (the determination of ability to return to driving is multifactorial and neuropsychological findings are one part), and ability to manage personal financial matters (this requires assessment of skills that are not part of a routine clinical or forensic assessment.). A neuropsychologist is also often called on to assess an individual regarding their cognitive capacity for competence in probate hearings or for living alone in their home. The APA and the American Bar Association (ABA) have collaborated to develop a document to provide a framework for these evaluations in older adults (ABA/APA, 2008). The overall methodology requires not only that one address cognitive capabilities but also link those capabilities to functional tasks. Most of these evaluations are completed in the person's home.

The Neuropsychological Examination

While most neuropsychologists rely largely on standardized test data, these data alone do not provide all of the information needed to fully assess an individual. There is a need to consider information from subjective sources, objective sources, and collateral sources. Subjective information includes information provided by the patient, family members, and caregivers, which cannot be verified with other data. It often includes complaints of physical, emotional, and/or cognitive difficulties. Family members and caregivers often relate the patient's complaints of their feelings or physical distress but may also provide, or be able to provide, with appropriate questioning, objective data. Beyond relating what they have been told about how the patient feels, they may have extensive knowledge of patterns of behavior, sleeping habits, eating habits, personality changes, and interpersonal relationship changes. Objective information includes information from school records, medical records, vocational records, neuropsychological and psychological test data, and other data sources from either before the injury, where available, or post-injury. The individual's social history, including educational and work experiences, provides information about premorbid cognitive potential. Marital history also provides relevant information and may provide information about emotional stability, social judgment, and relationship stability over time. Assessment of the individual's current life circumstances also provides information about current functioning and how they are adapting to changes. A concordance of data from the individual, family or caregivers, and medical records also provides for a non-quantitative behavioral measure of self-awareness.

Comparison of an individual's functioning pre- and post-injury helps to delineate the changes since the injury and helps in treatment planning. Medical history and current medical status provide some degree of information about the individual's premorbid history. Medications that have been prescribed, or dosage modifications required, may also provide some understanding of how functioning has changed over time. Another important source of information is the observation of the examinee during the testing process. While testing may be performed by either a psychometrist or the neuropsychologist, there is often a large amount of information gathered during the examination process, which lasts from several hours to days in some instances. For instance, how the individual approaches a task may give a significant amount of information beyond that provided by the test score alone. For example, any disruptive behaviors in a quiet, one-to-one setting are likely to be magnified in a work, school, social, or home environment. How an individual responds to success or failure on testing provides information regarding the potential for perseverance in the face of frustrating tasks and may speak to awareness of deficits. Behaviors that occur during the testing, again in a setting designed to obtain the person's best performance, are highly important in understanding the ability to function in the real-world environment. While some neuropsychologists break up the testing sessions over several days to minimize the effects of fatigue, how the person functions early in the day versus when they are tired may be more useful in predicting overall ability to return to school or work unless these settings will be asked to accommodate fatigue effects. Using all available data allows the neuropsychologist to develop a picture of how the person functioned before and after an injury or illness. Failure to consider this information may lead to spurious conclusions by the neuropsychologist. For example, this author tested an individual who reported being an average student and a high school graduate. On testing, his intellect was measured to fall in the third percentile (standard score 72) and academic assessment revealed reading in the extremely low range (no school records were available prior to the examination). When school records were provided, it was determined he had a certificate of attendance and not a diploma. He had also been in special education with an IEP beginning in elementary school. If results of testing had been the only consideration, his deficits would have been overstated. The converse may also occur if the neuropsychologist is not aware of past history; an individual with a high level of functioning may not be identified as having changes in cognitive abilities if there is no attempt to determine the premorbid level of function. It is important to note that there is expected variability in scores when multiple measures are administered. This variability must be considered by the neuropsychologist in interpretation of test results.

Answering Questions with Neuropsychological Test Results

The assessment dynamics should be predicated on the referral questions. It is often the case that the referral questions are related to an individual's ability to drive or return to work or school. Questions regarding the ability to manage financial affairs or make other high-complexity cognitive decisions are also often asked of neuropsychologists. Neuropsychologists are often asked to address diagnostic questions when the etiology of cognitive or behavioral problems is unknown. These are typically questions related to differential diagnosis (e.g., depression versus dementia). Questions regarding specific abilities often arise in vocational and educational planning. The answers to these questions are especially important if the referral involves withdrawal or return of normal adult rights and privileges, such as driving or legal competence. In these cases, the neuropsychological examination will focus heavily on the relevant skills and functions. Other areas of assessment include awareness of one's condition and capacity to incorporate new information and skills.

Tests are typically selected that meet criteria for reliability and validity and have norms appropriate for the individual being assessed. There are some neuropsychologists who use a fixed battery approach; this approach is exemplified by the Halstead–Reitan Battery. Most neuropsychologists use a flexible battery approach to address the referral question(s). In a flexible battery, a selection of tests to measure the various domains of cognitive functioning are combined. Rabin et al. (2016) have a list of the tests most commonly used by neuropsychologists. Typically, multiple measures in each cognitive domain are employed. The cognitive domains that are typically assessed include intellectual abilities, attention/concentration, speed of cognitive information processing, memory and learning in verbal and visual modalities, speech and language, academic functioning, motor and sensory functioning, visual spatial functioning, response bias and effort, executive function, mood, personality, and adaptive functioning. In the Rabin et al. (2016) study, participants reported a lack of ecological validity and difficulty comparing the meaning of obtained standard scores across measures as the primary challenges associated with the selection of neuropsychological instruments and interpretation of test data.

The most commonly used tests for measuring intellect are the intellectual scales which were originated by David Wechsler (e.g., Wechsler Adult Intelligence Scales). Others in the top five are the Wechsler Memory Scales, the Trailmaking Test, the California Verbal Learning Test, and the Wechsler Intelligence Scale for Children (Rabin et al., 2016). Another element of the examination is determining the pre-injury baseline of the individual. It is relatively unusual to have someone who has had a previous neuropsychological examination unless they have suffered a previous injury or neurological illness. Neuropsychologists must try to ascertain how the person might have functioned in the past to develop a benchmark to which current test scores are compared. While most of the general population functions in the average range, the individuals whose scores premorbidly fall closer to the ends of the distribution pose a challenge. If an individual functioned at the upper end of the score distribution, even milder changes may affect their ability to function, at least in a vocational sense. For example, a neurosurgeon with mild injuries is likely to have greater difficulty vocationally than an individual who does not deal with tasks of the complexity of a neurosurgeon on a daily basis. An individual who was functioning marginally pre-injury, may have greater difficulty coping than would be the case for someone who functions at an average level. Individuals with fewer cognitive reserves do not have the cognitive resources to adapt as efficiently. There are several regression equations that have been developed to estimate premorbid intellect (e.g., the Barona equation). Another method frequently used is reading ability (Johnstone et al., 1996). There is an obvious difficulty in using this method in cases of premorbid reading difficulties or where the person has sustained damage to reading centers of the left hemisphere. However, given that reading is learned relatively early in development, and is then overlearned as part of the education process, it provides one measure of premorbid abilities in many cases.

Consideration must also be given to factors other than brain damage which may affect test results. These include motivation, fatigue, pain, depression, anxiety, medications, and litigation. These factors, either singly or in combination, may affect results of testing to varying degrees. Neuropsychologists are encouraged to use measures of performance validity to assess, to the degree possible, the person's performance validity, particularly as part of a neuropsychological examination performed in a forensic context (NAN position paper).

Use of an interpreter is another issue that may impact test results. There are limited tests that are available in other languages, for example Spanish, with appropriate norms for populations of individuals who speak the language. In the Rabin et al. (2016) study, the majority of most commonly used test instruments lacked appropriate normative data for Spanish-speaking populations in the U.S. Additionally, some the most frequently reported difficulties associated with selection of testing instruments included a "lack of adequate normative data" (33.5% of survey respondents) and that "tests are culturally biased" (11.5%). Additionally, 15.9% of the respondents noted, "lack of norms for additional demographic groups" as an issue in data interpretation.

The use of an interpreter to administer test questions translated from English into another language should be applied judiciously, if at all, since it enhances the potential for errors such as those described in the Rabin et al. (2016) study. There is a high likelihood that the test will not render fully valid or reliable results. The problem is multifactorial. First, the accuracy of the translation of test questions cannot be monitored. Second, the tests often have inherent cultural biases. Finally, having a third person present during an evaluation has the potential to change the dynamics creating unknown amounts of error variance. A recent study (Suárez et al., 2021) also provided evidence regarding the effects of bilingualism on testing, underscoring the importance of gathering thorough information about an examinee's level of second-language ability in neuropsychological assessments, to assess the need to take into account Spanish-English bilingualism as part of the interpretation of testing. There has been a concerted effort to develop more extensive norms for Spanish-speaking individuals in the United States; however, according to a review by Paredes et al. (2021), the information remains limited. The greater the difference between the individual being tested and the normative sample, the less reliance one may place on the outcome. However, there are situations where it is not possible to find a neuropsychologist who fluently speaks the language of the examinee. In these cases, the choice becomes one of either making no attempt to assess the individual or using an interpreter. Some authors have argued there are ethical considerations in testing someone whose language we do not speak (Artiola & Mullaney, 1998); this should be given due consideration before attempting an assessment. It is the practice of this author to refer to a neuropsychologist who speaks the language of the examinee. If this is not possible, a clinical interview is completed using an interpreter. Testing is rarely attempted and if so is limited. Even with these cautions, the results are not considered fully reliable or valid but may provide some useful clinical information regarding function. Knowledge of the individual's culture becomes highly important in these situations as behaviors may be misinterpreted. When assessing an individual who is hard of hearing, American Sign Language (ASL) is considered a language. Given the small populations of hard of hearing individuals in many communities, the interpreter may have had personal interactions with the individual being assessed leading to an unknown degree of confounds in the results of testing in addition to the above-described caveats.

There are multiple neurobehavioral variables and diagnostic issues to be considered in the neuropsychological evaluation (Lezak et al., 2004). These variables include lesion characteristics, subject variables, and psychosocial variables. For example, there are changes in cognitive abilities related to the aging process. The relationship between moderate to severe TBI and later development of dementia has been documented in the research literature; most of the evidence seems to suggest there is a greater magnitude of risk to develop a neurodegenerative disorder than in the general population (Fleminger et al., 2003; Shively et al., 2012). Other epidemiological studies do not reach this conclusion (Smith et al., 2013). Thus, the findings remain equivocal to some extent regarding the degree of risk based on age at injury and individual genetics. An individual's premorbid personality and social adjustment also play a role in outcome following TBI. Research has shown that premorbid personality is not so often changed as it is exaggerated by brain injury. It is easy to see how the impulsivity, difficulty with anger management, and disinhibition associated with frontal lobe damage are complicated in an individual whose premorbid self-regulation of behavior was poor. Emotional difficulties, such as depression, may also complicate the clinical presentation of an individual with brain injury. It is important that the neuropsychologist identify depression, both premorbid and postmorbid, as it may complicate recovery; in addition, the patient may lack the initiative or cognitive ability to seek help on their own. The partial or complete loss of independence experienced by an individual with brain injury may also complicate testing, for example, due to uncooperative behavior, passive-aggressive behavior, fear of failure, or fear of additional loss of independence.

Questions Life Care Planners Should Ask Neuropsychologists

It is helpful to provide a series of questions for the neuropsychologist to address. There are a series of questions included in Chapter 4 of *The Life Care Planning and Case Management Handbook* (Berens & Weed, 2018) to be asked of a neuropsychologist. These include a description of areas of damage to the brain, the effects of the injury on functioning, and the opinion of the neuropsychologists with respect to intellect (pre and postmorbid), personality style, particularly as related to the workplace and home, stamina, functional limitations and assets, potential for education and retraining, insight, ability to compensate for deficits, initiation, visual and verbal short term and long-term memory and learning, recognition and correction of errors, recommended compensation strategies, and need for a companion or attendant. The questions included in the chapter by Berens and Weed (2018) also address a proposed treatment plan with specific questions regarding psychotherapy, family counseling, re-evaluations, referrals to physicians and others, as well as the duration, intensity, and cost for services. The answers to these questions are detailed as part of this chapter. Providing the most accurate and helpful responses to these questions requires pre-injury records, particularly school records and medical records. As previously mentioned, vocational records may be beneficial in answering some of the questions regarding vocational implications of the injury but need to include detailed information, which, if possible, would include records from human resources. This allows a finer-grained analysis of previous work performance (e.g., work attendance, productivity, interactions with peers). While absence of negative information does not ensure that there were no pre-existing problems, presence of premorbid problems is important in terms of assessment and potentially prediction of areas where problems may recur. A comprehensive neuropsychological examination will address issues related to intellectual capacity, attention and speed of information processing, memory, and learning for visual and verbal modalities (as well as remotely through the clinical interview). Stamina, in the opinion of this writer, is best assessed through behavioral observations during testing that is administered in one long setting where possible. An individual's ability to compensate is often multifactorial and includes self-awareness, the ability to develop problem solving strategies and/or utilize techniques that have been or will be a part of therapy, memory at a level to recall the steps, and/or ability to routinely utilize external cues to compensate. Younger patients often use their cellular phone as a tool for recall and some older individuals prefer small note pads. Not all neuropsychologists treat patients and provide neurocognitive rehabilitation. If they are able, a compensatory program may be delineated within the report. The treatment plan is also based on multiple factors, including the patient's age, willingness to participate in psychotherapy, or remediation. Too often, this author reads reports documenting that an individual has told the therapist they are there only because they were forced to come. This posture toward therapy does not bode well for participation in or benefit from therapy. In individual cases, the neuropsychologist may be able to intervene and help the patient gain a greater understanding of the process and potential outcomes.

Ensuring that questions for the neuropsychologist can be appropriately answered is paramount to increasing the utility of the examination. Receiving a report that documents the potential location of the lesion (without descriptors of what this means functionally) is not likely to be beneficial in determining life care planning needs as would be a report detailing the effects of both cognitive strengths and weaknesses on functional abilities of the individual with brain injury. One way to obtain the needed information is to ask the neuropsychologist a series of specific questions. Uomoto (2000) states that it is easier for a neuropsychologist to answer whether a person can perform a specific task for a specific job than to answer whether the same individual can return to work.

One of the most salient issues in answering questions posed has to do with the ecological validity of testing. Sbordone (1997, p. 368) defines ecological validity as the "functional and predictive relationship between the patient's performance on a set of neuropsychological tests and behavior in a variety of real-world settings." Providing the neuropsychologists with information regarding the demands of the environment allows for a better assessment of how the demands interact with the individual's cognitive strengths and weaknesses, premorbid abilities and skills, and future goals. Without this information, the predictions made based on test data alone have a significant likelihood of being inaccurate and unhelpful. In his article on ecological validity, Sbordone (1997) further notes the importance of obtaining a detailed history and interviewing collateral sources, the importance of behavioral observations, using appropriate norms, and the relevance of test scores to real-world settings. Sbordone cites the review of Acker in 1990, which examined the question of how neuropsychological tests relate to real-world behavior. Acker reportedly found moderate correlations between test results and various functional assessments. She also noted the findings varied according to what point during the recovery period the tests were administered. When attempts are made to correlate neuropsychological test results with activities of daily living, the complex tests appear to be better predictors. It seems that the most effective method to increase predictive ability is to ascertain the degree to which test data are consistent with data from other sources (medical records, family observations, academic records, vocational records, and observation of the patient's behavior in a variety of settings). The degree of agreement between these sources then provides an "operational estimate of our test data" (Sbordone, 1997). If the test data do not fit with the other data, then the ecological validity would be considered low. Neuropsychological test data with a higher level of concordance would be considered to have higher ecological validity. It is worth noting that the study by Rabin et al. (2016) supports the issues of ecological validity and testing.

Even with these issues related to ecological validity, it is possible to obtain ecologically valid predictions from neuropsychological and psychological testing results. The value of a neuropsychological examination is enhanced when it is designed to answer specific referral questions. When a patient is referred by a physician for a clinical evaluation (particularly an outpatient evaluation), the examination may not include review of the objective information and supplemental records listed earlier in this chapter (e.g., educational records, medical records). The neuropsychologist is in the role of treating neuropsychologist and often completes the examination without collateral information other than that provided by a family member who accompanies the patient (if the patient allows their participation). It is often the case, particularly early in the recovery process, that the family is overwhelmed by changes that have occurred in their lifestyle. This may lead to faulty information being provided. For example, the family may not be able to accurately assess deficits due to their own emotional overload. If the patient lacks insight, their view of self has a high probability of being inaccurate. This being the case, records should be provided to the neuropsychologist prior to the testing and reviewed by the neuropsychologist prior to answering the referral questions. The greater the specificity of the question, the more beneficial the examination can be. It is important to note that the setting (quiet, one-to-one setting) in which neuropsychological testing is performed is designed to elicit the best performance of the examinee. The individual post-TBI may be able to sustain attention in an environment with minimal, or even moderate, distractions but have difficulty if they are asked to perform in a work cubicle-type environment where multiple telephone conversations are taking place simultaneously. Describing the environment to the neuropsychologist is likely to increase their ability to make accurate predictions.

When asked about the need for supervision, it is often helpful to ask rehabilitation neuropsychologists this question in terms of Functional Independence Measure Scores (FIMS). For neuropsychologists who are unfamiliar with FIMS, using the descriptors from the scale (e.g., unable to perform an activity or independence in performing an activity) may be useful in translating a score from a categorial score or a percentile into a functionally based score. Another issue in interpretation is the use of different categorical referents in describing test results. The AACN encourages greater uniformity in labeling of test scores to assist in test comparisons and in communicating results (Guilmette et al., 2020).

It may also be useful to ask about specific tasks that may require supervision such as the self-administration of medications, the ability to be left alone with, or care for, a child who needs supervision, ability to manage finances, ability to make financial decisions, or ability to make safety decisions. Another avenue would be to ask questions that would be necessary to answer if the person were being evaluated with regard to civil competence.

In summary, when choosing a neuropsychologist for referral, determine the best person for the referral based on education and expertise in the area of interest. Ask specific questions. Rather than "Can they return to work?"—ask questions about specific tasks and demands in the environment. Provision of a job description may be helpful but often is too general to be useful. Also, ask about potential barriers, such as those imposed by fatigue or behavioral issues. Ask the neuropsychologist to address how test findings of cognitive strengths or weaknesses relate to behavior in naturalistic environments (e.g., the ecological validity of the test measures). When deficits are noted, the neuropsychologist should be able explain how the deficits are correlated with, and likely to interfere with, specific work demands in a specific job position. When asking about the ability to live independently, focusing on specific areas requiring independence rather than a global question of independence is likely to yield more precise information.

To avoid receiving a report that does not answer your questions, provide the referral questions in advance of neuropsychological examination. If not, you may receive a report that relates the person's cognitive strengths and deficits and behavioral deficits, which may not be easily extrapolated into life care plan recommendations. In many cases, the neuropsychologist may be able to answer your questions after the fact; however, having the questions beforehand should help guide test selection and interview questions. For example, knowing that answers to questions regarding independent living skills are needed may lead test selection in a different direction. It also ensures that the neuropsychologist does not, after the fact, tell the life care planner they have insufficient data to provide specific answers to the questions. The same general process is recommended in asking questions of the treating neuropsychologist. If the neuropsychologist has been involved in the care during either at an inpatient rehabilitation facility, or a specialized outpatient facility, they should be able to correlate behaviors with testing results more readily than a neuropsychologist who has seen the individual for a one-time evaluation. When the patient lives near the rehabilitation facility, they often return to the neuropsychologist at the setting for the serial testings during the natural recovery period. If the patient lives distant to the rehabilitation facility, referral may be made by the rehabilitation facility to a local neuropsychologist; at that point, the process employed may be driven by the payor source rather than being needs based. While there is an identified need to be able to complete neuropsychological examinations remotely, at present there are no large-scale studies demonstrating the equivalence of face-to-face versus videoconference administration of neuropsychological testing. The results from a meta-analysis by Brearly et al. (2017), documents overall consistency between scores obtained during face-to-face and video conferencing for selected measures. However, neuropsychological test instruments are not normed for use in remote testing. Another testing issue is the need for both the examiner and the examinee to physically manipulate some of the test materials. There are also technical and environmental issues to be considered. Technical problems may ensue due to issues with equipment and connectivity. Environmentally, there needs to be a quiet, distraction free, space for the testing to be administered. Preventing interruptions is often more difficult in a home environment. When the testing is referred to a local neuropsychologist, this author recommends meeting with the rehabilitation neuropsychologist (who may not have read all medical records but would have been involved in team conferences) and the neuropsychologist who examined the individual post-discharge (after providing them, if appropriate, at a minimum the team conference reports, and any neuropsychological testing performed prior to discharge).

When should neuropsychological testing be administered for use in a life care plan? Most of the natural recovery following acquired brain injury occurs in the first 6–12 months after an injury

(Fleminger & Ponsford, 2005). The degree of recovery is affected by a number of factors including premorbid abilities, age, and family support. It is generally the case that an adult with brain injury is re-evaluated every six months until the end of two years or until the treating neuropsychologist determines the patient's deficits are unlikely to change significantly. Research tends to support permanence of deficits at the end of two years (Lezak et al., 2004). However, there are studies documenting significant cognitive improvement in some people over longer intervals post-injury when cognitive treatment is provided post-injury (Whiteneck et al., 2018).

The course of recovery is more complex in children. Children with moderate to severe brain injury have been shown to have cognitive and behavioral deficits that can persist over a span of several years. As the child matures, and additional cognitive skills and behaviors are expected to develop, a secondary impact of the brain injury may become apparent. In these cases, in addition to follow-up for two years post-injury, having evaluations completed at academic transition periods is recommended. Specifically, this author recommends evaluations at the end of third grade, fifth grade, eighth grade, and tenth grade as they are likely to be helpful in guiding academics. For those individuals for whom postsecondary education is expected, additional neuropsychological examination is recommended after completion of high school. In the situation where a child is in special education, the results of neuropsychological evaluation may help in developing and/or implementing the IEP. The Individuals with Disabilities Act (IDEA) requires retesting every three years for children who have an IEP (performed by the school). The results of testing can also help to determine services needed, beyond those mandated by IDEA and provided by the school system, to maximize the child's ability to benefit from education. For more information on this technical topic, go to: www2.ed.gov/parents/needs/speced/iepguide/index.html). Once the patient's deficits have reached a level where significant additional change is not anticipated, neuropsychological examination is included as the patient ages. There are declines in cognition that occur as a function of normal aging. In addition to these normal changes, those individuals who have experienced a more severe brain injury are found to be at higher risk for developing dementia in some studies (e.g., Fleminger et al., 2003; Shively et al., 2012). Neuropsychological evaluation at approximately 65–70 years of age is likely to provide information regarding these potential cognitive changes. Given that 8.8% of the population beyond age 65 has been diagnosed with a neurodegenerative process, this is the age range at which changes in cognition might be expected to show the greatest impact (Langa et al., 2017).

Psychotherapy, either with a neuropsychologist or other mental health professional with training and experience in acquired brain injury, is likely to be needed. In adults, this is likely to be required periodically throughout their life expectancy, especially during periods of stress or when they are confronted with situations that are changed by the impact of their injury and subsequent deficits. An example would be a parent who loses custody of a child because of a brain injury or the stress for an adult having to move in with family after living independently.

The disruptive effect of acquired brain injury has been well-documented in the literature (Kreutzer et al., 1992). Family members and other caregivers, particularly in the cases where there are negative behavioral changes, will require education, support, and therapy to cope. Rosenthal and Geckler (1997) in an historical article, note that the primary focus, until more recently, was on the physical aspects of the injury. The issues of psychosocial and family adjustment have since been recognized with regard to the effect on progress in rehabilitation and overall recovery. Family support and pre-injury family environment have been shown to have significant effects on outcome in children following TBI(Max et al., 1999; Ryan et al., 2016; Wade et al., 2016; Yeates et al., 1997). Anecdotally, it is the experience of this author that families may have a prolonged period of grief related to the changes that accrue following a brain injury. This may result in their attributing deficits in executive function exhibited by the individual who has residual symptoms of brain damage to volitional behavior. Conversely, feelings of guilt, empathy, or fear may lead them to reinforce negative behaviors to avoid confrontation. There are myriad other family and social difficulties where psychological intervention may help improve the quality of life for the patient and family or caregivers.

In the case where the person with the injury is a child, parents benefit from therapy to help with parenting skills, as well as help in adjusting to changes in the child's current behavior and future goals and aspirations. In the Wade et al. (2016) study, the authors found that either overly permissive or overly strict parenting resulted in poorer outcomes. This may be an area where intervention is beneficial. Additional psychotherapy sessions may be needed during puberty and through the teenage years when sexual issues need to be addressed and, if no injury or illness had occurred, the child would have been expected to have become increasingly independent.

Mild Traumatic Brain Injury

Mild TBI has not been addressed in this chapter in great detail. The rationale is that research demonstrates that most cases resolve in weeks to months without cognitive consequences (Carroll et al., 2014; Karr et al., 2014; Rohling et al., 2011; Silverberg et al., 2020). When there are persisting symptoms, they are typically related to an emotional reaction to the injury (Carroll et al., 2014). Evaluation by a neuropsychologist can elucidate the findings and recommend whether coping assistance is needed and if so, recommend a treatment plan.

Clinical Practice Guidelines

The following clinical practice guidelines may be useful to the practicing life care planner in addressing issues related to the populations served by neuropsychologists. The full citation may be found in the references:

> *A Systematic Review and Quality Analysis of Pediatric Traumatic Brain Injury Clinical Practice Guidelines* (Appenteng et al., 2018)
> American Academy of Clinical Neuropsychology (AACN) *Practice Guidelines for Neuropsychological Assessment and Consultation* (2007)
> Veterans Affairs/Department of Defense *Clinical Practice Guideline for Management of Post-Traumatic Stress* (2017)
> *One- and Five-Year Outcomes After Moderate-to-Severe Traumatic Brain Injury Requiring Inpatient Rehabilitation: Traumatic Brain Injury Report.* Centers for Disease Control and Prevention; National Center for Injury Prevention and Control; Administration for Community Living; National Institute on Disability, Independent, Living and Rehabilitation Research (Whiteneck et al., 2018)

Case Study

The following tables are excerpted from a life care plan for a woman who sustained a severe TBI in a motor vehicle collision. Since the accident, she has had multiple cognitive symptoms, consistent with diffuse brain injury and specific injury to the right frontal lobe. She also has significant physical limitations that impair her abilities in performance of activities other than basic activities of daily living (ADLs). The recommendations were obtained through consultations with her treating physiatrist and neuropsychologist. Consultation was also held with a medical case manager to determine appropriate recommendations for Ms. Smith's ongoing needs in this domain. The life care planning tables are displayed in SaddlePoint Software, LLC format (format reprinted by permission, William Walker).

Modified Life Care Plan
for
Jane L. Smith

Highway 41265

Houston, AL 35579

Date of Birth: 04/28/1984

Event Date: 09/30/2020

Primary Disability: Multiple Trauma

Preparation Date: July 6, 2022

NeuroLife, LLC
Carol P. Walker, PhD, ABPP-CN, CLCP
PO Box 4647
Huntsville, AL 35815

256-535-2322

Copyright 2000 - 2005, SaddlePoint Software, LLC - All Rights Reserved.

Prepared By: Carol P. Walker PhD, ABPP-CN, CLCP

Projected Evaluations

Item or Service	Purpose	Replacement Schedule	Start / End	Costs
Case Manager 1 Options 1, 2	The case manager will assist in appointment scheduling and other activities associated with medical care. The case manager will also assist in hiring and monitoring attendant care.	1 Time Only	# Start Age/Year 38 2022 # End Age/Year 38 2022	Cost/Unit $90.00 to $105.00 Cost/Year $360.00 to $420.00

Cost/Year = 4/1 x $90.00 = $360.00
Cost/Year = 4/1 x $105.00 = $420.00
Cost/Year Average = ($360.00 + $420.00) ÷ 2 = $390.00

Family/Guardian Counseling and Education 2 Options 1, 2	Assist immediate family with coping skills.	1 Time/Year	# Start Age/Year 38 2022 # End Age/Year 38 2022	Cost/Unit $125.13 to $125.13 Cost/Year $125.13 to $125.13
Home Assessment 3 Option 1	Professional assessment of home for safety issues.	1 Time Only	# Start Age/Year 38 2022 # End Age/Year 38 2022	Cost/Unit $161.25 to $161.25 Cost/Year $645.00 to $645.00

This is for four hours of either a PT or an OT to assess her home for safety issues that may be addressed in addition to home modifications. Additional assessment may be needed if she moves to another home.
Cost/Year = 4/1 x $161.25 = $645.00

Modified Life Care Plan for Jane L. Smith
Copyright 2000 - 2005, SaddlePoint Software, LLC - All Rights Reserved.

Growth Trends to be determined by an Economist.
*LE = Life Expectancy **U = Unknown   N/A = Not Applicable
All Ages and Dates are Inclusive, e.g. 2000-2006 = 7 Years

Prepared By: Carol P. Walker PhD, ABPP-CN, CLCP

Projected Evaluations

Item or Service	Purpose	Replacement Schedule	Start / End	Costs
Psychologist 4 Options 1, 2	Evaluation in anticipation of therapy and to develop a plan of care.	1 Time Only	# Start Age/Year 38 2022 # End Age/Year 38 2022	Cost/Unit $198.42 to $198.42 Cost/Year $198.42 to $198.42
Occupational Therapy Evaluation 5 Option 1	Assess ongoing equipment needs and ADLs.	1 Time/Year	# Start Age/Year 38 2022 # End Age/Year 72 2056	Cost/Unit $199.17 to $228.90 Cost/Year $199.17 to $228.90

Cost/Year Average = ($199.17 + $228.90) ÷ 2 = $214.04

Physical Therapy Evaluation 6 Option 1	Assess status and make recommendations regarding physical therapy needs.	1 Time/Year	# Start Age/Year 38 2022 # End Age/Year 72 2056	Cost/Unit $185.93 to $228.07 Cost/Year $185.93 to $228.07

Cost/Year Average = ($185.93 + $228.07) ÷ 2 = $207.00

350 ■ Carol P. Walker

Prepared By: Carol P. Walker PhD, ABPP-CN, CLCP

Projected Therapeutic Modalities

	Item or Service	Purpose	Replacement Schedule	Start End	Costs
1	Case Management - Home Care Setup Option 1	The case manager will assist in appointment scheduling and other activities associated with medical care. The case manager will also assist in hiring and monitoring attendant care.	1 Time Only	# Start Age/Year 38 2022 # End Age/Year 38 2022	Cost/Unit $90.00 to $105.00 Cost/Year $900.00 to $1,050.00

This recommendation was obtained from J. Bragg, a Certified Case Manager.
Cost/Year = 10/1 x $90.00 = $900.00
Cost/Year = 10/1 x $105.00 = $1,050.00
Cost/Year Average = ($900.00 + $1,050.00) ÷ 2 = $975.00

	Item or Service	Purpose	Replacement Schedule	Start End	Costs
2	Case Management Option 1	The case manager will assist in appointment scheduling and other activities associated with medical care. The case manager will also assist in hiring and monitoring attendant care.	2 - 4 Hours/ Month	# Start Age/Year 38 2022 # End Age/Year 72 2056	Cost/Unit $90.00 to $105.00 Cost/Year $2,160.00 to $5,040.00

Cost/Year = $90.00 x 2 x 12 = $2,160.00   Cost/Year = $105.00 x 4 x 12 = $5,040.00
Cost/Year = $105.00 x 2 x 12 = $2,520.00   Cost/Year Average = ($2,160.00 + $5,040.00) ÷ 2 = $3,600.00
Cost/Year = $90.00 x 4 x 12 = $4,320.00

Prepared By: Carol P. Walker PhD, ABPP-CN, CLCP

Projected Therapeutic Modalities

	Item or Service	Purpose	Replacement Schedule	Start End	Costs
3	Case Manager Facility Set Up Option 2	The case manager will assist in arranging aspects of facility care.	1 Time Only	# Start Age/Year 38 2022 # End Age/Year 38 2022	Cost/Unit $90.00 to $105.00 Cost/Year $540.00 to $630.00

This recommendation was obtained from J. Bragg, a Certified Case Manager.
Cost/Year = 6/1 x $90.00 = $540.00
Cost/Year = 6/1 x $105.00 = $630.00
Cost/Year Average = ($540.00 + $630.00) ÷ 2 = $585.00

	Item or Service	Purpose	Replacement Schedule	Start End	Costs
4	Case Manager Option 2	The case manager will assist in appointment scheduling and other activities associated with medical care. The case manager will also assist in hiring and monitoring attendant care.	6 Hours/ Year	# Start Age/Year 38 2022 # End Age/Year 72 2056	Cost/Unit $90.00 to $105.00 Cost/Year $540.00 to $630.00

Cost/Year = $90.00 x 6 = $540.00
Cost/Year = $105.00 x 6 = $630.00
Cost/Year Average = ($540.00 + $630.00) ÷ 2 = $585.00

Prepared By: Carol P. Walker PhD, ABPP-CN, CLCP   **Projected Therapeutic Modalities**

Item or Service	Purpose	Replacement Schedule	Start / End	Costs
Family/Guardian Counseling and Education 5 Options 1, 2	Assist family with coping skills.	17 - 23 Times/Year	# Start Age/Year 38 2022 # End Age/Year 38 2022	Cost/Unit $125.13 to $125.13 Cost/Year $14,890.47 to $20,145.93

This recommendation is based on consultation with Ms. Smith's treating neuropsychologist.
Cost/Year = 7/1 x $125.13 x 17 = $14,890.47
Cost/Year = 7/1 x $125.13 x 23 = $20,145.93
Cost/Year Average = ($14,890.47 + $20,145.93) ÷ 2 = $17,518.20

| Psychotherapy (Individual)

6   Options 1, 2 | This therapy is specifically to address adjustment to changes in her life secondary to her injuries and to address behavioral issues related to her brain injury. | 12 - 24 Times/Year | # Start Age/Year
38
2022
End Age/Year
38
2022 | Cost/Unit
$141.08 to $152.31
Cost/Year
$1,692.96 to $3,655.44 |

This recommendation is based on consultation with Ms. Smith's treating neuropsychologist. Ms. Smith was being treated for anxiety and depression prior to the injury.
Cost/Year = $141.08 x 12 = $1,692.96   Cost/Year = $152.31 x 24 = $3,655.44
Cost/Year = $152.31 x 12 = $1,827.72   Cost/Year Average = ($1,692.96 + $3,655.44) ÷ 2 = $2,674.20
Cost/Year = $141.08 x 24 = $3,385.92

Prepared By: Carol P. Walker PhD, ABPP-CN, CLCP   **Projected Therapeutic Modalities**

Item or Service	Purpose	Replacement Schedule	Start / End	Costs
Psychotherapy (Individual) 7 Options 1, 2	This therapy is specifically to address adjustment to changes in her life secondary to her injuries and to address behavioral issues related to her brain injury.	1 Time/Year	# Start Age/Year 39 2023 # End Age/Year 72 2056	Cost/Unit $1.00 to $1.00 Cost/Year $1.00 to $1.00

This recommendation is based on consultation with Ms. Smith's treating neuropsychologist. Ms. Smith was being treated for anxiety and depression prior to the injury.

| Physical Therapy

8   Options 1, 2 | Maintain physical capacity and address balance issues. | 12 - 16 Visits/Year | # Start Age/Year
38
2022
End Age/Year
72
2056 | Cost/Unit
$141.08 to $158.31
Cost/Year
$6,771.84 to $10,131.84 |

Recommended by Ms. Smith's treating physiatrist.
Cost/Year = 4/1 x $141.08 x 12 = $6,771.84   Cost/Year = 4/1 x $158.31 x 16 = $10,131.84
Cost/Year = 4/1 x $158.31 x 12 = $7,598.88   Cost/Year Average = ($6,771.84 + $10,131.84) ÷ 2 = $8,451.84
Cost/Year = 4/1 x $141.08 x 16 = $9,029.12

Projected Therapeutic Modalities

Prepared By: Carol P. Walker PhD, ABPP-CN, CLCP

Item or Service	Purpose	Replacement Schedule	Start / End	Costs
Occupational Therapy	Maintain ADLs.	12 - 16 Times/Year	# Start Age/Year: 38, 2022	Cost/Unit: $56.93 to $87.71
9 Options 1, 2			# End Age/Year: 72, 2056	Cost/Year: $2,732.64 to $5,613.44

Recommended by Ms. Smith's treating physiatrist.
Cost/Year = 4/1 x $56.93 x 12 = $2,732.64
Cost/Year = 4/1 x $87.71 x 12 = $4,210.08
Cost/Year = 4/1 x $56.93 x 16 = $3,643.52
Cost/Year = 4/1 x $87.71 x 16 = $5,613.44
Cost/Year Average = ($2,732.64 + $5,613.44) ÷ 2 = $4,173.04

Item or Service	Purpose	Replacement Schedule	Start / End	Costs
Bookkeeper/Financial Manager	Manage household expenses.	1 Time/Week	# Start Age/Year: 38, 2022	Cost/Unit: $22.31 to $22.31
10 Options 1, 2			# End Age/Year: 72, 2056	Cost/Year: $1,647.37 to $1,647.37

This service is based on consultations with and recommendations by Ms. Smith's treating physician and neuropsychologist as well as this consultant. The time and hourly costs are from the Dollar Value of a Day, Home Management which includes these services as well as others related to financial management.
Cost/Year = 1.42/1 x $22.31 x 52 = $1,647.37

Diagnostic/Educational Testing

Prepared By: Carol P. Walker PhD, ABPP-CN, CLCP

Item or Service	Purpose	Replacement Schedule	Start / End	Costs
Neuropsychological Evaluation	Monitor cognitive, emotional and behavioral status.	2 Times/Year	# Start Age/Year: 38, 2022	Cost/Unit: $1,366.24 to $1,366.24
1 Options 1, 2			# End Age/Year: 39, 2023	Cost/Year: $2,732.48 to $2,732.48

This item is based on consultation with her treating neuropsychologist.
Cost/Year = $1,366.24 x 2 = $2,732.48

Item or Service	Purpose	Replacement Schedule	Start / End	Costs
Neuropsychological Evaluation	Monitor cognitive, emotional and behavioral status.	1 Time Only	# Start Age/Year: 42, 2021	Cost/Unit: $1,366.24 to $1,366.24
2 Options 1, 2			# End Age/Year: 42, 2021	Cost/Year: $1,366.24 to $1,366.24

This item is based on consultation with her treating neuropsychologist.

Item or Service	Purpose	Replacement Schedule	Start / End	Costs
Neuropsychological Evaluation	Monitor cognitive, emotional and behavioral status.	1 Time/ 10 - 15 Years	# Start Age/Year: 52, 2036	Cost/Unit: $1,366.24 to $1,366.24
3 Options 1, 2			# End Age/Year: 72, 2056	Cost/Year: $364.33 to $546.50

This item is based on recommendation by her treating neuropsychologist for ongoing cognitive and behavioral screening. Four hours are included for these evaluations.
Cost/Year = 4/1 x $1,366.24 x 1÷ 10 = $546.50
Cost/Year = 4/1 x $1,366.24 x 1÷ 15 = $364.33
Cost/Year Average = ($364.33 + $546.50) ÷ 2 = $455.41

Item or Service	Purpose	Replacement Schedule	Start End	Costs
Head Injury Foundation 4 Options 1, 2	Provide support to Ms.Smith and her family.		# Start Age/Year # End Age/Year	Cost/Unit Cost/Year

References

Aguilar-Mediavilla, E., Pérez-Pereira, M., Serrat-Sellabona, E., & Adrover-Roig, D. (2022). Introduction to language development in children: Description to detect and prevent language difficulties. *Children (Basel, Switzerland)*, *9*(3), 412. https://doi.org/10.3390/children9030412

Akrout-Brizard, B., Limbu, B., Baeza-Velasco, C., & Deb, S. (2021). Association between epilepsy and psychiatric disorders in adults with intellectual disabilities: Systematic review and meta-analysis. *BJPsych Open*, *7*(3), e95. https://doi.org/10.1192/bjo.2021.55

American Academy of Clinical Neuropsychology. (2007). American Academy of Clinical Neuropsychology (AACN) practice guidelines for neuropsychological assessment and consultation. *The Clinical Neuropsychologist*, *21*(2), 209–231. https://doi.org/10.1080/13825580601025932

American Bar Association/American Psychological Association Assessment of Capacity in Older Adults Project Working Group. (2008). *Assessment of older adults with diminished capacity: A handbook for psychologists*. American Bar Association and American Psychological Association. https://www.apa.org/pi/aging/programs/assessment/capacity-psychologist-handbook.pdf

American Board of Clinical Neuropsychology (1989). Definition of a clinical neuropsychologist. *Clinical Neuropsychologist*, *3*(1), 22. https://doi.org/10.1080/13854048908404071

American Psychiatric Association. (2022). *Diagnostic and statistical manual of mental disorders* (5th ed., text rev.). Author.

American Psychological Association. (2017). *Ethical principles of psychologists and code of conduct* (2002, amended effective June 1, 2010, and January 1, 2017). www.apa.org/ethics/code/

Appenteng, R., Nelp, T., Abdelgadir, J., Weledji, N., Haglund, M., Smith, E., Obiga,O., Sakita, F.M., Miguel, E.A., Vissoci, C.M., Rice, H., Vissoci, J.R.N., & Staton, C. A systematic review and quality analysis of pediatric traumatic brain injury clinical practice guidelines. (2018 Aug 2). *PLoS One*, *13*(8):e0201550. doi: 10.1371/journal.pone.0201550.

Aram, D. M., & Eisele, J. A. (1992). Plasticity and recovery of higher cognitive functioning following brain injury. In I. Rapin & S. Segalowitz (Eds.), *Handbook of neuropsychology* (Vol. 10, p. 73). Elsevier.

Artiola i Fortuny, L., & Mullaney, H. A. (1998). Assessing patients whose language you do not know: Can the absurd be ethical? *The Clinical Neuropsychologist, 12*, 113–126.

Bandura, A., Ross, D., & Ross, S., (1961). Transmission of aggression through imitation of aggressive models. *The Journal of Abnormal and Social Psychology, 63*(3), 575–582.

Benitez, A., Hassenstab, J., & Bangen, K. J. (2014). Neuroimaging training among neuropsychologists: A survey of the state of current training and recommendations for trainees. *The Clinical Neuropsychologist, 28*(4), 600–613.

Ben-Yishay, Y., & Diller, L. (2011) *Handbook of holistic neuropsychological rehabilitation*. Oxford Press.

Berens, D. E., & Weed, R. O. (2018). The role of the vocational rehabilitation counselor in life care planning. In R. O. Weed & D. E. Berens (Eds.), *Life care planning and case management handbook* (4th ed., pp. 41–60). Routledge.

Berman, M. G., Jonides, J., & Nee, D. E. (2006). Studying mind and brain with fMRI. *Social Cognitive and Affective Neuroscience, 1*(2), 158–161. https://doi.org/10.1093/scan/nsl019

Bigler, E. D. (1996). *Neuroimaging: I basic science; I clinical applications*. Plenum Press.

Bijlenga, D., Vollebregt, M. A., Kooij, J., & Arns, M. (2019). The role of the circadian system in the etiology and pathophysiology of ADHD: Time to redefine ADHD? *Attention Deficit and Hyperactivity Disorders, 11*(1), 5–19. https://doi.org/10.1007/s12402-018-0271-z

Bilder, R. M. (2011). Neuropsychology 3.0: Evidence based science and practice. *Journal International Neuropsychological Society, 17*(1), 7–13.

Brearly, T. W., Shura, R., Martindale, S. L., Lazowski, R. A., Luxton, D.D., Shenal, B. V., & Rowland, J. A. (2017). Neuropsychological test administration by videoconference: A systematic review and meta-analysis. *Neuropsychology Review, 27*, 174–186.

Brown, R. B., & Milner, P. M. (2003). The legacy of Donald O. Hebb: More than the Hebb synapse. *Nature Reviews Neurology*, 1013–1019. https://doi.org/10.1038/nrn1257

Carroll, L. J., Cassidy, J. D., Cancelliere, C., Cote, P., Hincapie´, C. A., Kristman, V. L., Holm, L. W., Borg, J., de Boussard, C. N., & Hartvigsen, J. (2014). Systematic review of the prognosis after mild traumatic brain injury in adults: Cognitive, psychiatric, and mortality outcomes: Results of the international collaboration on mild traumatic brain injury prognosis. *Archives of Physical Medicine and Rehabilitation, 95* (3 Suppl 2), Si52–73.

Cicerone, K. D., Goldin, Y., Ganci, K., Rosenbaum, A., Wethe, J. V., Langenbahn, D. M., Malec, J. F., Bergquist, T. F., Kingsley, K., Nagele, D., Trexler, L., Fraas, M., Bogdanova, Y., & Harley, J. P. (2019). Evidence-based cognitive rehabilitation: Systematic review of the literature from 2009 through 2014. *Archives of Physical Medicine and Rehabilitation, 100*(8), 1515–1533. https://doi.org/10.1016/j.apmr.2019.02.011

Commission for the Recognition of Specialties and Proficiencies in Professional Psychology. (n.d.). www.apa.org/ed/graduate/specialize/neuro.aspx

Damasio, H., & Damasio, A. R. (1989). *Lesion analysis in neuropsychology*. Oxford Press.

Dehorter, N., & Del Pino, I. (2020). Shifting developmental trajectories during critical periods of brain formation. *Frontiers in Cellular Neuroscience, 14*, 283. https://doi.org/10.3389/fncel.2020.00283

Department of Veterans Affairs/Department of Defense. (June 2017). *Clinical practice guideline for management of post-traumatic stress*. www.ptsd.va.gov/professional/treat/txessentials/cpg_ptsd_management.asp

Fitzhardinge, P. M., Flodmark, O., Fitz, C. R., & Ashby, S. (1981). The prognostic value of computed tomography as an adjunct to assessment of the term infant with post asphyxial encephalopathy. *The Journal of Pediatrics, 99*(5), 777–781. https://doi.org/10.1016/s0022-3476(81)80410-6

Fitzhugh-Bell, K. B. (1997). Historical antecedents of clinical neuropsychology. In A. M. Horton, D. Wedding, & S. J. Webster (Eds.), *The neuropsychological handbook: Volume 1. Foundations and assessment* (2nd ed., pp. 67–90). Macmillan.

Fleminger, S., & Ponsford, J. (2005). Long term outcome after traumatic brain injury. *BMJ, 331*(7539), 1419–1420.

Fleminger, S., Oliver, D., Lovestone, S., Rabe-Hesketh, S., & Giora, A. (2003). Head injury as a risk factor for Alzheimer's disease: The evidence 10 years on; A partial replication. *Journal Neurology, Neurosurgery & Psychiatry, 74*, 857–862.

Freemon, F. R. (1994). Galen's ideas on neurological function. *Journal of the History of the Neurosciences, 4*, 263–271.

Freud, A. (1963). The concept of developmental lines. *Psychoanalytic Study of the Child*, 18, 245.

Goisis, A., Özcan, B., & Myrskylä, M. (2017). Decline in the negative association between low birth weight and cognitive ability. *Proceedings of the National Academy of Sciences of the United States of America, 114*(1), 84–88. https://doi.org/10.1073/pnas.1605544114

Greenberg, S. A., & Shuman, D. W. (1997). Irreconcilable conflict between therapeutic and forensic roles. *Professional Psychology: Research and Practice, 28*, 50–57.

Guarini, A., Pereira, M. P., van Baar, A., & Sansavini, A. (2021). Special issue: Preterm birth: Research, intervention, and developmental outcomes. *International Journal of Environmental Research and Public Health, 18*(6), 3169. https://doi.org/10.3390/ijerph18063169

Guilmette, T. J., Sweet, J. J., Hebben, N., Koltai, D., Mahone, E. M., Spiegler, B. J., Stucky, K., Westerveld, M., & Conference Participants. (2020). American Academy of Clinical Neuropsychology consensus conference statement on uniform labeling of performance test scores. *The Clinical Neuropsychologist, 34*(3), 437–453. https://doi.org/10.1080/13854046.2020.1722244

Gur, R. E., McGrath, C., Chan, R. M., Schroeder, L., Turner, T., Turetsky, B. I., Kohler, C., Alsop, D., Maldjian, J., Ragland, J. D., & Gur, R. C. (2002). An fMRI study of facial emotion processing in patients with schizophrenia. *The American Journal of Psychiatry, 159*(12), 1992–1999. https://doi.org/10.1176/appi.ajp.159.12.1992

Hannay, H. J., Bieliauskas, L. A., Crosson, B. A., Hammeke, T. A., Hamsher, K. deS., & Koffler, S. P. (1998). Proceedings: The Houston Conference on specialty education and training in clinical neuropsychology. *Archives of Clinical Neuropsychology, 13*(2), 1–8.

Hebb, D. O. (1980) *Essay on mind*. Psychology Press.

Heilbronner, R. L., Sweet, J. J., Attix, D. K., Krull, K. R, Henry, G. K., & Hart, R. P. (2010). Official position of the American Academy of Clinical Neuropsychology on serial neuropsychological assessments: The utility and challenges of repeat test administrations in clinical and forensic contexts. *The Clinical Neuropsychologist, 24*(8), 1267–1278. https://doi.org/10.1080/13854046.2010.526785

Heilman, K. M., & Valenstein, E. (1993). Introduction. In K. M. Heilman & E. Valenstein (Eds.), *Clinical neuropsychology* (3rd ed., pp. 1–16). Oxford Press.

Helmstaedter, C., & Elger, C. E. (2009). Chronic temporal lobe epilepsy: A neurodevelopmental or progressively dementing disease? *Brain: A Journal of Neurology, 132*(Pt 10), 2822–2830. https://doi.org/10.1093/brain/awp182

Hermann, B. P., Struck, A. F., Dabbs, K., Seidenberg, M., & Jones, J. E. (2021). Behavioral phenotypes of temporal lobe epilepsy. *Epilepsia Open, 6*(2), 369–380. https://doi.org/10.1002/epi4.12488

Johnstone, B., Callahan, C. D., Kapila, C. J., & Bowman, D. E. (1996). The comparability of the WRAT-R Reading Test and NAART as estimates of premorbid intelligence in neurologically impaired patients. *Archives of Clinical Neuropsychology, 11*, 513–519.

Josephson, C. B., Lowerison M., Vallerand I., Sajobi, T. T., Patten, S., Jette, N., & Weibe, S. (2017). Association of depression and treated depression with epilepsy and seizure outcomes: A multicohort analysis. *JAMA Neurology, 74*(5), 533–539. https://doi.org/10.1001/jamaneurol.2016.5042

Kaaden, S., & Helmstaedter, C. (2009). Age at onset of epilepsy as a determinant of intellectual impairment in temporal lobe epilepsy. *Epilepsy & Behavior, 15*(2), 213–217. https://doi.org/10.1016/j.yebeh.2009.03.027

Kang, S. K., & Kadam, S. D. (2015). Neonatal seizures: Impact on neurodevelopmental outcomes. *Frontiers in Pediatrics, 3*, 1–9. www.frontiersin.org/article/10.3389/fped.2015.00101

Karr. J. E., Areshenkoff, C. N., & Garcia-Barrera, M. C. (2014). The neuropsychological outcomes of concussion: A systematic review of meta-analyses on the cognitive sequelae of mild traumatic brain injury. *Neuropsychology, 28* (3), 321–336.

Kaufman, A. S. (1999). Genetics of childhood disorders: Genetics and intelligence. *Journal of the Academy of Child and Adolescent Psychiatry, 38*, 48.

Kendler, H. H., & Kendler, T. S. (1962). Vertical and horizontal processes in problem solving. *Psychological Review*, 69, 1.

Kennedy, M. R., Coelho, C., Turkstra, L., Ylvisaker, M., Moore Sohlberg, M., Yorkston, K., Chou, H. & Kan, P. F. (2008). Intervention for executive functions after traumatic brain injury: A systematic review, meta-analysis and clinical recommendations. *Neuropsychological rehabilitation*, 18(3), 257-299

Khan I., & Leventhal B. L. (2021). *Developmental delay*. StatPearls Publishing. www.ncbi.nlm.nih.gov/books/NBK562231/

Kiff, C. J., Lengua, L. J., & Zalewski, M. (2011). Nature and nurturing: Parenting in the context of child temperament. *Clinical Child and Family Psychology Review*, 14(3), 251–301. https://doi.org/10.1007/s10567-011-0093-4

Koehler, R., Wilhelm, E., & Shoulson, I. (Eds.). (2011). *Cognitive rehabilitation therapy for traumatic brain injury: Evaluating the evidence*. Committee on Cognitive Rehabilitation Therapy for Traumatic Brain Injury: Institute of Medicine. http://nap.edu/13220

Kolb, B., & Gibb, R. (2011). Brain plasticity and behaviour in developing brain. *Journal of the Canadian Academy of Child and Adolescent Psychiatry*, 20(4), 265–276)

Kreutzer, J., Marwitz, J., & Kepler, K. (1992). Traumatic brain injury: Family response and outcome. *Archives of Physical Medicine and Rehabilitation*, 73, 771–778.

Langa, K. M., Larson, E. B., Crimmins, E. M., Faul, J. D., Levine, D. A., Kabeto, M. U., & Weir, D. R. (2017). A comparison of the prevalence of dementia in the United States in 2000 and 2012. *JAMA Internal Medicine*, 177, 51–58.

Lashley, K. S. (1960). *The neuropsychology of Lashley: Selected papers of K. S. Lashley*, McGraw-Hill.

Lee, B. L. & Glass, H. C. (2021). Cognitive outcomes in late childhood and adolescence of neonatal hypoxic-ischemic encephalopathy. *Clinical and Experimental Pediatrics*, 64(12), 608-6018.

Leon-Carrion, J., Machuca-Murga, F., Solís, M. I., Leon-Dominguez, U., & Domínguez-Morales, M. (2013). The sooner patients begin neurorehabilitation, the better their functional outcome. *Brain Injury: Early Online*, 1–5.

Lezak, M. D., Howieson, D. B., & Loring, D. W. (2004). *Neuropsychological assessment* (4th ed.). Oxford Press.

Libon, D. J., Swenson, R., Ashendorf, L., Bauer, R. M., & Bowers, D. (2013). Edith Kaplan and the Boston process approach. *The Clinical Neuropsychologist*, 27(8), 1223–1233. https://doi.org/10.1080/13854046.2013.833295

Linsell, L., Johnson, S., Wolke, D., O'Reilly, H., Morris, J. K., Kurinczuk, J. J., & Marlow, N. (2018). Cognitive trajectories from infancy to early adulthood following birth before 26 weeks of gestation: A prospective, population-based cohort study. *Archives of Disease in Childhood*, 103(4), 363–370. https://doi.org/10.1136/archdischild-2017-313414.

Lord, C., Brugha, T. S., Charman, T., Cusack, J., Dumas, G., Frazier, T., Jones, E., Jones, R. M., Pickles, A., State, M. W., Taylor, J. L., & Veenstra-VanderWeele, J. (2020). Autism spectrum disorder. *Nature Reviews. Disease Primers*, 6(1), 5. https://doi.org/10.1038/s41572-019-0138-4

Lu, E., Pyatka, N., Burant, C. J., & Sajatovic, M. (2021). Systematic literature review of psychiatric comorbidities in adults with epilepsy. *Journal of Clinical Neurology (Seoul, Korea)*, 17(2), 176–186. https://doi.org/10.3988/jcn.2021.17.2.176

Luria, A. R. (1970). Functional organization of the brain. *Scientific American*, 222, 66.

Luria, A. R. (1973). *The working brain: An introduction to neuropsychology*. Penguin.

Marlow, N., Rose, A. S., Rands, C. E., & Draper, E. S. (2005) Neuropsychological and educational problems at school age associated with neonatal encephalopathy. *Archives of Disease in Childhood, Fetal and Neonatal Edition*, 90(5), 380–7. https://doi.org/10.1136/adc.2004.067520

Martin, B. S., & Huntsman, M. M. (2012). Pathological plasticity in fragile X syndrome. *Neural Plasticity*, 2012, 275630. https://doi.org/10.1155/2012/275630

Max, J. E., Roberts, M. A., Koele, S. L., Lindgren, S. D., Robin, D. A., Arndt, S., Smith, W. L., Jr., & Sato, Y. (1999). Cognitive outcome in children and adolescents following severe traumatic brain injury: Influence of psychosocial, psychiatric, and injury-related variables. *Journal of the International Neuropsychological Society*, 5, 58–68.

Miller, P. H. (1983). *Theories of developmental psychology*. W. H. Freeman & Company.

Modabbernia, A., Velthorst, E., & Reichenberg, A. (2017). Environmental risk factors for autism: An evidence-based review of systematic reviews and meta-analyses. *Molecular Autism*, *8*, 13. https://doi.org/10.1186/s13229-017-0121-4

National Academy of Neuropsychology. (2001). *Definition of a neuropsychologist*. https://nanonline.org/nan/Professional_Resources/Position_Papers/NAN/_ProfessionalResources/Position_Papers

Norbury, C. F., Gooch, D., Wray, C., Baird, G., Charman, T., Simonoff, E., Vamvakas, G., & Pickles, A. (2016). The impact of nonverbal ability on prevalence and clinical presentation of language disorder: Evidence from a population study. *Journal of Child Psychology and Psychiatry*, *57*, 1247–1257. https://doi.org/10.1111/jcpp.12573

Núñez-Jaramillo, L., Herrera-Solís, A., & Herrera-Morales, W. V. (2021). ADHD: Reviewing the causes and evaluating solutions. *Journal of Personalized Medicine*, *11*(3), 166. https://doi.org/10.3390/jpm1103016

Paredes, A. M., Gooding, A., Artiola i Fortuny, L., Mindt, M. R., Suárez, P., Scott, T. M., Heaton, A., Heaton, R. K., Cherner, M., & Marquine, M. J. (2021) The state of neuropsychological test norms for Spanish-speaking adults in the United States. *The Clinical Neuropsychologist*, *35*(2), 236–252. https://doi.org/10.1080/13854046.2020.1729866

Pascal, A., Govaert, P., Oostra, A., Naulaers, G., Ortibus, E., & Van den Broeck, C. (2018). Neurodevelopmental outcome in very preterm and very-low-birthweight infants born over the past decade: A meta-analytic review. *Developmental Medicine and Child Neurology*, *60*(4), 342–355. https://doi.org/10.1111/dmcn.13675

Plomin, R., & von Stumm, S. (2018). The new genetics of intelligence. *Nature Reviews. Genetics*, *19*(3), 148–159. https://doi.org/10.1038/nrg.2017.104

Puderbaugh, M., & Emmady, P. D. (2022). *Neuroplasticity*. StatPearls Publishing. www.ncbi.nlm.nih.gov/books/NBK557811/

Rabin, L. A., Paolillo, E., & Barr, W. B. (2016). Stability in test-usage practices of clinical neuropsychologists in the United States and Canada over a 10-year period: A follow-up survey of INS and NAN Members. *Archives of Clinical Neuropsychology*, *31*(3), 206–230. https://doi.org/10.1093/arclin/acw007

Reitan, R. M. (1988). Integration of neuropsychological theory, assessment, and application. *Clinical Neuropsychologist*, *2*(4), 331–349. https://doi.org/10.1080/13854048808403272

Roalf, D. R., & Gur, R. C. (2017). Functional brain imaging in neuropsychology over the past 25 years. *Neuropsychology*, *31*(8), 954–971. https://doi.org/10.1037/neu0000426

Rohling, M. L., Binder, L. M., Demakis, G. J., Larrabee, G. J., Ploetz, D. M., & Langhinrichsen-Rohling, J. (2011). A meta-analysis of neuropsychological outcome after mild traumatic brain injury: Re-analyses and reconsiderations of Binder et al., (1997), Frencham et al., (2005), and Pertab et al. *The Clinical Neuropsychologist*, *25*, 608–623.

Rosado, D. L., Buehler, S., Botbol-Berman, E., Feigon, M., León, A., Luu, H., Carrión, C., Gonzalez, M., Rao, J., Greif, T., Seidenberg, M., & Pliskin, N. H. (2018). Neuropsychological feedback services improve quality of life and social adjustment. *The Clinical Neuropsychologist*, *32*(3), 422–435. https://doi.org/10.1080/13854046.2017.1400105

Rosenthal, M., & Geckler, C. (1997). Family intervention in neuropsychology. *Brain Injury*, *11*, 891–906.

Ryan, N. P., van Bijnen, L., Catroppa, C., Beauchamp, M. H., Crossley, L., Hearps, S., & Anderson, V. (2016). Longitudinal outcome and recovery of social problems after pediatric traumatic brain injury (TBI): Contribution of brain insult and family environment. *International Journal of Developmental Neuroscience: The Official Journal of the International Society for Developmental Neuroscience*, *49*, 23–30. https://doi.org/10.1016/j.ijdevneu.2015.12.004

Sbordone, R. J. (1997). The ecological validity of neuropsychological testing. In A. M. Horton, Jr., D. Wedding, & S. J. Webster (Eds.), *The neuropsychology handbook* (Vol. 1, pp. 365–393). Springer Publishing.

Sbordone, R. J., Saul, R. E., & Purisch, A. D. (2007). *Neuropsychology for psychologists, health care professionals, and attorneys*. CRC Press.

Seltzer, L. E., & Paciorkowski, A. R. (2014). Genetic disorders associated with postnatal microcephaly. *American Journal of Medical Genetics. Part C, Seminars in Medical Genetics*, *166C*(2), 140–155. https://doi.org/10.1002/ajmg.c.31400

Shively, S., Scher, A. I., Perl, D. P., & Diaz-Arrastia, R. (2012). Dementia resulting from traumatic brain injury: What is the pathology? *Archives of Neurology, 69*(10), 1245–1251. https://doi.org/10.1001/archneurol.2011.3747

Silverberg, N. D., Iaccarino, M. A., Panenka, W. J., Iverson, G. L., McCulloch, K. L., Dams-O'Connor, K., Reed, N., & McCrea, M. (2020). American Congress of Rehabilitation Medicine Brain Injury Interdisciplinary Special Interest Group Mild TBI Task Force. Management of concussion and mild traumatic brain injury: A synthesis of practice guidelines. *Archives of Physical Medicine and Rehabilitation, 101*(2), 382–393. https://doi.org/10.1016/j.apmr.2019.10.179

Simeonsson, R. J. (1983). Theories of child development. In C. E. Walker & M. C. Roberts (Eds.), *Handbook of child clinical psychology*. John Wiley & Sons.

Smith, D. H., Johnson, V. E., & Stewart, W. (2013). Chronic neuropathologies of single and repetitive TBI: Substrates of dementia? *Nature Reviews Neurology, 9*. https://doi.org/10.1038/nrneurol.2013.29

Spreen, O., Risser, A. H., & Edgell, D. (1995). *Developmental neuropsychology*. Oxford University Press.

Stavljenić-Rukavina A. (2008). 1. Prenatal diagnosis of chromosomal disorders – Molecular aspects. *eJIFCC, 19*(1), 2–6. https://doi.org/10.1016/j.dcn.2017.05.006

Steward, K. A., & Kretzmer, T. (2021). Anosognosia in moderate-to-severe traumatic brain injury: A review of prevalence, clinical correlates, and diversity considerations. *The Clinical Neuropsychologist*, 1–19. https://doi.org/10.1080/13854046.2021.1967452

Strahle, J. M., Triplett, R. L., Alexopoulos, D., Smyser, T. A., Rogers, C. E., Limbrick, D. D., & Smyser, C. D. (2019). Impaired hippocampal development and outcomes in very preterm infants with perinatal brain injury. *NeuroImage: Clinical, 22*, [101787]. https://doi.org/10.1016/j.nicl.2019.101787

Suárez, P. A., Marquine, M. J., Díaz-Santos, M., Gollan, T., Artiola i Fortuny, L., Mindt, M. R., Heaton, R., & Cherner, M. (2021). Native Spanish-speaker's test performance and the effects of Spanish-English bilingualism: Results from the neuropsychological norms for the U.S.-Mexico Border Region in Spanish (NP-NUMBRS) project. *The Clinical Neuropsychologist, 35*(2), 453–465. https://doi.org/10.1080/13854046.2020.1861330

Substance Abuse and Mental Health Services Administration. (2016). *A collaborative approach to the treatment of pregnant women with opioid use disorders*. HHS Publication No. (SMA) 16–4978. Author. http://store.samhsa.gov/

Temple, C. (1997a). *Developmental cognitive neuropsychology*. Psychology Press.

Tripathi, A., Kar, S. K., & Shukla, R. (2018). Cognitive deficits in schizophrenia: Understanding the biological correlates and remediation strategies. *Clinical Psychopharmacology and Neuroscience: The Official Scientific Journal of the Korean College of Neuropsychopharmacology, 16*(1), 7–17. https://doi.org/10.9758/cpn.2018.16.1.7

Uomoto, J. M. (2000). Application of the neuropsychological evaluation in vocational planning after brain injury. In R. T. Fraser & D. C. Clemmons (Eds.), *Traumatic brain injury rehabilitation: Practical vocational, neuropsychological, and psychotherapy interventions* (pp. 1–94). CRC Press.

Vallar, G., & Caputi, N. (2022). The history of human neuropsychology. *Encyclopedia of behavioral neuroscience* (2nd ed., Vol. 1). Elsevier.

van Handel, M., Swaab, H., de Vries, L. S., & Jongmans, M. J. (2007). Long-term cognitive and behavioral consequences of neonatal encephalopathy following perinatal asphyxia: A review. *European Journal of Pediatrics, 166*(7), 645–654. https://doi.org/10.1007/s00431-007-0437-8

Wade, S. L., Zhang, N., Yeates, K. O., Stancin, T., & Taylor, H. G. (2016). Social environmental moderators of long-term functional outcomes of early childhood brain injury. *JAMA Pediatrics, 170*(4), 343–349. https://doi.org/10.1001/jamapediatrics.2015.4485

Wang, K., Gaitsch, H., Poon, H., Cox, N. J., & Rzhetsky, A. (2017). Classification of common human diseases derived from shared genetic and environmental determinants. *Nature Genetics, 49*(9), 1319–1325. https://doi.org/10.1038/ng.3931

Watson, J.B. (n.d.). *Behaviorism*. Kegan Paul, Trench, Trubner, & Company.

Weerasinghe-Mudiyanselage, P., Ang, M. J., Kang, S., Kim, J. S., & Moon, C. (2022). Structural plasticity of the hippocampus in neurodegenerative diseases. *International Journal of Molecular Sciences, 23*(6), 3349. https://doi.org/10.3390/ijms23063349

Whiteneck, G. G., Eagye, C. B., Cuthbert, J. P., Corrigan, J. D., Bell, J. M., Haarbauer-Krupa, J. K., Miller, A. C., Hammond, F. M., Dams-O'Connor, K., & Harrison-Felix, C., (2018). *One- and five-year outcomes after moderate-to-severe traumatic brain injury requiring inpatient rehabilitation: Traumatic brain injury report.* Centers for Disease Control and Prevention; National Center for Injury Prevention and Control; Administration for Community Living; National Institute on Disability, Independent Living and Rehabilitation Research. www.cdc.gov/traumaticbraininjury/pdf/cdc-nidilrr-self-report-508.pdf

Yantz, C. L., Gavett, B. E., Lynch, J. K., & McCaffrey, R. J. (2006). Potential for interpretation disparities of Halstead–Reitan neuropsychological battery performances in a litigating sample. *Archives of Clinical Neuropsychology, 21*(8), 809–817.

Yeates, K. O., Taylor, H. G., Drotar, D., Wade, S. L., Klein, S., & Stancin, T. (1997). Preinjury family environment as a determinant of recovery from traumatic brain injury in school-age children. *Journal of the International Neuropsychological Society, 3,* 617–630.

Zhang, J., Luo, W., Li, Q., Xu, R., Wang, Q., & Huang, Q. (2018). Peripheral brain-derived neurotrophic factor in attention-deficit/hyperactivity disorder: A comprehensive systematic review and meta-analysis. *Journal of Affective Disorders, 227,* 298–304. https://doi.org/10.1016/j.jad.2017.11.012

Chapter 13

The Role of the Neurologist in Life Care Planning

Stephen L. Nelson

The neurologist functions as a generalist and a specialist and may be one of several physicians involved in the case management and life care plan of an individual with a neurological condition. Despite there being a shortage of neurologists, and even more so pediatric neurologists, a neurologist is often required for diagnosis and management of neurological conditions. In these cases, the neurologist tends to become the primary physician for patients with complicated neurological conditions of which generalists have little familiarity or experience.

Origins of the Discipline of Neurology

The roots of modern neurology are traditionally traced to the European schools of Jean-Martin Charcot, John Hughlings Jackson, William Gowers, and Gordon Holmes. American neurology, however, began in the late nineteenth century with William Hammond, Silas Weir Mitchell, and William Osler. The Neurological Institute of New York in 1909 became the first hospital dedicated to the care of patients with nervous conditions (Columbia University, 2022). The American Board of Psychiatry and Neurology (ABPN) was founded in 1934 for board certification in neurology and psychiatry (American Board of Psychiatry and Neurology [ABPN], n.d.-a).

The beginning of pediatric neurology dates back to the 1600s and 1700s, where conditions such as chorea, hydrocephalus, spina bifida, and poliomyelitis were described. Formal designation of pediatric neurology as a medical subspecialty did not occur until the 1950s even though early descriptions of childhood seizures and other neurological conditions can be traced back to Hippocrates (Ashwal & Rust, 2003). Specialists in neurologic diseases of children were increasingly identified in the 1950s, and by the mid-1970s, most medical schools had pediatric neurologists on their faculty. Early pioneers of pediatric neurology in the early twentieth century included Bernard Sachs, Frank Ford, and Bronson Crothers (Ashwal, 1990; Ashwal & Rust, 2003). In 1959, the ABPN began offering board certification in pediatric neurology. Professional societies for child neurologists were established in multiple countries, including the Child Neurology Society in the

United States in 1972. Journals dedicated to academic work in pediatric neurology were founded, including Developmental Medicine and Child Neurology in 1958, Neuropediatrics in 1969, Brain and Development in 1979, Pediatric Neurology in 1985, and the Journal of Child Neurology in 1986 (Ashwal & Rust, 2003).

The Process of Becoming an Adult or Pediatric Neurologist

To become an adult neurologist, a four-year residency in neurology is typically required upon completion of medical school. To become a pediatric neurologist, the residency is typically at least two years of pediatrics in addition to a three-year pediatric neurology residency, of which one year is adult neurology. For initial board certification through the ABPN, adult or pediatric neurologists take the same written examination, thus ensuring that all neurologists have at least some knowledge regarding both pediatric and adult neurological conditions. There are numerous additional fellowships available for adult and pediatric neurologists to complete to gain further subspecialty training such as clinical neurophysiology, neurocritical care, sleep medicine, epilepsy, and others with the opportunity to become board-certified through the ABPN.

Kinds of Patients and Problems Usually Seen and Addressed

Adult and pediatric neurologists evaluate and treat patients with conditions that can affect multiple different areas including the central (i.e., brain, spinal cord) and peripheral (i.e., plexus, motor and sensory peripheral nerve, neuromuscular junction, muscles) nervous systems, as well as other organ systems including the eyes, kidneys, skin, and liver. The signs and symptoms that lead to a neurology evaluation can include altered mental status, possible seizure, weakness, dizziness or vertigo, memory concerns, pain, abnormal movements, and others. Common conditions that an neurologists may see include epilepsy, migraines, stroke, dementia such as Alzheimer's, movement disorders such as Parkinson's disease, autoimmune conditions such as multiple sclerosis, acute or chronic encephalopathy, and many others, depending upon the age of the patient

Common reasons for a patient to be referred to a pediatric neurologist include epilepsy, intellectual disability, learning disabilities, autism spectrum disorder, cerebral palsy, migraines, developmental delay, genetic and metabolic disorders, and movement disorders such as Tourette syndrome. Pediatric neurology also encompasses the fields of fetal and neonatal neurology, which include abnormalities of brain development during pregnancy; *in utero* infections and toxic exposures; hypoxic–ischemic encephalopathy (HIE) occurring prenatally, perinatally, and postnatally; and intracranial hemorrhages.

Advances in neonatology have led to remarkably improved survival rates in premature infants. However, the resulting increased risk of intraventricular hemorrhage, periventricular leukomalacia (PVL), and cerebral palsy each impact the pediatric neurology patient population. Additionally, therapeutic hypothermia has had a tremendous impact on the outcome of neonatal HIE.

Birth defects such as spina bifida (myelomeningocele) require the involvement of multiple specialists, but the pediatric neurologist often serves as the fulcrum for such multidisciplinary clinics. This analogy probably serves as the best example of the role of the pediatric neurologist in caring for a child with a serious chronic disease that requires highly specialized medical services and life care planning (acting as a "fulcrum"). Pediatric neurologists also care for children with infectious and inflammatory diseases of the nervous system, including meningitis, encephalitis, transverse myelitis, poliomyelitis, multiple sclerosis, and Guillain–Barré syndrome. Conditions traditionally associated with adult neurology, such as stroke, also occur in childhood and adolescence, especially in certain populations such as patients with sickle cell anemia. In addition, pediatric neuro-oncology has emerged as a field with dramatic and steady advances in diagnosis, therapy, and modalities to reduce toxicity from the radiation and chemotherapy.

There also are a multitude of genetic–metabolic disorders with associated multisystem involvement that require pediatric neurology involvement. Prime examples include the neurocutaneous disorders, which manifest on the skin but also affect the nervous system in addition to other organ systems. These disorders include several well-known entities, such as neurofibromatosis types I and II, tuberous sclerosis complex, Sturge–Weber syndrome, von Hippel–Lindau syndrome, and ataxia telangiectasia.

The diagnosis of genetic or neurological syndromes by phenotype has been replaced by next generation sequencing and comparative genomic hybridization techniques to identify genetic mutations and chromosomal alterations. These advances in genetic technology have led to new classification systems to correct inappropriate grouping or separation of disorders. Examples of the former include neurofibromatosis types I and II, now recognized as separate entities mapped to chromosome 17 and chromosome 22, respectively. Another example is the reclassification of the types of Charcot-Marie-Tooth disease. Examples of the latter include the seemingly unrelated entities of adrenoleukodystrophy, Refsum disease, and Zellweger syndrome, now grouped together as peroxisomal dysfunction disorders. Other examples are genetic epilepsies and neurodevelopmental disorders, where a single mutation can give rise to variable spectrums of seizures and developmental disabilities.

As knowledge about the basic biochemical and genetic controls of the nervous system increases, it leads to increasingly sophisticated classification and ultimately treatment approaches to neurological disease. Initial description of clinical syndromes based on localization of neurological signs and symptoms (e.g., spasticity, ataxia, proximal weakness) or anatomic areas of involvement (e.g., gray matter, white matter, basal ganglia, cerebellum, selective long tracts) remains a time-honored process of "localization of the lesion." More detailed evaluations such as neuroimaging, muscle biopsy, genetic or metabolic testing, and neurodiagnostic testing provide greater localization of the lesion as well as potential identification of the specific affected cellular structures (lysosomes, mitochondria, peroxisomes, and the Golgi body). Current research is leading to attribution of clinical disorders to channelopathies, neurotransmitter metabolism, and genetic changes in membrane proteins, and previously unknown epigenetic phenomena. For example, the day-to-day practice of neurologists has been dramatically impacted by the recent discoveries in epilepsy genetics, such as the identification of sodium channel mutations in both severe myoclonic epilepsy of infancy (Dravet syndrome) and the syndrome of generalized epilepsy with febrile seizures plus other seizure types (GEFFS+). Understanding the underlying genetic cause of epilepsies or other conditions provides opportunities for new treatments or modifications of treatment, proactive rather than reactive management of complications, and counseling regarding occurrence risk in other family members.

Medical Issues Confronted by a Neurologist

Long ago, neurology was deemed a specialty of diagnostic intellectualism and therapeutic nihilism. This has changed radically. The 1990s were hailed as the "Decade of the Brain" and were associated with a dramatic proliferation of therapeutic agents for patients with neurological conditions.

Routine therapeutics in the daily life of a practicing neurologist include medications for epilepsy, attention deficit/hyperactivity disorder, movement disorders, cerebral palsy, as well as mood and behavioral manifestations of neuropsychiatric disorders. New understanding and therapy in neuroimmunology have led to the use of plasmapheresis, immunoglobulins, interferons, steroids, and other immunosuppressives in conditions ranging from multiple sclerosis to postinfectious encephalomyelitis, as well as a legion of neuropathies, myopathies, and neuromuscular junction disorders. The importance of early identification of a treatable number of disorders by dietary modification or enzyme replacement such as inborn errors of metabolism has led to expanding newborn screening tests. New therapies such as gene replacement therapy or modulation of transcription and translation have been instrumental in extending the lives of patients with inherited conditions, improving the quality and quantity of life.

At the same time, alternative therapies for a number of conditions are often tried by parents or patients, such as dietary modifications, heavy metal chelation, herbs or supplements, or hyperbaric therapy. Although in general neurologists do not want to discourage parents and patients trying to learn more about their conditions and potential alternative treatments, at the same time some treatments may actually cause harm to the patient or be chosen as an alternative to a proven therapy.

Ethical Issues Confronted by the Neurologist

Ethics plays a central role in many of the truly difficult decisions in neurology. Principle ethics (see Chapter 5) span across bioethics, medicine, and allied services, including neurology in helping the neurologist navigate ethical dilemmas such as working with the care team and providing care based on shared decision-making (Dan et al., 2017). Ethical choices are not always clear and obvious, especially in this setting of potentially serious and often devastating conditions affecting a particularly vulnerable population, such as our children. Bodensteiner and Ng (2011) explored the ethics of working with children with Duchenne Muscular Dystrophy and epilepsy, particular in light of the financial and human costs of treating such conditions and concluded that "physicians should let third parties worry about fighting among themselves and simply consider and propose the best medical and surgical therapies to … patients" (p. 602). Neurologists regularly confront the difficulties associated with the long-term prognosis of the critically ill or the minimally conscious state and must constantly walk the thin line between heroic care and futility. For example, when is it appropriate to discontinue "life support"? The criteria for brain death, defined as irreversible loss of all brain and brainstem functions, have been established, but can raise ethical concerns especially in vulnerable populations, particularly in the very young such as neonates, infants, and children (Dan et al., 2017), or in the very elderly. In fact, the American Academy of Neurology (AAN) Code of Professional Conduct (2009/2010) contains a section (3.3) regarding brain death as a guide to practicing neurologists (Russell et al., 2021). It can be much more difficult to predict prognosis when families are trying to decide on whether to continue care, agree to certain procedures, and attempt to understand what the future holds (Bodensteiner & Ng, 2011)

Clinical Practice Guidelines

Clinical practice guidelines for neurology exist to assist physicians in making decisions about patient care, which is especially crucial in creating life care plans for individuals with complex life issues. Formal guidelines have become increasingly promoted by professional organizations and government agencies to organize and disseminate information regarding evidence-based and cost-effective diagnostics and therapeutics. Guidelines are not laws that are set in stone, but rather, ever-evolving parameters based on current research and methods. They are meant to guide rather than mandate clinical decision-making.

Clinical practice guidelines stem from a larger movement known as evidence-based medicine. The Cochrane database (2022) is a repository that summarizes the evidence associated with specific medical conditions (www.cochranelibrary.com). Both evidence-based medicine and clinical practice guidelines strive to standardize healthcare using current knowledge and research. Physicians use these standards of practice to make educated medical decisions about the care of individual patients, while courts use them as standards of care to gauge the reasonableness of a neurologist's actions in a particular case. Evidence-based medicine should always be balanced by clinical experience, ethics, and the beliefs and wishes of patients and their families. This balance is essential in creating a life care plan for individual children, especially those with chronic or complex life care issues. The American Academy of Neurology (2022a) presently publishes 56 endorsed or affirmed guidelines on its website (www.aan.com) on topics including brain injury, epilepsy, stroke, geriatric neurology, headache, and multiple sclerosis that may be helpful to life care planners.

While guidelines can be helpful, they are not infallible. The American Academy of Neurology (AAN) notes that such guidelines do "… not mandate any particular course of medical care …" (AAN, 2022b, para. 3). Limitations in pediatric guidelines include a lack of clinical research in many areas of care, varying levels of usage or adherence to guidelines, the existence of multiple guidelines for each topic, and the fact that guidelines are impermanent (Bauchner et al., 1997). Patient care extends beyond the span of existing guidelines. However, these guidelines remain a resource that can be helpful for physicians and parents caring for children with chronic neurological issues or terminal disease.

The Role of the Neurologist in Life Care Planning

As mentioned above, the neurologist can be integral for a life care plan being developed for someone with neurological impairments. While the individual with a chronic health condition may follow closely with their primary care provider and may have involvement with other specialists such as psychiatrists or psychologists, the neurologist is the specialist who will likely oversee the long-term treatment plan for neurologically necessary care.

Guidelines, as described above, can be useful in the process of life care plan development. Included below is a summary of guidelines recommended for common pediatric neurological conditions:

- Early intervention services for possible movement disorders or developmental delays.
- Neuroimaging (there is an entire guideline dedicated solely to this topic).
- Routine neuromotor and sensory screening throughout the child's development.
- Education of and partnering with a patient's parents/family to make decisions about care.
- Referral to a geneticist or neurologist (if the primary provider is not a neurologist).
- Regular preventative healthcare (e.g., watching for development of comorbid conditions, such as seizures, learning difficulties, or nutritional deficits).
- Managing spasticity with the least invasive procedures (e.g., oral baclofen) and only choosing more invasive management (e.g., Botox injections or implantation of a baclofen pump) where necessary.

- Verifying that patients have adequate resources and services in their school environment, such as nursing and occupational, physical, and speech therapy.
- Making referrals for state services to which the child may be entitled.
- Seeking feedback for how to better achieve some of the previously mentioned goals.
- Making a "medical home" for the patient (as discussed below).
- Developing a plan for the child's future beginning no later than 12 years of age (Cooley, 2004).

These recommendations come from a collection of guidelines written by the American Academy of Pediatrics (2022) and are useful for physicians, parents, and can also inform the life care planner. Familiarity with such guidelines can assist the life care planner when conducting collaborative discussions with a neurologist.

What Should a Life Care Planner Ask a Neurologist?

Below are suggested questions that the life care planer may ask a neurologist in the process of life care plan development:

- Does the evaluee need to be seen by a neurologist in the future as a result of conditions arising from the incident?
- Are there other specialists who should evaluate the evaluee now or into the future?
- How often does the evaluee need to be seen by the neurology provider and for how long?
- What imaging studies or other diagnostic tests are needed (e.g., MRI, EEG)?
- What is the probability that the individual develops a seizure disorder or another condition as the evaluee ages?
- What medications are required to manage the neurological symptoms? Will the use of these medications change over the evaluee's lifespan and, if so, in what way and when?
- If spasticity is involved, what long-term management strategies are anticipated?
- What other specialists should the evaluee see (e.g., neurosurgery for shunt management, PMR (physical medicine and rehabilitation physician) for spasticity)?
- Based upon their condition, would you anticipate a reduction in life expectancy?
- Are there therapies from which the patient would benefit?
- Do you expect hospitalizations in the future, given the individual's diagnosis?
- What will likely be emerging medical issues the evaluee will face over the lifespan that need to be considered while aging with the diagnosis?
- How will the condition affect the individual's ability to participate in activities of daily living and instrumental activities of daily living now and in the future?
- Are there any invasive or aggressive medical treatments or procedures the evaluee will likely benefit from?
- What level and amount of supervision will the evaluee require over their lifetime (if any)? Will they be able to graduate high school, live independently, or be gainfully employed?

As noted in the treatment guidelines above, it is recommended that individuals with neurological (and other) conditions have a medical home. This "home" should provide a forum for coordination of all aspects of patient care, including clinical care as well as emotional, spiritual, and social support for patients and their families. A medical home is an approach to care designed to be comprehensive, culturally sensitive, and family centered (Kondrad, 2009). For a discussion of the medical home, the reader is referred to Chapter 7.

Conclusion

Because neurologists function as generalists and specialists, they can be critically important in the development of a life care plan for individuals with neurological conditions. Neurological conditions in pediatric, adult, and elderly individuals can be multifactorial requiring various modalities and management of medication, durable medical items, and medical services as the individual ages with these conditions. In cases where a neurological diagnosis is made, consultation with a treating or consulting neurologist over current and ongoing routine and episodic care may be vital to ensure a comprehensive individualized assessment by the life care planner.

References

American Academy of Neurology. (2009/2010). *Code of professional conduct.* American Academy of Neurology. https://www.aan.com/globals/axon/assets/7708.pdf

American Academy of Neurology. (2022a). *Practice guidelines.* www.aan.com/practice/guidelines

American Academy of Neurology. (2022b). *Endorsed or affirmed guidelines.* www.aan.com/Guidelines/Home/ByStatusOrType?status=affirmed

American Academy of Pediatrics. (2022). *Pediatric clinical practice guidelines & policies* (22nd Edition). Author.

American Board of Psychiatry and Neurology. (n.d.-a). *History.* www.abpn.com/about/mission-and-history/

Ashwal, S. (1990). *The founders of child neurology.* Normal Publishing.

Ashwal, S., & Rust, R. (2003). Child neurology in the 20th century. *Pediatric Research, 53,* 345–361.

Bauchner, H., Homer, C., Salem-Schwartz, S. R., & Adams, W. (1997). The status of pediatric practice guidelines. *Journal of Pediatrics, 99,* 876–878.

Bodensteiner, J. B., & Ng, Y. T. (2011). Ethical considerations in pediatric neurology: Neuromuscular disease and epilepsy. *Journal of Paediatrics and Child Health, 47*(9), 599–602.

Cochrane Library. (2022). www.cochranelibrary.com/

Columbia University. (2022). *Our history.* www.neurosurgery.columbia.edu/about-us/our-history

Cooley, W. C. (2004). Providing a primary care home for children and youth with cerebral palsy. *Pediatrics, 114*(4), 1106–1113.

Dan, B., Rosenbaum, P. L., Ronen, G. M., Johannsen, J., & Racine, E. (2017). Ethics in paediatric neurology. *Journal of International Child Neurology Association, 17,* 1–5.

Kondrad, M. (2009). Completing the circle: Providing comprehensive care to children with special healthcare needs. *Nursing Administration Quarterly, 33*(1), 70–72.

Russell, J. A., Hutchins, J. C., Epstein, L. G., & AAN Ethics, Law and Humanities Committee. (2021). American Academy of Neurology code of professional conduct. *Neurology, 97,* 489–495.

Chapter 14

The Role of the Occupational Therapist in Life Care Planning

Sarah Brown, Amy Thompson, and Sarah Malloy

"Occupational therapy is defined as the therapeutic use of everyday life occupations with persons, groups, or populations (i.e., the evaluee) for the purpose of enhancing or enabling participation" (AOTA, 2020b, p. 1). Occupational therapists use activities and occupations, the things people "want to, need to, and are expected to do," (World Federation of Occupational Therapy [WFOT], 2012 as cited in WFOT, 2018) as therapeutic interventions to support their evaluees' participation within the relevant environment. Clinical reasoning within the occupational therapy process aligns closely with the World Health Organization's International Classification of Functioning, Disability, and Health (2002) in that both consider how personal and environmental factors interact with an individual's health condition(s) to impact bodily functions, activity performance, and participation.

In the United States and Canada, the occupational therapy profession originated during World War I (AOTA, 2017; Lewis et al., 2021). Occupational therapy reconstruction aides (AOTA, 2017) and war aids (Lewis et al., 2021) worked with nurses to provide handicrafts and vocational activities to returning wounded soldiers as a means of improving their physical function and morale. According to these sources, societal shifts and historical events, such as the Great Depression, World War II, the polio epidemic, and new laws, shaped the profession's expansion, direction, and focus. Additionally, occupational therapy officially expanded its global reach with the inauguration of the World Federation of Occupational Therapy in 1952, with the United States and Canada among the first ten member associations (WFOT, n.d.).

Dr. Florence Clark's famous quote "Occupational therapy practitioners help people live life to its fullest-no matter what …" (Stromsdorfer, 2020, para. 6) not only inspires many occupational therapists but also mimics some of the basic tenets of life care planning which stress the importance of maximizing the individual's potential through the consideration of individualized, proactive, multidimensional recommendations that span life expectancy (Deutsch, n.d.). Furthermore, occupational therapists throughout the world have been establishing their role as expert witnesses in a variety of capacities for decades (DeMaio-Feldman, 1987; Harris et al., 1994; Klinger et al., 2004; Royal College of Occupational Therapists, 2018). This chapter provides an overview of occupational therapy, including key references within the field, occupational therapy educational requirements, the profession's scope of practice, the types of patients commonly treated, as well as problems, interventions, and recommendations occupational therapists often provide throughout the life span. Because occupational therapists are well suited and often called upon to complete home assessments, that aspect of practice is described. Finally, questions the life care planner should consider asking an occupational therapist are discussed.

Review of the Literature

In the video, *Celebrating AOTA's Centennial: A Historical Look at 100 Years of Occupational Therapy* (AOTA, 2017), Ruth Brunyate Wiemer opined that occupational therapists claim that the domain and impact of occupation on people, was staked in 1917. The American Occupational Therapy Association (2019a, p. 74–75) "reaffirmed its commitment to occupation-based practice" and reiterated the distinct value of occupational therapy as being improved health and quality of life through evaluation, intervention, and outcomes that focus on enhanced participation and successful engagement in evaluee-centered occupations. The American Occupational Therapy Association's Vision 2025 reinforces this concept and emphasizes the profession's inclusive nature and focus on service to people, populations, and communities (AOTA, 2021a). The *Occupational Therapy Practice Framework: Domain and Process* (4th Ed.) [OTPF-4], (AOTA, 2020c) presents a summary of the complex and interrelated components that create the fabric of occupational therapy and is a cornerstone reference for occupational therapists in the United States. The document highlights that occupational therapists differentiate themselves from other allied health professionals in that their interventions rely upon the therapeutic use of carefully selected occupations to achieve evaluee-centered outcomes. Engagement in various occupations is interwoven into the occupational therapy process of evaluation, intervention, and outcomes. Additionally, occupational therapists' therapeutic use of self, wherein therapists develop a relationship with evaluees that enhances collaboration, professional and clinical reasoning skills, distinguishes occupational therapy from other professions.

The *Profile of Practice of Occupational Therapists in Canada* (Canadian Association of Occupational Therapists [CAOT], 2012) is a similar guiding document for occupational therapists in Canada. The document describes a vision for occupational therapy practice that aligns with their professional direction of enabling occupation. It also identifies the "practice context, scope of practice, interprofessional practice, advanced competencies and career mobility" (CAOT, 2012, p. 1). The *Profile of Practice* emphasizes that the key role of an occupational therapist is as an "expert in enabling occupation," from which several other professional roles stem. The degree to which an occupational therapist engages in each role depends on the practice context, which describes the interplay between the evaluee, therapist, and practice environment. According to CAOT, a key mandate for occupational therapists is to enable occupation among the people of their nation.

In Canada, each college of occupational therapy identifies their standards of practice. However, the Association for Canadian Occupational Therapy Regulatory Organization (ACOTRO), the Association for Canadian Occupational Therapy University Programs (ACOTUP), and the CAOT (2021) recently created a framework outline, the first joint set of competencies for Canadian occupational practitioners. In the United States, AOTA (2019b) has established standards of practice for the profession of occupational therapy. These standards outline the expectations for behavior, the minimum standards, as well as the best practices for provision of occupational therapy services. The standards also provide the profession a means to control and direct its course from within.

Both CAOT (2007) and AOTA (2020a) have developed a code of ethics for occupational therapists in their respective countries. These documents are based on the core values of occupational therapy, its principles, and standards of conduct. There are variations between the organization's documents, but several concepts overlap, including the values of dignity, professional integrity, therapeutic relationships, the evaluee's right to autonomy, maintenance of confidentiality, professional competence, and communication. Within AOTA's code of ethics, an ethics commission, and the process for dealing with cases of breaches of ethics, are identified.

Professional organizations in Canada, the United States, as well as many other countries globally have established documents which emphasize core values and beliefs and guide the provision of occupational therapy services. While occupational therapists primarily provide occupation-based interventions to individuals, groups, or populations with the focus of enhancing life participation, their professional scope and holistic perspective may also make them valuable as expert witnesses who speak to an individual's occupational needs throughout the lifespan. DeMaio-Feldman (1987) highlights the value of an occupational therapist to the jury and the judge in providing an objective assessment of the evaluee's functional limitations and residual capacity, specifically regarding work. The Royal College of Occupational Therapists (2018) identifies several areas where the expertise of an occupational therapy expert witness may prove valuable including: commenting on past and future care costs, therapy, equipment and adaptation needs, work-related skills and abilities, and ability/support requirements for an evaluee to resume roles and responsibilities. Harris et al. (1994) and Klinger et al. (2004) note that occupational therapists, through their education and experience, specialize in studying the effects and etiology of disease and chronic and acute impairments on a person's self-care, leisure, and vocational function within their personal environment. This evaluee-centered focus on function makes occupational therapists suited to formulate, in collaboration with other professionals, present and future cost analyses and life care plans.

Educational Requirements

Educational requirements and curricula for occupational therapists in the United States and Canada are similar. Foundational courses include physical and biological sciences, kinesiology, biomechanics, sociology, anthropology, and developmental psychology. To apply this knowledge to human development across the lifespan, an understanding of behavioral sciences, social sciences, and the science of occupation in addition to quantitative and qualitative analysis, is needed. Finally, using evidence-based practice, occupational therapy education applies this broad knowledge to understand the impact of societal, economic, and other diverse factors to meet the needs of various groups, persons, and populations (Accreditation Council for Occupational Therapy Education [ACOTE], 2018).

To work as an occupational therapist, the practitioner must earn an entry-level master's or professional doctorate in occupational therapy from a school that is accredited by ACOTE. Included in these entry-level programs are a minimum of 24 weeks of full-time Level II fieldwork. Additionally, post professional masters and doctorate degrees are offered by some schools to accommodate those returning to obtain a higher degree of education. Recently, there has been robust discussion throughout the occupational therapy profession regarding the advancement of entry-level practice to a doctorate level. However, in 2019, the AOTA Representative Assembly voted for dual entry degrees (AOTA, 2019c). For practical purposes, this means occupational therapists can earn either an entry-level master's or doctorate degree and occupational therapy assistants can earn either an entry-level associates or bachelor's degree (AOTA, 2019c). Additionally, after degree completion from an ACOTE accredited school, occupational therapists must successfully complete the national certification examination administered by the National Board for Certification of Occupational Therapy, Inc. (NBCOT). Following the completion of those requirements, state licensure is required in all 50 states, the District of Columbia, Puerto Rico, and Guam, with continuing education requirements and timelines for renewal that vary between states.

According to Willmarth and Conway (2022), in 2019, AOTA and NBCOT announced a joint initiative to develop an Occupational Therapy Licensure Compact (Occupational Therapy Compact) with the purpose of facilitating interstate occupational therapy practice while maintaining consumer safeguards and state regulatory authority. Throughout the following year, advisory groups were formed, drafts were developed, stakeholder reviews were completed, and the Occupational Therapy Compact legislation was finalized. Twenty states have enacted the Occupational Therapy Compact thus far, with legislation pending in several others (Eliassen, 2022b). Member states will develop an interstate commission which will draft rules and bylaws and establish a start-up process. The first Occupational Therapy Licensure Compact privileges may be issued beginning in mid-2023 (Eliassen, 2022a).

Canadian educated occupational therapists attend one of the 14 accredited educational institutions. The Academic Credentialing Council, whose role is to establish standards and evaluate these educational programs, submits their recommendations to the CAOT. Based on adherence to established procedures, CAOT then provides approval of the programs. These programs offer entry-level masters educational programs (CAOT, ACOTRO, ACOTUP, COTF, PAC, 2013), and include a required 1,000 hours of field work. According to ACOTRO, ACOTUP, and CAOT (2021), occupational therapy practitioners, except those in Quebec, must successfully complete the National Occupational Therapy Certification Examination. Additionally, all Canadian provinces require occupational therapists to be registered to practice, whereas the territories do not require registration.

Due to occupational therapists' wide scope of practice, many therapists choose to advance their practice with specialized training. In the United States, AOTA offers Advanced Certification Programs in gerontology, physical rehabilitation, and pediatrics. These programs have rigorous qualifications. Additionally, AOTA offers continuing education in the form of micro credentials and professional certificates.

Outside of AOTA, there are a multitude of specialty certifications that occupational therapists pursue. This list is not exhaustive, but examples include Certified Hand Therapist, Certified Driving Rehabilitation Specialist, Certified Aging in Place Specialist (CAPS), Assisted Technology Professional, Seating and Mobility Specialist, Certified Industrial Ergonomic Evaluation, Certified Case Manager, Certified Life Care Planner™, and Certified Canadian Life Care Planner™. These certifications should be sought after when looking for an appropriate occupational therapist to provide consultation on a case. Online directories are available to locate a certified professional.

Scope of Practice

In the United States, the scope of occupational therapy practice is based on an official document set forth by AOTA (2021c). In this document, AOTA opines that a referral is unnecessary for the delivery of occupational therapy services, but the organization reiterates that occupational therapy practitioners must comply with state and federal laws and regulations, the profession's code of ethics, and payor policies. Occupational therapists' scope of practice includes the domains of occupation and the process of service delivery. The OTPF-4 identifies nine domains of occupation, activities of daily living (ADLs), instrumental activities of daily living (IADLs), health management, rest and sleep, education, work, play, leisure, and social participation (AOTA, 2020c).

Activities of daily living (ADLs) are defined as "activities oriented toward taking care of one's own body and completed on a routine basis" (AOTA, 2021c, p.3). The OTPF-4 describes the following occupations which fall under this domain (AOTA, 2020c):

- *Bathing, showering, toileting*, and *toilet hygiene* include obtaining and using all necessary supplies, as well as transferring to and from and/or maintaining any necessary positions to complete the task.
- *Dressing* involves selecting and obtaining appropriate clothing and all aspects of putting it on and taking it off.
- *Eating and swallowing* addresses the manipulation of food and liquid within the mouth and throat while feeding involves the actions of setting up the food and drink and bringing it to/from the mouth.
- *Functional mobility* considers movement to and from necessary positions or places in the performance of an activity.
- *Personal grooming and hygiene* encompass all aspects of daily hair, skin, nail, and oral care appropriate to an individual.
- *Sexual activity* encompasses various means for sexual expression (AOTA, 2020c).

Instrumental activities of daily living (IADLs) are "activities to support daily life within the home and community that often require complex interactions" (AOTA, 2021c, p. 3), which require a combination of motor, cognitive, and psychosocial skills. The OTPF-4 articulates the following types of activities and the components included within each of them (AOTA, 2020c):

- *Care of others* and *care of pets and animals* may entail providing, arranging, or supervising either paid or informal care.
- *Child rearing* activities support the "developmental and physiological needs of a child" (AOTA, 2020c, p. 31).
- *Communication management* is the "sending, receiving, and interpreting of information using systems and equipment" appropriate to the individual and their needs (AOTA, 2020c, p. 31). Assistive technology, such as augmentative and alternative communication, Braille writers, and others, are included in this category.
- *Driving and community mobility* includes transportation and the methods by which people plan and move around the community.
- *Financial management* is the process of using fiscal resources to establish and achieve short- and long-term goals.
- *Home establishment and management* involves obtaining, maintaining, and using resources to repair possessions and environments.
- *Meal preparation and cleanup* includes all tasks related to food provision.
- *Religious and spiritual expression* describes engagement in activities, organizations, and practices that aim for self-fulfillment, such as attending services, praying, chanting, contemplating, and contributing to a cause.
- *Safety and emergency maintenance* includes taking precautions, assessing, and reducing potential risks, recognizing and responding to hazardous situations.

- *Shopping*, whether in person or online, involves making lists, obtaining desired items, and paying for them (AOTA, 2020c).

The OTPF-4 describes health management as "activities relating to developing, managing, and maintaining health and wellness routines…with the goal of improving or maintaining health to support participation in other occupations" (AOTA, 2020c, p. 32) and outlines the following occupations that comprise it:

- *Social and emotional health promotion and maintenance* includes identifying personal strengths, self-advocacy, managing emotions, identifying, choosing, and engaging in occupations to support health, wellness, and participation.
- *Symptom and condition management* involves taking care of physical and mental health needs, pain, and disease by using various strategies and supports available in the community and the healthcare system.
- *Communication with the healthcare system* describes the use of various modalities to convey information between the evaluee, providers, and payor sources.
- *Medication management* requires communicating about, filling, interpreting instructions, and taking prescriptions as they were intended.
- *Physical activity* is taking part in exercise to optimize health outcomes.
- *Nutrition management* describes the process of following nutrition and hydration, meal preparation, and diet recommendations to support health.
- *Personal care device management* requires the procurement, use, and maintenance of the device (AOTA, 2020c).

The OTPF-4 describes rest and sleep as "activities related to obtaining restorative rest and sleep to support healthy, active engagement in other occupations" (AOTA, 2020c, p. 32):

- *Rest* requires identification of the need to engage in activities that interrupt and reduce activity to restore, calm, and renew.
- *Sleep preparation* includes establishing routines, patterns, and environments that prepare people for sleep, determining appropriate sleep and wake cycles, and managing sleep-related devices.
- *Sleep participation* requires taking care of personal needs to ensure successful onset and sustainment of sleep (AOTA, 2020c).

The OTPF-4 defines education as "activities needed for learning and participating in the educational environment"(AOTA, 2020c, p. 33):

- *Formal educational participation* includes academic, nonacademic, extracurricular, technological, and vocational pursuits.
- *Informal personal educational needs or interests' exploration* and *informal educational participation* are also considered occupations within the education domain (AOTA, 2020c).

Work includes "activities for engaging in employment or volunteer activities with financial and nonfinancial benefits" (AOTA, 2021c, p. 3). The OTPF-4 encourages occupational therapists to consider the following activities as they relate to work (AOTA, 2020c):

- *Employment interests and pursuits* should be consistent with personal strengths, limitations, and goals.
- *Employment seeking and acquisition* involves preparation and the completion of all tasks required to secure employment.
- *Job performance and maintenance* requires the completion of employment duties, negotiating relationships with people in the workplace, and complying with employment expectations.
- *Retirement preparation and adjustment* considers exploration of interests, securing necessary resources, and lifestyle adaptation to shifting roles.
- *Volunteer exploration* and *volunteer participation* describe learning about volunteer opportunities and participating in unpaid work (AOTA, 2020c).

Both occupational therapists and vocational counselors address paid and unpaid work with individuals with disabilities. For occupational therapists, work is one of the nine domains of "occupation" that can be addressed. Occupational therapists utilize occupations as a treatment modality and outcome while engaging evaluees in their paid and unpaid work. Many occupational therapists utilize task analysis and assist individuals with ergonomic modifications as well as work hardening and return to work. Similarly, vocational counselors also assist evaluees with disabilities to return to work by engaging them in the counseling process. This process entails "communication, goal setting, and beneficial growth or change through self-advocacy, psychological, vocational, social, and behavioral interventions" (Commission on Rehabilitation Counselor Certification, n.d.)

The AOTA (2021c, p. 3) describes play as "activities that are intrinsically motivated, internally controlled, and freely chosen" and leisure as "nonobligatory and intrinsically motivated activities during discretionary time." In the OTPF-4, *play* and *leisure* both involve the *exploration* of various activities that suit a person's interests, skills, and opportunities, as well as *participation* in those activities through planning, obtaining, and maintaining necessary resources, and balancing the demands of other occupations (AOTA, 2020c):

- Play is often considered a childhood occupation.
- Leisure is usually considered an adolescent/adult occupation.

Social participation includes "activities that involve social interaction with others and support social interdependence" (AOTA, 2021c, p.3).

Community, *family*, and *peer group participation* are considered separate occupations that require engagement in activities and interacting with others based on different aims or roles within the group.

Friendships require engagement in activities that support mutually beneficial relationships between two people.

Intimate partner relationships describe engagement in activities that foster and maintain closeness, affection, and role fulfillment (AOTA, 2020c).

Similarities and overlap exist between case management, life care planning, and occupational therapy. Occupational therapists' scope of practice resembles the broad view that case managers take of their evaluees and similarly, the holistic view a life care plan takes of its evaluee. An occupational therapist acting as a case manager or as a life care planner brings a tremendous amount of knowledge and ability to opine about recommendations in the life care plan. Table 14.1 correlates common life care plan categories with occupational therapy's nine domains and their constituent occupations to highlight recommendations that are within the profession's scope of practice.

Table 14.1 Occupational Therapist Contributions to Life Care Plan Recommendations

Care Category	Can Occupational Therapist Make Recommendation?
Physician (MD, DO, DC, DDS) referral to evaluate/consult	Can refer to some specialists within scope of practice, otherwise collaborative
Physician (MD, DO) ongoing visits	Outside of scope of practice
Chiropractic visits	Outside of scope of practice
Dentist ongoing visits and sedation	Outside of scope of practice
Ancillary (non-physician professionals) referrals	Within scope of practice to recommend referrals
Ancillary ongoing visits	Within scope of practice for occupational therapy, otherwise not within scope of practice
Diagnostic testing	Outside of scope of practice
Surgery	Outside of scope of practice
Aggressive interventions (e.g., invasive procedures, specialty programs)	Outside of scope of practice, except that acupuncture may be performed by Canadian occupational therapists with training
Wheelchairs, including features and accessories	Within scope of practice
Other mobility equipment	Within scope of practice
Orthotics	Within scope of practice
Prosthetics	Collaborative
Other medical equipment	Collaborative for some equipment or outside of scope of practice
Adaptive aids for independent function	Within scope of practice
Drugs requiring prescription	Outside of scope of practice
Over-the-counter drugs	Outside of scope of practice
Disposable supplies	Outside of scope of practice
Home care skill level (to attend to person) (i.e., unlicensed aide, licensed nurse)	Within scope of practice to identify need for assistance and level of assistance
Home care hours	Within scope of practice
Household (housekeeping, yard care, house repairs) services and hours	Within scope of practice
Adapted transportation (evaluation, training, equipment)	Within scope of practice
Alternative transportation	Within scope of practice
Architectural modification	Within scope of practice but most often collaborative
Home furnishings	Within scope of practice
Health maintenance	Within scope of practice for exercise programs
Adaptive or therapeutic recreation	Within scope of practice or collaborative with therapeutic recreation specialist
Potential complications	Within scope of practice or collaborative

Source: Boniface, G., Smith, J., Mitchell, C., & Bowles, H. L. (2019). What life care planners need to know about the professional discipline of occupational therapy. *Journal of Life Care Planning*, *17*(1), 7–12. Reprinted with permission.

Kinds of Patients and Problems Usually Seen and Addressed

Occupational therapists work with all types of people across the lifespan. Any person experiencing difficulty completing their "occupations" can receive occupational therapy. Occupational therapists work in collaboration with their patients to address occupational needs in areas such as mental health; work and industry; participation in education; rehabilitation, disability, productive aging; and health and wellness (AOTA, 2021c). With this broad understanding of occupations in mind, an occupational therapist evaluates a person considering not just the motor and process skills required to complete meaningful occupations but also considers contextual factors. Contextual factors include environmental factors and personal factors that may be impeding a person's ability to complete their occupation (AOTA, 2020c). A person does not need to have a specific diagnosis to receive occupational therapy services. Rather, an individual who is having difficulties completing their occupations may be a candidate for occupational therapy services.

Occupational therapists are trained to administer a variety of standardized and non-standardized assessments. An occupational therapist uses clinical reasoning to choose the assessment method most appropriate for the individual evaluee. An occupational therapy assessment may add valuable information to a life care plan about a person's strengths and areas that need support.

Pediatric Service Provision

For young children, two of the main occupations are play and eating. Other common problems that impact childhood occupational domains include fine, visual, and sensory motor delays that impede play and completion of chores, dressing, or school activities. Children with cerebral palsy, traumatic brain injury, autism, brachial plexus injuries, and other diagnoses may have difficulty in these areas.

Children can receive occupational therapy services in a variety of settings. In the United States, between the ages of birth through age two, a child typically will participate in occupational therapy through an early intervention program. Early intervention programs are overseen by the U.S. Department of Education. Early intervention programs are for children experiencing developmental delays in one or more of the following areas: cognitive, physical, social, emotional, communication, or adaptive development. Also, a child who has a diagnosed physical or mental condition that has a high probability of resulting in developmental delay may receive early intervention (U.S. Department of Education, n.d.-a). While these programs are federally mandated, each state has the ability to structure the program in a way that best suits the people of that state. Therefore, when completing a life care plan, it is important to understand the specific state guidelines regarding early intervention services. It is possible to receive outpatient occupational therapy services in addition to occupational therapy provided through early intervention services. Typically, early intervention services are provided in a child's natural environment which could include the home or a daycare setting.

Once a child turns three years old, they can be evaluated for school-based occupational therapy services. Under the IDEA (Individuals with Disabilities Education Act) law, occupational therapy services are classified as a related service (U.S. Department of Education, n.d.-b). Occupational therapy services provided in the school setting need to be educationally relevant and support a child's needs identified in their Individualized Education Plan (IEP) (Thompson, 2021).

Children may also receive occupational therapy as an outpatient, and this is often considered medically-based therapy. Thompson (2021, p.16) noted:

> In a medically-based setting, a child is often seen 1–3 times/week, for 30–60-minute sessions. While some children are seen weekly for years, this setting offers opportunities for episodes of care in which a child is seen for a finite period to address specific functional deficits. Therapy intensives might be possible wherein a child is seen multiple times per week for several hours at a time to focus on acquisition of a specific skill (e.g., constraint induced movement therapy).

It is important for life care planners to understand that it is not uncommon for children to have both educationally and medically-based occupational therapy services.

Adult Service Provision

While occupational therapists who work with adults and older adults focus on "occupations," the occupations must be appropriate to their evaluees' phase of life. Individuals in adulthood and older adults may encounter occupational therapy if they experience a medical, physical, or mental health issue or are having difficulties in any of the nine domains of occupational therapy. An understanding of their values, beliefs, spirituality, bodily functions, and structures are factors which are assessed to form the basis of the intervention. Similarly, a thorough understanding of personal and environmental factors is required to fully comprehend the impact of the condition on the evaluee's current state of occupation. An evaluee-centered assessment is completed using standardized and non-standardized methods. Individualized and/or family-centered occupational therapy goals flow from the knowledge gained from the assessments. Assessment tools vary by region, availability, clinician preference, and training.

Although occupational therapists can intervene wherever a deficit in function exists, common medical conditions which result in impairment include, but are not limited to spinal cord injury, traumatic brain injury, cerebral vascular accidents, complex medical conditions, poly-trauma, mental health conditions, dementia, Parkinson's disease, oncology, muscular-skeletal and orthopedic deficits. Individuals may be referred for occupational therapy services because of one condition and receive occupational therapy intervention focusing on a co-morbid or chronic condition which is impeding progress in their daily function. These individuals will be seen for interventions focused on any skills negatively impacting their habits, roles, routines, and rituals (AOTA, 2020c). A body of research is accumulating in the form of systematic reviews evaluating the impact of occupational therapy interventions with individuals who have a variety of impairments. The Occupational Therapy Practice Guideline for Adults with Chronic Conditions was published by Fields and Smallfield (2022) outlining occupational therapy professionals' role in using a preventative, collaborative goal setting approach to help individuals with heart disease, chronic lung disease, kidney disease, and diabetes in establishing habits and routines. Additionally, Practice Guidelines for Adults with Stroke was published in 2015 (Wolf & Nilsen). Generally speaking, therapy treatment planning includes short- and long-term goals. Goals should be measurable, attainable, and reasonable (James & Pitonyak, 2019). Outcomes, including personal goals, flow from the assessment and intervention provided. The occupational therapy process emphasizes evidence and occupationally based practice with targeted outcomes (Chisholm & Schell, 2019). Additionally, if any other areas impede progress toward outcomes, they should be addressed.

Adults and older adult treatment settings consist primarily of acute care hospitals, skilled nursing facilities, acute rehabilitation hospitals, long-term acute care hospitals, specialty hospitals, group homes, outpatient clinics, assisted living facilities, and home care. An emerging setting for occupational therapists is primary care physician offices with evidence to support its efficacy (AOTA, 2020b).

With the onset of aging, individuals develop a greater deterioration of their ADLs and IADLs (Edemekong et al., 2022). This fundamental knowledge of the functional impact of aging benefits the occupational therapy life care planner to effectively incorporate services across the evaluee's lifespan. According to Mitchell (2014), individuals with a disability experience normal age-related changes 20–30 years earlier compared to the normal trajectory commonly seen in aging. Combining this longitudinal understanding with the educational background of disability enables the life care planner to rely on an occupational therapist's expertise to opine upon life care plan items.

Home Assessment

Karl and Weed (2018) outlined the importance of home assessment in life care planning. Life care planners are equipped to assess evaluees' environmental needs related to customized spaces, housing, and home modifications. Evaluees with spinal cord injury, brain injury, amputation, or the elderly may require a more complex and in-depth assessment. In these instances, a professional with the education and training to handle more complex situations should be sought. These individuals come from various backgrounds but obtain additional credentials related to home evaluation and modifications, such as Certified Environmental Access Consultant (CEAC) (www.vgmliveathome.com/membership-privileges/education), Certified Home Assessment and Modification Professional (CHAMP) (https://champcertification.com/), and Certified Aging in Place Specialist (CAPS) (www.nahb.org/education-and-events/education/designations/Certified-Aging-in-Place-Specialist-CAPS). Additionally, some licensed general contractors and architects specialize in accessible construction (Karl & Weed, 2018).

Karl and Weed (2018) state that the home assessment should provide an overview of the current space and encompass all the evaluee's needs and goals to allow the life care planner to make appropriate recommendations. When a home assessment professional is consulted, it is important for the life care planner to share as much information as possible about the evaluee's equipment, skills, needs, strengths, and level of required support so the assessor can determine the most appropriate solution(s) (Karl & Weed, 2018). The evaluee and/or their family should be involved in the home assessment to facilitate a clear understanding of the evaluee's needs and the recommendations being made. Karl and Weed (2018) suggest that a home assessment report should identify all necessary living spaces and whether modifications are or are not recommended to avoid the perception that a space was overlooked. A life care planner or home assessment specialist might choose to develop a checklist based on the following considerations.

The U.S. Access Board (n.d.) promotes equality for people with disabilities and fulfills many duties. While they do enforce accessibility standards for federally funded facilities, they also develop accessibility guidelines and provide technical assistance. The U.S. Access Board is a leading source of information regarding accessible design. While personal properties are not required to comply with the Americans with Disabilities Act ([ADA], 1990) or its subsequent amendment, the Americans with Disabilities Act Amendment Act ([ADAAA], 2008) accessibility standards, the standards can be useful when considering home modifications to support function and improve quality of life in the home.

When considering the entrance to the home, the rise of the entrance should be measured (Karl & Weed, 2018). The U.S. Access Board (n.d.) iterates that the maximum rise for any ramp should be 30" (405.6), with a maximum slope of 1:12 (405.2). Compliant handrails are required for ramps that rise 6" or more (405.8) and they should have at least 36" between them (405.5). Additionally, an appropriate landing should be available at the top and bottom of the ramp (405.7). Ramps and landings that have a vertical drop off of ½" or more should have compliant edge protection (Table 405.9). The board also provides guidance regarding the minimum maneuvering clearance, dependent upon the direction of the approach, and the type and position of the door. (Table 404.2.4.1; Table 404.2.4.2).

Karl and Weed (2018) note that entrances with an inaccessible rise and limited space, such as a garage or carport, may accommodate a lift. When assessing the garage and approach to the home for an evaluee who requires a wheelchair, Karl and Weed (2018) recommend measuring the height of the garage door, as modified vehicles may be larger to accommodate equipment. Further, the size of the chair, as well as the function and the age of the evaluee should be examined (Karl & Weed, 2018).

A variety of additional safety features must be assessed. At the primary entrance to the home, the U.S. Access Board (n.d.) draws attention to the need for accessible doorbells (809.5.5.1) for people with certain sensory deficits and an accessible means for an evaluee to identify a visitor (809.5.5.2). When considering storm protection for a person with limited mobility, a ramp or a lift might be viable options for access from a deck to a basement (Karl & Weed, 2018). While porch lifts may increase accessibility in tight spaces, the home assessor must remember that another permanent, safe option must be available in the event of an equipment failure (Karl & Weed, 2018). Karl and Weed (2018) further iterate that safety exits should not pass through a kitchen, carport, garage, or past gas heaters because these areas are most likely to be inaccessible in the event of a fire. A safe egress from every required living space must be a priority. The U.S. Access Board (n.d.) guidelines also note that at least one accessible route should connect all living spaces (809.2.1) and those living spaces should have an acceptable turning space (809.2.2). They provide additional guidance regarding accessible fire alarm and smoke detection systems (809.5.1), an important aspect to consider for those with sensory impairments.

Karl and Weed (2018) suggest that a variety of lifts and/or an elevator might be considered if access is required to more than one level of the home. The style and placement of furniture, type of flooring, trip hazards, and location of controls within rooms must be evaluated (Karl & Weed, 2018). The U.S. Access Board (n.d.) provides guidance regarding accessible design elements which could be considered in a home assessment, especially for an evaluee who uses a wheelchair for mobility, including door openings (404.2.3), height of thresholds (404.2.5), and turning spaces (304.3.1, 304.3.2). Karl and Weed (2018) indicate that the size and layout of each required living space will be affected by the evaluee's mobility, required equipment, and caregiving needs, and should be assessed with these factors in mind.

Karl and Weed (2018) highlight several considerations for the evaluee's bedroom. Space around the bed should accommodate the evaluee's transfer needs in terms of necessary equipment and caregiver assistance. Adequate lighting, heat sources, and electric outlets must be appropriately situated. For those with life supporting equipment, space must be available for a backup generator. Various lift systems, some of which allow an evaluee to move between rooms and/or decrease the level of assistance needed for transfers, might be explored. Custom designed closets and dresser drawers may ease clothing retrieval and storage (Karl & Weed, 2018).

Karl and Weed (2018) emphasize the importance of communication with the evaluee's, healthcare providers, and family members to assess and develop the bathroom design and recommendations. Karl and Weed (2018) recommend a minimum bathroom size of 10' by

10'. They suggest the type of flooring must also be considered because spills and water on the floor are likely. Extra storage space for equipment and supplies, additional space under the sink to roll a wheelchair, and easy to maneuver faucet handles should also be considered (Karl & Weed, 2018).

The size and location of required bathing equipment, as well as the need for space for an attendant, will affect the size and layout of the bathroom redesign. In general, the more assistance a person needs for bathing and toileting, the larger the bathroom needs to be (Karl & Weed, 2018). The U.S. Access Board (n.d.) recommends a 60-inch turning diameter in a bathroom space. Grab bar placement will need to be assessed for both toilet and bathing transfers. Most walls will require backing material installation to properly anchor the grab bar (Karl & Weed, 2018). For individuals who require an elevated toilet seat, either a stand-alone high-rise toilet or a toilet riser that fits over an existing toilet might be installed. The assessor must consider how an individual performs toilet transfers (e.g., using a lift, stand pivot transfer with attendant assistance, overhead lift system) as this will determine how much space is needed around the toilet for safe transfers. Open bottom shower chairs may serve as a toileting aid as well as a shower chair (Karl & Weed, 2018). Using a single chair for showering and toileting can also help decrease the numbers of transfers needed during the day.

For individuals who can step up approximately three inches, walk-in showers with built-in seats improve safety (Karl & Weed, 2018). Roll-in showers require a recommended minimum space of 4' by 5' and can be used with a shower chair (Karl & Weed, 2018). The U.S. Access Board (n.d.) recommends grab bars on three walls for a roll-in shower without a seat. Shower controls must be located at least 1½ inches above a grab bar so they do not impede use of the grab bar (U.S. Access Board, n.d.). Other specialized bathing equipment, such as shower trolleys or therapeutic bathtubs, may be considered.

For buildings that are required to comply with the ADA and subsequent ADAAA, the U.S. Access Board (n.d.) requires pass-through kitchens to have two entrances/exits and have a minimum of 40" clearance between opposing cabinets or walls (804.2.1) and U-shaped kitchens should have a minimum of 60" clearance (804.2.2). This can also provide a guideline for personal home modifications. Individuals in wheelchairs should consider roll-in sinks and roll-in electric work tops (Karl & Weed, 2018). Multiple surface levels may be beneficial to accommodate people who are seated, alternate family members, or caregivers who are standing with open areas for roll-under capability. Raised appliances including the dishwasher, built-in wall oven and microwave, front mounted switch controls, and base cabinets with pull out extension drawers provide easier access and increased safety (Karl & Weed, 2018). Heat resistant, solid surface worktops may be required. As with other rooms in the home, adequate room size to accommodate wheelchair radius or other assistive mobility devices needs to be considered (Karl & Weed, 2018).

The laundry room may be designed for a care attendant or for the evaluee. For an individual in a wheelchair, a front-loading washer and dryer, roll-under work surfaces, accessible rods for hanging clothes, accessible storage areas, and maneuvering space may promote independence (Karl & Weed, 2018).

The home assessment and resultant life care recommendations frequently occur as a result of a sudden illness or accident; therefore, preemptive design elements are not feasible. Also, Karl and Weed (2018) noted that some evaluees require such extensive home modifications whose costs for remodeling may outweigh the benefits, resulting in the decision to build a new accessible home or purchase a different pre-existing home. When this occurs, the evaluee should consider homes that follow universal design concepts, a term coined by Ron Mace (North Carolina State University, 1985–2001). Universal design is defined as the creation of "environments to be usable to the greatest extent possible by people of all ages and abilities" (Story et al., 1998, pp. 2).

With funding through the Department of Education's National Institute on Disability and Rehabilitation Research, Bettye Rose Connell, Mike Jones, Ron Mace, Jim Mueller, Abir Mullick, Elaine Ostroff, Jon Sanford, Ed Steinfeld, Molly Story, and Gregg Vanderheiden, in conjunction with universal design researchers and United States based practitioners, developed the seven Principles of Universal Design.[1] The following principles should serve as a guide when considering projected items, assisted devices, durable medical equipment, aides for independent living, or major home modification recommendations for a life care plan. Equitable use encourages builders to make the space useful and marketable to people with varied ability. Flexibility in use means the space accommodates a wide range of preferences and abilities. The principle of simple and intuitive use makes the space easy to understand. The next principle, perceptible information, suggests that the design effectively conveys necessary information to the user, regardless of their abilities. Tolerance for error encourages builders and designers to minimize hazards and potential adverse consequences for users. The principle of low physical effort encourages creation of spaces that can be efficiently and comfortably used. Finally, appropriate size and space should be allowed for easy approach and use regardless of the person's physical characteristics.[2]

Standard Treatment Recommendations

Through the evaluation process, the occupational therapist identifies difficulties in a person's occupational performance. The occupational therapist then collaborates with the evaluee to develop an intervention plan that includes the use of personalized and meaningful occupations and therapeutic activities to achieve a desired outcome. Occupational therapy standard treatment, for all ages and types of evaluees, includes the use of "occupations" and "activities" (AOTA, 2020c). Because occupations are viewed broadly, occupational therapy treatment can be broad in scope as well. For a child with cerebral palsy who has difficulty writing, treatment could explore assistive technology to help compensate for motor deficits or work on skill development to improve the child's fine motor skills. For an adult with a traumatic brain injury, the occupational therapist could work on community mobility by teaching them how to use public transportation safely. For an older adult with chronic back pain, occupational therapy could focus on ADL retraining using adaptive equipment such as a raised toilet seat and shower tub bench to reduce pain.

The OTPF-4 (AOTA, 2020c) outlines several interventions occupational therapists use to support a person's occupation. Occupational therapists can use physical agent modalities and mechanical modalities to decrease pain, assist with wound healing, edema control, or to prepare muscles for movement. Occupational therapists can fabricate or order and fit orthotics and prosthetics (AOTA, 2020c), often for the upper extremity. For example, an occupational therapist could fabricate a resting hand splint to prevent contractures for an individual who had a stroke. Occupational therapists complete assessments, choose equipment, and provide education and training in the use of high- and low-tech assistive devices (AOTA, 2020c). On the low-tech end, an occupational therapist might create a visual support for a child; while on the high-tech end, an occupational therapist might train an older adult to use environmental controls that allow them to age in place. Occupational therapists are often part of a wheelchair seating and positioning team and make recommendations for seating and positioning systems (AOTA, 2020c). Occupational therapists are trained to use self-regulation programs and sensory integration techniques with people throughout the lifespan. They often assist people with self-regulation by educating families, caregivers, and school staff on strategies to help people maintain an appropriate level of alertness for task completion (AOTA, 2020c). Advocacy, group, and virtual interventions (e.g., telehealth) are also treatment options for occupational therapists (AOTA, 2020c).

AOTA defines telehealth as "the application of evaluative, consultative, preventative, and therapeutic services delivered through information and communication technology" (AOTA, 2018, p. 1). Telehealth allows improved and timely access to services, providers, and specialists as well as remote collaboration among professionals. Clinical reasoning and professional ethics guide the selection of the appropriate technology for the provision of services, as well as the determination of which evaluees may be effectively served using this service delivery model. Therapists are responsible for ensuring their understanding and compliance with each state's regulations and the payor source policies surrounding telehealth practice. AOTA has developed a guiding resource which lists the citations, provisions, and special notes regarding the provision of occupational therapy via telehealth for all 50 states (AOTA State Affairs Group, 2022).

After completing an evaluation, an occupational therapist determines which of five intervention approaches or combinations of approaches is most appropriate for the evaluee (AOTA, 2020c). Health promotion is one intervention approach. An example of this intervention approach would be an occupational therapist training home health attendant staff on fall prevention in an evaluee's home. The restorative intervention approach works to establish a skill that has not yet been developed or to restore a skill that has been impaired (AOTA, 2020c). This could include improving a person's upper extremity range of motion so they can reach the items in the upper cupboards of the kitchen. An occupational therapist using the maintenance approach focuses on preserving a person's performance capacities. The assumption with this approach is that without continued maintenance intervention, performance would decrease (AOTA, 2020c). The compensatory approach centers on finding ways to change the environment or activity demands to improve a person's performance (AOTA, 2020c). This could include training in adaptive equipment and recommending home modifications such as toilet riser, shower benches, grab bars, etc. Finally, the disability prevention approach for occupational therapy treatment might include preventing social isolation by connecting an evaluee with a card playing group.

Occupational therapy has a holistic and wide-ranging approach to treatments making it a useful therapeutic modality to include in many life care plans. In fact, inpatient occupational therapy treatment has been shown to lower hospital readmission rates, supporting the life care plan's aim of preventing complications. (Rogers et al., 2017). The outcomes of occupational therapy intervention are directed toward "achieving health, well-being, and participation in life through engagement in occupations" (AOTA, 2020c, p. 5). The successful implementation and results of occupational therapy intervention are congruent with successful life care plans as well.

Questions Life Care Planners Should Ask the Occupational Therapist When Developing a Life Care Plan

In general, occupational therapists think about an evaluee's needs in terms of their current therapy episode of care. They may require prompting from a life care planner to think about an evaluee's lifelong needs, as is necessary in a life care plan. Few occupational therapists have forensic experience, and most are not familiar with litigation issues. Occupational therapists may need education from a life care planner to feel comfortable opining on life care plan recommendations (Mitchell & Mitchell, 2018). Frequency and duration of an occupational therapy episode of care can be impacted by the payor source. Occupational therapists can become accustomed to a frequency and duration of therapy that is determined by outside payor reimbursement. The same can be true when an occupational therapist considers replacement intervals of durable medical equipment. Therefore, occupational therapists may need education from a life care planner to consider the optimal frequency and duration of therapy as well as the optimal replacement intervals of durable medical equipment rather than basing their opinion on payor source coverage. As mentioned earlier in the chapter, occupational therapists can specialize in an area of practice (e.g., driving rehabilitation, pediatrics, geriatrics, home assessments). Therefore, it may be necessary and add depth, and detail to a life care plan when more than one occupational therapist is involved (Mitchell & Mitchell, 2018).

Case Study

Using the Boniface et al. (2019) chart as a guide, occupational therapists, given their education and functional focus, may opine upon items in many different life care plan categories. In the following case study, the role of occupational therapy is highlighted.

Evaluee History

Mr. Smith is a 65-year-old man who was physically assaulted, fell, and was eventually diagnosed with central cord syndrome. He underwent an emergency cervical fusion to stabilize his spine. As a result of the spinal cord injury, he has spasticity, pain, limited range of motion, a neurogenic bladder, and decreased standing and dynamic balance. He attended inpatient rehabilitation followed by home based therapies and nursing. His past medical history consisted of substance abuse and benign prostatic hyperplasia. He was unemployed and lived alone in a one-bedroom apartment at the time of the life care plan assessment.

Prior to the initiation of life care planning services, Mr. Smith had frequent falls and a hospitalization because of injuries sustained in those falls. He required assistance with ADLs and IADLs. His current services included physical therapy, occupational therapy, a personal care attendant, and a registered nurse. Mr. Smith ambulated with a straight cane, was incontinent of bladder function, and had an adjustment disorder with anxiety.

Life Care Plan Recommendations Within an Occupational Therapist's Scope of Practice

Projected Evaluations

- Physical therapy to assess current mobility status and balance
- Occupational therapy to assess basic and instrumental ADLs
- Case Management
- Counseling

Projected Therapeutic Modalities

- Occupational therapy visits to maximize independence with daily activities and provide compensatory strategies throughout the aging process

Aids for Independent Living

- Bathtub seat, bench, or stool depending on evaluee's needs
- Grab bars, 2, for shower
- Raised toilet seat with arms to assist with transfers
- Lifeline due to falls
- T-Pull door closer to assist with opening and closing front door
- Air conditioning/heating unit to assist with thermoregulation

Durable Medical Equipment

- Adjustable hospital bed
- Straight cane
- Electric recliner to assist with sit to stand transfers
- Ramp to access front door to use electric wheelchair

Orthotics, Prosthetics

- Hand orthotic to assist with neutral positioning due to increased spasticity and decreased range of motion

Wheelchairs

- Electric wheelchair for community mobility
- Wheelchair cushion
- Wheelchair maintenance
- Replacement battery
- Wheelchair cup holder

Home Care

- Attendant care, 6 hours per day beginning now
- Attendant care, 8 hours per day, beginning at age 70
- Nursing to assist with medication set up and management
- Housekeeping

Leisure

- Local community resources for adapted recreation
- Strength maintenance
- Local community YMCA membership with pool access for aqua therapy

Summary

Occupational therapists are trained to evaluate nine domains of a person's occupations and consider the environmental factors which might impact a person's ability to complete their occupations. Occupational therapy treatment is always evaluee centered. Treatment may use a restorative approach, teach compensatory strategies, or focus on maintaining a person's current skills. Occupational therapy treatment can also include health promotion and disability prevention. With a lens on evaluating and treating difficulties in completing life's "occupations," occupational therapy is well suited as a recommendation in many life care plans. Additionally, occupational therapists are qualified to opine on recommendations for a variety of life care plan categories and items, including non-physician referrals, ongoing occupational therapy visits, wheelchairs and mobility equipment, orthotics, adaptive aids for independent function, home care, and household services and hours (Boniface et al., 2019).

Notes

1 Copyright © 1997 NC State University, The Center for Universal Design.
2 Copyright © 1997 NC State University, The Center for Universal Design.

References

Accreditation Council for Occupational Therapy Education (ACOTE'). (2018). Standards and interpretive guide. *American Journal of Occupational Therapy*, *72*(Suppl. 2), 7212410005p1–7212410005p83. https://doi.org/10.5014/ajot.2018.72S217

American Occupational Therapy Association State Affairs Group. (2022, February). *Telehealth state statutes regulations regulatory board*. www.aota.org/-/media/Corporate/Files/Advocacy/State/telehealth/Telehealth-State-Statutes-Regulations-Regulatory-Board-Statements.pdf

American Occupational Therapy Association. (2017, April 20). *Celebrating AOTA's centennial: A historical look at 100 years of occupational therapy* [Video]. YouTube. www.youtube.com/watch?v=DbCwf2CzGvw

American Occupational Therapy Association. (2018). Telehealth in occupational therapy. *American Journal of Occupational Therapy*, *72*(Suppl.2). https://research.aota.org/ajot/article-abstract/72/Supplement_2/7212410059p1/6514/Telehealth-in-Occupational-Therapy?redirectedFrom=fulltext

American Occupational Therapy Association. (2019a). *Reaffirmation of commitment to occupation-based practice*. [Policy manual]. https://www.aota.org/-/media/corporate/files/aboutaota/officialdocs/policies/policy-e13-20190812.pdf

American Occupational Therapy Association. (2019b). *Standards of Practice*. [Policy manual]. https://research.aota.org/ajot/article/75/Supplement_3/7513410030/23113/Standards-of-Practice-for-Occupational-Therapy

American Occupational Therapy Association. (2019c). 2019 representative assembly summary of minutes. *American Journal of Occupational Therapy*, *73*(Suppl. 2), 7312420015. https://doi.org/10.5014/ajot.2019.73S211

American Occupational Therapy Association. (2020a). AOTA 2020 occupational therapy code of ethics. *American Journal of Occupational Therapy*, *74*(Suppl. 3), 7413410005. https://research.aota.org/ajot/article/74/Supplement_3/7413410005p1/6691/AOTA-2020-Occupational-Therapy-Code-of-Ethics

American Occupational Therapy Association. (2020b). Role of occupational therapy in primary care. *American Journal of Occupational Therapy*, *74*(Suppl. 3). 7413410040p1–7413410040p16. https://research.aota.org/ajot/article-abstract/74/Supplement_3/7413410040p1/6696/Role-of-Occupational-Therapy-in-Primary-Care?redirectedFrom=fulltext

American Occupational Therapy Association. (2020c). Occupational therapy practice framework: Domain and process (4th ed.). *American Journal of Occupational Therapy*, *74*(Suppl. 2), 7412410010. https://research.aota.org/ajot/article-abstract/74/Supplement_2/7412410010p1/8382/Occupational-Therapy-Practice-Framework-Domain-and?redirectedFrom=fulltext

American Occupational Therapy Association. (2021a, June). *AOTA strategic framework*. www.aota.org/-/media/corporate/files/aboutaota/2021-aota-strategic-framework.pdf

American Occupational Therapy Association. (2021b). *Definition of occupational therapy practice for the AOTA Model Practice Act*. www.aota.org/Advocacy-Policy/State-Policy/Resource-Factsheets.aspx

American Occupational Therapy Association. (2021c). Occupational therapy scope of practice. *American Journal of Occupational Therapy*, *75*(Suppl. 3), https://research.aota.org/ajot/article/75/Supplement_3/7513410020/23136/Occupational-Therapy-Scope-of-Practice

Americans with Disabilities Act Amendments Act of 2008, 42 U.S.C 12101 note. (2008). www.eeoc.gov/statutes/ada-amendments-act-2008

Americans with Disabilities Act of 1990, 42 U.S.C. § 12101 et seq. (1990). www.ada.gov/pubs/adastatute08.htm

Association for Canadian Occupational Therapy Regulatory Organization, Association for Canadian Occupational Therapy University Programs, and the Canadian Association of Occupational Therapists. (2021). *Competencies for occupational therapists in Canada*. https://acot.ca/wp-content/uploads/2021/12/Competencies-for-Occupational-Therapists-in-Canada-2021-Final-EN-web.pdf

Boniface, G., Smith, J., Mitchell, C., & Bowles, H. L. (2019). What life care planners need to know about the professional discipline of occupational therapy. *Journal of Life Care Planning*, *17*(1), 7–12.

Canadian Association of Occupational Therapists, Association of Canadian Occupational Therapy Regulatory Organizations, Association of Canadian Occupational Therapy Programs. (2021). *Competencies for occupational therapists in Canada*. https://acotro-acore.org/sites/default/files/uploads/ot_competency_document_en_web.pdf

Canadian Association of Occupational Therapists, Association of Canadian Occupational Therapy Regulatory Organizations, Association of Canadian Occupational Therapy University Programs, Canadian Occupational Therapy Foundation, Occupational Therapy Professional Alliance of Canada. (2013). *Position Statement: Professional identity, individual responsibility and public accountability through the use of title in occupational therapy*. https://caot.ca/document/3712/P%20-%20Prof%20Identity,%20Individual%20Responsibility%20&%20Public%20Accountability%20through%20OT.pdf

Canadian Association of Occupational Therapists. (2007). *Code of ethics*. https://caot.in1touch.org/document/4604/codeofethics.pdf

Canadian Association of Occupational Therapists. (2012). *Profile of practice of occupational therapists*. www.caot-ace.ca/document/3653/2012otprofile.pdf

Chisholm, D., & Schell, B. A. B. (2019). Overview of the occupational therapy process and outcomes. In B. A. B. Schell, & G. Gillen (Eds.), *Willard & Spackman's occupational therapy* (13th ed. p. 353–368), Wolters Kluwer.

Commission on Rehabilitation Counselor Certification. (n.d.) *Rehabilitation counseling scope of practice*. https://crccertification.com/wp-content/uploads/2020/11/Scope-of-Practice.pdf

DeMaio-Feldman, D. (1987). The occupational therapist as an expert witness. *The American Journal of Occupational Therapy*, *41*(9), 590–594. https://doi.org/10.5014/ajot.41.9.590

Deutsch, P. (n. d.). *Publications – life care planning. Tenets of life care planning*. www.paulmdeutsch.com/LCP-tenets-of-life-care-planning.htm

Edemekong, P., Bomgaars, D. L., Sukumaran, S., & Levy, S. B. (2022, February). *Activities of daily living*. StatPearls Publishing. www.ncbi.nlm.nih.gov/books/NBK470404/

Eliassen, I. (2022a, March 9). *West Virginia and Alabama enact OT compact*. Occupational Therapy Licensure Compact. https://otcompact.org/west-virginia-and-alabama-enact-ot-compact/

Eliassen, I. (2022b, May 16). *South Carolina becomes 20th OT compact member state*. Occupational Therapy Licensure Compact. https://otcompact.org/south-carolina-becomes-20th-ot-compact-member-state/

Fields, B., & Smallfield, S. (2022). Occupational therapy practice guidelines for adults with chronic conditions. *American Journal of Occupational Therapy*, *76*(2), https://doi.org/10.5014/ajot.2022/762001

Harris, I., Henry, A., Green, N., & Dodson, J. (1994). The occupational therapist as an expert analyst on the cost of future health care in legal cases. *Canadian Journal of Occupational Therapy*, *61*(3), 136–140.

James, A. B., & Pitonyak, J. S. (2019). Activities of daily living and instrumental activities of daily living. In B. A. B. Schell & G. Gillen (Eds.), *Willard & Spackman's occupational therapy* (13th ed., p. 353–368), Wolters Kluwer.

Karl, J., & Weed, R. O. (2018). Home assessment in life care planning. In R. O. Weed & D. E. Berens (Eds.), *Life care planning and case management handbook* (4th ed., pp. 787–798). Routledge.

Klinger, L., Baptiste, B., & Adams, J. R. (2004). Life care plans: An emerging area for occupational therapists. *Canadian Journal of Occupational Therapy, 71*(2), 88–99. https://doi.org/10.1177/000841740407100204

Lewis, K. E., Lehman, M. J., & Cockburn, L. (2021). Looking back to move forward: Canadian occupational therapy in public health, 1914–2019. *Canadian Journal of Occupational Therapy, 88*(1), 48–58. https://doi.org/10.1177/0008417421992617

Mitchell, N. (2014) Aging with cerebral palsy, spinal cord injury, and amputation: Implications for life care planners. *Journal of Life Care Planning, 3,* 163–175.

Mitchell, N. L., & Mitchell, C. V. (2018). The role of the occupational therapist in life care planning. In R. O. Weed & D. E. Berens (Eds.), *Life care planning and case management handbook* (4th ed., pp. 105–133). Routledge.

North Carolina State University, College of Design, Center for Universal Design Records 1985-2001, North Carolina State University, UA 110.052, Special Collections Research Center, NC State University Libraries.

Rogers, A. T., Bai, G., Lavin, R. A., & Anderson, G. F. (2017). Higher hospital spending on occupational therapy is associated with lower readmission rates. *Medical Care Research and Review, 74*(6) 668–686. https://doi.org/10.1177/1077558716666981

Royal College of Occupational Therapists. (2018). *Acting as an expert witness guidance for occupational therapists* (2nd Ed.). Lavenham Press.

Story, M. F., Mueller, J. L., & Mace, R. L. (1998). *The universal design file: Designing for people of all ages and abilities.* The Center for Universal Design, North Carolina State University.

Stromsdorfer, S. (2020, August 4). The 11 best occupational therapy quotes. *myOT Spot.* www.myotspot.com/occupational-therapy-quotes/

The Center for Universal Design. (1997). *The principles of universal design, Version 2.0.* North Carolina State University.

Thompson, A. (2021). Pediatric therapy service delivery 101: What's the difference and why does it matter to life care planners? *Journal of Life Care Planning, 19*(2), 17–24.

U.S. Access Board. (n.d.) *American with Disabilities Act accessibility standards.* U.S. Access Board. www.access-board.gov/ada/

U.S. Department of Education. (n.d.-a) *Early intervention program for infants and toddlers with disabilities.* www2.ed.gov/programs/osepeip/index.html

U.S. Department of Education. (n.d.-b). *Related services. IDEA: Individuals with Disabilities Education Act.* https://sites.ed.gov/idea/regs/b/a/300.34

Willmarth, C., & Conway, S. (2022). AOTA–NBCOT® joint initiative: Developing the occupational therapy licensure compact. *The American Journal of Occupational Therapy, 76*(1). https://research.aota.org/ajot/article/76/1/7601070010/23148/AOTA-NBCOTR-Joint-Initiative-Developing-the

Wolf, T. J., & Nilsen, D. M. (2015). *Occupational therapy practice guidelines for adults with stroke.* AOTA Press.

World Federation of Occupational Therapy. (2018). *Definitions of occupational therapy from member organizations* (May 2018 rev.). www.wfot.org/resources/definitions-of-occupational-therapy-from-member-organisations

World Federation of Occupational Therapy. (n.d.). *History.* https://wfot.org/about/history

World Health Organization. (2002). *Towards a common language for functioning, disability, and health: ICF.* https://cdn.who.int/media/docs/default-source/classification/icf/icfbeginnersguide.pdf

Chapter 15

The Role of the Physical Therapist in Life Care Planning

Diana Bubanja

History and Development of Physical Therapy

The profession of physical therapy began with reconstruction aides who were civilian employees of the Medical Department of the United States Army during World War I (American Physical Therapy Association [APTA], 2022a). Marguerite Sanderson oversaw the first reconstruction aides and established the Division of Physical Reconstruction. Mary McMillan was the first female appointed as the first reconstruction aide in February 1918. She organized the Physiotherapy Department at Walter Reed General Hospital. Of the original 18 Aides, 16 formed the American Women's Physical Therapeutic Association, which is now known as the American Physical Therapy Association (APTA, 2022a).

Physical Therapist Education

Over the decades, physical therapy evolved from a Bachelor of Science to a Master of Science degree. In 2015, all accredited and developing physical therapist programs evolved into a post-baccalaureate three-year Doctor of Physical Therapy (DPT) degree (APTA, 2015). In 2000, the APTA passed its Vision 2020 statement, which advocated for direct access to physical therapy evaluation and treatment without a physician's referral (APTA, 2022b).

The basic physical therapy curriculum includes, but is not limited to, the following courses: functional, neuromuscular, and musculoskeletal anatomy with dissection lab; neuroanatomy and neurophysiology; exercise physiology; musculoskeletal disorders; neurorehabilitation; pharmacology for physical therapy practice; principles of disease; radiology and diagnostic imaging in physical therapy practice; motor control/therapeutic modalities (therapeutic intervention skills including manual skills, exercise, and neuro rehab intervention); differential diagnosis; prosthetics and orthotics; evidence based practice; health promotion and wellness and clinical skills; psychosocial/behavioral content; ethics; human development/life span; and business principles.

DOI: 10.4324/9781003388456-18

Though the clinical practice of physical therapy is very similar in the United States and Canada, the access to physical therapy and licensing practices differ, due to the differences in the health systems. Differences in settings and salaries exist within each country based on area of the country and demand for physical therapists

Scope of Practice

Physical therapists are trained and experienced in collaboratively working with a multi-disciplinary team, consisting of, but not limited to, physicians, psychotherapists, occupational and speech therapists, orthotists, prosthetists, nurses, vocational evaluators, massage therapists, acupuncturists, social workers, personal trainers, attendant and companion caregivers in settings such as home care, skilled nursing, and intermediate and assistive care facilities, as well as hospitals, school systems, and outpatient practices. Physical therapists treat clients using various modalities. They teach clients how to use medical and durable medical equipment including walkers, canes, wheelchairs and accessories, power scooters, shower benches, grab bars, TENS units, braces, splints, and exercise equipment safely and effectively. It is within a physical therapist's scope of practice and clinical experience as a rehabilitation professional and educator to provide recommendations related to these types of rehabilitation equipment with reasonable replacement schedules. For an in-depth discussion of replacement schedules, the reader is referred to chapter 33 in this text.

The role of a physical therapist overlaps that of other medical professionals. In the area of activities of daily living (ADLs), occupational and physical therapists work closely together. Occupational therapists usually have more training in specific adaptive equipment. In some settings, occupational therapists prescribe wheelchairs, and in others physical therapists make those recommendations. In most settings with both professions, a physical therapist will make the recommendations for equipment related to walking, transfers, and gross motor mobility. An occupational therapist will make recommendations for equipment related to self-care.

Orthotists and physical therapists can overlap as well. Some physical therapists are specially trained in evaluating for and providing orthotics. It is more typical that a physical therapist would evaluate the functional impairments and communicate the improvements desired from an orthotic. The orthotist would then fit and provide the product, with the physical therapist making the final assessment of the benefits gained. Physical therapists working in home care settings provide functional mobility strengthening and balance training, teach energy conservation techniques, and offer recommendations for architectural modifications. As rehabilitation professionals and educators, it is within the physical therapy scope of practice to provide recommendations for adaptive aids used for cooking, bathing, and grooming, as well as widening of doors and installation of ramps for wheelchair accessibility, railings for stair navigation, and walk-in showers for safe bathing. Physical therapists evaluate critical work-related physical demands by providing job-site analyses and functional capacity evaluations.

Kinds of Patients and Problems Usually Seen and Addressed by Physical Therapists

Physical therapy services are provided with the goal of maintaining or regaining maximum movement, strength, and function of clients of all ages who have sustained an injury, experience pain, or have a chronic disease. Physical therapists evaluate and treat adult and pediatric clients who have sustained brain injuries, spinal cord injuries, traumatic amputations, orthopedic injuries, neurological conditions, and chronic pain and other physical impairments related to musculoskeletal function. Physical therapists are equipped to advise patients/clients on issues related to general health and wellness, in addition to pathological conditions, in the realm of functional mobility. Physical therapists also have the breadth of knowledge to serve as an advocate or case manager for individuals who have multiple and diverse needs best provided by a team of specialized healthcare providers. Commonly seen conditions in adults include strokes, brain injuries, spinal cord injuries, multiple sclerosis, Parkinson's disease, heart attacks, and arthritis, with the goal of improving and/or maintaining one's strength, mobility, and balance. Pediatric physical therapists evaluate and treat orthopedic, neurologic conditions, and delays in motor skills (large scale movements of the legs, arms, and trunk), taking into consideration the unique developmental stages of children and youth, specifically early childhood (birth to age 5 years), middle childhood (ages 6–12 years), and adolescence (ages 13–18 years). Pediatric diagnoses include cerebral palsy, autism, Down syndrome, muscular dystrophy, spina bifida, juvenile rheumatoid arthritis, torticollis, cardiopulmonary disorders, cystic fibrosis, cancer, hypotonia, traumatic brain injury, as well as scoliosis, back pain, and sports injuries.

The role of a pediatric physical therapist is to specifically assist each child to reach their maximum level of function at home, in school, and in the community. The pediatric physical therapist will also assist the child and family with coordination of ancillary services and items like adaptive equipment, custom wheelchair seating systems, and adaptive technology, as well as orthotics or prosthetics. Generally speaking, the services provided by pediatric physical therapists should be provided in the facility that the child spends their time in. For example, if the child spends time in the home, then the therapy services should be provided in the home.

If the child attends school, physical therapy services should be provided in the school, as long as the child meets the school criteria for school-based therapy. The Individuals with Disabilities Education Act (IDEA) provides school-based physical therapy for children from birth to age 21 years; however, children must be eligible for the program and meet criteria for the program. The advantage of school-based physical therapy is that it teaches and provides children with the necessary skills and tools required in an academic environment in order to reduce or overcome learning and physical barriers and functional limitations. For an in-depth discussion of special education service provision, the reader is referred to Chapter 31 in this text.

Physical Therapy Service Delivery

Physical therapy treatment begins with an evaluation which includes an interview of the client or caregiver. Through careful questioning and listening, the primary problems, impairments, co-existing conditions, past medical and surgical history, medications, support systems, functional goals, pain levels, psychosocial and cognitive issues, and previous or current medical and social services are identified. Limitations in functional mobility can be due to both objective and subjective impairments. During this initial interview, any pain, dizziness, or other reported discomfort is identified and documented, often with ratings by the client using to a numerical scale. Commonly used devices include dynamometry which measures grip strength, as well as inclinometry which measures spinal range of motion, and goniometry which measures upper and lower extremity range of motion.

The objective portion of the physical therapy evaluation includes general system screens, more in-depth exams, and special tests. General screens include basic soft tissue evaluation, range of motion, strength, sensory systems, gait analysis, flexibility, balance, and functional mobility such as transfers. With the information obtained from the subjective reporting, as well as findings on general screens, a physical therapist knows what areas to further examine/treat. More specific exams include, but are not limited to a neurological exam, joint mobility, an in-depth soft tissue exam, detailed gait analysis, cardiovascular fitness testing, vestibular testing, specific manual muscle testing, and functional capacity testing. Some of these are very extensive, such as vestibular and post-concussion testing or functional and work capacity testing and may require a second visit in order to fully complete the evaluation. Within these more detailed examinations, physical therapists have a wide range and depth of specialized standardized tests and measures in order to identify the originating and contributing causes of impairment, measure the disabilities, and provide baseline levels from which to establish goals and treatment plans. In addition to these goals and treatment plans, physical therapists make recommendations for equipment, make referrals to other professionals (i.e., physician specialist or orthotist), and provide information related to general health, safety, and condition related precautions or restrictions. In many situations, a physical therapist is one of the most qualified professionals to make recommendations related to return to work, school, or athletic activities.

According to the APTA (2012), the physical therapist's responsibility in the diagnostic process is to organize and interpret information collected through taking a relevant history, conducing a systems review, and selecting and administering specific tests and measures (APTA, 2012). In doing so, a physical therapist may order appropriate tests to be performed by themselves or other healthcare professionals (APTA, 2012). Physical therapist interventions include therapeutic exercises, manual therapy (including mobilization/manipulation); electrotherapeutic and ultrasound modalities; functional activity training; transfer and gait training; training in the use of assistive technology; home care, including ADL training; community integration; fabrication of devices and equipment; teaching safe patient handling techniques to families and health providers; and providing airway clearance. The goals of physical therapy include mobility restoration, pain reduction, home exercise program and self-care implementation, increasing physical fitness, increasing endurance, regaining or maintaining maximal or functional independence, and reducing or preventing potential illness or injury. In summary, physical therapy intervention focuses on improving, maximizing, or maintaining an individual's independence.

Pediatric Physical Therapy Service Delivery

Unlike an adult or geriatric physical therapy session, a pediatric physical therapy session often looks like play. Colorful exercise tools and equipment, like various sized therapy balls for positioning, stretching, and balance; small trampolines for hopping and jumping; foam rollers for positioning and stretching; and toys to promote reaching or head turning are typically employed. The goals of these tools are to develop a child's gross motor movement which positively impacts a child's functional mobility.

Functional Capacity Evaluations

A Functional Capacity Evaluation (FCE) is a comprehensive battery of performance-based tests that is used to measure a worker's safe physical capacities, as well as limitations in respect to work, activities of daily living, or leisure activities. The FCE is designed to measure tasks that an individual can do safely and reliably on a dependable basis with the goal of predicting one's ability to sustain tasks over a defined period of time. Physical therapists who are trained in FCEs provide objective and clinical data that can be integrated into services related to gardening, handyman services, and heavy housecleaning. For example, if a client exhibits trunk flexion range of motion and strength limitations, poor grip, and manual and finger dexterity, and the FCE demonstrates that the client is unable to lift/carry more than three pounds, the physical therapist can provide recommendations for assistance with activities of daily living and household services. Because the FCE is an evaluation, it provides the life care planner with an individual's physical abilities and limitations for both work-related tasks and ADLs and identifies task modifications. The FCE also provides the life care planner with what a person is able to do safely and repetitiously, which assists in determining the level of needed care and assistance.

Standard Treatment Recommendations

Physical therapists are healthcare professionals who maintain, restore, and improve movement, activity, and health enabling individuals of all ages to have optimal functioning and quality of life (APTA, 2011). Physical therapist interventions include therapeutic exercises, manual therapy (including mobilization/manipulation); electrotherapeutic and ultrasound modalities; functional activity training; transfer and gait training; training in the use of assistive technology; home care, including ADL training; community integration; fabrication of devices and equipment; teaching safe patient handling techniques to families and health providers; and providing airway clearance.

The goals of physical therapy include mobility restoration, pain reduction, home exercise program and self-care implementation, increasing physical fitness, increasing endurance, regaining or maintaining maximal or functional independence, and reducing or preventing potential illness or injury. In summary, physical therapy intervention focuses on improving, maximizing, or maintaining an individual's independence, activity level and health well-being, as well as preventing injuries.

Physical Therapists in Life Care Planning

An important role of the physical therapist in life care planning is the assessment of future needs. When there is a disability or impairment in some aspect or multiple aspects of mobility, the wear and tear on the body is altered from that of a typically aging individual. The systems which were possibly once injured in isolation from other body systems, with time can affect the health of other parts. Art Peddle (2010) describes an example of an individual who is unable to use her lower body and requires a wheelchair for mobility. Over time, she experiences wear and tear on her upper body and therefore may in the future require medical attention which might not have otherwise been required. This same individual may have had no integumentary problems initially, but because of the inability to move out of a chair, is at much greater risk of pressure related issues in the future. Because of the in-depth training and education in musculoskeletal, neurological, and biomechanical systems, a physical therapist is able to predict and advise on potential secondary system impairments which might require care in the future. The individual who has a life care plan will likely be one who will have physical therapy treatment as part of that plan. Generally, physical therapy treatment is episodic. These episodes begin with an evaluation for one or more specific problems. Treatment goals, a plan, and an estimated time frame are established. The patient is discharged from physical therapy at the conclusion of this sequence of treatment visits.

Length of visits, frequency, and total duration of the episode of care varies greatly based on the impairments, treatment goals, and prognosis. An individual with a chronic condition will likely require at least one episode of care per year, and often several. There are instances when it is determined that ongoing maintenance care provided by a skilled physical therapist is the only option available to provide the treatment needed to prevent a decline in function. These ongoing treatment plans are not typical, but at times necessary to prevent more costly future treatment. According to Paul Ramos (2021, p. 6), "maintenance therapy differs from traditional, restorative, therapy in that improvement is not expected and return to one's prior level of function is not anticipated." He states that maintenance therapy is:

> …intended to stabilize or slow the natural course of deterioration with a progressive condition or to prevent potential sequelae that may occur. These services are typically delivered at a decreased frequency but with a much longer duration (e.g. one time a week for 50 weeks/year).
>
> (Ramos, 2021, p. 6)

Other life care planning considerations on which a physical therapist is capable of advising may include predicted replacement of mobility equipment, a change of equipment due to predicted mobility changes of the client/evaluee over time, home adaptations for increased safety and independence, amount and frequency of caregiver assistance required, and transportation needs and adaptations.

According to Deutsch (n.d.), the tenants of life care planning include the consideration of many elements. Listed below are considered areas with additional comments by the author related to the role of physical therapy in life care planning (Bubanja & Conover, 2019):

- Projected Evaluations: Physical therapists are able to project the frequency of physical therapy evaluations for the evaluee, as well as aid the life care planner in suggestions of the likelihood of various other medical evaluations which might be required. The life care planner would need input from disciplines outside of physical therapy.
- Projected Therapeutic Modalities: Physical therapists are able to project the frequency of physical therapy treatments for the evaluee, as well as help the life care planner in suggestions of the likelihood of various other medical evaluations which might be required. The life care planner would need input from disciplines outside of physical therapy.
- Diagnostic Testing and Educational Assessments: Physical therapists are able to advise on, but not order, diagnostic testing. Those physical therapists working in the U.S. military system are legally able to order limited diagnostic tests.
- Wheelchair, Accessories, and Maintenance: Physical therapists have the skill, education, and legal ability to advise, fit, and prescribe wheelchairs. Due to physical therapist specialization, some physical therapists might defer to other professionals for this area.
- Orthopedic Equipment: In most cases, physical therapists have the skill, education, and training to advise and collaborate with others in this area.
- Orthotic or Prosthetic Requirements: Due to the immense advances in prosthetic technology, a physical therapist typically will work with a prosthetist to make decisions about prosthetic limbs. The physical therapist is the functional mobility expert as well as the one projecting the future needs and capabilities for the client/evaluee. The prosthetist is able to provide expertise on how best to meet those needs with the prosthetic device. Training of the client/evaluee is also usually a collaborative effort. Orthotics are similar, however, at times can be handled solely by the physical therapist.

- Home Furnishings and Accessories and Aids for Independent Function: Physical therapists can provide a wide variety of recommendations in this category.
- Medication: Physical therapists have the education to make recommendations for consults with physicians, physicians' assistants, or nurse practitioners on impairments which might be improved by certain classes of medication. For example, a physical therapist might recommend that the evaluee discuss with the physician the possibility of a muscle relaxer to improve mobility.
- Supply Needs: Physical therapists are able to recommend supplies related to physical therapy treatments and those conditions requiring care from a physical therapist.
- Home Care or Facility-Based Care Needs: Because they are highly skilled in determining the independence and safety of the evaluee in terms of physical mobility, physical therapists have valuable recommendations and considerations for this area. Collaboration with physiatry, occupational therapy, and possibly neuropsychology is beneficial.
- Projected Routine Future Medical Care: Physical therapists would, in some cases, have input in this area; however, the therapist would likely defer to physicians.
- Projected Surgical Treatment or Other Aggressive Medical Care: Physical therapists would, in most cases defer to physicians and surgeons.
- Transportation Needs: Some physical therapists have advanced knowledge in this area. Occupational therapists typically are in these care roles.
- Architectural Renovations: Physical therapists are able to provide a wide variety of recommendations in this category. Collaborating with a carpenter skilled in making home modifications, allows for the evaluee's needs to be matched with the ability of the home to be modified in such ways as to provide the necessary safety and independence.
- Leisure or Recreational Equipment: Many physical therapists are highly skilled in this area. Occupational and recreational therapists are as well. While also following the methodology of consultation with the client's team and lead physician, physical therapists who are practicing as life care planners may consider projected therapeutic evaluations and modalities, wheelchair needs, orthopedic equipment needs, home furnishings and accessories, aids for independent functions, recreational equipment, durable medical supplies, transportation needs, architectural renovations, and home care versus facility-based care among the items and services that they can recommend when preparing a life care plan.

Questions Life Care Planners Should Ask a Physical Therapist When Developing a Life Care Plan

Whether the life care planner is preparing a life care plan for a child, adult, or elder individual, the components of an individual's life care plan across all ages include the same domains, such as medical, environmental, psychological, cognitive, and cultural. The goal of a life care plan is to describe an individual's deficits and offer medical and ancillary services and procedures to ensure the highest quality and dignity of life and make the individual as whole as possible.

Physical therapy evaluations and treatment relative to pediatric, youth, adult, and geriatric age groups all across the lifespan, address flexibility, mobility, strength, posture, gait, balance, and motor sensory function, endurance in the context of ADLs, work and recreational abilities and limitations specific to an individual's injury, diagnosis, and congenital conditions. The physical therapy evaluation, treatment, and discharge note can provide the life care planner with data points that translate functional abilities and limitations into life care recommendations. Physical therapists use ADL inventories to measure pre- and post-incident ADL function. It is essential for the life care planner to identify the pre and post injury ADL function in order to determine the loss of physical or cognitive abilities and services due to the incident.

Activities of Daily Living (ADL) and Instrumental Activities of Daily Living (IADL)

When preparing a life care plan, the life care planner should gather the following ADL and IADL categories of information from the physical therapist. The activities of daily living are classified into basic ADLs and IADLs). The physical ADLs are those skills required to manage one's basic physical needs, including personal hygiene or grooming, dressing, toileting, transferring, ambulating, and eating. The physical ADLs are those skills required to manage one's basic physical needs, including personal hygiene or grooming, dressing, toileting, transferring, ambulating, and eating.

Activities of Daily Living (ADL)

- Personal Hygiene or Grooming: Personal hygiene and grooming activities range from washing and drying oneself; transferring in and out of a tub or shower; as well as care for a catheter or colostomy bag.
- Dressing: Dressing includes donning and doffing clothes, socks, shoes, braces, and prostheses.
- Toileting: Toileting refers to reaching to wipe oneself and getting on and off the toilet or commode or shower chair with or without grab bars or assistive devices.
- Transferring: Transferring refers to getting in and out of a bed, chair, car, and wheelchair. For example, taking into consideration safety and reliance on assistive devices like a cane, walker, crutches, braces and level of assistance needed.
- Ambulation: Ambulation refers to gait on flat surfaces, uneven or inclined terrain, and stairs, while taking into consideration safety and reliance on assistive devices like a cane, walker, crutches, braces, and level of assistance needed.
- Eating: Eating refers to using utensils, or reliance on feeding tube or intravenous feeding.

The IADLs include more complex activities related to the ability to live independently in the community, such as managing finances and medications, food preparation, housekeeping, shopping, laundry, transportation, and caring for pets.

Instrumental Activities of Daily Living (IADLs)

- Managing Medications: Taking medications safely and remembering to take them at the correct time of day or do they need reminders or assistance with medications.
- Preparing Food: Preparing food refers to whether the person is able to plan and cook full meals; are they able to use a microwave, heat up food or prepare only light meals by themselves; or are they unable to prepare any food at all.
- Housekeeping: Housework and chores identify whether the individual can do heavy housework like moving furniture; vacuuming; cleaning the floors, tubs, and showers; and, taking out the trash; can they only do light housework, but may need help with heavy housecleaning; or are they not capable of doing any housework and chores.

- Managing Personal Finances: Managing finances refers to paying bills, taxes, and balancing one's own checkbook.
- Shopping for Groceries or Clothes: Shopping needs to address whether a person can select and buy food and clothing by themselves or are they not capable of shopping.
- Accessing Transportation: Transportation refers to whether a person is able to drive neighborhood distances; on freeways; in the evenings and/or travel independently on buses or taxis or with a companion; or are they not able to travel at all.
- Caring for pets.

The physical therapist will also evaluate the level of assistance needed to complete ADLs and IADLs, another critical component of preparing a life care plan. The definition of levels of assistance required for ADL's and IADL's are as follows:

Maximal Assist: Maximal assist is when the assisting person(s) or device(s) are required to perform approximately 75 percent of the work of a mobility task while you perform 25 percent of the work (O'Sullivan, 2019).

Moderate Assist: Moderate assist is when the assisting person(s) or device(s) are required to perform approximately 50 percent of the work of a mobility task while you perform 50 percent of the work.

Minimal Assist: Minimal assist is when the assisting person(s) or device(s) are required to perform approximately 25 percent of the work of a mobility task while you perform 75 percent of the work.

Contact Guard Assist: With contact guard assist, the assisting person has one or two hands on your body but provides no other assistance to perform the functional mobility task. The contact is made to help steady your body or help with balance.

Standby Assist or Supervision: During standby assist, the assisting person does not touch you or provide any assistance but needs to be close by for safety in case you lose your balance or need help to maintain safety during the task being performed.

Supervision: Patient requires no more help than standby, cueing, or coaxing, without physical contact, or someone is needed to set up needed items or apply orthoses; requires supervision and/or verbal cues to complete activity (may not always be done safely or correctly).

Independent: Independent status means that you can perform the functional task with no help and that you are safe during the task.

An example of an ADLs' inventory for a 75 year-old widower, with a cervical discectomy and lumbar fusion is illustrated below. Prior and current levels of ADLs' function are necessary in measuring the quantitative and qualitative change when determining the level, frequency, and duration of home care and housework assistance.

	Prior Level of Function	Current Level of Function
Dressing:		
Upper Extremity	Independent	Minimal Assist
Lower Extremity	Independent	Maximal Assist

Notes: Client/evaluee needs to sit when dressing and undressing due to pain and balance issues. He needs assistance with donning/doffing socks and shoes due to lumbar range of motion limitations and right hip external rotation. He uses a reacher to pull up his pants.

Transfers		
Bed	Independent	Minimal Assist
Chair Independent	Independent	Minimal Assist
Car	Independent	Moderate Assist
On and off Floor	Independent	Maximal Assist
Toilet	Independent	Minimal Assist
Tub	Independent	Moderate Assist

Notes: When transferring from sit to stand, he was observed to move slowly, tilt his pelvis posteriorly (compromised mechanics), and stand for a few seconds to regain his neutral stance before initiating his gait. He needed to hold onto the armrests of a chair when lowering himself to sit down.

Gait

Pre-incident, the client/evaluee was an independent community ambulator. Post-incident, the client/evaluee ambulates with a rollator walker with a poor heel strike phase of gait due to left knee extensor lag (unable to straighten his knee to full range), decreased push off, and decreased stride length x 200 feet before needing to take a seated break due to lumbar pain, burning in his thighs, as well as fatigue. He needs assistance to navigate a flight of stairs in his home. He uses a singe point cane for short household ambulation and walker for community ambulation.

Balance

The Tinetti (Berg et al., 1992; Tinetti et al., 1986) assessment tool is an easily administered task-oriented test that measures an individual's gait and balance abilities.

Scoring

A three-point ordinal scale, ranging from 0–2. A "0" indicates the highest level of impairment and a "2" indicates the individual's independence.

Total Balance Score =16
Total Gait Score =12
Total Test Score =28

Interpretation: 25–28 = Low Fall Risk
19–24 = Medium Fall Risk
< 19 = High Fall Risk

The client/evaluee scored in the Medium Fall Risk category, with a score of 20/28.

Spine Range of Motion (ROM)

The client's active range of motion was objectively evaluated with Tracker ROM from JTECH Medical Industries (2022) using inclinometry protocols outlined in the AMA Guides to the Evaluation of Permanent Impairment.

The question that the life care planner should ask the physical therapist is, "Is the client's active range of motion functional?"

Table 15.1 Lumbar ROM

Lumbar ROM	Norm	Result	Difference	% Norm
Lumbar Flexion	60°	25°	35°	42%
Lumbar Extension	25°	17°	8°	68%
Lumbar Lateral Left	25°	15°	10°	60%
Lumbar Lateral Right	25°	18°	7°	72%

Table 15.2 Lower Extremity Muscle Tests

	Result		CV		
Lower Extremity Muscle Tests	Left	Right	Left	Right	Difference
Hip Flexion	2.1 lbs.	1.2 lbs.	4%	8%	−42% R
Knee Extension	1.5 lbs.	< 1 lb.	10%		−
Ankle Plantar Flexion (Knee Neutral)	12.4 lbs.	6.3 lbs.	2%	5%	−49% R

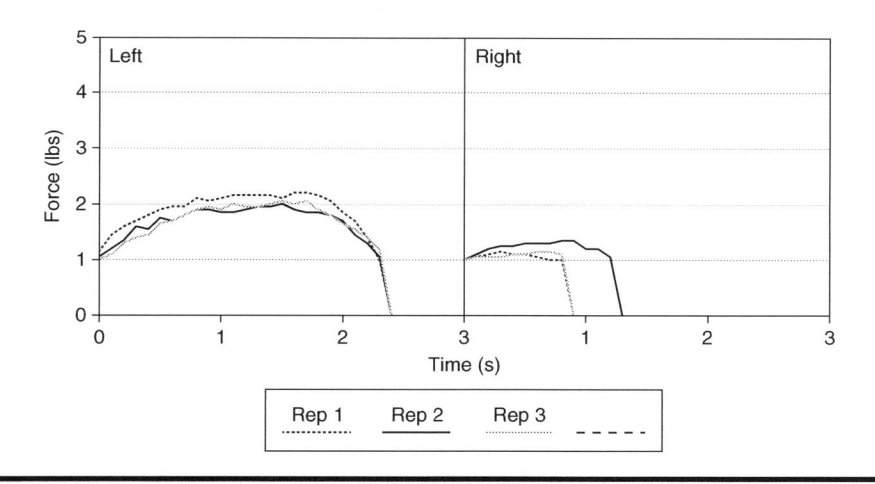

Figure 15.1 Hip Flexion

Muscle Strength Testing:

The client/evaluee was tested using the JTECH Tracker system, a computerized muscle strength evaluation system. When compared to the opposite side, a strength difference greater than 15% is generally recognized as an indication of motor deficit.

The question that the life care planner should ask the physical therapist is, "Is the individual's strength functional?"

Based on the range of motion and strength measurements, the question then arises, "Will the individual need therapeutic exercises and therapeutic activities now or in the future to maintain and/or improve his range of motion and strength and/or upgrade his home exercise program?"

Based on the physical therapy findings, the following items will be included in the life care plan.

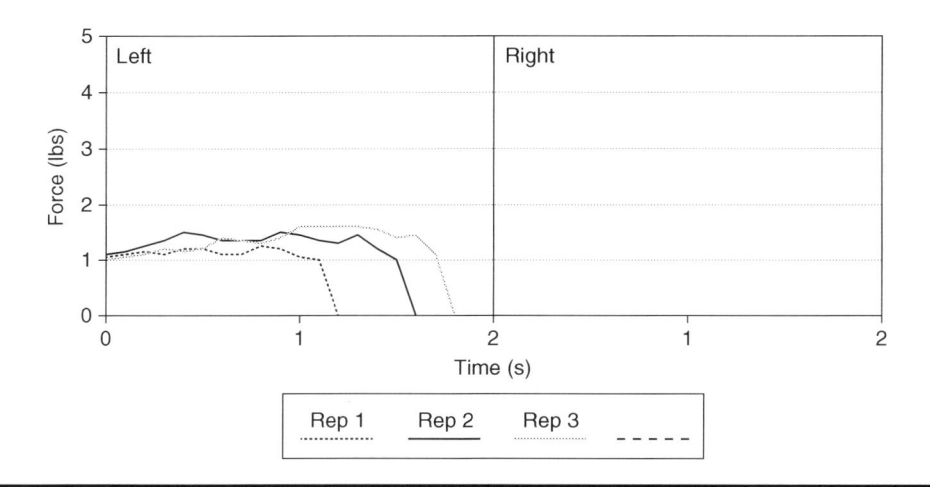

Figure 15.2 Knee Extension: Right Knee Extension (ibid.)

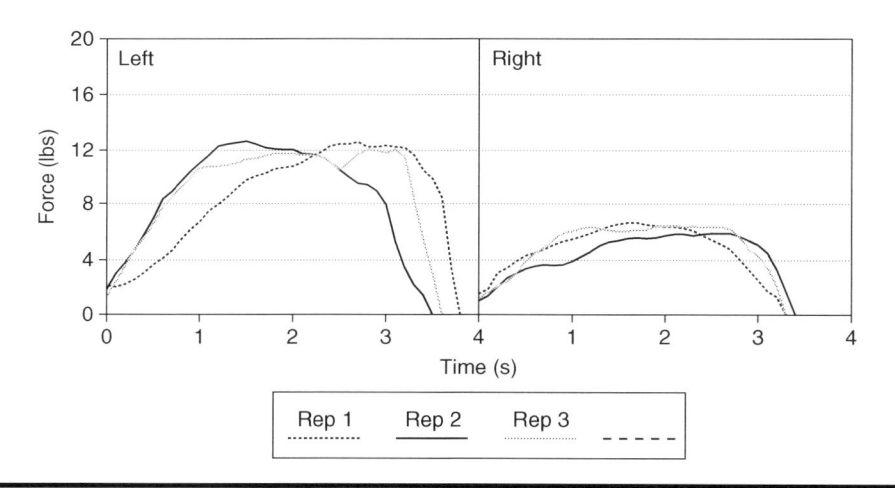

Figure 15.3 Ankle Plantar Flexion (Knee Neutral)

As a result of the measures obtained in Tables 15.1 and 15.2 and Figures 15.1, 15.2, and 15.3, as well as other information obtained from the evaluee, a life care plan for physical therapy needs is found in Table 15.3.

Table 15.3 PT Article Tables Adult

EVALUATIONS*

Item or Service	Duration	Frequency	Purpose	Estimated Cost/ Cost Obtained From	Recommended By
Physical Therapy	Lifetime	1x/yr.	Assess strength, function, range of motion and endurance; treat pain flare-ups.	$258/eval. $258/yr. PFR 2022	Diana Bubanja, DPT, CLCP, CFCE

*These evaluations will probably result in additional future care recommendations.

(*Continued*)

Table 15.3 (Continued)   PT Article Tables Adult

THERAPEUTIC MODALITIES

Item or Service	Duration	Frequency	Purpose	Estimated Cost/ Cost Obtained From	Recommended By
Physical Therapy	Lifetime	8-12x/yr.	Improve and maintain strength, function, range of motion and endurance; treat pain flare-ups.	$347/visit $2,776-4,164/yr. ($3,470/avg.)	Diana Bubanja, DPT, CLCP, CFCE
Acupuncture Trial	Lifetime	8 sessions; then to be determined	Treat/relieve pain.	$198/initial visit; then $90/visit $828/total	Diana Bubanja, DPT, CLCP, CFCE

DURABLE MEDICAL EQUIPMENT

Item or Service	Duration	Frequency	Purpose	Estimated Cost/ Cost Obtained From	Recommended By
Single-Point Cane	Lifetime	1x/7-10 yrs.	Provide ambulation assistance.	$19-21/ea. $2-3/yr. ($3/avg.) walgreens.com: $20 riteaid.com: $21 walmart.com: $19	Diana Bubanja, DPT, CLCP, CFCE
Front-Wheeled Walker with Seat	Lifetime	1x/5 yrs.	Provide ambulation assistance.	$75-90/ea. $15-18/yr. ($17/avg.) walmart.com: $75 simplymedical.com: $90 riteaid.com: $90	Diana Bubanja, DPT, CLCP, CFCE
Reacher	Lifetime	1x/yr.	Aid reaching.	$10-11/ea. $10-11/yr. ($11/avg.) healthproductsforyou.com: $11 carewell.com: $11 jamilink.com: $10	Diana Bubanja, DPT, CLCP, CFCE
Adjustable Bed Base (King)	Lifetime	1x/10 yrs.	Improve sleeping comfort.	$2,300-3,600/ea. $230-360/yr. ($295/avg.) mattressfirm.com: $2,300 sleepgalleria.com: $3,600 rcwilley.com: $2,300	Diana Bubanja, DPT, CLCP, CFCE
Adjustable Bed Mattress (King)	Lifetime	1x/8 yrs.	Improve sleeping comfort.	$4,000-5,100/ea. $500-638/yr. ($569/avg.) mattressfirm.com: $5,100 sleepgalleria.com: $4,000 rcwilley.com: $4,000	Diana Bubanja, DPT, CLCP, CFCE

DURABLE MEDICAL EQUIPMENT

Item or Service	Duration	Frequency	Purpose	Estimated Cost/ Cost Obtained From	Recommended By
Handheld Shower	In next yr.	1 x only	Provide personal hygiene safety and assistance.	$33-50/ea. $33-50/total ($42/avg.) Bedbathandbeyond.com: $50 Spinlife.com: $33 Homedepot.com: $50	Diana Bubanja, DPT, CLCP, CFCE
Shower Chair	In next yr.	1 x only	Provide personal hygiene safety and assistance.	$38-57/ea. $38-57/total ($48/avg.) Allegromedical.com: $38 Spinlife.com: $47 4mdmedical.com: $57	Diana Bubanja, DPT, CLCP, CFCE
Grab Bars (2)	In next yr.	1 x only	Provide personal hygiene safety.	$21-31/ea. $42-62/pair $42-62/total ($52/avg.) Harneyhardware.com: $21 Healthproductsforyou.com: $31 Grabbarspecialists.com: $27	Diana Bubanja, DPT, CLCP, CFCE

(Continued)

Table 15.3 (Continued)   PT Article Tables Adult

CARE PROVIDERS

Item or Service	Duration	Frequency	Purpose	Estimated Cost/ Cost Obtained From	Recommended By
Attendant/ Chore Services	Lifetime	8-12 hrs./wk. (52 wks./yr.)	Provide assistance and supervision with Activities of Daily Living (ADLs) including cooking/meal preparation, grocery shopping, light housecleaning, laundry, transportation, running errands, etc.	$34.50-39/hr. $276-468/wk. $14,352-24,338/yr. ($19,344/avg.) 24 Hour Home Care: $36 Alegre Home Care: $34.50 All Seasons Homecare: $35-39 Genworth Cost of Care Survey $38.37	Diana Bubanja, DPT, CLCP, CFCE

HOME MODIFICATIONS*

Item or Service	Duration	Frequency	Purpose	Estimated Cost/ Cost Obtained From	Recommended By
Bathroom Modifications	Lifetime	1 x only	Improve safety and mobility within bathroom.	$20,387/total	Diana Bubanja, DPT, CLCP, CFCE

*Absent a contractor estimate regarding the cost for such bathroom modifications, we are utilizing the Department of Veteran's Affairs (VA) Loan Guaranty Service as a standard. Modifications include a walk-in shower with seat, handheld shower, grab bars, etc. The maximum dollar amount allowable for the Special Housing Adaptation (SHA) grant in fiscal year 2022 is $20,387 (https://www.benefits.va.gov/homeloans/adaptedhousing.asp). The SHA benefit amounts is set by law, but may be adjusted upward annually based on a cost-of-construction index. The cost for the client's future home modifications will likely be higher than this estimate, but more information is needed in order to refine the recommendation.   He will require similar renovations if he changes residences in the future.

Cost research is proprietary and confidential and not for public dissemination   6

Expected costs in this case study are for illustration purposes only. Actual costs will be determined by individualized therapy needs and the geographic location of where the client/evaluee resides or receives care.

Physical Therapy Considerations for Pediatric Life Care Plans

The life care plan for children is dependent upon several factors: age, diagnosis, and the impact of development through an individual's life from birth through childhood. Certain developmental stages in the pediatric population are characterized by physical, cognitive, and psychological changes, such that physical therapy should be considered to maximize a child's independence and positive passage through the various developmental stages. An interview with the child and family is critical. A child's growth, motor development, interactions with family and staff/students in school, and ability to perform age-related ADLs are key components when preparing a pediatric life care plan.

Pediatric and young adult clients will generally require more medical and therapy services than adult clients in lieu of developmental milestones including physical and cognitive changes, as well as accelerated age-related changes and overuse symptoms. Pediatric developmental milestones also play a role in life care planning and provide a baseline for age-appropriate ADL function. For example, a child is able to lace their shoes at age 4 years and able to dress independently at age 5 years (Center for Disease Control, 2022). These pediatric age markers assist the life care planner in determining whether the ADL assistance is needed because of developmental delay, orthopedic, or neurologic condition.

Pediatric clients will also need more frequent monitoring screening related to orthopedic conditions due to growth plate changes and spurts. The frequency of replacing orthotics, braces, splints, and prosthetics in youth with disabilities is projected to be as low as every six months to two years in children who are growing and use the appliances on a daily basis. Due to a child's growth spurts, replacement of assistive gait devices for children should be estimated at every three years, compared to adults being every five years (Marini & Harper, 2006).

Consideration of durable medical equipment (DME) replacement, such as a walker or wheelchair for children, should consider that children will more likely use DME more often each day as compared to middle aged adults and elderly adults who are active. Children may replace wheelchairs on a yearly basis due to changes in size of wheelchairs resulting from growth and weight changes.

Children may be more active than adults and may volitionally or without care be rough on DME equipment or let other kids play with equipment, which affects the replacement scheduling of DMEs.

Regarding range of motion testing, the same question is raised with pediatrics as it is with adult and geriatric cases, that is, does the child's range of motion interfere with his/her ADLs? For example, if a child or adult has limited shoulder internal rotation, he/she would have difficulty performing hygiene (wiping their bottom) and would need assistance.

The life care planner must consider the layout of the home for accessibility and safety for the child, adult, or geriatric client/evaluee.

If using an ankle foot orthosis (AFO) to prevent drop foot, the physical therapist, in the author's experience, will need to provide needs training and instructions to the family and child at 3 x a week for 3 weeks; then two sessions per week for three months; followed by one session per week for another three months. The AFO for a child would need to be replaced every two years with 1–2 sessions for evaluation and fitting. On the other hand, an adult or geriatric client/evaluee will need an AFO every two years.

Pediatric Case Study

A ten-year-old female, who lives with her parents and was involved in an MVA.
   Medical Diagnosis: Traumatic brain injury (TBI)—closed.
   Therapy Diagnosis: Spastic quadriplegic

1. Client/evaluee is unable to independently perform any ADLs
2. Client/evaluee requires maximum care.
3. Physical therapy to decrease hypertonicity and increase range of motion; develop head and trunk control to assist with independent sitting; and promote development of assisted transfers.

Range of Motion: No active range of motion was noted. It took great effort to passively bring her head to midline. Both upper extremities were held in flexion at the elbows and wrists while the shoulders were in extension and fingers in strong flexion. Neck and trunk muscle tone is hypotonic, with her head falling forward. All four extremities are hypertonic.

Positioning:
Lying: She can be placed on side lying, but she is unable to roll. The prone position was not tolerated well.

Sitting: She cannot get to sitting independently. Once placed in sitting, she is unable to maintain without maximum support. Quadruped, standing, balance/equilibrium are not possible at this time.

Sensory: It is not possible to determine what sensory information she is receiving and processing at this time. She does not respond to light touch, deep pressure, or auditory stimulation.

Oral Motor: She is being fed through a G-tube.

Cognition and Awareness: She is vegetative state.

ADLs She is dependent for all care, has a gastrostomy tube for feeding.

Impairments:

1. Hypotonia, neck and trunk
2. Hypertonia, all four extremities
3. Decreased range of motion, all extremities, with contractures
4. Reflex—Asymmetric Tonic Neck Reflex
5. Visual impairment
6. Oral motor dysfunction

Based on the physical therapy findings, the following items will be included in the life care plan as found in Table 15.4.

Table 15.4   PT Tables Pediatric

THERAPEUTIC MODALITIES

Item or Service	Duration	Frequency	Purpose	Estimated Cost/ Cost Obtained From	Recommended By
Physical Therapy	Lifetime	1-2x/wk. for 1 yr.; then 10 courses @ 2x/wk. for 8 wks. over lifetime (52 wks./yr.)	Provide gentle stretching and range of motion exercises in lower extremities; train caregivers in appropriate exercises and monitor PT status.	$165-273/visit $8,580-28,392/1 yr. ($18,486/avg.); then $2,640-4,368/course $26,400-43,680/10 courses total ($35,040/avg.) PFR '18	Diana Bubanja DPT, CLCP, CFCE
Occupational Therapy	Lifetime	1-2x/wk. for 1 yr.; then 10 courses @ 2x/wk. for 8 wks. over lifetime (52 wks./yr.)	Provide gentle stretching and range of motion exercises in Upper extremities; train caregivers in appropriate care and monitor skin, contractures and bracing and/or splinting as appropriate.	$168-269/visit $8,736-27,976/1 yr. ($18,356/avg.); then $2,688-4,304/course $26,880-43,040/10 courses total ($34,960/avg.) PFR '18	Diana Bubanja DPT, DPT, CLCP, CFCE
Speech Therapy	Lifetime	1-2x/wk. for 1 yr.; then 10 courses @ 2x/wk. for 8 wks. over lifetime (52 wks./yr.)	Improve and maintain oral motor control, speech, voice and communication ability; monitor and train caregivers in appropriate care. Monitor and update speech therapy needs, adaptive communication equipment/supply needs, and cognitive functioning.	$126-288/visit $6,552-29,952/1 yr.; then $18,252/avg.); then $2,016-4,608/course $20,610-46,080/10 courses total ($33,345/avg.) PFR '18	Diana Bubanja DPT, DPT, CLCP, CFCE

(Continued)

Table 15.4 (Continued) PT Tables Pediatric

DURABLE MEDICAL EQUIPMENT*

Item or Service	Duration	Frequency	Purpose	Estimated Cost/ Cost Obtained From	Recommended By
Pediatric Rifton Wave Bath and Shower Chair	To age 18	1x/5 yrs.	Provide personal hygiene safety and assistance.	$1,710/ea. $342/yr. Rifton.com	Diana Bubanja DPT, CPCP, CFCE
Pediatric Rifton Wave Bath and Shower Chair Maintenance	To age 18	1x/yr.	Maintain Rifton bath and shower chair.	$171/yr. Rifton.com	Diana Bubanja DPT, CPCP, CFCE
Adult Reclining Shower Chair with Custom Seating**	Begin age 18	1x/3-4 yrs.	Provide personal hygiene safety and assistance.	$2,942-2,995/ea. $736-998/yr. ($867/avg.) southwestmedical.com: $2,995 vitalitymedical.com: $2,942 medicaleshop.com: $2,995	Diana Bubanja DPT, CPCP, CFCE

**Actual shower wheelchair costs will likely be higher as the estimates above are base costs and do not include various options and upgrades. In addition, costs will likely change as she transitions from a pediatric to adult shower wheelchair in the future; however, more information is needed in order to refine this recommendation.

Item or Service	Duration	Frequency	Purpose	Estimated Cost/ Cost Obtained From	Recommended By
Reclining Shower Maintenance	Begin age 18	1x/yr.	Maintain shower chair.	$294-300/yr. ($297/avg.) southwestmedical.com: $300 vitalitymedical.com: $294 medicaleshop.com: $300	Diana Bubanja DPT, CPCP, CFCE
Handheld Shower	Lifetime	1x/5-7 yrs.	Provide personal hygiene safety and assistance.	$29-70/ea. $4-14/yr. ($9/avg.) spinlife.com: $29-33 performancehealth.com: $35-45 homedepot.com: $30-70	Diana Bubanja DPT, CPCP, CFCE

DURABLE MEDICAL EQUIPMENT

Item or Service	Duration	Frequency	Purpose	Estimated Cost/ Cost Obtained From	Recommended By
Fully Electric Hospital Bed with Rails	Lifetime	1x/15 yrs.	Provide sleeping comfort, positioning and transfer assistance.	$6,400-13,275/ea. $427-885/yr. ($656/avg.) spinlife.com: $6,400-13,275 vitalitymedial.com: $6,400-13,275	Diana Bubanja DPT, CPCP, CFCE
Hospital Bed Maintenance	Lifetime	1x/yr.	Maintain hospital bed.	$640-1,328/yr. ($984/avg.) spinlife.com: $640-1,328 vitalitymedial.com: $640-1,328	Diana Bubanja DPT, CPCP, CFCE
Hospital Bed Mattress Replacement	Begin in 4 yrs. for life	1x/4 yrs.	Provide sleeping comfort, positioning and transfer assistance.	$650-971/ea. $163-243/yr. ($203/avg.) rehabmart.com: $971 spinlife.com: $650	Diana Bubanja DPT, CPCP, CFCE
Power Hoyer Lift	Begin age 18	1x/5 yrs.	Provide transfer safety and assistance.	$1,799-3,534/ea. $360-707/yr. ($534/avg.) spinlife.com: $1,799-3,534 rehabmart.com: $2,213 vitalitymedical.com: $2,233	Diana Bubanja DPT, CPCP, CFCE
Power Hoyer Lift Slings (2)	Begin age 18	2 slings/3 yrs.	Transfer safety.	$75-408/ea. $150-816/2 slings $50-272/yr. ($161/avg.) spinlife.com: $75-214 rehabmart.com: $408 performancehealth.com: $234	Diana Bubanja DPT, CPCP, CFCE

HOME MODIFICATIONS*

Item or Service	Duration	Frequency	Purpose	Estimated Cost/ Cost Obtained From	Recommended By
Home Modifications**	Lifetime	1-2x/total	Provide wheelchair accessible housing to properly provide care.	$85,845/home $85,645-171,290/total ($128,468/avg.)	Diana Bubanja DPT, CLCP, CFCE

**The client currently lives with her family in a non-wheelchair accessible home but requires various home modifications for safety and mobility within the home. The physical therapist has recommended various home modifications including wheelchair accessible ramping for two entry/exit points, overhead transfer/transport track system, and an environmental control unit (ECU) on iPad, etc. Other home modifications include a roll-in shower, widened doorways, storage for supplies, covered parking for van, etc.

(Continued)

Table 15.4 (Continued)   PT Tables Pediatric

HOME CARE OPTION I (AT HOME)

Item or Service	Duration	Frequency	Purpose	Estimated Cost/ Cost Obtained From	Recommended By
Licensed Vocational Nurse (LVN)	Lifetime	24 hrs./day	Monitor medical status (vitals, skin, respiratory status, suctioning, etc.); gastric tube feedings; setup and administer medications.	$50/hr. $1,200/day $438,000/yr. Maxim Healthcare Services: $50 BrightStar Care: $50	Diana Bubanja DPT, CLCP, CFCE
Registered Nurse	Lifetime	1x/mo.	Monitor medical status; supervise LVN.	$165/mo. $1,980/yr. BrightStar Care	Diana Bubanja DPT, CLCP, CFCE

FACILITY CARE - OPTION II*

Item or Service	Duration	Frequency	Purpose	Estimated Cost/ Cost Obtained From	Recommended By
Subacute Brain Injury Rehabilitation Facility (e.g. Care Meridian)**	Lifetime	24 hrs./day	Provided skilled nursing and rehabilitative services.	$1,100/day $401,500/yr. Care Meridian: $1,100	Diana Bubanja DPT, CLCP, CFCE

**A subacute brain injury rehabilitation facility will not be required during periods of acute rehabilitation hospitalization (20 weeks total).

**The subacute brain injury rehabilitation facility daily rate includes room and board, 24-hour nursing assistance, rehabilitative services, nutritionist, housekeeping, case management, daily supplies (i.e. diapers and enteral supplies), as well as equipment such as a hospital bed, transfer manual wheelchair, shower chair, Hoyer lift, suction machine (and related supplies). Specialty equipment and supplies, medications, physician visits, and diagnostic and laboratory studies are not included in the daily rate.

*Option II assumes that the will transfer to a subacute brain injury rehabilitation facility for the remainder of her lifetime.

Cost research is proprietary and confidential and not for public dissemination

Conclusion

Many of the core components of a life care plan fall under the professional education, scope of practice, professional experience, and domain of the physical therapist. As rehabilitation specialists, physical therapists focus on maximizing functional abilities of individuals with disabilities of all ages with the goal of restoring patients or clients to their maximum level of function, the basis for life care planning. Those life care planners whose primary professional discipline is not physical therapy should consider consultation with a physical therapist in the areas of the life care plan that involve functional mobility and physical independence. The process of evaluation and treating a patient has strong parallels to the methodology used in life care planning. Physical therapists are well prepared to make valuable contributions to the life care planning profession for individuals from birth to childhood, adolescence to adulthood, and adult to aging adult.

References

American Physical Therapy Association. (2011). *Today's physical therapist: A comprehensive review of a 21st-century health care profession.* http://www.scottsevinsky.com/pt/todays_pt.pdf

American Physical Therapy Association. (2012). *Diagnosis by physical therapists.* https://www.apta.org/siteassets/pdfs/policies/diagnosis-by-physical-therapist.pdf

American Physical Therapy Association. (2022a). *APTA 100 years 1921–2021 100 milestones of physical therapy.* https://centennial.apta.org/home/timeline/

American Physical Therapy Association. (2022b). *Vision, mission, and strategic plan.* www.apta.org/vision2020/

Berg, K. O., Wood-Dauphinée, S. L., Williams, J. I., & Maki, B. (1992). Measuring balance in the elderly: Validation of an instrument. *Canadian Journal of Public Health*, *83*(suppl 2), S7–S11.

Bubanja, D., & Conover, S. M. (2019). What life care planners need to know about the professional discipline of physical therapy. *Journal of Life Care Planning*, *17*(1), 13–17

Center for Disease Control. (2022). *CDC's developmental milestones.* www.cdc.gov/ncbddd/actearly/milestones/index.html

Deutsch, P. M. (n.d.). *Tenants of life care planning.* www.paulmdeutsch.com/LCP-tenets-of-life-care-planning.htm

JTECH Medical Industries. (2022). *Functional status assessment tools.* www.jtechmedical.com

Marini, I., & Harper, D. Empirical validation of medical equipment replacement values in life care plans. *Journal of Life Care Planning*, *4*(4), 173–182.

O'Sullivan, S. B., Schmitz, T. J., & Fulk, G. (2019). *Physical rehabilitation*. FA Davis.

Peddle, A. (2010). The role of the physical therapist in life care planning. In Weed, R. O., & Berens, D. E. (Eds.) *Life care planning and case management handbook* (3rd ed., pp. 123–138). CRC Press.

Ramos, P. (2021). Reinventing therapy frequency: Recommendations for the medically complex patient. *Journal of Life Care Planning*, *19*(3), 5–16.

Tinetti, M. E. (1986). Performance-oriented assessment of mobility problems in elderly patients. *Journal of the American Geriatrics Society*, *34*(2), 119–26.

Chapter 16

The Role of the Speech-Language Pathologist and Audiologist in Life Care Planning

Carolyn Wiles Higdon

Speech-Language Pathology

The SLP is defined as the professional who engages in professional practice in the areas of communication and swallowing across the life span. Communication and swallowing are broad terms encompassing many facets of function. Communication includes speech production and fluency, language, cognition, voice, resonance, and hearing. Swallowing includes all aspects of swallowing, including related feeding behaviors. Throughout this document, the terms communication and swallowing are to reflect all areas.

The American Speech-Language-Hearing Association (ASHA) is the leading professional credentialing and scientific organization representing over 200,000 SLPs , speech-language and hearing scientists, audiology and speech-language support personnel, and students in the United States (ASHA, 2020). The ASHA has been a leader of these professions for almost 100 years, initiating the development of national standards for audiologist and speech-language pathologist certification since 1952. Canada's Speech-Language-Hearing organization is Speech-Language & Audiology Canada), formerly known as the Canadian Association of Speech-Language Pathologists and Audiologists). This is a national organization supporting and representing SLPs, audiologists, and communication health assistants. The association adopted its new name and logo in 2014. Other countries have similar associations.

Kinds of Patients and Problems Usually Seen and Addressed

This list of practice areas and the bulleted examples are not comprehensive. Current areas of practice, such as literacy, have continued to evolve, whereas other new areas of practice are emerging.

Fluency

- Stuttering
- Cluttering

Speech Production

- Motor planning and execution
- Articulation
- Phonological

Language

Spoken and written language (listening, processing, speaking, reading, writing, pragmatics)

- Phonology
- Morphology
- Syntax
- Semantics
- Pragmatics (language use and social aspects of communication)
- Prelinguistic communication (e.g., joint attention, intentionality, communicative signaling)
- Paralinguistic communication (e.g., gestures, signs, body language)
- Literacy (reading, writing, spelling)

Cognition

- Attention
- Memory
- Problem solving
- Executive functioning

Voice

- Phonation quality
- Pitch
- Loudness
- Alaryngeal voice

Resonance

- Hypernasality
- Hyponasality
- Cul-de-sac resonance
- Forward focus

Feeding and Swallowing

- Oral phase
- Pharyngeal phase
- Esophageal phase
- Atypical eating (e.g., food selectivity/refusal, negative physiologic response)

Auditory Habilitation/Rehabilitation

- Speech, language, communication, and listening skills impacted by hearing loss, deafness
- Auditory processing

Potential Etiologies of Communication and Swallowing Disorders Include

- Neonatal problems (e.g., prematurity, low birth weight, substance exposure)
- Developmental disabilities (e.g., specific language impairment, autism spectrum disorder, dyslexia, learning disabilities, attention-deficit disorder, intellectual disabilities, unspecified neurodevelopmental disorders)
- Disorders of aerodigestive tract function (e.g., irritable larynx, chronic cough, abnormal respiratory patterns or airway protection, paradoxical vocal fold motion, tracheostomy)
- Oral anomalies (e.g., cleft lip/palate, dental malocclusion, macroglossia, oral motor dysfunction)
- Respiratory patterns and compromise (e.g., bronchopulmonary dysplasia, chronic obstructive pulmonary disease)
- Pharyngeal anomalies (e.g., upper airway obstruction, velopharyngeal insufficiency/incompetence)
- Laryngeal anomalies (e.g., vocal fold pathology, tracheal stenosis)
- Neurological disease/dysfunction (e.g., traumatic brain injury, cerebral palsy, cerebrovascular accident, dementia, Parkinson's disease, and amyotrophic lateral sclerosis)
- Psychiatric disorder (e.g., psychosis, schizophrenia)
- Genetic disorders (e.g., Down syndrome, fragile X syndrome, Rett syndrome, velocardiofacial syndrome)
- Orofacial myofunctional disorders (e.g., habitual open-mouth posture/nasal breathing, orofacial habits, tethered oral tissues, chewing and chewing muscles, lips and tongue resting position).

This list of etiologies is not comprehensive but may also include transgender communication, verbal and nonverbal communication, preventive vocal hygiene, business communication, accent/dialect modification, and professional voice use.

Practice settings include private practices, physicians' offices, hospitals, schools, colleges and universities, rehabilitation centers, and long-term and residential healthcare facilities.

SLP Credentials and Licensure/Certification Requirements

The generally accepted national standard for practice in speech-language pathology (communication sciences and disorders) is the ASHA certificate of clinical competence in speech-language pathology (CCC-SLP). The ASHA CCC-SLP credential, at the entry level, requires a master's degree in speech-language pathology, completion of a one-year clinical fellowship, and successful passage of the national examination to practice in clinical and school settings. For states with licensure, the legal right to practice will vary with the individual licensing acts. Most licensure laws were modeled after the ASHA CCC standard (ASHA, 2022a). Licensure, unlike certification, is mandatory for those states that regulate the practice of audiology and speech-language pathology. In many states, licensure requirements parallel those of ASHA certification. Furthermore, ASHA certification will satisfy many of the requirements of state licensure when one applies for reciprocity. When services are supported by third party funding streams, third party intermediaries in most instances require the ASHA CCC and state licensure.

In addition, the SLP clinical doctorate, the Doctor of Philosophy (PhD), and the Doctor of Education (EdD) are distinct terminal degrees with the PhD and EdD as terminal research degrees, advanced from the entry-level master's degree in speech-language pathology. Typically, a doctoral level SLP with any of the terminal degrees (SLPD, PhD, EdD) will have the needed expertise to contribute and consult for a life care plan and thus, the best choice to include in the life care planning team.

Often, the state education agency requirements do not equate to the national standard, requiring only a bachelor's degree and education certification in some states to practice. There are 31 states that allow or require state licensure for school-based SLPs. There are 37 states that require a master's degree for school-based SLPs. There are 15 states that require ASHA certification for school-based SLPs (ASHA, 2020).

Scope of Practice/Code of Ethics

The ASHA *Scope of Practice* (ASHA, 2022a) in speech-language pathology comprises five domains of professional practice and eight domains of service delivery. Professional practice domains include advocacy and outreach, supervision, education, administration and leadership, and research. Service delivery domains include collaboration, counseling, prevention and wellness, screening, assessment, treatment, modalities/technology/and instrumentation, and population and systems. The domains of speech-language pathology service delivery complement the International Classification of Functioning, Disability, and Health, the World Health Organization's (2022) multipurpose health classification for the description of functioning and health.

The Audiology and Speech-Language Pathology Interstate Compact (Universal Licensure) (ASHA, 2022g) is an occupational licensure compact that allows professionals to practice in multiple states without having to obtain additional state licensures. The compact addresses increased demand to provide/receive audiology and speech-language pathology services and authorizes in-person and telepractice across state lines. States participating in the compact share information, including verification of licensure and disciplinary sanctions; however, compact states retain the ability to regulate practice in their state. The ASLP-IC will certify that audiologists and speech-language pathologists have met the standards of practice, promote communication about licensure and regulation, and offer a higher degree of consumer protection across state lines. Licensed SLPs and audiologists will be able to practice in-person or through telepractice, increasing access and continuity of care for clients, patients, and student care. This also facilitates services to underserved or geographically isolated populations as well as allowing military personnel and spouses to maintain their profession when relocating.

Table 16.1 ASHA Special Interest Groups (SIGs)

1 Language learning and education
2 Neurophysiology and neurogenic speech and language disorders
3 Voice and voice disorders
4 Fluency and fluency disorders
5 Speech science and orofacial disorders
6 Hearing and hearing disorders: research and diagnostics
7 Aural rehabilitation and its instrumentation
8 Hearing conservation and occupational audiology
9 Hearing and hearing disorders
10 Issues in higher education
11 Administration and supervision
12 Augmentative and alternative communication
13 Swallowing and swallowing disorders (dysphagia)
14 Communication disorders and sciences in culturally and linguistically diverse populations
15 Gerontology
16 School-based issues
17 Global issues in communication sciences and related disorders
18 Telepractice
19 Speech science

The speech-language pathology scope of practice covers 19 special interest areas (see Table 16.1).

Speech-language pathologists and audiologists must comply with the code of ethics for their discipline. The ASHA *Code of Ethics* (ASHA, 2022a) sets forth the fundamental principles and rules considered essential to the preservation of the highest standards of integrity and ethical conduct to which members of the profession of speech-language pathology and audiology are bound. All professional activity must be consistent with the code of ethics.

The SLP who is consulting on a life care plan should demonstrate an advanced knowledge and understanding of healthcare and educational facility practices; the common diseases and conditions affecting human communication, swallowing, and development across the life span; and medical, educational, surgical, and behavioral treatment as they relate to communication disorders. The SLP should be able to demonstrate advanced skills and abilities in diagnostics, treatment, and service delivery. The SLP should be able to review medical records and conduct succinct clinical case histories and interviews to gather relevant information related to communication and swallowing, and to select and administer appropriate diagnostic tools and procedures and treatment for communication and swallowing disorders that are functionally relevant, family-centered, culturally sensitive, and theoretically grounded. Readers may want to refer to Higdon (2019) in the *Journal of Life Care Planning*.

The ASHA (2022a, 2022c) formally recognizes independent Specialty Certification Boards who have met the criteria outlined by the Council for Clinical Certification in Audiology and Speech-Language Pathology (CFCC). Clinical specialty certification enables an audiologist or speech-language pathologist with advanced knowledge, skills, and experience beyond the Certificate of

Clinical Competence (CCC) to be formally identified as a Board Certified Specialist (BCS) in a specific area of clinical practice. Professionals must have their CCC-A or CCC-SLP credential to apply for specialty certification. The BCS designation also helps consumers easily identify professionals who have advanced knowledge and skills in a certain specialty. Specialty certification is currently available through the: American Audiology Board of Intraoperative Monitoring; American Board of Child Language and Language Disorders; American Board of Fluency and Fluency Disorders; and the American Board of Swallowing and Swallowing Disorders. Several new board specialty certifications are pending including the American Board of Augmentative and Alternative Communication, the American Board of Voice and Upper Airway Disorders, the American Board of Autism Spectrum Disorder, and the American Board of Clinical Instruction and Supervision.

SLP Assessment Process

There are four methods of gathering and interpreting quantitative and qualitative information about the client that should be used in the communication sciences and disorders' assessment process by the SLP. These four measures are a collection of the initial database, interview procedures, clinical assessment, and formal assessment procedures (Dunn & Dunn, 1991). Often more than one method is used to gather information about the same aspect of a client's skills and abilities, the context, the activity, or the use of technology or equipment. Information collected should include the reason and need for referral, medical diagnosis, and educational and vocational background information. This information is collected during the referral and intake phase, and its purpose is to provide preliminary data for planning the assessment. The interview takes place during the identification phase as a means of gathering information regarding the consumer and their needs. It is important that the consumer, family members, rehabilitation or education professionals, and other care providers be interviewed.

Formal assessment procedures are administered in a prescribed way and have set methods of scoring and interpretation. Therefore, they can be duplicated and analyzed. They may or may not be standardized. Clinical assessment techniques involve skilled observation of the consumer and are used throughout the assessment process. These techniques may be structured so that a series of steps is followed to determine specific skills, or they may be intentionally left unstructured to see what takes place. Observation can be done during a simulated task in a clinic setting or in a context familiar to the consumer such as a classroom or workplace. Differential diagnosis is an ongoing and essential component of the assessment process and one that requires an advanced level of understanding and perspective about the trauma or injury.

Pediatric and Adolescent Assessments

Evaluating children (pediatric and adolescent) presents complex and challenging issues, complicated by the catastrophic nature of the disease, disability, or trauma, and frequently challenged by the almost insurmountable task of planning a child's life. For these reasons, it is critical to make accurate and thorough projections and careful analysis of the disability, educate team members and caregivers about the pediatric disabilities, and develop a differential diagnostic therapeutic approach to service delivery to the child. The list of pediatric and adolescent considerations in the communication sciences and disorders assessment is lengthy, detailed, and can be complex. It is important to disclose that the list is not all-inclusive, because changes occur as research and science enhance the process. Readers should see Appendix 1 for a developmental speech and language checklist for birth to 24 months.

There are areas that warrant consideration when performing a communication evaluation for a pediatric or adolescent individual that are not considered, or at least not in the same detail, when evaluating an adult. Chronological age and pre-trauma development are used as the normal benchmarks against which to measure the disability issues. Routine medical needs must be addressed to the pediatric specialists who would provide the information that impacts a child's communication development. These include pediatric physiatry, otolaryngology, pediatric neurology, developmental medicine, audiology, dental/orthodontic, prosthodontist, and pediatric neuro-ophthalmology and ophthalmology. It should be noted here that there is a trend in the medical specialty fields to identify specialists who work solely with adolescents. Additional cognitive and educational information is gathered from the following sources:

- Educational consultants to private and public educational programs
- Personal caregivers and attendants
- Pediatric neuropsychological assessment
- Occupational and physical therapy
- Vision and hearing specialists
- Evaluators of driving
- Programs for the development of social and pragmatic skills
- Prevocational and vocational training programs

One area receiving an increased amount of attention at this time is autism. Autism (autistic disorders) is within the broader diagnostic category of autism spectrum disorder (ASD). Other diagnoses in the category include Asperger's syndrome, pervasive developmental disorder (PDD) (sometimes referred to as PDD-NOS), and childhood disintegrative disorder. These disorders occur in males approximately four times more often than in females. In earlier years, autism affected one in 500 children; however, with the explosive increase in the United States (and apparently in other countries), whether because of better diagnoses or actual increases in cases, it is now estimated that one in 150 children aged 10 years and younger are classified as having some form of ASD (Bishop, 1989; Gillberg, 1991; Owens, 2004, Prelock, 2020; Tonge, 2002). Speech-language pathologists are aggressively involved in treating children and adolescents with ASD.

At the completion of the assessment, the SLP must be able to provide a written report, documenting the test results, observations, and conclusions with clear recommendations. These recommendations must be detailed to include a projection of future care costs, frequency of service or treatment, duration, base cost, source of information, and recognized vendors or manufacturers, current prices, collaborative sources, and categories of information. It is recommended that the consulting SLP be knowledgeable about the local sources and costs of these recommendations, either through direct contact with suppliers or through catalog and desktop/computerized research. Recommendations from the SLP should be discussed with the client and family, treatment team members, and other life care team members if they directly impact the final recommendations and the cost analysis of the plan by the economist. Any coordination and agreement needed between team members including the economist should occur at this time. A draft of the communication sciences and disorders' assessment and recommendations report should be written and distributed to the life care planner for review relative to the accuracy and completeness of the information. The SLP must be able to explain, from a life care planning perspective, the reasons and rationales that are relative to their recommendations. These must be lifelong recommendations and objectives, developed in an integrated format. Once the document is correct and complete, a final draft should be compiled and distributed to the life care planner and the referral source. It should be determined, by these two parties, whether the written documentation should be sent to other internal life care planning team members, including the family and client, and to external individuals. Bauby (1998) described, following his stroke, how he communicated when he was dictating his memoirs. Rizzo (1999) discussed the speech and communication needs of Jenny Craig, the well-known cofounder of weight-loss centers. Both vignettes are described in the box locations in this chapter.

> In December 1995, Jean-Dominique Bauby, the 43-year-old editor of the French magazine *ELLE* (published in many languages), suffered from a severe stroke in his brain stem that left him permanently paralyzed from head to toe, although his mind was intact—a victim of locked-in syndrome. Where once he had been renowned for his gregariousness and wit, Bauby now found himself imprisoned in an inert body, able to communicate only by blinking his left eye. It is remarkable that in doing so he was able to compose an eloquent memoir, which was published two days before his death in 1996 and went on to become an international bestseller. Bauby was able to accomplish this time-consuming and tedious task through the help of an assistant from his publisher. For each letter of every word of the 132-page book, the assistant would begin with the letter A and proceed through the alphabet until she reached the correct letter, at which time Bauby would make his only possible response, the blink of his left eye, to indicate that was the letter he wanted. In this manner he dictated his memoir, *The Diving Bell and the Butterfly*.
>
> (adapted from Bauby, 1998; Rizzo, 1999)

> Jenny Craig, the well-known cofounder of weight-loss centers, had a bizarre accident in 1995. She was watching television while sitting on a couch with no headrest. She fell asleep and her head fell forward with her chin on her chest. A loud noise from the TV startled her and her head jerked up, causing the mandible to snap over her maxilla. She had to pry her teeth apart and began to speak with a lisp because of trying to keep her lower teeth from hitting her upper teeth. She immediately saw her dentist, who referred her to a temporal mandibular joint (TMJ) specialist who told her that she had dislocated her jaw. The TMJ specialist recommended she try dental appliances, none of which helped. Her speech problem became worse and chronic. She was diagnosed with focal dystonia of the mandible (involuntary muscle contractions that induce abnormal movements and postures caused by the trauma of the sudden jerking of her mandible). She received Botox injections in her cheeks, which had no beneficial effect on her speech. Three years after the accident, she saw a reconstructive surgeon who specialized in cleft lip and palate and was able to repair some of the damaged muscle tissue that had been caused by the years of abnormal mandibular movements. In addition, the surgeon was the first person to recommend speech therapy. Craig began working with an SLP 5 days a week, 1 hour per day plus speech exercises in between appointments. Although her speech is not the same as it had been before the unusual accident, Craig is thankful she can communicate with people.
>
> (Rizzo, 1999)

The critical information obtained from a thorough communication sciences and disorders' assessment must be considered within all the parameters of the life care plan itself. In other words, any and all areas that are impacted by deficits in communication and swallowing must be addressed with recommendations, if deemed appropriate by the evaluating SLP. These parameters include projected evaluation, projected therapeutic modalities, diagnostic testing and educational assessment, mobility (including accessories and maintenance of mobility technology), aids for independent functioning, orthotics and prosthetics, home furnishing and accessories, pharmacology needs, home/facility care, future medical care, transportation, health and strength maintenance, architectural renovations, potential complications, orthopedic equipment needs, vocational/educational planning, AT in the areas of sensory deficits, cognitive challenges, and communication disorders (including hearing and processing difficulties needing assistive listening devices). See Appendices 2 and 3 at the end of the chapter for an outline.

Glossary Terminology in the Field of Communication Sciences and Disorders

The importance of terminology relative to our communication with other professionals and the public, as well as the very special needs of international and transdisciplinary communication and development, has become increasingly apparent. In addition to improved consistency in the use of terms, there is the need to carefully examine what meanings the developing jargon may have to other individuals who rely primarily on a dictionary and common sense. Although many people in the field may know what is meant by a given term, others may not share the same meaning. Some terms used by people in one country may not easily translate into other languages. Even more apparent, with the diversity of people in the world today, care must be exercised to consider multiple interpretations of a term, sometimes affected by the perspective of one's culture.

Because of the transdisciplinary nature of the medical-legal-clinical world, there are also problems of various disciplines using other jargon to describe essentially the same phenomenon, act, or characteristic. These problems reflect the need for an emerging field like life care planning to develop an internally consistent and logical terminology that will facilitate the international and transdisciplinary development of the field. It is important to actively educate individuals on the life care planning team concerning specific terminology that defines and describes areas of assessment and treatment within the field of communication sciences and disorders. Refer to Appendix 4 for a list of communication sciences and disorders (both audiology and speech-language pathology) acronyms.

Medical Coding and Billing for Speech-Language Pathology

Medical coding is useful to life care planners and SLPs for documentation and billing purposes. *Current Procedural Terminology* ([CPT®] (American Medical Association, 2022; ASHA, 2022d) is a systematic listing and coding of procedures and services performed by physicians, based upon the procedure being consistent with contemporary medical practice and being performed by many physicians in clinical practice in multiple locations. Each procedure is identified with a five-digit CPT® code. International Classification of Diseases-10-Clinical Modification (ICD-10-CM) (CMS, 2022b) is an indexing of medical information by disease and operations. Within the ICD-10-CM classification system are V codes that may be used in any healthcare setting. These

V codes may be used as either a first listed (principal diagnosis code in the inpatient setting) or secondary code, depending on the circumstances of the encounter. The V codes indicate a reason for an encounter and are not procedure codes. A corresponding procedure code must accompany a V code to describe the procedure performed. Readers should refer to the ASHA website (ASHA, 2022a, 2022c, 2022e) for listings of all SLP CPT®, ICD-10 codes, and V codes. Table 16.2 gives the links to coding and billing resources. The Model Superbill for SLPs (ASHA, 2022e) is another point of reference for SLP medical coding. Appendix 6 offers readers an example of life care plan entries with costs for speech-language pathology.

Table 16.2 Comprehensive List of SLP Billing Resources

Resource Link
CPT® Coding (2022) www.asha.org/practice/reimbursement/coding/slpcpt ICD-10-CM Codes (2022) www.asha.org/Practice/reimbursement/coding/ICD-10/ Model Super Bill for SLPs www.asha.org/practice/reimbursement/coding/superbill-templates-for-audiologists-and-speech-language-pathologists/

Research in Communication Sciences and Disorders

Research in the field of speech-language pathology (and audiology has received increased attention over the past several years. Trending research includes looking at children with specific language impairments, increased use of technology to treat individuals with communication impairments, the use of brain reading techniques to identify neural representations of social thoughts, possibly establishing the first biological based diagnostic tool to detect autism, the increased risk to individuals with traumatic brain injuries of developing neurodegenerative diseases, ways to prevent noise-induced hearing loss, the use of innovative prostheses, and new tests and treatments for communication disorders by using new drugs and new diagnostic procedures. Today, research and developments in this field are based on application and patient needs and funded accordingly. Health economy considerations will play a major role in all new speech and language pathology and audiology developments in the field of communication sciences and disorders in the future. Life care planners need to be current and knowledgeable about trial research, as well as emerging research and the application to patient treatment in the field of communication sciences and disorders to uphold the responsibility to the life plan recipients of providing the best and most current life care plan possible as the template for treatment, future needs, and economic planning for the individual. The research in communication sciences and disorders changes daily, the outcomes improve the services of speech-language pathologists and audiologists, and the patients' communication disorders' outcomes improve as a result. Life care planners are encouraged to improve their understanding of the field of communication sciences and disorders and to critically assess the information they include in their life care plan to assure that they are offering the best plan available for individuals with communication disorders. This author encourages all readers to promote this concept as they develop their future life care plans. It is important for life care planners to understand the roles, responsibilities, certifications, and credentials, and to be able to critically evaluate the skills and knowledge the speech-language pathologists (and audiologists) bring to the development of the life care plan. Life care planners are challenged to be aware of emerging research in the areas of communication sciences and disorders so they can determine if there are technologies or procedures that will enhance the delivery of services in the present or in the future for the recipient of the life care plan.

The following is a list of current research topics in the field of speech-language pathology/communication disorders. These topics will continue to develop over the next several years, affecting recommendations in life care plans. Life care planners are encouraged to monitor these topics and to be assured that they are always at the cutting edge of this information as they develop strong well-written and well-researched life care plans.

- Development of assessment and treatment guidelines for autism spectrum disorders
- Development of assessment and treatment guidelines for central auditory processing disorders
- Development of specific treatment guidelines in neurological treatment of communication disorders (e.g., cognitive communication, aphasia, apraxia, dysarthria, and dementia)
- Development of research in gastroesophageal reflux disease (GERD)
- Efficacy and evidence-based studies to determine what treatments are effective
- Development of a stronger presence with funding streams and sources
- Improving treatment outcomes with all areas of treatment
- Development of instrumentation to improve diagnostic and treatment measures (fiber endoscopy, e-stimulation, cervical auscultation, deep pharyngeal stimulation)
- Increased inclusion as a member of medical surgical teams for management of head and neck issues (e.g., laryngectomies, palatal surgeries, vocal cord surgeries) and brain surgeries (e.g., removal of tumors, control postcerebral vascular accidents, seizure controls)
- Increased research and treatment of progressive neurological diseases such as Parkinson's, dementia, Alzheimer's, and multiple sclerosis
- Increased research participation with neurotrophic cortical electrode implantation
- Increased research with speech-language treatment post-cochlear implants
- Research with pharmacological therapeutic interventions to improve communication in patients with communication disorders
- Use of Vital Stimulation to correct swallowing problems
- Collaborative surgical and prosthetic intervention for craniofacial anomalies
- Assessment and treatment through telepractice
- Artificial intelligence
- Brain computer interface development for augmentative communication systems

The Role of the SLP in Life Care Planning

The life care plan identifies the comprehensive and individualized needs of a person as they relate to a disability or chronic illness with relevant associated cost considerations. These needs are the operational components of a life care planning process. They should never be compromised or manipulated. The costs assigned to these needs are determined by the geographical consumer rate for the identified services and equipment. The costs can be developed through understanding the range of available funding streams, creative and innovative ways of negotiating, available resources, and the cost projection analyses that accompany such planning.

The SLP must be well-grounded in the theory of normal development in all ages, in any previous learning or developmental problems affecting the individual, and in the current status of the individual, and must be able to predict future functioning of the individual. Many times, SLPs will practice in the treatment of either the pediatric or the adult population. This frequently precludes the SLP from being able to look backward or beyond to make accurate recommendations about future functioning needs. An SLP who takes on the role to assess, accepts a leadership role to collaborate and counsel; to interpret and apply research, perhaps as researcher or as a knowledgeable consumer of research; and to advocate and educate about an area of specialization, particularly clinical specializations.

It is always useful for the SLP, who is consulting in the life care planning process, to be able to actively engage in the clinical treatment of individuals and their families. This enhances the SLP's credibility, because the SLP should have realistic estimates of current needs and prognostic predictions. However, it is also imperative that the consulting SLP have a fluid understanding of the current literature and research that directly or indirectly impacts the area of communication sciences and disorders. This includes knowledge of the most current assessment procedures, state-of-the-art assistive technology, trends in pharmacology and medical care, and possible needs in the areas of residential and geriatric care (ASHA, 2022a, 2022d).

The SLP should be able to perform an independent case intake, consisting of talking with the referral source, determining the time frames needed to complete testing, arranging the financial and billing agreements, and arranging for a release of all pertinent information. Additional testing needed may be identified at this time or during the initial interview arrangements.

The SLP will review the medical, educational, and vocational records. This includes nursing and medical notes, doctor's orders, day-in-the-life videos, and other relevant documentation, depending on the etiology and diagnosis. A thorough assessment battery is then administered, gathering information from the spouse, family, or other relatives, including the clients themselves. This step may also include the opportunity for the SLP to consult and interview other team members whose information may have a bearing on final recommendations of the SLP. See Appendix 5 at the end of the chapter for additional SLP resources. See Appendices 2 and 3 for checklists of SLP considerations in preparing assessment and treatment information for a life care plan.

Audiology

Review of the Literature: Impact of Hearing Loss

Life care planners and other individuals should be aware of the impact that hearing loss, and particularly untreated hearing loss, can have. Hearing loss affects people differently, depending on the degree and type of loss, their personality type, the demands of their individual hearing environment, and the type of intervention they receive. However, there is almost always some negative impact associated with a hearing loss. This includes not only effects on the ability to communicate with others, but often more wide-ranging consequences, impacting physical functioning, quality of life, cognitive functioning, and even mental health.

Generally, the effects of a conductive (outer or middle ear) hearing loss, which cannot be medically remediated, can be effectively eliminated by making sound louder. In conductive hearing loss, the inner ear is normal, so amplifying sound provides functionally normal hearing, in the same way that eyeglasses provide normal vision for most visual problems. It must be cautioned that young children commonly experience conductive hearing loss due to ear and upper respiratory infections. Although these episodes are usually self-limiting or respond to medical intervention, when necessary, some children persist with conductive hearing loss, which may affect their speech and language development. These children should be referred to an audiologist as well as a SLP.

An individual with a sensorineural (inner ear) hearing loss, however, can be expected to experience some degree of difficulty understanding speech, particularly when the listening environment is less than ideal. This means that when a person with a sensorineural hearing loss is greater than three to four feet from the source of the sound or when there is noise in the background (there almost always is some noise in the background), that person will likely misunderstand some of what is being said. This is because the pattern of hearing with a sensorineural hearing loss is typically worse in the high frequencies or pitches and better in the low frequencies or pitches. In order to understand speech clearly, we must hear all the pitches equally well. The vowels are generally low in pitch (and loud) compared to consonants, which are high in pitch (and soft). Also, damage to sensory cells and nerve fibers create more than just loudness loss. There are varying degrees of distortion present in the damaged ear that cannot be overcome by simply raising the volume.

A properly fitted hearing aid can be extremely beneficial. However, it is important for all to recognize that even with appropriate amplification, individuals with sensorineural hearing loss will still frequently have difficulty understanding what is being said, particularly with noise in the background.

Research studies have examined the potential functional consequences of hearing loss (Jiam, 2016; Lin & Ferrucci, 2012). Hearing loss has been shown to be associated with increased fall risk in the elderly. Since the peripheral organs for hearing and balance share space in the cochlea diseases affecting one may affect the other. Hearing loss has been shown to affect spatial orientation and postural stability in the elderly and may contribute to an increased fall risk (Viljanen, 2009). When people have trouble hearing, they must spend more energy trying to understand what is coming from their ears. Older people also have less functional reserve that they can allocate to this task. As a result, they can have trouble dealing with a separate but simultaneous task, such as walking or dealing with a sudden obstacle (Ferrucci & Studenski, 2012). Several studies suggest that hearing aid use may improve postural stability and by inference may reduce risk of falls (Lacerda, 2012; Rumalla, 2015).

Accumulating research evidence points to a link between age-related hearing loss and cognitive decline (Wayne & Johnsrude, 2015). Several possible mechanisms have been offered. The information-degradation hypothesis suggests that higher level cognitive processes suffer when more mental resources are used to deal with impaired perception, such as hearing loss. The sensory deprivation hypothesis implies these perceptual changes may cause permanent cognitive declines through neuroplastic changes because of long-term sensory deprivation. These changes may disadvantage general cognition in favor of processes supporting speech perception (Lin, 2013).

Hearing loss has also been associated with social isolation and poor perceived quality of life. Weinstein and Ventry (1982) found that people who were socially isolated had a greater self-perceived hearing disability, worse auditory processing difficulties, and poorer hearing. The people who were most subjectively and most objectively isolated were the ones with the worst-measured hearing, the greatest self-perceived hearing disability, and the most challenges in auditory processing. A more recent study analyzed results of 50 studies in the literature which compared quality of life of the hearing impaired and non-hearing impaired (Ciorba et al., 2012). For individuals who are not hearing impaired, 68 percent rated their quality of life as excellent as compared to only 39 percent of the individuals with hearing loss.

The literature shows a relationship between hearing loss and depression. A 2010 and a 2020 meta-analysis reviewed the results of studies published between 1997–2010 and in 2020 to determine the association between chronic disease and depression in old age (Chang-Quan, 2010; Jiang et al., 2020). Seven of these studies compared poor hearing with good hearing individuals. Results showed that poor hearing is an important risk factor for depression. In a study from Canada, MacDonald (2011) found a strong relationship between self-reported hearing problems and depression. Saito et al. (2010), in a study conducted in Japan, found that the odds of depressive symptoms were high in people with self-reported hearing disability as compared to those without hearing disability. Gopinath (2012) also found an independent association between hearing disability and the presence of depressive symptoms. ASHA (2021) (www.asha.org/practice/connecting-audiologists-and-speech-language-pathologists-with-mental-health-resources/) discusses the growing need to address mental health issues for individuals with speech, language, and hearing impairments.

Audiology, an autonomous profession that encompasses healthcare and educational professional areas of practice, is the study of hearing, balance, and related disorders. The audiologist is the independent hearing healthcare professional who provides comprehensive diagnostic and habilitative/rehabilitative services for all areas of auditory, balance, and related disorders. These services are provided to individuals across the entire age span from birth through adulthood (which is in concert with the goals of a life care plan); to individuals from diverse language, ethnic, cultural, and socio-economic backgrounds; and to individuals who have multiple disabilities. Within life care planning, the audiologist should be involved in pediatric and adult rehabilitation efforts when individuals experience decreased hearing sensitivity, auditory processing problems, auditory neuropathy (auditory dys-synchrony), or balance problems. Clients may experience auditory or balance deficits due to genetic or natural aging factors, ear disease, physical trauma, brain injury, environmental noise exposure, or reactions to medications that are toxic to the auditory or balance system. Services provided by audiologists include the ability to:

- Test for and diagnose hearing and balance disorders
- Select, fit, and dispense hearing aids and assistive devices
- Provide audiological/aural (re)habilitation services
- Educate consumers and professionals on prevention of hearing loss
- Participate in hearing conservation programs to help prevent workplace-related and recreational hearing loss
- Consult for federal, state, and local agencies in reducing community noise
- Conduct research

Audiology services are available in the following work settings:

- Colleges and universities
- Community-based hearing and speech centers
- Hospitals
- Industry
- Military
- Nursing care facilities
- Private practices
- Public and private schools
- Rehabilitation centers
- State and federal governmental agencies
- State and local health departments

Audiology can be categorized by either the setting in which one practices or the population one serves. The pediatric audiologist concentrates on the audiological management of children of all ages. The pediatric audiologist is often employed in a children's hospital or a healthcare facility primarily serving children. The medical audiologist works with patients of all ages and is more concerned with establishing the site and cause of a hearing or balance problem. Medical audiologists are typically employed in hospitals as part of either a hearing and speech department or a department of otolaryngology (i.e., ear, nose, and throat). Some audiologists who work in a medical environment perform intraoperative monitoring, which involves monitoring central and peripheral nerve function during surgical procedures. The rehabilitative/dispensing audiologist focuses on the management of children or adults with hearing impairment. Rehabilitative audiologists are often in private practice and may specialize in the direct dispensing of hearing aids in addition to offering other audiological rehabilitation services. Rehabilitative audiologists are also employed by a variety of healthcare facilities (e.g., hospitals and nursing homes). The industrial audiologist provides consultative hearing conservation services to companies whose workers are exposed to high noise levels. The industrial audiologist may be in private practice or work on a part-time basis. The forensic audiologist serves as an expert witness in legal issues related to hearing and balance. The forensic audiologist may serve as an expert witness for the plaintiff or defense in compensation cases and may also serve as a consultant in community or environmental noise issues. Finally, the educational audiologist serves children in schools and is employed or contracted by the educational system. Many audiologists, not just those in academic environments, engage in basic and applied research that is not only essential to understanding human auditory function but also necessary to develop testing materials and procedures and improved amplification systems.

Audiology Credentials/Scope of Practice/Code of Ethics and Licensure/Certification Requirements

As health professionals concerned with the welfare of the patients they serve, audiologists must possess certain credentials to practice audiology. These credentials signify a specific level of education and competence that serve to protect consumers. Certification and licensure are the two most common credentials possessed by audiologists.

To be certified by ASHA and licensed/registered/certified by a particular state regulatory board or agency to practice audiology, one must possess a doctoral degree earned from an accredited college or university audiology graduate (doctoral) program (note: this requirement is relatively new, so one may encounter audiologists who do not possess doctoral degrees). College and university graduate audiology programs seek accreditation from the Council on Academic Accreditation of the ASHA. This ensures that graduates of these programs are eligible for the certificate of clinical competence (CCC) issued by the Council for Clinical Certification of ASHA. The U.S. Department of Education and the Council on Recognition of Postsecondary Accreditation have approved ASHA as a credentialing agency. The standard on which the certificate of clinical competence in audiology (CCC-A) is based has served as the foundation for most states' licensing laws. ASHA's national certification standards have undergone costly scientific tests of validity (ASHA, 2022a. ASHA-certified audiologists possess specific knowledge and competencies and must pass a national examination as well as maintain currency through continuing education.

Readers are referred to the ASHA *Scope of Practice in Audiology* (2018) for updates in the current audiology scope of practice, including telehealth, a discussion of hearing technologies beyond traditional hearing devices (e.g., over the counter [OTC]), and information about personal sound amplification products (PSAPs). Advancements in hearing device implantation, vestibular assessment and rehabilitation, hearing preservation, educational audiology, and interoperative monitoring practice are also included.

Most states require audiologists to be licensed, registered, or certified to practice audiology in that particular state. Each state's licensing or regulatory board has specific educational and competency requirements, which are assessed through examination. Renewal of state credentials usually requires maintenance of currency through continuing education. Details per state for regulations of audiology can be researched at www.asha.org/advocacy/state (ASHA, 2022h).

Causes of Hearing Loss (Perinatal and Postnatal)

Hearing loss can occur at any age, from birth through adulthood. Causative factors include genetics, systemic diseases and infections, vascular events, tumors, localized and generalized trauma, and environmental toxins. These factors can affect one or more of the components of the auditory system (outer/middle ear, inner ear, or central nervous system). The resulting hearing loss can vary in terms of degree, prognosis for recovery and response to intervention depending on the age of onset, and the components of the auditory system affected.

Perinatal causes of hearing loss are those that occur during the birth process. Infants who must be admitted to neonatal intensive care units (NICUs) are 20 times more likely to have hearing problems than infants in normal newborn nurseries (Simmons et al., 1980). Hearing loss in infants who were in NICUs is often associated with the identifiable disorders that caused the need for the NICU or treatment for the disorders. Respiratory distress syndrome (RDS/hyaline membrane disease) is the most common respiratory disease in premature infants. Infants with RDS receive treatment by invasive procedures such as intubation and suctioning, putting them at an additional risk of infections. If infants become septic (generalized infection), general treatment is with antibiotics with potential ototoxic properties, placing them at a higher risk for hearing loss.

Congenital heart disease is among the most common birth defects, affecting as many as 1 in 100 newborns (Fogle, 2008), and the patient may exhibit cyanosis, respiratory distress, congestive heart failure, or a combination of these. In addition, these infants frequently exhibit failure-to-thrive and feeding problems. Congenital heart disease is often associated with syndromes such as growth deficiencies, mental retardation, Down syndrome, and external ear anomalies. Again, ototoxic drugs may be needed to fight infections.

Central nervous system disorders may have hearing loss as one component of the disorder, including cerebral hemorrhage, hydrocephalus, hypoxic encephalopathy, and neonatal seizures. Any individual who experiences hypoxia may have compromised neurological status and hearing abilities.

Postnatal causes of cochlear hearing loss are factors occurring after birth. These include bacterial meningitis, measles, mumps, chicken pox, influenza, and viral pneumonia. Most viral-producing hearing losses are bilateral, except for mumps. The body's natural reaction to infection is elevation of temperature; however, when fever becomes excessive, cellular damage can occur, including cells of the cochlea. Treatments may warrant ototoxic antibiotics. Diabetes mellitus and kidney disease have been implicated in sensorineural hearing loss, as have head traumas, which cause both neurological disorders and hearing loss (Fogle, 2008). As noted previously, Table 16.3 lists some of the risk factors for hearing loss in infants and young children.

In older children (and adults), one of the most preventable is noise-induced hearing loss. Most people will have reduced hearing as they grow older (especially after the age of 60); however, there are things individuals can do to try to preserve their hearing. Noise-induced hearing loss, once called "blacksmith's deafness" from the continual clanging of metal on metal, dates back hundreds of years. During World War II, it received much more attention because of the heavy artillery used in the war. Acoustic trauma from a single exposure may cause permanent hearing loss. Gradual hearing loss from repeated exposure to excessive sound can damage or destroy the delicate hair cells in the cochlea. Hearing conservation programs and hearing research programs (Nicholson et al., 2022) have developed public education campaigns to alert people, especially adolescents and teenagers, to the damage caused to hearing by loud music. Wearing ear plugs or earmuffs to help block the loud sounds or music, limiting the time of an iPod session with breaks to allow your hearing to rest, and keeping the volume reduced are just a few suggestions included in a hearing conservation program.

Table 16.3 Risk Factors for Hearing Loss in Infants and Young Children

Family history of childhood hearing loss
Congenital infections (TORCH)[a]
Craniofacial anomalies
Low birth weight (less than 3.5 lbs. or 1.6 kg.)
Hyperbilirubinemia requiring blood exchange
Bacterial meningitis
Asphyxia
Ototoxic medication
Mechanical ventilation of more than 10 days
Syndromes that include hearing loss

[a] TORCH is an acronym describing congenital perinatal infections, including toxoplasmosis, other infections (like syphilis), rubella, CMV, and herpes simplex.

Some common causative factors associated with hearing loss include:

- Bacterial meningitis and other infections associated with sensorineural hearing loss
- Birth weight less than 1,500 grams (3.3 pounds)
- Craniofacial anomalies, including those with morphological abnormalities of the pinna and ear canal
- Family history of hearing loss
- Head trauma associated with loss of consciousness or skull fracture
- Hyperbilirubinemia at a serum level requiring exchange transfusion
- *In utero* infection (e.g., cytomegalovirus, rubella, syphilis, or toxoplasmosis)
- Neurofibromatosis type II and neurodegenerative disorders
- Ototoxic medications, including, but not limited to, chemotherapeutic agents, or aminoglycosides used in multiple courses or in combination with loop diuretics
- Parent/caregiver concern regarding hearing, speech, language, or developmental delay
- Prolonged mechanical ventilation of five days or longer (e.g., persistent pulmonary hypertension)
- Recurrent or persistent otitis media with effusion for at least three months
- Severe depression at birth with Apgar scores of 0–4 at 1 min. or 0–6 at 5 min.
- Stigmata or other findings associated with a syndrome known to include a sensorineural or conductive hearing loss

Audiological Assessment Procedures

When referring a patient to an audiologist for evaluation, one may expect certain procedures to be conducted to quantify and qualify hearing loss based on responses to acoustic stimuli and to screen for other associated communication disorders. These procedures include a pure tone hearing test (ASHA, 2022i, 2022k, 2022l), speech audiometry (ASHA, 2022i, 2022k, 2022l), and acoustic immittance (ASHA, 2022i, 2022k, 2022l) procedures accomplished in accordance with American National Standards Institute standards (ANSI, 2022). These audiological procedures may be modified depending on the age or level of cooperation of the patient.

Pure Tone Audiometry

Pure tone audiometry is performed to determine if hearing is normal or impaired. An audiologist, using a calibrated electronic device, called an audiometer, and standardized procedures, measures hearing sensitivity. The individual being tested initially wears earphones and the audiologist presents tones of varying frequencies and intensities to each ear. When the individual hears the tone, they respond by raising their hand or pressing a response button. The lowest intensity level at which the tone is heard two out of three times is called the threshold. This process is then repeated with the individual wearing a bone vibrator placed on the mastoid bone. When thresholds using earphones are outside the normal range, a comparison with the bone vibrator thresholds will indicate which part of the auditory system is responsible for the hearing loss.

The audiogram is a graphic representation of hearing sensitivity. It shows an individual's threshold for tones of different frequencies. Frequency, measured in hertz (Hz), is plotted along the abscissa and intensity, measured in decibels (dB), is plotted along the ordinate. Thresholds for the left ear are plotted with an *X* and thresholds for the right ear are plotted with a *0*. Normal hearing is considered to be between −10 and +20 dB HL. Hearing level (HL) is the number of decibels relative to normal hearing, which is 0 dB HL on the audiogram. The audiogram shown in Figure 16.1 indicates normal hearing in the left ear and a hearing loss in the right ear. The area enclosed by the two wavy lines is called the speech banana. This area represents the frequencies and intensities of spoken English and assists the audiologist in explaining how a given hearing loss may affect a person's ability to understand speech. In the example audiogram, the person will not be able to hear speech sounds above 1,000 Hz in the right ear because his/her thresholds are out of the speech banana. Were this person to have this degree of hearing loss in both ears, he may be expected to have difficulty understanding high-frequency speech sounds such as *s*, *f*, *th*, *p*, *t*, *k*, *sh*, and *ch*, for example. In addition, he may be expected to have considerable difficulty understanding conversational speech in the presence of background noise, such as in a cafeteria. Figure 16.1 shows the frequency of various speech sounds, as well as the intensity of some common environmental sounds.

Audiograms indicate presence of a hearing loss and the type and degree of loss. There are three types of hearing loss directly associated with the peripheral auditory mechanism:

1. Conductive (a problem in the outer or middle ear)
2. Sensorineural (a problem in the inner ear or the eighth cranial nerve, which carries the auditory signals to the brain)
3. Mixed conductive and sensorineural loss

As mentioned earlier, comparison of earphone (air conduction) and bone vibrator (bone conduction) hearing provides the necessary information for determination of type of hearing loss.

Speech Audiometry

Audiological assessment also includes speech audiometry. The audiologist evaluates how well a person can hear and understand speech. Speech audiometry consists of speech threshold and

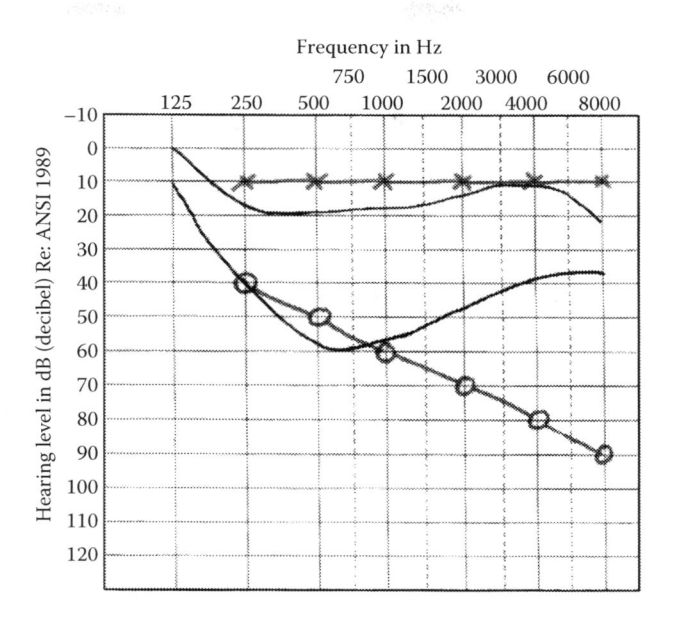

Figure 16.1 Audiogram

Source: (From Northern, J. L., & Downs, M. (2014). Hearing in children (6th ed.), Plural Publishing, Inc. With permission.)

word recognition (understanding) or speech discrimination testing. Speech threshold testing determines how soft a speech sound a person can recognize, whereas word recognition testing tells the audiologist what percentage of conversational speech is correctly understood at a particular intensity level.

Most people understand conversational speech maximally at approximately 40 dB above their speech threshold. The evaluator starts by presenting the speech level at 40 dB above the patient's speech threshold and reading a list of 50 single-syllable words with the person instructed to repeat back each word.

The percentage correct score at 40 dB above a person's threshold is then plotted. If 100 percent correct is not achieved, the test is repeated using a similar list of words at 50 dB above the person's threshold, and that score is plotted. This procedure is repeated until the person's best score is obtained.

Acoustic Immittance/Impedance

Acoustic immittance, sometimes referred to as acoustic impedance, measures the mobility of the middle ear system. The middle ear is basically a vibratory system consisting of the eardrum and the three middle ear bones: the malleus, incus, and stapes. The middle ear is responsible for taking acoustic energy (sound) and transferring it via mechanical energy from the outer ear to the fluids in the inner ear. The functioning of the middle ear affects the way people hear. Tympanometry is a measure of the mobility of the middle ear (compliance) as a function of middle ear pressure,

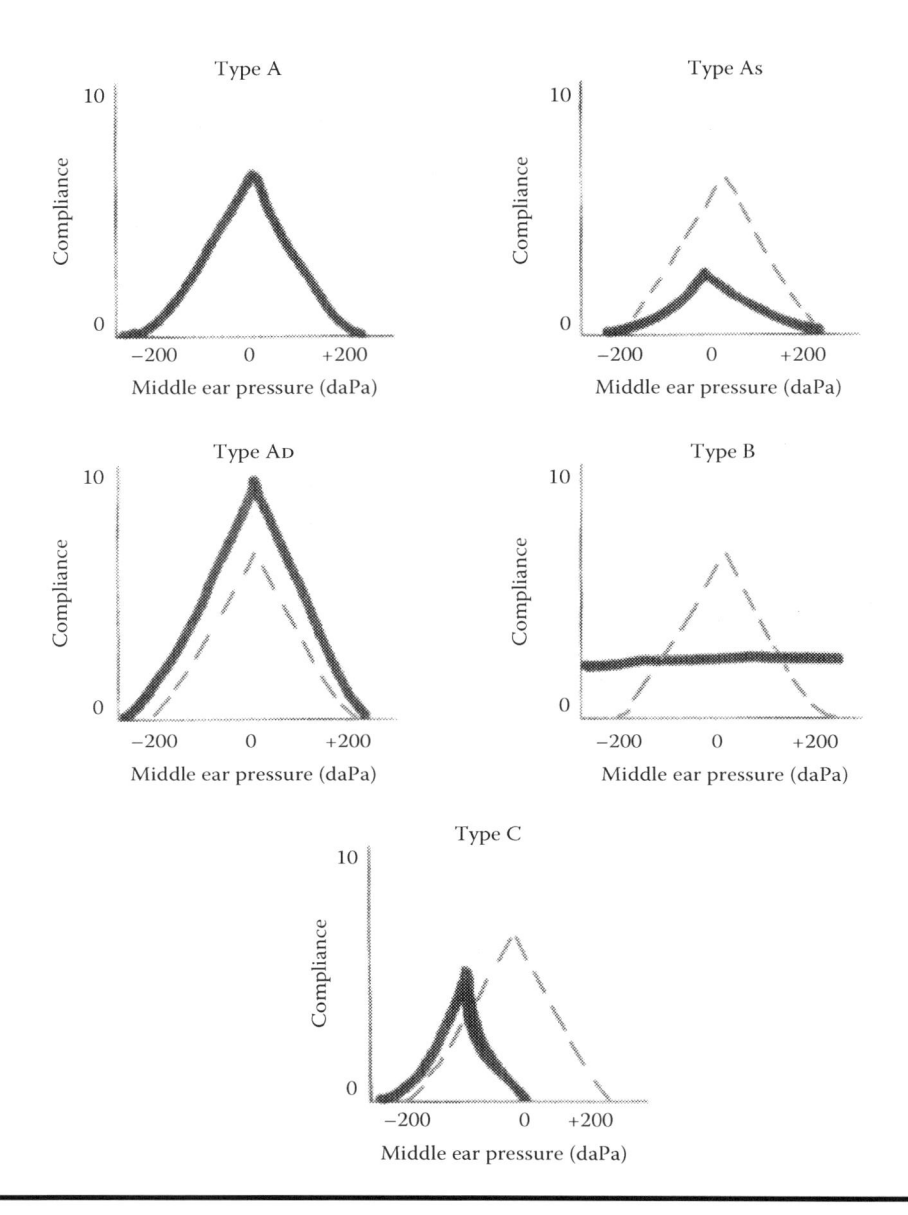

Figure 16.2 Tympanograms

measured in da pascals (daPa). The results are displayed on a graph called a tympanogram (Figure 16.2), and interpretation of these results can help indicate the site of the lesion or the part of the auditory system causing a hearing loss (ASHA, 1991).

An electroacoustic immittance meter is used to measure the middle ear function. A plug is inserted into the ear canal, and the instrument takes the measurements and graphs the information.

Tympanograms can be classified into five types based on the peak pressure and where, in terms of pressure, the peak occurs. Although tympanometry does not provide direct evidence of hearing loss, abnormal results are often associated with a temporary or conductive type hearing loss.

Otoacoustic Emissions

Otoacoustic Emissions (OAEs) are acoustic signals generated by the inner ear of healthy ears in normal hearing individuals. The acoustic signals are by-products of the activity of the outer hair cells in the cochlea. The clinical significance is that they are evidence of a vital sensory process arising in the cochlea, and OAEs only occur in a normal cochlea with normal hearing.

The OAE evaluation is relatively quick (approximately 5 minutes per ear) and is noninvasive. A soft rubber tip is inserted in the ear canal and a series of comfortably loud tones or clicks are presented. No response is necessary from the patient; he only needs to sit quietly while the test is being conducted. Otoacoustic Emissions can be completed at any age from shortly after birth to above 90.

In addition to applications for pediatric hearing assessment, OAEs are powerful diagnostic tools that assist audiologists in ruling out unusual auditory disorders, where there are unexplained differences in hearing between two ears, when a sudden hearing loss occurs, in medical-legal cases, and in cases of questionable validity of hearing test results.

Auditory Evoked Response (AER)

An AER assessment describes the clinical status of the auditory neural pathway and associated sensory elements and assists in differential diagnosis and in estimating threshold sensitivity. The assessment may also be conducted with patients who are difficult to test by conventional behavioral methods and for the purposes of site of lesion identification or in resolution of conflicting data. The AER of greatest value in nonbehavioral hearing assessment is the auditory brain stem response (ABR) (ASHA, 2022m). This procedure can provide physiological evidence of audibility for frequency specific stimuli and effectively rule out significant hearing loss. It forms the basis for universal newborn hearing screening, which will be discussed in the next section.

Identification of Hearing Loss in the Newborn

Hearing loss significant enough to affect the understanding of speech creates a potential handicap and adversely affects quality of life, regardless of age of onset. However, hearing loss present at birth or occurring during the newborn period has even greater implications. Normal hearing, particularly during the first three years of life, is essential to the development of speech and language. Children affected with congenital or newborn hearing loss may lose their ability to acquire fundamental speech, language, cognition, and social skills required for later schooling and success in society. Therefore, early identification and intervention for newborn hearing loss has been a priority for audiologists for decades. However, the fact that newborns show little behavioral responses to sound makes early identification of hearing loss in this population particularly challenging.

Although the vast majority of newborns in the United States receive hearing screening before hospital discharge, problems remain in assuring a proper diagnosis for screening failures and in the provision of appropriate and timely intervention to those diagnosed with hearing loss. According to recent Joint Committee on Infant Hearing (2019) between 25 and 35 percent of newborn screening failures are "lost to follow-up," either because they do not receive the indicated post-screening diagnosis and intervention services, or services provided are not tracked effectively. Also, certain conditions can make a newborn at risk for late onset hearing loss (see Table 16.4). Per Joint Committee recommendations, an infant with any of these "red flags" (Table 16.4) should receive audiological follow-up, even if they pass the newborn hearing screening.

Table 16.4 Birth to 24 Months: Red Flags

Birth to 28 days
1. An illness or condition requiring admission of 48 hours or greater to a neonatal intensive care unit (NICU).
2. Stigmata or other findings associated with a syndrome known to include sensorineural or conductive hearing loss.
3. Family history of permanent childhood sensorineural hearing loss.
4. Craniofacial anomalies, including morphological anomalies of the pinna and ear canal.
5. *In utero* infection such as cytomegalovirus, herpes, toxoplasmosis, or rubella.
29 days to 24 months
All the above, plus the following:
1. Parent or caregiver concern regarding hearing, speech, language, developmental delay, or a combination of these.
2. Postnatal infections associated with sensorineural hearing loss, including bacterial meningitis.
3. Recurrent or persistent otitis media with effusion for at least 3 months.
4. Neonatal indicators—specifically, hyperbilirubinemia at a serum level requiring blood exchange transfusion, persistent pulmonary hypertension of the newborn associated with mechanical ventilation, and conditions requiring the use of extracorporal membrane oxygenation.
5. Syndromes associated with progressive hearing loss such as neurofibromatosis, osteoporosis, and Usher's syndrome.
6. Neurodegenerative disorders such as Hunter's syndrome, kyphosis, gargoylism, or sensorimotor neuropathies such as Friedreich's ataxia and Charcot-Marie-Tooth syndrome.
7. Recurrent or persistent otitis media with effusion for at least 3 months.
8. Head trauma.

Pediatric Audiological Assessment

Audiological assessment of infants and young children (under 5 years of age) (ASHA, 2022k) and other individuals with developmental delay may preclude the use of standard adult audiological assessment procedures. Valid assessment of hearing in this population typically requires an audiologist skilled in pediatric assessment and may involve multiple office visits. The assessment may include one or more assessment tools (acoustic immittance measures, audiological (re)habilitation and education needs assessment, otoacoustic emissions [OAE], electrophysiological assessment, and developmentally appropriate behavioral procedures).

Behavioral testing measures make use of operant conditioning and include the following:

- Visual Reinforcement Audiometry (VRA)
- Conditioned Play Audiometry
- Tangible Reinforcement Operant Conditioning Audiometry (TROCA)
- Behavioral Observation Audiometry (BOA)

Nonbehavioral Hearing Assessment

The behavioral assessment techniques listed previously are usually successful with developmentally normal infants and young children, beginning at age 6–7 months. However, when behavioral testing fails to confirm hearing status, several nonbehavioral assessment procedures are available. These "objective techniques" measure various physiological aspects of normal auditory function which are associated with normal hearing. They require no active participation from the individual being assessed and can often be recorded during sleep or if necessary, under sedation.

Pressure-Equalizing (PE) Tubes

Many infants and children have repeated ear infections requiring pressure-equalizing (PE) tubes. The surgical procedure is called a myringotomy, performed with a small surgical incision into the tympanic membrane to relieve pressure and release fluid or pus from the middle ear. A small suction device may be inserted through the incision to delicately suction out the fluid and pus. Antibiotics are given before and continued afterward to manage infection (Mosby, 2006).

Following the myringotomy and cleaning of the middle ear, the otolaryngologist may insert a PE tube through the incision in the tympanic membrane. The tube is plastic, tiny, and hollow with a flange on each end that prevents the tube from falling into the middle ear or falling out of the tympanic membrane prematurely. The tube allows direct ventilation of the middle ear and functions as an artificial Eustachian tube to maintain normal middle ear pressure. The tube may remain in place from several weeks to several months, after which time it extrudes (pushes out) naturally into the external auditory canal, usually without the child noticing. Newer-designed tubes may remain in place indefinitely.

Audiological (Re)habilitation for Children

Specific services for children depend on individual needs as dictated by the current age of the child, the age of onset of the hearing loss, the age at which the hearing loss was discovered, the severity of the hearing loss, the type of hearing loss, the extent of hearing loss, and the age at which amplification was introduced. The audiological rehabilitation plan is also influenced by the communication mode the child is using. Examples of communication modes are speaking/listening/looking, cued speech, manually coded English, total communication, auditory-oral, auditory-verbal, and American Sign Language.

The most debilitating consequence of onset of hearing loss in childhood is its disruption in learning speech and language. The combination of early detection of hearing loss and early use of amplification has been shown to have a dramatically positive effect on the language acquisition abilities of a child with hearing loss. In fact, infants identified with a hearing loss by six months can be expected to attain language development on a par with hearing peers if appropriately managed.

Neurophysiologic Intraoperative Monitoring

Audiologists do many specialized assessments and treatments. These include neurophysiologic intraoperative monitoring and vestibular system access.

Neurophysiologic intraoperative monitoring involves continuous direct or indirect measurement and interpretation of myogenic and neural responses to intraoperative events or modality-specific, controlled stimulation during surgery on or in the vicinity of those structures. The important aspect of intraoperative monitoring is the online moment-to-moment correlation between the changes in neurophysiologic responses and intraoperative events.

The principal objectives of neurophysiologic intraoperative monitoring are: (1) to avoid intraoperative injury to neural structures; (2) to facilitate specific stages of the surgical procedure; (3) to reduce the risk of permanent postoperative neurological injury; and (4) to assist the surgeon in identifying specific neural structures (ASHA, 1992).

Although neurophysiologic intraoperative monitoring is within the scope of practice of audiology, it requires knowledge and skills not routinely acquired during the academic preparation of most audiologists. Audiologists may acquire board certification through the American Audiology Board of Intraoperative Monitoring (American Audiological Board of Interoperative Monitoring, 2018).

Balance (Vestibular) System Assessment

The clinical assessment process may include some or all the following:

- Electronystagmography (ENG): Surface electrodes are placed around the eyes to record vestibular initiated eye movements (nystagmus), in particular the vestibular ocular reflex (VOR). These electrodes record changes in the electrical potential between the cornea and the retina, which are used to measure eye movement. Subtests of the ENG battery include tests of coordinated eye movement (saccadic eye movement, smooth pursuit eye movement, and optokinetic-induced eye movement) and tests for the presence of nystagmus under a variety of conditions (horizontal and vertical gaze, static head and body position change, and rapid position change). A physical stimulus, usually cool and warm water, or air, is also presented to each ear in order to generate a VOR and determine the relative strength of response from each ear (bithermal caloric test).
- Videonystagmography (VNG): Most clinical vestibular laboratories no longer use surface electrode recording of eye movement, but rather employ newer, computerized, video-based recording techniques. The patient wears goggles that house an infrared camera. This camera sends a real-time video recording of the eyes to a computer where eye movement analysis is performed. This technology provides a more precise measurement of eye movement and allows video storage for later analysis, consultation with colleagues, and teaching purposes. The subtests for VNG are the same as those for ENG assessment.
- Rotary Chair: Video technology is used to record eye movements in response to computer-controlled chair rotation around the Earth's vertical axis. This rotation provides stimulation of the vestibular system and produces a VOR, which is computer analyzed regarding gain, phase, and symmetry.
- Computerized Dynamic Posturography (CDP): Postural stability can be assessed under simulated real-life conditions using dynamic force plate technology. The patient stands on a pressure-sensitive force plate, which measures lateral and vertical forces. This can be used to quantify postural sway under static and dynamic conditions. The Sensory Organization Test isolates the principal components of balance (vestibular, visual, and somatosensory) and analyzes the patient's ability to use each alone and in combination to maintain standing posture. The Motor Control Test evaluates a patient's ability to react to unpredictable surface perturbations (up, down, backward, and forward). CDP is helpful in evaluating patients with complaints of unsteadiness and disequilibrium, neurological or orthopedically compromised patients, or symptomatic patients with negative or equivocal findings on VNG/ENG

assessment. It can also be used as a quantitative method for evaluating the efficacy of vestibular rehabilitation.
- Vestibular Evoked Myogenic Potentials (VEMPS): Until recently, procedures for evaluating the vestibular system have focused on the semicircular canals, the part of the balance system which detects angular movement. There were no procedures to assess the otolithic system, which detects linear movement. In the early 1990s, several research groups demonstrated a sound evoked modification in the activity of contracted muscles in the neck. This myogenic evoked potential has been shown to originate from the otolithic system and now enjoys widespread use as a vestibular assessment tool. This same response can be recorded from the muscles around the eyes and is called the ocular vestibular evoked myogenic potential or OVEMP.
- Video Head Impulse Test (VHIT): The newest addition to the vestibular test battery is the VHIT. This procedure assesses eye movements produced by rapid head thrusts. It makes use of video-based recording and allows evaluation of all six semicircular canals, as opposed to the caloric test which only evaluates the horizontal canal. The addition of the VEMP and VHIT to the traditional vestibular test battery now allows assessment of the entire balance system.

Ototoxic Drug Therapy (Audiological Management)

Audiologic treatment and management also includes management of individuals who have taken drugs with the potential to cause toxic reactions to structures of the middle ear, including the cochlea, vestibule, semicircular canals, and otoliths, considered ototoxic (Altissimi et al., 2020; Govaerts et al., 1990). Drug-induced damage affecting the auditory and vestibular systems can be called, respectively, cochleotoxicity and vestibulotoxicity. Over 200 drugs have been labeled ototoxic (Altissimi et al., 2020; Govaerts et al., 1990; Lien et al., 1983; Rybak, 1986). Different ototoxic drugs can cause either permanent or temporary structural damage of varying degrees and reversibility (Bendush, 1982; Brummett, 1980; Dufner-Almeida et al., 2019). The actual frequency of occurrence of cochleotoxicity associated with specific drugs is unclear because of inconsistencies in reported data (Kopelman et al., 1988; Lord, 2019; Pasic & Dobie, 1991; Powell et al., 1983).

Permanent hearing loss or balance disorders caused by ototoxic drugs can have serious vocational, educational, and social consequences. These effects may be minimized or even prevented if the ototoxic process is detected early in treatment.

Although the role and responsibility for designing and implementing an auditory monitoring program for ototoxicity rest with the audiologist, the implementation and continuation of such a program require an interprofessional effort between the audiologist, physician, and other medical center personnel. The relationship between ototoxicity and drug administration parameters such as dosage, duration of treatment, and serum concentration is highly variable (ASHA, 2022j; Barza & Lauermann, 1978; Fausti et al., 1990). An attending physician, therefore, cannot rely solely on dosage or serum concentration to predict the risk of ototoxicity. The prospective assessment of hearing function remains the only reliable method for detecting the presence of cochleotoxicity prior to symptomatic hearing loss. Evidence suggests that high-frequency audiometry is the method of choice for the earliest detection of ototoxic hearing loss (Frank, 1990; Ganesan et al., 2018; Govaerts et al., 1990; Valente et al., 1992).

Audiological Rehabilitation

Audiological rehabilitation assessment evaluates and describes the receptive and expressive communication skills of individuals with a hearing loss or related hearing disorders. Individuals of all ages are assessed based on results from the audiological assessment, hearing aid or assistive system/device assessment, fitting, or orientation; sensory aid assessment; and assessment of communication needs or preferences.

The assessment includes an evaluation of the impact of the loss of hearing on the individual and his/her family/caregiver. The assessment may result in the development of a culturally appropriate audiological rehabilitation management plan (ASHA, 2022l).

Audiological rehabilitation is provided to persons of all ages who have any degree or type of hearing loss based upon the results of the audiological rehabilitation assessment. Audiological rehabilitation facilitates receptive and expressive communication of individuals with a hearing loss or related hearing disorders, and results in achievement of improved, altered, augmented, or compensated communication processes. Performance in both clinical and natural environments is considered. The family/caregiver plays an integral part in the rehabilitation process.

Auditory Processing Disorders Assessment (as Performed by an Audiologist)

Auditory processing disorder (APD) is the current terminology for what was referred to in earlier literature as central auditory processing disorder . With current research and improved diagnostic tools, we now know that not all APDs can be related to a central origin. An APD assessment helps to define the functional status of the central auditory nervous system (CANS) and central auditory processes. The assessment is indicated for individuals of all ages who have symptoms or complaints of hearing difficulty with documented normal peripheral auditory function, have a central nervous system disorder potentially affecting the central auditory system, or have learning problems possibly related to auditory difficulties. The APD assessment requires a team approach and is to be conducted with other audiological, speech, and language tests, as well as neuropsychological tests, to evaluate the overall communication behaviors, including spoken language processing and production, and educational achievement of the individual (ASHA, 1999).

In the *American Journal of Audiology*, Schow et al. (2000) defined central APDs as a problem in one or more of six areas:

1. Sound localization and lateralization (knowing where in space a sound source is located)
2. Auditory discrimination (usually with reference to speech, but the ability to tell that one sound is different from another)
3. Auditory pattern recognition (musical rhythms are one example of an auditory pattern)
4. Temporal aspects of audition (auditory processing relies on making fine discriminations of timing changes in auditory input, especially differences in timing by the way input comes through one ear as opposed to the other)
5. Auditory performance decrements with competing acoustic signals (listening in noise)
6. Auditory performance decrements with degraded acoustic signals (listening to sounds that are muffled, missing information, or for some reason not clear—the best example is trying to listen to speech taking place on the other side of a wall; the wall filters or blocks out certain parts of the speech signal, but a typical listener can often understand the conversation)

The interpretation of results is derived for multiple tests; there is no single test to determine the presence of an APD. The APD battery of tests may involve a series of appointments over a period. The test results will be measured against age-appropriate norms and knowledge of the CANS in normal and disordered states. The procedures in an APD battery should be viewed as separate entities for purposes of service delivery and reimbursement. Once identified by an audiologist, an SLP can work on specific treatment remediations or modifications.

Assistive Listening Devices (ALDs)

An ALD is any type of device that can help a person function better in day-to-day communication situations. An ALD can be used with or without hearing aids to overcome the negative effects of distance (sound fades as distance increases, or speech may become unintelligible for someone with a hearing impairment), background noise (classrooms and meeting areas tend to be noisy, and noise can come from within the room, such as heating and cooling, or from outside the room, such as hallways and traffic), and poor room acoustics (reverberation: sound waves reflect off walls and hit other walls repeatedly, and multiple reflection/reverberation disrupts speech understanding by causing echoes). So, even though a patient has a hearing aid, ALDs can offer greater ease of hearing (and therefore reduced stress and fatigue) in many day-to-day communication situations.

Examples of ALDs include personal frequency-modulated (FM) systems and FM systems. Personal FM systems are useful in a variety of situations such as listening to a travel guide, in a classroom lecture, in a restaurant, in a sales meeting, to a book review, in nursing homes, in senior centers, etc. Personal FM systems are also especially useful for children with auditory processing disorders (or ADD/ADHD) who are distracted by classroom noise or other background noise. The teacher wears the microphone, taking the sound of her voice directly into the child's ears. FM systems are also used in theaters, places of worship, museums, public meeting places, corporate conference rooms, convention centers, and other large areas for gathering. In this situation, the microphone/transmitter is built into the overall sound system. Patients are provided with an FM receiver that can connect to their hearing aid or to a headset. Additional systems include infrared systems, induction loop systems, and one-to-one communicators.

Personal sound amplification products or PSAPs are a relatively new category of ALDs. A PSAP is an electronic device that is worn behind the ear or inside the ear. Although it looks similar to a hearing aid, it is not considered a hearing aid and is intended to provide amplification to help normal hearing individuals in unfavorable listening situations. There are many other ALDs such as telephone amplifying devices for cordless, cell, digital, and wired phones; amplified answering machines; amplified telephones with different frequency responses; paging systems; computers; and wake-up alarms; There are also alerting devices that signal when a sound occurs. For example, there are doorbell, knock-at-the-door, or phone-alerting devices; fire alarm/smoke alarm devices; baby-cry devices or room-to-room sound alerting systems; vibrating clock alarms; vibrating paging systems; vibrating watch alarms; and so on. Many use strobe light or conventional light to alert; others use vibrating systems to alert. There are other ALDs such as closed captioning, a device for an individual with a hearing impairment used to provide written text to match spoken words on a TV program (Fogle, 2008). A telephone text (TTY) transmits text messages through the telephone line. A telecommunication device (TDD) has a visual display of typed messages over the phone, available also for printed messages.

Hearing Aid Selection and Fitting

Any individual who subjectively reports and audiometrically demonstrates hearing loss of a degree that interferes with communication should be considered for fitting with amplification. The clinical process is initially the same as that for a basic audiological assessment. The complete audiological assessment and needs assessment is necessary to initiate a treatment plan that may include amplification. The process of the hearing aid selection in conjunction with determination of the treatment plan is necessary prior to initiating the selection regimen. The U. S. Food and Drug Administration (FDA) regulates the conditions for sale of medical devices, including hearing aids, and requires a recent medical clearance by a licensed physician prior to purchase of a hearing aid. The medical clearance can be waived if the prospective hearing aid user is over 18 years of age.

Prior to hearing aid selection and fitting, the patient must be counseled regarding the potential benefits and limitations associated with personal amplification. Hearing aids do not restore hearing to normal. Just as eyeglasses do not cure vision problems, hearing aids do not cure hearing loss. Like eyeglasses, hearing aids provide benefit and improvement. They can improve hearing and listening abilities, and they can substantially improve quality of life.

The fitting of a personal amplification system and verification of its appropriateness for the communication needs of the patient, family, and caregiver are necessary requisites. There must be validation of the benefit to and satisfaction of the patient, family, and caregiver. In many cases it is necessary to demonstrate that a support system is in place to assist in maximizing the use and maintenance of the personal amplification system. The clinical decision-making process is based on professional judgment and individual patient characteristics that may significantly influence the nature and course of the selection and fitting process. The process may vary by audiologist and may vary based on the patient needs, cooperation, comprehension, and process setting. The hearing aid fitting procedures require the completion of an audiological assessment within the prior six months. Most audiologists will require their own assessment at the time of the hearing aid selection process.

In-the-canal and completely-in-the-canal) are aids contained in a tiny case that fits partly or completely into the ear canal. In-the-ear (aids are contained in a shell that fills in the outer part of the ear. Behind the ear) aids are contained in a small plastic case that rests behind the ear. Contralateral Routing of Signal (CROS) hearing aids are used for patients with one unaidable ear, due to the severity of loss, and one normal hearing ear on the contralateral side.

Today, microchips, computerization, and digitized sound processing are used in hearing aid design. Conventional analog hearing aids are designed with a particular frequency response based on the individual's audiogram. Analog programmable hearing aids have a microchip that allows the aid to have settings programmed for different listening environments such as quiet conversation in the home, noisy situations like a restaurant, or large areas like a theater. Some aids can store several programs. As the listening environment changes, a wearer can change the hearing aid settings by pushing a button on the hearing aid or by using a remote control to switch channels. The aid can be reprogrammed by the audiologist if hearing or hearing needs change. These aids are more expensive than conventional analog hearing aids, but generally have a longer life span and may provide better hearing in different listening situations. Most modern high-quality hearing aids have a life expectancy average between three and seven years (Healthy Hearing, 2020).

Digital programmable hearing aids have all the features of analog programmable aids but use digitized sound processing to convert sound waves into digital signals. A computer chip in the aid analyzes the signals of your environment to determine if the sound is noise or speech and then makes modifications to provide a clear, amplified distortion-free signal. Digital hearing aids are usually self-adjusting. The digital processing allows for more flexibility in programming the aid so that the sound it transmits matches a specific pattern of hearing loss. This digital technology is the most expensive, but it allows for improvement in programmability, greater precision in fitting,

Table 16.5   Cochlear Implant Candidacy Criteria (Cochlear, 2022)

Be at least one-year of age (with anticipation of even younger in near future)
• Have severe to profound bilateral sensorineural deafness
• Demonstrate no significant benefit from traditional amplification
• Have strong family support
• Have no medical contraindications to surgery
• For children, have a supportive school system
• For adults, have appropriate expectations

management of loudness discomfort, control of acoustic feedback (whistling sounds), and noise reduction. For additional information on types of hearing aids, readers are referred to the FDA website (2018).

For profound hearing loss, conventional hearing aids may not have sufficient gain to make sound audible. In these cases, electrical stimulation of the auditory nerve by electrodes implanted in the cochleacan produce sound awareness. With time and training, this can lead to speech understanding. Cochlear implants (ASHA 2022b) have external (outside) and internal (surgically implanted) parts. The external parts include a microphone, a speech processor, and a transmitter. The microphone looks like a behind the ear hearing aid. It picks up sounds—just like a hearing aid microphone does—and sends them to the speech processor. The speech processor may be housed, with the microphone, behind the ear, or it may be a small box worn in a chest pocket. The speech processor is a computer that analyzes and digitizes the sound signals and sends them to a transmitter worn on the head just behind the ear. The transmitter sends the coded signals to an implanted receiver just under the skin. The internal (implanted) parts include a receiver and electrodes. The receiver is just under the skin behind the ear. The receiver takes the coded electrical signals from the transmitter and delivers them to the array of electrodes that have been surgically inserted into the cochlea. The electrodes stimulate the fibers of the auditory nerve, and sound sensations are perceived (ASHA 2022b). Criteria for candidacy are shown in Table 16.5.

Some insurance companies and Medicare/Medicaid may pay for cochlear implants (see www.cochlear.com/us/home/take-the-next-step/insurance-resource-center). The average cost of cochlear implants can range from $30,000 to $50,000 with insurance, and $30,000 to $100,000 without insurance. Costs vary a great deal depending on the type of coverage a patient has available as well as the location and medical setting for the surgery.

Costs include the cochlear implant evaluation, a determination of candidacy by the physician, a CT temporal bone evaluation, a review of the cochlear implant evaluation and CT with the physician, surgery (surgeon, anesthesia, hospital/surgery center fees), prescription pain medication and antibiotic, the cochlear implant activation, multiple months of programming and reprogramming (post op at 2 weeks, 1 month, 2 months, 3 months, 6 months, and 12 months), then an annual or as needed reprogramming, two rechargeable batteries for processor of one ear (2 years postop), new external processors at 5 years post op, and new warranty if no processor purchased at 5 years post op.

Young children: 12 months to 2 years
- Profound sensorineural hearing loss (nerve deafness) in both ears
- Lack of progress in development of auditory skill with hearing aid or other amplification

- High motivation and realistic expectations from family
- Other medical conditions, if present, do not interfere with cochlear implant procedure

Children: 2–17 years
- Severe to profound sensorineural hearing loss (nerve deafness) in both ears
- Receive little or no benefit from hearing aids
- Lack of progress in the development of auditory skills
- High motivation and realistic expectations from family

Adults: 18 years and over
- Severe to profound sensorineural hearing loss in both ears
- Receive little or no useful benefit from hearing aids

Qualified candidates are those scoring, with a hearing aid, 50 percent or less on sentence recognition tests in the ear to be implanted and 60 percent or less in the nonimplanted ear or bilaterally.

There are various cochlear implant centers around the country. Teams of professionals work together with adults and children from start to finish. Team members include an audiologist, otologist/surgeon, medical specialists as needed, psychologist, counselors, and SLPs. They work with potential candidates and their families to determine candidacy for an implant, perform the surgery, and provide follow-up care both through the center and through local agencies or school districts near the cochlear implant recipient.

If the cochlea is congenitally absent or severely damaged by disease, or if the auditory nerve is damaged during surgery to remove a tumor, a cochlear implant is of no value. In these rare cases of profound deafness, an auditory brain stem implant may be indicated. The auditory brain stem implant uses technology like that of the cochlear implant, but instead of electrical stimulation being used to stimulate the cochlea, it is used to stimulate the brain stem.

Bone anchored devices are used to help people with chronic ear infections, congenital external auditory canal atresia, and single sided deafness who cannot benefit from conventional hearing aids. The system is surgically implanted and allows sound to be conducted through the bone rather than via the middle ear—a process known as direct bone conduction. The bone anchored device consists of three parts: a titanium implant, an external abutment, and a sound processor. The system works by enhancing natural bone transmission as a pathway for sound to travel to the inner ear, bypassing the external auditory canal and middle ear. The titanium implant is placed during a short surgical procedure and over time naturally integrates with the skull bone. For hearing, the sound processor transmits sound vibrations through the external abutment to the titanium implant. The vibrating implant sets up vibrations within the skull and inner ear that finally stimulate the nerve fibers of the inner ear, allowing hearing.

Tinnitus Management

Tinnitus, more commonly spoken of as ringing in the ear or head noise, has been experienced by almost everyone at one time or another. It is defined as the perception of sound in the head when no external sound is present. In addition to ringing, head noises have been described as hissing, roaring, pulsing, whooshing, chirping, whistling, and clicking. Ringing and head noises can occur in one ear or both ears and can be perceived to be occurring inside or outside the ear.

Tinnitus can accompany hearing loss (ASHA, 2022f). It can exist independent of a hearing loss. Tinnitus cannot be measured objectively. Rather, the audiologist relies on information provided in describing the tinnitus. Unfortunately, in many cases the cause of tinnitus cannot be identified, or medical or surgical treatment is not the appropriate course of action. In these cases, the tinnitus itself may need to be treated. Drug therapy, vitamin therapy, biofeedback, hypnosis, electrical stimulation, relaxation therapy, counseling, habituation therapies, and tinnitus maskers are among many forms of management available. Audiologists and otolaryngologists routinely collaborate in identifying the cause and providing treatment. Readers are referred to ASHA (2022f) for more information.

Costs Related to Amplification

The cost of hearing aids varies from approximately $500 to $2,500 per instrument depending upon type and options. A single behind the ear instrument may be as little as $500 (as high as $2500), while a digital instrument will typically cost $1000 to $6,000. Middle ear implantable instruments may run $30,000 to $50,000, plus $5,000 per year for technical support. Many patients with disabilities may need manufacturer support to ensure they can operate the volume control and other instrument options. Digital hearing aids often have an external control much like a television remote control. Care must be given to ensure appropriate fitting and follow-up services. Pitfalls that must be avoided are indiscriminate fitting of patients with amplification not appropriate for their loss and insufficient follow-up and audiological/aural rehabilitation.

Just immediately prior to the printing of this book, the Food and Drug Administration (FDA, 2022) released its final rule establishing a regulatory category for OTC hearing aids. Access to OTC hearing aids is intended to increase the availability and affordability for adults age 18 and over with mild to moderate hearing loss. Companies may begin selling these devices as early as mid-October. These hearing aids do not require a hearing exam or prescription from a physician or a hearing healthcare professional. Although not required, any consumer can get a hearing test from an audiologist before buying OTC hearing aids. It needs to be noted that not all hearing loss is the same. Through an office visit (which is usually not covered by insurance), the audiologist can also provide support on how to use the OTC hearing aids. Over the counter hearing aids are meant to be less expensive than professionally fitted hearing aids with reasons including technology differences, buying only the device without professional services. It should also be noted that basic hearing tests found online or through apps need to be used with caution. It should also be noted that your hearing and the demands on your hearing change with time. Current estimates indicate that the hearing aid will cost between $300 and $600.

The OTC hearing aids will have to follow certain rules including how loud the devices can be, what labeling will be required on the inside and outside of the box, and what requirements are related to the sale of the devices. Again, at the time of press, the ASHA and the American Academy of Audiology (AAA) as well as other hearing health associations are concerned that the OTCs will not include a gain limit and there is no mention of the benefit of seeking consultation from an audiologist prior to a hearing aid or if the user does not experience the expected benefit from the device www.audiology.org/consumers-and-patients/managing-hearing-loss/consumers-and-otc-hearing-aids (AAA, 2022; ASHA, 2022n).

Some states require health benefit plans in their states pay for hearing aids for children. These states include Colorado, Delaware, Georgia, Kentucky, Louisiana, Maine, Maryland, Massachusetts, Minnesota, Missouri, New Jersey, New Mexico, North Carolina, Oklahoma, Oregon, Tennessee, Texas, Vermont, and Virginia. Arkansas, Connecticut, Illinois, New Hampshire, and Rhode Island require coverage for both children and adults. Wisconsin requires coverage for both hearing aids and cochlear implants for children. Requirements vary state by state for ages covered, amount of coverage, benefit period, and provider qualifications. One example is that in March 2022, the Mississippi Legislature removed the prohibition in state health insurance, allowing hearing aids now to be paid for by state health insurance. Readers are referred to the State Insurance Mandates for Hearing Aids section of the American Speech-Language-Hearing Association website at www.asha.org/advocacy/state/issues/ha_reimbursement/ for further information on the individual state statutes. Laws, regulations, and policies may change at any time, so updates are necessary.

Another source of funding, if the individual qualifies, is to have vocational rehabilitation (VR) services pay for hearing-assistive technologies. State-federal VR programs have different implementation and service delivery models that vary state by state, but the VR program is an eligibility program for which an applicant must be determined eligible based on specific criteria. The individual must have a physical or mental impairment that is a substantial impediment to employment, or requires VR services to become employed and or can benefit from those VR services in terms of employment outcome. With a greater need than available resources, individuals considered the most significantly disabled (determined by state by state guidelines) must be served first. A series of necessary evaluations (audiologic, otologic, communication assessment, psychosocial among others) must be completed to make an eligibility decision.

In terms of replacement, a hearing aid should be effective for 3–7 years before replacement is necessary. It is wise to purchase replacement and repair warranties. A standard factory warranty will be 1–2 years. If an instrument is out of warranty, the cost of repair is approximately $150 to include a one-year warranty.

Children under 21 are entitled to mandatory hearing services, including hearing aids, under Medicaid. Hearing aid coverage for adults is optional and varies from state to state. A list of state Medicaid office contacts can be found at www.medicaid.gov/about-us/contact-us/index.html (Centers for Medicaid and Medicare [CMS], 2022a).

Communicating with Individuals with Hearing Impairments

The following suggestions are examples of effective strategies for communicating with individuals with hearing impairment:

Positioning

Be sure the light, whether natural or artificial, falls on your face. Do not stand with the sun to your back or in front of a window. If you are aware that the hard-of-hearing person has a better ear, stand, or sit on that side. Avoid background noise to the extent possible.

Method

Get the person's attention before you start talking. You may need to touch the person to attract attention. Speak to the hard-of-hearing person from an ideal distance of 36 feet in face-to-face visual contact. Speak as clearly as possible in a natural way. Speak more slowly to the hard-of-hearing person. Pausing between sentences will assist the listener. Do not shout. Shouting often results in distortion of speech and it displays a negative visual signal to the listener. Do not drop your voice at the end of the sentence. If the person does not understand what you said, rephrase it. When changing the subject, indicate the new topic with a word or two or a phrase.

Physical

Do not obscure your mouth with your hands. Do not chew or smoke while talking. Facial expressions and lip movements are important clues to the hard-of-hearing person. Feelings are more often expressed by nonverbal communication than through words.

Attitude

Do not become impatient. Stay positive and relaxed. Never talk about a hard-of-hearing person in their presence. Talk *to* them, not *about* them. Ask what you can do to facilitate communication.

How to Communicate with People Who Are Deaf

Be facially expressive when communicating. Do not break eye contact when communicating with people who are deaf; lack of eye contact is considered rude when communicating with a visually oriented person. Get the attention of a person who is deaf by tapping the shoulder. Do not take offense at direct questions regarding qualifications or personal life; direct questions between one person who is deaf and another person who is deaf are culturally quite common and can spill over into interactions with hearing people with no attempt to be rude. Be conscious of hearing-loss terminology; within the culture of the deaf, the norm is profound deafness, and a mild hearing loss may mean "hard-of-hearing" to the person who is deaf. While a person who is deaf is signing, do not touch their hands. Define individuals who are deaf by their abilities, rather than their disabilities. Do not talk with another hearing person in the presence of a person who is deaf without signing or ensuring a clear line of sight for speech reading. Just as those with acquired hearing loss may be suspicious when they do not understand what others are saying, so may individuals who are deaf. Use sign language, written communication, or ensure that the individual who is deaf can speech read (lip read) what is said. Do attempt to use sign language with an individual who is deaf; any attempt is appreciated, but if you are not fluent, the services of an interpreter should be obtained. Do not use the term oral as it implies oral ideologies (oralists). Rather, use the term spoken English or spoken communication. Similarly, communication training may be preferred to aural rehabilitation because the former implies improvements in aspects of communication, such as written communication, that are not aurally based.

In Table 16.6 is a link to a superbill that could be used by an audiology practice when billing private health plans. This sample is not meant to dictate which services should or should not be listed on the bill. Most billable codes are from the American Medical Association CPT® Prosthetic and durable medical equipment codes, such as hearing aid codes, are published by the CMS as the Healthcare Common Procedure Code System (HCPCS). The superbill is a standard form that health plans use to process claims. For the professional who is rendering services, it provides a time-efficient means to document services, fees, codes, and other information required by insurance companies (i.e., certification and licensure).

Table 16.6 Comprehensive List of Audiology Billing Resources

State Requirements for Audiology: www.asha.org/advocacy/state/
Degree of Hearing Loss: www.asha.org/public/hearing/degree-of-hearing-loss/
Audiology Superbill: www.asha.org/practice/reimbursement/coding/superbill-templates-for-audiologists-and-speech-language-pathologists/

The Role of the Audiologist in Life Care Planning

Early identification of a hearing impairment is important. For life care planners, the opportunity to identify a hearing impairment in an individual, pediatric or adult, is important and then the life care planner has the opportunity to plan and support the individual with his or her healthcare needs over the life span. The first step is to look for evidence of possible hearing loss or hearing needs, by asking some of the questions in Appendix 4.

In many life care plans, audiological services can be a critical component. In personal injury litigation, common sequelae from head trauma can destroy or reduce hearing, disrupt balance, and produce serious ringing in the ears (tinnitus). In medical illness, malpractice, or mistakes, the audiologist is commonly an important member for diagnosis and treatment of hearing dysfunction. Of particular interest is the role the audiologist can play regarding children. Hearing deficits can seriously hamper educational achievement, resulting in poor social adjustment and a poor vocational outlook. Indeed, many deaf children are initially termed as "mentally retarded," or more appropriately, diagnosed as a person with an intellectual disability, and do not receive services during critical developmental periods. The audiology section of this chapter should assist the life care planner by providing information related to the roles and responsibilities of the audiologist and provides resources for information, services, and products to assist the individual with a hearing impairment. Appendix 8 gives readers an example of the audiology components of a life care plan.

Standards must be placed on what the industry expects from its consultants for the consultants to provide strong, useful, and accurate assessments and recommendations. It is time for life care planners to set a level of accountability, responsibility, and recognition for the consultants that they use to develop the hearing, speech, language, and swallowing areas of the life care plan, and it is time for SLPs and audiologists to empower themselves for this process

Conclusion

SLPs and audiologists can supply crucial and detailed information about all areas of communication (hearing, swallowing, voice, fluency, articulation, pragmatics, oral motor, as well as receptive and expressive language abilities). This requires professionals who are respected among their peers for their hard work, diligent study, research, data collection and use, expert testimony, and even ability to explain their results and information in written form. It also requires a strong understanding of interprofessional practice, of diagnostics and treatments of other professions. It requires an ability to understand normal development, the disease process, the neurology and rehabilitation issues, and prognostic indicators. Life care planners need to understand and support the range of information available from both of these disciplines, and how that information is measurable and useful in many ways to the life care plan. Inclusion of strong communication information in a life care plan is life changing for many individuals. The opportunity to participate in the life care planning process should not be taken lightly. It has been one of the most rewarding parts of the audiology and speech-language pathology professions for this author.

References

Altissimi, G., Colizza, A., Cianfrone, G., De Vincentiis, G. A., Taurone, S., Musacchio, A., Ciofalo, A., Turchetta, R., Angeletti, D., & Ralli, M. (2020). Drugs inducing hearing loss, tinnitus, dizziness, and vertigo: An updated guide. *European Review for Medical and Pharmacological Sciences, 24,* 7946–7952.

American Academy of Audiology. (2022). www.audiology.org/consumers-and-patients/managing-hearing-loss/consumers-and-otc-hearing-aids

American Audiological Board of Interoperative Monitoring. (2018). www.aabiom.com

American Medical Association. (2022). *What is a CPT° code?* www.ama-assn.org/practice-management/cpt/cpt-overview-and-code-approval

American National Standards Institute. (2022). www.ansi.org

American Speech-Language-Hearing Association. (2022a). *ASHA practice policies.* www.asha.org/policy/

American Speech-Language-Hearing Association. (2022b). *Cochlear implants.* www.asha.org/practice-portal/professional-issues/cochlear-implants/

American Speech-Language-Hearing Association (2022c). *Coding for reimbursement.* www.asha.org/practice/reimbursement/coding

American Speech-Language-Hearing Association. (2022d). *Current Procedural Terminology (CPT°) codes: Speech-language pathology.* www.asha.org/practice/reimbursement/coding/slpcpt

American Speech-Language-Hearing Association. (2022e). *Superbill templates for audiologists and speech-language pathologists.* www.asha.org/practice/reimbursement/coding/superbill-templates-for-audiologists-and-speech-language-pathologists/

American Speech-Language-Hearing Association. (2022f). *Tinnitus and hyperacusis.* www.asha.org/practice-portal/clinical-topics/tinnitus-and-hyperacusis/

American Speech-Language-Hearing Association. (2022g). *Audiology and speech-language pathology interstate compact (ASLP-IC).* www.asha.org/advocacy/state/audiology-and-speech-language-pathology-interstate-compact

American Speech-Language-Hearing Association. (2022h). *ASHA state by state.* www.asha.org/advocacy/state/

American Speech-Language-Hearing Association. (2022i). *Degree of hearing loss.* www.asha.org/public/hearing/degree-of-hearing-loss/

American Speech-Language-Hearing Association. (2022j). *Ototoxic medications (medication effects).* www.asha.org/public/hearing/ototoxic-medications

American Speech-Language-Hearing Association. (2022k). *Permanent childhood hearing loss.* www.asha.org/practice-portal/clinical-topics/permanent-childhood-hearing-loss/#:~:text=Permanent%20childhood%20hearing%20loss%20can,screening%20conducted%20shortly%20after%20birth.

American Speech-Language-Hearing Association. (2022l). *Hearing loss in adults.* www.asha.org/practice-portal/clinical-topics/hearing-loss/#collapse_5

American Speech-Language-Hearing Association. (2022m). *Auditory brainstem response (ABR).* www.asha.org/public/hearing/auditory-brainstem-response/

American Speech-Language-Hearing Association. (2022n). www.asha.org/news/2022/asha-responds-to-fda-on-proposed-rule-for-otc-hearing-aids/

American Speech-Language-Hearing Association. (2021). *Connecting audiologists and speech-language pathologists with mental health resources.* www.asha.org/practice/connecting-audiologists-and-speech-language-pathologists-with-mental-health-resources/

American Speech-Language-Hearing Association. (2020). *Annual workforce data: 2020 ASHA-certified audiologist and speech-language pathologist-to-population ratios.* www.asha.org/siteassets/surveys/audiologist-and-slp-to-population-ratios-report.pdf

American Speech-Language Hearing Association. (2018). *Scope of practice in audiology.* www.asha.org/policy/sp2018-00353/

American Speech-Language-Hearing Association. (1999). *Joint audiology committee clinical practice statements and algorithms: Guidelines.* www.asha.org/policy/gl1999-00013/

American Speech-Language-Hearing Association. (1992). *Neurophysiologic intraoperative monitoring: Position statement.* www.asha.org/policy/ps1992-00036/#:~:text=The%20principal%20objectives%20of%20neurophysiologic,the%20surgeon%20in%20identifying%20specific

American Speech-Language-Hearing Association. (1991). *Acoustic immittance: A bibliography. ASHA, 33*, 1–44.

Barza, M., & Lauermann, M. (1978). Why monitor serum levels of gentamicin? *Clinical Pharmacokinetics, 3*, 202–215.

Bauby, J. D. (1998). *The diving bell and the butterfly: A memoir of life in death.* Éditions Robert Laffont.

Bendush, C. L. (1982). Ototoxicity: Clinical considerations and comparative information. In A. Whelton & H. C. Neu (Eds.), *The aminoglycosides: Microbiology, clinical use and toxicology* (pp. 235–268). Marcel Dekker, Inc.

Bishop, D. V. M. (1989). Autism, Asperger's Syndrome and semantic-pragmatic disorder: Where are the boundaries? *British Journal of Disorders of Communication*, *24*, 107–121. https://doi.org/10.3109/13682828909011951

Brummett, R. E. (1980). Drug-induced ototoxicity. *Drugs*, *19*, 412–428.

Chang-Quan, H. (2010). Chronic diseases and risk for depression in old age: A meta-analysis of published literature. *Ageing Research Reviews*, *9*(2), 131–141.

Centers for Medicare and Medicaid Services. (2022a). *Medicaid*. www.medicaid.gov/about-us/contact-us/index.html

Centers for Medicare and Medicaid Services. (2022b). *When to contact your state Medicaid office*. www.cms.gov/medicare/icd-10/2022-icd-10-pcs

Ciorba, A., Bianchini, C., Pelucchi, S., & Pasteore, A. (2012). The impact of hearing loss on the quality of life of elderly adults. *Clinical Interventions in Aging*, *7*, 159–163. https://doi.org/10.2147/CIA.S26059

Cochlear. (2022). www.cochlear.com/us/en/professionals/products-and-candidacy/candidacy/cochlear-implant

Dufner-Almeida, L.G., Cruz, D. B. D., Mingroni Netto, R. C., Batissoco, A. C., Oiticica, J., & Salazar-Silva, R. (2019). Stem-cell therapy for hearing loss: Are we there yet? *Brazilian Journal of Otohinolaryngology*, *85*, 520–529.

Dunn, L., & Dunn, L. (1991). *Peabody picture vocabulary test* (Rev. ed). American Guidance Service.

Fausti, S. A., Frey, R. H., Henry, J. A., Knutsen, J. M., & Olson, D. J. (1990). Reliability and validity of high frequency (8–20 kHz) thresholds obtained on a computer based audiometer as compared to a documented laboratory system. *Journal of the American Academy of Audiology*, *1*, 162–170.

Ferrucci, L., & Studenski, S. (2012). Clinical problems of aging. In D. Kasper, A. Fauci, S. Hauser, D. Longo, J. Jameson, & J. Loscalzo (Eds.), *Harrison's principles of internal medicine*. McGraw Hill.

Food & Drug Administration. Medical Devices; Ear, Nose, and Throat Devices; Establishing Over-the-Counter Hearing Aids, 87 Fed. Reg. 50698-50762 (October 17, 2022) (to be codified as 21 C.F.R. 800, 801, 808, & 874). https://www.federalregister.gov/documents/2022/08/17/2022-17230/medical-devices-ear-nose-and-throat-devices-establishing-over-the-counter-hearing-aids

Fogle, P. (2008). *Foundations of communication sciences & disorders*. Thomson Delmar Learning.

Frank, T. (1990). High frequency hearing thresholds in young adults using a commercially available audiometer. *Ear and Hearing*, *11*, 450–454.

Ganesan, P., Schmiedge, J., Manchaiah, V., Swapna, S., Dhandayutham, S., & Kothandaraman, P. P. (2018). Ototoxicity: A challenge in diagnosis and treatment. *Journal of Audiology and Otology*, *22*(2), 59–68. https://doi.org/10.7874/jao.2017.00360

Gillberg, C. (1991). Clinical and neurobiological aspects of Asperger syndrome in six family studies. In U. Frith (Ed.), *Autism and Asperger syndrome* (pp. 122–146). Cambridge University Press.

Gopinath, B. (2012). Hearing-impaired adults are at increased risk of experiencing emotional distress and social engagement restrictions five years later. *Age and Ageing*, *41*(5), 618–623.

Govaerts, P. J., Claes, J., Van De Heyning, P. H., Jorens, P. G., Marquet, J., & De Broe, M. E. (1990). Aminoglycoside-induced ototoxicity. *Toxicology Letters*, *52*, 227–251.

Healthy Hearing. (2020). www.healthyhearing.com/report/30926-Long-do-hearing-aids#

Higdon, C. W. (2019). What life care planners need to know about the professional discipline of speech-language pathology. *Journal of Life Care Planning*, *17*(1), 45–72.

Jiam, N. (2016). Hearing loss and falls: A systematic review and meta-analysis. *The Laryngoscope*. https://onlinelibrary.wiley.com/doi/abs/10.1002/lary.25927

Jiang, Ch., Zhu, F., & Qin, T. T. (2020). Relationships between chronic diseases and depression among middle-aged and elderly people in China: A prospective study from CHARLS. *Current Medical Science*, *40*, 858–870. https://doi.org/org/10.1007/s11596-020-2270-5

Joint Committee on Infant Hearing. (2019). *Position statements from the Joint Committee on Infant Hearing*. https://digitalcommons.usu.edu/jehdi/vol4/iss2/1/

Kopelman, J., Budnick, A. S., Sessions, R. B., Kramer, M. B., & Wong, G. Y. (1988). Ototoxicity of high dose cisplatin by bolus administration in patients with advanced cancers and normal hearing. *Laryngoscope, 98*, 858–864.

Lacerda, C. (2012). Effects of hearing aids in the balance, quality of life, and fear to fall in elderly people with sensorineural hearing loss. *International Archives of Otorhinolaryngology, 16*(2), 156–162.

Lien, E. J., Lipsett, L. R., & Lien, L. L. (1983). Structure side effect sorting of drugs. VI. Ototoxicities. *Journal of Clinical and Hospital Pharmacy, 8*, 15–33.

Lin, F., & Ferrucci, L. (2012). Hearing loss and falls among older adults in the United States. *Archives of Internal Medicine, 172*(4), 369–371.

Lin, F. (2013). Hearing loss and cognitive decline in older adults. *JAMA Internal Medicine, 173*(4), 293–299.

Lord, S. G. (2019). Monitoring protocols for cochlear toxicity. *Seminar Hear, 40*, 122–143.

MacDonald, M. (2011). *The association between degree of hearing loss and depression in older adults.* [Master's thesis, University of British Columbia, Vancouver].

Mosby. (2006). *Mosby's dictionary of medicine, nursing, & health professions* (7th ed.). Mosby Elsevier.

Nicholson, N., Rhoades, E., & Glade, R. (2022), Analysis of health disparities in the screening and diagnosis of hearing loss: Early hearing detection and intervention hearing screening follow-up survey. *American Journal of Audiology*, reprint ASHA Wire. https://doi.org/10.1044/2022_AJA-21-00014

Northern, J. L., & Downs, M. P. (2014). *Hearing in children* (6th ed.). Plural Publishing, Inc.

Owens, Jr. R. E. (2004). *Language development: An introduction* (5th ed.). Allyn & Bacon.

Pasic, T. R., & Dobie, R. A. (1991). Cis-platinum ototoxicity in children. *The Laryngoscope, 101*, 985–991.

Powell, S. H., Thompson, W. L., & Luthe, M. A. (1983). Once daily vs. continuous aminoglycoside dosing: Efficacy and toxicity in animal and clinical studies of gentamicin, netilmicin, and tobromycin. *Journal of Infectious Diseases, 147*, 918–932.

Prelock, P. (2020) *Autism Spectrum Disorder: Issues in assessment and intervention.* Pro-Ed.

Rizzo, M. (May 3, 1999). *Painful silence.* People.com. http://people.com/archive/painful-silence-vol-51-no-16/

Rumalla, K. (2015). The effect of hearing aids on postural stability. *The Laryngoscope, 125*, 720–723.

Rybak, L. P. (1986). Drug ototoxicity. *Annual Review of Pharmacology and Toxicology, 26*, 79–99.

Saito, H., Nishiwaki, Y., Michikawa, T., Kikuchi, Y., Mizutari, K., Takebayashi, T., & Ogawa, K. (2010). Hearing handicap predicts the development of depressive symptoms after 3 years in older community-dwelling Japanese. *Journal of the American Geriatrics Society, 58*(1), 93–97.

Schow, R., Seikel, J. A., Chermak, G. D., & Berent, M. (2000). Central auditory processes and test measures: ASHA 1996 revisited. *ASHA Leader.* https://doi.org/10.1044/1059-0889(2000/013

Simmons, F. B., McFarland, W. H., & Jones, F. R. (1980). Patterns of deafness in newborns. *Laryngoscope, 90*, 448–453.

Tonge, B. J. (2002). Autism, Autistic Spectrum and the need for a better definition. *The Medical Journal of Australia, 176*(9), 412.

U. S. Food and Drug Administration. (2018). *Types of hearing aids.* www.fda.gov/medical-devices/hearing-aids/types-hearing-aids

Valente, M. L., Gulledge-Potts, M., Valente, M., French-St. George, J., & Goebel, J. (1992). High frequency thresholds: Sound suite versus hospital room. *Journal of the American Academy of Audiology, 3*, 287-294.

Viljanen, A. (2009). Hearing acuity as a predictor of walking difficulties in older women. *Journal of the American Geriatric Society, 57*, 2282–2286.

Wayne, R., & Johnsrude, I. (2015). A review of causal mechanisms underlying the link between age-related hearing loss and cognitive decline. *Ageing Research Reviews, 23*, 154–166.

Weinstein, B., & Ventry, I. (1982). Hearing impairment and social isolation in the elderly. *Journal of Speech, Language, and Hearing Research, 25*(4), 593–599.

World Health Organization. (2022). *International classification of functioning, disability and health.* www.who.int/standards/classifications/international-classification-of-functioning-disability-and-health

Appendix One
Developmental Milestone Checklist

	Yes	No
Birth to 5 months		
Reacts to loud sounds		
Turns head toward a sound source		
Watches your face when you speak		
Vocalizes pleasure and displeasure sounds (laughs, giggles, cries, or fusses)		
Makes noise when talked to		
6 to 11 months		
Understands "no-no"		
Babbles (says "ba-ba-ba" or "ma-ma-ma")		
Tries to communicate by actions or gestures		
Tries to repeat your sounds		
12 to 17 months		
Attends to a book or toy for about 2 minutes		
Follows simple directions accompanied by gestures		
Answers simple directions nonverbally		
Points to objects, pictures, and family members		
Says two or three words to label a person or object (pronunciation may not be clear)		
Tries to imitate simple words		
18 to 23 months		
Enjoys being read to		
Follows simple commands without gestures		
Points to simple body parts such as "nose"		
Understands simple verbs such as "eat," "sleep"		
Correctly pronounces most vowels and n, m, p, b, words. Also begins to use other speech sounds		
Says 8 to 10 words (pronunciation may still be unclear)		
Asks for common foods by name		
Makes animal sounds such as "moo"		
Starts to combine words such as "more milk"		
Begins to use pronouns such as "mine"		

Appendix Two
Communication Sciences and Disorders/SLP Assessment Process

1. *Who* is a qualified SLP for life care planning purposes?
  A Training, licensure, certification, and practice settings
  B Ability to network
  C Integrated transdisciplinary model
  D Knowledge of funding streams and creative funding
  E Knowledge of state and federal policy, laws, and procedures
  F Knowledge of the development of collaborative sources

2. *What* will a qualified SLP need?
  A Review of all pertinent medical, vocational, educational, pharmacological, and sociological information
  B Differences between a staff speech-language pathology evaluation and the type of data needed to support a life care plan and to support the medical-legal challenges
  C Time needed to complete a communication sciences and disorders assessment
  D Understanding of related professional information and how it impacts and affects the speech-language information and plans
  E An ability to understand future trends and their application to the life care plan

3. *Components* of a communication disorders assessment
  A Oral and pharyngeal swallowing (dysphagia) assessment to include modified barium swallows, videostroboscopy evaluations, prostodontic intervention, and palatal prostheses
  B Cognitive communication information
  C Audiological information to include central auditory processing information
  D Augmentative communication assessment information
  E Assistive technology (AT) assessment information
  F Voice (to include videostroboscopy, Botox assessment information, etc.)
  G Oral peripheral motor information
  H Hearing acuity information
  I Assistive listening device or cochlear implant information

4. *Written* documentation prepared in a defensible but understandable plan with functional milestones and goals
  A Ability to determine lifelong goals and functional outcomes
  B Ability to understand how to develop services and technology needs over time
  C Ability to explain how decisions within other areas of the life care plan will impact assessment, treatment, and technology needs within the communication sciences and disorders part of the plan
  D Ability to explain present data in terms of future impact

Appendix Three
Communication Sciences and Disorders: Checklist for SLP Life Care Planning

1. Does the funding source understand the purpose and usefulness of a complete evaluation from an SLP?
2. Check qualifications, credentials, and areas of expertise of the SLP you have selected to provide the information.
3. Does the SLP understand the concepts of the life care planning process and how the information provided by him will be used?
4. Is the SLP aware of the professional content areas within communication sciences and disorders that must be included/considered in the report to the life care planner?
A. Expressive language
B. Receptive language
C. Cognitive communication
D. Oral and pharyngeal dysphagia
E. Augmentative communication
F. Assistive technology (AT)
G. Hearing and auditory processing as it relates to communication
H. Voice and voicing aspects
I. Fluency and rate
5. Can the SLP provide the results in a timely manner that meets deadlines?
6. Has the SLP been provided access to all available and necessary records, including medical, educational, vocational, and specialized testing?
7. Are the client and family available for a thorough test battery? Are there access restrictions?
8. Once information is gathered, is the SLP able to provide thorough written documentation with clear recommendations?
9. Have the questions in the following areas been considered during the communication sciences and disorders assessment?
Evaluations/Assessments
Have all the necessary assessments in the areas of communication sciences and disorders (language, speech, swallowing, augmentative communication, AT, hearing, central auditory processing, videostroboscopy, modified barium swallow studies) been considered?
When will reassessments be scheduled?
At what ages or levels of functioning will these reassessments (or additional assessments) be considered?

(Continued)

Therapy
How will necessary therapies be identified?
How will collaborative sources be used?
AT
How will technology recommendations for augmentative communication be integrated with other AT recommendations or other AT that is already present?
Consider the use of low and high technology to include wheelchairs, environmental controls, vision equipment, hearing aids, computers, adaptive aids, and assistive listening systems.
Have maintenance schedules, maintenance contracts, extended warranties, and replacement schedules been considered?
What is the range of AT that is needed?
Have the following been considered: computers, means of access, size of screens, assisted listening, low-technology communication needs, high-technology communication needs, memory aids, swallowing program equipment, necessary software, ancillary battery power, systems to integrate augmentative communication with computers for complete system development, adapted phones, variety of synthetic and digitized voices, amount of memory needed in computerized systems, and positional items for mounting and portability?
Home Furnishing/Accessories
How will AT within the existing home and environment be included?
Have probable versus potential environmental changes been considered?
Drug Supplies and Needs
Is there a need for medications for saliva control?
Have all pharmacological interventions been recommended for motor control (ataxia, tremors, etc.), for memory enhancement, for seizure control?
Have potential side effects of drugs or pharmacological intervention plans been considered in relationship to all areas of communication, swallowing, or auditory processing? These drug recommendations directly impact treatment recommendations and must be aggressively considered in the plan.
Future Medical Care
What annual evaluations will be needed?
What specialties will need to repeat the evaluations for specific treatment needs and recommendations?
Potential Complications
What complications could potentially occur because of poor treatment or no treatment in the areas where recommendations have been made?
What complications in speech, language, swallowing, communication, cognitive communication, oral motor, hearing, and processing could occur with this etiology during the life span?

(Continued)

Vocational Planning
How will communication, hearing, and language/speech recommendations, as well as augmentative communication and AT recommendations, integrate with vocational plans and needs at this time and in the future?
Educational Planning
How will communication, hearing, and language/speech recommendations as well as augmentative communication and AT recommendations, integrate with educational plans and needs at this time and in the future?
What systems and equipment are available within educational programs (primary, secondary, and postsecondary)?
Is the software appropriate for cognitive needs and projections in the future?
Have specialized camps, summer training programs, specialized preschools, and specialized short-term programs for upgrading and improvement, as well as further training needs in the future, been considered?
10. Is the SLP able to explain from a life care planning perspective the reasons and rationales relative to the recommendations?
11. Does the SLP understand how to develop lifelong recommendations and objectives? An integrated plan?
12. Is the SLP able to give detailed specifications in the written documentation that allow the life care planner the ability to develop life care plan specifics (i.e., vendors, dates, current prices, specific individuals, collaborative sources, and categories of information)?
13. Once the draft of the life care plan is complete, is the SLP furnished a draft for careful review relative to the accuracy and completeness of the information?
14. Is the SLP aware that the data collection and analysis (evaluation) information may be presented to an insurance carrier, in testimony through deposition, or at a trial?

Appendix Four
Communication Sciences and Disorders: Check list for Audiology Life Care Planning

1. Are there anatomic deformities and other disorders, which affect Eustachian tube or function?
2. Does the individual constantly request that information be repeated?
3. Does the individual exhibit behavior problems?
4. Does the individual give inconsistent responses to auditory stimuli?
5. Does the individual give slow or delayed responses to verbal stimuli?
6. Does the individual have difficulty following oral instructions?
7. Does the individual have difficulty listening in the presence of background noise?
8. Does the individual have difficulty with phonics and speech sound discrimination?
9. Does the individual have poor auditory attention?
10. Does the individual have poor auditory memory (span and sequence)?
11. Does the individual have poor receptive and expressive language?
12. Does the individual have reading, spelling, and other learning problems?

13. Is the individual easily distracted?
14. Does the individual learn poorly through the auditory channel?
15. Does the individual says "Huh?" or "What?" frequently?
16. Does the individual turn up the volume of the television, radio, or stereo?
17. Does the individual often misunderstand what is said?
18. Degrees of hearing loss are noted at asha.org/public/hearing/degree-of-hearing-loss/ (ASHA, 2022i)

The next step is to ask...

1. Do you have a medical history that identifies a hearing loss or hearing impairment?
2. Do you have ear pain?
3. Are you worried about an ear wax blockage?
4. Do you have noises in your ears (such as ringing, buzzing, clicking, humming)?
5. Do you have dizziness or trouble with balance?
6. Do your friends and family tell you that your TV is too loud?
7. Do you have trouble hearing on the telephone?
8. Do you hear better in one ear than the other?
9. Do you have trouble hearing in restaurants or large groups?
10. Do you ask people to repeat themselves?
11. Do you respond inappropriately in conversation?
12. Do family members or co-workers say that you misunderstand what they said?
13. Do many people you talk to seem to mumble (or not speak clearly)?
14. Do you have trouble understanding women and children?
15. Do people get upset because you don't hear what they say?
16. Do you take medications that may affect your hearing?
17. Do you currently wear hearing aid(s) or a hearing device?
18. Have you had a cochlear implant in your life?
19. What is your main hearing problem?

Appendix Five
Key Acronyms and Phrases Used in Communication Sciences and Disorders

AAA	American Academy of Audiology
AAS	American Auditory Society
ABD	All but dissertation
ACPCA	American Cleft Palate Craniofacial Association
ADA	Americans with Disabilities Act
AIC	Asian Indian Caucus
ANCDS	Academy of Neurological Communication Disorders and Sciences
APA	American Psychological Association

(Continued)

API	Asian Pacific Islander
ARO	Association for Research in Otolaryngology
ASA	Acoustical Society of America
ASHA	American Speech-Language-Hearing Association
ASHF	American Speech-Language-Hearing Foundation
ASL	American Sign Language
AuD	Doctorate of Audiology
BA	Bachelor of Arts
BBS	Bachelor of health sciences
BHSM	Better Hearing and Speech Month
BS	Bachelor of Sciences
CAOHC	Council for Accreditation in Occupational Hearing Conversation
CAPCSD	Council for Academic Programs in Communications Sciences and Disorders
CCC	Certificate of Clinical Competence
CEU	Continuing education unit
CF	Clinical fellowship
CLD	Culturally and linguistically different
CSD	Communication sciences and disorders
CV	Curriculum vitae
DIVISIONS	Special interest divisions
EB	Executive board
EC	Executive council
FAFSA	Free Application for Federal Student Aid
GPA	Grade point average
GSF	Graduate school fair
GUR	General university requirement
IDEA	Individuals with Disabilities Education Act
IEP	Individual Education Plan
IRB	Institutional Review Board
LC	Legislative council
LSA	Linguistic Society of America
MA	Master of Arts
MS	Master of Science
NAFDA	National Association of Future Doctors of Audiology
NAPP	National Association of Preprofessional Programs

(Continued)

NBASLH	National Black Association for Speech-Language Pathology and Hearing
NBGSA	National Black Graduate Student Association, Inc.
NESPA	National Examination in Speech-Language Pathology and Audiology
NIH	National Institute of Health
NSF	National Science Foundation
NSSLHA	National Student Speech-Language-Hearing Association
OT	Occupational therapist *or* occupational therapy
PAC	Political action committee
PET	Positron emission topography
PhD	Doctor of Philosophy
PT	Physical therapist *or* physical therapy
Quals	Qualifying examinations
RC	Regional counselor
SHS	Speech, language, and hearing scientist
SLP	Speech-language pathologist
SLP-A	Speech-language pathology assistant

Appendix Six
Speech-Language Pathology, Augmentative, and Alternative Communication, and Assistive Technology Resources

- *Ability Hub*
  AbilityHub.com's purpose is to help users find information on adaptive equipment and alternative methods available for accessing computers. Ability Hub's founder is Dan Gilman, a certified assistive technology practitioner (ATP) with RESNA.
  www.abilityhub.com/index.html

- *ABLEDATA:*
  A national database of information on more than 17,000 products that are currently available for people with disabilities.
  www.tandfonline.com/doi/abs/10.1300/J115v10n03_01?needAccess=true&journalCode=wmrs20

- *Access Board:* An independent federal agency. Contains information on Section 508 of the Rehabilitation Act, as amended requiring that electronic and information technology developed, procured, maintained, or used by the federal government be accessible to people with disabilities. In 1998, the board established an Electronic and Information Technology Access Advisory Committee (EITAAC) to help the board develop standards under Section 508.
  www.access-board.gov/

- *Accessible Website Design Resources*
  Connects to a Government Services Administration (GSA) site with links to several organizations with "how-tos" on designing websites for accessibility for people with disabilities, including a link to "Top Ten Mistakes in Web Design."

(Continued)

■ Adaptive Solutions Assistive Technology Tracker www.adaptive-sol.com
■ Alexander Graham Bell Association for the Deaf www.agbell.org
■ ALS Association www.alsa.org
■ American Association on Intellectual and Developmental Disabilities https://aaidd.org/
■ American Foundation for the Blind, Technology Center www.afb.org
■ American Medical Association www.ama-assn.org
■ American Physical Therapy Association www.apta.org
■ American Speech-Language-Hearing Association www.asha.org
■ *Apple's Disability Solutions* Information on computer access solutions for individuals with disabilities.
■ *Assistive Technology Funding and Systems Change Project (ATFSCP)* AT funding and systems change information.
■ *AT Quick Reference Series* This TechConnections resource provides quick reference guides for work-related accommodations, such as Voice Input Systems, accessible calculators, mouse alternatives, one-handed keyboards, and other assistive technologies.
■ Audible, Inc. www.audible.com
■ Augmentative Communication On-Line User Group (ACOLUG) (must join, members only) https://listserv.temple.edu/cgi-bin/wa?A0=ACOLUG and click on the third link "join or leave the list" and then follow the instructions provided.
■ *AZtech, Inc.* Information on transforming inventions into products for individuals with disabilities.
■ Brain Actuated Technologies, Inc. www.brainfingers.com
■ *Breaking New Ground Resource Center* Provides information and resources on AT for agricultural workers and agricultural worksites. In 1990, the Outreach Center of Breaking New Ground became a part of the USDA AgrAbility program. www.agrability.org/
■ California Relay Service 800-735-2929

(*Continued*)

■ California State University–Northridge, Center on Disabilities www.csun.edu/cod/
■ *Center for Information Technology Accommodation (CITA)* Legislation and policies on information systems accessibility, including the Assistive Technology Act of 1998.
■ Center for International Rehabilitation Research Information and Exchange (CIRRIE) http://cirrie-sphhp.webapps.buffalo.edu/
■ Centers for Disease Control and Prevention www.cdc.gov
■ *Closing the Gap* Closing the Gap's role is to provide information on microcomputer materials and practices that can help enrich the lives of persons with special needs. www.closingthegap.com/
■ *Consortium for Citizens with Disabilities (CCD)* CCD is a working coalition of more than 100 national consumer, advocacy, provider, and professional organizations working together with and on behalf of the 54 million children and adults with disabilities and their families living in the United States. The CCD has several task forces on various disability issues, such as employment and training, developmental disabilities, health, Social Security, long-term services and supports, telecommunications and technology, rights, etc. www.c-c-d.org/index.php
■ *Cornucopia of Disability Information (CODI)* A wealth of information relating to disabilities, including topics such as aging, statistics, computing, centers for independent living, and universal design. This site is based at the State University of New York–Buffalo.
■ Council for Exceptional Children www.cec.sped.org
■ Council for Licensure Enforcement and Regulation (CLEAR) www.clearhq.org
■ *CPB/WGBH National Center for Accessible Media* "Making Educational Software Accessible: Design Guidelines, Including Math and Science Solutions." These guidelines represent an ambitious initiative to capture access challenges and solutions and present them in a format specifically designed to educate and assist educational software developers. The detailed guidelines and solutions specific to math and science are unique to this document. This work is the result of a 3-year project funded by the National Science Foundation's Program for Persons with Disabilities. The CPB/WGBH National Center for Accessible Media developed this document with input from a distinguished board of advisers with expertise in accessible design, AT, and the education of students with disabilities. www.wgbh.org/foundation/what-we-do/ncam
■ Department of Veterans Affairs www.va.gov
■ Design to Learn www.designtolearn.com

(Continued)

- *DISABILITY Resources on the Internet*
  This site was created and is maintained by Jim Lubin, a person with quadriplegia.
  www.makoa.org/

- *Do-It Internet Resources*
  Resources are listed in many categories, including general resources, education, technology, legal, social, and political issues.
  www.washington.edu/doit/resources/curricula/do-it-internet-lessons

- Doug Dodgen and Associates
  AAC Feature Match Software
  www.dougdodgen.com

- Dragon Dictate Systems
  www.nuance.com/support.html

- Eisenhower National Clearinghouse for Math and Science Education
  www.goenc.com/

- *Equal Access to Software and Information (EASI)*
  EASI is part of the Teaching, Learning, and Technology Group, an affiliate of the American Association of Higher Education. EASI's mission is to promote the same access to information and resources for people with disabilities as everyone else.
  www.easi.cc/

- *Federal Communications Commission (FCC)*
  Contains the Telecommunications Act of 1996 and links to FCC's Disabilities Issues Task Force that contain press releases and reports that affect telecommunications and technology issues for people with disabilities.

- Food and Drug Administration
  www.fda.gov

- Greater Detroit Agency for the Blind and Visually Impaired
  Technology Information and Resources Services
  www.lifebeyondsight.org/

- Guillain-Barre Fact Sheet
  www.ninds.nih.gov/Disorders/Patient-Caregiver-Education/Fact-Sheets/Guillain-Barr%C3%A9-Syndrome-Fact-Sheet

- Harris Communications
  15159 Technology Dr.
  Eden Prairie, MN 55344-2277
  www.harriscomm.com/

- HMS School for Children with Cerebral Palsy
  Philadelphia, PA
  www.hmsschool.org

- Human Factors and Ergonomics Society (HFES)
  HFES is one of the major professional organizations for practitioners and researchers in ergonomics and human factors.
  http://hfes.org

(Continued)

- *IBM Special Needs Solutions*
  Information on IBM computer access solutions for persons with disabilities.
  www.ibm.com/able/about.html

- Institute of Medicine
  www.nas.edu/iom

- *International Center for Disability Resources on the Internet*
  The center will collect and present best practices in areas related to disability and accessibility issues. The center will collect disability-related Internet resources, including resources that may be helpful to the disability community.

- International Society for Augmentative and Alternative Communication (ISAAC)
  www.isaac-online.org

- *Job Accommodation Network (JAN)*
  A service of the U.S. Department of Labor's President's Committee on Employment of People with Disabilities, JAN provides information about job accommodation and the employability of people with functional limitations. Publishes quarterly reports on the number of cases handled by information and ADA-related concerns, among many other outcome data statistics.
  https://askjan.org/

- Krown Manufacturing, Inc.
  www.krownmfg.com

- *Kurzweil Applied Intelligence*
  www.kurzweiltech.com/kai.html

- *Learning Disabilities OnLine*
  Interactive guide to learning disabilities for parents, teachers, and children.
  www.ldonline.org/

- *LifeSpan Access Profile*
  Don Johnston Company
  www.donjohnston.com

- Muscular Dystrophy Association (MDA)
  www.mda.org

- *National Clearing House of Rehabilitation Training Materials (NCHRTM)*
  Download AT-related documents from this site. Sample titles include "Assistive Technology: Practical Intervention Strategies"; "ADA: Train the Trainer Program"; and "Reasonable Accommodations in the Workplace."
  https://ncrtm.ed.gov/

- National Easter Seal Society
  www.easterseals.com/

- National Federation of the Blind (NFB)
  www.nfb.org

- *National Institute on Disability and Rehabilitation Research (NIDRR)*
  NIDRR, part of the U.S. Department of Education, manages and funds more than 300 projects on disability and rehabilitation research, including 56 state and U.S. territory AT projects and several Rehabilitation Engineering Research Centers.

(Continued)

■ National Institutes of Health www.nih.gov
■ National Organization on Disability www.nod.org
■ *National Rehabilitation Information Center (NARIC)* NARIC is a library and information center on disability and rehabilitation. More than 50,000 National Institute on Disability and Rehabilitation Research (NIDRR)-funded, other federal agency, and private disability-related publications are held and abstracted by NARIC in its REHABDATA database, searchable online. www.naric.com/
■ National Technical Institute for the Deaf www.ntid.rit.edu
■ Oklahoma Able Tech www.okabletech.org/
■ *On a Roll—Talk Radio* Talk Radio focusing on life and disability news, updated daily. While at the site, check out the RealAudio archives of this award-winning radio talk show.
■ *One-Hand Typing* Information on free downloads, how-to manuals, therapists, and more.
■ Prentke Romich Company (PRC) www.prentrom.com
■ Quality Indicators for Assistive Technology Services https://qiat.org/
■ Rehabilitation Engineering and Assistive Technology Society of North America (RESNA) RESNA is an interdisciplinary association of people with a common interest in technology and disability. This association promotes research, development, education, advocacy, and the provision of technology. www.resna.org
■ Social Security Disability Administration Disability Information www.ssa.gov
■ Speech to Speech www.speechtospeech.org
■ *TeamRehab Report* A monthly magazine for professionals in rehabilitation technology and services. https://team-rehab.com/
■ Texas Commission for the Blind www.tsl.texas.gov/tbp/index.html
■ The Arc (of the United States) www.thearc.org

(Continued)

- *Trace Research & Development Center*
  The Trace Center conducts research aimed at improving technology that can benefit individuals with disabilities by making it more accessible in four main areas: communication, control, computer access, and next-generation communication information and transaction systems.
  www.trace.umd.edu/

- U.S. government site for Medicare information
  www.medicare.gov

- United Cerebral Palsy, Funding for Assistive Technology
  www.ucp.org/resources/assistive-technology

- United Spinal Association
  www.spinalcord.org

- United Way of America home page
  www.unitedway.org

- University of Nebraska–Lincoln
  AAC Vendors Information
  http://aac.unl.edu/

- University of Washington Speech and Hearing Sciences Department
  UW AugComm
  This site has been established as part of the UW Tele-Collaboration Project to provide information and resources for professionals and community members with an interest in AAC.
  https://depts.washington.edu/sphsc

- USSAAC (U.S. Chapter of ISAAC)
  USAAC@aol.com
  /www.ussaac.org/

- *West Virginia Rehabilitation Research and Training Center (WVRRTC)*
  Information resources on vocational rehabilitation, including links to the Job Accommodation Network and Project Enable.
  www.wvdrs.org/

- *WheelchairNet*
  WheelchairNet is a continuously developing resource for a broad community of people who are interested in wheelchairs: consumers, clinicians, manufacturers, researchers, funders. It contains resources for lifestyle, wheelchair technology and research developments, discussions, products, industry product standards, funding, services, etc.
  https://wheelchairnetwork.org/

- Wisconsin Assistive Technology Initiative
  http://aac-rerc.com
  http://wati.org

- World Health Organization
  www.who.ch

(Continued)

■ *World Wide Web Consortium (W3C)* The W3C, an international industry consortium, was founded in October 1994 to lead the World Wide Web to its full potential by developing common protocols that promote its evolution and ensure its operability. The W3C also includes the World Accessibility Initiative, which provides guidelines on website accessibility. www.w3.org/
■ *Wynd Communications* www.Purplevrs.com
■ *YAACK (Augmentative Communication Connecting Young Kids)* http://cehs.unl.edu/aac/connecting-young-kids-yaack/
■ *Yuri Rubinsky Insight Foundation: webABLE!* Contains an accessibility database that provides links to an extensive list of Internet resources related to disability and accessibility. Resources include mailing lists, websites, and newsgroups.

Appendix Seven
Speech-Language Pathology Portion of the Life Care Plan Example Case

Case Study

The client, Sam Hall, age 22, sustained a brain injury following a motor vehicle accident. His traumatic brain injury (TBI) resulted in physical and mental deficits that required AT. A complete series of tests were administered, including cognitive and oral motor (results will not be included in this brief example) assessments as appropriate, and the client clearly appeared capable of participation in speech and language therapy, as well as swallowing therapy and therapy to address his AT needs. The partial life care plan shown in the following was part of a comprehensive life care plan; however, only the appropriate topics for the SLP are included.

Recommendation	Medical Needs	Dates	Frequency	Expected Cost
	Swallow study with fiber endoscopy	2022–2025	Every 6 months through 2025, then optional depending on complications and need	$500
	Swallow study with MBS	2022–life	Yearly for life	$400
	Otolaryngology	2022–life	Yearly for life, more if additional respiratory complications occur	$400
	Nutrition consult	2022–life	Yearly for life because of the traumatic injury nutrition is a crucial part of the lifelong plan	$350
	Audiological evaluation	2022–life	Yearly for life expectancy, because of the traumatic injury and later aging	$520
	Optional: pulmonology	Only if complications	Unknown	Unknown
Home and Accessories				
	Environmental control unit	2022–life expectancy	Replace every 5 years	$1,800 plus $200 per year maintenance and updates
AT Equipment and Supplies				
	Augmentative and alternative communication	2022–life expectancy	Replace or upgrade every 5 years for life Initial AAC device may need to be basic, but the system will either have to increase in complexity with the client's recovery or be replaced with a new device of increasing complexity	Initially, $2,500, later at $7,000
	Wheelchair mount and latching system for AAC	2022–life expectancy	When power chair is replaced but at 5 years as a maximum replacement time	$1,800
	Computer, desktop, and printer	2022–life expectancy	For integration of the AAC device, to increase communication and therapy options initially, later for independent living purposes	$2,500

(Continued)

Recommendation	Medical Needs	Dates	Frequency	Expected Cost
	Assisted listening device to include earphone, speaker's microphone	2022–2028	For auditory processing in therapy and in the community, enhancing listening ability and minimizing "noise" in the environment	$1900
	MyoTrac 2 biofeedback portable unit for swallowing and motor speech	2022–2026	For biofeedback of swallowing, motor speech in therapy	$2500 every 5 years (with 1-year warranty), pack of 10 sensors $75 (replace one every 3 years)
	Low-technology and no-technology assistive devices for communication and cognition	2022–life expectancy	For quick communication (basic AAC devices) for attention, to communicate immediate needs quickly	$400 per year
	Memory aids	2022–life expectancy	Initially will start with low-tech device such as a card, simple voice output, then progress to an electronic calendar and organizer	$350 per year
	Adapted phone for AAC	2022	One time only, but upgrades in the technology will be needed	Phone: $1200 with upgrades at $200 every 5 years
	Work/study station (electronic)	2022–2057	Update every 5 years, needs to be electronic with the necessary adapted equipment	$8,000 for initial, then $1,000 every 5 years for electronic upgrade and $500 per year for maintenance of the electronics on the desk.
Speech Pathology Services				
	Assessment to include swallowing, cognition, speech (motor), auditory processing, and reading/writing	2022–life expectancy	Yearly assessment (reassessment) until 2028, then every 5 years for life	$3000 per year

(Continued)

Recommendation	Medical Needs	Dates	Frequency	Expected Cost
	Assessment for augmentative communication system and additional AT	2022–life expectancy	Yearly reassessment until 2028, then every 5 years for life Note: the SLP evaluation and the AT evaluation may be combined, completed by one person; however, the expected cost should then be combined (i.e., $2,000–$3,000) yearly, etc.	$2500.00
	SLP therapy	2022–2034, then dependent upon the re-evaluation every 5 years	First year: 5 hours per week. Second year: 3 hours per week. Third year: 2 hours per week. Fourth/fifth years: 1 hour per week if progress continues without further complications (illnesses, other accidents, etc.)	$300 per hour
	SLP (AT/AAC) technology training	2022–2024, then dependent upon the AT re-evaluation and the AT devices	First year: 5 hours per week. Second year: 3 hours per week. Third year: 2 hours per week. Fourth/fifth years: 1 hour per week if progress continues without further complications (illnesses, other accidents, etc.) Will need 2 hours per week for 4 weeks every 5 years if new technology is introduced and/or when aging issues complicate the use of the technology (typically at age 50 and 70 for someone with a disability)	$150 per hour
Vocational program and independent living program		2022–2047	Job training, and/or independent living training	No additional cost
Rehabilitation engineering; tech support and home/transportation access		2048–2067	Technology support, home modifications as needed, transportation modifications as needed. First year: 10 hours per month; second year: 4 hours per quarter (16 hours for the year); third/fourth/fifth years: 10 hours per year. Every year after 2013, 5 hours as needed.	$100 per hour

(Continued)

Appendix Eight
Audiology Portion of the Life Care Plan Example Case

The following is an example *portion* of a plan for a six-year-old child, with a severe sensorineural hearing loss due to meningitis at the age of one, who met the criteria for a cochlear implant. His parents were very bright based on educational achievements and testing. Both were employed by the school system. The child and an older sibling were both judged to be intellectually gifted.

Area	Recommendation	Dates	Frequency	Expected Cost
Medical/ Surgery	Cochlear implant device[a]	2022	Replacement 1x in life	$50,000
	Overnight hospital stay	2022	1x	$1500
	Surgeon fees	2022	1x	Included in the device cost
	Audiologist fees	2022	1x for the implant itself	Included in the device cost
Assessment/ Therapy	Speech pathology	2022 to 2033	Intensive speech perception training and additional language and speech therapy for the first 5 years, then weekly until age 22	Provided by school system under IDEA for school year, 5x/week for 5 years. If private pay during summer months, expected cost at $250 per hour
	Audiology for programming, mapping, adjustments, general maintenance, tuning[b]	2022 to life	Seen after the first 4–6 weeks for calibration, then seen monthly for the year, then yearly recheck, unless complications	$250 per hour
	ENT	2022 to life	First 4–6 weeks, seen weekly, then monthly for the first year, then yearly thereafter for life unless complications	$300 per visit
Assistive Technology	TTY (text phone); SuperPrinter 4425 recommended (includes printer, auto answer, ring, and flasher)[c]	2022 to life	Every 10 years	$1000 (includes 1-year warranty)

(Continued)

Role of Speech-Language Pathologist/Audiologist in Life Care Planning ■ 465

Area	Recommendation	Dates	Frequency	Expected Cost
	TTY paper refill (3 pack of 2.5 inch thermal paper)	2022 to life	Every 3 months or as needed depending on the use	$24 per year (estimate)
	TTY batteries (6)	2022 to life	Yearly or more depending on use	$35 for a pack of two
	Sonic Alert or Silent Call Alerting System, including receiver, transmitters, and rechargeable battery	2022 to life	Sonic Alert: 1x only. Silent Call: every 10 years	Sonic Alert: $360 with 1-year warranty. Silent Call: $640 with vibrating unit and 2-year warranty
	Door knock signaler with light	2022 to life	Every 10 years	$75 for package
	Portable smoke detector	2022 to life	Every 10 years	$175
	Allowance for batteries, light bulbs, etc.	2022 to life	Batteries: monthly Bulbs: yearly depending on use	$75 per year (estimate)
	Baby-cry alerter (assumes child)	Estimate 2048	1x (assumes child)	Sonic Alert: $60 (may also be used as smoke detector)
	Replacement cords and batteries for implant device	$1,000 to life	Every 3 months for two cords at $10 each. One time per year for 2 pack batteries at $50 per year	$100 per year
	Replacement headset	2022 (after 3-year warranty to life)	Project 3–4 upgrades over life	$750 every 3 years
	Upgrade external processor	2023	1x	$6,000
	Silent Call or Sleep Alert charger unit	2022	Every 10 years	$110
	Service contract for external speech processor and headset (internal device has a 99-year warranty)	2022 to life	Every 2 years	$850 for 2 years (after 3-year manufacturer warranty expires)
Education	Public school	2022 to 2035	School year	$0 provided under IDEA

(Continued)

Area	Recommendation	Dates	Frequency	Expected Cost
Interpreter		2022 to life	6 hours/day, 5 days/wk., August to June until 2037, then 2–4 hours/wk. average to life	$0 for school hours until age 18 (2034), then $25 per hour for medical, dental, contracts, legal, and other noneducation-related activities
Counseling	Parents	2022	1 hr./wk.	$250 per hr.
	Child/adult	2022 to 2024, then weekly until age 18, then as needed to life	2x per week from 2022 to 2024. Weekly to 2034 as needed	$0 with school counselor. $250 per hour privately. $0 should be paid by vocational rehabilitation

[a] No provision for technology advances.
[b] Economist to determine present value.
[c] TTY unit uses regular phone lines; however, units are unable to distinguish between incoming TTY call or voice calls. A separate phone line dedicated to TTY calls may be appropriate. Cost for additional phone line installation is estimated between $100 and $110 plus monthly charge of $35. Does not include long-distance charges that are usually higher due to length of time to transmit written words rather than spoken words. Cost cannot be projected. Internet access cost is $25/month.

Chapter 17

The Role of the Prosthetist in Life Care Planning

LeRoy Oddie

The development of a life care plan requires extensive clinical knowledge and experience of the evaluee's diagnoses and functional outcomes. Rarely does a life care planner individually have comprehensive expertise necessary to develop a life care plan without collaboration. Just as patient care requires team effort, the development of a life care plan similarly requires the joint effort of various clinical experts, particularly in cases involving amputations.

One of the tenets of life care planning is for the life care planner to stay within their area of expertise (Preston & Johnson, 2012; Weed, 2019). It is important to note that patient care experience with a specific patient cohort, such as amputees, does not in and of itself qualify a life care planner in all aspects of amputee management. One of the consensus statements derived from Life Care Planning Summits specifically advises: "Life Care Planners [shall] seek recommendations from other qualified professionals and/or relevant sources for inclusion of care items/services outside the individual life care planner's professional scope(s) of practice" (Johnson et al., 2018, p. 17). Thus, in the development of a life care plan for amputees, the life care planner should seek the expertise of a qualified and experienced physician (preferably a physiatrist) and prosthetist, unless the life care planner is already appropriately experienced and qualified in the detailed prescription of prostheses.

Prosthetists play a significant and integral role in the lifelong care of amputees.[1] While other clinicians, particularly those in the interdisciplinary rehabilitation team, also provide essential clinical services to maximize the potential outcomes of amputees, the prosthetist has the unique qualifications and experience to have a deep and detailed understanding of the lifelong prosthetic components required. Subsequently, prosthetists can be a valuable resource for the formation of amputation life care plans and other aspects of medicolegal cases involving amputation. This chapter provides a discussion of the prosthetist's scope of practice, credentialing and qualifications, clinical and coding practices, and valuable contributions relevant to life care planning.

DOI: 10.4324/9781003388456-20

Review of the Literature

Historically, the role of the prosthetist has evolved significantly (Pettengill & Pettengill, 2020). In the Civil War and World Wars I and II, the skills of "limb makers" or "fitters" were highly technical, primarily limited to the craft of fabricating "artificial limbs" using metal, wood, and leather (Boone, 2020). While fabrication of prostheses is still an essential element of the discipline of prosthetics, this skill is now typically relegated to prosthetic technicians. The role of the prosthetist has evolved from mechanical skills to a focus on management of clinical care (Mackenzie et al., 2018) and "is unique as there are very few disciplines where there is such a wide demand of knowledge areas and skill sets" (Blocka, 2008, p. 282). A prosthetist must not only have technical expertise, but also knowledge of engineering, medical, therapeutic, biomechanical, and psychosocial disciplines.

While the prosthetist is frequently described as a member of the rehabilitation team (de Laat et al., 2019; Donaghy et al., 2020; Keszler et al., 2020; Latour, 2022), there is a dearth of current scientific literature discussing the role of the prosthetist regarding amputee management. Perhaps a more pragmatic approach to understanding the role of the prosthetist is to review the resources of American Board for Certification in Orthotics, Prosthetics and Pedorthics (ABC), the current credentialing body for prosthetists. The ABC defines the prosthetist's role in the care of amputees as including "patient assessment, formulation of a treatment plan, implementation of the treatment plan, follow-up and practice management" (ABC, 2022, p. 9). Furthermore, the ABC states that "prosthetic care includes patient evaluation and the design, fabrication, fitting, modification, maintenance and repair of prostheses to restore physiological function and/or cosmesis" (ABC, 2022, p. 3).

Over the past century, prosthetists have struggled to educate other clinicians that the prosthetist's role is much more than simply fitting an artificial body part (Blocka, 2008). It was not until 2018 when Congress finally acknowledged that the clinical documentation of the prosthetist "shall be considered part of the individual's [amputee's] medical record to support documentation created by eligible professionals" for "purposes of determining the reasonableness and medical necessity of orthotics and prosthetics" (U. S. Congress, 1934, Section 1834(h) of the Social Security Act (42 U.S.C. 1395m(h)).

The role of the prosthetist extends beyond that of mechanic, technologist, and treating clinician. The prosthetist as a member of the multidisciplinary rehabilitation team often plays the role of educator, from advising surgeons of the residual limb length for an imminent amputation surgery to educating physical and occupational therapists of the unique biomechanical functions of individual prosthetic components (Etchegaray et al., 2019). The prosthetist's role as educator also extends to life care planners and referral sources, regardless of if the amputation case is on the behalf of the plaintiff or the defense.

The prosthetist's role in the development of life care plans is lacking in the scientific literature. However, several authors have written non-peer reviewed articles discussing how a prosthetist may be a valuable resource for the life care plan. Weed (2001) describes the prosthetist as "an extremely important consultant" in personal injury cases and encourages the life care planner to include a prosthetist in the development of a life care plan. Weed (1992) also provides guidance of how a prosthetist can effectively collaborate with a life care planner. Fairley (2010) provides an overview of how prosthetists participate in the legal process and includes feedback from several prosthetists' experience in life care plan consultation. Supan (2022) outlines a practical guidance for prosthetists to develop a consultation practice with discussion of life care plan methodology. Pettengill and Pettengill (2020) provide an overview of the qualification requirements of prosthetists, stating that: "life care planners must work collaboratively with prosthetists" (p. 18).

Scope of Practice

In comparison to many clinical disciplines, the prosthetist's scope of practice is rather limited to catastrophic injury cases as prosthetists exclusively treat amputees.[2] However, in catastrophic injury cases involving amputation(s), prosthetists may play both a critical and major role when an amputee elects to utilize a prosthesis. Not all amputees use a prosthesis while others may try, yet ultimately reject them. In amputation cases in which a prosthesis is not currently used nor are there future plans to do so, there is no need to consult with a prosthetist. On rare occasions, the evaluee may not currently be an amputee but may plan to have a future elective amputation due to various health related needs. In such cases, consultation with a prosthetist would be beneficial. In reference to the life care plan, the prosthetist's scope of practice is usually limited to the orthotics and prosthetics section.

A limitation of the prosthetist's scope of practice is the prosthetic prescription. A prescription is required for a prosthesis, which, from a regulatory perspective, is the exclusive domain of the physician. As many physiatrists manage clinical care for amputees, frequently in amputee clinics with attending prosthetists, they are the preferred source for the prosthetic prescription. However, most physiatrists' knowledge of prosthetics is limited to a high level of understanding and they frequently defer to the expertise of the prosthetist. Subsequently, the prosthetist may fill the knowledge gap of the physiatrist and provide vital guidance for the detailed prosthetic prescription, ultimately selecting the individual modular prosthetic components such as suspension, interface (socket) type, joint(s) type(s) (e.g., prosthetic feet, knees), etc. The prosthetist's role in the formulation of the prosthetic prescription was recognized decades ago by Bechtol who stated:

> His [the prosthetist's] consultation is particularly valuable at the time of prescription of the prosthesis. Using the medical data supplied him by the physician and the therapist, he [the prosthetist] can give excellent advice as to the relative degree of function that can be offered by different artificial-limb components. With cooperation in this respect, later changes in the prosthesis can be held to a minimum and possibly avoided entirely.
>
> (Bechtol, 1954, p. 10)

The roles of the physiatrist and prosthetist similarly extend to the life care plan, with the physiatrist who is skilled in amputation being the ideal clinician to establish the medical foundation for prostheses and the prosthetist collaboratively providing a detailed list of prosthetic needs (Bonfiglio, 2018).

Prosthetist Credentialing and Qualifications

In the United States, the qualifications and credentialing of prosthetists have evolved over time. While national certification is available, a national requirement to hold credentials to practice as a prosthetist does not currently exist, nor does an international credentialing organization exist (Clarke et al., 2021). However, currently fifteen states require licensure for prosthetists, three states do not issue prosthetist licenses yet require certification, and two states require facility accreditation for provision of prosthetics (see Figure 17.1) (ABC, 2022).[3] In the remaining thirty states, individuals may practice as prosthetists without any formal education, training, residency experience, or clinical experience.

| Has state licensure
| Has facility accreditation requirements for the provision of custom fabricated orthoses or prostheses
| Has certification requirements, but does not issue licenses for O,P&P

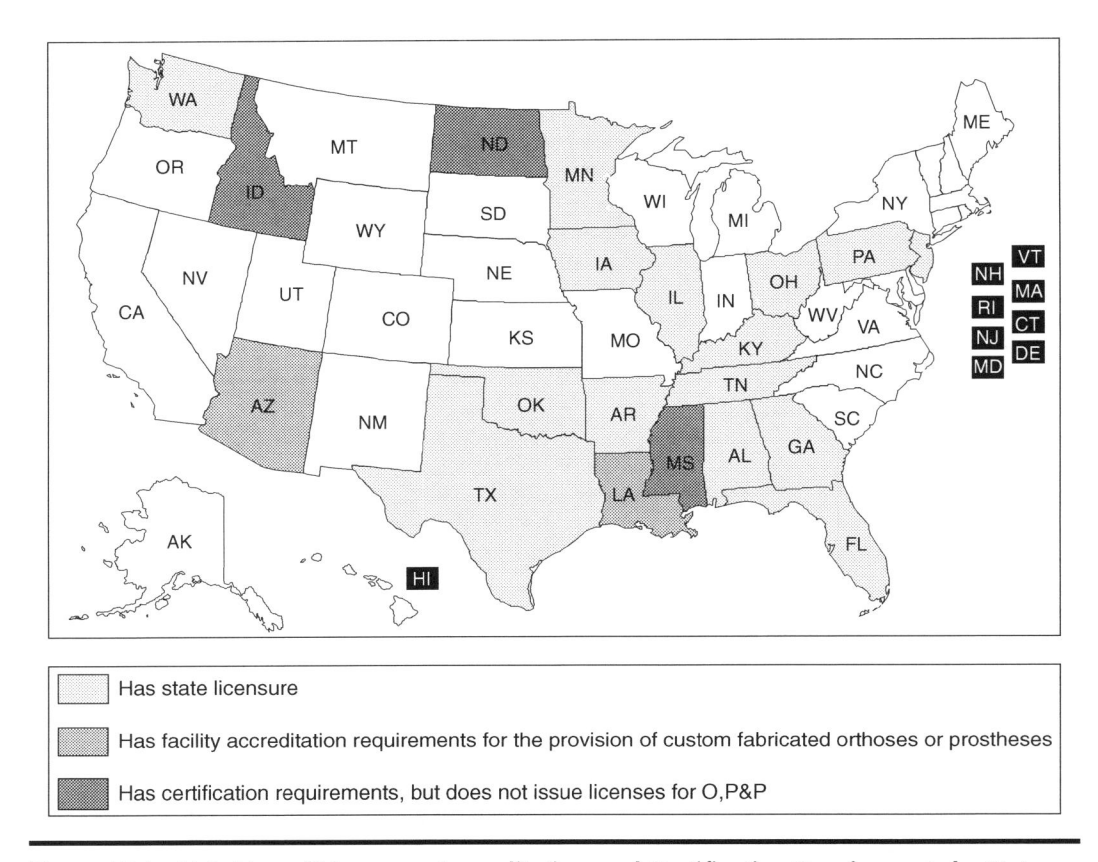

Figure 17.1 U.S. Map of Licensure, Accreditation, and Certification Requirements by State

In the past, numerous organizations have provided credentialing for prosthetists. However, as of July 2016, the American Board for Certification in Orthotics, Prosthetics & Pedorthics (ABC) is the only organization which offers new prosthetist credentials as a Certified Prosthetist (CP) or Certified Prosthetist Orthotist (CPO). The Board of Certification/Accreditation (BOC) still maintains the credentials of BOC Prosthetist (BOCP) and BOC Prosthetist Orthotist (BOCPO) but does not accept new applicants (Board of Certification/Accreditation, n.d.).[4] It worth noting that for a period, ABC "grandfathered" clinicians who lacked formal education or training and thus the credentials of CP or CPO do not provide assurance that a prosthetist is qualified in manner consistent with other allied health professions. Thus, it would behoove individuals, particularly referral sources or life care planners, to consider a prosthetist's qualifications beyond their certification credentials.

Currently, a master's degree from a Commission on Accreditation of Allied Health Education Programs (CAAHEP) accredited prosthetics program is required for prosthetist certification. After successful completion of a qualified master's degree, fulfillment of a National Commission on Orthotic and Prosthetic Education (NCOPE) accredited 12-month residency[5] is required to be eligible to sit for the ABC prosthetist certification exam (U.S. Department of Labor, 2022). The eligible master's degree may be either a Master of Prosthetics and Orthotics or Master of Science in Prosthetics and Orthotics. As part of their didactic education, prosthetists also receive training in mechanics, biomechanics, material science, anatomy, physiology, pathophysiology, and administrative topics in addition to amputee care knowledge.

In Canada, Orthotics Prosthetics Canada provides national credentials for prosthetists. Certification may be as a Certified Prosthetist in Canada (CP(c)) or as a Certified Prosthetist and Orthotist in Canada (CPO(c)). A bachelor's degree is required for admittance to an accredited two-year post graduate Prosthetics and Orthotics Clinical Methods program and a residency must be completed to be eligible for certification (Orthotics Prosthetics Canada, n.d.).

Areas of Specialty

In contrast to many other medical professions, prosthetists generally do not specialize in a specific area of practice within prosthetics. The profession of prosthetics overlaps with many aspects of the profession of orthotics and the study of both disciplines is currently mandatory for master's-level prosthetic programs. Subsequently, many prosthetists maintain dual certification in both prosthetic and orthotic disciplines and are often referred to as a CPO (ABC Certified Prosthetist Orthotist). Depending on the practice of employment, a prosthetist may spend much more time providing orthotic care than prosthetic care due to a higher demand for orthoses. Thus, many prosthetists may be considered a "jack-of-all trades" providing various types of orthoses and prostheses for many differing diagnoses. Life care planners are thus advised to consult with prosthetists who spend a significant portion of their time as prosthetists, not orthotists.

Unlike some medical professions, fellowships or formal certifications do not exist for subspecialties within the prosthetic profession. However, prosthetists may join specialized scientific societies and/or informally specialize in specific amputations areas such as pediatrics, upper limb, high-activity amputees, or complex multiple amputations (Pettengill & Pettengill, 2020).

Kinds of Patients/Problems Usually Managed

Unlike other clinicians who frequently treat a large variety of diagnoses, prosthetists exclusively provide care to amputees who utilize prostheses. The primary focus of the prosthetist is to provide and maintain prostheses provided for mobility, daily function, and/or cosmetic restoration. For lower limb amputees, the primary goal is to safely and efficiently restore mobility, including transfers, single or variable speed ambulation, and the ability to negotiate stairs/ramps, and traverse uneven terrain. For upper limb amputees, the primary focus is the restoration of functional deficits for activities of daily living (ADLs) and instrumental activities of daily living (IADLs). In addition to restoring lost mobility and function, prosthetists also strive to maximize the quality of life of amputees.

The functional deficits of amputees vary greatly from the loss of a partial digit to the loss of multiple limbs. Subsequently, the complexity of amputation cases and corresponding functional deficits may also vary greatly depending on the level of amputation(s). It is worth noting that approximately four out of five amputations are due to complications of dysvascular disease (Pasquina et al., 2014) and the functional abilities and needs of dysvascular amputees may vary significantly from those of traumatic amputees. As the etiology of amputations in life care plans are very often traumatic, a prosthetist with traumatic amputee management experience is desirable for life care plan consulting.

Prosthetists treat many levels of amputation. In the lower limbs, prosthetists typically treat partial foot, ankle disarticulation (Symes), transtibial, knee disarticulation, transfemoral, hip disarticulation, and hemipelvectomy amputations, with transtibial and transfemoral being the most common. In the upper limb, prosthetists typically treat partial digit, partial hand, wrist disarticulation, transradial, elbow disarticulation, transhumeral, shoulder disarticulation, and forequarter amputations. Due to the nature of the injury, some amputees may have multiple amputations with various combinations of upper and lower limbs, which may impact both mobility and daily function (ADLs/IADLS).

Some amputations do not affect mobility or daily function (ADLs/IADLS) and yet may have a significant cosmetic impact, such as the loss of a nose, ear, or partial digit. In such cases, a cosmetic restoration specialist known as an anaplastologist may be a valuable resource for the life care planner (Rimmer & Caruso, 2011). Anaplastologists often focus exclusively on passive facial, ocular or somatic prostheses, typically fabricated of tinted silicone with hair and/or veins to achieve life-like cosmetic restoration. While both prosthetists and anaplastologists provide cosmetic prostheses, anaplastology is a distinct discipline with its own board certification and is beyond the scope of this chapter.

Ethical Issues Confronted by the Prosthetist

Similar to any medical or allied health professional, a prosthetist is expected to exhibit ethical behavior in all professional endeavors. While the credentials of prosthetists provide an enforceable means of encouraging ethical behavior, neither the ABC Code of Professional Responsibility (American Board for Certification in Orthotics, Prosthetics & Pedorthics, 2020) nor the BOC Code of Ethics (Board of Certification/Accreditation, n.d.) specifically address behavior related to consulting services, life care planning, and/or expert witness reports and testimony. Furthermore, as previously discussed, prosthetist credentials are not required in a majority of states and in such jurisdictions, absent voluntary prosthetist credentials, a means of encouraging ethical behavior, and disciplining unethical behavior do not exist.

Prosthetists financially benefit directly from the clinical services they provide which may present ethical concerns. Generally, the more advanced a prosthesis is, the more profitable it is for the prosthetist and/or their employer. Additionally, employers may offer profit sharing or bonus programs to prosthetists with incentives to maximize revenue. Thus, prosthetists may be financially motivated to provide more functional prosthetic component capacity than is necessary ("over-prescribe"), replace prosthetic components more frequently than necessary, submit claims exceeding the fair value provided, or conduct other means of maximizing revenue. The Centers for Medicare & Medicaid Services (CMS) establishment of the Recovery Audit Contractor Program (CMS, n.d.) and various reports indicate some prosthetists are willing to engage in unethical behaviors to maximize personal financial gain (Department of Veterans Affairs, 2018; Grimm, 2021; Levinson, 2011; Mamuya et al., 2016). Such ethical concerns related to financial gain extend to life care planning activities, as prosthetists employed by the plaintiff legal team may be pressured to maximize the lifetime prosthetic needs costs while a defense team may conversely exert pressure to minimize such costs (Weed, 1992).

The ethical principle of non-maleficence, the obligation to not harm a patient, is particularly challenging in prosthetics. While prosthetic technology has made significant advancements, prostheses are still inadequate replacements of the natural, intact healthy human limb, despite the overly optimistic glorification of prosthetics in the media. In other words, prosthetic sockets may induce harm to the residual limb and the use of a prosthesis can induce secondary complications (Gailey et al., 2008). While such induced harm may not be unethical considering the limitations of prosthetic options currently available, non-maleficence may become unethical when harm could be avoided with alternative solutions. For example, a prosthetist may recommend a heavy electronic prosthesis for a very young developing congenital amputee as it may provide the most advanced function. However, such prosthetic prescription could disrupt normal bone growth and further complicate the existing deformity while other prosthetic solutions may not (Kulkarni, 2010). Given the aforementioned limited deterrent and disciplinary mechanisms to prevent unethical behavior within the profession of prosthetics, and the frequently-present financial pressures, the life care planning team should carefully vet prosthetists to ensure that their testimony and/or any written reports will be ethically robust and unbiased.

Standard Treatment Recommendations

Unlike other durable medical devices such as orthoses, all prostheses are custom made specifically for one individual amputee. While custom made, most prostheses are modular, assembled from a variety of interchangeable prosthetic components from various manufacturers and/or custom-made components. While other clinical disciplines have standard treatment recommendations, the prosthetics profession is not regulated, providing prosthetists with the flexibility to select the most appropriate combination of prosthetic components to meet the amputee's individual needs for mobility, daily function, and/or cosmetic restoration.

To further complicate standardized clinical practice, prosthetists effectively treat many varying diagnoses. In other words, each amputation level is essentially a differing diagnosis. With hundreds of prosthetics components available for each diagnosis, there is a significant number of possible prosthetic interventions and, thus, standard treatment recommendations do not apply to prosthetics domestically. While the World Health Organization (WHO) has provided standards for prosthetics (WHO, 2017), the sixty published standards are primarily aimed at improving prosthetic standards in countries lacking appropriate prosthetic care.

Clinical Practice Guidelines

Due to the custom nature and high number of prosthetic solutions, the prosthetic profession lacks comprehensive clinical practice guidelines, deferring instead, to the clinical judgment and expertise of the prosthetist. A further contributing factor to the lack of clinical practice guidelines is insufficient evidence in the form of qualified published prosthetics clinical research, such as literature reviews and meta-analyses. Most clinical practice guidelines for amputation management are specific to surgical and rehabilitation protocols, most notable the rehabilitation protocols provided by the Veterans Affairs and Department of Defense (Department of Veterans Affairs/Department of Defense, 2017).

The Steeper Group has published comprehensive clinical practice guidelines specific to the selection of lower limb prosthetic components (Steeper Group, n.d.). However, the Steeper Group is based in the United Kingdom, where it manages prosthetic clinics, and the United Kingdom's socialized healthcare system may not align with best clinical practice in the United States due to public health funding. Furthermore, many of the Steeper Group guidelines lack supporting evidence or are of sufficient quality necessary to meet the evidentiary standards for clinical practice guidelines.

A few authors have provided clinical practice guidelines for specific prosthetic topics (O'Brien et al., 2021; Stevens et al., 2018; Stevens & Wurdeman, 2019; Stevens et al., 2019.) However, as prosthetics is a vast discipline, a comprehensive review of individual clinical practice guidelines for each amputation level and prosthetic component would fill a large volume and is beyond the scope of this chapter.[6] For best clinical practice recommendations, the reader is advised to consult Chapter 19 in this text.

The Prosthetist's Role in Life Care Planning

The Prosthetist as an Expert Witness/Consultant

The core prosthetics component of the life care plan falls within the professional domain of the prosthetist. The cost of prostheses and associated supplies may be a significant portion of the overall projected lifetime need costs of the evaluee and, as a result, may become a focused source of scrutiny by opposing counsel. While the projected prosthetic costs may seem similar in various life care plans, typically prosthetists can most effectively provide the rationale behind the selected combination of individual prosthetic components (Pettengill & Pettengill, 2020).

A prosthetist may be a resource for medicolegal amputation cases via several pathways, each having advantages and disadvantages. The evaluee's treating prosthetist may serve as a resource for the referral source. For example, in legal cases, the evaluee's treating prosthetist may be employed directly by the legal team or as a consultant to the life care planner. While the evaluee's treating prosthetist is knowledgeable of the evaluee's clinical treatment and needs, there may be a perceived financial conflict of interest which should be avoided whenever possible (Fairley, 2010). Furthermore, many prosthetists are not familiar with life care planning nor the associated rigors of the legal process. Thus, an alternative pathway is to employ an independent prosthetist as a prosthetic expert, either as a consultant or expert witness. Such prosthetic experts may be familiar with the objectivity required of the life care planning and medicolegal processes yet may also be portrayed as a "hired gun." As the referral source may not be aware of the benefits of including a prosthetist in amputation cases, the life care planner may educate them on the potential contributions a prosthetist may provide and the advantages and disadvantages of each pathway.

Selecting a Prosthetist

For the life care planner seeking the most defensible life care plan, careful selection of a prosthetic expert is advised. As described previously, the certifications/qualifications of prosthetists may not be representative of complete education and training. Furthermore, there are several ethical concerns within the profession of prosthetics, particularly as the cost of prosthetic components can vary greatly and impact the prosthetist's revenue. See list below for desirable traits a life care planner should seek when selecting a prosthetist to be a prosthetic expert.

Desirable Traits for Prosthetists

- Graduated from an accredited prosthetist program
- Completed an NCOPE accredited residency
- Obtained ABC board certification
- Obtained state license credentials (if applicable)
- Spends more time as a prosthetist than orthotist (if applicable)
- Experienced with traumatic amputee care

- Has not been disciplined by credentialing organization or state board
- Familiar with litigation process
- Experienced as an expert witness
- Is not a full-time expert witness or retired from clinical practice
- Recognized by rehabilitation peers for expertise
- Published author on prosthetic/amputee topics
- Reputable for objectivity, comprehensive consultation, and ethical behavior
- Stays within expertise/scope of practice
- Possesses verbal and analytical reasoning skills
- Communicates effectively with life care planning team
- Exhibits effective educator skills
- Pays attention to details
- Maintains meticulous records and is well organized

Questions to Ask of a Prosthetist

The effectiveness of a prosthetic expert can impact the reputation of a life care planner. Even after careful selection, the life care planner should ensure the prosthetic expert's contributions are objective, effective, and defensible. Below is a list of questions life care planners should consider asking prosthetists in the development of a life care plan. Note that the list is not exhaustive, as each case presents unique circumstances. Also note some questions may also be posed to the physician providing medical foundation to ensure there is alignment of the prosthetic treatment plan:

- Has the prosthetist evaluated all of the available applicable records/resources?
- Has the prosthetist evaluated the amputee?
- Has medical foundation been established for the prosthetic items?
- Do the prosthetist and physician agree on the future prosthetic treatment plan?
- What are the appropriate prostheses?
- What is the frequency of prosthesis replacement?
- Has the appropriate life expectancy been used?
- What is the duration of need over the amputee's lifespan?
- What is the total cost per prosthesis and supplies?
- What is the itemized cost per prosthesis and supplies?
- What fee schedule was used to determine the prosthetic costs?
- Do any projected prosthetic items have specific needs which may impact other sections of the life care plan (e.g., specific therapy needs)?
- Are the projected prosthetic needs inclusive of vocational/therapeutic goals/activities?
- Is there potential conflict with projected wheelchair needs and the prostheses projected (when applicable)?
- Do any of the projected prosthetic needs conflict with the evaluee's comorbidities (when applicable)?
- Are there any foreseeable complications due to prosthesis use?
- Are any of the projected prosthetic needs unreasonable/indefensible?
- Have alternative technologies or surgical interventions been considered (e.g., osseointegration)?
- Billing and coding for prostheses

The methodology for determining the costs of future lifetime prosthetic needs may differ from other portions of the life care plan. For example, while prosthetists evaluate amputees in the provision of care, the cost of evaluation is included in the cost of a prosthesis, not as a separate line item. Other cost differences exist due to the billing/coding structure, extended warranties, inclusive repairs, etc. Furthermore, there are hundreds of modular prosthetics' components with various coding requirements, used in various combinations with unique inclusion/exclusion criteria to form a complete prosthesis. Thus, consultation with a prosthetist may be particularly useful in projecting future prosthetic needs, as they are unlike other types of goods and services that may be found throughout the life care plan.

The costs for prosthetic devices are based upon the CMS Healthcare Common Procedure Coding System (HCPCS) codes. More specifically, the Durable Medical Equipment, Prosthetics/Orthotics & Supplies (DMEPOS) L-codes and the associated fee schedules are the industry standard for determining prosthetic costs. It is noted, however, that L-codes often serve simply a reference cost and may differ from the actual billed cost.

In prosthetics, there are effectively three fee schedules. The first fee schedule is the aforementioned durable medical equipment (DME) L-codes published by the Medicare Administrative Contractor (MAC) of CMS. Currently, four MACs provide national coverage divided into four jurisdictions (A, B, C, and D), with each geographical region having its own fee schedule. This fee schedule is commonly referred to as the "Medicare rate" and is the reference for other fee schedules. When submitting a reimbursement claim to CMS, prosthetists reference the DMEPOS L-codes. These rates may also be used for other payors such as workers' compensation programs and may be applicable to some life care plans where adherence to specific fee schedules are required in medicolegal proceedings.

The second effective fee schedule for prosthetics is the negotiated (or "discounted") rate. Prosthetic providers typically contract with third party healthcare payors as a means of ensuring business volume. In return for increased volume, prosthetic providers negotiate a discounted contract rate lower than the "Medicare rate," which typically varies as a 10–40% discount. The negotiated rate is often not applicable to life care plans as there is no guarantee the discount will be available in the future nor are such discounted rates typically available if an amputee pays "out-of-pocket" (also referred to as "cash pay").

The third effective fee schedule for prosthetics is *usual and customary* (U&C) rate (Berry, 2020). The U&C rate is the price an amputee must pay to a prosthetics provider when paying "out-of-pocket" ("cash pay"). Unlike Medicare or private insurance, individual amputees do not provide any assurance of business volume for prosthetists. Thus, amputees paying "out-of-pocket" usually pay the U&C rate which is typically 20–30% higher than the Medicare rate (Berry, 2020). Unless stipulated by individual state regulations, the U&C rate is the most relevant cost for prosthetic components for life care plans as it represents the rate an amputee must pay "out-of-pocket" for prosthetic services (Weed, 1992; Weed, 2001).

It is beyond the scope of this chapter to provide a comprehensive discussion of determining various prosthetic component costs as there many modular options. However, an overview of various cost factors is warranted to advise the life care planner and/or referral source of the methodology of prosthetic consultants. While numerous factors influence the treatment plan and subsequent selection of prosthetic components, a few key factors are discussed below.

The functional capabilities of prosthetic components may vary greatly. For example, a prosthetic knee may simply provide the basic function of manually locking when standing and swinging freely when ambulating. Conversely, a technologically-advanced prosthetic knee may include a microprocessor with various sensors to provide sophisticated control of a hydraulic cylinder for advanced functions such as variable cadence adaption, stair/ramp descent, task specific modes, etc. Subsequently, as the functional capabilities of prosthetic components vary, so does the cost.

For example, the former basic prosthetic knee may only cost hundreds of dollars while the latter advanced prosthetic knee may cost $80,000 or more.

To accommodate the significant range of functional and cost differences of lower limb prosthetic components, amputees are classified by their potential functional levels. The industry standard for determining amputee functional potential is the CMS Medicare Functional Classification Levels (MFCL), established in 1995 (see Table 17.1) (Dillon et al., 2018). The MFCL is divided into five varying levels of function, commonly referred to as "K levels" (e.g., K0, K1, K2, K3, or K4). Physiatrists and/or prosthetists may determine an amputee's K level using standardized outcome measures. Once the K level has been determined, the potential applicable prosthetic components are narrowed. For example, for a transfemoral amputee classified as a K1 level amputee who will only use a prosthesis to transfer and/or ambulate at a fixed cadence in the household, it would not be appropriate to provide such an individual with a highly advanced powered prosthetic knee as many if not most of its features would not be utilized. For upper limb amputees, restrictions equivalent to K levels do not exist.

The regulations that payors impose for insurance plans may not always apply to life care plan costs. For example, while the guidance related to L-codes and MFCL K levels is applicable to life care plans, it may not apply rigidly to all scenarios. An objective of a life care plan is to provide sufficient resources for an amputee to reasonably return to the previous functional level prior to the catastrophic amputation(s). The regulations of MFCL K levels and prosthetic coding are not always based upon clinical practice as they may be intended to limit costs rather than reasonably and necessarily restore functional deficits. For example, CMS regulations limit an amputee to one prosthesis per amputation and thus, an auxiliary prosthesis for specific activities such as sports are not covered. If coding regulations conflict with recommended clinical practice for financial reasons, the life care plan should not be limited and preference should be given to restoring the evaluee's

Table 17.1 Medicare Functional Classification Levels (MFCLs)/K Levels

Medicare Functional Classification Levels (MFCL)		
	K Level	Description
	0	Does not have the ability or potential to ambulate or transfer safely with or without assistance and a prosthesis does not enhance their quality of life or mobility.
	1	Has the ability or potential to use a prosthesis for transfers or ambulation on level surfaces at fixed cadence, typical of the limited and unlimited household ambulator.
	2	Has the ability or potential for ambulation with the ability to transverse low level environmental barriers such as curbs, stairs, or uneven surfaces. This level is typical of the limited community ambulator.
	3	Has the ability or potential for ambulation with variable cadence, typical of the community ambulator who has the ability to transverse most environmental barriers and may have vocational, therapeutic, or exercise activity that demands prosthetic utilization beyond simple locomotion.
	4	Has the ability or potential for prosthetic ambulation that exceeds the basic ambulation skills, exhibiting high impact, stress, or energy levels typical of the prosthetic demands of the child, active adult, or athlete.

function (Berry, 2020). Additionally, many insurance plans limit an amputee to one prosthesis or cap annual/lifetime expenses related to prosthetic components. Such limitations should not be extended to a life care plan, particularly when an amputee may benefit from a second prosthesis intended for a specific activity or vocation (Pettengill & Pettengill, 2020).

Conclusion

Just as medical professions have become more specialized, the life care planning team has also expanded to include specialized expertise. In amputation life care plans, the prosthetist may provide a vital role for developing the future lifetime itemized costs of prosthetic needs with consideration of associated factors such as replacement frequency, warranties, repairs, etc. While the scope of the prosthetist is a narrow focus in the life care plan in comparison to other clinical members of the rehabilitation team, the prosthetist has the unique experience and knowledge to provide a detailed treatment plan specific to the needs of individuals with limb loss, particularly as the prosthetic options have significantly expanded in volume and complexity over the past several decades. If a consulting prosthetist is desired, the retaining referral source should carefully vet the prosthetist's qualifications to ensure the prosthetist's expertise will objectively add to the life care plan.

Glossary

Amputee	An individual with limb loss or limb deficiency
BOCP	A BOC Prosthetist credentialed by Board of Certification/Accreditation (BOC)
BOCPO	A BOC Prosthetist Orthotist credentialed by Board of Certification/Accreditation (BOC)
Cash pay	When a patient directly pays a clinician for services rendered
CMS	Centers for Medicare & Medicaid Services
CP	A Certified Prosthetist credentialed by the American Board for Certification in Orthotics, Prosthetics & Pedorthics (ABC)
CPO	A Certified Prosthetist Orthotist credentialed by the American Board for Certification in Orthotics, Prosthetics & Pedorthics (ABC)
K levels	Five classification levels of mobility for lower limb amputees as defined by the CMS Medicare Functional Classification Levels (MFCL)
L-codes	Reimbursement codes specific to orthotics and prosthetic components
O&P	The professions of orthotics and prosthetics
Prosthetic technician	An individual who fabricates and assembles prosthetic components, maintains prostheses, typically under the supervision of a prosthetist. A technician is not involved in the clinical care of an amputee.

Resources

Prosthetic Organizations

American Board for Certification in Orthotics, Prosthetics & Pedorthics (ABC)
330 John Carlyle Street, Suite 210, Alexandria, Virginia 22314
Phone: (703) 836-7114
Fax: (703) 836-0838
Email: info@abcop.org
Website: www.abcop.org

American Academy of Orthotists and Prosthetists (AAOP)
8116 Arlington Blvd
PMB214
Falls Church, VA 22042
United States
Phone: (202) 380-3663
Fax: (202) 380-3447
Website: www.oandp.org

American Orthotic and Prosthetic Association (AOPA)
330 John Carlyle Street, Suite 200
Alexandria, VA 22314
Phone: (571) 431-0876
Fax: (571) 431-0899
Email: info@aopanet.org
Website: www.aopanet.org

Amputee Coalition of America
601 Pennsylvania Avenue NW, Suite 420, South Building
Washington, DC 20004
Phone: (888) 267-5669
Website: www.amputee-coalition.org

Board of Certification/Accreditation (BOC)
10461 Mill Run Circle | Suite 1250 Owings Mills, MD 21117-5575
Phone: (410) 581-6222
Fax: (410) 581-6228
Website: www.bocusa.org

International Society for Prosthetics and Orthotics (ISPO)
Rue du Luxembourg 22-24
1000 Brussels
Belgium
Phone: +32 (2) 213 13 79
Email: ispo@ispoint.org
Website: www.ispoint.org

National Commission on Orthotic and Prosthetic Education (NCOPE)
330 John Carlyle St., Suite 200
Alexandria, VA 22314
Phone: (703) 836-7114
Fax: (703) 890-2425
Email: info@ncope.org
Website: https://ncope.org

Orthotics Prosthetics Canada (OPC)
1 Eglinton Ave. E., Suite 705
Toronto, ON M4P 3A1
Phone: (416) 623-6687
Email: info@opcanada.ca
Website: www.opcanada.ca

Commission on Accreditation of Allied Health Education Programs (CAAHEP)
9355 – 113th St. N, #7709
Seminole, FL 33775
Phone: (727) 210-2350
Fax: (727) 210-2354
Email: mail@caahep.org
Website: https://caahep.org

Notes

1. For purposes of this chapter, the term amputee is synonymous with an individual with limb loss, individual with congenital limb deficiency, congenital amputee, evaluee, or other similar relevant terminology.
2. It is worth noting many prosthetists are also orthotists and thus may treat many diagnoses which, however, are not within the scope of this chapter.
3. www.abcop.org/state-licensure
4. www.bocusa.org/bocs-board-approves-program-changes-for-orthotic-prosthetic-and-pedorthic-certifications/
5. Or 18 months if combined with an orthotics residency.
6. For example, the concisely written Steeper Group clinical practice guidelines exceed 100 pages.

References

American Board for Certification in Orthotics, Prosthetics, & Pedorthics. (2020). *The code of professional responsibility and rules & procedures*. American Board for Certification in Orthotics, Prosthetics & Pedorthics. www.abcop.org/docs/default-source/publications/code-of-professional-responsibility.pdf?sfvrsn=d38e7a1a_3

American Board for Certification in Orthotics, Prosthetics, & Pedorthics. (2022). *Orthotic prosthetic & pedorthic scope of practice*. American Board for Certification in Orthotics, Prosthetics, & Pedorthics. www.abcop.org/publication/scope-of-practice

Bechtol, C. O. (1954). The prosthetics clinic team. *Artificial. Limbs, 1*, 9–14. O&P Library. www.oandplibrary.org/al/pdf/1954_01_009.pdf

Berry, D. (2020). Expert consult: Prosthetic criteria and. considerations for life care planning. *Journal of Nurse Life Care Planning, 20*(2), 21–30.

Blocka, D. (2008). Moving the profession. *Prosthetics and Orthotics International, 32*(3), 282–286.

Board of Certification/Accreditation. (n.d.). *Code of ethics*. Board of Certification/Accreditation. www.bocusa.org/wp-content/uploads/Code_of_Ethics.pdf

Bonfiglio, R. P. (2018). The role of the physiatrist in life care planning. In R. O. Weed & D. E. Berens (Eds): *Life care planning and case management handbook* (4th ed., pp. 21–28). Routledge.

Boone, D. (2020). Prosthetists and orthotists: An evolution from mechanic to clinician. *Prosthetics and Orthotics International, 44*(6), 368–372.

Centers for Medicare & Medicaid Services. (n.d.). *Medicare fee for service recovery audit program*. Centers for Medicare & Medicaid Services. www.cms.gov/Research-Statistics-Data-and-Systems/Monitoring-Programs/Medicare-FFS-Compliance-Programs/Recovery-Audit-Program

Clarke, L., Puli, L., Ridgewell, E., Dillon, M. P., & Anderson, S. (2021). Regulation of the global orthotist/prosthetist workforce, and what we might learn from allied health professions with international-level regulatory support: A narrative review. *Human Resources for Health, 19*(1), 1–14.

de Laat, F. A., van Heerebeek, B., & van Netten, J. J. (2019). Advantages and disadvantages of interdisciplinary consultation in the prescription of assistive technologies for mobility limitations. *Disability and Rehabilitation: Assistive Technology, 14*(4), 386–390.

Department of Veterans Affairs, Office of Audits and Evaluations, Office of Inspector General. (2018). *Use of not otherwise classified codes for prosthetic limb components*. Author. https://www.va.gov/oig/pubs/VAOIG-16-01913-223.pdf

Department of Veterans Affairs/Department of Defense (2017). *VA/DoD clinical practice guideline for rehabilitation of individuals with lower limb amputation*. www.healthquality.va.gov/guidelines/rehab/amp/index.asp

Dillon, M. P., Major, M. J., Kaluf, B., Balasanov, Y., & Fatone, S. (2018). Predict the Medicare Functional Classification Level (K-level) using the Amputee Mobility Predictor in people with unilateral transfemoral and transtibial amputation: A pilot study. *Prosthetics and Orthotics International, 42*(2), 191–197.

Donaghy, A. C., Morgan, S. J., Kaufman, G. E., & Morgenroth, D. C. (2020). Team approach to prosthetic prescription decision-making. *Current Physical Medicine and Rehabilitation Reports, 8*(4), 386–395.

Etchegaray, J. M., Krull, H., Holliday, S. B., Xenakis, L., Rostker, B. D., Beyene, N. M., & Clague, A. (2019). *Core competencies for amputation rehabilitation*. Rand Arroyo Center.

Fairley, M. (2010, June). Expert witness in litigation, life care planning: Should this be part of your practice? *The O&P Edge*. www.oandp.com/articles/2010-06_01.asp

Gailey, R., Allen, K., Castles, J., Kucharik, J., & Roeder, M. (2008). Review of secondary physical conditions associated with lower-limb amputation and long-term prosthesis use. *Journal of Rehabilitation Research & Development, 45*(1), 15–29.

Grimm. (2021). Medicare improperly paid supplier an estimated $117 million over 4 years for durable medical equipment, prosthetics, orthotics, and supplies provided to hospice beneficiaries. Department of Health and Human Services. https://oig.hhs.gov/oas/reports/region9/92003026.pdf

Johnson, C. B., Pomeranz, J. L., & Stetten, N. E. (2018). Consensus and majority statements derived from Life Care Planning Summits held in 2000, 2002, 2004, 2006, 2008, 2010, 2012, 2015 and 2017 and updated via Delphi study in 2018. *Journal of Life Care Planning, 16*(4), 5–13.

Keszler, M. S., Wright, K. S., Miranda, A., & Hopkins, M. S. (2020). Multidisciplinary amputation team management of individuals with limb loss. *Current Physical Medicine and Rehabilitation Reports, 8*(3), 118–126.

Kulkarni, J. (2010). Ethical and medico-legal issues in amputee prosthetic rehabilitation. In C. Murray (Ed.), *Amputation, prosthesis use, and phantom limb pain*. (pp. 23–31). Springer. https://doi.org/10.1007/978-0-387-87462-3_3

Latour, D. (2022). Advances in upper extremity prosthetic technology: Rehabilitation and the interprofessional team. *Current Physical Medicine and Rehabilitation Reports*, 1–6.

Levinson. (2011). *Questionable billing by suppliers of lower limb prostheses*. Department of Health & Human Services. https://oig.hhs.gov/oei/reports/oei-02-10-00170.pdf

Mackenzie, R. L., Morris, M. E., Murphy, G., & Hodge, M. C. (2018). The prosthetist role expectations scale: Development and initial validation of a scale for clinical settings. *Prosthetics and Orthotics International, 42*(2), 171–178.

Mamuya, E., Hoover, R. D. Jr., Brennan, S. V., & Gurk, P. J. (2016). *Documentation of artificial limbs.* www.cgsmedicare.com/jb/mr/pdf/dear_physician_artificial_limbs.pdf

O'Brien, E., Stevens, P. M., Mandacina, S., & Jackman, C. (2021). Prosthetic management of unilateral transradial amputation and limb deficiency: Consensus clinical standards of care. *Journal of Rehabilitation and Assistive Technologies Engineering, 8,* 20556683211065262.

Orthotics Prosthetics Canada. (n.d.). *Certification pathway.* https://opcanada.ca/OPC-Member/02_The-Profession-Section/Profession-Overview.aspx?New_ContentCollectionOrganizerCommon=3&54c5d5ba1599=2#54c5d5ba1599

Pasquina, P. F., Miller, M., Carvalho, A. J., Corcoran, M., Vandersea, J., Johnson, E., & Chen, Y. T. (2014). Special considerations for multiple limb amputation. *Current Physical Medicine and Rehabilitation Reports, 2*(4), 273–289.

Pettengill, A., & Pettengill, C. (2020). Know your prosthetist. *Journal of Nurse Life Care Planning, 20*(2), 14–20.

Preston, K., & Johnson, C. (2012). Consensus and majority statements derived from Life Care Planning Summits held in 2000, 2002, 2004, 2006, 2008, 2010 and 2012. *Journal of Life Care Planning, 11*(2), 9–14.

Rimmer, R., & Caruso, D. M. (2011). Life care planning for the pediatric burn patient. In S. Riddick-Grisham & L. M. Deming (Eds.), *Pediatric life care planning and case management* (2nd ed., pp. 581–606). Routledge.

Steeper Group. (n.d.). *Prosthetic best practice guidelines.* www.steepergroup.com/SteeperGroup/media/SteeperGroupMedia/Additional%20Downloads/Steeper-Prosthetic-Best-Practice-Guidelines.pdf

Stevens, P. M., Rheinstein, J., & Wurdeman, S. R. (2018). Prosthetic foot selection for individuals with lower-limb amputation: A clinical practice guideline. *Journal of Prosthetics and Orthotics, 30*(4), 175.

Stevens, P. M., & Wurdeman, S. R. (2019). Prosthetic knee selection for individuals with unilateral transfemoral amputation: A clinical practice guideline. *Journal of Prosthetics and Orthotics, 31*(1), 2.

Stevens, P. M., DePalma, R. R., & Wurdeman, S. R. (2019). Transtibial socket design, interface, and suspension: A clinical practice guideline. *JPO: Journal of Prosthetics and Orthotics, 31*(3), 172–178.

Supan, T. J. (2022). The role of an O&P expert witness. *The O&P Edge Magazine, 21*(3), 58–64.

U.S. Congress. (1934). United States code: Social Security Act, 42 U.S.C. §§ 301- Suppl. 4 www.loc.gov/item/uscode1934-005042007/

U.S. Department of Labor, Bureau of Labor Statistics. (2022). Orthotists and prosthetists. *Occupational outlook handbook.* www.bls.gov/ooh/healthcare/orthotists-and-prosthetists.htm

Weed, R. (1992). Orthotist and prosthetist roles in life care plans. *Orthotist & Prosthetist Business News, 1*(4).

Weed, R. O. (2001). Contemporary life care planning for the amputee. *Orthotics and Prosthetics Business News, 10*(23), 20–30.

Weed, R. O. (2019). A brief history of life care planning. *Journal of Life Care Planning, 17*(3), 5–14.

World Health Organization. (2017). *WHO standards for prosthetics and orthotics.* Author. https://www.who.int/publications-detail-redirect/9789241512480

Chapter 18

The Role of the Economist in Life Care Planning

Frederick A. Raffa and Matthew B. Raffa

Economics is the study of scarcity and choice. It is a social science that studies how best to use limited resources (e.g., land, labor, and capital) given unlimited wants, needs, and desires. Economics is an integral part of our lives. Whether we are consciously aware of the forces of supply (and all aspects of production and distribution of goods and services) and the forces of demand (or the consumption of goods and services), we are constantly impacted by the interaction of these primal economic forces. The interaction of supply and demand in a market economy serves to establish prices and the market value of goods and services. These market values influence the choices that we make and determine in large part the level of want satisfaction that we experience as consumers.

A forensic economist will have an advanced degree (i.e., MS, MBA, or PhD) in Economics (or possibly in accounting or finance). Some will have a background in academia (as a college professor) while others will have spent years working as an economic consultant.

There is no licensure or certification required to work as a forensic economist. In addition to an advanced degree, they will need years of experience. Some will gain that experience through research projects at universities, while other will find employment with an economic consulting firm.

In life care planning, the life care planner, in collaboration with healthcare professionals, provides the forensic economist with the foundation from which a present value lifetime needs assessment can be undertaken. For example, assume that the life care planner, using the protocols for life care planning, has determined that an injured 50-year-old non-Hispanic white male needs to follow-up with a physiatrist each year for the rest of his life. Moreover, by researching the prices charged by such providers, the life care planner has determined that the current cost is $200 per visit. Using the 2019 United States Life Tables (National Center for Health Statistics, 2022), the economist determines that the individual in question has a remaining life expectancy of 29.9 years.

Given that inflation must be considered in determining the future cost of this care, the economist will examine historical data specific to the cost of physician services (published as part of the U.S. Department of Labor's Consumer Price Index, n.d.) to determine that an annual inflation adjustment equal to 2.89% per year should be incorporated into the calculation of the future cost of follow-up visits to a physician. In turn, once a projection of the future annual costs associated with the future follow-up care by a physician has been accomplished, the economist must adjust the future cost of these physician services for the ability to invest money today in an interest-bearing account such that the amount invested plus the interest earned would be used to pay for the future follow-up care by a physician. Based on current after-tax yields on U.S. Treasury Bonds (ranging from 0.79% to 2.01%), the present value or the present amount of financial funding that would be needed today to fund the future follow-up physician care, is calculated to be $6,826.

This hypothetical present value assessment of the cost of future physician services illustrates an important example of perhaps what not to do in evaluating the present value of future care needs identified in a life care plan. Many life care planners, likely in an effort to facilitate the attorney's understanding of the potential value of the life care needs' claim, include in their reports a summary of the future life care needs wherein they multiply the current cost by the future time period over which the care plan item will be needed. In this example, the $200 per year would be multiplied by the remaining life expectancy of 30 years and the life care planner's "summary" would show the cost of future follow-up care by a physician as having a present value of $6,000. As demonstrated in this hypothetical evaluation, the "multiplication method" understates the true present value by $826.

The Life Care Plan as a Predicate for Future Economic Losses

Any present value analysis of the future cost of care required by an injured individual must begin with a precise assessment of the items of future care that will be required to facilitate the injured individual's rehabilitation and recovery. This means that a life care plan must contain a precise list of the medical and rehabilitative items that will be required by the injured individual, together with the cost specific to each of the care plan's goods or services, as well as the specific time frame and frequency over which the care plan goods or services will be needed.

Most economists create a spreadsheet in which they undertake a present value analysis of each item in a life care plan. It is important that each item of future care is clearly identified, so that the proper inflation rate can be established. For example, the inflation rate for physicians' services is different (higher) than the inflation rate for physical therapy treatments. The inflation rate for prescription drugs is different (higher) than the inflation rate for nonprescription or over-the-counter drugs. The same can be said for nursing care and home health aide services. If there is a medical procedure in which there is a surgical facility required, a physician to perform the procedure, a nurse to assist the physician, and perhaps post-procedure physical therapy required, there would potentially be four separate inflation rates to be considered.

The life care plan is the source for the current cost of each item of care. Since most economists have at best a cursory understanding of medical cost billing, they are relying on the care planner and the life care plan to determine the cost of each item of need. Economists evaluate the present value of an individual's care needs on an annual cost basis. This means that it is imperative that the life care plan permit the identification and/or specification of an annual cost for each distinct life care plan item. In some cases, the life care planner will cite a need that is to be fulfilled as a single event each year. The life care planner in this case will obviously quote the cost of this care plan item on an annual cost basis. For example, the life care plan may project an annual follow-up visit with a physician with the cost of the annual follow-up care as $200.

In other care plans, we might see the life care planner call for two to four visits a year at a cost of $200 per visit. In the first example, the annual cost is clearly $200, while in the second example, the annual cost would be based on an average of three visits per year (the mid-point of the range given by the life care planner) at a cost of $200 per visit or an annual cost of $600. In other cases, the life care planner will specify an initial need of perhaps two to four physician visits per year for the first five years, to be followed by one-time annual visits for the balance of the individual's remaining life expectancy. An economist will always seek to analyze each year's need, based on the cost and frequency of need per annum.

The life care plan must also provide precise information about the frequency of need. This frequency of need may vary over an injured individual's life expectancy and the specific date at which the frequency is anticipated to change must be identified. For example, the follow-up care by a physician may begin as an annual need; however, based upon the successful utilization of the treatment modalities prescribed in the life care plan, the follow-up care may go from requiring annual care initially and for the first five-year period, to perhaps every other year or even every three years, beginning with year six. Often, a change in the frequency of need may occur after a surgical event, which alters the level of function and, in turn, the frequency of care. Certain equipment needs will have an expected replacement schedule that may require the purchase of new equipment every five years. Where there is an annual maintenance schedule attached to the equipment in question, the economist must know if the maintenance is suspended or omitted during the year that the new equipment is purchased or if the maintenance is required every year, regardless.

The last essential element to the economist's analysis is the time frame of need. In certain care plans, there is a treatment schedule that is expected to accomplish certain rehabilitation needs and as such has a specific time frame identified by the life care planner. For example, a prosthetic package need may be initially identified for an amputee as a K2 ambulator. With a program of physical therapy over say three to five years (typically interpreted as a four-year time frame) it is anticipated that the plaintiff amputee will progress to a prosthetic package for a K3 ambulator. Thus, the economist will be relying on the care planner to provide both the initial time frame and frequency for the K2 ambulator package, the likely time frame for the change from the K2 to the K3 ambulator package, as well as the costs associated with both the K2 and K3 ambulator packages. In many cases, the care plan items will have been assigned a specific time frame over which a particular item will be needed, such as 5 years, 10 years, 20 years, etc.

In most life care plans, there will be items for which the need is expected to be lifetime in nature. In these cases, the economist will adopt the standard life expectancy table called for by statute if there is one, or a standard adopted by many states, and which is deemed to be admissible under "Self-authentication" in Federal Court, known as the *United States Life Tables*. The latest *United States Life Tables*, based on the United States mortality experience in 2019, were published on March 22, 2022 (National Center for Health Statistics, 2022). The *United States Life Tables* provide cumulative statistical probabilities of living, based on the age, race, and gender of the injured plaintiff. The *United States Life Tables* are a compilation of the mortality experience in the United States, taken from death certificates that by law are required to be completed upon the death of an individual. The current *United States Life Tables* provide cumulative probabilities of living for males and females; Hispanic males and Hispanic females; for non-Hispanic black males and non-Hispanic black females; for non-Hispanic white males and non-Hispanic white females; and for non-Hispanic Asian males and non-Hispanic Asian females. The *United States Life Tables* can be found at www.cdc.gov/nchs/products/index.htm

In certain catastrophic injury cases, there may be medical testimony offered about the probable remaining life expectancy of the specific plaintiff. Where unanimity about the remaining life expectancy of an injured plaintiff is typically lacking between medical experts, the economist may be asked to evaluate the present value of the injured plaintiff's life care needs using alternative life expectancies.

Present Value Analysis of Plaintiff's Future Life Care Needs

With a life care plan in hand, and with all clarification questions asked by the economist and answered by the care planner, the economist must make essentially two adjustments to arrive at a present value determination of the future life care needs of an injured plaintiff. While the life care plan provides a detailed analysis of the program of care and the cost of the future care required by the injured plaintiff in today's prices, the need for care is likely to exist for much of the remaining life expectancy of the injured plaintiff. Thus, the first issue that an economist must contend with is the matter of establishing the likely rate of inflation or the anticipated rate at which the current life care plan prices are going to increase as the needs of the injured plaintiff move from today to tomorrow and to the many days over the remaining life expectancy of the injured plaintiff. Thus, once a life care plan is in hand, the economist must begin an analysis of the inflation rates that will be used to project the future cost of the life care needs of the injured plaintiff.

Inflation/Growth Rate

Most economists make use of the U.S. Department of Labor's Consumer Price Index or CPI. The CPI-U reports the price changes experienced by approximately 93% of the United States population. Using data obtained by the U.S. Department of Labor's 2021 Consumer Expenditure Survey (U.S. Department of Labor, Bureau of Labor Statistics, 2021) to establish the weights for each CPI item, the U.S. Department of Labor surveys prices for over 8,000 categories of goods and services that are combined into almost 300 individual price categories that fall within eight principal inflation categories, including food and beverages, housing, apparel, transportation, medical care, recreation, education, and communication. The categories used by most economists, include the CPI categories that are summarized in Table 18.1.

Table 18.1 Categories Used by Most Economists

Inflation/ Growth Rates	CPI Component	Data Range
0.39%	New Vehicles	1990–2021
0.63%	Personal Care Products	1990–2021
0.64%	Nonprescription Drugs/	2009–2021/
	Internal and Respiratory Over-the-Counter Drugs	1990–2008
0.75%	Medical Equipment and Supplies/	2009–2021/
	Nonprescription Medical Equipment and Supplies	1990–2008
1.56%	Eyeglasses and Eye Care	1990–2021
1.80%	Vehicle Parts and Equipment	1990–2021
2.03%	Private Transportation	1990–2021
2.13%	Lodging Away from Home Including Hotels & Motels	1990–2021

(Continued)

Table 18.1 (Continued) Categories Used by Most Economists

Inflation/ Growth Rates	CPI Component	Data Range
2.17%	Care of Invalids and Elderly at Home	1998–2021
2.29%	All Items	1990–2021
2.33%	Services by Other Medical Professionals	1990–2021
2.38%	Domestic Services	1997–2021
2.46%	Food	1990–2021
2.72%	Shelter	1990–2021
2.74%	Medical Care Commodities	1990–2021
2.80%	Pets, Pet Products and Services	1997–2021
2.88%	Motor Vehicle Maintenance and Repair	1990–2021
2.89%	Physicians' Services	1990–2021
2.96%	Household Operations	1997–2021
3.03%	Fuels and Utilities	1990–2021
3.16%	Health Insurance	2005–2021
3.22%	Gardening and Lawncare Services	1997–2021
3.29%	Financial Services	1990–2021
3.52%	Prescription Drugs	1990–2021
3.67%	Average of Services by Other Medical Professionals & Physicians' Services & Hospital Services	1990–2021 & 1990–2021 & 1996–2021
3.78%	Nursing Homes and Adult Day Services	1996–2021
3.80%	Legal Services	1990–2021
3.96%	Dental Services	1990–2021
4.35%	Average of Hospital Services & Physicians' Services	1996–2021 & 1990–2021
4.48%	Repair of Household Items	1997–2021
4.67%	Education	1997–2021
5.80%	Hospital Services	1996–2021

Source: Consumer Price Index, U.S. Department of Labor, Bureau of Labor Statistics.

Using the past three business cycles, ranging from 1990 through 2021, the rates of increase in the prices of the goods and services most likely to be found in a life care plan are listed in the above inflation rate summary. For example, if the life care plan calls for various therapies, the economist would likely use the inflation rate for Services by Other Medical Professionals, or 2.33%. If the plan calls for follow-up by a physician, the economist will likely use the CPI category of Physicians' Services or 2.89%.

The selection of the historic time frame for examining the itemized rates of inflation is based in part on the economist's perception of the current state of the economy. Until the inflation experience of 2021 emerged from the U.S. Department of Labor's monthly price surveys beginning mid-year, there were a number of economists who were of the opinion that inflation had been brought under control by increased productivity, such that the ten-year period of relatively low levels of inflation for 2010 through 2020 were suggestive of the rates of inflation that should be anticipated going forward in time. Table 18.1 contains a summary of inflation or growth rate expectations based on an historical time frame of 1990–2021. In general, economists who were of the opinion that inflation was under control would have relied on the 2010–2020 inflation rates; while those who were of the opinion that inflation was still an issue to be dealt with would have relied on the 1990–2021 inflation rates, i.e., incorporating three complete business cycles. Until the current surge in inflation brought about by supply shortages and increased labor costs (sometimes referred to as cost-push inflation) has been brought under control, most economists appear to be relying on historical price level data taken from either the 2000–2020 or 1990–2020/2021 historic time frames.

Once the economist receives the life care plan, the work initially focuses on reviewing the time frames and frequencies (and inquiring of the care planner if there are any questions) and then identifying the appropriate inflation rate for each of the goods and/or services that comprise the life care plan. Indeed, many economists use matrix formatted care plans as a worksheet and place the inflation rates for each item in or adjacent to the matrix boxes containing the itemized cost of care and will always be looking for any notes or information that should be considered in the evaluation by the economist. Often, these "notes" will explain that a particular item of equipment was originally purchased three years ago and will need to be replaced every five years going forward in time. This type of notation allows the economist to begin the analysis of this item in two years from the present and, once begun, provide for the replacement of the equipment on a five-year cycle. As always, the costs included in the life care plan are the marginal or additional costs that will be incurred by the injured plaintiff over and above what might considered a "normal" purchase. Any item for which the life care plan notation states that the item is "if needed" or "as needed" will be omitted by the economist, due to the lack of specificity and the lack of a statement of probability.

With a life care plan in hand, and with inflation rates identified for each item in the life care plan, the economist can forecast of the future value or future cost of the care needs of the plaintiff. After projecting the annual cost of the future care needs of the plaintiff, the economist must adjust the projected future values for the ability to invest a smaller sum of money today and allow the current investment to earn interest, so that the plaintiff will be able to purchase every item in the life care plan at the projected future cost, leaving a zero balance in the investment account as of the end of the plaintiff's statistical life expectancy. This last step in the analysis is often referred to as "reduction to present value."

Interest/Discount Rate

The essential ingredient in the reduction to present value process is the establishment of an interest rate that can be earned on a sum of money invested today and from which withdrawals will be made using both the invested funds and the interest earned on the investment account. By following exactly the guidance and direction of the life care plan, the plaintiff should be able to fund the cost of all future care needs and will have a zero balance left in the investment account at the end of the statistical life expectancy of the plaintiff. There are numerous investment alternatives but in 1983, the U.S. Supreme Court in a case styled as *Jones and Laughlin Steel vs. Pfeifer* (143 S. Ct. 241, 1983) stated that the discount rate should be based on the rate of interest that would be earned on "the best and safest investments" (p. 491). The Court also stated that "the discount rate should also represent the after-tax rate of return" (p. 462 U.S. 523). Following the ruling of the Court, there is only one investment that meets the criteria of "safest and best" and that is the U.S. Treasury Bond. Each month, the Board of Governors of the Federal Reserve System (2022) publishes the monthly yields on U.S. Treasury Bonds with maturities of 1, 2, 3, 5, 7, 10, 20, and 30 years. Given the month-to-month variability of yields on U.S. Treasury Bonds due to money moving into and out of either the bond or the equities markets, which is unrelated to expectations as concerns long-term inflation rates, most economists use an average of these yields to essentially smooth the series of yields and to capture the long-term inflation expectations of the market. Table 18.2 provides a

Table 18.2 Summary of the Yields on U.S. Treasury Bonds from November 2021 to April 2022

Year	Discount rate
2022	0.79%
2023	1.21%
2024	1.42%
2025	1.51%
2026	1.60%
2027	1.66%
2028	1.71%
2029	1.72%
2030	1.73%
2031	1.74%
2032	1.77%
2033	1.81%
2034	1.84%
2035	1.87%

(*Continued*)

Table 18.2 (Continued) Summary of the Yields on U.S. Treasury Bonds from November 2021 to April 2022

Year	Discount rate
2036	1.91%
2037	1.94%
2038	1.98%
2039	2.01%
2040	2.04%
2041	2.08%
2042	2.07%
2043	2.06%
2044	2.06%
2045	2.05%
2046	2.04%
2047	2.04%
2048	2.03%
2049	2.02%
2050	2.01%
2051	2.01%
2052	2.01%

summary of the yields on U.S. Treasury Bonds, using a six-month look back from April 2022 to November 2021. Bond yields for which the Federal Reserve does not publish a specific yield are estimated by interpolation using yields that are available. For example, we have a three-year and a five-year U.S. Treasury Bond yield but lack a four-year yield. Using an average of the yield on the three-year bond and the five-year bond, we can estimate the yield on a four-year bond by taking a simple average. In addition, a conservative 10% tax rate has been applied to conform to the Supreme Court's after-tax requirement as concerns the interest/discount rate used to reduce future values to a present value equivalent.

In Table 18.2, we observe that the yield summary stops at the 30-year bond or the year 2052. This reflects that the U.S. Treasury does not borrow money (and sell bonds) beyond a 30-year maturity. Since we have no accurate way to predict interest rates beyond the 30-year maturity, most economists use the 30-year maturity bond to discount all future costs that are 30 or more years into the future.

Exemplar Present Value Analysis

Plaintiff John Doe was a 57.27 year old white male at the time of his February 6, 2020 motor vehicle accident. As a result of the accident in question, Mr. Doe sustained back and neck injuries. As of a May 9, 2022 trial date, Mr. Doe will be 59.52 years of age with a statistical average remaining life expectancy of 22.08 years, which equates to a maximum age of 81.60 years.

A basic 20-item life care plan was developed to address Mr. Doe's rehabilitation and medical care needs. An economist was retained to undertake a present value analysis of the future cost of the plaintiff's care. The life care plan in question is available in Table 18.3. Using inflation/growth rates reflecting the 1990–2021 rate of increase in the cost of the individual life care items, the economist determined that the future cost of care totaled $603,456 (see Table 18.4). Finally, using

Table 18.3 Life Care Plan for Mr. Doe

Life Care Plan: Orthopedic Injuries from Motor Vehicle Accident			
Category/Need	Period Over Which Services Provided	Frequency	Cost
Medical Care			
Orthopedic Spine Surgeon	Life	1x/Year for the Next 5yrs	$200–800/Visit
Physiatrist	Life	2–6 Visits/Year	$50–200/Visit
MRI Scan—Cervical	Life	1x Every 5–10 Years	$325–400/Scan
MRI Scan—Lumbar	Life	1x Every 5–10 Years	$325–400/Scan
Therapy			
Physical Therapist Evaluation	Life	2 Visits/Year	$100/Visit
Physical Therapy Treatments	Life	24 Visits/Year	$190–275/Visit
Trigger Point Injections			
Trigger Point Injections	Life	1–10x/Year—Cervical	$150/Injection

(Continued)

Table 18.3 (Continued) Life Care Plan for Mr. Doe

Life Care Plan: Orthopedic Injuries from Motor Vehicle Accident			
Category/Need	Period Over Which Services Provided	Frequency	Cost
Trigger Point Injections	Life	1–10x/Year—Lumber	$150/Injection
Epidural Steroid Injections			
Epidural Steroid Injections	Life	9x/Life—Cervical	$2,000–3,000/Injection
Epidural Steroid Injections	Life	9x/Life—Lumber	$2,000–3,000/Injection
Surgical Needs			
Conversion of Disc to Fusion	Life	1x	$80,000–100,000
Lumber Spinal Fusion	Life	1x	$100,000–150,000
Arthroscopic Hip Repair	Life	1x	$20,000–30,000
Rehabilitation			
Physical Therapy Evaluation	Life	1 Visit After Each Surgery	$100/Visit
Postoperative Protocol	Life	5 Days/Week for 16–20 Weeks After Each Surgery	$190–275/Day
Medications			
Ultracet	Life	2 Pills/Day for 4 Months/Year @ $15 for 60 Pills	$60.88 Per Year

Table 18.4 Economist's Present Value Table

Summary of the Present Value Analysis of the Cost of Future life Care Needs of Mr. John Doe

Category	Start Date	Age	End Date	Age	Freq	Base Amount	Base Year	Growth Rate	Future Value	Present Value
Cost of Medical Care										
Orthopedic Surgeon	05.09.22	59.52	05.09.26	63.52	1 year	$500.00	2022	2.89%	$2,648	$2,584
Physiatrist	05.09.22	59.52	06.08.44	81.60	Annual	$500.00	2022	2.89%	$15,314	$12,450
MRI—Cervical	05.09.22	59.52	06.08.44	81.60	8 years	$362.50	2022	3.67%	$1,492	$1,275
MRI—Lumbar	05.09.22	59.52	06.08.44	81.60	8 years	$362.50	2022	3.67%	$1,492	$1,275
Total Cost of Medical Care									**$20,946**	**$17,584**
Cost of Therapy										
Physical Therapy Evals	05.09.22	59.52	06.08.44	81.60	Annual	$200.00	2022	2.33%	$5,739	$4,687
Physical Therapy Treatments	05.09.22	59.52	06.08.44	81.60	Annual	$5,580.00	2022	2.33%	$160,112	$130,764
Total Cost of Therapy									**$165,851**	**$135,451**
Cost of Trigger Point Injections										
Cervical	05.09.22	59.52	06.08.44	81.60	Annual	$825.00	2022	2.91%	$25,326	$20,588
Lumbar	05.09.22	59.52	06.08.44	81.60	Annual	$825.00	2022	2.91%	$25,326	$20,588
Total Cost of Trigger Point Injections									**$50,652**	**$41,176**
Cost of Epidural Steroid Injections										
Cervical	05.09.22	59.52	11.01.39	77.00	2 years	$2,500.00	2022	3.64%	$30,462	$26,386
Lumbar	05.09.22	59.52	11.01.39	77.00	2 years	$2,500.00	2022	3.64%	$30,462	$26,386

(Continued)

Table 18.4 (Continued) Economist's Present Value Table

Summary of the Present Value Analysis of the Cost of Future life Care Needs of Mr. John Doe

Category	Start Date	Age	End Date	Age	Freq	Base Amount	Base Year	Growth Rate	Future Value	Present Value
Total Cost of Epidural Steroid Injections									**$60,924**	**$52,772**
Cost of Surgical Needs										
Conversion Disc to Fusion	05.09.22	59.52	05.09.22	59.52	Onetime	$90,000.00	2022	0.00%	$90,000	$90,000
Lumbar Spinal Fusion	05.09.22	59.52	05.09.22	59.52	Onetime	$125,000.00	2022	0.00%	$125,000	$125,000
Arthroscopic Repair Hip	05.09.22	59.52	05.09.22	59.52	Onetime	$25,000.00	2022	0.00%	$25,000	$25,000
Total Cost of Surgical Needs									**$240,000**	**$240,000**
Cost of Rehabilitation										
PT Eval—Conversion to Fusion	05.09.22	59.52	05.09.22	59.52	Onetime	$100.00	2022	0.00%	$100	$100
PT Eval—Microdiscectomy/Fusion	05.09.22	59.52	05.09.22	59.52	Onetime	$100.00	2022	0.00%	$100	$100
PT Eval-Arthroscopic Repair Hip	05.09.22	59.52	05.09.22	59.52	Onetime	$100.00	2022	0.00%	$100	$100
Protocol—Conversion to Fusion	05.09.22	59.52	05.09.22	59.52	Onetime	$20,925.00	2022	0.00%	$20,925	$20,925
Protocol—Microdiscectomy/Fusion	05.09.22	59.52	05.09.22	59.52	Onetime	$20,925.00	2022	0.00%	$20,925	$20,925

(Continued)

Table 18.4 (Continued) Economist's Present Value Table

Summary of the Present Value Analysis of the Cost of Future life Care Needs of Mr. John Doe

Category	Start Date	Age	End Date	Age	Freq	Base Amount	Base Year	Growth Rate	Future Value	Present Value
Protocol—Arthroscopic Repair Hip	05.09.22	59.52	05.09.22	59.52	Onetime	$20,925.00	2022	0.00%	$20,925	$20,925
Total Cost of Rehabilitation									**$63,075**	**$63,075**
Cost Of Medications										
Ultracet	05.09.22	59.52	06.08.44	81.60	Annual	$60.88	2022	3.52%	$2,008	$1,623
Total Cost Of Medications									**$2,008**	**$1,623**
Life Care Plan Totals									**$603,456**	**$551,681**

after-tax yields on U.S. Treasury Bonds covering the plaintiff's 22-year remaining life expectancy (see Table 18.2), the present value of Mr. Doe's future care needs is calculated to be $551,681 (see Table 18.4).

Table 18.4 reflects the blending of the expertise of the life care planner and the economist. The start date will usually be tied to the trial date and the first age reference is to the plaintiff's age as of the trial date. The second age reference is to the plaintiff's age as of the end of the time period for which the life care item is to be provided. In the Doe case, where we see 81.60, we would be observing the plaintiff's age as of the end of his statistical life expectancy.

Moving from left to right, we observe the information provided in the life care plan being used to calculate the present value of each life care plan item. The very first item, follow-up by an orthopedic surgeon, is to be provided once now and once per year for each future year, for a total of five visits over five years. The life care plan (Table 18.3) indicates that the cost of this orthopedic surgeon follow-up will range from $200 to $800 per visit. Lacking an indication that one price is more likely than the other, the economist will take an average of the two prices (as our market economy will do over time) to obtain a price of $500 per visit.

Since the item of need is to be provided by a physician, we will need to apply an inflation rate reflecting the market increases in the price of physician services. Reviewing the available data from the U.S. Department of Labor's CPI, we observe that the category which reflects the rate of increase in the price of a doctor visit is the CPI category of physician services. Reviewing Table 18.1, we find that over the past three business cycles, the rate of inflation for physician services is 2.89%. Applying a 2.89% inflation rate to the base cost or base amount of $500, we obtain $2,648 as the future value of the cost of orthopedic surgeon follow-up care for Mr. Doe.

Finally, applying a series of interest rates or yields on U.S. Treasury Bonds ranging from one to five years of maturity (0.79% to 1.60%, per Table 18.2) we obtain $2,584 as the present value of the cost of orthopedic surgeon follow-up required by Mr. Doe.

We notice that in this basic 20-item life care plan, the economist has followed several different time frames, and has used five different inflation rates to prepare an item-by-item analysis. It is important that the life care plan be evaluated by the economist on an item-by-item basis, as Table 18.4 will potentially be presented to a jury who will weigh the appropriateness of the individual plan items and possibly adjust their opinions accordingly.

Conclusion

Economists rely upon the life care planner to provide a precise listing of the goods and services required to maximize the functioning of an injured individual over time. The specific costs, frequencies, and durations must be provided in order for the economist to apply the appropriate inflation/growth rate and to reduce the projected cost to a present value equivalent. To help facilitate this relationship and avoid annoying phone calls from frustrated economists, it is worth remembering the following:

- Different items and services have different growth rates. For example, a *catheter* falls under "Medical Equipment and Supplies" while *skin lotion* falls under "Personal Care Products." Rather than put both of those items into a generic "Supplies" category, place them into a relevant category with similar items.
- Another example of this is medications. Please specify if a medication is prescription or nonprescription. Save us a trip to Google. Or, better yet, put all prescription medications under a prescription category. Same for nonprescription.

- Avoid using script symbols (TID or BID). Likewise, avoid making the economist determine how many puffs are in 100 ml for a nebulizer. We are not pharmacists. Rather, provide the appropriate frequency along with the relevant cost or better yet provide the annual cost.
- Some life care planners use "through" and some use "to" and some use them interchangeably without alerting the economist. For example, if an item is needed until age 18, some life care planners will write "Now–17" (meaning through age 17 or to age 18); other life care planners write "Now–18" (meaning to age 18); while some do both in the same plan. Please pick one or the other and stick to it.
- Be specific when listing prices (as in "per visit" or "per day" or "per month" or "per item" or "per year"). For example, assume a plan says "*grab bars (2x)*" are needed at a cost of $250. Is that $250 per grab bar or $250 for both?
- Keeping in mind that all costs posted to a life care plan should be costs specific to the injury at hand, it should be noted that in certain cases this may involve identifying the marginal or incremental/additional cost associated with a life care plan item. For example, if a particular prescription medication, already being taken by the plaintiff, is prescribed at a higher dosage by a physician, the life care plan needs to be specific as to the incremental or marginal cost of the medication so as to not overstate the life care needs that are specific to the incident at issue.
- Similar issues present themselves when a handicap equipped van is called for in the life care plan. If this vehicle is for a specific need or used by the injured party, the van may be an additional family vehicle without any type of offset for the family automobile that most families own. However, if the van is to be used as the family's principal vehicle, the life care planner should specify whether the economist is to offset the cost of the handicap equipped vehicle by the cost of a traditional family four door sedan. This same matter is at issue when a life care plan calls for handicap modified home—should there be an offset using the value of the injured party's currently owned home? In most cases the life care planner will instruct the economist as to what adjustment is appropriate with regards to include the new home.
- When updating a life care plan, it is helpful to identify for the economist the changes that were made. Some life care plans have hundreds of items on almost as many pages. You can save the economist a lot of time by saying, "We changed the cost of the wheelchair on p. 45." Or, if you updated all the costs just say that. The more specific the better.

References

Board of Governors of the Federal Reserve System. (2022). *H.15 Selected interest rates*. Economic Research & Data. Statistical Releases and Historical Data. www.federalreserve.gov/releases/h15/current/default.htm

Jones & Laughlin Steel Corp. v. Pfeifer, 462 U.S. 523 (1983). https://supreme.justia.com/cases/federal/us/462/523/

National Center for Health Statistics, National Vital Statistics Systems. (2022). *United States life tables, 2019* (National Vital Statistics Reports, Vol. 70, No. 19). U.S. Department of Health and Human Resources, Centers for Disease Control and Prevention. www.cdc.gov/nchs/data/nvsr/nvsr70/nvsr70-19.pdf

U.S. Department of Labor, Bureau of Labor Statistics. (2021, December 2). *Consumer expenditure survey*. www.bls.gov/cex/tables.htm

U.S. Department of Labor, Bureau of Labor Statistics. (2022). *Consumer price index*. www.bls.gov/cpi/

SELECTED DIAGNOSES, FORENSIC, LEGAL, AND OTHER ISSUES 4

Chapter 19

Life Care Planning for the Patient with an Amputation

Robert H. Meier, Liesl Meier Rose, and Christian D. Meier

The physiatrist has been trained in the team approach to provide rehabilitative care to persons with simple and complex disabilities and is an excellent resource to provide rehabilitative care and determine appropriate equipment needs and how appropriate they may be, as a physician is usually required to prescribe equipment, including prosthetics. For the pediatric population, congenital or complications associated with diseases/or adverse reactions to medications, can be a source resulting in amputation (Meier, 2011). For the person with an amputation, the physiatrist should have the ability to provide meaningful information for the life care plan, especially in the following areas (Meier et al., 2013):

1. Adaptive equipment needs and costs
2. Architectural modifications for function
3. Attendant care hours and level of service
4. Costs of prosthetic devices
5. Expected functional outcomes
6. Frequency of prosthetic replacement
7. Future medical needs, potential medical problems and their treatment options
8. Future surgical needs
9. Life expectancy
10. Point of maximum medical improvement
11. Psychosocial needs
12. Quantity and types of rehabilitation services and their costs
13. Vocational and avocational expectations and modifications
14. Work restrictions

There is a network of local and national specialized physiatrists who have years of experience in working with the rehabilitation of specific areas of disability. These physiatric specialists can be located through the life care planner network. They should have extensive experience in providing healthcare for a person with an amputation, representing the level(s) specific for a particular case.

Demographics of Limb Amputation

Amputation varies in prevalence and incidence by limb, period over the lifespan, and also geography. Lower limb amputation in children, for example, including the indications, revisions, and complications is so different between locations to create research complications for inter-group comparisons (Horsch et al., 2022). In the United States, the Amputee Coalition reports that 507 people lose a limb daily, 185,000 experience an amputation annually, and 2.1 million are living with amputations (Amputee Collation, 2021). The Amputee Coalition (2021) further reports that the vast majority of amputees are male (69%), between the ages of 45–64 years (46%) and then 65–84 years (36%), have lower limb loss (65%), lost the limb due to vascular disease (54%), trauma (45%), or cancer (2%), and about one in three (36%) experience depression. In Canada, between 2006 and 2012, there were over 44,000 lower limb amputations with a mean patient age of 65.7 years, mostly male (68.8%), and about two in three amputations (65%) were due to diabetes (Imam et al., 2017).

Amputation of the leg is more common than amputation of the arm and occurs in a 3:1 ratio. The leg amputee is usually a person in the sixth or seventh decade of life who sustains the amputation because of occlusive arterial vascular disease. Often this person also has associated diabetes mellitus. In addition to vascular disease in the legs, there is often accompanying arterial disease in the coronary and cerebral arteries. With associated diabetes, the complications can include peripheral neuropathy, renal disease, and diminished eyesight. All of these comorbid factors can diminish the functional outcomes in prosthetic rehabilitation.

The arm amputee is usually a young man who has sustained a work-related injury. The amputation most frequently involves the right arm and most often results in a below-elbow amputation of the dominant arm. The arm amputee, unlike the leg amputee, can function independently with the use of one arm. Functional prosthetic restoration in the arm amputee is less successful than in the leg amputee.

Essential Differences Between Children and Adults with Amputations

A child is not a little adult. Most health professionals experienced in working with pediatric amputees understand that the principles of prosthetic fitting and rehabilitation for a child amputee are not those used in an adult amputee (Meier, 2011). For this reason, it is important that the prosthetist and rehabilitation team work with a significant number of pediatric amputees annually, and not just an occasional case of a child. Whenever possible, the pediatric amputee clinic at a large pediatric hospital should be used for prosthetic fitting and training. This type of setting is most likely to provide the experience necessary in working with pediatric amputees to assure the best type of prosthesis and the ideal functional outcome for the child and their family.

It is also essential to remember that the child with a congenital or acquired limb deficiency is not an ill or a sick child, unless there is another condition that fits this description. They may be physically challenged but are healthy in all aspects. The family should be encouraged to mainstream the child and treat them as any other member of the family or community.

The child who is born with a limb deficiency matures knowing only their body as it has been since birth and does not need to make a major life change in order to adapt to the limb loss (Meier & Atkins, 2004). This is less true for the child with an acquired amputation. However, there are times of difficulty for the congenitally limb-deficient child when other children may make fun of them, or as they reach adolescence and their limb difference becomes a concern as they begin to date.

A child who has a traumatic limb loss or amputation secondary to a tumor may benefit from short-term counseling to assist with the life adaptation as a new amputee. Most commonly, these formal sessions or even group therapy might require six to eight visits with a pediatric counselor.

The most common congenital limb deficiency is a left-sided below-elbow (transradial) amputation. In some cases, there may be a hereditary factor that caused the limb deficiency, or there may have been constricting bands present in the uterus that resulted in the limb alteration. On rare occasions, there may be an external agent or medication that could have caused the limb change.

Other causes of limb amputation in children are trauma, tumor, infection, and vascular etiologies. Vehicular accidents top the list for traumatic amputations in children. When a tumor is the cause of limb amputation, it is seen more often in the second decade of life. However, there are excellent limb salvage procedures in the presence of tumor, and often a limb can be spared and reconstructed without risking greater mortality, and without undergoing an extremity amputation (Setoguchi & Patton, 2004).

An infectious-related cause of amputation is seen in persons with systemic meningococcemia who require such large quantities of vasopressor medications over a sustained period of time that they develop gangrene in one or more extremities and ultimately require an amputation as a result. Also, the "flesh-eating" bacterium, streptococcus, can require extensive debridement to get rid of the involved tissues, and this may result in extremity amputation. Occasionally, frostbite or snakebite will lead to an extremity amputation. Neurofibromatosis and lymphangiomatosis may also require limb amputation to remove involved tissue and provide an extremity that might retain some functionality. In addition, some congenital limb anomalies of the arms and legs may lead to amputation because the functional outcome following amputation and prosthetic restoration can be superior to trying to salvage or reconstruct the anomalous anatomy. Burns, whether thermal or high voltage in etiology, may result in loss of one or more extremities. High-voltage electric injury often leads to loss of the arms with extensive soft tissue loss and the need for staged plastic surgical reconstruction.

One of the most significant differences in life care planning for the child amputee when contrasted with the adult amputee is the child's expected rate of growth and motor development (Horsch et al., 2022; Meier & Atkins, 2004; Patton, 1989). In the adult, there may be soft tissue shape and size changes, but the pediatric extremity changes in length and size, requiring frequent prosthetic socket and component changes when compared with the adult. As a general rule, the life care plan should account for a major prosthetic replacement, at least of the socket, every two years during the growth years until the child is 18 years old.

In the child with an arm deficiency, the components chosen and the system for their functional use are related to the child's developmental milestones and their physical size. However, with experience, it has become increasingly the practice to apply myoelectric components earlier in life than had been done previously. In the past, myoelectric componentry was not applied until the child was four years of age, and now it is applied as early as two years of age. There is an adage that if the child has not become a prosthetic user by the time they are four years old, they will not be likely to wear a prosthesis through the remainder of their life.

The unilateral arm amputee can become independent in almost every activity of life except for bimanual fine motor skills. Children are especially adaptable to their congenital condition and usually develop their own styles of substitution for their altered anatomy.

Initial Prosthetic Device

Typically, the first arm prosthetic device is fabricated when the child has achieved good sitting balance, reaches to the midline, and is actively exploring their immediate environment—perhaps at 6–9 months. The terminal device utilized is often a passive mitt that does not have individual fingers but is concave, so that it can be used for bimanual holding and play activities. At this age, the child is too immature to learn to use a cable or myoelectric control but can become accustomed to wearing the prosthetic socket and begin to explore bimanual activities using the passive prosthesis. Obviously, the prosthesis is kept as lightweight as possible to encourage the child's wearing and use of this initially "foreign" object. A pediatric occupational therapist and, in some settings, a physical therapist should be involved in training the child to use the prosthesis (and to compensate for any postural abnormalities that the child may develop).

As the child with an arm amputation matures socially, skeletally, and motorically, prosthetic componentry is changed as well as prosthetic operating systems. On average, the socket may need a change every two years. The terminal device will last an average of three years until the skeleton is mature, for example, at least by age 18. The entire list of prosthetic components will not be listed here since they are constantly changing; and the prosthetic prescription should be a collaborative team effort between the child, parents, physician, prosthetist, and therapists experienced in working with child amputees. In determining the life care plan, the treating physician, prosthetist, and therapist should be suggesting the appropriate evolution of prosthetic fitting for the child.

For the child with a leg amputation, the first prosthesis is provided when the child begins to pull up in order to stand. This often occurs between 6–12 months. Therapy training with a leg prosthesis is important, but the instinct to stand and walk is inherent in most children (with normal motor development). In the leg amputee, frequent socket changes or prosthetic leg lengthening is important to ensure equal leg lengths and comfortable prosthetic fitting. The frequency of socket change varies during growth spurts but probably averages every two years until the child has reached skeletal maturity around age 18. Again, the life care plan recommendations for prosthetic provision are best made with input from an experienced physiatrist or orthopedic surgeon, a pediatric-experienced prosthetist, and therapists.

Treating the Parents in Addition to the Child

For the child with congenital or acquired amputation(s), in the lead author's experience, the rehabilitation team may be more involved in treating the parents than they are in treating the child itself. The presence of guilt in the parents regarding their role in the congenital or acquired loss may lead to a need to cover up the amputation with a prosthesis so the amputation is less evident. However, even young children are interested and can understand at least some of the education and information that are provided to the parents. It is important that the health practitioner include the child in the discussion, even if they are (as young as) 24 months of age.

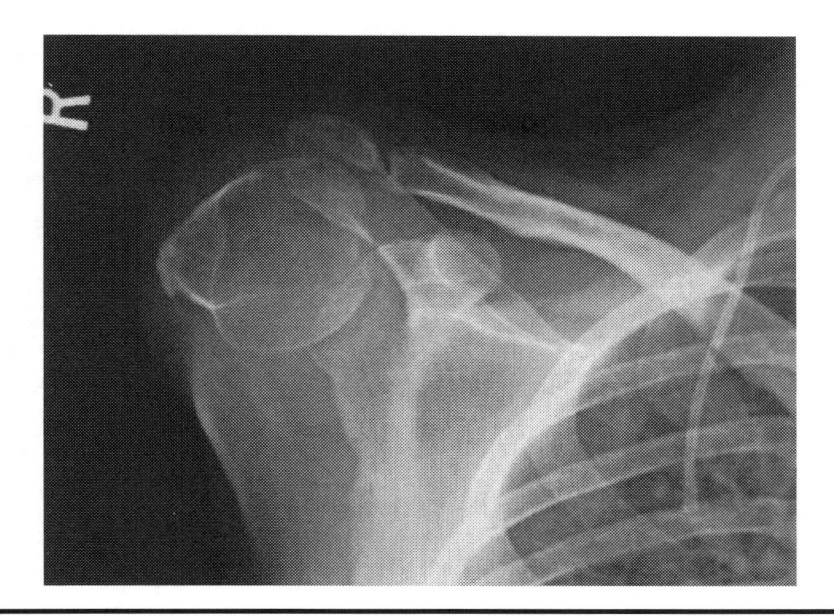

Figure 19.1 X-Ray Showing Extremely Short Above-Elbow Amputation Post Electrical Burn With Nothing Remaining Other Than Humeral Head

Source: Meier's chapter in 2011 Pediatric and Case Management Handbook (Grisham & Deming.)

Levels of Limb Amputation

In general, the longer the length of the residual limb, the better the prosthetic function that can be expected. In the leg, amputation below the knee provides for lower energy expenditure than the use of an above-knee prosthesis. Salvaging the leg at a below-knee level is now the goal of leg amputation surgery in the United States (Moore & Malone, 1989). Disarticulation levels for the arm and leg have certain relative contraindications and should be carefully considered on an individual basis. Full thickness skin and soft tissue coverage are also helpful in achieving ideal prosthetic functional outcomes. However, with the new gel interfaces, scarred skin and poor soft tissue coverage can be dealt with in a more satisfactory manner than in the past.

Phases of Amputation Rehabilitation

The loss of a body part(s) is an emotionally traumatic experience that affects quality of life across the lifespan (Meier & Heckman, 2014; Young et al., 2019). Yet, most persons who sustain an amputation can look forward to a fulfilling life of meaningful function using contemporary prosthetic designs. The key to successful prosthetic rehabilitation is understanding the desired functional outcome and the process of achieving that outcome. Recent critical appraisal literature demonstrated the positive effects of physical rehabilitation with amputees as early as possible to significantly impact restoration of one's function (Ülger et al., 2018). Special issues for the amputee, such as sexual health, can be an important part of the rehabilitation process (Brooks et al., 2021).

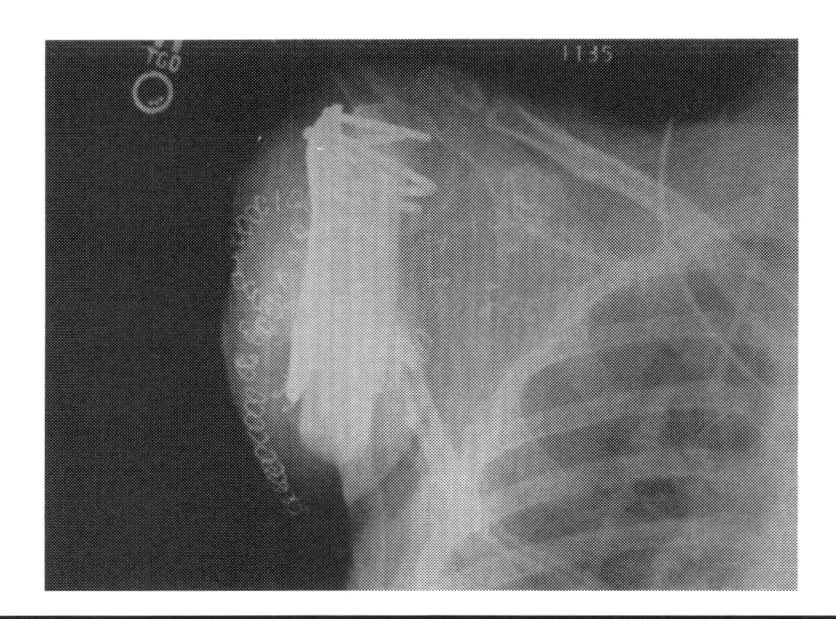

Figure 19.2 X-Ray Showing Same Arm With lengthening Using Allograft Bone Plated into the Residual Humeral Head. A Pedicle Graft of Latissimus Dorsi Muscle and Overlying Soft Tissue Were Used to Cover the Added Bone Length. Amputee is Now Able to Wear and Use an Above-Elbow Prosthesis

Source: Meier's chapter in 2011 Pediatric and Case Management Handbook (Grisham & Deming.)

In addition, the physiatrist should provide a time framework for the achievement of the ideal outcome. The physiatrist can also outline the most cost-efficient array of rehabilitative services to achieve the desired rehabilitation goals.

To understand the rehabilitative process for a person with an amputation, it is best to consider the following phases of amputation rehabilitation. These phases, while somewhat artificial, do interweave and flow from one to the next. By knowing the phase of the amputation rehabilitative process, the life care planner can identify the issues to be considered in each phase and assist the amputee toward the next phase. The U. S. Department of Veterans Affairs/Department of Defense (2017, 2019, 2022) and a systematic review for the World Health Organization (Heyns et al., 20021) developed useful clinical practice guidelines for amputees to assist the practitioner. The hallmarks of each phase can be used to determine if the amputee is successfully moving through the phases or is delayed in a phase. Being delayed in a phase of rehabilitative care can detract from the best functional or psychosocial outcome and will also add to the costs of healthcare.

The phases for amputation rehabilitation staging are:

1. Preoperative
2. Surgical
3. Acute postsurgical
4. Preprosthetic
5. Prosthetic prescription and fabrication
6. Prosthetic training
7. Community reentry

8. Vocational/avocational
9. Follow-up

Hallmarks of each phase have been assigned to measure the progress of the person with an amputation from one phase to the next (Table 19.1). There is usually some overlap from one phase to the next and the person may move more quickly through one phase than another (Meier, 1994). The focus throughout all these phases is on the needs and desires of the amputee. The person's ability to adapt to an altered body image and in some cases, an altered lifestyle, is essential for achieving the idealized outcome. Paying attention to and providing service for their psychosocial well-being is paramount to successful rehabilitative outcomes.

Table 19.1 Medical and Rehabilitation Progression of Amputation

Phase		Hallmarks
1	Preoperative	Assess body condition, patient education; discuss surgical level, postoperative rehabilitation, and prosthetic plans
2	Amputation surgery	Length, myoplastic closure, soft tissue coverage, nerve reconstruction handling, rigid dressing
3	Acute postoperative	Wound healing, pain control, proximal body motion, emotional support
4	Preprosthetic	Shaping and shrinking amputation stump, increasing muscle strength, restoring patient locus of control
5	Prosthetic fabrication	Team consensus on prosthetic prescription, experienced prosthetic fabrication
6	Prosthetic training	Increase wearing of prosthesis, mobility, and ADL skills
7	Community reintegration	Resume roles in family and community activities; regain emotional equilibrium and healthy coping strategies; pursue recreational activities
8	Vocational rehabilitation	Assess and plan vocational activities for future. May need further education, training, or job modification
9	Follow-up	Provide lifelong prosthetic, functional, medical, and emotional support; provide regular assessment of functional level and prosthetic problem solving

Preoperative

On a few occasions, the patient is delayed in the decision for an amputation. This is an ideal time for the rehabilitation team to assess and begin a treatment plan focusing on function of the remaining extremities. This is also an appropriate time to practice preventive care to maintain full range of motion and strength in the proximal limb muscles of the side to be amputated and also in the intact limb. An aerobic conditioning program should be provided during this phase since this type of exercise will hasten the postoperative functional recovery.

Amputation Surgery and Reconstruction Phase

Amputation surgery should proceed as a reconstructive surgery that will provide a residual limb with the best function, whether or not a prosthesis is likely to be prescribed. A reconstructive philosophy of amputation is best accomplished by a surgeon who has performed a number of amputations and understands contemporary prosthetic options and functional outcomes.

Acute Postoperative Phase

This is a time for wound healing and pain control. Usually there is wound care necessary until the sutures are removed. Potential complications at this phase could be chronic wounds (Jarbrink et al., 2016). The rehabilitation focus is on the remaining limbs and instructing the amputee in preventive exercise for the amputated limb and the opposite limb. Psychosocial support is essential during this period of loss for the individual.

Preprosthetic Phase

This period is usually accomplished on an outpatient basis. Once the sutures are removed, attention is paid to shaping and shrinking the residual limb in preparation for prosthetic casting. This is a good time to educate the amputee and the family regarding the prosthetic options available, and to develop and review the rehabilitation plan, if it has not previously been accomplished. At this time careful therapeutic attention should be paid to aerobic conditioning and strength training. Emotional stresses should be anticipated that surround change in body image, function, family roles, and income. Helping the amputee regain the locus of control in their life is important during this phase.

Prosthetic Fabrication

At this phase, the team, including the amputee, should decide on a prosthetic prescription that best meets the person's needs and desires (Meier, 1995). More and more, the prosthetic prescription is also dependent on what a third-party payer will sponsor. It is preferable that a prosthetist who is frequently experienced in fitting the specific level of amputation be used to fabricate the prosthesis. The time framework from prosthetic casting until final fitting should be presented to the amputee and the rehabilitation team for planning purposes. Please see Chapter 17 for more in-depth discussion on this topic.

As a general rule, the lower limb amputee should be fitted within eight weeks of amputation and the arm amputee fitted within four to six weeks of amputation surgery. If the upper limb amputee is delayed in fitting, their chances of using a prosthesis for bimanual activities decreases significantly. They become accustomed to performing activities in a one-handed manner and, therefore, do not find the prosthesis to be of much assistance in performing their daily activities.

Prosthetic Training

This phase is best accomplished in an outpatient therapy setting by therapists who have trained many amputees with similar levels and types of prostheses. This phase should continue until the

Table 19.2 Functional Expectations for the Below-Knee Amputee

1.	Can fall safely and arise from the floor
2.	Can hop without the prosthesis
3.	Can run (if cardiovascular status permits)
4.	Climbs stairs step over step
5.	Does not use any gait aid
6.	Drives a car (if desired)
7.	Has returned to same or modified work
8.	Independent in ADL
9.	Knows how to buy a correctly fitting shoe for the remaining foot
10.	Knows how to change stump socks to accommodate for soft tissue changes
11.	Knows how to inspect skin of the amputated and nonamputated legs and foot
12.	Participates in avocational interests
13.	Performs aerobic conditioning exercise (if cardiovascular system permits)
14.	Understands the necessity of follow-up
15.	Walks on level and uneven surfaces
16.	Wears the prosthesis during all waking hours

expected level of functional outcome has been achieved. The length of treatment time will vary depending on the level of amputation, the amputee's health, level of function prior to the amputation, associated injuries, and medical problems. The rehabilitation team should proceed with gradual prosthetic wearing and functional training with the goal of achieving the idealized functional outcomes listed in Tables 19.2 and 19.3. The rehabilitation treatment plan should focus on the level of function necessary for community reintegration, vocational, and avocational outcomes.

Community Reintegration

The person with the amputation should begin to resume their roles in the family and the community as quickly as possible following the amputation. Prosthetic training can assist with community reintegration by providing meaningful function. A psychologist or social worker should assist the amputee in developing productive social interactions with their family, friends, peers, and other persons in their community.

Vocational Rehabilitation

The physiatrist should be closely involved during this phase of amputee rehabilitation. The physiatrist is most knowledgeable in the expected level of prosthetic use in a variety of vocational settings. The physiatrist is also best suited to place the work restrictions in relation to the level of amputation

Table 19.3 Functional Expectations for the Above- and Below-Elbow Amputee

1.	Can tie laces with one hand or with the remaining hand and the prosthesis
2.	Can write legibly with remaining hand
3.	Drives (if desired)
4.	Has been shown adaptive equipment for the kitchen and ADLs
5.	Has performed carpentry and automotive maintenance (if desired)
6.	Has prepared a meal in the kitchen
6.	Has returned to work (same or modified job)
7.	Has successfully switched dominance (if necessary)
8.	Independent in activities of daily living
9.	Independent in donning and doffing the prosthesis
10.	Understands the necessity of follow-up
11.	Uses a button hook easily
12.	Uses the prosthesis for bimanual activities
13.	Wears prosthesis during all waking hours

and functional outcome. Working as a team, the case manager, the physiatrist, and the vocational rehabilitation specialist can provide an excellent support system for the amputee and enhance their successful return to the workplace (Weed & Atkins, 2004).

While vocational rehabilitation should begin shortly after the amputation, return to the workplace may require a functional capacity evaluation, worksite evaluation, and perhaps worksite modification. Generally, it is ill advised to provide a vocational prognosis until the person has achieved maximum functional outcome with or without the prosthesis.

(Greater energy expenditure than for below-knee prosthetic use)	
1.	A few can run with high-level training
2.	Can fall safely and arise from the floor
3.	Can hop without the prosthesis
4.	Climbs stairs step over step (some may do one step at a time)
5.	Does not use any gait aid (some may need a cane)
6.	Drives a car (if desired)
7.	Has returned to same or modified work
8.	Independent in ADLs
9.	Knows how to buy a correctly fitting shoe for the remaining foot
10.	Knows how to inspect skin of the amputated and nonamputated leg and foot
11.	Participates in avocational interests
12.	Performs aerobic conditioning exercise (if cardiovascular system permits)

(Continued)

	(Greater energy expenditure than for below-knee prosthetic use)
13.	Understands the necessity of follow-up
14.	Walks on level and uneven surfaces
15.	Wears the prosthesis during all waking hours

Follow-Up

To ensure the most appropriate level of prosthetic function, prevent prosthetic problems, and address emotional adjustment to amputation, a regular and periodic program of rehabilitation follow-up should be provided for the amputee. Once the ideal level of function has been achieved and the amputee is wearing a definitive prosthesis, the person should be seen in regular follow-up on an annual or every-other-year basis. This schedule permits measurement of the functional outcomes of amputation rehabilitation. It also serves to enhance the education of the amputee regarding preventive care and further prosthetic needs.

Amputation Related Complications

Amputation related complications are dependent on the reason for the amputation (trauma, electrocution, diabetes, cancer, cardiovascular disease, etc.), fit of prosthesis (if one is used), work demands, living environment, quality of medical treatment, and other factors. However, common considerations include (Weed & Sluis, 1990):

1. Some of the most common complications are psychological. In many cases, psychological counseling will be provided while the client is an inpatient and may be continued following discharge from acute care. If psychological counseling is offered, the costs for this should be placed on the Projected Therapeutic Modalities page. In the example case, the client experienced significant depression, was hospitalized for suicidal ideation, and had undergone a significant amount of psychological counseling following discharge. In this case, the family unit fell apart and a number of family counseling issues were raised.
2. In the event of amputations where the client wears a prosthesis, one would expect the probability of occasional skin breakdown. In one case, the client suffered amputations as a result of an electrocution injury. In this situation, the skin loses its integrity due to the burn. The client may require surgical intervention to repair skin breakdown.
3. Bone spurs occasionally become a problem and may require surgery.
4. Phantom pain or sensations are very common, at least during acute recovery, and may need some sort of treatment.
5. Other complications include osteoarthritis, which may be experienced in the knees and lower back, as well as back pain that may be experienced due to an abnormal gait. Fit of the prostheses is of paramount importance to avoid these kinds of complications. In addition to proper fit, specific gait training to educate the client as to proper body mechanics will be important.
6. Another often overlooked complication has to do with weight gain. Weight gain affects the fit of the prostheses, requiring either adjustment or a complete refabrication of the socket (Bouldin et al., 2016).

7. Complicated recoveries from other injuries may result in the inability of the client to manage self-care during periods of injury or illness. For example, an individual who is a triple amputee (bilateral below knee and dominant arm at the shoulder) may be unable to take care of himself for even bowel and bladder care or other survival needs should he injure his other arm.
8. Knee problems when not wearing the prosthesis is often a complication for bilateral below-knee amputees. It is sometimes much easier to avoid the time it takes to put on a prosthesis by simply walking on one's knees to get around the house, such as going to the bathroom at night or trying to get out of the house in case of an emergency. After years of using this method to move around, it is not uncommon for clients to experience knee problems.
9. While working in hot environments or having to exert considerable effort to walk or engage in physical activity with a prosthesis, sweating can become an irritating problem. Prostheses tend to feel heavy and awkward. Although earlier studies suggested that prostheses require a 10% increase in energy for a single below-knee amputation and much more energy expenditure with multiple amputations (Friedmann, 1981), more recent research suggests a wide range of expenditure based on a different variables such as surface or the use of mobility aids, but generally the higher the level of amputation, the higher the energy expenditure (van Schaik et al., 2019; Vllasolli et al., 2014). It does not take an educated observer to understand that a bilateral above-knee amputee will expend considerable energy simply getting from one place to another. In fact, many amputees may prefer to use a wheelchair to do things quicker. In addition, an upper-extremity amputee, such as a shoulder disarticulation, requires the addition of a mechanical arm or a Utah arm, which also requires considerable effort. This may result in excessive sweating and irritation as well. In addition, working in a hot environment, such as outdoors in the summertime in the south or in a boiler room indoors, may become intolerable.
10. Neuromas are also fairly frequent and can be quite irritating if the prosthesis impacts on the area where the neuroma resides. Often surgery is the treatment of choice.
11. Overuse syndromes are now seen for the amputee who leads an active lifestyle and usually involve the remaining, intact extremity. For the arm amputee, a common issue would be the development of carpal tunnel syndrome from repetitive use of the hand and wrist which is compensation for the loss of the hand and arm from the other side. Another commonly seen arm issue is earlier degenerative joint disease or impingement at the shoulder of the intact arm. Again this comes from increased stress and strain on the joints of the intact arm.

Phantom and Residual Limb Pain

This phenomenon occurs in most patients immediately following the amputation surgery and subsides during the first 4–6 weeks after the amputation (Uustal & Meier, 2014). A recent systematic review and meta-analysis covering 40 years and nearly 13,000 subjects found that "six out of every 10 people with amputation report [phantom limb pain]" (Limakatso et al., 2020, p. 1) and that depression post injury and stump pain were "consistently positively associated with [phantom limb pain]" (p. 17). In only a few amputees does phantom limb pain become so problematic that it interferes with the quality of life. It should not be treated with narcotics other than during the acute postoperative period (Davis, 1993). Today, a variety of medications can be used to alleviate this pain. Popular at this time are tricyclic antidepressants, gabapentin, and carbamazepine (Uustal & Meier, 2014). These medications affect the way the body processes pain messages in the peripheral and central nervous systems. Other physical modalities have been utilized but have met with varied success depending on the individual amputee. If the phantom pain interferes greatly with the quality of life and/or prosthetic function, an amputee pain specialist should be consulted.

Pain in the residual limb should be differentiated from phantom pain. Often, residual limb pain is caused by a poorly fitting prosthesis and can be alleviated with socket modifications. Residual limb pain may also be caused by the development of a neuroma from a peripheral nerve that was severed at the time of the amputation. There are a variety of conservative and surgical methods to attempt to decrease the pain from a neuroma (Sherman et al., 1980), such as pulsed radiofrequency ablation (West & Wu, 2010) and Targeted Sensory Reinnervation (TSR)-based surgical technique (Garetto et al., 2021).

Prosthetic Prescription

There has been an explosion of available prosthetic components in the past ten years and it is hard to keep up with the constant barrage of new options for the amputee. Many of the new components have added to the expense of the prosthesis without scientific demonstration that they have enhanced the functional outcome (Donnelley et al., 2021). Many of the new components are lighter weight and therefore more comfortable to wear. Globally, the prosthetics and orthotics market was projected to grow from $7.32 billion to $7.65 billion between 2021 and 2022 per the *Prosthetics and Orthotics Global Market Report 2022* (Research and Markets, 2022). Contemporary research and development in prosthetic technology is aimed at creating the sense of touch (Bumbasirevic et al., 2020, Hamilton, 2022). The use of electric components for the arm amputee has not been universally applied in the United States. In the prosthetics author's experience this technology remains less frequently prescribed than the conventional body-powered designs. The prices of prostheses, especially those using the new socket designs and components, have risen dramatically. With costs at these levels, it is imperative that the amputee be treated in a comprehensive interdisciplinary center of amputee rehabilitative excellence.

The usual components required for a prosthetic leg include the socket, a foot/ankle complex, and a means of suspension. Of course, for the above-knee prosthesis, a knee component is also prescribed.

For the arm amputee, there is a socket that fits onto the residual limb and for the below-elbow amputee, a wrist joint, a terminal device, and a suspension system are required elements of the prescription. Terminal devices can be a hook or a hand (Sear, 1991). The hand can be passive or it can move. For the above-elbow amputee, an elbow joint is prescribed. In considering the arm prosthetic prescription, the team needs to consider the three basic prosthetic designs available. They are a passive prosthesis that provides mainly cosmetic restoration, one that is cable controlled by body power, or one that has electric moving parts. A comparison of these types of arm prostheses is presented in Table 19.4 (Esquenazi et al., 1989), a comparative reference that is still used today.

Prosthetic options are generally between a body-powered, myoelectric, or hybrid options. Uellendahl (2017) compares these options including the indications, benefits, contraindications, and drawbacks with each option. Trent et al. (2019) emphasize that while much of the current research about upper limb prostheses focuses on technology, "successful rehabilitation hinges on awareness of new components, the functional efficacy of these components, and the evolved techniques used in prosthetic design and fabrication" (p. 1).

Table 19.4 Advantages and Disadvantages of Various Upper Limb Prostheses

Type	Pros	Cons
Cosmetic (passive)	Most lightweight	High cost if custom made
	Best cosmesis	Least functional
	Least harnessing	Low-cost gloves stain easily
Body powered	Moderate cost	Most body movement to operate
	Moderately lightweight	Most harnessing
	Most durable	Least satisfactory appearance
	Highest sensory feedback	
Externally powered (myoelectric and switch control)	Moderate or no harnessing	Heaviest
	Least body movement to operate	Most expensive
	Moderate cosmesis	Most maintenance
	More function-proximal levels	Limited sensory feedback
Hybrid (cable elbow/ electric TD)	All cable excursion to elbow	Electric weights forearm
	Increased TD pinch	(harder to lift)
		Good for elbow disarticulation
		(or long above elbow)
Hybrid (electric elbow/ cable TD)	All cable excursion to TD	Least cosmesis
	Low effort to position TD	Lower pinch force for TD
	Low maintenance TD	

Source: Esquenazi et al., 1989.

Partial Hand

This level of amputation can be handled in several ways. Many partial hand amputees choose to not wear any prosthetic restoration. However, if cosmesis is desired, a cosmetic glove can be fabricated. This is usually made from a mold taken of the residual hand. A custom-made silicone glove that is hand-colored can provide excellent cosmesis and is reasonably durable. However, if it is worn at work, a protective glove should be worn. Another manner to prosthetically handle this level is to make an opposition bar that can provide improved prehension between the prosthetic bar and the residual moving parts of the hand. If the thumb has been amputated, an excellent prosthetic thumb can be fabricated. The functional and cosmetic results from this prosthesis often decrease the need for surgical reconstruction of the amputated thumb.

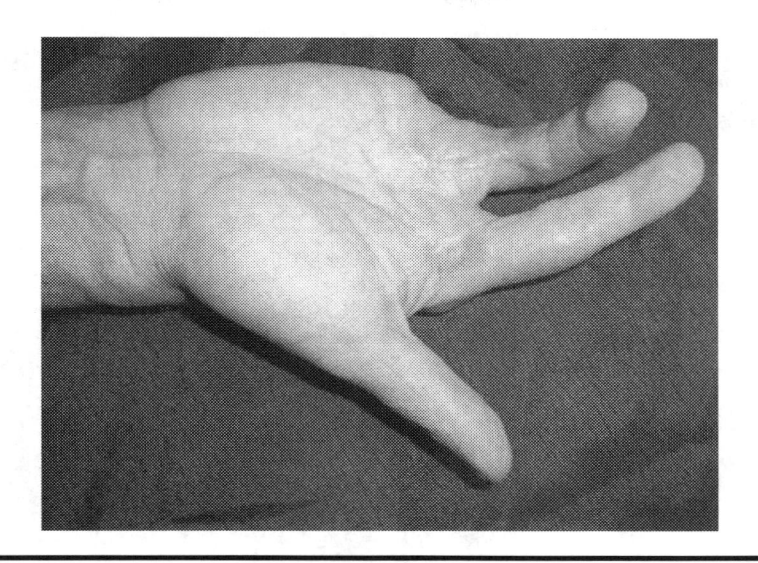

Life Care Planning for the Patient with an Amputation ■ 515

Figure 19.3   Traumatic Amputations of the Ring and Little Fingers with Cosmetic Deformity

Source: *Meier's chapter in 2011 Pediatric and Case Management Handbook (Grisham & Deming.)*

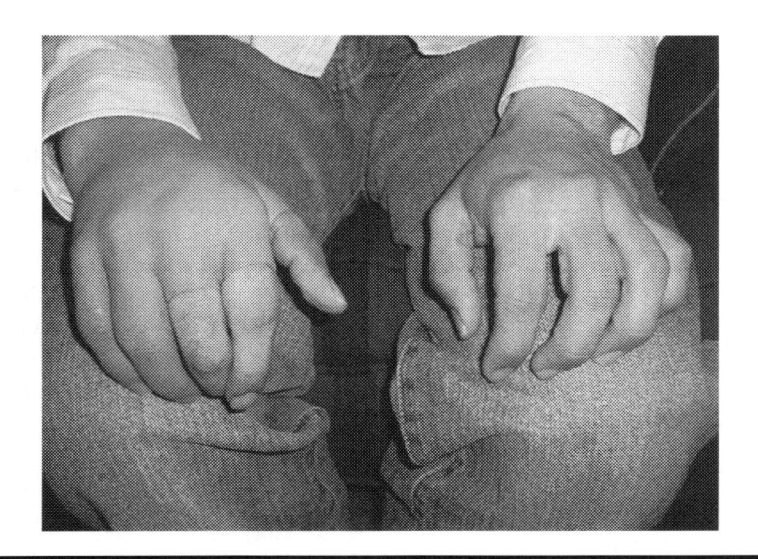

Figure 19.4   Finger Amputations now Covered with a Passive Cosmetic Glove Replacing the Ring and Little Fingers that Permits use of the Residual Thumb, Index, and Long Digits

Source: *Meier's chapter in 2011 Pediatric and Case Management Handbook (Grisham & Deming.)*

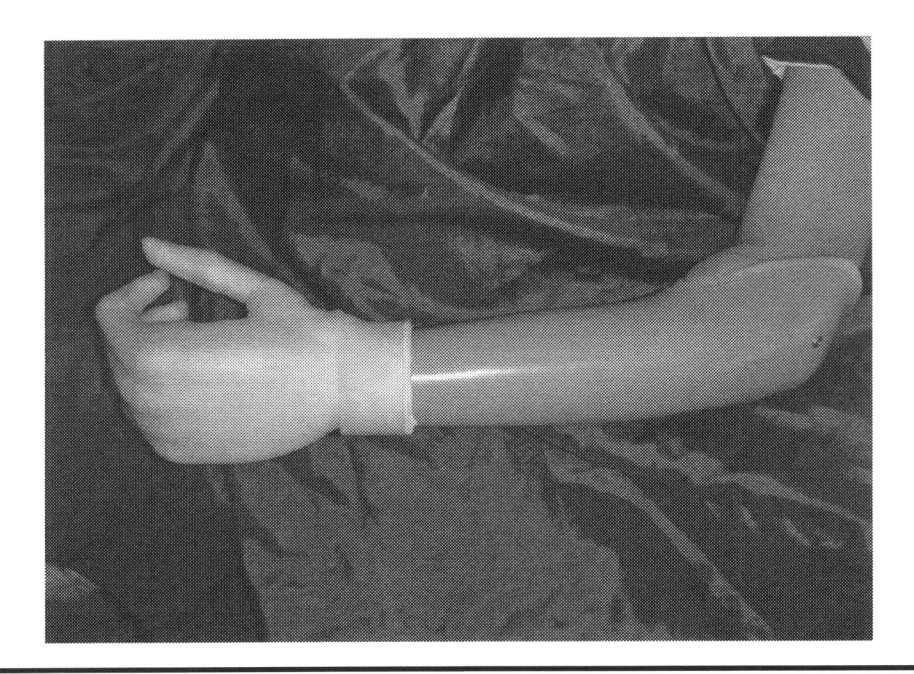

Figure 19.5 "I-Hand" Without Coverage of a Cosmetic Glove. Individual Fingers Move Using Myoelectric Signals

Wrist Disarticulation/Below Elbow (Transradial)

The below-elbow prosthesis is usually composed of a double-walled plastic laminate socket that fits intimately over the residual limb. A locking, quick-change wrist unit is commonly prescribed through which the terminal device is attached to the forearm shell. This wrist unit permits ease of change of various terminal devices and locks the terminal device in a position of function when handling heavier objects. For most men who will return to heavy-duty work, a body-powered prosthesis will be useful. For the businessman or white-collar worker, a myoelectric or a passive cosmetic prosthesis may be preferable (Meier, 1996).

Elbow Disarticulation/Above Elbow (Transhumeral)

The prosthetic options at this level of restoration are body-powered or electric control. The electric prosthesis is many times the expense of the body-powered arm. For a very short above-elbow level of amputation, an electric prosthesis may be the only functional restoration that is reasonable.

Shoulder Disarticulation

This level can be fitted with a lighter weight endoskeletal design with a passive elbow joint and a moving terminal device. At this proximal level of amputation, an electric prosthesis will permit more functional motion of the component parts. However, it is heavy to wear and very expensive.

Partial/Hindfoot

Often this level of amputation can be fitted with a full-length insole with toe filler that fits inside the shoe. This insole can usually be interchanged between various shoes. The bottom of the shoe may need to be modified to provide a more normal gait pattern.

Below Knee (Transtibial)

The prosthesis that is currently used for this level of amputation was popularized in the mid-1950s. It is called a patellar tendon bearing design. It was originally designed to place superincumbent body weight on the remaining anatomic landmarks that were pressure tolerant. It relieves pressure from the pressure-intolerant areas of the residual stump. For this level, the prosthetic prescription includes the design of the prosthetic socket, a foot/ankle complex, and a means of suspending the prosthesis on the residual leg. A current popular suspension design is called the triple "S" system or the silicone sleeve suspension. A silicone sleeve is worn against the skin and a knurled pin extends from the distal end. This pin locks inside a coupling in the distal end of the prosthetic socket. The silicone sleeve provides additional padding to the inside of the socket against the skin. Other types of gel liners are in vogue today and have made prosthetic leg wearing more comfortable. These liners reduce the number of skin problems seen with prosthetic wear and function.

Knee Disarticulation/Above Knee (Transfemoral)

The contemporary socket design for the above-knee amputee changed in the 1980s and 1990s (Leonard & Meier, 1993). There are a number of designs available but the one in greatest use is a narrow mediolateral, ischial containment design. In the prosthetics author's practice, new socket designs also include thermoplastic inner liners that have improved the comfort of prosthetic wearing. Gel liners are also available for this level of amputation. A variety of knee units are also available that provide differing degrees of knee stability and cosmesis with gait.

Hip Disarticulation

This is a difficult level to fit comfortably and to have the amputee walk successfully with the prosthesis. This level of amputation should be handled by a prosthetist who makes ten or more of this type of prosthesis a year. More important, for best success, this amputee should have their rehabilitation in a center that has trained a number of amputees to wear this type of prosthesis with good results.

Prosthetic Cost & Replacement

Because of the high cost of prosthetics, a team of experienced amputee rehabilitation specialists should develop a prescription. To have the prosthetist develop the prescription in a vacuum is almost a conflict of interest and should be avoided.

Within the first two years following the amputation, several socket changes are usually necessary to accommodate the rapid soft tissue changes that occur. These changes improve the prosthetic fit and comfort of wearing. Usually after this time, a prosthesis should last the amputee from three to five years before a replacement prosthesis is prescribed. Certainly, the level of activity in using the prosthesis will affect the frequency with which these replacements are needed. Modifications to the prosthesis are usually needed once every six months on average.

A well-fitted prosthesis is in intimate contact with the skin of the residual limb. There are shearing forces applied to the skin in arm and leg prostheses. In the leg amputee, there are also direct pressures applied from the prosthesis to the skin of the residual leg. These forces can create skin pressure problems. These issues are usually addressed with prosthetic socket modifications or the use of gel-skin interfaces. A differing socket design may also be necessary to change the forces applied to the skin. A recent systematic review identified four implications for rehabilitation for prosthesis satisfaction (Luza et al., 2020):

- Adjustment to amputation and prosthesis use involves both physical and psychosocial issues.
- The adaptation to the prosthesis and recovery of walking capacity are important goals in the rehabilitation process.
- Well-adjusted, comfortable, and easy-to-use prostheses are of great importance as they enable the patient to perform their daily activities and maintain their independence.
- It is important to encourage participation of the individual in both rehabilitation and choice of prosthesis (p. 582).

From co-author, Christian Meier, CPO, in today's world (2022), prosthetic pricing can be quite varied and is dependent on the prosthetic laboratory used. Pricing is also varied because of new technology coming into use and advances in prosthetic design, and things are changing rapidly. Prices range from $25,000 to $300,000 in today's marketplace (see www.utaharm.com/ for the many options and specifications). It might be useful for the life care planner to have contacts in the prosthetic industry who can be used to provide contemporary pricing even if that prosthetist will not be making the prosthesis in question. Always cite the source of any pricing that is included in the plan. Sometimes, pricing from a couple or several sources is safest.

While a life care plan can be a one time document, the individual's life is dynamic and may represent a variety of geographic moves, marital situations, vocational settings, and health-related issues. It is expected that the life care plan can cover most life instances for the limb loss person and can be updated as needed. Please develop your life care plan focusing on the emotional well-being for the future life of the client. With this intent, the life care plan should provide the most ideal outcomes for the amputee and their future life.

When assembling the prosthetic costs of the life care plan, it is essential that the life care planner understand what estimate the prosthetist is providing. There are at least three ways of pricing a prosthesis. There is a usual and customary cost of a prosthesis. This cost would be the full, non-discounted, non-Medicare allowable cost that usually will have significant mark-up built into the numbers provided from the prosthetic laboratory. Almost never is this price paid to the prosthetist for the final prosthetic device. Rather, the Medicare allowable rate is the usual amount at which a prosthesis will be paid. Some managed care and insurance providers will discount from the Medicare allowable fee schedule or will provide an add on amount that will be a specific percentage above the Medicare allowable reimbursement schedule.

Also, if the life care planner is obtaining price quotations from a variety of prosthetic facilities, it is imperative that the same "L" codes be utilized when comparing the various pieces of the prosthesis. The "L" code is the Medicare system of providing specific numbers for specific prosthetic components. If specific "L" codes are not used in obtaining the variety of quotes, it will be like comparing apples and oranges. However, it may be of benefit to obtain a variety of prosthetic price quotes and provide a range in the life care plan using a high estimate, a low estimate, and the median price. Prosthetic pricing does vary from laboratory to laboratory for the exact same prosthesis. Prosthetic price quotes can also vary dramatically from one region of the United States to another geographic region.

The life care planner should be expected to support each of the major L codes included in the prosthetic prescription. This would likely include the major components of the prescription. A way to do this would be to explain the major components in the life care plan. Also be certain to indicate why the physician who generated the prescription had included those particular components. This should provide the basis for prosthetic costs that have been increasing with this new technology.

Aging with an Amputation

As the amputee matures and reaches age 60–65 years, it is expected that prosthetic use decreases. This decreased use should increase the length of time between essential prosthetic replacement. It is likely that an average replacement for a new prosthesis would occur every five years instead of the previously recommended four years. Also the use of alternative mobility may come into play usually at age 65 and above. So, at this point in time, a motorized scooter may enter the life care plan or a powered stair lift may be placed in the home for safe stair negotiation. As functional use of the prosthesis decreases, it should also be expected that additional assistance for essential household function should be provided in the life care plan. In the male amputee, this sort of assistance would include outdoor home maintenance and yard work. For the female amputee, additional assistance with the heavier housework would be appropriate. This would include items such as bed making, laundry, housecleaning, mopping, vacuuming, etc. Also, the incidence of low back pain in the more mature amputee has been found in about 75% of lower limb amputees. This pain is generally secondary to biomechanical issues but should be evaluated and treated on a regular basis.

Also, aging with disability research has shown the onset of additional disabling changes in body systems within 20–30 years from the onset of the initial disability (Widerstrom-Noga & Finlayson, 2010). In the amputee, issues of overuse and biomechanical stress and strain do occur over years of altered biomechanics. Often, these changes are seen in the extremity opposite to the amputated one and also in the more proximal body segments which take additional stress and strain to compensate for the amputation.

Scope of Practice

The physiatrist who specializes in amputation can play a valuable role in assisting in the development of the life care plan for the person who has sustained an amputation. The physiatrist can be of great service to the life care planner in indicating the appropriate level of function and future needs for the amputee, as well as which phase of amputation rehabilitation the person has already achieved and what is yet to be achieved.

There are three differing scenarios for physiatric involvement with life care planning. The ideal scenario is when the physiatrist to be involved with the life care plan has been the treating physiatrist throughout the individual's rehabilitation process. In this scenario, the physiatrist has become quite involved with directing the amputee's rehabilitation treatment goals and plan. Having worked with the amputee through the phases of amputation rehabilitation, they can give individualized prognostic information. The physiatrist will have a clear picture of the amputee's psychosocial support system and their needs and desires, as well as the amputee's pre-amputation lifestyle and how likely it will be to achieve that quality of life post-amputation.

Another scenario is the physiatrist who has been asked to participate in a life care plan but has not been involved with the amputee's rehabilitation program. This physiatrist has agreed to evaluate the individual to provide meaningful information for a life care plan. Often, this requires a visit from the amputee to the physiatrist for a thorough assessment. This may be accomplished over a one to several day process, depending on the complexity of the case. Almost always, this evaluation will be performed during an outpatient visit. The evaluation usually includes the physiatric assessment and visits with an occupational therapist, a physical therapist, a psychologist, and a prosthetist. Other rehabilitation professionals and consultants may be included in this evaluation depending on other areas of disability or comorbid factors. The product of this evaluation should be a report that provides all the information that a life care planner will include in the final plan (Meier et al., 2013). For this reason, it is essential that the life care planner pose all of the important questions they wish the physician to address before the evaluation process begins.

The evaluation process by the physiatrist should include the following elements that are clearly delineated during the evaluation and the physiatrist's opinions that are to be included in the life care document.

These items should include:

1. History
2. Past medical history
3. Review of systems
4. Medications
5. Psychosocial history
6. Activity status
7. Vocational history
8. Avocational history
9. Prosthetic history
10. Adaptive equipment used
11. Achievement of maximum medical improvement
12. Future needs
    - prosthetic
    - emotional
    - rehabilitative
    - medical
    - surgical
    - equipment
    - architectural modifications
    - attendant care
    - vocational options
    - follow-up plan
    - health maintenance and preventive care

A third manner for physiatric involvement in life care planning is the "curbside consultation." In this instance, the physiatrist does not have the advantage of evaluating the amputee but instead reviews the case records and provides input into the life care plan based on the physiatrist's experience with similar patients. This manner of physiatric involvement can be very useful to the life care planner in helping to assure that important life care planning issues for a person with an amputation are not overlooked.

For the person with an amputation, the physiatrist should have the ability to provide meaningful information for the life care plan, especially in the following areas:

1. Point of maximum medical improvement
2. Life expectancy
3. Expected functional outcomes
4. Costs of prosthetic service
5. Frequency of prosthetic replacement
6. Adaptive equipment needs and costs
7. Architectural modifications for function
8. Attendant care hours and level of service
9. Psychosocial needs
10. Vocational and avocational expectations and modifications
11. Future medical needs
12. Future surgical needs

Case Study

Below is a case study involving a life care plan prepared for an individual with an amputation. It is noted that this case study is reprinted from the fourth edition of this text and material contained therein has not been updated.

Mr. AK Amputee is a 35-year-old man who, as a commercial truck driver, was severely injured in a head-on collision while driving his 18-wheel truck carrying a heavy load of steel. He was urgently taken to a Level 1 trauma-designated hospital in Houston, Texas. His life was salvaged despite nearly severing his right leg above the knee. Significant attempts to save the right leg were successful after eight surgeries. However, 12 months after his injury, the hardware in his right leg became infected with methicillin resistant staphylococcus aureus (MRSA) and threatened his life. It was decided to perform a mid-femoral amputation. Following the amputation, he healed primarily but was significantly deconditioned. He was prepared and fitted for an above-knee prosthesis with input from a full array of rehabilitation health professionals.

Mr. AK Amputee has been married and in a stable relationship for 10 years. He and his wife have two children ages 6 and 8. He has a high school diploma and has periodic pain well-controlled with an occasional nonsteroidal tablet. He does have Type II diabetes that is controlled with oral medication. He is otherwise healthy with no other complaints. Before the amputation, he was active in his community through his children's school activities. He enjoyed swimming and playing golf on weekends. He wants to return to these activities. He and his family live in a ranch style home with all major living areas on one floor.

He has been told he cannot return to work. He is concerned about future vocational options and whether his education will be enough to become employed again.

After completing the life care plan tables, it is useful to provide supportive explanation for each line contained in the life care plan. This explanation can be supported by a professional recommendation, literature citation, or standard of practice. If an item is recommended by a health care professional, that name should be listed on that same line. It is helpful to indicate the first draft is not for distribution until discussed with the appropriate parties and any questions have been answered.

Life Care Plan Narrative for Mr. AK Amputee

The narrative below is an attempt to explain the recommended items in the Life Care Plan (LCP) charts. I will list my reasons for suggesting the items listed. The recommendations made in the LCP are based on the assumption that this person will elect to wear and use a prosthetic leg for the above-knee level of amputation. Some persons with above-knee amputations do not do this and instead opt to use a wheelchair for their mobility. Some items in the LCP may have been recommended by other persons. In these cases, a thorough explanation of why this item is essential should be made.

The other important component to include in a life care plan is what the idealized outcome should be for function, future health needs, anticipated equipment needs, pain control, and emotional well-being. Potential life complications should also be projected and any costs associated with that health care.

An above-knee amputee without other comorbidities should be expected to achieve the following functions:

1. Ambulation with prosthesis on all surfaces
2. No gait aids
3. Independent in donning and doffing prosthesis
4. Standing up to two continuous hours
5. Walking up to two continuous hours
6. Get up from kneeling
7. Return to recreational activities (hunting, fishing, golfing, jogging, skiing), if performed prior to amputation
8. Return to previous work
9. Comfortable with falling techniques
10. Perform cardiovascular conditioning program safely
11. Drive
12. Shop
13. Perform housework, gardening, home maintenance
14. Independent in Activities of Daily Living (ADL)
15. Know how to purchase correct footwear
16. Can inspect skin and nails for remaining foot
17. Ascend and descend stairs one step at a time usually
18. Can run (if patient desires and has adequate cardiopulmonary reserve)

The ability to perform all of these functions often requires a coordinated team effort of various health professionals who have had significant experience in working with other persons with aboveknee amputation and have followed those persons back into the community with full function. Usually, this team will be facilitated by a physiatrist or orthopedic surgeon with significant amputation experience.

Projected Rehabilitation Program

These rehabilitation modalities are recommended for Mr. AK Amputee in order to take him through the adaptive process of leg amputation and prosthetic restoration to maximum function with an artificial leg. This process normally takes some 12–18 months from the time of the amputation. Returning to work and successful integration into the workplace may take a bit longer. This program does not just focus on use of a prosthetic leg but pays close attention to the issues of pain, emotional well-being, weight control, recreation, and integration back into the family and his community. It should involve more than a surgeon, a prosthetist, and the amputee.

Projected Evaluations

It is anticipated that with his weight and an above-knee amputation, he will develop low back pain at age 65 that will require ongoing conservative orthopedic back care. This treatment is usually nonsurgical.

Projected Therapeutic Modalities

He will also require periodic evaluations and therapy from occupational therapy, physical therapy, and psychology as his prosthesis needs maintenance and replacement. New componentry and changes in his own anatomy require periodic and regular follow-up with these therapists. Often physical therapy is useful when a new prosthesis is fabricated, often every 3 to 5 years since the fit. New components take a period of accommodation before achieving ideal function.

Diagnostic Testing

I do anticipate the need for periodic MRI studies of his low back related to the low back pain that I anticipate will have an onset about age 65.

Wheelchair Needs

An ultra lightweight manual wheelchair is often used when he does not wear his prosthesis or needs to go long distances beyond his capability to use the prosthesis for walking. A wheelchair cushion should also be provided and replaced once every 3 years.

Wheelchair Accessories and Maintenance

He needs an allowance for regular and periodic wheelchair maintenance. This equates to 10 percent of the original cost of the wheelchair that is required every 2 years for the 7-year life of the wheelchair.

Aids for Independent Function

He should have a shower commode chair that can be used in the shower for safety reasons. The replacement schedule is listed.

Orthotics/Prosthetics

With the transfemoral (above-knee) level of amputation, he will require a contemporary design of above-knee prosthesis. The price for this will vary depending on the prosthetic components that are prescribed and also on the prosthetic laboratory that makes the prosthesis. A cost range should be provided by the prosthetic laboratory but, at times, it may be helpful to know the price range from other prosthetic laboratories or elsewhere in the United States. The price of the prosthesis will vary depending on the components used which are usually designated by "L" codes used for Medicare pricing. Routine prosthetic maintenance is recommended and costs 10 percent annually of the base price of the prosthesis. This maintenance cost is incurred once the warranty of the prosthesis has expired, generally at the end of the first year following fabrication.

Gel liners that are used to pad the skin are replaced on an annual basis and stump socks must be used as the size of the amputated leg and soft tissues change in shape and volume. These socks also need to be replaced annually.

Often, a custom-made foot insole orthotic is appropriate for the remaining foot. This is an attempt to distribute weight more evenly over the plantar aspect of the remaining foot. Hopefully, this will maintain skin and bone architecture through the remainder of life. This is especially important if the amputee has diabetes.

Home Furnishings and Accessories

This will vary depending on the amputee but most often few items are required following the amputation.

Drug/Supply Needs

This depends on what may be prescribed because of the amputation. It most likely will be pain medication, at least for a short period of time. Most amputees should not complain of long term pain issues.

Home/Facility Care

It is anticipated that he should have assistance with the heavier housework and with outside home maintenance. I do not assume that a spouse is available for providing assistance. I therefore always include some home assistance in order to try to avoid excess wear and tear on the remaining body parts which are essential for future functioning.

Future Medical Care—Routine

See under Potential Complications. Future medical care may be related to comorbid diagnoses such as diabetes mellitus, peripheral arterial disease, or cardiac abnormalities.

Transportation

He will need to drive an automatic transmission motor vehicle and it could be outfitted with a left-footed accelerator, if a right-leg amputee.

Health and Strength Maintenance

He should regularly participate in an exercise program to maintain his cardiopulmonary status essential for leg prosthetic use. A YMCA or similar health club would be excellent for this type of aerobic conditioning. Swimming is also an excellent exercise regimen for a person with an aboveknee amputation.

It should be assumed that function will change as he ages and therefore prosthetic replacement may be less frequent. Thus, he might need a 3-year replacement schedule between ages 35–65 but then with less strenuous activity, replacement would go to every 5 years.

Often, the socket will need more frequent replacement than all of the lower prosthetic leg components (knee, foot/ankle). A new socket is often desirable every 2 years while the entire leg replacement is less frequent, every 3 to 5 years.

Architectural Renovations

He may need to have a bathroom modified for functional safety. Occasionally, a walk-in shower is desirable but not essential for safe bathing activity. Some multi-level homes benefit from the addition of a Stairglide if climbing stairs is difficult. Bathroom modifications for wheelchair access may also be desirable.

Potential Complications

He is likely to develop a minor skin infection from time to time with prosthetic wear and use. This infection should be easily treated with not wearing the prosthesis for a few days and the use of oral antibiotics. Crutches are necessary for this period of time. Low back pain is an expected complication for him to develop at age 65. This should be managed conservatively by an orthopedic back specialist and may require medication to decrease the pain. He may also need periodic MRI evaluation of his spine.

Vocational/Educational Plan

Because he has been out of work for so long, I believe that he will need a formal vocational assessment and a vocational plan to be developed. I also believe he will benefit from formal job coaching as he returns to work in order to enhance the likelihood he will be successful in the chosen occupation and that the ergonomics of the workplace fit his disability needs.

Future Medical Care—Aggressive Treatment

This is unlikely unless medical issues develop related to the cause of the amputation and may complicate future prosthetic function.

Orthopedic Equipment Needs

He should have ergonomically designed crutches available for use on a periodic basis.

These items listed in the LCP more probably than not will return Mr. AK Amputee to his most full function and to assure the best quality of life in his future.

Robert H. Meier, III, MD
Director
Amputee Services of America
NAME: Mr. AK Amputee
DOB: 09/15/1982
DOI: 11/12/2015
AGE: 35 yrs.
REPORT DATE: 12/16/2017

FUTURE CARE PLAN

For purposes of this plan, the following initials are placed in parentheses according to their respective recommendations:
(XYZ) = Dr. XYZ, physician

Routine Future Medical Care—Physician Only

Recommendation (by whom)	Frequency and Duration	Purpose	Expected Cost
Amputation Rehabilitation Physician—PM&R	Every 2 yrs. after initial rehabilitation program is completed	Assess prosthetic function, fit, maintenance, and quality of life	$325
Orthopedic Surgeon	Every 2 yrs.	Assess issues related to prior fractures, bone surgery, and low back issues	$325

Projected Evaluations—Nonphysician (Include all allied health evals)

Recommendation (by whom)	Year Initiated/ Suspended	Frequency/Duration	Expected Cost
Physical Therapy	2020	1 visit every 3 yrs. with new prosthesis	$350 for eval and $175 for therapy visits
Psychology	2022	Every 5 yrs. for 5 visits	$225/visit for assessment of coping skills, parenting, emotional adaptation to life changes, and disabilities
Occupational Therapy	2020	Every 3 yrs.	$350 for evaluation of ADL skills and need for adaptive equipment

Projected Therapeutic Modalities

Recommendation (by whom)	Year Initiated/ Suspended	Frequency/Duration	Expected Cost
Physical Therapy	2020	4 visits every 3 yrs. with new prosthesis	$175 for therapy visits

(Continued)

Diagnostic Testing/Educational Assessment			
Recommendation (by whom)	Year Initiated/ Suspended	Frequency/Duration	Expected Cost
Potentially consider for future work			
Assistive Technology			
Recommendation (by whom)	Year Initiated	Frequency	Expected Cost
Consider if usual for employment			
Wheelchair Needs			
Recommendation (by whom)	Year Purchased	Replacement Schedule	Expected Cost
Ultra-lightweight wheelchair	2017	Every 7 yrs. until age 65 then every 5 yrs.	$2,800
Powered scooter	Age 65 or 2055	Every 5 yrs.	$3,500
Wheelchair Maintenance and Accessories			
Recommendation (by whom)	Year Purchased	Replacement Schedule	Expected Cost
Annual maintenance	2017	Annual	$280
Annual scooter maintenance	2055	Annual	$350
Battery replacement	2058	Every 3 yrs.	
Independent Aids for Functioning			
Recommendation (by whom)	Year Purchased	Replacement Schedule	Expected Cost
Commode chair	2017	Every 7 years	$246 (no wheels) to $1001 (with wheels)
Prosthetics			
Recommendation (by whom)	Year Purchased	Replacement Schedule	Expected Cost
Above knee prosthesis for general duty	2017	Every 3 yrs. until age 65 then every 5 yrs. for life	Per prosthetic laboratory
Socket replacement	2019	Every 1½ yrs. until age 65 then every 2½ yrs. For life	Per prosthetic laboratory
Above-knee prosthesis for high performance activities such as running, golf, etc.			Per prosthetic laboratory
Possible water leg for showering, water sports, or beach activities			Per prosthetic laboratory

(*Continued*)

Home Furnishings and Equipment			
Recommendation (by whom)	Year Purchased	Replacement	Expected Cost
Depending on home design			Potentially use VA housing allowance for modification
Health and Strength Maintenance (Leisure Time Activities)			
Recommendation (by whom)	Year of Purchase	Replacement Schedule	Expected Cost
Gym Membership til age 72	2017	Annual membership fee	
Transportation			
Recommendation (by whom)	Year Purchased	Replacement Schedule	Expected Cost
None unless vehicle is to be modified			
Drug Needs			
Drug needs and costs are representative of the client's current need and may change from time to time.			
Recommendation (by whom)	Purpose	Cost per Unit	Cost per Year
None at present			
Supply Needs			
Supply needs and costs are representative of the client's current need and may change from time to time.			
Recommendation (by whom)	Purpose	Cost per Unit	Cost per Year
Prosthetic liners	Cushion fit of prosthetic socket	$1,600/pr with annual replacement	$1600
Vocational/Educational Plan			
Recommendation (by whom)	Initiated/ Suspended	Purpose	Expected Cost
Depends on whether plan is to include potential for return to work?			Depends on what potential there may be for useful employment
Architectural Considerations			
Consider whether VA allowance is to be used.			
Home/Facility Care			
Recommendation (by whom)	Initiated/ Suspended	Hours/Shifts/Days	Expected Cost
Homemaking assistance	2017 until 2056	4 hrs. three times a week for heavier duty housework	$20/hr. to include Social Security, health insurance, etc.

(Continued)

Homemaking assistance	2056 until 2066	6 hrs. three times a week for heavier housework	Same
Homemaking assistance	2066 for lifetime	4 hrs./day every day	Assistance with ADL, all housework and shopping
Future Medical Care, Surgical Intervention, Aggressive Treatment			
Recommendation (by whom)	**Year Initiated/ Suspended**	**Frequency**	**Expected Cost**
Because of Mr. AK Amputee's extensive bony injuries and multiple surgeries, I am anticipating the following medical problems to be more likely than not: 1. Total hip replacement 2. Low back pain 3. Degenerative joint disease in arm, legs, and lower back			Chances are that he will require regular and ongoing medical and orthopaedic assessments for long term medical problems. I also expect he will require a total hip replacement, nonsurgical low back treatments, multiple pain, and arthritis medications.
Potential Complications			
Potential complications are included for information only. *No frequency or duration of complications is available.*			
He is likely to develop a minor skin infection from time to time with prosthetic wear and use. This infection should be easily treated with not wearing the prosthesis for a few days and the use of oral antibiotics. Crutches are necessary for this period of time.			
Lower back pain is an expected complication for him to develop at age 65. This should be managed conservatively by an orthopedic back specialist and may require medication to decrease the pain. He may also need periodic MRI evaluation of his spine.			

At the conclusion, a Life Care Planning Narrative is useful to explain every line item of recommended service or equipment as it relates to the individual for whom the care plan is developed.

Conclusion

An emphasis should be placed on the amputee achieving the ideal level of function with an appropriate rehabilitation program. Providing a prosthesis is not the same as providing an integrated rehabilitation program that includes a prosthesis. The emphasis should be placed on the amputee's needs and desires. Measuring the functional outcome, the success of community reintegration, and the individual's emotional adaptation to the changes in their life are important in developing an accurate life care plan. The physiatrist can serve as an invaluable collaborator with the life care planner to develop the most accurate and comprehensive life care plan. As noted above, for pediatric cases, family inclusion in the process can be vital.

Amputation rehabilitation and prosthetic options are changing so quickly that it is important that the life care planner use rehabilitation professionals who have access to the most current information and practices. The annual quantity of particular levels of amputation and prosthetic services should be a known component when using a source of clinical information. An example could be: if the prosthetist does not fit at least 25 of a particular level of amputation per year, that prosthetist is not particularly experienced to render an opinion. The same could be said for any other rehabilitation team professional whether it be surgeon, physician, or therapist. The number 25 is plucked from the air since perhaps treating ten would be sufficient. The point for the life care planner is to assess how many amputees of a particular level the person providing the information for the life care plan does actually treat in a year's time and which they might use when queried in a deposition or on a witness stand. It is also essential that the person providing input to the life care plan is current in their understanding of contemporary amputation techniques and amputee rehabilitation practices.

References

Amputee Coalition. (2021). *Limb loss in the U.S.* https://3w568y1pmc7umeynn2o6c1my-wpengine.netdna-ssl.com/wp-content/uploads/2021/04/llam-infographic-2021.pdf

Bouldin, E. D., Thompson, M. L., Boyko, E., & Morgenroth, D. C. (2016). Weight change trajectories following incident lower limb amputation. *Archives of Physical Medicine and Rehabilitation, 97*(1), 1–7e1. https://doi.org/10.1016/j.apmr.2015.09.0117

Brooks, S. G., Atkinson, S. L., Cimino, S. R., MacKay, C., Mayo, A. L., & Hitzig, S. L. (2021). Sexuality and sexual health in adults with limb loss: A systematic review. *Sexuality and Disability, 39*, 3–21. https://doi.org/10.1007/s11195-020-09665-w

Bumbasirevic, M., Lesic, A., Palibrk, T., Milovanovic, D., Zoka, M., Kravic-Stevovic, T., & Raspopovic, S. (2020). The current state of bionic limbs from the surgeon's viewpoint. *EFORT Open Reviews, 5*(2), 65–72. https://doi.org/10.1302/2058-5241.5.180038

Davis, R. (1993). Phantom sensation, phantom pain and stump pain. *Archives of Physical Medicine & Rehabilitation, 74*(70), 79–84.

Donnelley, C. A., Shirley, C., von Kaeppler, E. P., Hetherington, A., Albright, P. D., Morshed, S., & Shearer, D. W. (2021). Cost analyses of prosthetic devices: A systematic review. *Archives of Physical Medicine and Rehabilitation, 102*(7), 1401–1415. https://doi.org/10.1016/j.apmr.2021.02.010

Esquenazi, A., Leonard, J. A., & Meier, R. H. (1989). Prosthetics. *Archives of Physical Medicine & Rehabilitation, 70* (suppl.), 207.

Friedmann, L. (1981). Amputation. In W. Stolov & M. Clowers (Eds.), *Handbook of severe disability* (pp. 169–188). U.S. Department of Education, Rehabilitation Services Administration.

Garetto, A., Baur, E. M., Prahm, C., Smekal, V., Jeschke, J., Peternell, G., Pedrini, M. T., & Kolbenschlag, J. (2021). Reduction of phantom limb pain and improved proprioception through a TSR-based surgical technique: A case series of four patients with lower limb amputation. *Journal of Clinical Medicine, 10*(17), 429. https://doi.org/10.3390/jcm10174029

Hamilton, J. (2022, June 13). *Researchers work to create a sense of touch in prosthetic limbs.* National Public Radio. www.npr.org/sections/health-shots/2022/06/09/1103884757/researchers-are-developing-prosthetics-that-have-a-sense-of-touch

Horsch, A., Gleichauf, S., Lehner, B., Ghandour, M., Koch, J., Alimusaj, M., Renkawitz, T., & Putz, C. (2022). Lower-limb amputation in children and adolescents – A rare encounter with unique and special challenges. *Children, 9*, 1–11. https://doi.org/10.3390/children9071004

Heyns, A., Jacobs, S., Negrini, S., Patrini, M., & Rauch, A. (2021). Systematic review of clinical practice guidelines for individuals with amputation: Identification of best evidence for rehabilitation to develop the WHO's package of interventions for rehabilitation. *Archives of Physical Medicine and Rehabilitation, 102*(6), 1191–1197. https://doi.org/10.1016/j.ampr.2020.11.019

Imam, B., Miller, W. C., Finlayson, H. C., Eng, J. J., & Jarus, T. (2017). Incidence of lower limb amputation in Canada. *Canadian Journal of Public Health, 108*(4), 374–380.

Jarbrink, K., Gao, N., Bajpai, R., Car, J., Soonergren, H., Schmidtchen, A., & Pang, C. (2016). Prevalence and incidence of chronic wounds and related complications: A protocol for a systematic review. *Systematic Reviews*, *5*, 1–6. https://doi.org/10.1186/s13643-016-0329-y

Leonard, J. A., & Meier, R. H. (1993). Upper and lower extremity prosthetics. In J. A. DeLisa (Ed.), *Rehabilitation medicine: Principles and practices* (pp. 507–525). J. B. Lippincott.

Limakatso, K., Bedwell, G. J., Madden, V. J., & Parker, R. (2020). The prevalence and risk factors for phantom limb pain in people with amputations: A systematic review and meta-analysis. *PLoS ONE*, e0240431. https://doi.org/10.1371/journal.pone.0240431

Luza, L. P., Ferreira, E. G., Minsky, R. C., Pires, G. K. W., & da Silva, R. (2020). Psychosocial and physical adjustments and prosthesis satisfaction in amputees: A systematic review of observational studies. *Disability and Rehabilitation: Assistive Technology*, *15*(5), 582–589.

Meier, R. H. (1994). Upper limb amputee rehabilitation. In A. Esquenazi (Ed.), *Prosthetics: State of the art reviews* (pp. 165–185). Hanley & Belfus.

Meier, R. H. (1995). Rehabilitation of the person with an amputation. In R. B. Rutherford (Ed.), *Vascular surgery* (pp. 2227–2248). W.B. Saunders.

Meier, R. H. (1996). Upper limb prosthetics: Design, prescription and application. In C. A. Peimer (Ed.), *Surgery of the hand and upper extremity* (pp. 2453–2468). McGraw-Hill.

Meier, R. H. (2011). Life care planning for the child with an amputation. In S. Riddick-Grisham & L. Deming (Eds.). *Pediatric life care planning and case management handbook* (2nd ed., pp. 591–620). CRC Press.

Meier, R. H., & Atkins, D. J. (2004). *Functional restoration of adults and children with upper extremity amputation*. Demos Medical Publishing.

Meier, R. H., Choppa, A. J., & Johnson, C. B. (2013). The person with amputation and their life care plan. *Physical Medicine and Rehabilitation Clinics of North America*, *24*(3), 467–489.

Meier, R.H. & Heckman, J.T. (2014). Principles of contemporary amputation rehabilitation in the United States, 2013. *Physical Medicine and Rehabilitation Clinics of North America*, *25*(1), 29-33.

Moore, W. S., & Malone, J. M. (Eds.). (1989). *Lower extremity amputation*. W.B. Saunders.

Patton, J. G. (1989). Developmental approach to pediatric prosthetic evaluation and training. In: Atkins, D.J., & Meier, R.H. (eds) *Comprehensive management of the upper-limb amputee*. Springer, New York, NY. https://doi.org/10.1007/978-1-4612-3530-9_13

Research and Markets. (2022). *Prosthetics and Orthotics Global Market Report 2022*. Author.

Sear, H. H. (1991). Approaches to prescription of body-powered and myoelectric prosthetics. In L. W. Friedmann (Ed.), *Prosthetics: Physical medicine and rehabilitation clinics of North America* (pp. 361–371). W.B. Saunders.

Sherman, R. A., Sherman, C. J., & Gail, N. A. (1980). Survey of current phantom limb treatment in the United States. *Pain*, *8*, 85–99.

Setoguchi, Y., & Patton, J. (2004). Training the child with a unilateral upper-extremity prosthesis. In R. H. Meier & D. J. Atkins (Eds.), *Functional restoration of adults and children with upper extremity amputations*. Demos Medical Publishing.

Trent, L., Intintoli, M., Prigge, P., Bolinger, C., Walters, L. S., Conyers, D., Miguelez, J., & Ryan, T. (2019). A narrative review: Current upper limb prosthetic options and design. *Disability and Rehabilitation: Assistive Technology*. https://doi.org/10.1080/17483107.2019.1594403. www.researchgate.net/profile/Lisa-Walters-7/publication/332366308_A_narrative_review_current_upper_limb_prosthetic_options_and_design/links/5e68611f92851c7ce05b2e1b/A-narrative-review-current-upper-limb-prosthetic-options-and-design.pdf

Uellendahl, J. (2017). Myoelectric versus body-powered upper-limb prosthesis: A clinical perspective. *Journal of Prosthetics and Orthotics*, *29*(45), 25–29. https://journals.lww.com/jpojournal/fulltext/2017/10001/myoelectric_versus_body_powered_upper_limb.5.aspx

Ülger, O., Yildirim Sahanm, T., & Celik, S. E. (2018). A systematic literature review of physiotherapy and rehabilitation approaches to lower-limb amputation. *Physiotherapy Theory & Practice*, *34*(11), 821–834. https://doi.org/10.1080/09593985.2018.1425938

U. S. Department of Veterans Affairs, Department of Defense. (2022). *VA/DoD clinical practice guidelines: The management of upper limb amputation rehabilitation (ULA)*. www.healthquality.va.gov/guidelines/rehab/ula/

U. S. Department of Veterans Affairs, Department of Defense. (2019). *Lower limb amputation: An update*. https://pubmed.ncbi.nlm.nih.gov/31419214/

U. S. Department of Veterans Affairs, Department of Defense. (2017). *VA/DoD clinical practice guidelines: Rehabilitation of lower limb amputation*. www.healthquality.va.gov/guidelines/rehab/amp/

Uustal, H., & Meier, R. H. (February, 2014). Pain issues in amputee rehabilitation. *Physical Medicine Clinics of North America*, 25(1), 45–52.

van Schaik, L., Geertzen, J. H. B., Dijkstra, P. U., & Dekker, R. (2019). Metabolic costs of activities of daily living in persons with a lower limb amputation: A systematic review and meta-analysis. *PLoS ONE*, e0123256. https://doi.org/10.1371/journal.pone.0213256

Vllasolli, T. O., Zafirova, B., Orovcanec, N., Poposka, A., Muretzani, A., & Krasniqi, B. (2014). Energy expenditure and walking speed in lower limb amputees: A cross sectional study. *Ostopedia, Traumatologia, Rehabilitacja*, 161(4), 419–426. https://doi.org/10.5604/15093492.1119619

Weed, R., & Atkins, D. (2004). Return to work issues for persons with upper extremity amputation. In R. Meier and D. Atkins (eds.). *Functional restoration of adults and children with upper extremity amputation*, 337–351. Demos Publishing.

Weed, R., & Sluis, A. (1990). *Life care plans for the amputee: A step by step guide*. CRC Press.

West, M., & Wu, H. (2010). Pulse radiofrequency ablation for residual and phantom limb pain: A case series. *Pain Practice*, 10(5), 485–491. https://doi.org/10.1111/j.1533-2500.2009.00353.x

Widerstrom-Noga, E., & Finalyson, M. (2010). Aging with a disability: Physical impairment, pain, and fatigue. *Physical Medicine and Rehabilitation Clinics of North America*, 21, 321–337.

Young, M., McKay, C., Williams, S., Rouse, P., & Bilzon, J. L. J. (2019). Time-related changes in quality of life in persons with lower limb amputation or spinal cord injury: Protocol for a systematic review. *Systematic Reviews*, 8(191), 1–6. https://doi.org/10.1186/s13643-019-1108-3

Chapter 20

Life Care Planning for Acquired Brain Injury

David L. Ripley

Traumatic brain injury (TBI) is one of the leading causes of neurological impairment in the United States. In a 2015 report to Congress, between 2002–2010, TBI accounted for over 2.2 million visits to the emergency room each year with 50,000 deaths and 280,000 hospitalizations (Centers for Disease Control and Prevention [CDC], 2015). By 2019, average annual TBI-related hospitalizations had decreased to 223,135 while related deaths escalated to 64,362 by 2020 (CDC, 2022a). Data from 2019 indicate that more than 611 hospitalizations and 176 deaths occur due to brain injury every day in the United States (CDC, 2022a). Acquired brain injury (ABI) is the leading cause of neurological impairment for individuals between the ages of 16 and 30 years of age. It is estimated that about 5.3 million people are living with the consequences of TBI in the United States (CDC, 2021a, 2021b).

The brain, as the neurological control center for the body, affects almost every aspect of physiological functioning (Kaufman et al., 1993; Macciocchi et al., 1993; National Institute of Neurological Disorders and Stroke, 2022; Piek, 1995; Rosenthal, 1990). Practitioners in the field of brain injury rehabilitation must be prepared to deal with problems in essentially every organ system in the body, as well as a variety of cognitive and behavioral problems (CDC, 2015; Uomoto & Brockway, 1992; Wood, 1987).

Because many people who sustain a brain injury are young at the time of their injury, it is difficult in many circumstances to estimate lifetime earning capacity and needs (Chan et al., 2020; Corthell, 1993; Dikmen et al., 1994; Goodall et al., 1994; Horn & Zasler, 1996; Ip et al., 1995; Stapleton et al., 1989; Wehman et al., 1988; Zasler & Faadep, 1997). Additionally, as acute trauma management and medical and rehabilitation care improve, the survival of persons with brain injury will continue to increase (High et al., 1996; Kreutzer et al., 2001; Shi et al., 2014). The result is that many more people survive with increasingly complex medical and rehabilitation problems. Creating an appropriate life care plan for an individual with ABI can be a formidable challenge. Due to the variability in recovery following brain injury, life care planners are often forced to develop, in a sense, multiple care plans to accommodate the different potential outcomes that may occur in a single individual.

Epidemiology

There are several factors associated with a higher risk for TBI. Males are nearly twice as likely as females to be hospitalized and three times more likely to die from a TBI (CDC, 2022a). Also, persons with brain injury tend to be from racial and ethnic minorities, service members, individuals who experience homelessness or are in correctional facilities, those living in rural areas and survivors of intimate partner violence (CDC, 2022b). (CDC, 2020b). Additionally, individuals with brain injury are more likely to be homeless and have lower access to health insurance and medical care.

Brain injury generally follows a *bimodal* distribution with respect to age. Adolescents between the ages of 15–19 years and adults 65 years and older are the most likely to sustain a TBI (Georges & Das, 2022). When preparing life care plans for individuals with brain injuries, lifelong concerns must be taken into consideration, including aging and aging issues, education, vocational rehabilitation, and community reintegration. Age may also be correlated with outcomes, as older individuals (over age 65) tend to have a slower recovery and worse outcomes following brain injury (Caplan, et al., 2018; Coronado et al., 2005; Gardner et al., 2018; Harrison-Felix et al., 2012).

Costs

Estimating the economic impact of TBI is difficult primarily due to methodological variations. However, most studies have suggested that the costs associated with treating TBI in the United States range from $37.8 to $60 billion annually (Brown et al., 2008; Humphreys et al., 2013; Miller et al., 2021).

Etiology

The etiology of brain injuries occurring in the United States has been changing over time. In data from the Traumatic Brain Injury Model Systems National Data and Statistical Center (National Data and Statistical Center Traumatic Brain Injury Model System, 2022), vehicular crash (49%) followed by falls (29%), violence (11%), and other (11%) are cited as the most frequent causes of TBI for individuals who receive inpatient rehabilitation.

Anatomy of the Brain Coverings

The brain is protected by a number of layers of differing tissue. A layer of skin is the outermost covering, followed by a layer of connective tissue and muscle. The bony calvarium, or skull, provides the greatest protection for the brain. Fractures of the skull are present concomitantly with many brain injuries and are generally associated with a more severe injury. Under the skull are three distinct layers that provide the direct cover of the brain. The outermost, thickest layer is called the *dura mater* and is attached to the inner layer of the skull in many places. Underneath this layer is the *arachnoid mater*, which derives its name from its similarity in appearance to a spider web. The arachnoid mater follows the surface of the brain closely but does not follow the surface down deep into the crevices, or *sulci*, on the surface of the brain. The innermost layer of covering is called the *pia mater*, and this layer does follow the brain into the sulci.

Cerebral Cortex

The outer surface of the brain is called the cerebral cortex. There are many convolutions of the surface of the brain, which serve to increase the surface area of the outside of the brain. The bulges are referred to as *gyri*, and the involutions are referred to as *sulci*. The origination of neural messages to the rest of the body, for the most part, occurs on the surface of the brain. In most cases, seizure activity also originates at the level of the cortex.

The cortex of the brain is divided into lobes that represent areas of specific functioning (see Figure 20.1). The *frontal lobe* is responsible for higher cognitive processes, such as planning, organization, and problem solving. It is also the part of the brain responsible for control of impulsive and instinctual behavior (Blair, 2016; Grafman et al., 1996). Last, the origination of motor activity occurs in the most posterior portion of the frontal lobe.

The *parietal lobe* is predominately involved in the registration of sensory information, particularly the ability to sense when something has touched the skin. Other types of sensory information are processed in this area, and the parietal lobe gives us the ability to orient objects in space, follow a map, and appreciate music. Individuals with injury to the parietal lobe will often exhibit *neglect*, or lack of awareness of part of their own body.

The *temporal lobes* are located on the sides of the brain. These lobes are critical in the registration of auditory information and are critical in the understanding and formulation of language. They are also involved in other aspects of communication, such as interpretation of emotional components of communication. The inner portion of the temporal lobes also contains structures that are responsible for memory formation, as well as the origination of emotions.

The *occipital lobe* is located on the most posterior aspect of the brain. Visual information is registered and processed here. Individuals with injury to this area may have *cortical blindness*, which is an inability to see because of failure of the brain to recognize the neural signals sent from the eyes.

Deeper Brain Structures

The *basal ganglia* are a group of structures deeper in the brain. The primary function of the basal ganglia is to regulate motor function, predominantly by providing feedback to other structures to regulate motor activity, as well as being implicated in behavior, especially involved in risk and reward. Injury to the basal ganglia can result in disorders of movement, as well as problems in learning decision making and motivation (Chakravarthy et al., 2010; Dudman & Karkauer, 2016; Fix, 2008; Ikemoto et al., 2015; Maaike & van Swieten, 2020; Stocco et al., 2010; Turner & Desmurget, 2010; Yahya, 2021).

The *thalamus* is another deep brain structure. The thalamus is primarily thought of as a "relay station" for sensory information coming into the brain from the sensory organs. Part of the role of the thalamus involves processing the sensory information to determine what information is of greatest significance at a particular moment, then passing that information on to higher cortical structures for registration and processing. In this respect, it plays a large role in determining what information the brain's attention is directed to at a given moment. Because of its connection to many other structures as well as its critical role in sensory information processing, injury to the thalamus can result in impairment of almost any neurological function (Schmitt et al., 2017; Sherman & Guillery, 2006; Ward, 2016).

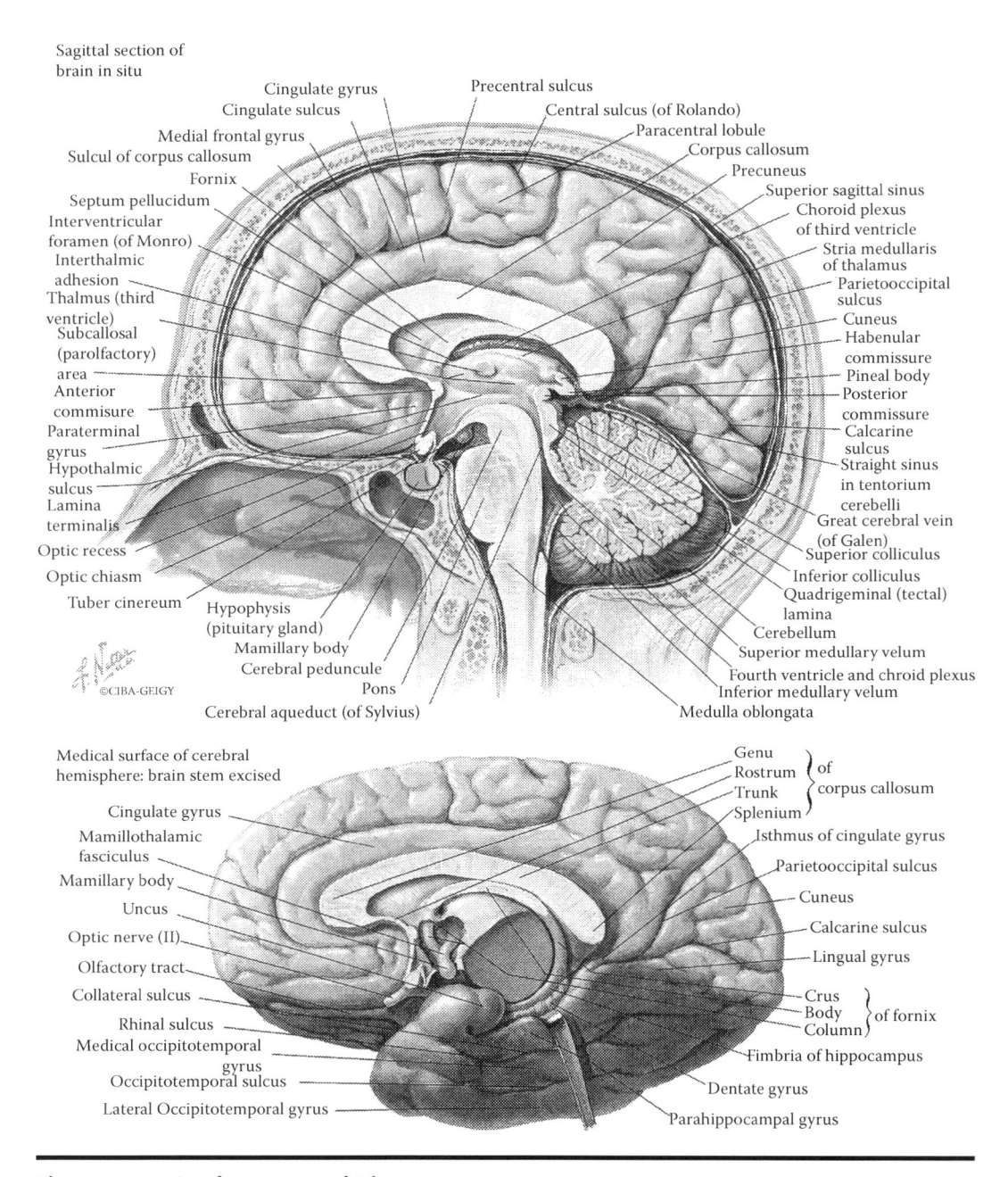

Figure 20.1 Cerebrum, Lateral Views

Source: (From Netter, F. H. (1997). *Atlas of human anatomy* (2nd ed.). Icon Learning Systems. With permission.)

Cerebellum

The *cerebellum* is an area of the brain that facilitates coordinated motor movements. There are extensive neural pathways between the cerebellum and other areas of the brain concerned with motor movement. Individuals with injury to the cerebellum exhibit *ataxia*, or lack of control of smooth coordinated movements. Interestingly, persons with brain injury with ataxia often have no problems with strength and often have the muscle strength to carry out any activity you ask. However, they lack an ability to control their limbs' movements, such that it is often difficult or impossible for them to perform basic activities like picking up a glass or walking.

Brain Stem

The *brain stem* (Figure 20.2) is the most inferior portion of the brain. This part of the brain is critical for basic life-sustaining functions, as it is responsible for regulating breathing and heart rates. Most of the cranial nerves exit here, so the brain stem is intimately involved in the transmission and reception of sensory and motor information of the head, such as tongue movement, facial movement, and sensation. Because all sensory and motor information to and from the body and brain must travel through the brain stem, even a very small area of injury to the brain stem can have devastating effects on the person with the injury. The brainstem is also the location of the *reticular formation*, a structure inherently involved in wakefulness. Most individuals who have a disorder of consciousness following TBI have injury to the brainstem. The brainstem is further divided into three sections: the midbrain, the pons, and the medulla oblongata.

Midbrain

The *midbrain* contains a number of structures that help to control movement, interpret sensory information, and also help with such activities as controlling our level of consciousness. The structures in the midbrain are involved in motor control, as well as transmission of information for vision and hearing, The substantia nigra, located within the midbrain, is the primary site of dopamine production in the brain, which is involved in attention, excitation, and motivation, along with its role in motor control. Injury to the midbrain may produce impairments similar to those seen in Parkinson's disease (Damier et al., 1999; Haines, 2012; Sciacca et al., 2019)

Pons

The *pons* is the middle portion of the brainstem. It is defined by its connections with the cerebellum, which is located posteriorly and inferiorly to the pons. The cranial nerves that control eye movements, hearing, and balance originate in the pons, as well as those responsible for movement and sensation of the face (Rahman & Tadi, 2021; Sciacca et al., 2019). Injury to the pons can result in a wide variety of problems with facial and oromotor function, and individuals with injury to the pons may have difficulty with speaking and swallowing.

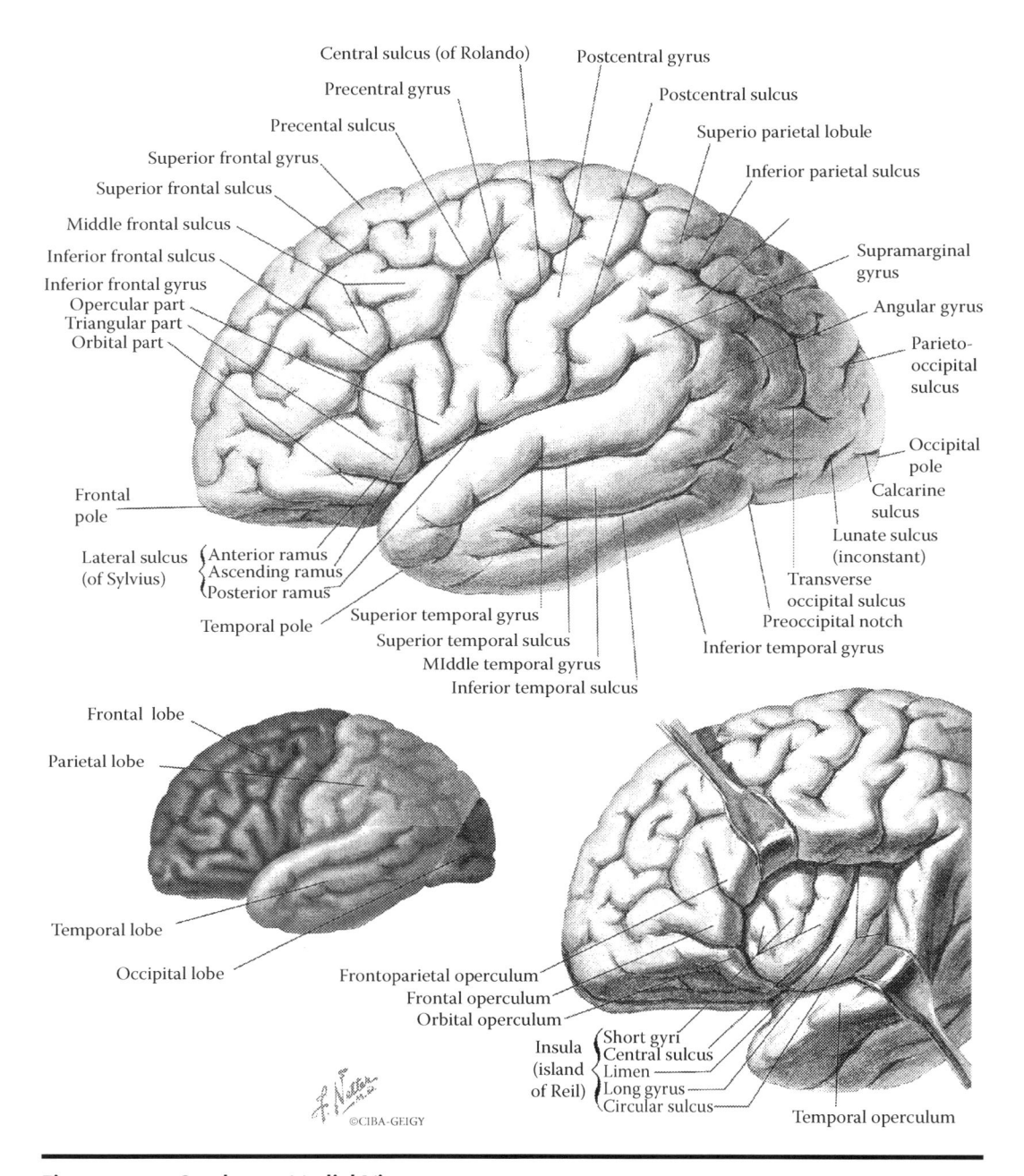

Figure 20.2 Cerebrum, Medial Views

Source: (From Netter, Netter, F. H. (1997). *Atlas of human anatomy* (2nd ed.). Icon Learning Systems. With permission.)

Medulla Oblongata

The *medulla oblongata*, (or just "medulla") is the most inferior portion of the brainstem and continues inferiorly as the spinal cord. The medulla is the site of origin of control centers for breathing and cardiac function (Sciacca et al., 2019). Because of this, many individuals who have injury to the medulla do not survive.

Brain Injury Classification

Brain injuries can be classified by several methods (Marshall et al., 1992; O'Neil et al., 2013; Teasdale et al., 1992; van Ierssel et al., 2018). Acquired brain injuries are generally classified as traumatic, anoxic/hypoxic-ischemic, vascular, or other. Anoxic or hypoxic-ischemic brain injuries occur when areas of the brain do not receive enough oxygen. This is frequently the cause of secondary injury after a traumatic injury but may also occur independently of trauma. The most frequent cause of hypoxic-ischemic brain injury is secondary to myocardial infarction. During resuscitative efforts for a heart attack, the brain may be deprived of oxygen for several minutes. Vascular brain injuries, commonly called strokes, most commonly occur as a result of thromboembolic phenomena. However, other types of vascular brain injuries include aneurysms, arteriovenous malformation, and spontaneous intracranial hemorrhages. Finally, injury to the brain may occur as a result of viral or bacterial infections, metabolic derangements, or tumors.

Traumatic brain injuries, the broadest category of ABI, may be further subdivided in a number of ways. One of the most basic methods of subcategorization is to divide them between *open* or *closed*. Open injuries are those injuries in which there is disruption of the scalp and skull, creating the possibility that the brain may be contaminated by material from the outside environment. Penetrating brain injuries are a type of open injury, in which a foreign body (such as a bullet) passes through the skull and outer coverings of the brain into the brain tissue itself. Closed head injuries are those in which the skull remains intact, and the brain is not exposed to the outside environment, although significant injury may occur from the impact of the brain against the inner part of the skull, or from shearing of axons secondary to rotational forces.

Medical professionals caring for survivors of brain injury will also classify the injuries based on severity. The most common, widely utilized method of classification is the *Glasgow Coma Scale*, a method that classifies injuries based on clinical presentation (see Table 20.1). A medical professional will rate the person with brain injury's response in three separate areas: eye opening, motor response, and verbal response. The scale gives scores for each of the areas, which are summed to give a total score that can be used to rank the severity of the injury. Individuals who score 3–8 are said to have a severe injury, from 9–12 a moderate injury, and from 13–15 a mild injury. This information may be useful to predict the outcome and likelihood of long-term impairments (Clifton et al., 1993; Li et al., 2021; Teasdale et al., 1998; Wan-Ting et al., 2020; Zafonte et al., 1996).

Other methods of rating injury severity are available but not as widely utilized. One alternative method of injury classification uses duration of *post-traumatic amnesia* as the best method of predicting outcomes following TBI (Briggs et al., 2015; Zafonte et al., 1997). Other methods of classification have tried to use radiographic findings, such as location and size of lesions on computed tomography (CT) or magnetic resonance imaging (MRI) (Firsching et al., 2001; Teasdale et al., 1992; Yadav et al., 2016), with new classification systems emerging (Hu et al., 2022; Wilson et al., 2022). Other techniques, including diffusion tensor imaging, functional MRIs (fMRI), and brain perfusion single photon emission computed tomography are used in the evaluation of TBI (Edlow & Wu, 2012; Georges & Das, 2022; Smith et al., 2019).

Table 20.1 The Glasgow Coma Scale

Person with brain injury's response		Score
Eye opening		
	Spontaneously	4
	To voice	3
	To painful stimulus	2
	No eye opening	1
Motor		
	Follows commands	6
	Localizes to pain	5
	Withdraws from pain	4
	Flexor response	3
	Extensor response	2
	No motor response	1
Verbal		
	Oriented	5
	Converses but disoriented	4
	Inappropriate words	3
	Incomprehensible verbal utterances	2
	Not vocalizing	1
Total		
	(Sum of score from each of three areas)	(3–15)
	Injury classification:	
	Severe	3–8
	Moderate	9–12
	Mild	13–15

Note: A score with a T (e.g., 8T) means the person with brain injury was intubated for airway purposes and may be unable to fully respond.

Another broad categorization of brain injury is based on the anatomy of the injury to the brain. Two broad anatomical categories are *diffuse* and *focal* brain injuries. Diffuse injuries are generally due to shearing injury of the axons and generally occur across broad areas of the brain. Focal injuries occur with trauma to one specific region of the brain. These two types of injury may occur concomitantly. In general, focal injuries result in shorter periods of unconsciousness than diffuse injuries. Individuals with diffuse injury, sometimes referred to as diffuse axonal injury (DAI), may have prolonged periods of unconsciousness from several days to weeks. In general, individuals with DAI have a prolonged recovery period compared to those with focal injuries (Berker, 1996; Bontke & Boake, 1991; Viera et al., 2016).

Disorders of Consciousness

Many individuals with severe brain injuries may experience at least a transient disruption in systems of the brain that are responsible for arousal or alertness. Due to a variety of descriptions used by medical professionals throughout the years, and the problems this caused with communication, the American Congress of Rehabilitation Medicine (ACRM) in 1993 proposed a uniform nomenclature for brain injury. The following definitions are part of the ACRM's recommendations (Mild Traumatic Brain Injury Committee, American Congress of Rehabilitation Medicine Head Injury Interdisciplinary Special Interest Group, 1993). These criteria were reviewed and updated by the American Academy of Neurology in 2018 (Giacino et al., 2018).

- *Coma*: A state of being completely unconscious. The person is not awake, and the eyes remain constantly closed. Also, there is no behavior suggesting the person is aware of self or surroundings
- *Vegetative State (VS) or Unresponsive Wakefulness Syndrome (UWS)*: A state of being awake, with eyes open, and of not showing signs of behavior suggesting the person is aware of self or surroundings
- *Persistent VS*: A VS or UWS that persists longer than one month
- *Minimally Conscious State (MCS):* A state in which the person has definite signs of behavior showing awareness of self or surroundings Often these behaviors may not be obvious or may not happen regularly.

Initial Treatment

When a person with brain injury presents to the emergency room following TBI, the initial activities focus on life preservation. Often, concomitant injuries preclude addressing the brain injuries until later in the course of treatment. However, for those persons with severe brain injuries, the initial protocols involve rating the person with brain injury's level of arousal using the Glasgow Coma Scale, and some form of neuroradiographic imaging. Computed tomography scans remain the preferred type of image, due to the faster speed with which images can be obtained and the fact that the types of injury that require emergency surgical intervention show much more readily on CT than MRI. However, MRI techniques are more sensitive to intracranial injury (Gerber et al., 2004; Horn & Zasler, 1996; Levin, 1992; Marshall et al., 1992; Piek, 1995; Rappaport et al., 1992; Schweitzer et al., 2019).

Once the person with brain injury is stabilized, a more detailed assessment of the injury will occur, and further treatment may be recommended. For severe injuries, assessment by a neurosurgeon will usually occur. If there is evidence of specific, severe types of bleeding or increased pressure inside the head, surgery may be performed to evacuate the blood or alleviate the pressure. Sometimes an intracranial pressure monitor will be placed to accurately measure the pressure inside the brain.

Persons with more severe brain injuries frequently require assistance with basic life functions. They may be placed on a mechanical ventilator to help them breathe. For prolonged management, sometimes a tracheotomy is performed to facilitate prolonged ventilator support. Additionally, for persons with brain injury who are unconscious for prolonged periods, or have prolonged difficulty with swallowing, a feeding tube may be surgically introduced. Many persons with severe brain injury have sustained injuries to other parts of their body as well. Surgical attention, for either children or adults, is often necessary during the early hospitalization to address fractures, damaged internal organs, internal bleeding, and other medical concerns.

Rehabilitation Care

While persons with brain injury are still in the hospital, physical and occupational therapy referrals should occur to maintain joint range of motion and strength and to begin working on activities of self-care. The more severely injured persons with brain injury should be referred to a rehabilitation facility following their acute hospitalization to begin the work of trying to be restored to their highest level of functioning. An assessment by a physiatrist, a medical doctor with training in physical medicine and rehabilitation (PM&R), is important during this phase to facilitate the coordination of services and medical treatment to promote the best outcome following TBI (Almli & Finger, 1992; Berker, 1996; Bontke et al., 1993; Greiss et al., 2016; Kreitzer et al., 2019; Rosenthal, 1990; Semlyen et al., 1998).

Persons with brain injury will often require further medical and rehabilitation care after medical issues are stabilized (Cope, 1995). Rehabilitation services may be provided in a number of different settings. The most appropriate level of care depends on the nature of the concomitant medical issues, as well as the level of functioning of the person with brain injury (Evans & Ruff, 1992; Hall & Cope, 1995; Levine & Flanagan, 2010; Mazmanian et al., 1993; Patrick et al., 2012; Schmidt, 1997). The most common level of rehabilitation care is in an *inpatient rehabilitation facility* (IRF), where persons with brain injury receive three or more hours of therapy a day from several different therapy disciplines (i.e., physical therapy, occupational therapy, speech therapy), as well as ongoing medical attention, usually by a physician who specializes in PM&R (Laker et al., 2019; Malec & Basford, 1996). Some IRFs have programs specifically tailored for the rehabilitation of individuals with brain injury. These centers often provide greater expertise in the care of individuals with TBI.

Once individuals with brain injury are medically stable and safe to be managed at home, therapy efforts transition to an outpatient setting. *Rehabilitation Day Programs* are therapy programs designed for individuals who still need therapy from several different disciplines in a team format, but no longer need as close medical attention as individuals in the acute inpatient setting. Some individuals will not need the interdisciplinary model of therapy, but only require therapy from one or two disciplines; then single-service outpatient therapy is indicated. In some cases, if medical issues prohibit active participation in therapy, persons with brain injury may be sent to other settings, such as long-term acute care hospitals or skilled nursing facilities. In these settings, rehabilitation services may be provided, but generally not to the extent and intensity of that provided in IRFs, and generally not with the same level of medical and rehabilitation oversight. Another option for persons with brain injury is treatment in a post-acute rehabilitation program. These programs, commonly referred to as *Community Reintegration Programs*, *Residential Brain Injury Programs*, or *Transitional Care Programs*, are residential programs where the patient stays in a community setting, like a house, apartment, or dormitory, and receives therapy service much like inpatient rehabilitation. These programs require that the patient be medically stable and ready to work on higher functional activities, such as eating out, shopping, meal management, and pre-vocational activities.

Medical Complications

An adept life care planner who works with survivors of brain injury must be aware of the potential medical complications that arise following brain injury and their impact on recovery, long-term function, and reintegration in the community. As the brain is the control center for all neurological processes in the body, injury to the brain can result in complications to almost every organ system. It is beyond the scope of this chapter to discuss all complications, although there are several common complications that we will describe (Bigler, 1989; Bloomfield, 1989; Bontke et al., 1993; Cifu et al., 1996a; Corrigan & Mysiw, 1988; Goya et al., 2018; Jorge et al., 1993; Katz & Alexander, 1994; Kaufman et al., 1993; Kraus et al., 1984; Piek, 1995; Pilitsis & Rengachary, 2013; Russell-Jones & Shorvon, 1989; Uomoto & Brockway, 1992).

Cranial Complications

Injury to the cranial nerves frequently occurs following TBI. As a result, persons with brain injury may have difficulty with basic sensory functions, such as vision, hearing, smell, and taste. Facial paresis is frequently seen, with resultant difficulty in oromotor functions, such as speaking and eating. It is very common for the olfactory nerve (cranial nerve I), the cranial nerve that controls sense of smell, to be damaged, resulting in problems with eating and appetite. Fractures of the temporal bone, a part of the skull, can result in disruption of the acousticovestibular nerve (cranial nerve VIII), resulting in hearing impairment. Injury to structures involved in balance, such as the acousticovestibular nerve may result in dizziness and balance disorders. This by itself may lead to problems with standing, walking, and transfers.

Many persons with brain injury will have significant difficulty with vision problems following brain injury. Problems may range from inability to see objects in certain parts of the field of vision (sometimes referred to as a field cut) to blurry or double vision. This may be due to injury to the visual pathways within the brain, to injury to the nerves that control eye movements, or to injury to the eye itself.

Endocrine Disorders

Endocrinology is the study of hormones and their function. Many hormones are regulated or secreted by the pituitary gland, a structure at the base of the brain. The pituitary can frequently be damaged during injury to the brain due to its location and structure. Common endocrine disorders following brain injury include syndrome of inappropriate diuretic hormone, growth hormone deficiency, and irregularities of gonadal steroid production, and thyroid dysfunction. Endocrinopathies are much more evident in women, because menstrual irregularities, as a result of altered pituitary-gonadal axis functioning, may persist for a year or longer after brain injury (Duncan & Garijo-Garde, 2021; Ripley et al., 2008; Snook et al., 2017).

Pulmonary Complications

Persons with brain injury with severe TBI frequently have respiratory failure as sequelae of the initial trauma. As a result, persons with brain injury often require mechanical ventilation with a breathing machine (ventilator). Sometimes physicians must perform a tracheotomy, or a surgically created hole, to allow the person with brain injury to breathe and to help prevent complications from prolonged ventilator management. Persons with brain injury who are immobile for prolonged periods are at a higher risk for developing pneumonia. A pulmonary embolus, or a blood clot that lodges in the blood vessels of the lungs, is also a potential complication of prolonged immobility.

Cardiovascular Complications

Direct effects of brain injury on the cardiovascular system are infrequent. However, a complication that may lead to cardiovascular injury is called paroxysmal sympathetic hyperactivity, sometimes referred to as "central storming," in which abnormally high levels of stimulant hormones are released into the bloodstream, resulting in fevers, high heart rates, and high blood pressure (Chen et al., 2017; Perkes et al., 2010). This phenomenon can result in heart injury to people who are susceptible. In addition, immobility may lead to cardiovascular complications over time. The most common is the formation of deep vein thromboses or blood clots in the veins. These clots can be potentially life threatening, as they can break free and lodge in the lung vessels causing a pulmonary embolus, as noted previously. Deep vein thromboses may also result in post-phlebitic syndrome, or a painful condition of inflammation of the veins.

Neurological Complications

Typical neurological problems include weakness, sensory deficits, and the previously mentioned cranial nerve problems. Persons with brain injury are also at increased risk of seizures. The risk of seizures increases with more severe injury, increased age, prolonged coma, hydrocephalus, presence of a penetrating brain injury, skull fracture, or significant amounts of subarachnoid blood (Annegers & Coan, 2000; Zhang et al., 2021a) Hydrocephalus which occurs when the system for reabsorption of cerebrospinal fluid is not functioning properly, can interfere with recovery and neurological progress, and often must be treated with a surgically implanted device called a *shunt* (Chen et al., 2019). Another neurological complication is the upper motor neuron syndrome, with its constellation of symptoms of weakness, spasticity, and increased reflexes. Spasticity is a velocity-dependent increase in motor tone that is seen frequently following injury to motor nerves in the central nervous system. This is such a profound problem after brain injury that it will be discussed in detail later in the chapter. Additionally, cognitive and behavioral problems are frequent neurological complications and will also be discussed in more detail later.

Gastrointestinal Complications

Persons with brain injury frequently exhibit dysphagia, or impairment in the ability to swallow, as a result of weakness of the pharyngeal muscles. Often, persons with brain injury require the placement of a feeding tube to prevent aspiration of food and to allow for feeding while the pharyngeal muscles remain weak. Additional gastrointestinal problems may include incontinence secondary to neurological impairment of the muscles controlling bowel function or alternatively from cognitive impairment. Constipation is frequently seen due to immobility or due to medications, particularly opioid analgesics.

Genitourinary Complications

Neurological control of the bladder may be impaired, resulting in incontinence. However, most cases of incontinence following brain injury are a result of disinhibition instead of injury to urological structures. Persons with brain injury with neurological impairment of bladder function may retain urine, which can lead to other problems, including frequent infections of the urinary tract, infection of the kidneys, and renal and bladder stones. Sexual dysfunction may also be an issue. Persons with brain injury may have sexual dysfunction as a result of hormonal abnormalities, psychological issues, or behavioral control problems. Although the predominant lay viewpoint is that persons with brain injury exhibit inappropriate sexual behavior or sexual disinhibition, frequently the opposite is the case. Sexual inhibition may occur as a result of altered body image due to impairments in physical function or changes in physical appearance due to the injury (Kreutzer et al., 1998; Ponsford, 2003; Sander et al., 2013). Sexual functioning is an area that is frequently overlooked by medical professionals (Calabrò et al., 2017; Deschênes et al., 2019; Khajeei et al., 2019; O'Shea et al., 2020; Simpson et al., 2017). In women, infertility may occur secondary to the endocrine changes mentioned earlier (Ripley et al., 2008).

Musculoskeletal Complications

Musculoskeletal complications are very common following brain injury. Injury to the motor nerves in the brain may result in upper motor neuron syndrome, which consists of a constellation of symptoms of spasticity, weakness, and hyperreflexia. Areas of weakness can vary depending on where the injury is located in the brain. Due to the brain's structural organization, injury on one side of the brain results in weakness on the opposite side of the body. Additionally, the weak side is frequently associated with spasticity. If unchecked, spasticity and immobility may ultimately result in *contractures*, which is tightening of the soft tissues and shortening of tendons around a joint resulting in a reduction in the person with brain injury's mobility. As a result of associated trauma, persons with brain injuries also frequently have associated fractures, peripheral nerve injuries, or soft tissue injury that can also make rehabilitation difficult. An interesting musculoskeletal problem that sometimes occurs following TBI is *heterotopic ossification*, a condition in which bone is formed inappropriately in soft tissue areas. This problem, if left untreated, can result in ankylosis, or fusion of a joint, such that moving it is impossible. Extremity pain may also be a problem, due to inherent injury to the extremity or from neurological damage to the sensory pathways.

Cognitive Problems

Injury to the brain can result in any number of changes in mental function, including changes in personality. The specific changes, of course, depend on the specific structures damaged. Very commonly, individuals with brain injury experience problems with memory, attention, and arousal, as well as difficulties with language and communication (Seel et al., 1997). Even persons with brain

Table 20.2   Potential Cognitive Problems after TBI

Aggression	Bizarre ideation	Impulsivity	Silliness
Anasognosia	Denial	Irritability	Slovenliness
Anxiety	Depression	Lability	Social problems
Apathy	Fatigue	Memory problems	Spatial neglect
Attention deficit	Forgetfulness	Sexual problems	Substance abuse

Table 20.3   Rancho Los Amigos Scale of Cognitive Functioning: Variable Outcomes Dependent on Nature and Severity of Injury

I	No response: Unresponsive to any stimulus
II	Generalized response: Limited, inconsistent, non-purposeful responses, often to pain only
III	Localized response: Purposeful responses; may follow simple commands; may focus on presented object
IV	Confused, agitated: Heightened state of activity; confusion, disorientation, aggressive behavior
V	Confused, inappropriate, non-agitated: Appears alert; responds to commands; distractible; does not concentrate on task
VI	Confused, appropriate: Good directed behavior, needs cuing; can relearn old skills; serious memory problems; some awareness of self and others
VII	Automatic, appropriate: Robot-like appropriate behavior, minimal confusion; shallow recall, poor insight into condition; initiates tasks, but needs structure; poor judgment, problem-solving, and planning skills
VIII	Purposeful, appropriate: Alert, oriented; recalls and integrates past events; learns new activities and can continue without supervision; independent in home and living skills; capable of driving; defects in stress tolerance, judgment, abstract reasoning persist; many functions at reduced levels in society

injury who experience a relatively good recovery will often have subtle cognitive deficits that make returning to work or living independently difficult. A list of potential cognitive problems after TBI can be found in Table 20.2 (Groswasser & Stern, 1998; Whyte et al., 2011).

Recovery from TBI

Recovery from brain injury is a highly variable process. Severely injured persons with brain injury recover *in general* along a set of stages, classified as the Rancho Los Amigos Scale of Cognitive Functioning (see Table 20.3). Persons with brain injury do not always progress through each stage in a stepwise fashion; some persons with brain injury may skip one or more stages. This scale has its greatest usefulness in communicating with other team members about the condition of the person with brain injury, although at times it is helpful for family members, particularly when persons with brain injury are in an agitated state. Some families find it somewhat comforting to know that the agitated state is part of a normal recovery process following TBI.

A common perception is that the time it takes for completion of neurological recovery of the brain following a severe injury is approximately one year. Although this is a good estimate for many persons with brain injury, there are certainly exceptions, and some persons with brain injury have demonstrated significant recovery even after one year. Researchers are learning more about the process of neuroplasticity and factors affecting better outcomes (Ginsberg et al., 1997; Mateos-Aparicio & Rodríguez-Moreno, 2019; Pike & Hamm, 1997).

Long-Term Impairments

Impairments following brain injury may include almost any complication imaginable. However, there are certain impairments that occur with such regularity after TBI that they warrant special mention. These impairments are the main issues that cause long-term problems after brain injury. Any life care plan for a person with brain injury who is traumatically, severely injured should be sure to address these particular issues:

- *Weakness*: Injury to the motor cortex or motor pathways may lead to weakness. Severe enough injury will result in paralysis. Weakness is usually the biggest factor affecting a person's ability to perform activities of self-care, such as dressing, grooming, and feeding. It may also impair an individual's ability to walk and move about and, in extreme cases, may lead to the necessity of assistance with transfers.
- *Spasticity*: Spasticity, defined as "velocity-dependent increase in motor tone," as mentioned earlier in the chapter, often remains a huge obstacle to independence after a brain injury. Spasticity is manifested clinically as an involuntary "tightening" of the muscles, resulting in difficulty moving a joint through normal range of motion. Spasticity is often associated with weakness and further complicates the person with brain injury's ability to move and perform activities of self-care. Furthermore, severe spasticity places the person with brain injury at risk for several other complications, such as contractures and skin breakdown. Much of the medical treatment following TBI centers around the prevention and treatment of spasticity. A number of medical interventions in the treatment of spasticity are available. Aside from oral medications and therapeutic interventions such as splinting, casting, bracing, and range-of-motion exercises, persons with brain injury are frequently treated with a variety of injections for spasticity. These may include nerve blocks using ethanol or phenol or botulinum toxin injections. A surgically implanted device, the intrathecal pump, may provide a higher concentration of medicine for spasticity directly at the level of the spinal cord, where it is most effective. The advantage to this technique is that it allows greater control over the administration of medicine, while avoiding many of the side effects associated with oral administration of medication, such as sedation (Enslin et al., 2020; Stecco et al., 2014). Finally, various surgical techniques may be used, usually as last-resort efforts, for treatment of spasticity. These include various tendon-lengthening procedures, rhizotomy, or cordotomy.
- *Behavioral problems*: Although other issues may be more of a focus of medical treatment, it is often behavioral issues that prevent successful community reintegration and return to gainful employment. Persons with brain injury may have low frustration tolerance, impaired judgment, and, in many cases, emotional lability or aggression that hinder successful rehabilitation outcomes. Behavioral problems are usually addressed on a number of levels, including

psychological counseling, behavior modification plans, medications, and, in some cases, inpatient neurobehavioral treatment programs.
- *Cognition*: The most common complaint at one year after injury is problems with memory (Machamer et al., 2022). Areas of the brain associated with memory formation are particularly susceptible to injury following trauma, due to their proximity to bony protuberances inside the skull. Additionally, these structures are particularly susceptible to anoxic injury as well, which can occur secondarily following trauma. Deficits in attention, motivation, and sensory input can also secondarily result in memory problems.
- *Aging*: As noted in the vocational category that follows, adults aging with a brain injury experience a faster than average decline physically, as well as cognitively. Reduced physical skills and judgment can also result in additional injury as time passes. Additionally, once a person has experienced a brain injury, they are much more likely to have a second injury than people without a brain injury. Also, for some mild to moderately brain-injured individuals, social isolation and awareness of deficits eventually erode the hope and optimism that occur while progress is being made, and behavior and emotional problems may arise several years after the original insult. These problems are not as much related to aging as to the passage of time and the slow realization that they will never achieve their pre-injury levels and may be unable to enjoy normal social and love relationships (Gardner et al., 2018; Trudel & Purdum, 1998).

Community Reintegration

Successful return to the community remains a significant challenge given all of the potential barriers a person with brain injury may face due to the impairments sustained as a result of the injury (Berens, 2008; Braunling-McMorrow et al., 2010; Novack et al., 2010; Oral, 2018; Smith-Knapp et al., 1996; Therriault et al., 2016; Wall et al., 1998). With changes in personality and behavioral problems, interpersonal relationships often become difficult. Many persons with brain injury require ongoing supervision for safety reasons, which interferes with social activities. Driving a motor vehicle is a significant concern, and a formal driving evaluation should be performed by a therapist trained to look for the specific problems that may interfere with safe driving (McKerral et al., 2019; Novack et al., 2010).

An additional issue frequently seen is the return to recreational activities. A high percentage of individuals with brain injury engaged in high-risk activities prior to their injury (Chesnut et al., 1993). In fact, it is often engagement in high-risk activities that led to the brain injury in the first place. It is extremely important that individuals protect themselves against a second injury, particularly while the brain is healing. The *second impact syndrome*, in which a person healing from one injury is exposed to a second injury, may result in exponentially worse or even fatal outcomes, even with a relatively minor second injury. It is therefore extremely important that the person with brain injury be restricted from engaging in activities that may place them at risk for another injury. A therapeutic recreation specialist may be helpful in identifying and developing appropriate leisure interests after brain injury as well as helping develop techniques to pursue those interests when physical and cognitive impairments make them difficult. In addition, substance abuse may adversely affect recovery and ultimate outcome, further complicating the vocational and life care planning needs (Corrigan, 1995).

For the young adult or pediatric evaluee, an educational consultant can be very important to maximize the individual's educational potential. Under the Individuals with Disabilities Education Act, the public school system is responsible for providing specialized services to children with disabilities. However, many of these individuals are unserved for a variety of reasons. One reason is that the individual has not been adequately assessed to identify deficits that would meet the criteria for specialized education. Another reason is that the individual may meet the definition, but the school's funding is inadequate, and the school will fail to provide appropriate support. Educational consultants who are familiar with the rules often can negotiate the appropriate education protocol.

Vocational Rehabilitation

Return to gainful employment after brain injury remains a significant challenge (Cifu et al., 1997; Cuthbert et al., 2015; Dikmen et al., 1994; Goodall et al., 1994; Ip et al., 1995; Ma et al., 2020; Mani et al., 2017; O'Keefe et al., 2019; Stapleton et al., 1989; Wehman et al., 1988, 1993; Zasler & Faadep, 1997). A systemic review of 49 studies examining return to work rates following ABI found that approximately 40% of individuals with traumatic or non-traumatic ABI returned to work within one- to two-years post-injury (Van Velzen et al., 2009). Even with milder brain injuries, work-related issues often become a major problem due to significant problems with interpersonal relationships and behavioral changes (Baker, 1990; Chwalisz, 1992; DePompei & Williams, 1994; Harvey et al., 2020; Paice et al., 2020). Many TBIs occur in individuals between the ages of 16–30 years, a time in most people's lives when education is being completed and career goals established. For those who have completed their education, the cognitive problems often prohibit the use of previously gained knowledge. Additionally, memory problems may make further education or training impossible, in the worst cases.

It is strongly recommended that individuals undergo a neuropsychological evaluation to determine their capacity for education and work (Macciocchi et al., 1993; Soble et al., 2017; Weed, 1996, 1998). A proper, thorough neuropsychological evaluation will give information about how the person with brain injury learns and processes information and will help the vocational rehabilitation counselor in establishing appropriate return to work goals (Uomoto, 2000) (also see Table 20.4 for a checklist of recommended questions to the neuropsychologist). Many individuals are unable to return to competitive employment due to their impairments or need significant support and assistance to do so. A significant proportion of persons with brain injury have no difficulty obtaining employment but have a great deal of trouble maintaining employment due to impaired social awareness or interpersonal skills.

To adequately assess the vocational and life planning needs of a person with a brain injury, it is recommended that, as clinical judgment dictates, other allied health professionals be consulted. The occupational therapist may be an appropriate referral for an assessment for seating and positioning, adaptive aids, and other vocationally related issues. For some individuals, activities of daily living training, including household safety, would be included. The speech and language pathologist will be instrumental in determining augmentative communications and assistive technology for individuals with more severe injuries, as well as in providing an assessment of receptive and expressive speech and language. They also often offer cognitive remediation strategies. A physical therapist can be important in determining the individual's true physical capabilities by compiling a functional capacity assessment (or physical capacity assessment). These reports can provide more detailed information about work-related capacities than physicians.

Several methods of vocational assistance have been developed, including enclaves and supported employment. The supported employment model involves a job coach who spends time with the person with brain injury at the worksite and assists with training the person with brain injury for the job, accommodations of the workspace if necessary, and helping with problems that may occur if needed. Much of the support involves educating the employer about the nature of brain injury (Graham et al., 2016; McMahon & Shaw, 1991; Wehman et al., 1993). Another intervention

Table 20.4 Neuropsychologist Questions

	In addition to the standard evaluation report, add the following questions as appropriate:
1.	Please describe, in layman's terms, the injury to the brain
2.	Please describe the effects of the accident on the client's ability to function
3.	Please provide an opinion to the following topics: a. Intelligence level (include pre- vs. post-incident if able)? b. Personality style with regard to the workplace and home? c. Stamina level? d. Functional limitations and assets? e. Ability for education/training? f. Vocational implications—style of learning? g. Level of insight into present functioning? h. Ability to compensate for deficits? i. Ability to initiate action? j. Memory impairments (short-term, long-term, auditory, visual, etc.)? k. Ability to identify and correct errors? l. Recommendations for compensation strategies? m. Need for companion or attendant care?
4.	What is the proposed treatment plan? a. Counseling (individual and family)? b. Cognitive therapy? c. Reevaluations? d. Referral to others (e.g., physicians)? e. Other?
5.	How much and how long (include cost per session or hour and reevaluations)?

Source: © 1996 Roger O. Weed With permission, with acknowledgment to Robert Frasier, PhD for some content.

method that has met with some success is the Clubhouse Model. The advantage of this model is that it allows peer feedback for interpersonal interaction in a more real-world way. This is particularly useful with patients with TBI who often lack insight into their own behaviors and are less open to feedback from professionals (Tyerman, 2012).

Aging with Brain Injury

The effects of aging with a brain injury may affect work life expectancy (Weed, 1998). Data reveal that many clients with a brain injury cognitively or physically deteriorate at a faster rate and appear years older than their chronological age; it is not uncommon for individuals to depart from work (i.e., retire early) at an age younger than that of most able-bodied workers. Because of reduced physical capacity, persons with brain injury may reach the threshold of dependence at an earlier age. There also may be earlier onset of dementia due to reduced neurological reserve, leading to loss of independence earlier than with the average person (Chandra et al., 1989; Cifu et al., 1996b; Gedye et al., 1989; Li et al., 2017; O'Meara et al., 1997; Rosenthal, 1990; Zhang et al., 2021b). For example, it may be appropriate to phase out work and phase in a day program or volunteer activities by the time the individual is in his or her fifties. The decline in work life can also be a result of moving from full-time to part-time work, as well as earlier retirement.

Life Care Plan Case Study

A 32-year-old evaluee was riding a motorcycle that was hit by a car. At the time of the interview, three years post-injury, he stated that he did not remember the incident or anything "a couple of weeks" prior to the incident. Following the incident, his first consistent memory is approximately two to three months post-injury. He was treated for two months in an acute care hospital and then for five months in a brain injury rehabilitation hospital. The evaluee was diagnosed with severe TBI with physical and cognitive deficits, including ventriculoperitoneal shunt and orthopedic injuries requiring extensive care.

Neuropsychological testing results concluded that the evaluee sustained a very severe TBI. Testing revealed reduced intellectual capacity of one standard deviation, perhaps slightly more, below pre-injury levels. His primary deficit is in visual/motor problem solving. He is able to read beyond a high school level. He has significant deficits in mathematical calculations, with overall performance at a level much lower than expected given his pre-injury educational level. No anomia was noted, and he is able to mildly retrieve words without perseveration or intrusive errors. He has significant difficulty with fine motor coordination, with reduced range in the left upper extremity. He has significantly improved executive function from prior testing, which is the most promising part of the overall evaluation, although he continues to exhibit occasions of temper outbursts. He has moderately to severely impaired short-term memory, especially with verbal short-term memory given the absence of consolidation of information. He has a positive effect, although he has times of unhappiness/frustration, and is basically functioning in a more adaptive manner.

He has a young daughter and must be supervised when with her. His wife is supportive and has quit work to be his caregiver. He must have someone available for assistance with judgment, safety, food preparation, and financial commitments. Work is not a reasonable goal, although volunteer activities part-time would be therapeutic.

LIFE CARE PLAN
Note: For purposes of this plan, the following initials are placed in parentheses according to their respective recommendations: JP = physiatrist MC = psychiatrist RH = ophthalmologist IR = hand surgeon WW = internist AP = physical therapist JH = neuropsychologist RW = life care planner

(Continued)

Routine Future Medical Care—Physician Only			
Recommendation (by whom)	Initiated/Duration	Purpose	Expected Cost
Physiatrist (JP) X-rays: left hip, knee, or shoulder (JP) Head CT scan (JP) Head MRI (JP) EEG (JP)	4 times/year to life expectancy 3 times/year to life expectancy 1 time/year to life expectancy Every 5 years to life, 1 time/year to life expectancy	Monitor overall rehabilitation program and prevent/reduce complications, etc. Monitor development of expected degenerative joint disease. Assess integrity of shunt. Monitor structural changes to brain. Assess brain wave activity due to high risk of seizures	$276–$320/year at $69–$80/visit (see Note 1) Range: $609–$1,365/year at $203–$455 each, 3 times/year to life. CT scan: $2,173–$2,296/year to life. MRI: $3,016–$4,370 every 5 years to life. EEG: $854/year to life
Note 1: Cost for physiatrist does not include one-time new patient evaluation at $100 to $150 required by one physiatrist. Note 2: Costs for X-rays, CT scan, MRI, and EEG include both diagnostic study and physician interpretation fee. Cost range for MRI depends on whether the study is done with or without contrast. If done with contrast, an additional fee for the contrast dye will incur.			
Neurologist (JP)	2 times/year to life expectancy	Monitor neurological status	$148–$460/year at $74–$115/visit
Orthopedic surgeon (JP)	2 times/year to life expectancy	Monitor orthopedic status and development of expected degenerative joint disease	New patient: $180, 1 time only Follow-up: $120–$160/year to life at $60–$80/visit
Note: See also expected future left knee and hip replacement surgery recommended by Dr. Preston.			
Neuro-ophthalmologist (RH)	2 times/year to life expectancy	Monitor visual impairments	$160/year at $80/visit
Note: Economist to deduct cost of routine ophthalmology or optometry follow-up since it is recommended for the general population.			
Psychiatrist (MC)	4–6 times/year for 2–3 years, then 2–3 times/year to life expectancy	Medication management	$288–$432/year for 2–3 years, then $144–$216/year to life at $72/visit
Hand surgeon (IR)	1 time/year to life expectancy	Monitor left-hand problems related to neurological disorder	$60/year to life expectancy
Internist (WW)	4 times/year to life expectancy	General medical care and treatment	$424/year at $106/visit
Note 1: The internist reports the evaluee is expected to require more frequent visits and at a higher level per visit than typically expected of the general population. Visits included in the plan are *over and above* recommendations for the general population. Note 2: The evaluee also may need evaluation and follow-up by specialists, including neurosurgeon, urologist, and others as needed depending on complications and at the discretion of his treating physicians. See also Potential Complications.			

(Continued)

Projected Evaluations—Nonphysician (Include all allied health evaluations)			
Recommendation (by whom)	*Dates*	*Frequency/Duration*	*Expected Cost*
Physical therapy evaluation to assess gait changes (JP)	2022 to life expectancy	1 time/year to life expectancy	$200–$250/year to life expectancy
Note 1: According to the records, the evaluee was discharged from physical therapy in April 2022 and transitioned to a home exercise program. The therapist recommended physical therapy reevaluation in 3 to 4 months to determine maintenance of his function and carryover of skills. *Note 2:* See also Health and Strength Maintenance for ongoing fitness program.			
Occupational therapy evaluation to evaluate for and monitor adaptive equipment needs (JP)	2022 to life expectancy	1 time/year to life expectancy	$300–$350/year to life expectancy
Note: According to the physiatrist, speech therapy does not appear to be indicated for the evaluee and no recommendations are made for yearly speech evaluations or therapy to monitor his status and provide recommendations depending on needs.			
Home accessibility evaluation by qualified occupational therapist (RW)	2022	1 time only	$200 (average) for in-home occupational therapy evaluation with recommendations
Note: Although the evaluee's home generally appears appropriate for him at this time, a home accessibility evaluation is reasonable and appropriate to evaluate the home and make recommendations for additional modifications to ensure the evaluee maintains his highest level of independence and function in his home, especially given an expected further decline in physical functioning as he ages.			
Projected Therapeutic Modalities			
Recommendation (by whom)	*Year Initiated*	*Frequency/Duration*	*Expected Cost*
Physical therapy to develop, monitor, and supervise fitness program and home exercise program (JP)	2022	4 times/year to life expectancy	$988/year to life for four 1-hour sessions/year at $247/session
Note: See also Health and Strength Maintenance for ongoing fitness program.			
Neuropsychologist consultation for coping strategies, adjustment issues, cognitive remediation, and behavior management strategies (JH)	2022	4–6 times/year to life expectancy	$392–$840/year to life at $98–$140 (depends on length of visit)

(Continued)

Note 1: It is likely the evaluee also will need counseling episodically throughout his lifetime, especially during transitional times in his life (i.e., mid-30s, middle age, elderly, etc.), as well as during life-changing events that may occur (i.e., birth of second child, expected in January 2023, etc.). Frequency and duration of counseling are unknown, and no additional cost is included in plan totals.

Note 2: The evaluee's wife/family also may need counseling as needed throughout their life expectancy depending on circumstances. The neuropsychologist states he is available to the evaluee and wife as needed, typically for telephonic intervention related to various issues/questions that arise, at no additional cost to the evaluee. The physiatrist also states the evaluee's family/wife may need counseling intervention at some time in the future.

Case manager experienced in working with clients with a brain injury to problem solve, coordinate care, client advocate, etc. (RW)	2022	2 hours/month (average) to life expectancy	$1,800–$2,136/year (average) to life expectancy at $75–$89/hour (does not include mileage to appointments and to meet with evaluee)
Financial planner/consultant (JH)	2022 to life expectancy	2 hours/month (average)	$1,920–$2,499/year (average) to life expectancy at $80–$100/hour (estimate)

Note: The evaluee requires assistance and oversight with legal and business contracts, budgeting, financial planning, major decision making, and other money management decisions. Although his wife currently performs these activities, it is recommended a financial consultant, independent from the family, be utilized.

Diagnostic Testing/Educational Assessment

Recommendation (by whom)	Year Initiated	Frequency/Duration	Expected Cost
Neuropsychology evaluations (JH)	2022–2025	2 times over course of lifetime	$1,200–$1,600 total at $600–$800/evaluation

Wheeled Mobility Needs, Accessories, and Maintenance

Recommendation (by whom)	Year Purchased	Replacement Schedule	Expected Cost
Power scooter (JP), Scooter maintenance (RW)	2022 to life expectancy	Scooter: Every 5 years (average) Batteries: 1 time/year (average) to life expectancy 1 time/year after warranty expires	Scooter: $2,700–$2,900 every 5 years average. Batteries (2): $180/year at $89.95 each. Maintenance: $100/year (average estimate)

Note 1: The physiatrist recommends a power scooter for prolonged mobility assistance and extended outings in the community. See also scooter lift for vehicle in the following sections.

Note 2: The evaluee states (and records confirm) that he previously used a manual wheelchair for mobility assistance and no longer requires the chair. For purposes of future care planning, it is presumed the wheelchair is available in the home for his use in the future, if needed, and no cost for replacement is included in plan totals.

(Continued)

Home Furnishings/Aids for Independent Function			
Recommendation (by whom)	*Year Purchased*	*Replacement Schedule*	*Expected Cost*
Shower/tub bench with back (JP)	2022	Every 5 years (average) to life expectancy	$48.95–$59.95 every 5 years (average) to life expectancy
Elevated toilet seat (JP)	2022	N/A; see note	N/A; see note
Note: The evaluee states he no longer uses this item; however, for purposes of future care planning, it is presumed the elevated toilet seat is available in the home for his future use, if needed, and no cost for replacement is included in plan totals.			
Allowance for daily planner/scheduler, memory book and other compensatory tools, handheld shower, cellular phone, etc. (JH, RW)	2022 (already has some items)	1 time/year allowance to life expectancy	$50/year (average) to life expectancy
Orthotics/Prosthetics			
Recommendation (by whom)	*Year Purchased*	*Replacement Schedule*	*Expected Cost*
Custom left ankle, foot orthosis (AFO) (JP)	2022	Every 2–3 years (average) to life expectancy	$600–$1,000 every 2–3 years (average) to life (includes measuring, molding, casting, fittings, and adjustments)
Note 1: The physiatrist states the evaluee also may benefit from custom insoles or orthopedic footwear due to his altered gait; however, no information is available regarding specific type or kind of orthopedic supply and no additional cost is included in plan totals. See Potential Complications. *Note 2:* The orthotist suggests replacement every 1 to 2 years (average) depending on wear and tear, maintenance, and need or changes in the evaluee's mobility and musculoskeletal structure.			
Orthopedic Equipment Needs			
Recommendation (by whom)	*Year Purchased*	*Replacement Schedule*	*Expected Cost*
Cane with offset handle (JP, WW)	2022 (already has)	Every 10 years (average) to life expectancy	$20–$25 every 10 years (average) to life expectancy
Standard folding walker (JP, WW)	2022	Every 10 years (average) to life expectancy	$70–$85 every 10 years (average) to life expectancy
Note 1: The evaluee currently uses a cane with offset handle for mobility assistance primarily in the community. The physiatrist recommends both a cane and walker be available to him throughout his life expectancy. If a rolling walker is needed, cost is $200 to $270 each. *Note 2:* The physiatrist also recommends a power scooter for long-distance outings in the community (see scooter).			
Drug Needs			

(Continued)

Drug needs and costs are representative of the evaluee's current need and may change from time to time.			
Recommendation (by whom)	Purpose	Cost per Month	Cost per Year
Clonazepam (Klonopin), 0.5 mg, 2 times/day (MC) Oxybutynin (Ditropan), 5 mg, 3 times/day (WW)	Seizure prevention Bladder control and management	$21.12–$43.59 for 60 tablets/month, $17.11–$25.79 for 90 tablets/month, $34.27–$42.59 for 90 tablets/month	$257–$530/year to life expectancy, $208–$314/year to life expectancy, $730–$907/year to life expectancy
Zanaflex, 4 mg, ½ tablet in A.M., ½ tablet at noon, 1 tablet at bedtime (1½ tablets/day) (WW) Baclofen, 20 mg, 3 times/day (WW) Propranolol LA (Inderal), 60 mg, 2 times/day (WW)	Reduce spasticity/ataxia. Reduce spasticity/ataxia. Reduce spasticity/ataxia	30 tablets/month, $25.92–$47.69 for 90 tablets/month, $47–$61.79 for 60 tablets/month	$315–$580/year to life expectancy, $572–$752/year to life expectancy
Note: According to the physiatrist, the evaluee is expected to require these or similar medications throughout his life expectancy. The internist also states medications are expected to be needed throughout his lifetime.			
Supply Needs			
Supply needs and costs are representative of the evaluee's current need and may change from time to time.			
Recommendation (by whom)	Purpose	Replacement Schedule	Cost per Year
Prism glasses (RH)	Reduce double vision	Expect replacement every 1–2 years (average)	$283 for frames and lenses every 1–2 years (average) to life expectancy
Note 1: According to the ophthalmologist, the evaluee's vision impairment as related to the brain injury is expected to remain the same over his lifetime. He states there will probably be no new problems with his vision assuming no additional or further ocular trauma occurs. See also Potential Complications. Note 2: The evaluee states he does not use other supplies related to injuries received in the incident.			
Home/Facility Care			
Recommendation (by whom)	Year Initiated/Suspended	Hours/Shifts/Days of Attendance or Care	Expected Cost
Competent companion for assistance, safety, and supervision in the home (JP, JH) Child care assistance (JP, JH)	2022	10–12 hours/day, 7 days/week, 365 days/year to life expectancy. As needed	$35,953–$65,700/year to life expectancy at $9.85–$15/hour. Defer to economist for loss of child care services

(Continued)

Note 1: The evaluee's wife currently performs the function of a live-in caregiver.

Note 2: Of the nine home health agencies contacted in the evaluee's local area, only one agency offered a live-in caregiver and the service currently was not available due to staffing shortages and difficulty in hiring and retaining live-ins. When and if available, live-in at the one agency is $139.20/day.

Note 3: The neuropsychologist states the evaluee does not require overnight *awake* care and should be able to summon emergency assistance if needed.

Note 4: Both the neuropsychologist and physiatrist state the evaluee is expected to have difficulty with child-raising activities with his 2-year-old daughter and his expected second child in January 2023 and requires childcare assistance. Economic value of time that a father normally spends in child-rearing and child-raising activities and that which is lost due to the evaluee's injury are deferred to the economist.

Yard care and interior/exterior home maintenance and repairs (per interview)	2022	N/A	Defer to economist as part of loss of household services

Note: The evaluee's home is in obvious need of repair due to injury caused by maneuvering the wheelchair in the home (i.e., injury to doorways, flooring, walls, etc.). The evaluee states he is unable to do the repairs and is unable to paint or do other interior/exterior home maintenance tasks since the injury.

Transportation			
Recommendation (by whom)	*Year Purchased*	*Replacement*	*Expected Cost*
Cellular telephone for emergency communication (RW)	2000 (already has)	Every 5 years (estimate)	N/A (had pre-injury)
Scooter lift for vehicle (RW)	2022 or when scooter purchased; see scooter	Every 5–7 years (average) to life expectancy or at time of vehicle replacement	$2,500 every 5–7 years (average) for hoist arm scooter lift

Note: Although the evaluee received satisfactory scores in the behind-the-wheel adapted driving evaluation in July 2022, the neuropsychologist opines that driving is not recommended due to judgment impairments and slow processing that impair his ability to act quickly or in emergencies.

Health and Strength Maintenance (Leisure Time Activities)			
Recommendation (by whom)	*Year of Purchase or Attendance*	*Replacement or Attendance Schedule*	*Expected Cost*
Fitness program: Option 1 Gym membership (JP) Option 2 Home exercise equipment to include treadmill, parallel bars, and multi-station exercise machine	2022 to life expectancy	N/A; already has equipment; plan for 2-time replacements (estimate) over his lifetime	N/A; no additional cost over general population 2011: $3,000 (estimate) 2021: $3,000 (estimate)

(Continued)

Note 1: The physiatrist recommends a physical conditioning/exercise program under the supervision of a physical therapist to monitor and oversee/supervise fitness program. See also physical therapy for recommended four times/year physical therapist supervision. *Note 2:* The physical therapist suggests a recumbent stationary bicycle also may be useful for the evaluee.			
Membership to National Brain Injury Association and local support groups/networking (RW)	2022 to life expectancy	Yearly membership	$35/year to life expectancy

Vocational/Educational Plan

Recommendation (by whom)	Year Initiated/Suspended	Purpose	Expected Cost
Computer with monitor, printer, Internet access, software package, and other features (RW)	1-time-only replacement estimated in 2026 (approximately 4 years after purchase of current computer)	Increase independence for educational and recreational activity	$2,000 (average) for 1-time-only replacement in approximately 2026

Note 1: Dr. Preston states in his deposition that a personal computer is medically indicated for the evaluee to include possible access for environmental control unit or adaptive devices integration in the future.
Note 2: A one-time-only replacement cost for computer and related equipment/supplies is included in plan. Replacement after that is presumed to be consistent with use of a personal computer by the general population.

Note: The evaluee has no competitive vocational potential. Volunteer activity is a best option for him to increase his sense of productivity and self-worth, and provide a sense of purpose. If professional services are required in the future to develop or cultivate an alternate volunteer program for the evaluee, expect 20 to 40 hours for vocational counseling and related services, including vocational evaluation, labor market research, job site analysis, etc., at $75 to $89/hour. However, costs for these services are not included in the plan.

Architectural Considerations

(List considerations for home accessibility and modifications.)
The evaluee currently lives with his wife and 2-year-old daughter in a ranch-style house that has been modified to accommodate him and generally appears appropriate for his current needs. A ramp has been constructed to the back door, which is the entrance the evaluee uses to enter and exit the home, and grab bars have been installed in the bathroom. The front entrance has steps leading to the front door, although no handrail is available and the evaluee demonstrates he generally is able to ascend and descend the stairs with difficulty in a modified fashion and with altered gait.

The evaluee requires a one-story home with accessibility features and minimal, if any, stairs. If stairs, he requires handrails. See also home accessibility evaluation for one-time-only evaluation to assure the home is accessible both now and for the future as he ages and experiences an expected reduction in his physical capabilities.

Future Medical Care, Surgical Intervention, Aggressive Treatment

Recommendation (by whom)	Year Initiated	Frequency	Expected Cost*
Eye muscle surgery (RH)	2002–2003 (age 32–33)	1 time only, if successful	$5,000 (approximate)

(Continued)

Life Care Planning for Acquired Brain Injury ■ 559

Left total knee replacement (JP) Left knee revision (JP)	2020 (age 50) Approximately 2030–2032 and every 10–12 years (average) thereafter to life expectancy	Initial knee replacement in 2020, then every 10–12 years (average) knee revision to life expectancy	Replacement in approximately 2020: $30,948, 1st revision: $35,608, 2nd revision: $34,378
Left total hip replacement (JP) Left hip revision (JP)	2020 (age 50) Approximately 2030–2032 and every 10–12 years (average) thereafter to life expectancy	Initial hip replacement in 2020, then every 10–12 years (average) hip revision to life expectancy	Replacement in approximately 2020: $31,568, 1st revision: $39,811, 2nd revision: $37,479
*Expected cost for knee and hip replacement/revision includes surgeon fee and average hospital charges and does not include surgeon assistant fee, if applicable, anesthesiologist fee, or subacute or rehab unit stay. One case of an evaluee similar in age to this evaluee with diagnosis of degenerative joint disease required total knee replacement at a cost of $40,733, inclusive.			
Note 1: The physiatrist states he expects the evaluee to require joint replacement in both left hip and left knee due to altered gait and increased wear and tear on his lower-extremity joints, as well as expected degenerative joint disease. He states the severity of the degenerative joint disease depends on maintenance of the evaluee's weight and overall health and fitness. *Note 2:* According to one orthopedic surgeon who performs knee and hip replacement surgeries, knee and hip prostheses last on average 10 to 12 years (based on geriatric population); however, the evaluee may require more frequent revision due to his young age at the time of projected initial replacement and expected increased activity level (more so than geriatric activity level). See also Potential Complications. *Note 3:* For purposes of future care planning and based on the physiatrist's recommendation for initial hip and knee joint replacement at approximately age 50, presume two hip and knee revisions over the evaluee's lifetime at approximately age 60 to 62 and age 72 to 74. *Note 4:* The orthopedic surgeon states joint revision surgeries are more difficult than the initial replacement surgery and each subsequent revision is more difficult than the previous one. Recovery also tends to take longer. However, no additional cost for extended recovery is included in plan totals for revision surgeries.			
Note 5: Pain medication is expected to be needed following each joint revision surgery, as well as probable anti-inflammatory medication. Exact kind, dose, and duration of medication are unknown and no additional cost for medications is included in plan totals. *Note 6:* Orthopedic visits following joint replacement/revision generally include one post-op visit (at no cost) plus three other visits at 3, 6, and 12 months post-replacement/post-revision at $60 to $80/visit. Routine follow-up also includes AP and lateral X-rays of hip at $174.25/X-ray and knee at $261.25/X-ray at each post-op visit. Additional medical needs following joint replacement/revision likely include postoperative physical therapy and probable long-term need for cane or walker for mobility assistance. Aqua therapy also may be indicated following joint replacement/revision.			
Ventriculoperitoneal (VP), shunt revision (JP)	Approximately 2011 (15 years after initial shunt placement)	1 time only, assuming no complications	Neurosurgeon evaluation: $286 Revision surgery: $28,927

(Continued)

Note 1: The evaluee was released from the care of his neurosurgeon in February 2022 to be followed by the physiatrist and return as needed if there were complications with his shunt or changes in his neurologic status. The physiatrist states it is probable the evaluee will require at least one shunt revision over his lifetime due to expected complications. *Note 2:* Expected cost for VP shunt revision includes surgeon fee and hospital charges only and does not include diagnostic studies that may be needed such as abdominal X-rays or head CT scan, or anesthesiology charges. See head CT scan, which may be used for diagnostic purposes at time of shunt revision.
Potential Complications
Note: Potential complications are included for information only. No frequency or duration of complications is available. No costs are included in the plan.
Neurologic problems, including increased risk of seizures, shunt complications, increased spasticity that is expected to get worse over time, etc., which require aggressive treatment (including Botox injections), diagnostic tests, and prescription medication. Psychological difficulties, including poor adjustment to disability, anger, aggression, irritability, depression, poor social behavior, increased social isolation, increased risk of suicide if not getting adequate care, etc., which could require medication and psychotherapy or hospitalization to treat. The psychiatrist states the evaluee is at higher risk of affective symptoms. Additionally, the neuropsychologist states an anger management program may be an option in the future. Increased risk for early onset of dementia due to the effect of TBI and the aging process, as well as more prone to earlier onset of memory problems and overall decline in cognitive abilities associated with aging. Increased risk for falls and additional injuries (i.e., bone fractures, secondary brain injury, etc.) due to spasticity, impulsivity, poor balance, and reduced physical abilities. The physiatrist states there is a very high probability of the evaluee experiencing falls with resultant fractures. The neuropsychologist states a second brain injury would be devastating and the evaluee would not recover to the extent he has recovered from the primary brain injury.
Musculoskeletal and mobility problems due to altered gait. May require custom orthopedic footwear and insoles. May also experience additional hand problems, depending on his neurological status, that require surgical correction. May require more frequent hip or knee revisions than normally expected or have longer than expected recovery following joint revisions. Urology problems if Ditropan medication becomes ineffective and urology services are needed, including evaluation, diagnostic studies, other medications, surgery, etc. Visual problems, including additional or further ocular trauma or need for other aggressive treatment/surgery to correct or improve his double vision caused by left trochlear nerve palsy and partial oculomotor palsy. More extensive or expensive medical care and equipment than expected. Adverse reaction to long-term use of medication(s).

Conclusion

Millions of Americans experience a brain injury each year. The more knowledgeable one is about this specialized problem, the better equipped one is to obtain effective treatment while controlling costs and complications. Life care plans can effectively help ask the right questions and guide the individual and their family members and funding source through the complex maze of rehabilitation and long-term care. Effective vocational rehabilitation can help children with injuries plan for the future (e.g., development stages and pre-vocational evaluations) as well as integrate working age persons back into the community, perhaps as an employed, productive individual and students back into educational institutions. To accomplish these monumental tasks, numerous professionals and family members, with assistance of a qualified life care planner, must work together in a collaborative fashion to achieve common goals.

References

Almli, C. R., & Finger, S. (1992). Brain injury and recovery of function: Theories and mechanisms of functional reorganization. *Journal of Head Trauma Rehabilitation*, 7(2), 70–77.

Annegers, J. F., & Coan, S. P. (2000). The risks of epilepsy after traumatic brain injury. *Seizure*, 9(7), 453–457. https://doi.org/10.1053/seiz.2000.0458

Baker, J. E. (1990). Family adaptation when one member has a head injury. *The Journal of Neuroscience Nursing: Journal of the American Association of Neuroscience Nurses*, 22(4), 232–237.

Berens, D. E. (2008). *The ABI Clubhouse outcomes measurement tool: Instrument development and pilot study*. Unpublished Manuscript.

Berker, E. (1996). Diagnosis, physiology, pathology, and rehabilitation of traumatic brain injuries. *International Journal of Neuroscience*, 85(3-4), 195–220.

Bigler, E. D. (1989). Behavioural and cognitive changes in traumatic brain injury: A spouse's perspective. *Brain Injury*, 3(1), 73–78.

Blair, R. J. R. (2016). The neurobiology of impulsive aggression. *Journal of Child and Adolescent Psychopharmacology*, 26(1), 4–9. https://doi.org/10.1089/cap.2015.0088

Bloomfield, E. L. (1989). Extracerebral complications of head injury. *Critical Care Clinics*, 5(4), 881–892.

Bontke, C. F., & Boake, C. (1991). Traumatic brain injury rehabilitation. *Neurosurgery Clinics of North America*, 2(2), 473–482.

Bontke, C. F., Lehmkuhl, D. I., Englander, J., Mann, N., Ragnarsson, K. T., Zasler, N. D., Graves, D. E., Thoi, L. I., & Jung, C. (1993). Medical complications and associated injuries of persons treated in the traumatic brain injury model systems programs. *Journal of Head Trauma Rehabilitation*, 8(2), 34–46.

Braunling-McMorrow, D., Dollinger, S. J., Gould, M., Neumann, T., & Heiligenthal, R. (2010). Outcomes of post-acute rehabilitation for persons with brain injury. *Brain Injury*, 24(7–8), 928–938.

Briggs, R., Brookes, N., Tate, R., & Lah, S. (2015). Duration of post-traumatic amnesia as a predictor of functional outcome in school-age children: A systematic review. *Developmental Medicine & Child Neurology*, 57(7), 618–627.

Brown, A. W., Elovic, E. P., Kothari, S., Flanagan, S. R., & Kwasnica, C. (2008). Congenital and acquired brain injury. Epidemiology, pathophysiology, prognostication, innovative treatments, and prevention. *Archives of Physical Medicine and Rehabilitation*, 89(3), S3–S8.

Calabrò, R. S., Russo, M., & Naro, A. (2017). Discussing sexual health after traumatic brain injury: An unmet need! *Innovations in Clinical Neuroscience*, 14(1–2), 11–12.

Caplan, B., Bogner, J., Brenner, L., Malec, J., Kumar, R. G., Juengst, S. B., Wang., Z. Dams-O'Connor, K., Dkimen, S. S., O'Neil-Pirozzi, T. M., Dahdah, M. N., Hammond, F. M., Felix, E. R., Arenth, P. M., & Wagner, A. K. (2018). Epidemiology of comorbid conditions among adults 50 years and older with traumatic brain injury. *Journal of Head Trauma Rehabilitation*, 33(1), 15–24.

Centers for Disease Control and Prevention. (2021a). *National Center for Health Statistics. About the National Vital Statistics System*. www.cdc.gov/nchs/nvss/about_nvss.htm

Centers for Disease Control and Prevention, National Center for Injury Prevention CDC and Control. (2021b). *TBI data*. www.cdc.gov/traumaticbraininjury/data/

Centers for Disease Control and Prevention. (2022a). *Surveillance report: Traumatic brain injury-related deaths by age group, sex, and mechanism of injury – United States, 2018 and 2019*. Centers for Disease Control and Prevention, US Department of Health and Human Services. www.cdc.gov/traumaticbraininjury/pdf/TBI-surveillance-report-2018-2019-508.pdf

Centers for Disease Control and Prevention. (March 21, 2022b). *Facts about TBI*. www.cdc.gov/traumaticbraininjury/get_the_facts.html

Centers for Disease Control, National Institutes of Health. (2015). *Report to Congress: Traumatic brain injury in the United States: Epidemiology and rehabilitation. Centers for Disease Control and Prevention*. www.cdc.gov/traumaticbraininjury/pdf/TBI_Report_to_Congress_Epi_and_Rehab-a.pdf

Chakravarthy, S., Joseph, D., & Bapi, R. S. (2010). What do the basal ganglia do? A modeling perspective. *Biological Cybernetics, 103*(3), 237–253.

Chan, F., Rumrill, P., Wehman, P., Iwanaga, K., Wu, J.-R., Rumrill, S., Chen, X., & Lee, B. (2020). Effects of postsecondary education on employment outcomes and earnings of young adults with traumatic brain injuries. *Journal of Vocational Rehabilitation, 53*, 159–166. https://doi.org/10.3233/JVR-201093

Chandra, V., Kokmen, E., Schoenberg, B. S., & Beard, C. M. (1989). Head trauma with loss of consciousness as a risk factor for Alzheimer's disease. *Neurology, 39*(12), 1576–1576.

Chen, K. H., Lee, C. P., Yang, Y. H., Yang, Y. H., Chen, C. M., Lu, M. L., Msg, L., Yi-Chen, P., & Chen, V. C. H. (2019). Incidence of hydrocephalus in traumatic brain injury: A nationwide population-based cohort study. *Medicine, 98*(42). https://doi.org/10.1097/MD.0000000000017568

Chen, Z., Venkat, P., Seyfried, D., Chopp, M., Yan, T., & Chen, J. (2017). Brain-heart interaction: Cardiac complications after stroke. *Journal of Circulation Research, 121*(4), 451–468.

Chesnut, R. M., Marshall, L. F., Klauber, M. R., Blunt, B. A., Baldwin, N., Eisenberg, H. M., Janes, J. A., Marmarou, A., & Foulkes, M. A. (1993). The role of secondary brain injury in determining outcome from severe head injury. *The Journal of Trauma, 34*(2), 216–222.

Chwalisz, K. (1992). Perceived stress and caregiver burden after brain injury: A theoretical integration. *Rehabilitation Psychology, 37*(3), 189.

Cifu, D. X., Kaelin, D. L., & Wall, B. E. (1996a). Deep venous thrombosis: Incidence on admission to a brain injury rehabilitation program. *Archives of Physical Medicine and Rehabilitation, 77*(11), 1182–1185.

Cifu, D. X., Keyser-Marcus, L., Lopez, E., Wehman, P., Kreutzer, J. S., Englander, J., & High, W. (1997). Acute predictors of successful return to work 1 year after traumatic brain injury: A multicenter analysis. *Archives of Physical Medicine and Rehabilitation, 78*(2), 125–131.

Cifu, D. X., Kreutzer, J. S., Marwitz, J. H., Rosenthal, M., Englander, J., & High, W. (1996b). Functional outcomes of older adults with traumatic brain injury: A prospective, multicenter analysis. *Archives of Physical Medicine and Rehabilitation, 77*(9), 883–888.

Clifton, G. L., Kreutzer, J. S., Choi, S. C., Devany, C. W., Eisenberg, H. M., Foulkes, M. A., Janes, J. A., Marmarou, A., & Marshall, L. F. (1993). Relationship between Glasgow Outcome Scale and neuropsychological measures after brain injury. *Neurosurgery, 33*(1), 34–39.

Cope, D. N. (1995). The effectiveness of traumatic brain injury rehabilitation: A review. *Brain Injury, 9*(7), 649–670.

Coronado, V. G., Thomas, K. E., Sattin, R. W., & Johnson, R. L. (2005). The CDC traumatic brain injury surveillance system: characteristics of persons aged 65 years and older hospitalized with a TBI. *The Journal of Head Trauma Rehabilitation, 20*(3), 215–228. https://doi.org/10.1097/00001199-200505000-00005

Corrigan, J. D. (1995). Substance abuse as a mediating factor in outcome from traumatic brain injury. *Archives of Physical Medicine and Rehabilitation, 76*(4), 302–309.

Corrigan, J. D., & Mysiw, W. J. (1988). Agitation following traumatic head injury: Equivocal evidence for a discrete stage of cognitive recovery. *Archives of Physical Medicine and Rehabilitation, 69*(7), 487–492.

Corthell, D. W. (1993). *Employment outcomes for persons with acquired brain injury*. Research and Training Center WU-SMW, National Institute on Disability and Rehabilitation and Research.

Cuthbert, J. P., Harrison-Felix, C., Corrigan, J. D., Bell, J. M., Haarbauer-Krupa, J. K., & Miller, A. C. (2015). Unemployment in the United States after traumatic brain injury for working-age individuals: Prevalence and associated factors 2 years postinjury. *The Journal of Head Trauma Rehabilitation, 30*(3), 160.

Damier, P., Hirsch, E. C., Agid, Y., & Graybiel, A. M. (1999). The substantia nigra of the human brain II. Patterns of loss of dopamine-containing neurons in Parkinson's disease. *Brain, 122*(8), 1437–1448. https://doi.org/10.1093/brain/122.8.1437

DePompei, R., & Williams, J. (1994). Working with families after TBI: A family-centered approach. *Topics in Language Disorders, 15*, 68–81.

Deschênes, P. M., Lamontagne, M. E., Gagnon, M. P., & Moreno, J. A. (2019). Talking about sexuality in the context of rehabilitation following traumatic brain injury: An integrative review of operational aspects. *Sexuality and Disability, 37*(3), 297–314. https://doi.org/10.1007/s11195-019-09576-5

Dikmen, S. S., Temkin, N. R., Machamer, J. E., Holubkov, A. L., Fraser, R. T., & Winn, H. R. (1994). Employment following traumatic head injuries. *Archives of Neurology, 51*(2), 177–186.

Dudman, J. T., & Krakauer, J. W. (2016). The basal ganglia: From motor commands to the control of vigor. *Current Opinion in Neurobiology, 37*, 158–166. https://doi.org/10.1016/j.conb.2016.02.005

Duncan, K. A., & Garijo-Garde, S. (2021). Sex, genes, and traumatic brain injury (TBI): A call for a gender inclusive approach to the study of TBI in the lab. *Frontiers in Neuroscience, Section of Neuroendocrine Science.* www.frontiersin.org/articles/10.3389/fnins.2021.681599/full

Edlow, B. L., & Wu, O. (2012). Advanced neuroimaging in traumatic brain injury. *Seminars in Neurology, 32*(4), 374–400. https://doi.org/10.1055/s-0032-1331810

Enslin, J. M., Rohlwink, U. K., & Figaji, A. (2020). Management of spasticity after traumatic brain injury in children. *Frontiers in Neurology, 11*, 126.

Evans, R. W., & Ruff, R. M. (1992). Outcome and value: A perspective on rehabilitation outcomes achieved in acquired brain injury. *Journal of Head Trauma Rehabilitation, 7*, 24–36.

Firsching, R., Woischneck, D., Klein, S., Reissberg, S., Döhring, W., & Peters, B. (2001). Classification of severe head injury based on magnetic resonance imaging. *Comparative Study, 143*(3), 263–271. https://doi.org/10.1007/s007010170106

Fix, J. D. (2008). Basal ganglia and the striatal motor system. *Neuroanatomy (Board Review Series)* (4th ed.). Wulters Kluwer & Lippincott Williams & Wilkins.

Gardner, R. C., Dams-Connor, K., Morrissey, M. R., & Manley, G. T. (2018). Geriatric traumatic brain injury: Epidemiology, outcomes, knowledge gaps, and future directions. *Journal of Neurotrauma, 35*(7), 889–906.

Gedye, A. B. H. A. E., Beattie, B. L., Tuokko, H., Horton, A., & Korsarek, E. (1989). Severe head injury hastens age of onset of Alzheimer's disease. *Journal of the American Geriatrics Society, 37*(10), 970–973.

Georges, A., & Das, J. M. (2022). *Traumatic brain injury.* StatPearls. StatPearls Publishing, LLC.

Gerber, D. J., Weintraub, A. H., Cusick, C. P., Ricci, P. E., & Whiteneck, G. G. (2004). Magnetic resonance imaging of traumatic brain injury: Relationship of T2 SE and T2* GE to clinical severity and outcome. *Brain Injury, 18*(11), 1083–1097.

Giacino, J. T., Katz, D. I., Schiff, N. D., Whyte, J., Ashman, E. J., Ashwal, S., Barbano, R., Hammond, F. M., Laureys. S., Ling, G. S. F., Nakase-Richardson, R., Seel, R. T., Yablon, S., Getchius, T. S. D., Gronseth, G. S., & Armstrong, M. J. (2018). Comprehensive systematic review update summary: Disorders of consciousness: Report of the Guideline Development, Dissemination, and Implementation Subcommittee of the American Academy of Neurology; the American Congress of Rehabilitation Medicine; and the National Institute on Disability, Independent Living, and Rehabilitation Research. *Neurology, 91*(10), 461–470. https://doi.org/10.1212/WNL.0000000000005928

Ginsberg, M. D., Zhao, W., Back, T., Belayev, L., Stagliano, N., Dietrich, W. D., & Prado, R. (1997). Three-dimensional autoradiographic image-processing strategies for the study of brain injury and plasticity. *Advances in Neurology, 73*, 239–250.

Goodall, P., Lawyer, H. L., & Wehman, P. (1994). Vocational rehabilitation and traumatic brain injury: A legislative and public policy perspective. *The Journal of Head Trauma Rehabilitation, 9*(2), 61–81.

Goya, K., Hazarika, A., Khandelwal, A., Sokhal, N., Bindra, A., Kumar, N., Kedia, S., & Rath, G. P. (2018). Non-neurological complications after traumatic brain injury: A prospective observational study. *Journal of Critical Care Medicine, 22*(9), 632–638. https://doi.org/10/4103/jccm.IJCCM_156_18/

Grafman, J., Schwab, K., Warden, D., Pridgen, A., Brown, H. R., & Salazar, A. M. (1996). Frontal lobe injuries, violence, and aggression: A report of the Vietnam Head Injury Study. *Neurology, 46*(5), 1231–1231.

Graham, C. W., West, M. D., Bourdon, J. L., Inge, K. J., & Seward, H. E. (2016). Employment interventions for return to work in working aged adults following traumatic brain injury (TBI): A systematic review. *Campbell Systematic Reviews, 12*(1), i–133.

Greiss, C., Yonclas, P. P., Jasey, N., Lequerica, A., Ward, I., Chiaravalloti, G. F., Dabaghian, L., & Livingston, D. H. (2016). Presence of a dedicated trauma center physiatrist improves functional outcomes following traumatic brain injury. *Journal of Trauma and Acute Care Surgery, 80*(1), 70–75.

Groswasser, Z., & Stern, M. J. (1998). A psychodynamic model of behavior after acute central nervous system damage. *The Journal of Head Trauma Rehabilitation, 13*(1), 69–79.

Haines, D. E. (2012). *Neuroanatomy: An atlas of structures, sections, and systems* (7th ed.). Lippincott Williams & Wilkins.

Hall, K. M., & Cope, D. N. (1995). The benefit of rehabilitation in traumatic brain injury: A literature review. *The Journal of Head Trauma Rehabilitation*, *10*, 1–13.

Harrison-Felix, C., Kolakowsky-Hayner, S. A., Hammond, F. M., Wang, R., Englander, J., Dams-Connor, K., Kreider, S. E. D., Novack, T. A., & Diaz-Arrastia, R. (2012). Mortality after surviving traumatic brain injury: Risks based on age groups. *The Journal of Head Trauma Rehabilitation*, *27*(6), E45–E56.

Harvey, K., Ockerese, T., & Fady, J. (2020). A literature review pertaining to vocational rehabilitation for people experiencing adult-acquired neurological conditions. *New Zealand Journal of Occupational Therapy*, *67*(3), 15–22.

High Jr., W. M., Hall, K. M., Rosenthal, M., Mann, N., Zafonte, R., Cifu, D. X., Boake, C., Bartha, M., Ivanhoe, C., Yablon, S., Newton, C. N., Sherer, M., Silver, B., & Lehmkuhl, L. D. (1996). Factors affecting hospital length of stay and charges following traumatic brain injury. *The Journal of Head Trauma Rehabilitation*, *11*(5), 85–96.

Horn, L. J., & Zasler, N. D. (1996). *Medical rehabilitation of traumatic brain injury*. Hanley & Belfus.

Hu, L., Yang, S., Jin, B., & Wang, C. (2022). Advanced neuroimaging role in traumatic brain injury: A narrative review. *Frontiers in Neuroscience*. https://doi.org/10.3389/fnins.2022.872609 www.frontiersin.org/articles/10.3389/fnins.2022.872609/full

Humphreys, I., Wood, R. L., Phillips, C. J., & Macey, S. (2013). The costs of traumatic brain injury: a literature review. *ClinicoEconomics and Outcomes Research*, *5*, 281.

Ikemoto, S., Yang, C., & Tan, A. (2015). Basal ganglia circuit loops, dopamine, and motivation: A review and enquiry. *Behavioural Brain Research*, *290*, 17–31.

Ip, R. Y., Dornan, J., & Schentag, C. (1995). Traumatic brain injury: Factors predicting return to work or school. *Brain Injury*, *9*(5), 517–532.

Jorge, R. E., Robinson, R. G., Starkstein, S. E., & Arndt, S. V. (1993). Depression and anxiety following traumatic brain injury. *The Journal of Neuropsychiatry and Clinical Neurosciences*, *5*, 369–374.

Katz, D. I., & Alexander, M. P. (1994). Traumatic brain injury: Predicting course of recovery and outcome for patients admitted to rehabilitation. *Archives of Neurology*, *51*(7), 661–670.

Kaufman, H. H., Timberlake, G., Voelker, J., & Pait, T. G. (1993). Medical complications of head injury. *Medical Clinics of North America*, *77*(1), 43–60.

Khajeei, D., Smith, D., Kachur, B., & Abdul, N. (2019). Sexuality re-education program logic model for people with traumatic brain injury (TBI): Synthesis via scoping literature review. *Sexuality and Disability*, *37*(1), 41–61. https://doi.org/10.1007/s11195-018-09556-1

Kraus, J. F., Black, M. A., Hessol, N., Ley, P., Rokaw, W., Sullivan, C., Bowers, S., Knowlton, S., & Marshall, L. (1984). The incidence of acute brain injury and serious impairment in a defined population. *American Journal of Epidemiology*, *119*(2), 186–201.

Kreitzer, N., Rath, K., Kurowski, B. G., Bakas, T., Hart, K., Lindsell, C. J., & Adeoye, O. (2019). Rehabilitation practices in patients with moderate and severe traumatic brain injury. *The Journal of Head Trauma Rehabilitation*, *34*(5), E66.

Kreutzer, J. S., Kolakowsky-Hayner, S. A., Ripley, D., Cifu, D. X., Rosenthal, M., Bushnik, T., Zafonte, R., Englander, J., & High, W. (2001). Charges and lengths of stay for acute and inpatient rehabilitation treatment of traumatic brain injury 1990–1996. *Brain Injury*, *15*(9), 763–774.

Kreutzer, M., Dahllöf, A. G., Gudjonsson, G., Sullivan, M., & Siösteen, A. (1998). Sexual adjustment and its predictors after traumatic brain injury. *Brain Injury*, *12*(5), 349–368.

Laker, S. R., Adair, W. A., III, Annaswamy, T. M., Frank, L. W., Hatzakis, M., Jr., Hubbell, S. L., Ifejika, N. L., Ivanhoe, C. B., Jones, V. A., Lupinacci, M. F., Purcell, A. D., Standaert, C. J., & Dolak, M. A. (2019). American Academy of Physical Medicine and Rehabilitation position statement on definitions for rehabilitation physician and director of rehabilitation in inpatient rehabilitation settings. *American Journal of Physical Medicine & Rehabilitation*, 98–102.

Levin, H. S. (1992). Head injury and its rehabilitation. *Current Opinion in Neurology and Neurosurgery*, *5*(5), 673–676.

Levine, J. M., & Flanagan, S. R. (2010). Rehabilitation and traumatic brain injury. *The Psychiatric Clinics of North America*, *33*(4), 877–891.

Li, A., Atem, D. D., Venkatachalam, A. M., Barnes, A., Stutzman, S. E., & Olson, D. M. (2021). Admission Glasgow Coma Scale as a predictor of outcome in patients without traumatic brain injury. *American Journal of Critical Care*, *30*(5), 350–355. https://doi.org/10.4037/ajcc2021163

Li, Y., Li, Y., Li, X., Zhang, S., Zhao, J., Zhu, X., & Tian, G. (2017). Head injury as a risk factor for dementia and Alzheimer's Disease: A systematic review and meta-analysis of 32 observational studies. *PLoS ONE*, *12*(1), e0169650. https://doi.org/10.1371/journal.prone.0169650

Ma, Z., Dhir, P., Perrier, L., Bayley, M., & Munce, S. (2020). The impact of vocational interventions on vocational outcomes, quality of life, and community integration in adults with childhood onset disabilities: A systematic review. *Journal of Occupational Rehabilitation*, *30*(1), 1–21. https://doi.org/10.1007/s10926-019-09854-1

Maaike, M. H., & van Swieten, R. B. (2020). Modeling the effects of motivation on choice and learning in the basal ganglia. *PLOS Computational Biology*. https://doi.org/10.1371/journal.pcbi.1007465

Macciocchi, S. N., Reid, D. B., & Barth, J. T. (1993). Disability following head injury. *Current Opinion in Neurology*, *6*(5), 773–777.

Machamer, J., Temkin, N., Dikmen, S., Nelson, L. D., Barber, J., Hwang, P., Boase, K., Stein, M. B., Sun, X., Giacino, J., McCrea, M. A., Taylor, S. R., Jain, S. Manley, G., & TRACK-TBI Investigators. (2022). Symptom frequency and persistence in the first year after traumatic brain injury: A TRACK-TBI Study. *Journal of Neurotrauma*, *39*(5–6), 358–370.

Malec, J. F., & Basford, J. S. (1996). Postacute brain injury rehabilitation. *Archives of Physical Medicine and Rehabilitation*, *77*(2), 198–207.

Mani, K., Cater, B., & Hudlikar, A. (2017). Cognition and return to work after mild/moderate traumatic brain injury: A systematic review. *Journal of Prevention, Assessment, & Rehabilitation*, *58*(1), 51–62. https://doi.org/10.3233/WOR-172597

Marshall, L. F., Marshall, S. B., Klauber, M. R., Van Berkum Clark, M., Eisenberg, H., Jane, J. A., Luerssen, T. G., Marmarou, A., & Foulkes, M. A. (1992). The diagnosis of head injury requires a classification based on computed axial tomography. *Journal of Neurotrauma*, *9*(Suppl 1), S287–S292.

Mateos-Aparicio, P., & Rodríguez-Moreno, A. (2019). The impact of studying brain plasticity. *Frontiers in Cellular Neuroscience*, *13*, 66.

Mazmanian, P. E., Kreutzer, J. S., Devany, C. W., & Martin, K. O. (1993). A survey of accredited and other rehabilitation facilities: Education, training, and cognitive rehabilitation in brain-injury programmes. *Brain Injury*, *7*(4), 319–331.

McKerral, M., Moreno, A., Delhomme, P., & Gélinas, I. (2019). Driving behaviors 2-3 years after traumatic brain injury rehabilitation: A multicenter case control study. *Frontiers in Neurology*, *7*(10), 144. www.ncbi.nlm.nih.gov/pmc/articles/PMC6417438/

McMahon, B., & Shaw, L. (1991). *Work worth doing*. PMD Press.

Mild Traumatic Brain Injury Committee, American Congress of Rehabilitation Medicine, Head Injury Interdisciplinary Special Interest Group. (1993). Definition of mild traumatic brain injury. *The Journal of Head Trauma Rehabilitation*, *8*(3), 86–87.

Miller, G. F., DePadilla, L., & Xu, L. (2021). Costs of nonfatal traumatic brain injury in the United States, 2016. *Medical Care*, *59*(5), 451–455.

National Data and Statistical Center Traumatic Brain Injury Model System. (2022, June). *National Database: 2022 profile of people within the Traumatic Brain Injury Model Systems*. www.tbindsc.org/StaticFiles/Documents/2022%20TBIMS%20National%20Database%20Update.pdf

National Institute of Neurological Disorders and Stroke. (2022, July 25). *Brain basics: Know your brain*. www.ninds.nih.gov/health-information/public-education/brain-basics/brain-basics-know-your-brain

Netter, F. H. (1997). *Atlas of human anatomy* (2nd ed.). Icon Learning Systems.

Novack, T. A., Labbe, D., Grote, M., Carlson, N., Sherer, M., Carlos Arango-Lasprilla, J., Bushnik, T., Cifu, D., Powell, J. M., Ripley, D., & Seel, R. T. (2010). Return to driving within 5 years of moderate–severe traumatic brain injury. *Brain Injury*, *24*(3), 464–471.

O'Keefe, S., Stanley, M., Adam, K., & Lannin, N. A. (2019). A systematic scoping review of work interventions for hospitalised adults with an acquired neurological impairment. *Journal of Occupational Rehabilitation*, *29*(3), 569–584. https://doi.org/10.1007/s10926-018-9820-8

O'Neil, M. E., Carlson, K., Storzbach, D., Brenner, L., Freeman, M., Quiñones, A., Motu'apuaka, M., Ensley, M., & Kansagara, D. (2013). *Complications of mild traumatic brain injury in veterans and military personnel: A systematic review*. Evidence-based Synthesis Program (ESP) Center, Portland VA Medical Center. www.ncbi.nlm.nih.gov/books/NBK189784/table/appc.t1/

O'Shea, A., Frawley, P., Leahy, J. W., & Nguyen, H. D. (2020). A critical appraisal of sexuality and relationships programs for people with acquired brain injury. *Sexuality and Disability*, *38*(1), 57–83. https://doi.org/10.1007/s11195-020-09616-5

O'Meara, E. S., Kukull, W. A., Sheppard, L., Bowen, J. D., McCormick, W. C., Teri, L., Pfanschmidt, M., Thompson, J. D., Schellenberg, G. D., & Larson, E. B. (1997). Head injury and risk of Alzheimer's disease by apolipoprotein E genotype. *American Journal of Epidemiology*, *146*(5), 373–384.

Oral, A. (2018). Does cognitive rehabilitation improve occupational outcomes including employment and activities of daily living, as well as quality of life and community integration in individuals with traumatic brain injury? A Cochrane Review summary with commentary. *NeuroRehabilitation*, *43*(4), 525–528. https://doi.org/10.3233/NRE-189002

Paice, L., Aleligay, A., & Checklin, M. (2020). A systematic review of interventions for adults with social communication impairments due to an acquired brain injury: Significant other reports. *International Journal of Speech-Language Pathology*, *22*, 537–548. https://doi.org/10.1080/17549507.2019.1701082

Patrick, P. D., Savage, R. C., Cantore, L., Norwood, K., & Patrick, P. (2012). Medical aspects of pediatric rehabilitation after moderate to severe traumatic brain injury. *NeuroRehabilitation*, *30*(3), 225–234.

Perkes, I., Baguley, I. J., Nott, M. T., & Menon, D. K. (2010). A review of paroxysmal sympathetic hyperactivity after acquired brain injury. *Annals of Neurology*, *68*(2), 126–135.

Piek, J. (1995). Medical complications in severe head injury. *New Horizons*, *3*(3), 534–538.

Pike, B. R., & Hamm, R. J. (1997). Activating the posttraumatic cholinergic system for the treatment of cognitive impairment following traumatic brain injury. *Pharmacology Biochemistry and Behavior*, *57*(4), 785–791.

Pilitsis, J. G., & Rengachary, S. S. (2013). Complications of head injury. *Neurological Research*, *23*(2–3), 227–236. https://doi.org/10.1179/016164101101198389

Ponsford, J. (2003). Sexual changes associated with traumatic brain injury. *Neuropsychological Rehabilitation*, *13*(1–2), 275–289. https://doi.org/10.1080/09602010244000363

Rahman, M., & Tadi, P. (2021). *Neuroanatomy*. Pons.

Rappaport, M., Dougherty, A. M., & Kelting, D. L. (1992). Evaluation of coma and vegetative states. *Archives of Physical Medicine and Rehabilitation*, *73*(7), 628–634.

Ripley, D. L., Harrison-Felix, C., Sendroy-Terrill, M., Cusick, C. P., Dannels-McClure, A., & Morey, C. (2008). The impact of female reproductive function on outcomes after traumatic brain injury. *Archives of Physical Medicine and Rehabilitation*, *89*(6), 1090–1096.

Rosenthal, M. (1990). *Rehabilitation of the adult and child with traumatic brain injury* (2nd ed.). Davis.

Russell-Jones, D. L., & Shorvon, S. D. (1989). The frequency and consequences of head injury in epileptic seizures. *Journal of Neurology, Neurosurgery & Psychiatry*, *52*(5), 659–662.

Sander, A. M., Maestas, K. L., Nick, T. G., Pappadis, M. R., Hammond, F. M., Hanks, R. A., & Ripley, D. L. (2013). Predictors of sexual functioning and satisfaction 1 year following traumatic brain injury: A TBI model systems multicenter study. *The Journal of Head Trauma Rehabilitation*, *28*(3), 186–194.

Schmidt, N. D. (1997). Outcome-oriented rehabilitation: A response to managed care. *The Journal of Head Trauma Rehabilitation*, *12*(1), 44–50.

Schmitt, L. I., Wimmer, R. D., Nakajima, M., Happ, M., Mofakham, S., & Halassa, M. M. (2017). Thalamic amplification of cortical connectivity sustains attentional control. *Nature*, *545*(7653), 219–223.

Schweitzer, A. D., Niogi, S. N., Whitlow, C. T., & Tsiouris, A. J. (2019). Traumatic brain injury: Imaging patterns and complications. *Radiographics*, *39*(6). https://pubs.rsna.org/doi/pdf/10.1148/rg.2019190076

Sciacca, S., Lynch, J., Davagnanam, I., & Barker, R. (2019). *Midbrain, pons, and medulla: Anatomy and syndromes*. https://pubs.rsna.org/doi/pdf/10.1148/rg.2019180126

Seel, R. T., Kreutzer, J. S., & Sander, A. M. (1997). Concordance of patients' and family members' ratings of neurobehavioral functioning after traumatic brain injury. *Archives of Physical Medicine and Rehabilitation*, *78*(11), 1254–1259.

Semlyen, J. K., Summers, S. J., & Barnes, M. P. (1998). Traumatic brain injury: efficacy of multidisciplinary rehabilitation. *Archives of Physical Medicine and Rehabilitation*, *79*(6), 678–683.

Sherman, S. M., & Guillery, R. W. (2006) *Exploring the thalamus and its role in cortical function*. MIT Press.
Shi, H.-Y., Hwang, S.-L., Lee, I.-C., Chen, I.-T., Lee, K.-T., & Lin, C.-L. (2014). Trends and outcome predictors after traumatic brain injury surgery: A nationwide population-based study in Taiwan. *Journal of Neurosurgery*, *121*(6), 1323–1330.
Simpson, G., Simons-Coghill, M., Bates, A., & Gan, C. (2017). What is known about sexual health after pediatric acquired brain injury: A scoping review. *NeuroRehabilitation*, *41*(2), 261–280.
Smith, L. G., Milliron, E., Ho, M. L., Hu, H. H., Rusin, J., Leonard, J., & Sribnick, E. A. (2019). Advanced neuroimaging in traumatic brain injury: An overview. *Neurosurgical Focus*, *47*(6), E17.
Smith-Knapp, K. I. P., Corrigan, J. D., & Arnett, J. A. (1996). Predicting functional independence from neuropsychological tests following traumatic brain injury. *Brain Injury*, *10*(9), 651–662.
Snook, M. L., Henry, L. C., Sanfilippo, J. S., Zeleznik, A. J., & Kontos, A. P. (2017). Association of concussion with abnormal menstrual patterns in adolescent and young women. *JAMA Pediatrics*, *171*(9), 879–886.
Soble, J. R., Critchfield, E. A., & O'Rourke, J. J. (2017). Neuropsychological evaluation in traumatic brain injury. *Physical Medicine and Rehabilitation Clinics*, *28*(2), 339–350.
Stapleton, M., Parente, R., & Bennett, P. (1989). Job coaching traumatically brain injured individuals: Lessons learned. *Cognitive Rehabilitation*, *7*, 18–21.
Stecco, A., Stecco, C., & Raghavan, P. (2014). Peripheral mechanisms of spasticity and treatment implications. *Current Physical Medicine and Rehabilitation Reports*, *2*(2), 121–127.
Stocco, A., Lebiere, C., & Anderson, J. R. (2010). Conditional routing of information to the cortex: A model of the basal ganglia's role in cognitive coordination. *Psychological Review*, *117*(2), 541.
Teasdale, G. M., Pettigrew, L. E., Wilson, J. L., Murray, G., & Jennett, B. (1998). Analyzing outcome of treatment of severe head injury: A review and update on advancing the use of the Glasgow Outcome Scale. *Journal of Neurotrauma*, *15*(8), 587–597.
Teasdale, G., Teasdale, E., & Hadley, D. (1992). Computed tomographic and magnetic resonance imaging classification of head injury. *Journal of Neurotrauma*, *9*, S249–57.
Therriault, P.-Y., Lefebre, H., Guindon, A., Levert, M.-J., Briand, C., & Lord, M.-M. (2016). Accompanying citizen of persons with traumatic brain injury in a community integration project: An exploration of the role. *Work*, *(543)*, 591–600. https://doi.org/10.3233/WOR-162342
Trudel, T., & Purdum, C. (1998). Aging with a brain injury, long term issues. *The Rehabilitation Professional*, *6*, 37–41.
Turner, R. S., & Desmurget, M. (2010). Basal ganglia contributions to motor control: A vigorous tutor. *Current Opinion in Neurobiology*, *20*(6), 704–716.
Tyerman, A. (2012). Vocational rehabilitation after traumatic brain injury: Models and services. *NeuroRehabilitation*, *31*(1), 51–62.
Uomoto, J. M. (2000). Application of the neuropsychological evaluation in vocational planning after brain injury. In R. T. Fraser & D. C. Clemmons (Eds.), *Traumatic Brain injury rehabilitation* (pp. 1–94). Routledge.
Uomoto, J. M., & Brockway, J. A. (1992). Anger management training for brain injured patients and their family members. *Archives of Physical Medicine and Rehabilitation*, *73*(7), 674–679.
van Ierssel, J., Sveistrup, H., & Marshall, S. (2018). Identifying the concepts within health-related quality of life outcome measures in concussion research using the International Classification of Functioning, Disability, and Health as a reference: A systematic review. *Quality of Life Research*, *27*(12), 3071–3086. https://doi.org/10./1007/s11136-018-1939-8
Van Velzen, J. M., Van Bennekom, C. A. M., Edelaar, M. J. A., Sluiter, J. K., & Frings-Dresen, M. H. (2009). How many people return to work after acquired brain injury? A systematic review. *Brain Injury*, *23*(6), 473–488.
Viera, R. C. A., Paiva, WA. S., de Oliveira, D. V., Teixeira, M. J., de Andrade, A. F., & de Sousa, R. M. C. (2016). Diffuse axonal injury: Epidemiology, outcome, and associated risk factors. *Frontiers in Neurology*, *7*, 178. https://doi.org/10.3389/fneur.2016.00178
Wall, J. R., Rosenthal, M., & Niemczura, J. G. (1998). Community-based training after acquired brain injury: Preliminary findings. *Brain Injury*, *12*(3), 215–224.
Wan-Ting, C., Chin-Hsien, L., Cheng-Yu, L., Cheng-Yu, C., Chi-Chun, L., Keng-Wei, C., Jiann-Hwa, C., Wei-Lung, C., Chien-Cheng, H., Cherng-Jyr, L., & Jui-Yuan, C. (2020). Reverse shock index

multiplied by Glasgow Coma Scale (rSIG) predicts mortality in severe trauma patients with head injury. *Scientific Reports*, *10*(1), 1–7. https://doi.org/10.1038/s41598-020-59044-w

Ward, L. M. (2016). The thalamus: Gateway to the mind. https://cogsys.sites.olt.ubc.ca/files/2016/09/Ward-2013-WIRES-Thalamus.pdf

Weed, R. (1998). Aging with a brain injury: The effects on life care plans and vocational opinions. *The Rehabilitation Professional*, *6*(5), 30–34.

Weed, R. O. (1996). Life care planning and earnings capacity analysis for brain injured clients involved in personal injury litigation utilizing the RAPEL method. *NeuroRehabilitation*, *7*(2), 119–135.

Wehman, P., Kregel, J., Sherron, P., Nguyen, S., Kreutzer, J., Fry, R., & Zasler, N. (1993). Critical factors associated with the successful supported employment placement of patients with severe traumatic brain injury. *Brain Injury*, *7*(1), 31–44.

Wehman, P., Kreutzer, J., Wood, W., & Morton, M. V. (1988). Supported work model for persons with traumatic brain injury: Toward job placement and retention. *Rehabilitation Counseling Bulletin*, *31*, 298–312.

Whyte, E., Skidmore, E., Aizenstein, H., Ricker, J., & Butters, M. (2011). Cognitive impairment in acquired brain injury: A predictor of rehabilitation outcomes and an opportunity for novel interventions. *PM&R*, *3*(6), S45–S51.

Wilson, M. H., Ashworth, E., & Hutchinson, P. J. (2022). A proposed novel traumatic brain injury classification system – An overview and inter-rater reliability validation on behalf of the Society of British Neurological Surgeons. *British Journal of Neurosurgery*. https://doi.org/10.1080/02688697.2022.2090509

Wood, R. L. (1987). *Brain injury rehabilitation: A neurobehavioural approach*. Croom Helm.

Yadav, K., Sarioglu, E., Choi, H. A., & Cartwright, W. B. (2016). Automated outcome classification of computed tomography imaging reports for pediatric traumatic brain injury. *Journal of the Society for Academic Emergency Medicine*, *23*(2), 171–178.

Yahya, K. (2021). The basal ganglia corticostriatal loops and conditional learning. *Reviews in the Neurosciences*, *32*(2), 181–190.

Zafonte, R. D., Hammond, F. M., Mann, N. R., Wood, D. L., Black, K. L., & Millis, S. R. (1996). Relationship between Glasgow Coma Scale and functional outcome. *American Journal of Physical Medicine & Rehabilitation*, *75*(5), 364–369.

Zafonte, R. D., Mann, N. R., Millis, S. R., Black, K. L., Wood, D. L., & Hammond, F. (1997). Posttraumatic amnesia: Its relation to functional outcome. *Archives of Physical Medicine and Rehabilitation*, *78*(10), 1103–1106.

Zasler, N. D., & Faadep, R. (1997). The role of medical rehabilitation in vocational reentry. *The Journal of Head Trauma Rehabilitation*, *12*(5), 42–56.

Zhang, B., Huang, K., Karri, J., O'Brien, K., DiTommaso, C., Li, S., Schnakers, C., & Monti, M. (2021a). Many faces of the hidden souls: Medical and neurological complications and comorbidities in disorders of consciousness. *Brain Sciences*, *11*(5), 608. https://10.3390/brainsci11050608

Zhang, J., Zhang, Y., Zou, J., & Cao, F. (2021b). A meta-analysis of cohort studies: Traumatic brain injury and risk of Alzheimer's Disease. *PLoS ONE*, *16*(6), e0253206. https://doi.org10.1371/journal.pone.0253206

Chapter 21

Life Care Planning for the Patient with Burns

Ruth B. Rimmer and Kevin N. Foster

A well-documented and thorough life care plan plays an important role in the long-term recovery of a burn-injured individual. Serious burns cause a significant interruption of the patient's life, including physical, social, emotional, and financial stability (Spronk et al., 2018; Spronk et al., 2019). Therefore, it is vitally important that the life care plan for the burn patient is holistic and addresses concerns regarding the client's medical, emotional, social, and financial needs and well-being. The patient's family is also significantly impacted by the burn event. Life care planners and medical case managers should be familiar with the prevalence, etiology, and pathophysiology of burn injuries.

Burn Injury Prevalence

Over the past two decades, there has been a notable reduction in the total number of burn injuries in the United States; however, every year, approximately 486,000 persons in the United States continue to require medical attention for their burn injuries (American Burn Association, 2018). It is estimated that approximately 40,000 injured will be hospitalized, and approximately 3,275 individuals will die from their burns (American Burn Association, 2018). Survival is predicated based on a number of factors, including age, severity of the burn, comorbid trauma, inhalation injury, and premorbid health conditions. Burn patients between the ages of 5–20 years are among those most likely to have a favorable outcome. Infants and patients over age 70 have a marked increase for morbidity and mortality (Saffle et al., 1995).

The risk of being burned, as well as the etiology of the burn, is often related to a person's age, type of employment, economic status, type of recreational activities in which one engages, and location of residence. Although the number of burn injuries in the United States is unknown, individuals suffer from more minor than major burns. It is estimated that only 3–4% of burn-injured persons reporting to emergency rooms are admitted or transferred to a burn center/unit. However, burn injuries are still a significant problem and an expensive injury. According to the Centers for

Disease Control and Prevention (CDC), burns and fires are the third leading cause of death in the home. They are also the third leading cause of death in children (National Institute of General Medical Sciences, 2013). The economic cost of burn injury is high, with hospital bills for severe burns ranging from many thousands to millions of dollars for one patient. Ongoing reconstruction and rehabilitation are also costly, which is another reason why an accurate life care plan is so important (Jeschke et al., 2020).

Etiology of Burns

While burns can be caused in a variety of ways, the most prevalent cause of burn injuries requiring admission to the hospital are fire/flame, scalds (most common in young children and the elderly), and chemical, electrical, and radiation burns. Flame and scald burns account for the vast majority or approximately 43% of all reported cases. Scald burns account for the second most common cause at 36% (American Burn Association, 2018). The arms and hands, head and neck, and lower extremities are the areas of the body most likely to sustain burns. Of nonfatal burns, 45% involve the hand and arm, 25% involve the neck and head, and 16% result in burns to the leg and foot (Pruitt et al., 2007). The face, limbs, hands, and feet are vital to both physical and social function, and burns to these body parts, especially scarring across the joints, can be disfiguring as well as disabling (Demling & LaLonde, 1989).

Burn care has evolved dramatically over the past 25 years. Acute burn care has improved greatly and has resulted in dramatically higher survival rates (Brusselaers et al., 2005). Persons, especially children, with a large percentage of total body surface area burns (% TBSA) survive routinely (Sheridan et al., 2000). While it is encouraging that mortality has declined, an individual's survival of serious burn injury often results in lifelong challenges and complications for both the burn patient and their family.

Classification of Burns

The classification of the injury often determines the treatment of burns. Burn injuries are typically classified by etiology, depth of the burn (layers), location of the burn, and the % TBSA. Burn depth, which refers to the layers that have been damaged, is classified as superficial (first degree), superficial partial thickness (second degree), deep partial thickness (second degree), full thickness (third degree), and deep full thickness (fourth degree). Physicians will often defer the classification of a burn injury for several days to correctly determine the true depth of the burn:

- *Superficial (first degree) burns* involve only the superficial epidermis and usually require 3–7 days for healing with no scarring.
- *Superficial partial-thickness (second degree) burns* involve the epidermis and the dermis, excluding hair follicles, sweat glands, and sebaceous glands, and should heal in less than 21 days with minimal scarring.
- *Deep partial-thickness (also second-degree) burns* involve the epidermis and most of the dermis, requiring more than 21 days for healing, and may develop severe hypertrophic scarring.
- *Full-thickness (third degree) burns* result in the total destruction of the skin, both epidermis and dermis, and hypodermis, and may involve additional tissue. Full-thickness burns of any considerable size require skin grafting.

- *Deep full-thickness (fourth degree) burns* involve fat, nerve endings, muscle, and/or bone and are usually a result of prolonged contact with heat or an electrical injury and may require flap coverage or amputation (Fisher & Helm, 1984).

Burns are also categorized by the percentage of TBSA involved. It is customary to establish the percentage of partial- and full-thickness burns separately. The American Burn Association classifies burn injuries as mild, moderate, and major. Moderate and major burns require hospitalization.

- Minor burns are those that involve less than 15% TBSA and are partial thickness. In the elderly and pediatric populations, 10–20% full thickness is considered minor unless the eyes, ears, face, hands, or perineum are burned.
- Moderate burns include a TBSA of 15–25% (10–20% for pediatric patients less than age 10 or adults over age 40) without regard to the depth and 2–10% full-thickness burns unless the eyes, ears, face, or perineum are burned.
- Major burns include those partial-thickness burns that cover more than 25% of the body (20% for children and adults less than the age of 40) or those full-thickness burns that cover more than 10% of the TBSA, as well as all burns to the face, eyes, ears, feet, and perineum. Burns sustained from electricity or lightning or those involving inhalation injury are also considered major. Burns with comorbid trauma and all burns that present with premorbid illness or are in the very young or the elderly are also labeled as major burns (Hartford & Kealy, 2007).

Burn Severity

The severity of the burn is determined by a number of factors including the size of the burn injury, the need for skin grafting, and the presence or absence of an inhalation injury. The larger the percentage of TBSA burned, the less favorable the outcome is likely to be. The depth of the burn, including the degree of the burn, also influences the ultimate outcome, with deeper burns resulting in a less favorable prognosis and the need for the patient to receive skin grafts. Inhalation injury is another factor which often contributes to poorer outcomes. Burns may present with other trauma, which can also complicate survival and future care needs. Premorbid medical conditions can also have a negative influence on the patient's outcome (Hartford & Kealy, 2007). All these details are important to consider when developing the life care plan or managing a burn case; therefore, a thorough review of the patient's medical records and familiarity with the patient's medical history are imperative.

Pathophysiology and Treatment of Burns

The skin plays a major role in sustaining life since it makes up the largest organ system of the body. The main functions of the skin are:

- Protective barrier
- Body temperature regulation
- Fluid conservation
- Receives environmental stimuli

- Excretory gland
- Absorbs vitamin D
- Determines identity

Human skin is made up of several layers: the epidermis (10%), which is the outer layer, and the dermis (90%), which is the inner layer. The average thickness of adult skin is one to two millimeters. The top layer contains cells that determine skin color and make up the protective layer of skin. The dermis is found beneath the epidermis. The dermis contains connective tissue, capillaries, collagen, and elastic fibers. This layer supplies structure and nutrition to the epidermis, provides skin elasticity, and contains the hair follicles and excretory glands including the sweat and sebaceous glands. Sensory nerve endings are found throughout the skin; therefore, deeper burns may cause permanent changes (Cromes & Helm, 1993).

When both layers of the skin, the epidermis and dermis, are destroyed, the patient loses hair follicles, sweat, and sebaceous glands. A layer of fat and connective tissue is found under the dermis, and muscle, bone, and tendons are beneath this layer. Sensory nerve endings are distributed throughout the skin and subcutaneous layer. Therefore, burn injury, depending on the depth, may permanently change the burn victim's capacity to sense pain, touch, and temperature (Fisher & Helm, 1984).

Wounds

Wound care is a key component of acute and rehabilitative burn care. Wounds must be maintained in a manner that facilitates, and at the very least, does not impede re-epithelialization of the skin. This includes care designed to minimize infection, remove dead tissue, reduce heat loss, and prevent further tissue loss. A typical approach to wound care involves cleaning the wound and debriding it twice daily. The use of negative pressure wound dressings, i.e., dressings that draw out fluid and infection from the wound, helps with healing and may reduce the necessity of daily dressing changes (Lin et al., 2020; Pell, 2019). Donor site dressings must be changed once or twice a day. Wound care is extremely painful for the patient. If reconstructive surgery is a future recommendation for a patient, a provision for a home healthcare RN for wound care will likely be necessary.

Musculoskeletal Effects

A variety of musculoskeletal complications often accompany burn survival (Schneider & Qu, 2011). These may include scar contractures, bone loss, heterotopic ossification (HO), scoliosis, and arthritis. Other issues affecting the rehabilitation of individuals with burn injuries are impairment from muscle mass loss, scar contractures, HO, amputations, nervous system injury, and psychological problems, all of which present significant challenges for recovery from burns. Hypertrophic scarring and contractures, especially those involving the joints, mouth, and neck, can cause long-term functional problems. Scarring and hypertrophic ossification may lead to limited range of motion or joint fusion and much like amputations, may result in decreased function and the inability to engage in normal activity. It is important to document these problems in the life care plan as early identification and treatment of these problems should be considered as treatment goals in the recovery phase (Schneider & Qu, 2011).

St-Pierre et al. (1998) reported that patients who survived severe burns (TBSA of > 30%) had weak muscles for many years after the initial trauma, and this is likely due to incomplete recovery from the burns. The need exists for long-term musculoskeletal assessments in burn patients because their loss of lean body mass negatively affects rehabilitation and compromises successful community reintegration (Edelman et al., 2003). Other problems revealed by the Edelman study included joint pain, sleep disruption, fatigue, shortness of breath, heat and cold sensitivity, body image, and sexuality issues. Additionally, a disproportionate number of burn survivors have also been found to be physically unfit when compared to non-burned adults (Chaudhary et al., 2020; Chaudhary & Ahmad, 2021; Ganio at al., 2015). Therefore, the life care plan recommendations should include an exercise program designed to contribute to long-term rehabilitation and other interventions to address common complications of burn injury (Kowalske et al., 2015; Porter et al., 2015).

Recovery

A burn injury is complex and complicated from both a physical and a psychological standpoint, and survivors benefit from a multifaceted team approach to their care (Demling, 1995). Burn care is a highly specialized field of medicine. The burn care team is multidisciplinary and comprises an extensive array of medical professionals.

In the acute hospital setting, the patient is cared for by a team of burn care professionals, which includes burn surgeons, physician's assistants, nurses, burn techs, physical and occupational therapists, nutritionists, respiratory therapists, psychologists, social workers, and case managers. Patients often require additional care from specialists such as plastic/reconstructive surgeons, hand surgeons, cardiologists, neurologists, psychiatrists, and speech therapists. The acute medical care setting for burn patients is labor-intensive, and the care is expensive. It takes tremendous effort on the part of the entire burn care team, as well as an immense effort on the part of the patient and the patient's family, for basic survival to occur (Herndon & Blakeney, 2007). Rehabilitation begins in the hospital and is often extended in a specialized rehabilitation facility after discharge from the acute burn care setting for weeks or even months.

Recovery often necessitates post-acute care rehabilitation, for ongoing reconstructive surgeries with accompanying therapies, home healthcare, and the need for assistance with psychological, social, educational, financial, and vocational rehabilitation issues. A well-thought-out and comprehensive life care plan can provide the survivor and the family with a vital road map that will assist them in navigating the long and arduous road to recovery.

Common Acute and Reconstructive Surgical Procedures

There are several common surgical procedures in burn care. If the burn injury is circumferential, the skin can become very tight and stiff and stop the blood flow to the areas below the burn. An escharotomy, a cut made down through the burned skin (the eschar), may be performed. A fasciotomy, which is a deeper cut into the tissue below the skin (facia), may also be performed to expose the muscle. Medical records will document these procedures.

Grafting is a surgical procedure that involves the transplantation of skin. Grafting becomes necessary when the patient has burns that will not heal spontaneously. There are several types of skin grafts. The first is an autograft, created when the individual's skin is taken from an undamaged part of the body (donor site) and placed over the burned area.

If the burned area is not ready for an autograft, a temporary skin covering may be used, an allograft (homograft) or a xenograft (pigskin). This thin temporary covering is placed over the wound, allowing for better pain control and providing a barrier to infection. These temporary grafts stick to the skin and will be removed when the area is ready for a permanent skin graft (autograft). Skin grafts may take after the first surgery, but sometimes they fail, and the patient must be returned to the operating room, possibly several times, until all of the dead, burned skin has been removed (debrided or excised). A dermal replacement may also be used because it provides an outstanding barrier to infection, is easy to apply, and adheres well to lesions. It can be very costly, so it is important to inquire if dermal replacement will be necessary for any reconstructive surgeries. An additional encouraging solution that is being used for burn wound healing is the use of skin sprays, given their many benefits, such as their flexibility in delivering various cell types and materials. Skin sprays allow the transport of hydrogels and/or cells to the burn wound for healing (Pleguezuelos-Beltrán et al., 2022).

Tissue expansion with scar excision and tissue advancement is another procedure used to improve appearance and function. It has become a major reconstructive modality over the past three decades and is increasingly more popular in burn reconstruction. Tissue expansion has many advantages because the existing scarring can be excised, and the new expanded skin is advanced to cover the wound. The result is a great match in color and texture. It is a complicated 3–4-month process for the patient but can provide very effective results.

It is important to note the number and type of surgeries the burn patient has undergone in the narrative portion of the life care plan. It helps to illustrate just how burdensome and difficult the patient's acute care stay was.

Reconstruction

A seriously burned patient, especially a child, may need a great deal of post-acute care reconstructive surgery (Anthonissen et al., 2016; Jagdeo & Shumaker, 2017). Burn reconstruction aims to provide the patient with function, comfort, and improved appearance. In children, reconstruction may also be done to allow for growth. The burn patient will likely have a lifelong relationship with a reconstructive surgeon (Barret, 2004). This is particularly true for burns and scars of the face, head, and neck as they are subject to contractures and need for repeated reconstruction (Greenhalgh, 2020; Ryan et al., 2017; Sinha et al., 2019).

It is customary for definitive correction of burn scars to be postponed for at least a year or more. Scars mature over time, and some scars using pressure garments and splints may not need surgical correction. Scar contractures can be uncomfortable as well as unsightly. They may also impede function. Life care planners need to inquire as to which reconstruction procedures will be necessary and how often it is probable that they will be repeated over the life span. It is especially important to address those scar contractures that are present over joints, and skeletal deformities also need to be considered.

Once the surgery has been performed, the patient will likely need home healthcare, physical or occupational therapy, and pressure garments. These items are all important to the long-term success of any reconstructive surgery. The surgeries may also need to be repeated multiple times over the life span, especially when the burn is sustained in childhood or adolescence due to growth.

Laser Surgery

Laser surgery is playing an increasingly important role in reconstruction following burn injury. A burn injury can cause hypertrophic scarring, keloid scarring, and/or contractures, which may cause functional disability. Additionally, burn injury may cause pigment changes in the affected areas: healed or grafted skin can be lighter or darker than surrounding normal skin. Numerous laser types and treatment modalities have been used successfully in reconstructive efforts following burn injury. Laser therapy is complementary to traditional reconstructive surgery. In some cases, laser therapy may be utilized as an alternative to traditional surgery (Cohen et al., 2016; Ebid et al., 2017; Issler-Fisher et al., 2017). The burn surgeon will determine how many sessions are needed.

Pressure Garments and Splints

Burn injuries that destroy the dermis also cause the elimination of the normal pressure that these layers of skin provide. Absent this pressure, hypertrophic scars can form, causing deformities and impairment of function. Pressure garments help prevent and control hypertrophic scar formation by applying counter pressure to the wounded area. They also aid in reducing the effects of hypertrophic scarring, itching, and increased circulation to the area (Linares et al., 1972). Pressure garments are fitted by a specialist, usually before discharge from acute care.

Pressure garments can play a vital role in properly healing wounds and reducing the effects of scarring, but for the garments to perform their job properly, they need to fit tightly and be in good condition. Patients often wear their garments for anywhere from 12 to 24 months after initial discharge. They must typically be worn 23 hours per day. Therefore, patients are prescribed two sets with each fitting so that they may have one to wear and one to wash. Patients will often be fitted for new garments after reconstruction procedures.

Positioning is also very important for the burn patient. Patients are often sent home with splints. They are also often ordered after reconstruction. When discussing projected surgeries, the life care planner should inquire into the need and frequency of both garments and splints.

Prosthetics

A very severe burn, a fourth-degree or circumferential third-degree burn, may result in an amputation. This may involve a digit, hand, limb, nose, or ears (Fergason & Blanck, 2011; Riaz & Mehmood Bhatti, 2020). A prosthetist or orthotist can provide information regarding the patient's cost, replacement schedule, and need for other accessories. An anaplastologist, an individual who can create and customize highly individualized prosthetics for the face, can be consulted for information regarding prosthetic eyes, ears, noses, fingers, and so on. It is important to consider any additional physical or occupational therapy that will be needed with prosthetic/orthotic usage.

Nutritional Issues

Burn injuries affect the body's metabolic rate, and burn patients suffer from post-traumatic hypercatabolism. This well-known phenomenon causes the breakdown of tissue and exhausts the body's energy stores. The magnitude of the problem is defined by the TBSA and severity of the burns. Glucose uptake is compromised, cholesterol and lipoprotein concentrations are decreased, and protein catabolism causes patients to lose protein content. The increased metabolism is amplified by pain, anxiety, hypovolemia, and infection, as well as loss of body heat

(Gallal & Yousef, 2002). Burn patients' nutritional needs are of key importance, and patients are often given enteral feedings with a high caloric content to promote healing. Supplements are often prescribed after discharge from acute care and after reconstructive procedures to ensure proper healing. Significant weight gain after a severe burn injury can also be a problem. A weight loss program should be considered part of the life care plan if the client has experienced this complication.

Rehabilitation

Patient-specific rehabilitation services begin immediately during acute burn injury care and continue after, often long after, the patient is discharged from their initial hospitalization (Bayuo et al., 2020; Chin et al., 2018). The literature suggests that recovery from a major burn may take several years to return a patient to a satisfactory level of function (Ajoudani et al., 2018; Brown et al., 2004; Warden & Warner, 2007). The depth and location of the burn are key factors in determining the type and goals of immediate and aggressive therapeutic intervention. The preservation of function and mobility are the short-term goals of rehabilitation. Long-term goals involve returning the patient to independence through the ability to perform activities of daily living, compensation for functional loss, management of scars and pain, and reintegration into the home and community (Serghiou et al., 2007).

It is important to remember that discharge from the hospital does not mean that the patient is restored to good health (Pavoni et al., 2010). A burn patient's wounds have been covered, but they may have to return to the hospital for additional surgeries. They will likely have orders for outpatient physical therapy and/or occupational therapy, burn clinic visits, pain management, psychological care, as well as the need for pressure garment fittings (Brewin & Homer, 2018; Deflorin et al., 2020). Ongoing wound care, as mentioned previously, is also a facet of the rehabilitative phase of burn recovery.

Rehabilitation should begin immediately so that the scars do not mature and cause more severe contractions and limitations, which can increase complications, diminish function, and result in additional treatment and a greater cost of care. Burn scar maturation can vary from 6 to 18 months and longer. During this period, it is important to mobilize the burn area to decrease the likelihood of contractures, deformities, and hypertrophic scarring. Once scar maturation has occurred, correction of most deformities and cosmetic abnormalities involves costly surgical procedures with physical/occupational therapy, home healthcare, and burn clinic or doctor office follow-up for functional gains to be maintained (Cromes & Helm, 1993).

Massage Therapy

Scar massage has been found to be beneficial to burn patients and provides several important functions, including the promotion of collagen, the remodeling of scars, decreased itching, decreased anger, and decreased anxiety while providing moisture and pliability to the burned areas and donor sites (Ault et al., 2018; Cho et al., 2014; Field et al., 1998). It can also be a positive source of therapeutic touch. It should be considered after scar revision surgery and for ongoing pain, chronic itching, and scar management. Persistent, post-burn itching is estimated to affect about 87% of all patients and can persist for many years after the initial burn injury.

Outpatient Services

Over 75% of the 40,000 patients hospitalized annually for their burn injuries are admitted to the 125 hospitals with burn centers or units (DeFrances et al., 2003). Many of these specialized care centers are regional in nature. Therefore, patients must sometimes temporarily relocate to a burn center to receive ongoing and appropriate outpatient burn and rehabilitation care (Hartford & Kealy, 2007).

A comprehensive burn rehabilitation course may require as much as six hours of therapeutic intervention per day, five days per week. The frequency usually decreases gradually to three times per week and eventually to two times per week. The patient often requires attendant care from a family member or healthcare provider for dressing changes, exercise routines, and activities of daily living (ADLs). A severely burn-injured individual may need assistance for weeks or even months. If parents, spouses, or other family members are providing attendant care or transportation, an estimate of compensation for their time and effort should be considered for inclusion in the life care plan.

Physician follow-up visits are needed approximately every one to two weeks in the initial outpatient stage, with frequency decreasing to once or twice per month, if the patient is in physical therapy or occupational therapy, and for the first few weeks after treatment is stopped. Treatment typically lasts for anywhere from 12 to 16 weeks. To ensure that the patient is maintaining function after therapy has been discontinued, physician follow-up should continue but will likely gradually decrease to once every three months for 12 to 18 months, then biannually for another 12 to 18 months, then annually, unless unforeseen complications arise (Foster, 2022, personal communication, April 14, 2002). However, the number of weeks or months and the physician follow-up plan are always specific to the patient; therefore, a physician should make the actual recommendation.

Pediatric Life Care Plans Involving Burns

Life care plans for severely burn-injured children can be very complicated. Pediatric patients often need multiple reconstructive surgeries as they grow. Children may have cognitive problems due to trauma and/or inhalation injury, and there will be great demand placed on their parents and family to support them in their need for ongoing care. Educational needs should also be considered. Summer burn camp is a rehabilitation program that can bring great benefits to a burn-surviving child and should be considered for inclusion in the life care of a pediatric burn survivor (Kornhaber et al., 2020). The World Burn Congress, an annual rehabilitative event sponsored by the Phoenix Society, can also be beneficial for children and their families and can be extremely helpful for adult burn survivors and their families as well.

Psychological Issues

Psychological adjustment to a severe burn injury can often be profound (Bich et al., 2021; Rainey et al., 2014; Smith et al., 2006). A significant number of burn-injured patients will develop post-traumatic stress and experience intrusive memories related to the event during the acute care phase (Ehde et al., 1999; Macleod at al., 2016; Psychiatry.org, 2019; Quinn, 2014). Depression and anxiety on the part of the patient and/or the family may also occur (Stuart, 2022). If it was available, psychological intervention might have begun in the burn center during the acute care stage of hospitalization. However, not all burn centers or units provide psychological services as a regular part of their care protocol.

The medical chart should be reviewed to ascertain what psychological problems may have arisen during inpatient care and what psychiatric or psychological services if any, were delivered (Shepherd et al., 2019). Supportive services and crisis management care are often offered to patients' families in the burn center; however, as basic survival becomes the major goal during the initial phase of hospitalization, psychological matters may not have been addressed or may have been addressed inadequately.

Acute stress disorder may be diagnosed during acute hospitalization. Post-traumatic stress disorder, a complication that longitudinal studies have found to affect up to 45% of adults who were hospitalized for their burn injury one-year post-burn and nearly one-third of burn patients within two years of their burn, cannot be diagnosed until at least 30 days after the initial traumatic event (Perry et al., 1992; Weichman et al., 2001). Therefore, it is important to address the psychological issues of both the patient and the family, not only during the inpatient stay, but after discharge from the burn center or burn unit.

Many burn-injured patients persist with periods of fear and anxiety (Brubaker Rimmer et al., 2022). These symptoms often recur when the patient must return to the hospital for reconstructive surgeries. Adults may express their anxiety through physical symptoms such as palpitations, perspiration, nausea, and shaking. Children may become clingy or fearful, cry often, have headaches and stomach aches, or become disruptive and angry. The psychological impact of a burn injury has become a major focus of burn care. A variety of variables seem to influence the long-term emotional outcome. Therefore, constructing follow-up interventions tailored to the burn patient's individual circumstances is recommended (Gojowy et al., 2019).

A psychosocial survey should be performed for the specific patient (Kurian et al., 2019; Levi et al., 2018). As mentioned earlier, the patient and the patient's family may have been unable to address psychological and social issues such as post-traumatic stress disorder, financial pressures, or depression before discharge from acute care (Wiechman et al., 2018). They may be experiencing new problems at home such as sleep disturbance (Boeve et al., 2002; Masoodi et al., 2013), anxiety, sexual concerns (Connell et al., 2013), body image problems (Beaver et al., 2019; Cleary et al., 2020; Fauerbach et al., 2000; Pell, 2019; Stock et al., 2013), itching, identity issues, inability to return to work or school (Ohrtman et al., 2018; Schneider et al., 2020), and unresolved pain issues. If the patient or the family expresses concerns regarding any or all these matters, there should be an evaluation by a psychologist or psychiatrist. A neuropsychology evaluation, used to examine brain function and possible impairments, is often recommended for severely burned pediatric patients and may be ideal for any burn patient who has experienced an inhalation injury or trauma to the head concomitant with the burn injury.

Life care planners should inquire about any currently prescribed psychotropic drugs and the length of need for such medications. If medication is needed on an ongoing basis through life expectancy, the patient will likely need ongoing visits with a psychiatrist. Consideration should be made for immediate psychological intervention if problems are occurring, as well as the need for ongoing psychological care during major life shifts and periods of reconstructive surgery. Play therapy for children, individual therapy for adolescents and adults, and couples and family counseling for spouses, parents, and siblings should also be considered because a serious burn injury takes a toll on the entire family unit.

Vocational Rehabilitation

Limited literature is available on the details surrounding return to work following a serious burn injury (Dyster-Aas et al., 2007; Sheckter et al., 2021). One study revealed that most burn survivors return to work within two years with an average of 17 weeks off the job (Brych et al., 2001). However, there are several reported factors that tend to impede return to work. The most common risk factors associated with longer durations of work absence following serious injury and found to increase the unlikelihood of returning to work include the patient's admission to intensive care units, a lengthy hospitalization, and a low education level (Schulz et al., 2019). These are not unusual circumstances for individuals who have sustained severe burn injuries.

Other factors impeding return to work, which are related directly to burn injury, include TBSA, length of hospitalization, the thickness of burns, number of surgeries, age, presence of hand burns, reduced endurance, alcohol, or drug dependence, and prior psychological or psychiatric problems. The longer the time elapsed since the burn injury, the higher the likelihood of returning to work. Positive factors for the likelihood of returning to work include pre-employment status, age, good coping skills, and a higher level of education. However, having more full-thickness burn injuries is associated with a lower likelihood of returning to work (Dyster-Aas et al., 2007).

Several studies have shown that burn patients who can return to work report more satisfaction and a better overall quality of life than those who remain unemployed. Therefore, vocational rehabilitation issues should be considered during the early part of outpatient rehabilitation. Employers should be contacted regularly to keep them updated on the patient's status to encourage a good relationship and diminish the patient's fears that their former employment will be lost. A comprehensive job description can be used to determine therapy needs to assist the patient in maintaining job skills. Part-time employment or light duty should be discussed to diminish financial stress and avoid establishing a dependency pattern (Weed & Berens, 2005).

A majority of burn patients can return to work, but they are often unable to return to the job they had before their burn injury (Brych et al., 2001). If job modifications or return to the same type of employment is unlikely, vocational evaluation and training should be considered as soon as the patient is healthy enough to begin. Research from the University of Washington revealed that two years out from their injury, only 37% of survivors had returned to the same job and to the same employer without accommodation. Almost 50% had received disability benefits, not gone back to work, or had some degree of employment interruption (Brych et al., 2001).

Those individuals who have been deemed permanently impaired may benefit from the assistance of a knowledgeable rehabilitation counselor (a board-certified rehabilitation counselor/CRC is preferred) who has the necessary background to conduct an assessment of the person's physical, cognitive, and emotional functioning levels. A vocational evaluation by a qualified vocational evaluator may be justified. A psychological assessment and functional capacity evaluation should also be considered.

A burn patient's ability to return to work is highly individualized. The infirmity can range from no loss of function to living with an amputation and the need to adjust to a prosthesis. Life care planners are often confronted with electrical burns, which may have resulted in amputation, cognitive and emotional impairment, and vision problems. Early and ongoing physical, cognitive, psychosocial, and support factors may impact successful return to work after sustaining electrical injury. Specialized care and advocacy were found to be advantageous to a successful return to work (Stergiou-Kita et al., 2014). Productivity is a highly valued personal characteristic; therefore, helping clients with their return to work or assisting them in finding a new vocation or different form of recreation can be most helpful.

Complications

Complications after a burn injury can be extensive and wide-reaching, and they may affect many different body systems (Warden & Warner, 2007). It is important to ask the treating physician what the potential complications are for a particular patient. Table 21.1 includes common complications associated with burn injury. They have been divided by body systems with recommendations for intervention, the likely frequency and duration of treatment, and surgical options. The list includes the most significant and usual burn injury-related complications. The most common treatment options are also included.

Burn Injury: Damage Assessment Checklist

Serious burn injuries are considered catastrophic injuries. There is usually a significant cost associated with the recovery and rehabilitation of the burn patient, which can necessitate lifelong care. Pediatric burn patients often require extensive reconstruction and rehabilitation, especially during but not limited to their growth and developmental years. A burn injury impacts the entire family system, so it is important to consider the family's needs as well.

Patients may need a variety of physicians to care for them, including but not limited to plastic reconstructive surgeons, physiatrists, orthopedic surgeons, pediatric intensivists, cardiologists, internists, pulmonologists, and psychiatrists for lifelong care.

Allied healthcare, including psychological, physical, occupational, and vocational therapies, and the need for case management are important items to consider. In-home assistance, respite care, home maintenance and cleaning services, and assisted living in advanced years are also often a necessity.

Patients often have an ongoing need for pain medications, moisturizers, pressure garments, prosthetics and orthotics, splints, special makeup, and other supplies. Transportation and mobility assistance and exercise for optimum function should also be considered.

The following checklist can be utilized when meeting with care providers and considering future care needs.

Life Care Planning for the Patient with Burns ■ 581

Table 21.1 Complications Commonly Associated with Burn Injury

Complication	Location	Clinical presentation	Diagnosis	Nonsurgical options	Surgical options	Additional comments
Skin Complications						
Nonhealing wounds: acute	Can occur anywhere on burned, grafted, or donor site skin. Most often in poorly vascularized areas, areas under tension, or areas of contact or friction	Open, painful, wounds, often with bleeding or exudate	Clinical exam	Debridement of devitalized tissue and local wound care with a plethora of wound care products; improved nutrition; treatment of infections (which may not be clinically obvious); hyperbaric oxygen therapy (unproven)	Primary wound closure; partial-thickness skin grafting; full-thickness skin grafting; soft tissue rotation or flaps	Wound care is an art, not a science: what works for one patient may not work for another. A key element is patience. Assume wound closure of about 1 cm per month of therapy
Nonhealing wounds: chronic	As previous entry; often associated with infections such as MRSA or vascular insufficiency	As in previous entry; nonhealing or lack of progression over weeks or months; breakdown of a previously healed wound	Clinical exam; wound culture; non-invasive vascular studies	As in previous entry; antibiotics; good nutrition is key	As in previous entry	As in previous entry
Skin blistering	May occur anywhere; most often seen in freshly healed wound or donor sites	Superficial, pink, moist painful open wounds on a site that had been previously healed	Patient history; clinical exam	Local wound care with a variety of wound care products	Rarely requires split-thickness skin grafting	Usually heals with conservative care
Pigmentation changes	Can occur anywhere; most often seen in grafted skin especially on the face and head; may be seen in healed burns; rarely seen in healed donor sites	Skin that is darker (more common) or lighter (less common) than normal	Clinical examination	Makeup: can be difficult to locate and expensive to use	Tattooing and other pigmentation procedures; most only partially correct the abnormality	Pigmentation changes evolve over 6 to 24 months; it is important to wait until the wounds are completely stable

(Continued)

Table 21.1 (Continued) Complications Commonly Associated with Burn Injury

Complication	Location	Clinical presentation	Diagnosis	Nonsurgical options	Surgical options	Additional comments
Hypertrophic scars	Can occur anywhere; most often seen in grafted areas, but common in healed burns also; rarely seen in donor sites' deeper burns, burns that were open for a longer period of time, or burns that were infected tend to form worse hypertrophic scars. More common in persons with greater skin pigmentation	Thick, red, or purple, hard, nonpliable, raised scars; often itchy and/or painful	Clinical exam	Custom-fitted compression garments reduce and improve almost all of the symptoms associated with hypertrophic scars; silicone sheeting under the compression garment often is synergistic; custom plastic masks may be effective for face scars; garments must be worn 23½ hours per day to be truly effective; a variety of topical medications may improve symptoms: aloe, diphenhydramine lotion, aspirin cream, calcium channel blocker cream, ketamine lotion, and many others; some systemic medications may help: antihistamines, nonsteroidal anti-inflammatory drugs, and others; other therapy such as massage, ultrasound, etc., may be useful in selected cases	Scar excisions with primary closure; sequential excision and closure of a scar; excision and grafting; excision and soft tissue coverage following skin expansion	Wait for scars to mature to a stable point, usually 6 to 24 months after closure. This is the hardest part of burn care: waiting for the scars to mature. The most important factor in scar formation is genetics: some people are born to be good healers, and others are born to be scar formers
Keloids	As in previous entry	As in previous entry; tend to form in persons with high levels of skin pigmentation	Clinical examination	As in previous entry; steroid injection and/or radiation therapy may be useful	As in previous entry	Often recur following excision, regardless of treatment

(Continued)

Table 21.1 (Continued) Complications Commonly Associated with Burn Injury

Complication	Location	Clinical presentation	Diagnosis	Nonsurgical options	Surgical options	Additional comments
Painful scars	Can occur anywhere. More common on extremities than on torso or head	Painful scars, most sensitive to touch, heat, or cold; often make sleep difficult; can be unpredictable in extent and manifestation of pain; typically burning, may be sharp	Clinical examination of scar: palpation, and range of motion	As previously, for hypertrophic scars; desensitization and neuropathic pain medications may be useful (Neurontin, amitriptyline)	Scar excision may be helpful, but usually only temporarily, if at all, effective; surgery should be avoided if at all possible	This complication is very difficult to manage. Complete resolution is unusual; most patients have residual pain for many years
Wound contracture	Can occur anywhere that has been burned; usually seen with deep burns that have healed or been grafted. Most common: neck, axilla, hands, elbow, knees	Skin tightness, especially with extension, decreased range of motion, and decreased functionality	Clinical examination, and range-of-motion measurements	Aggressive physical or occupational therapy to prevent and treat; splinting in position of function; serious contractures may require serial splinting in progressive extension or flexion; massage, ultrasound may be useful adjuncts	Generally, depend upon therapy to prevent and treat; persistent contractures that interfere with function can be released surgically, with local soft tissue transfer or skin grafting	Wait until scar is mature and physical therapy and occupational therapy have been maximized before considering surgery. Therapy is very important after surgical release
Microstomia (small mouth)	Mouth	Face, lip, and neck burns, typically; neck and chest burn wound contracture can pull down on the lip, also	Clinical exam, mouth opening measurements	Prevention with a microstomia appliance; as in previous entry for hypertrophic scars; aggressive occupational therapy	Can be released surgically; usually quite successful	Prevention is key. A microstomia appliance must be worn at all times to effectively prevent or treat

(Continued)

Table 21.1 (Continued) Complications Commonly Associated with Burn Injury

Complication	Location	Clinical presentation	Diagnosis	Nonsurgical options	Surgical options	Additional comments
Ectropion (contraction of scar tissue of the eyelid or eversion of the eyelid caused by contraction of facial skin)	Occurs with deep facial burns or burns to the eye area; usually becomes obvious during acute hospitalization	Inability to close the eyes, thereby causing corneal damage due to drying	Clinical exam, ophthalmology consult	Therapy, including scar massage and stretching	Daily therapy until problem resolves	Surgical intervention for release and skin grafting is usually indicated
Skin infection	Can occur anywhere. May result from infection of ingrown hairs, ingrown glandular secretions, clogged pores, poor vascularization. Often caused by streptococcus or staphylococcus (including MRSA)	Skin redness, pain, erythema, swelling; may see pustules (especially with MRSA) or frank pus; may be subclinical	Skin examination and wound culture	Local wound care, pus drainage, debridement of devitalized tissue, removal of foreign body (staple or suture)	May require aggressive debridement, drainage, excision in the operating room	Do not forget to look for infections that are not obvious in wounds that are not healing
Fingernail loss	Occurs with deep hand burns	May see fingernail loss without regrowth, deformed nails, jagged nails	Clinical exam	Meticulous nail trimming and cleansing; massage	Can use toenails for reconstructive and cosmetic procedures	Often overlooked in a patient with other major burns
Hair follicle loss	Usually full-thickness burn to scalp with follicle destruction	Permanent hair loss and poor cosmesis	Clinical exam	Creative hair dressing, wigs, hairpieces, hats, glasses; no effective medications	Reconstruction with tissue expansion in nearby hair-bearing area with subsequent wound excision and soft tissue transfer	Scalp hair loss is recalcitrant; often requires multiple procedures. Eyebrows can be reconstructed with hair transfers or tattooing

(Continued)

Table 21.1 (Continued) Complications Commonly Associated with Burn Injury

Complication	Location	Clinical presentation	Diagnosis	Nonsurgical options	Surgical options	Additional comments
Ingrown hairs	Occurs on hair-bearing areas of the body that have been burned and grafted	Pain, itching, irritation, infection	Clinical examination	Local wound care, drainage of pus, topical antibiotics; may require systemic antibiotics	Surgical excision of the offending hair; may require reconstruction or skin grafting	Tends to occur on face and upper extremities in men
Loss of sebaceous and/or sweat glands	Almost always associated with deep burns that have been grafted; may occur in deep healed burns	Dry, scaly, itching skin; skin may be cracked or fissured	Clinical examination	Local wound care with lubrication creams/lotions/ointments	No effective surgery	Requires lifelong treatment, typically
Loss of or decreased skin innervation	Almost always associated with deep burns that have been grafted; may occur in deep healed burns	Loss of sensation to fine touch, temperature, vibration	Sensory testing	Reassurance of patient; wait for function to return; compression garments, silicone, massage may all help; avoid irritation, trauma; padded clothing	No effective surgery	Requires lifelong treatment, typically
Marjolin's ulcer (squamous cell carcinoma)	Typically develops in a healed or grafted burn that is chronically open; typically occurs 10–30 years after injury	Nonhealing wound with associated mass or growth	Wound biopsy	Nothing	Radical excision; possible adjuvant therapy	Relatively rare; occurs in far less than 1% of patients
Eye and Ear Complications						
Eyelid contracture	Burned upper or lower lids	Inability to close eyes; dry eyes; frequent tearing	Ophthalmologic examination	Tarsorrhaphy sutures	Reconstruction with full-thickness skin grafts	Prevention is key

(Continued)

Table 21.1 (Continued) Complications Commonly Associated with Burn Injury

Complication	Location	Clinical presentation	Diagnosis	Nonsurgical options	Surgical options	Additional comments
Ectropion (eversion of the eyelid caused by contraction of facial skin)	Usually occurs on upper or lower lid after serious facial burn	Pain, irritation, tearing, bleeding, inability to close eye	Clinical examination	Massage and passive stretching may help	Excision and grafting are usually required	Usually occurs acutely during initial hospitalization; difficult to prevent
Cataract	Occurs following electrical injury	Deteriorating visual acuity	Ophthalmologic examination	Usually none	Often requires operative intervention	Screening eye examination shoud be done on all patients with electrical injury
Loss of ear cartilage	Full-thickness burn to ear	Loss of normal anatomic appearance and contour of ear	Clinical examination	Massage and passive stretching may help minimally	Usually requires bone graft and skin grafting; occasionally requires soft tissue transfer	Cosmetic deformity primarily; hearing usually not affected
Lung and Heart Complications						
Tracheal stenosis	Tracheal narrowing as a result of prolonged intubation	Difficulty breathing; poor exercise tolerance; stridor	Clinical examination; bronchoscopy, laryngoscopy computerized tomography	Dilation	Usually requires surgical correction	Usually present at time of discharge from initial hospitalization
Pulmonary insufficiency	Results from inhalation injury (toxic effect of breathing products of combustion); may be exacerbated by pulmonary infections while hospitalized	Poor exercise tolerance; easy fatiguability; frequent pulmonary infections; cough	Clinical examination; pulmonary function testing; bronchoscopy	Exercise; bronchodilators	None	May not manifest until years after initial injury; usually present to some degree at time of discharge from initial hospitalization

(Continued)

Table 21.1 (Continued) Complications Commonly Associated with Burn Injury

Complication	Location	Clinical presentation	Diagnosis	Nonsurgical options	Surgical options	Additional comments
Cardiac dysrhythmias, cardiac dysfunction, coronary artery disease	Occurs following electrical injury	Chest pain, shortness of breath, poor exercise tolerance	Clinical examination, ECG, echocardiogram; Holter monitor	Exercise, diet, medications	Usually none; may rarely require coronary artery bypass grafting	Very rare complication seen only after electrical injury
Neurologic Complications						
Neuroma	Nerve or nerve ending that becomes hypersensitive following a burn; usually the result of the nerve or nerve ending getting caught up in the inflammatory process	Specific hypersensitive or painful and/or tender area usually on an extremity; may be hypersensitive to hot or cold or both	Clinical examination	Compression garments, silicone, topical analgesics, massage, ultrasound	May require surgical excision	Tends not to respond completely regardless of treatment modality
Complex Regional Pain Syndrome (CRPS) Type 1	Idiosyncratic pain syndrome that is poorly defined; usually occurs following serious burn; more common in extremities, especially lower extremity	Hypersensitive, painful, stiff, inflammatory skin; intolerance of cold or heat or both; may see redness and swelling; exam may be completely normal	Clinical examination	Compression garments, aggressive occupational or physical therapy; ganglion block may be helpful; a variety of medications have been used	Usually none	Difficult to diagnose—typically a diagnosis of exclusion; very difficult to treat successfully
Musculoskeletal Complications						
Heterotrophic ossification	Usually seen in large joints of burned extremities; elbow is the most commonly involved joint	Decreased range of motion; usually diagnosed by occupational therapists	Clinical examination; X-ray; bone scan	Passive and active range of motion to prevent and treat; dynamic and passive splints or casting; continuous passive range-of-motion devices	Excision and removal of heterotopic bone; postoperative therapy is very important	Difficult to treat conservatively in severe cases; usually requires surgery

(Continued)

Table 21.1 (Continued) Complications Commonly Associated with Burn Injury

Complication	Location	Clinical presentation	Diagnosis	Nonsurgical options	Surgical options	Additional comments
Joint subluxation	Typically seen in the small joints in hands, fingers, feet, and toes on burned extremities	Obvious deformity; decreased function and decreased range of motion	Clinical examination and X-rays	Prevention with range of motion and strengthening, splinting	Surgical release and reconstruction	Wait until scar is mature to surgically correct
Boutonniere deformity of finger	Dorsal aspect of burn hands involving extensor tendon	Obvious deformity; decreased function and decreased range of motion	Clinical examination and X-rays	Prevention with range of motion and strengthening, splinting	Surgical release and reconstruction	
Swan neck deformity of finger	Contracture of hand muscles and tendons	Obvious deformity; decreased function and decreased range of motion	Clinical examination and X-rays	Prevention with range of motion and strengthening, splinting	Surgical release and reconstruction	
Mallet finger deformity	Deep burns to the dorsum or back of hand; involves extensor tendons	Obvious deformity; decreased function and decreased range of motion; inability to extend the distal interphalangeal joint of finger	Clinical examination and X-rays	Prevention with range of motion and strengthening, splinting	Surgical release and reconstruction with tendon repair	
Exposed tendons	Deep burns, usually of hands or feet	Obviously exposed tendons with decreased function	Clinical examination	Local wound care; protection of tendon from desiccation	Soft tissue transfer and reconstruction	Usually requires surgery; may use skin substitutes

(Continued)

Life Care Planning for the Patient with Burns ■ 589

Table 21.1 (Continued) Complications Commonly Associated with Burn Injury

Complication	Location	Clinical presentation	Diagnosis	Nonsurgical options	Surgical options	Additional comments
Shortened extremity	Burn scars on extremities prevent normal bone growth	Obviously shortened extremity with decreased function	Clinical examination	Aggressive physical and occupational therapy	May require reconstruction for severe limitation of function	Usually requires wound contracture release simultaneously
Limb amputation	Full-thickness burns of extremities; often with compartment syndrome and/or vascular insufficiency	Obvious loss of extremity	None	Preoperative planning, if possible; immediate postoperative prosthesis if possible; maintenance of joint above amputation in neutral position; stump care; strengthening and balance training	Stump may require revision for chronic wound and/or poor soft tissue padding	Involvement of patient and family in care vital to success

Burn Life Care Plan Checklist

Annual Evaluations	
Physicians/Surgeons	
Primary Care	
Surgeries Related to Growth or Aging:	
Contracture Releases	
Dermabrasion	
Hand Surgeries	
Hypertrophic Scarring	
Heterotrophic Ossification	
Tissue Expansion	
Scar Excision	
Emergency Room Visits	
Physical Discomfort:	
Pain Control	
Itching	
Skin Breakdown	
Range-of-Motion Issues	
Sleep Problems	
Aesthetic Issues:	
Eyebrows	
Nipples	
Fingernails	
Eyelashes	
Special Makeup	
Breast Implants	
Special Bra	
Breast Prosthesis	
Pressure Garments:	
Face Mask	
Arms	
Trunk	
Back	
Legs	
Hands/Gloves	
Zippers	

(Continued)

Silicone Sheeting	
Splinting	
Occupational Therapy Needs	
Physical Therapy Needs	
Speech Therapy Needs	
Massage Therapy	
Lotions	
Dressing Change Materials	
Sun Protection Needs:	
Sunscreen	
Special UV-Protective Clothing	
Nutritional Needs	
Case Management	
Psychological Interventions:	
Psychiatry	
Play Therapy	
Neuropsychological Testing	
Family Therapy	
Individual Psychotherapy	
Support Group	
Burn Camp	
World Burn Congress	
Hypnosis	
Educational Needs:	
Private School	
Tutoring	
IEP Assistance	
Vocational Needs:	
Job Training	
Vocational Counseling	
Work Hardening	
Workplace Reintegration	
Recreational Issues:	
Recreation Therapy	
Home Care:	
Home Health	
Respite Care for Parents/Spouse	
Aids to Daily Living	
Assisted Living Needs	

(Continued)

Housekeeping	
Handyman	
Mobility:	
Wheelchair	
Scooter	
Walker	
Prosthetics	
Pulmonary Issues:	
Pulmonologist	
Breathing Treatments	
Humidifier	
Dressing Change Materials	
Pain Medications	
Other Medications	
Conservatorship	

Sample Life Care Plan for John Doe

Narrative Summary

Introduction

Mr. Attorney has requested that a life care plan be provided for John Doe regarding the severe 62% third-degree TBSA burn injuries that he sustained in a home explosion on XX/XX/2014. This life care plan will assist in determining John's long-term needs as they relate to his significant burn injuries. This document will outline a plan of care with the projected burn injury-related costs that John Doe will likely incur over his lifetime. The goal is to develop a personalized life care plan to help maintain John's medical stability, sustain or increase his functional status and quality of life, and assist in preventing further injury-related complications.

This life care plan report will consist of two parts, a narrative section and a table section. The narrative will include a summary of the available medical records, healthcare provider interviews, and details from two personal interviews with John Doe, his wife Jane, and this life care planner.

The second section of the life care plan will be presented in table form and will provide, in detail, the future injury-related projected care needs, costs, rationale, and recommenders of such care. This will include an itemized listing of likely future medical care expenses, with likely procedures/hospitalizations/surgeries, evaluations, therapies, diagnostic testing, medications, home care, transportation, and health and strength maintenance. Finally, it will outline potential complications. Costs will be broken down into annual and one-time expenses.

All prices quoted in this life care plan are present year and are calculated for a 12-month period. This plan will need to be re-evaluated if the evaluee becomes medically unstable, has a significant change in functional status, and/or his condition changes due to the burn disease process.

DEMOGRAPHIC INFORMATION:
Name: John Doe   Injury Date: XX/XX/2014
Address: City:
Phone: (757) XXX-XXXX   Birth Date: 9/22/XXXX
Gender: Male   Ethnicity: Caucasian
Education: High School Graduate
U. S. Citizen: Yes   Marital Status—Married—15 years   Glasses: No
                                  Dominant Hand: Right
Current Employment:
Family: Wife—Jane, 1 son—Jack—age—9, 1 daughter—Susie—age—7

Foundation for Report

Inpatient Medical Records................Burn Center Medical Center, Anytown, USA
Inpatient Medical Records.........Physical Rehabilitation Center
Outpatient Records Rehabilitation......................—Anytown, USA
Consultation—Dr. Surgeon, Burn Surgeon/Plastic Surgeon
Consultation—Dr. Surgeon, Burn/Plastic Surgeon
Email Consultation—2/24/2014- Dr. Surgeon
Phone Consultation—Dr.—Treating Psychiatrist—14/06/2013
Hanger Prosthetics—14/15/2013
Burn Center Medical Center Billing
Personal Interview with This Life Care Planner—John and Jane Doe

Medical Records and Reports Reviewed:

Burn Center Health System..........Medical Records
Best Rehabilitation Hospital........................Billing Records
Ms. Surgeon, MD, Plastic/Burn Surgeon................Billing Records
Physical and Occupational Therapy ....Medical Records
Physical and Occupational Therapy...............Billing Records

Summary: John Doe, a 32-year-old Caucasian male, sustained severe burns to 62% of his body at age 26. Specifically, he sustained deep burns to his neck, scalp, ears, both his upper and lower extremities, flanks, as well as bilateral hands, ankles, and feet.

Burn Injury

John Doe suffered multiple third-degree burns to 62% of his body. Many unburned areas of his body were harvested as donor sites for the multiple skin graft surgeries he underwent. Normal skin was harvested to provide coverage for the extensive third- and deep second-degree burns to his arms, scalp, forehead, buttocks, and legs. Therefore, damage to his skin far exceeds the 62% that was originally burned. A third-degree burn results in serious disruption of normal skin and creates the subsequent need for skin grafting. The harvesting of a skin graft from the individual's unburned skin often results in additional significant scarring as the body tries to diminish and "fix" the burn wounds. The hypertrophic scarring that now covers much of John's body impedes his function and physical activity level. It has also diminished his body's ability to regulate its temperature.

Injury Event

John Doe reports that he was burned at home on XX/XX/2014 when an explosion severely injured him. By helicopter, John Doe was rushed to Burn Center Medical Center in Anytown, State. He arrived lying on his abdomen, and this was due to the severe back pain he was experiencing due to deep and extensive burns. John also complained of pain in both hands and his lower extremities.

Burn Center, Anytown, USA
Problems documented during John's burn care hospitalization:
Primary Diagnosis: Full-thickness skin loss due to third-degree burns
Secondary Diagnosis:

1. 62% of body burned; 62% third degree
2. Acute kidney failure
3. Methicillin susceptible pneumonia due to staphylococcus aureus
4. Nutritional marasmus (severe malnutrition)
5. Hyperosmolality and/or hypernatremia—electrolyte problem—a rise in serum sodium
6. Full-thickness skin loss due to burns (third degree), multiple sites
7. Hypotension (low blood pressure)
8. Neutropenia (abnormally low white blood cell count)
9. Acute respiratory failure
10. Bacteremia (viable bacteria in the bloodstream)
11. Acute post-hemorrhagic anemia (anemia from bleeding)
12. Ventilator-associated pneumonia
13. Full-thickness skin loss due to burn (third degree, not otherwise specified), abdomen
14. Full-thickness skin loss due to burn (third degree), hands
15. Thrombocytopenia (abnormally low number of platelets)
16. Abnormal glucose (blood sugar level)
17. Constipation
18. Bacterial infection due to gram-negative bacteria
19. Leukocytosis (high white blood cell count)
20. Burns multiple sites (except with eye) of face/head/neck
21. Essential hypertension (high blood pressure with no identifiable cause)

Surgical and Invasive Procedure Details—John Doe was taken to the operating room 24 times for the following procedures as outlined below:

BURN CENTER—Surgical and Invasive Procedures
XX/19/2014– Burn Center Burn Center
Discharge Diagnosis

- 62% TBSA burns
- Acute blood loss with anemia that resolved

Consults during Burn Admission

- Plastic surgery
- Physical therapy
- Occupational therapy
- Nutrition
- Psychology

Burn Center—Surgical and Invasive Procedures

Procedure	Provider	Date
Excisional debridement of wound/infection/burn	Surgeon, MD	XX/XX/14
Temporary tracheostomy	Surgeon, MD	XX/XX/14
Continuous invasive mechanical ventilation for 84 consecutive days	Surgeon, MD	XX/07/14
Homograft to skin	Surgeon, MD	XX/19/14
Excisional debridement of wound/infection/burn	Surgeon, MD	XX/12/14
Excisional debridement of wound/infection/burn	Surgeon, MD	XX/15/14
Excisional debridement of wound/infection/burn	Surgeon, MD	XX/16/14
Skin graft	Surgeon, MD	XX/19/14
Skin graft	Surgeon, MD	XX/19/14
Skin graft	Surgeon, MD	XX/22/14
Homograft to skin	Surgeon, MD	XX/22/14
Excisional debridement of wound/infection/burn	Surgeon, MD	XX/26/14
Homograft to skin	Surgeon, MD	XX/26/14
Skin graft	Surgeon, MD	05/03/14
Homograft to skin	Surgeon, MD	05/03/14
Skin graft	Surgeon, MD	05/13/14
Homograft to skin	Surgeon, MD	05/13/14
Excisional debridement of wound/infection/burn	Surgeon, MD	05/31/14
Venous catheterization	Surgeon, MD	XX/03/14
Arterial catheterization	Surgeon, MD	XX/03/14
Bronchoscopy	Surgeon, MD	XX/07/14
Incision of skin and subcutaneous tissue	Surgeon, MD	XX/03/14
Non-excisional debridement of wound/infection/burn	Surgeon, MD	XX/19/14
Enteral infusion of concentrated nutritional substances	Surgeon, MD	XX/03/14
Transfusion of packed blood cells	Surgeon, MD	XX/13/14
Non-excisional debridement of wound/infection/burn	Surgeon, MD	XX/22/14
Non-excisional debridement of wound/infection/burn	Surgeon, MD	XX/26/14
Non-excisional debridement of wound/infection/burn	Surgeon, MD	XX/29/14
Non-excisional debridement of wound/infection/burn	Surgeon, MD	05/03/14

(Continued)

Procedure	Provider	Date
Non-excisional debridement of wound/infection/burn	Surgeon, MD	05/06/14
Non-excisional debridement of wound/infection/burn	Surgeon, MD	05/13/14
Hydrotherapy	Surgeon, MD	05/29/14
Non-excisional debridement of wound/infection/burn	Surgeon, MD	05/29/14
Non-excisional debridement of wound/infection/burn	Surgeon, MD	05/31/14

Upon discharge from the Burn Center, John Doe was transferred and admitted to Best Rehabilitation Hospital on XX/19/2014 for complex rehabilitation. He remained there for daily comprehensive inpatient rehabilitation until XX/10/2014.

After being discharged from Best Rehabilitation Hospital, John Doe returned to his home in Springfield, State. John Doe shared that he continued receiving physical/occupational therapy twice per week for more than a year after his discharge from rehab. He needed extensive therapy to regain many functions, including retaining the ability to put his shoes and socks on his feet.

Personal Interviews with John Doe and Jane Doe

August 09, 2019, in Springfield, State & January XX/XX/2020 in Springfield, State.

This interview aimed to ascertain to what extent John's multiple injuries are interfering with his ability to manage his activities of daily living.

Current Status and Disabling Problems: John Doe continues to suffer from physical and emotional problems related to his severe burn injuries. He remains highly anxious, has ongoing pain and itching, frequent headaches, sensitivity to hot and cold weather, dry skin, swelling of his hands and feet, fatigue, and decreased endurance and sleep disruption. He reported experiencing ongoing body image issues and reported that he no longer recognizes his own body.

John Doe also reported severe sleep problems and intermittent nightmares. He has been unable to return to his former job due to physical restraints. He acknowledged that he continues to feel depressed and anxious much of the time. John Doe shared that his relationship with his wife, Jane, has been strained due to his discomfort with having to lean on her so much and so often. He said she had been a constant support for him, but his role as husband, father, and head of the family has been compromised due to his lack of independence. His sex life has also been negatively affected since sustaining his injuries and disfigurement. John has been unable to continue with many of his other customary activities, especially sports, hunting, and fishing, due to his extensive arm and leg burns and the resulting physical limitations he continues to experience. Again, this is especially problematic due to his scar contractures and resulting disabilities, which have caused him significant physical and emotional challenges.

Burn and trauma injuries are complex and place great stress on the body's major organs. The skin is the body's largest organ, and when third-degree burns severely damage it, it causes physiologic and metabolic disruption of the entire body. Burns have been documented as the most injurious insult the human body can endure. John Doe's injuries were unexpected, creating a crisis situation. John, his wife Jane, his parents, and his children have all experienced emotional and psychological distress because of his extensive burns.

Medical History: John Doe reported enjoying good health before his injuries.

Family History: John Doe was born and raised in State by his mother and father, John and Joy Doe. His parents are both living, and he reports they are both healthy. He also has a brother, age 42, who is also healthy. John Doe has been married to his wife, Jane, for 15 years and has a seven-year-old son, Johnny, and a four-year-old daughter, Jill.

Social History: He was happy and felt fulfilled with close family relationships and good friends before the explosion. He was active in sports, hunting, and fishing and was happy with his marriage and children. John Doe shared that he loved his former job and is distressed because his doctor says it is highly likely that he will be unable to return to it due to the physical demands of his prior job.

Educational History: John Doe graduated from Anytown High School. Upon graduation he went to work directly in the plumbing business with his father. His wife Jane has a degree in accounting and was working as a CPA at the time of the explosion. She left her job to be with him throughout his lengthy hospitalization.

Employment History: John Doe started his career with Anytown Plumbing after graduating from high school.

Hobbies: John Doe loved going hunting and fishing in the past. He has been unable to engage in these activities since sustaining his physically limiting burn injuries.

Current Social Activities: John Doe reports that his social life is quite different now. He is uncomfortable going out in public and can no longer do many of the things he enjoyed doing prior to XX/XX/2014. He cannot be in the sun for an extended period, and this has greatly limited his activity. He reports being sensitive to both the heat and the cold, and laments being unable to even spend the day at the beach with his family, one of his favorite former pastimes.

Appearance Issues: Since sustaining his burns, John reports that he feels self-conscious about his body and wears long sleeve shirts and pants at all times because of his extensive scarring. He did try wearing short sleeve shirts in the summer due to the heat but felt uncomfortable when people looked at his scars. He shared that it is easier to stay at home rather than have he and his family subjected to people's comments and stares. His fatigue and pain also make it difficult for him to enjoy the activities he did in the past. John Doe always took good care of his body and tried to maintain a healthy physique. His physician, Dr. Surgeon, shared that his sound physical condition prior to the burns was probably why he survived. Prior to sustaining his burns, physical fitness was a top priority, and he said that he has not yet begun to adjust to the changes in his body; either his appearance or his diminished physical function. John Doe finds himself trying to hide his hands when he is outside of his home.

John Doe should continue to undergo psychological intervention to assist him in accepting the permanent, disfiguring changes to his arms, abdomen, neck, torso, hands, feet, and legs. He will benefit greatly from professional psychological/social interventions to better cope with the unwanted stares and questions he gets from acquaintances and strangers. The following recommended procedures will help decrease his itching, increase his range of motion, soften his scars, and reduce his pain; however, John's body will never look like it did before the fire.

"Sample Surgical Interventions"
Burn Reconstructive Surgery Consult
The Surgeon MD, —Burn Surgeon
Burn Center Burn Center

XX/15/2016

Dr. Surgeon reports that John Doe will likely require multiple surgical interventions to improve his range of motion and function.

He will require inpatient and outpatient occupational and physical therapy, home healthcare, laser surgery, medication, psychological intervention, pressure garments, splinting, and personal assistance. Much of the scarring on his body cannot be improved upon, and much of the scarring from his skin grafts will likely be permanent.

Dr. Surgeon has recommended the following reconstructive surgeries. The likely costs of these procedures can be found in the life care plan tables. Dr. Surgeon has also recommended allied healthcare related to the surgeries in the form of home healthcare for dressing changes and occupational therapy postoperatively. He has also recommended the number of hospital days associated with future operations. John Doe will need to be fitted for pressure garments and splinting after many surgeries.

Face and Neck

John Doe burned his face, scalp, and neck and has sensitivity in the residual scarring especially on his neck and scalp. Laser surgery is recommended for these areas.

Upper Extremities and Shoulders

John Doe has significant scarring to both of his upper arms. His shoulders have unburned skin, and this skin will be harvested during future surgeries to "fix" other severely scarred areas of his body. Dr. Surgeon will place tissue expanders under the unburned skin to correct the upper arm scarring. This will be done to improve function, diminish pain, and improve cosmesis. This intensive reconstruction will require a one-night inpatient surgical placement of a tissue expander in the shoulder area under general anesthesia. This type of surgery is challenging, as this is an uncomfortable location for expander placement, but necessary for effective correction. After the initial surgery, John Doe will return to the burn clinic, every week for between 7–10 weeks to have the expanders filled with saline solution. When the expanded skin is ready, John Doe will be taken to the operating room, again, as an inpatient. The expanders will be removed, and the new tissue and flap will be advanced to the area where the old scarring was excised. He will be hospitalized for 4–7 days after the second procedure and will need daily home healthcare for dressing changes for a month, with occupational therapy twice a week for 4–6 months. Each arm will be done separately. The entire process will take approximately four months.

Forearms, Elbows, and Wrists

He has a great deal of disfiguring and limiting scarring with hyperpigmentation on both his forearms and wrists. Both forearms are heavily scarred, and the scars are impeding full use and range of motion of his arms and hands. The scars are also painful and itchy. His surgeon will excise the scars, then apply skin grafts. Each arm will be operated on separately. This will be an inpatient procedure with a 4–7-day hospital stay. He will need a month of outpatient wound care and six months of occupational therapy post-surgery.

Web Space Releases

John Doe will need web space release surgery between all of the fingers on both hands. This will necessitate two separate surgeries (each hand will be done separately), under general anesthesia, for web spaces one, two, three, and four. These surgeries will be performed as an inpatient with a five-night hospital stay and two weeks of daily dressing changes at home, two visits to the plastic surgeon's office, and 6–12 months of outpatient occupational therapy. Dr. Surgeon said it is likely that the web space releases will need to be repeated every 10–12 years through life expectancy. He will need a hand splint and pressure glove after each surgery.

Legs—Thighs and Calves

The lower extremities present with extensive skin grafts, hyperpigmentation, and hypertrophic scarring. John Doe will likely need tangential excision of the hypertrophic scarring on the upper thighs with re-grafting. Both the front and back sides of each leg are heavily scarred. He will go to the operating room to have the scarring excised and have a skin substitute placed over the wound. He will then return to the operating room, three weeks later, for skin grafting to this area. Each thigh will be operated on separately. This lengthy process will include inpatient hospitalization, postoperative home healthcare, postoperative therapy, pressure garments, and splints.

Ankles and Feet

John Doe will also need ankle and foot contracture releases and skin grafting bilaterally to improve function and range of motion. Currently, John Doe is unable to bend his ankles far enough to put his feet in a pair of work boots. He has very little unscarred skin on his body; therefore Dr. Surgeon said that a dermal substitute will be used for this procedure. This process will require a 21-day hospital stay with use of a wound vac between surgeries. A second operation will then be performed to cover the skin substitute with an autograft (skin graft) and the two surgeries will require 21 days in the hospital with four weeks of outpatient wound care. Physical therapy would be required twice a week for up to 12 months. This process will likely need to be repeated on each ankle and foot every 10–15 years through his life expectancy to allow for range of motion and function.

The costs associated with all surgeries are listed in the life care plan tables. It should be noted that any surgical complications or infections could result in significantly higher medical costs for John Doe over his lifetime.

Laser Surgery

John Doe has a great deal of residual scarring from both his burn and donor sites. Dr. Surgeon has recommended laser therapy/surgery for John. Laser is a painful procedure; therefore, it is recommended that the laser procedures be performed under general anesthesia in an outpatient operating room. These surgeries will be performed on an outpatient basis. Recommendations are for John Doe to undergo six to eight sessions of laser therapy, after the recommended hand surgeries. Laser scar surgery can reduce and improve the appearance of scarring with a combination of steroid injections and laser therapy. The use of laser surgery for treating burn scars has increased in recent years particularly for scarring caused by third-degree burns. Research has also shown that the quality of life of patients has been found to improve significantly after laser surgery. This type of procedure is often preferred due to its ability to release contracted scars and provide unique chemical pathways that promote proper healing (Issler-Fisher et al., 2017; Waibel & Beer, 2009).

Skin Cancer

All burned areas and donor sites are at increased risk of skin cancer and must be protected by sunscreen daily.

Pressure Garments

John Doe will need to be fitted for pressure garments and gloves following his reconstruction surgeries. Although the garments can be uncomfortable, especially during the summer, they help flatten scars, increase blood supply, and decrease itching. They are typically worn for 10–12 months after each procedure. He should wear TED hose, through life expectancy, due to his history of deep vein thrombosis and the daily swelling of his lower legs.

Massage Therapy

John Doe will benefit from ongoing scar massage therapy, and he is recommended to have massage therapy 44–48 times per year throughout his life expectancy. Research has revealed that massage therapy can be an effective adjunct for improving function, reducing pain, diminishing itching, improving skin integrity, and helping burn patients to improve and maintain range of motion.

Ongoing Medical Needs
Burn Recovery Consult
Dr. Surgeon—1/27/2022
Burn/Plastic Surgeon
Burn Center Burn Center USA

The following are the ongoing medical evaluations and allied health services that John Doe will likely need according to Dr. Surgeon, his treating physician.

Burn Surgeon/Plastic Surgeon: John Doe should have an annual evaluation with a burn surgeon to monitor his burns, scars, and any potential complications which may arise through life expectancy.

Dermatologist: An annual visit should occur due to his heightened risk for skin cancer, through life expectancy.

Occupational Therapist: He should have an evaluation, once a year, through life expectancy. It is recommended 12 visits every two years to assist John Doe with management of activities of daily living (ADLs), function, and range of motion of hands, wrists, and arms.

Audiologist: He should have his hearing evaluated post-explosion.

Dietary Evaluation: John Doe has gained a significant amount of weight since sustaining his burn injuries. His doctor said that he must lose weight before surgery and will need to maintain his weight during the years of his major reconstruction. A weight loss program is recommended.

Physiatrist: He should have an evaluation and two to three visits annually with a physiatrist for pain management and functional issues through life expectancy.

Physical Therapist: He should have an evaluation once a year through life expectancy, as well as 12 visits per year from age 55 through life expectancy. He will need therapy to improve range of motion, balance, and function. He will be having ongoing physical therapy after recommended surgeries.

Pain Specialist: John Doe continues to see a pain specialist and should be evaluated annually for pain issues. He should have access to three additional visits, per year, for pain management through life expectancy.

Sleep Study: John Doe continues to have major problems with sleeping. Dr. X recommended a sleep study, but it has not been approved as of yet. Due to the long-term sleep issues of many burn patients, it is recommended that John Doe have access to a sleep study every five years through life expectancy.

Potential Complications: The aging process is accelerated in those with disabilities and causes them to age more quickly than the normal population. Skin breakdown, osteoporosis, arthritis, restricted range of motion, anxiety and depression, and the potential for vascular and immune problems can negatively affect burn patients as they age. John Doe is already experiencing compromised usage of his arms, wrists, and has ongoing problems with his legs and knees. John Doe will be forever saddled with many of these problems and will likely need much assistance with daily living activities in his advanced age. In summary, the life care planner should consider potential complications of arthritis, skin breakdown, major depression, systemic infection, surgical complications, osteoporosis, ongoing sexual dysfunction, chronic pain, range of motion, function issues, and dementia.

References

Ajoudani, F., Jasemi, M., & Lotfi, M. (2018). Social participation, social support, and body image in the first year of rehabilitation in burn survivors: A longitudinal, three-wave cross-lagged panel analysis using structural equation modeling. *Burns*, *44*(5), 1141–1150. www.sciencedirect.com/science/article/abs/pii/S0305417918302031?via%3Dihub

American Burn Association. (2018). *Burn injury fact sheet*. https://ameriburn.org/wp-content/uploads/2017/12/nbaw-factsheet_121417-1.pdf

Anthonissen, M., Daly, D., Janssens, T., & Van den Kerckhove, E. (2016). The effects of conservative treatments on burn scars: A systematic review. *Burns, 42*(3), 508–518. https://doi.org/10.1016/j.burns.2015.12.006

Ault, P., Plaza, A., & Paratz, J. (2018). Scar massage for hypertrophic burns scarring—A systematic review. *Burns, 44*(1), 24–38. https://doi.org/10.1016/j.burns.2017.05.006

Barret, J. P. (2004). Burns reconstruction. *BMJ, 329*, 274-276. https://doi.org/10.1136/bmj.329.7460.274

Bayuo, J., Wong, F. K., & Agyei, F. B. (2020). "On the recovery journey:" An integrative review of the needs of burn patients from immediate pre-discharge to post-discharge period using the Omaha System. *Journal of Nursing Scholarship, 52*(4), 360–368. https://doi.org/10.1111/jnu.12563

Beaver, K. M., Boccio, C., Smith, S., & Ferguson, C. J. (2019). Physical attractiveness and criminal justice processing: Results from a longitudinal sample of youth and young adults. *Psychiatry, Psychology and Law, 26*(4), 669–681. https://doi.org/10.1080/13218719.2019.1618750

Bich, C.-S., Kostev, K., Baus, A., & Jacob, L. (2021). Burn injury and incidence of psychiatric disorders: A retrospective cohort study of 18,198 patients from Germany. *Burns, 47*(5), 1110–1117. https://doi.org/10.1016/j.burns.2020.06.015

Boeve, S. A., Aaron, L. A., Martin-Herz, S. P., Peterson, A., Cain, V., Heimbach, D. M., & Patterson, D. R. (2002). Sleep disturbance after burn injury. *The Journal of Burn Care & Rehabilitation, 23*(1), 32–38. https://doi.org/10.1097/00004630-200201000-00007

Brewin, M. P., & Homer, S. J. (2018). The lived experience and quality of life with burn scarring—the results from a large-scale online survey. *Burns, 44*(7), 1801–1810. https://doi.org/10.1016/j.burns.2018.04.007

Brown, M., Helm, P., & Weed, R. (2004). Life care planning for the burn patient. In R. Weed (Ed.), *Life care planning and case management handbook* (2nd ed., pp. 351–380). CRC Press.

Brubaker Rimmer, R., Bay, R. C., Kalil, E. T., Chacon, D. W., & Foster, K. N. (2022). Anxiety disorder symptomology found to be prevalent in burn-injured youth. *Journal of Burn Care & Research, 43*(Supplement_1), S82–S83. https://doi.org/10.1093/jbcr/irac012.128

Brusselaers, N., Hoste, E. A. J., Monstrey, S., Colpaert, K. E., De Waele, J. J., Vandewoude, K. H., & Blot, S. I. (2005). Outcome and changes over time in survival following severe burns from 1985 to 2004. *Intensive Care Medicine, 31*(12), 1648–1654. doi: 10.1007/s00134-005-2819-6

Brych, S., Engrav, L., Rivara, F., Ptacek, J., Lezotte, D., & Esselman, P. (2001). Time off work and return to work after burns: Systematic review of the literature and a large two-center series. *Journal of Burn Care & Rehabilitation, 22*(6), 401–405.

Chaudhary, F. A., & Ahmad, B. (2021). The relationship between psychosocial distress and oral health status in patients with facial burns and mediation by oral health behaviour. *BMC Oral Health, 21*(1). https://doi.org/10.1186/s12903-021-01532-0

Chaudhary, F. A., Ahmad, B., Bashir, U., & Sinor, M. Z. (2020). Oral health-related quality of life and related factors among facial burn injury patients in Pakistan. https://doi.org/10.21203/rs.3.rs-26441/v1

Chin, T. L., Carrougher, G. J., Amtmann, D., McMullen, K., Herndon, D. N., Holavanahalli, R., Meyer, W., Ryan, C. M., Wong, J. N., & Gibran, N. S. (2018). Trends 10 years after burn injury: A burn model system national database study. *Burns, 44*(8), 1882–1886. https://doi.org/10.1016/j.burns.2018.09.033

Cho, Y. S., Joen, J. H., Hong, A., Yang, H. T., Yim, H., Cho, Y. S., Kim, D-H., Hur, J., Kim, J. H., Chun, W., Lee, B. C., & Seo, C. H. (2014). The effects of burn rehabilitation massage therapy on hypertrophic scar after burn: A randomized controlled trial. *Burns, 40*(8), 1513–1520.

Cleary, M., Kornhaber, R., Thapa, D. K., West, S., & Visentin, D. (2020). A quantitative systematic review assessing the impact of burn injuries on body image. *Body Image, 33*, 47–65. https://doi.org/10.1016/j.bodyim.2020.02.008

Cohen, S. R., Goodacre, A., Lim, S., Johnston, J., Henssler, C., Jeffers, B., Saad, A., & Leong, T. (2016). Clinical outcomes and complications associated with fractional lasers: A review of 730 patients. *Aesthetic Plastic Surgery, 41*(1), 171–178. https://doi.org/10.1007/s00266-016-0767-x

Connell, K. M., Coates, R., & Wood, F. M. (2013). Sexuality following burn injuries. *Journal of Burn Care & Research, 34*(5). https://doi.org/10.1097/bcr.0b013e31827819bf

Cromes, G. H., & Helm, P. A. (1993). Burn Injuries. In M. Eisenberg, R. Glueckauf, & H. Zaretsky (Eds.), *Medical aspects of disability* (pp. 121–136). Springer Publishing.

Deflorin, C., Hohenauer, E., Stoop, R., van Daele, U., Clijsen, R., & Taeymans, J. (2020). Physical management of scar tissue: A systematic review and meta-analysis. *The Journal of Alternative and Complementary Medicine*, *26*(10), 854–865. https://doi.org/10.1089/acm.2020.0109

DeFrances, C. J., Hall, M. J., Podgornik, M. N. (2003). *National Hospital Discharge Survey. Advance data from vital and health statistics; no 359*. National Center for Health Statistics.

Demling, R. H. (1995). The advantage of the burn team approach. *Journal of Burn Care & Rehabilitation*, *16*(6), 569–572.

Demling, R. H., & LaLonde, C. (1989). *Burn trauma, 4*. Thieme Publishing Group, 55–56.

Dyster-Aas, J., Kildal, M., & Willebrand, M. (2007). Return to work and health-related quality of life after burn injury. *Journal of Rehabilitation Medicine*, *39*(1), 49–55. https://doi.org/10.2340/16501977-0005

Ebid, A. A., Ibrahim, A. R., Omar, M. T., & El Baky, A. M. (2017). Long-term effects of pulsed high-intensity laser therapy in the treatment of post-burn pruritus: A double-blind, placebo-controlled, randomized study. *Lasers in Medical Science*, *32*(3), 693–701. https://doi.org/10.1007/s10103-017-2172-3

Edelman, L. S., McNaught, T., Chan, G. M., & Morris, S. E. (2003). Sustained bone mineral density changes after burn injury. *The Journal of Surgical Research*, *114*(2), 172–178. https://doi.org/10.1016/s0022-4804(03)00275-0

Ehde, D. M., Patterson, D. R., Weichman, S. A., & Wilson, L. G. (1999). Post-traumatic stress symptoms and distress following acute burn injury. *Burns*, *25*, 587–592.

Fauerbach, J. A., Heinberg, L. J., Lawrence, J. W., Munster, A. M., Palombo, D. A., Richter, D., Spence, R. J., Stevens, S. S., Ware, L., & Muehlberger, T. (2000). Effect of early body image dissatisfaction on subsequent psychological and physical adjustment after disfiguring injury. *Psychosomatic Medicine*, *62*(4), 576–582. https://doi.org/10.1097/00006842-200007000-00017

Fergason, J. R., & Blanck, R. (2011). Prosthetic management of the burn amputation. *Physical Medicine and Rehabilitation Clinics of North America*, *22*(2), 277–299. https://doi.org/10.1016/j.pmr.2011.03.00

Field, T., Peck, M., Krugman, S., Tuchel, T., Schanberg, S., Kuhn, C., & Burman, I. (1998). Burn injuries benefit from massage therapy. *Journal of Burn Care and Rehabilitation*, *19*, 242–244.

Fisher, S. V., & Helm, P. (1984). *Comprehensive rehabilitation of burns*. Williams & Wilkins.

Gallal, A. R. S., & Yousef, S. M. (2002) Our experience in the nutritional support of burn patients. *Annals of Burns and Fire Disasters*, *20*(3), 239–249

Ganio, M. S., Schlader, Z. J., Pearson, J., Lucas, R. A., Gagnon, D., Rivas, E., Kowalske, K. J., & Crandall, C. G. (2015, October 1). Nongrafted skin area best predicts exercise core temperature responses in burned humans. *Medicine and Science in Sports and Exercise*, *47*(10), 2224-2232.

Gojowy, D., Kauke, M., Ohmann, T., Homann, H.-H., & Mannil, L. (2019). Early and late-recorded predictors of health-related quality of life of burn patients on long-term follow-up. *Burns*, *45*(6), 1300–1310. https://doi.org/10.1016/j.burns.2019.03.016

Greenhalgh, D. G. (2020). Management of facial burns. *Burns & Trauma*, *8*. https://doi.org/10.1093/burnst/tkaa023

Hartford, C. E., & Kealy, G. P. (2007). Care of outpatient burns. In Herndon, D. N. (Ed.), *Total burn care* (3rd ed., pp. 67-80). Saunders Elsevier.

Herndon, D., & Blakeney, P. (2007). Teamwork for total burn care: Achievements, directions and hopes. In D. Herndon (Ed.), *Total burn care* (3rd ed., pp. 11–15). Saunders Elsevier.

Issler-Fisher, A. C., Fisher, O. M., Smialkowski, A. O., Li, F., van Schalkwyk, C. P., Haertsch, P., & Maitz, P. K. M. (2017). Ablative fractional CO^2 laser for burn scar reconstruction: An extensive subjective and objective short-term outcome analysis of a prospective treatment cohort. *Burns*, *43*(3), 573–582. https://doi.org/10.1016/j.burns.2016.09.014

Jagdeo, J., & Shumaker, P. R. (2017). Traumatic scarring. *JAMA Dermatology*, *153*(3), 364. https://doi.org/10.1001/jamadermatol.2016.5232

Jeschke, M. G., van Baar, M. E., Choudhry, M. A., Chung, K. K., Gibran, N. S., & Logsetty, S. (2020). Burn injury. *Nature Reviews Disease Primers*, *6*(1). https://doi.org/10.1038/s41572-020-0145-5

Kornhaber, R., Visentin, D., Kaji Thapa, D., West, S., Haik, J., & Cleary, M. (2020). Burn camps for burns survivors—realising the benefits for early adjustment: A systematic review. *Burns*, *46*(1), 33–43. https://doi.org/10.1016/j.burns.2018.12.005

Kowalske, K., Holavanahalli, R., Carrougher, G., Suman, O., & Dolezal, C. (2015). *Exercise after burn injury*. https://msktc.org/burn/factsheets/Exercise-After-Burn-Injury

Kurian, S., Padickaparambil, S., Thomas, J., Sreekumar, N. C., & James, A. R. (2019). Psychological evaluation of adult burn survivors: A pilot study. *International Surgery Journal, 6*(12), 4428-4434. https://doi.org/10.18203/2349-2902.isj20195407

Levi, B., Kraft, C. T., Shapiro, G. D., Trinh, N.-H. T., Dore, E. C., Jeng, J., Lee, A. F., Acton, A., Marino, M., Jette, A., Armstrong, E. A., Schneider, J. C., Kazis, L. E., & Ryan, C. M. (2018). The associations of gender with social participation of burn survivors: A life impact burn recovery evaluation profile study. *Journal of Burn Care & Research, 39*(6), 915–922. https://doi.org/10.1093/jbcr/iry007

Lin, D. Z., Kao, Y. C., Chen, C., Wang, H. J., & Chiu, W. K. (2020). Negative pressure wound therapy for burn patients: A meta-analysis and systematic review. *International Wound Journal, 18*(1), 112–123. https://doi.org/10.1111/iwj.13500

Linares, H. A., Kischer, C. W., Dobrkovsky, M., & Larson, D. L. (1972). The histiotypic organization of the hypertrophic scar in humans. *Journal of Investigative Dermatology, 59*, 323–331.

Macleod, R., Shepherd, L., & Thompson, A. R. (2016). Posttraumatic stress symptomatology and appearance distress following burn injury: An interpretative phenomenological analysis. *Health Psychology, 35*(11), 1197–1204. https://doi.org/10.1037/hea0000391

Masoodi, Z., Ahmad, I., Khurram, F., & Haq, A. (2013). Changes in sleep architecture after burn injury: 'Waking up' to this unaddressed aspect of postburn rehabilitation in the developing world. *Plastic Surgery, 21*(4). https://doi.org/10.4172/plastic-surgery.1000831

Ohrtman, E. A., Shapiro, G. D., Simko, L. C., Dore, E., Slavin, M. D., Saret, C., Amaya, F., Lomelin-Gascon, J., Ni, P., Acton, A., Marino, M., Kazis, L. E., Ryan, C. M., & Schneider, J. C. (2018). Social interactions and social activities after burn injury: A life impact burn recovery evaluation (libre) study. *Journal of Burn Care & Research, 39*(6), 1022–1028. https://doi.org/10.1093/jbcr/iry038

Pavoni, V., Gianesello, L., Paparella, L., Buoninsegni, L. T., & Barboni, E. (2010). Outcome predictors and quality of life of severe burn patients admitted to intensive care unit. *Scandinavian Journal of Trauma, Resuscitation and Emergency Medicine, 18*(1), 18-24. https://doi.org/10.1186/1757-7241-18-24

Pell, C. (2019). What to do when people stare: A workshop to teach individuals with disfiguring conditions to contend with staring and improve control of social interactions. *Journal of Burn Care & Research, 40*(6), 743–751. https://doi.org/10.1093/jbcr/irz117

Perry, S., Difede, J., Musngi, G., Frances, A., & Jacobsberg, L. (1992). Predictors of post-traumatic stress disorder after burn injury. *American Journal of Psychiatry, 149*, 931–935.

Pleguezuelos-Beltrán, P., Gálvez-Martín, P., Nieto-García, D., Marchal, J. A., & López-Ruiz, E. (2022). Advances in spray products for skin regeneration. *Bioactive Materials, 16*, 187–203. https://doi.org/10.1016/j.bioactmat.2022.02.023

Porter, C., Hardee, J. P., Herndon, D. N., & Suman, O. E. (2015). The role of exercise in the rehabilitation of patients with severe burns. *Exercise and Sport Sciences Reviews*. https://pubmed.ncbi.nlm.nih.gov/25390300/

Pruitt, B., Wolf, S. E., & Mason, A. (2007). Epidemiological, demographic and outcome characteristics of burn injury. In D. Herndon (Ed.), *Total burn care* (3rd ed., pp. 14–32). Saunders Elsevier.

Psychiatry.org (2019). *What is posttraumatic stress disorder (PTSD)?* www.psychiatry.org/patients-families/ptsd/what-is-ptsd

Quinn, D. K. (2014). "Burn catatonia." *Journal of Burn Care & Research, 35*(2), E135-E142. https://doi.org/10.1097/bcr.0b013e31828c73c7

Rainey, E. E., Petrey, L. B., Reynolds, M., Agtarap, S., & Warren, A. M. (2014). Psychological factors predicting outcome after traumatic injury: The role of resilience. *The American Journal of Surgery, 208*(4), 517–523. https://doi.org/10.1016/j.amjsurg.2014.05.016

Riaz, H. M., & Mehmood Bhatti, Z. (2020). Quality of life in adults with lower limb burn injury. *Journal of Burn Care & Research, 41*(6), 1212–1215. https://doi.org/10.1093/jbcr/iraa069

Ryan, C. M., Lee, A., Stoddard, F. J., Li, N. C., Schneider, J. C., Shapiro, G. D., Griggs, C. L., Wang, C., Palmieri, T., Meyer, W. J., Pidcock, F. S., Reilly, D., Sheridan, R. L., Kazis, L. E., & Tompkins, R. G. (2017). The effect of facial burns on long-term outcomes in young adults: A 5-year study. *Journal of Burn Care & Research, 39*(4), 497–506. https://doi.org/10.1093/jbcr/irx006

Saffle, J., Davis, B., & Williams, P. (1995). Recent outcomes in the treatment of burn injury: Burn Association Patient Registry. *Journal of Burn Care Rehabilitation, 16*, 219–230.

Schneider, J. C., Shie, V. L., Espinoza, L. F., Shapiro, G. D., Lee, A., Acton, A., Marino, M., Jette, A., Kazis, L. E., & Ryan, C. M. (2020). Impact of work-related burn injury on social reintegration outcomes: A life impact burn recovery evaluation (libre) study. *Archives of Physical Medicine and Rehabilitation*, *101*(1). https://doi.org/10.1016/j.apmr.2017.10.022

Schulz, J. T., Shapiro, G. D., Acton, A., Fidler, P., Marino, M. E., Jette, A., Schneider, J. E., Kazis, L. E., & Ryan, C. M. (2019). The relationship of level of education to social reintegration after burn injury: A libre study. *Journal of Burn Care & Research*, *40*(5), 696–702. https://doi.org/10.1093/jbcr/irz074

Serghiou, M. A., Ott, S., Farmer, S., Morgan, D., Gibson, P., & Suman, O. E. (2007). Comprehensive rehabilitation of the burn patient. In D. Herndon (Ed.), *Total burn care* (3rd ed., pp. 620-651). Saunders Elsevier.

Sheckter, C. C., Brych, S., Carrougher, G. J., Wolf, S. E., Schneider, J. C., Gibran, N., & Stewart, B. T. (2021). Exploring "return to productivity" among people living with burn injury: A burn model system national database report. *Journal of Burn Care & Research*, *42*(6), 1081–1086. https://doi.org/10.1093/jbcr/irab139

Shepherd, L., Reynolds, D. P., Turner, A., O'Boyle, C. P., & Thompson, A. R. (2019). The role of psychological flexibility in appearance anxiety in people who have experienced a visible burn injury. *Burns*, *45*(4), 942–949. https://doi.org/10.1016/j.burns.2018.11.015

Sheridan, R. L., Hinson, M. I., Liang, M. H., Nackel, A. F., Schoenfeld, D. A., Ryan, C. M., Mulligan, J. L., & Tompkins, R. G. (2000). Long-term outcome of children surviving massive burns. *JAMA*, *283*(1), 69–73.

Sinha, I., Nabi, M., Simko, L. C., Wolfe, A. W., Wiechman, S., Giatsidis, G., Bharadia, D., McMullen, K., Gibran, N. S., Kowalske, K., Meyer, W. J., Kazis, L. E., Ryan, C. M., & Schneider, J. C. (2019). Head and neck burns are associated with long-term patient-reported dissatisfaction with appearance: A burn model system national database study. *Burns*, *45*(2), 293–302. https://doi.org/10.1016/j.burns.2018.12.017

Smith, J. S., Smith, K. R., Rainey, S. L., & DelGiorno, J. (2006). The psychology of burn care. *Journal of Trauma Nursing*, *13*(3), 105–106.

Spronk, I., Legemate, C., Oen, I., van Loey, N., Polinder, S., & van Baar, M. (2018). Health related quality of life in adults after burn injuries: A systematic review. *PLOS ONE*, *13*(5), e0197507. https://doi.org/10.1371/journal.pone.0197507

Spronk, I., Polinder, S., van Loey, N. E. E., van der Vlies, C. H., Pijpe, A., Haagsma, J. A., & van Baar, M. E. (2019). Health related quality of life 5–7 years after minor and severe burn injuries: A multicentre cross-sectional study. *Burns*, *45*(6), 1291–1299. https://doi.org/10.1016/j.burns.2019.03.017

St-Pierre, D. M., Choiniere, M., Forget, R., & Garrel, D. R. (1998). Muscle strength in individuals with healed burns. *Archives of Physical Medicine & Rehabilitation*, *79*(2), 155–161.

Stergiou-Kita, M., Mansfield, E., Bayley, M., Cassidy, J. D., Colantonio, A., Gomez, M., Jeschke, M., Kirsh, B., Kristman, V., Moody, J., & Vartanian, O. (2014). Returning to work after electrical injuries: workers' perspectives and advice to others. *Journal of Burn Care & Research: Official Publication of the American Burn Association*, *35*(6), 498–507.

Stock, N. M., Whale, K., Jenkinson, E., Rumsey, N., & Fox, F. (2013). Young people's perceptions of visible difference. *Diversity and Equality in Health and Care*, *13*(10), 1–12.

Stuart, A. (2022). *How depression affects your body*. WebMD. www.webmd.com/depression/how-depression-affects-your-body

Waibel, J. & Beer, K. (2009). Ablative fractional laser resurfacing for the treatment of a third-degree burn. *Journal of Drugs in Dermatology, 8*(3):294–297.

Weed, R. O., & Berens, D. E. (2005). Basics of burn injury: Implications for case management and life care planning. *Lippincotts Case Management*, *10*(10), 22–29.

Weichman, S., Ptacek, J. T., Patterson, D. R., Gibran, S. N., Engrav, L. E., & Heimbach, D. M. (2001). Rates, trends, and severity of depression after burn injuries. *Burn Care Rehabilitation*, *22*, 417–424.

Chapter 22

Life Care Planning for the Patient with a Mental Health Disorder

Alexander Amit Missner and Shani Cohen Missner

The impact of mental illness on the cost of healthcare and productivity is considerably high. Mental Health America (MHA) released data showing that the number of people reporting signs of anxiety and depression since the start of the COVID-19 pandemic hit an all-time high in September 2021 (MHA, 2021). The new data accompany the release of the annual State of Mental Health in America report, showing that nationwide, 19% (47.1 million) of people in the U.S. are living with a mental health condition, a 1.5 million increase over last year's report. Nationwide, almost one in five people in the U.S. are living with a mental health condition. About 10% of youth in the U.S have severe depression and about 8% of people in the U.S. struggle with a substance use disorder (MHA, 2021). Furthermore, an estimated 4.2% of the American population has a serious mental illness resulting in significant impairments in daily functioning (Center for Behavioral Health Statistics and Quality, 2015). Psychiatric disorders are one of the leading causes of disability in the United States (U.S. Burden of Disease Collaborators, 2013).

Psychiatric illness programs have not traditionally used life care planners, while the legal system and other third parties increasingly do. Life care planning for mental illness requires reasonably predictable care and is lifelong (Hilligoss, 2003; Missner & Cohen, 2019). The prediction of expected care can be summarized in a life care plan (Weed & Berens, 2018; Weed & Field, 2001). To provide an accurate life care plan, it is important to consider the complexity of mental illness, including symptoms, treatment, and impact on functioning. Furthermore, mental illness may be the only medical concern, or may be a comorbid illness with chronic disease or trauma.

This chapter provides an overview of major depressive disorder, bipolar disorder, generalized anxiety disorder, obsessive-compulsive disorder, and schizophrenia. The role of mental health professionals as consultants to the life care plan is explored for the purpose of contributing to a strong medical and scientific foundation. At the end of the chapter, implications for life care planning are considered, including a checklist to help create the life care plan and an example of a life care plan for schizophrenia.

Life Care Planning for Comorbid Mental Health Concerns

Mental health is not a realm that is exclusive of other concerns, but rather often is comorbid with chronic illness and catastrophic injuries. Life care plans are created for a population that has suffered a range of catastrophic injuries or has chronic healthcare needs and therefore, comorbid psychiatric illnesses become part of the plan. The *Diagnostic and Statistical Manual of Mental Health Disorders* (5th ed., Text Revision) (APA, 2022) from the American Psychiatric Association (APA) contains the criteria that are used by mental health professionals to define mental disorders. Common comorbid psychiatric illnesses consist of anxiety disorders, mood disorders, trauma related disorders, neurocognitive disorders, and substance use disorders (Missner & Cohen, 2019). For example, the prevalence of major depression in the spinal cord injury cohort is estimated to be approximately 20%, more than double the prevalence in the primary care setting (Hoffman et al., 2011). The prevalence of clinically significant depressive symptomatology for young and middle-aged adults with vision loss is 40–45%, whereas 20% exhibit moderate to severe anxiety symptoms (Horowitz & Reinhardt, 2006). Depression is a common neuropsychiatric consequence of stroke, with up to 55% of stroke victims experiencing depression (Hama et al., 2011). The prevalence rates for depression in older patients with hip fractures was reported to be 9–47% (Holmes & House, 2000). Furthermore, studies have shown the incidence of new-onset psychiatric illness after a motor vehicle accident to be as high as 53%, wherein most illnesses are depression and post-traumatic stress disorder (PTSD), which are often comorbid (Matsuoka et al., 2008). Up to 80% of people who sustain a traumatic brain injury suffer from a psychiatric disturbance at some point in their recovery period (Rao, 2002). Of people experiencing a devastating disaster, 50–80% develop PTSD (Morina et al., 2018). Traumatic stress reactions are common following an acquired spinal cord injury (SCI), with 40% of adults reporting an acute symptom pattern of avoidance, heightened anxiety, and intrusive trauma memories (Pollock et al., 2017). In total, 4% experience these symptoms beyond one month after SCI, warranting a diagnosis of PTSD. Without treatment, the lifetime prevalence of PTSD for those with SCI remains high: up to 29% continue to report symptoms 30 years after injury. These findings illustrate that mental health may only be one aspect of a comprehensive life care plan for chronic illness or traumatic injury.

The comorbidity of psychiatric disorders with chronic medical illness and trauma causes disability and reduced quality of life and interferes with rehabilitation outcomes (Akechi, 2012; Halcomb et al., 2005; Steigelmar et al., 2001). Suicide is a significant concern in a population with serious emotional and physical illness. For example, it has been reported that patients with chronic pain have a 5–14% lifetime prevalence of suicide attempts and a suicide completion rate that is two to three times greater than that of the general population (Newton-John, 2014). The life care plan is a dynamic and multidimensional document that strives to encompass all relevant domains of a person's life, including mental healthcare.

Major Depressive Disorder (MDD)

The recent data from the 2020 National Survey on Drug Use and Health captures the prevalence of depression in the United States (National Institute of Mental Health [NIMH], 2022a).

These data show that an estimated 21.0 million adults in the United States had at least one major depressive episode representing 8.4% of all U.S. adults. The prevalence of adults with a major depressive episode was highest among individuals aged 18–25 (17.0%). In 2020, an estimated 14.8 million U.S. adults aged 18 or older had at least one major depressive episode with severe impairment in the past year, representing 6.0% of all U.S. adults. An estimated 4.1 million adolescents aged 12–17 in the United States had at least one major depressive episode, representing 17% of this age group. An estimated 2.9 million adolescents aged 12–17 in the United States had at least one major depressive episode with severe impairment in the past year, representing 12% of this age group. Major depressive disorder is a leading cause of disability worldwide (Ferrari et al., 2013).

Epidemiology and Course of Illness

A major depressive episode often occurs after an individual experiences a severe psychosocial stressor such as divorce or the death of a loved one. Major depressive disorder can occur at any age, but the average age of onset is in the twenties. The disorder may develop suddenly or take days or weeks to become clinically diagnostic. The duration of MDD is varied, and time to recovery can vary from a few months to a year or more (APA, 2022). Some individuals will later develop bipolar disorder after experiencing a hypomanic or manic episode. It is estimated that 50–85% of individuals with MDD will have another episode (Mueller et al., 1999). Risk factors for relapse include age of onset, the severity of the first episode, the number of episodes, family history of psychopathology, comorbid substance abuse, anxiety disorders, negative cognition styles, and stressful life events (Burcusa & Iacono, 2007). It is important to note that some people will have residual symptoms after an episode of depression resolves. The most common residual symptoms are anxiety, core mood symptoms, insomnia, and somatic symptoms (Romera et al., 2013).

Symptoms

Major depressive disorder is characterized by one or more major depressive episodes, with an absence of any hypomanic, manic, or mixed episodes. The fundamental feature of a major depressive episode is a persistent depressed mood that lasts at least two weeks or loss of interest or pleasure in almost all activities. Other symptoms of a major depressive episode include changes in sleep, appetite, weight, or psychomotor activity; lack of energy; feeling guilty or worthless; decreased ability to focus, think, or make decisions; and thoughts of death or suicidal thoughts, plans, or attempts (APA, 2022). At least five of these symptoms must be present and last for at least two weeks to meet the criteria of a major depressive episode. MDD can manifest a wide range of impairments, from mild to severe. In severe episodes, individuals with MDD can have psychotic symptoms, characterized by the presence of delusions (false, irrational beliefs) and hallucinations. Another severe manifestation of MDD is the presence of catatonic features, where there is a severe change in motor movements and behavior (e.g., an individual may remain motionless, engage in bizarre postures, or become mute) (APA, 2022).

Practice Guidelines for the Treatment of Depression

The APA and Department of Veterans Affairs/Department of Defense (VA/DoD) have established treatment guidelines for MDD (APA, 2010; VA/DoD, 2016). Treatment is conceptualized into three phases: (1) the acute phase, during which the goal is to induce remission and a return to baseline functioning; (2) the continuation phase, during which the goal is to preserve remission;

and (3) the maintenance phase, during which the goal is to prevent future episodes. Both pharmacotherapy and psychotherapeutic interventions are used to meet these goals. Treatment recommendations will vary based on the severity and characteristics of the depressive episodes and response to treatment.

Pharmacotherapy

Antidepressants

Antidepressant medications are utilized during all phases of treatment. Commonly prescribed first-line antidepressants include selective serotonin reuptake inhibitors (SSRIs), serotonin norepinephrine reuptake inhibitors (SNRIs), mirtazapine, and bupropion. Older agents such as tricyclics and monoamine oxidase inhibitors (MAOIs) may also be prescribed, most often when individuals fail first-line treatments. SSRIs include fluoxetine, fluvoxamine, sertraline, paroxetine, escitalopram, and citalopram. Common side effects of SSRIs include gastrointestinal distress, insomnia/agitation, sexual side effects, headaches, extrapyramidal side effects, effects on weight, falls, serotonin syndrome, and discontinuation syndrome (APA, 2010; VA/DoD 2016). SNRIs include venlafaxine, duloxetine, desvenlafaxine, and levomilnacipran. Common side effects of SNRIs include nausea, decreased appetite, headache, gastrointestinal distress, dizziness, dose-related hypertension, and discontinuation syndrome (APA, 2010; Keller et al., 2007). Tricyclic agents include amitriptyline, clomipramine, doxepin, and imipramine. Common side effects of tricyclics include cardiovascular and anticholinergic effects, weight gain, sedation, myoclonus, and seizures (APA, 2010; VA/DoD, 2016). MAOIs include phenelzine, tranylcypromine, and selegiline. Individuals taking MAOIs must avoid certain foods and beverages such as aged cheese and meats, fava beans, and red wine because a serious, life-threatening interaction (hypertensive crisis) may occur (Pies, 1998). Common side effects of MAOIs include cardiovascular effects, weight gain, sexual side effects, headaches, insomnia, and sedation (APA, 2010; VA/DoD, 2016).

Adjunctive Treatment

If an individual does not have an adequate response to antidepressant medications, other agents such as another antidepressant from a different class, mood stabilizers, and antipsychotics may be added in hopes of greater efficacy. There is evidence that adding bupropion, mirtazapine, or venlafaxine to an SSRI is an effective strategy (Trivedi et al., 2006). Lithium has demonstrated efficacy in up to 50% of individuals who do not respond to antidepressant therapy alone (Price et al., 1986). There is evidence that augmenting with an antipsychotic is also effective (Shelton et al., 2001; Papakostas et al., 2007). Electroconvulsive therapy (ECT) may be considered in moderate to severe depression, depression with psychotic or catatonic features, treatment refractory depression, and for suicidality. A meta-analytic review of ECT reports that it was more effective than all other pharmacologic treatments though lithium or antipsychotics were not included (Pagnin et al., 2004). Newer treatments that are approved by the Food and Drug Administration (FDA) for moderate to severe depression include transcranial magnetic stimulation (TMS), intravenous ketamine, or intranasal esketamine (Cohen et al., 2022; VA/DoD 2016).

Psychotherapeutic Interventions

First-line psychotherapeutic interventions that have demonstrated efficacy in treating depression include cognitive behavioral therapy (CBT), interpersonal psychotherapy, psychodynamic therapy, problem-solving therapy, mindfulness-based CBT, and acceptance and commitment therapy (ACT) (APA, 2010; VA/DoD, 2016). A core feature of many of the interventions is to enhance emotional regulation and these improvements correlate with improvements in psychopathology in both youth and adults (Moltrecht et al., 2021). Individuals with MDD often have marital and family issues, so therapy with the spouse or family may be helpful. Group therapy may also be beneficial to individuals with MDD. Depression-focused psychotherapy alone is recommended for people with mild to moderate depression and women who are pregnant, trying to become pregnant, or breastfeeding. For moderate to severe depression, psychotherapy plus antidepressant treatment is recommended (APA, 2010; VA/DoD, 2016).

Vocational Impact of MDD

For those with the primary diagnosis of mood disorder who receive effective employment and mental health services, there is a greater probability of employment when there is a recent work history, less time on the Social Security rolls, greater cognitive functioning, and a lower local unemployment rate (Metcalfe et al., 2018). Therefore, factors that determine employment for people with psychiatric disorders are complex and rely on treatments, personal factors related to the illness, and external factors such as local employment opportunities. Individuals with MDD experience a loss of interest in work activities, decreased motivation, poor initiative, lack of drive, changes in appetite, insomnia, fatigue, psychomotor agitation or retardation, negative thinking, and decreased ability to focus and concentrate, all of which can have a profound negative impact on work performance and work relationships (Fischler & Booth, 1999; Steadman & Taskila, 2015). These symptoms can make it difficult to learn new skills. Individuals with MDD may have irritability that negatively affects relationships with coworkers. They may be overly sensitive to criticism and have difficulty coping with others. The symptoms of MDD can make it difficult for an individual to stay on task or complete a project. Stress tolerance is decreased in MDD; therefore, a high-stress, fast-paced work environment may be inappropriate.

Reasonable Accommodations

Accommodations for an individual with MDD will depend on the severity of symptoms. It is important to offer flexibility in scheduling to allow for appointments for medication management or therapy. A quiet workstation away from distractions may improve attention and focus. A predictable routine can help minimize stress and maintain stamina. Hourly goals can help with maintaining work pace. Working in a team may decrease feelings of loneliness. Last, new information or new job skills may require extra instruction and additional time to learn. Providing written instructions can help to improve accuracy and aid in retention.

Cost of MDD

Major depressive disorder is a costly illness in terms of both direct costs (e.g., hospitalizations, doctor's visits, medications) and indirect costs (e.g., missed work, reduced productivity, quality of life). The economic burden of MDD in 2018 rose 38% since 2010, affecting 17.5 million adults at a total cost of $326 billion (Greenberg et al., 2021). The burden includes the direct medical costs of treating MDD, the costs from treating comorbidities, suicide-related costs, and workplace productivity impacts. A recent report by the World Health Organization estimated that MDD affects 322 million people globally, representing an 18.4% increase in the number of people living with MDD between 2005–2015. The American College of Occupational and Environmental Medicine

(ACOEM) reports that MDD has been shown to be equivalent to coronary heart disease in terms of reduced productivity. It is estimated that people with MDD function at an even lower rate than people with hypertension, diabetes, or arthritis (ACOEM, 2003). A large meta-analysis did not find evidence of cost-effectiveness differences between SSRIs, except for escitalopram, or of SSRIs versus TCAs (Pan et al., 2012).

Bipolar Disorder

Clinical classifications of bipolar disorder first appeared around the turn of the century, when Emil Kraepelin divided psychotic disorders into two major categories: manic-depressive insanity and dementia praecox (Kendler, 2020). These terms are the predecessors of bipolar disorder and schizophrenia, respectively. Bipolar disorder can be classified as bipolar I, bipolar II, and bipolar disorder not otherwise specified. Individuals with bipolar I have experienced at least one episode of mania, while individuals with bipolar II experience a milder form of mania termed *hypomania*.

Epidemiology and Course of Illness

Based on data from National Comorbidity Survey Replication (NCS-R), an estimated 2.8% of U.S. adults were diagnosed with bipolar disorder in the past year (NIMH, 2022b). An estimated 4.4% of U.S. adults experience bipolar disorder at some time in their lives. An estimated 82.9% of people with bipolar disorder had serious impairment. Furthermore, an estimated 2.9% of adolescents had bipolar disorder, and 2.6% had severe impairment (Kessler et al., 2005a, 2005b; NIMH, 2022b). The Epidemiologic Catchment Area (ECA) study reports the mean age of onset at 21 years of age (Robins & Reiger, 1991). There are generally an equal number of men and women affected with bipolar disorder, although their course of illness may be different. Women with bipolar disorder have higher rates of rapid cycling moods, mixed states, alcohol use disorder, depressive symptoms, and lifetime eating disorders (APA, 2022; Hirschfeld et al., 2003). Bipolar disorder is likely a result of a genetic predisposition combined with environmental influences, including stressful events (Rush, 2003).

Bipolar disorder can have a devastating impact on quality of life. When left untreated, an individual may experience ten or more episodes of mania and depression over a lifetime (Goodwin & Jamison, 1990). As many as 30–60% of individuals with bipolar disorder experience interpersonal and occupational impairments (Sanchez-Moreno et al., 2009). The divorce rates among these individuals are two to three times higher than those of the general population (Manning et al., 1997). The ECA study found that individuals with bipolar disorder were the most likely of all the mentally ill groups to have a history of previous suicide attempts. In fact, 25–60% of all individuals with bipolar disorder will attempt suicide at least once in their lifetime, and 18.9% succeed (Robins & Reiger, 1991). The lifetime suicide risk of people with bipolar disorder is 15 times higher than the general population (APA, 2022).

The course of illness in most individuals is chronic, often with alternating periods of depression and mania. Symptoms typically reduce for a period between these episodes; however, some individuals continue to have residual mood symptoms (Marangell et al., 2009). Approximately 10–15% of individuals with bipolar disorder have rapid cycling, which is defined as four or more episodes of mania, mixed mania, hypomania, or depression occurring in a 12-month period (Bowden, 1996).

Symptoms

To be diagnosed with bipolar disorder, a person must have experienced at least one episode of mania or hypomania (APA, 2022). Symptoms associated with bipolar disorder include mania, hypomania, depressive, and mixed states. Psychotic features may occur with all these states except hypomania. Psychotic features are defined as a break with reality characterized by delusions and hallucinations. The DSM-5-TR (2022) criteria for each of these mood states are detailed in the following section.

Mania

To be considered mania, the elevated, expansive, or irritable mood must last for at least one week and be present most of the day, nearly every day. To be considered hypomania, the mood must last at least four consecutive days and be present most of the day, almost every day. During this period, three or more of the following symptoms must be present and represent a significant change from usual behavior:

- Inflated self-esteem or grandiosity
- Decreased need for sleep
- Increased talkativeness
- Racing thoughts
- Distracted easily
- Increase in goal-directed activity or psychomotor agitation
- Engaging in activities that hold the potential for painful consequences, e.g., unrestrained buying sprees

Hypomania

Hypomania typically has milder symptoms than mania; however, functioning is still impacted. The symptoms are not severe enough to cause significant vocational or social impairment or to warrant hospitalization. Additionally, psychotic features are never present during a hypomanic episode (APA, 2022).

Depressive Episode

The criteria for a depressive episode are the same as for MDD and can be found in the corresponding section of this chapter.

Mixed Episode

A mixed episode occurs when the criteria for both a manic and depressive episode are met at the same time nearly every day for at least one week (APA, 2022). A mixed episode causes severe impairment and may lead to hospitalization. During a mixed state, it is common to have agitation, difficulty sleeping, significant changes in appetite, psychosis, and suicidal thoughts.

Practice Guidelines for the Treatment of Bipolar Disorder

Practice guidelines (British Association of Psychopharmacology, 2016; National Institute of Health [NIH], 2014) for the treatment of patients with bipolar disorder provide the following treatment goals: Perform a thorough diagnostic evaluation, evaluate the safety of the patient and others and determine a treatment setting, establish and maintain a therapeutic alliance, monitor the patient's psychiatric status, provide psychoeducation about bipolar disorder, enhance treatment compliance, promote regular patterns of activity and sleep, anticipate stressors, identify new episodes early, and minimize functional impairments. To achieve these goals, a combination of pharmacologic and psychotherapeutic interventions is required (British Association of Psychopharmacology, 2016; NIH, 2014).

Pharmacotherapy

Medications are used to treat acute manic symptoms, alleviate depression, and prevent future episodes. Common categories of drugs that are used to treat bipolar disorder include mood stabilizers/anticonvulsants, antipsychotics, and adjunctive agents. While lithium has been the most prescribed medication for the treatment of bipolar disorder for decades, the use of other mood stabilizers and atypical antipsychotics as first-line treatments has become increasingly common due to their perceived greater tolerability and mounting evidence of efficacy (British Association of Psychopharmacology, 2016; NIH, 2014).

Lithium

Lithium has been the mainstay of bipolar pharmacologic treatment. It was first found to have antimanic properties in 1949 but was not widely prescribed for bipolar disorder in the United States until the mid-1960s (Cade, 1999; Oruch et al., 2014). Lithium demonstrates efficacy in the treatment of acute mania, depressive episodes, and prevention of recurrent episodes. Lithium has demonstrated efficacy in suicide prevention, possibly from reducing "impulsive-aggressive" behavior (Benard et al., 2016). Side effects are reported in up to 75% of individuals that take lithium and is a source of noncompliance in 18–53%. Side effects of lithium include excessive thirst, excessive urination, memory problems, tremors, weight gain, and drowsiness/tiredness (Kamali et al., 2017). Toxic effects and overdose can occur and are more common with high serum levels. Monitoring of serum plasma levels is an important aspect of lithium treatment. Initially, close serum monitoring is required to find the optimal therapeutic dose and to avoid toxicity. It is recommended that renal and thyroid functions be tested regularly because lithium use may disrupt these processes (British Association of Psychopharmacology, 2016; NIH, 2014).

Other Mood Stabilizers

Valproate, an anticonvulsant, is another agent commonly used in the treatment of bipolar disorder. Valproate has demonstrated efficacy in the treatment of acute mania and some evidence of effectiveness in acute bipolar depression and maintenance (British Association of Psychopharmacology, 2016; NIH, 2014). Common side effects of valproate include sedation, gastrointestinal distress, tremors, increased appetite, and weight gain. There may be life-threatening adverse reactions, but such events are rare. Dosing is established through blood serum monitoring. Toxicity and overdose are not common with routine dosing. It is recommended that liver function and hematologic measures be assessed on a regular basis. Other commonly prescribed mood stabilizers include carbamazepine and lamotrigine.

Antipsychotics

Beginning with olanzapine in 1999, numerous atypical antipsychotics have FDA approval for the treatment of bipolar disorder except for paliperidone and iloperidone. This includes asenapine, lurasidone, aripiprazole, ziprasidone, risperidone, and quetiapine. The conventional antipsychotic chlorpromazine is indicated for the treatment of bipolar disorder. Traditionally, antipsychotics have been used to treat acute mania and psychotic symptoms. However, there is evidence that they can also treat depressive symptoms and prevent future episodes (Derry & Moore, 2007; Suppes et al., 2016). Unlike lithium and valproate, atypical antipsychotics do not require serum monitoring. Common side effects associated with the use of atypicals include drowsiness, sedation, dry mouth, constipation, dizziness, orthostatic hypotension, nausea, and possibly extrapyramidal symptoms (but reduced in comparison with conventional antipsychotics). Atypical antipsychotics can have negative metabolic effects such as an increased risk of weight gain, hyperglycemia, diabetes mellitus, and dyslipidemia. It is recommended that clinicians monitor weight, waist circumference, blood pressure, glucose, and lipids regularly in patients taking these medications (British Association of Psychopharmacology, 2016; NIH, 2014).

Adjunctive Medications

Other medications that are used to treat bipolar disorder include benzodiazepines, antidepressants, and other anticonvulsants. Benzodiazepines are used to treat acute mania because of their sedative effects. Antidepressants are used for bipolar depression; however, caution and close monitoring are required because these agents may induce mania (British Association of Psychopharmacology, 2016; National Institute for Health and Care Excellence [NICE], 2014). There have been investigations into the use of other anticonvulsants such as topiramate and gabapentin in treating bipolar disorder (Vasudev et al., 2006; Wang et al., 2002). Newer medications that show promise are being developed such as cariprazine and research in the field is ongoing (Edinoff et al., 2020).

Psychotherapeutic Interventions

Practice guidelines (British Association of Psychopharmacology, 2016; NICE, 2014) for the treatment of bipolar disorder recommend the use of psychoeducation and psychotherapeutic interventions. The primary goals of these treatments are to decrease distress, improve functioning, and reduce the risk and severity of future episodes. While psychotherapeutic interventions alone are typically not effective in the treatment of acute mania, they do demonstrate efficacy with bipolar depression (Vallarino et al., 2015; Zaretsky et al., 1999). Treating bipolar depression without antidepressants can be especially beneficial to individuals who have antidepressant side effects, antidepressant-induced mania, or rapid cycling. In addition to individual therapy, individuals with bipolar disorder may also benefit from family therapy, group therapy, and support groups.

Vocational Impact of Bipolar Disorder

Of those with bipolar disorder, 40–60% have challenges with independence in residence and gainful employment despite generally successful treatment of psychosis and mood dysregulation during the earliest phases of illness (Strassnig et al., 2018). Only half of people with bipolar disorder are employed (Marwaha et al., 2013). The known components of impairment in bipolar disorder include psychiatric symptoms, cognition, and functional skills. During a manic phase, symptoms such as grandiosity, distractibility, poor judgment, and excessive or inappropriate motivation can result in severe consequences on the job. A person experiencing manic symptoms has reduced interpersonal functioning, poor time management, difficulty maintaining attention, and may be distracting to coworkers. The individual may be unpredictable, unreliable, and irrational. At the most extreme, the individual experiencing mania can be dangerous to himself/herself and to others in the workplace. An individual experiencing a depressive episode may have a lack of motivation, lack of energy, social withdrawal, and decreased ability to attend and focus (Fischler & Booth, 1999). There are also physical contributors to disability such as weight gain due to medications and decreased physical endurance (Strassnig et al., 2018).

Reasonable Accommodations

Functional limitations and reasonable accommodations will vary according to the individual based on differences in episode, symptom severity, and effective coping strategies. Accommodations could include job sharing or job restructuring, putting all workplace communications in writing, and allowing time off for appointments and hospitalization, if needed. Increasing the structure of the workday and developing hourly goals can also be helpful. It is important to provide regular feedback on both job performance and interactions with others. Providing a quiet workstation with minimal distractions can improve attention and focus. Educating a supervisor or coworker about the early signs of mania could also be helpful in providing appropriate interventions early in the episode, thereby reducing functional impairment.

Costs of Bipolar Disorder

Studies in the U.S. population estimate the total annual costs of bipolar disorder at $219.1 billion, corresponding to an average of $88,443 per person per year (Cloutier et al., 2018). This figure includes $50.9 billion in direct healthcare costs (i.e., medical and pharmacy); $9.7 billion in direct non-healthcare costs (bipolar related substance use disorder, criminal justice involvement for those who commit or are victims of crime, prevention/research costs); and $158.5 billion in indirect costs (loss of work productivity or premature mortality). These data echo prior estimates of the total annual cost burden of bipolar I and bipolar II at $194.8 billion, including direct costs of $39.6 billion and indirect costs of $155.2 billion (Dilsaver, 2011).

It is estimated that 64% of individuals with bipolar disorder are noncompliant, meaning they do not take their medications as prescribed (Li et al., 2002). Direct healthcare costs rise in individuals who delay or do not take mood stabilizers during their first year of treatment (Li et al., 2002). Medication noncompliance can lead to relapse and rehospitalization which is a costly cycle. While newer medications may be more expensive, there is some evidence that shows that they help to reduce overall costs, due to improved efficacy (Bergeson et al., 2012).

Generalized Anxiety Disorder (GAD)

Generalized anxiety disorder is a condition characterized by persistent, excessive, uncontrollable, and unrealistic worry about everyday issues. Individuals meeting criteria for GAD mostly worry about the same issues that the average person worries about such as finances, health, and safety. However, a healthy person may worry up to an hour a day, whereas it is usually 3–10 hours per day for a person with GAD (Powers et al., 2015).

Epidemiology and Course of Illness

Anxiety disorders differ from normal feelings of nervousness or anxiousness and involve excessive fear or anxiety. Anxiety disorders are common mental disorders and affect nearly 30% of adults at some point in their lives (Gautam et al., 2017). Women are more likely than men to experience anxiety disorders. The occurrence of several negative life events greatly increases the likelihood that the disorder will develop. In any given year the estimated percent of U.S. adults with various anxiety disorders are specific phobia, 8–12%; social anxiety disorder, 7%; panic disorder, 2–3%; agoraphobia, 1–2.9% in adolescents and adults; GAD, 2%; and separation anxiety disorder, 0.9–1.9%.

Generalized anxiety disorder is usually regarded as a chronic illness, which fluctuates in severity over time. It typically emerges gradually and the onset of the full disorder is later than in other anxiety disorders. Outcome studies in community samples suggest a reasonable prognosis; for example, a 22-year follow-up study of individuals meeting criteria for GAD found that less than 20% had persistent GAD (Gautam et al., 2017). However, longitudinal studies in treatment seeking patients generally suggest a prolonged and fluctuating course of illness. Several effective treatments are available, and these help most people lead productive lives.

Symptoms

The DSM-5-TR (2022) criteria for diagnosing GAD are as follows: The presence of excessive anxiety and worry about a variety of topics, events, or activities which occurs often for at least six months and is clearly excessive. The worry is experienced as very challenging to control. The worry in both adults and children may easily shift from one topic to another. The anxiety and worry are accompanied by at least three of the following physical or cognitive symptoms (In children, only one of these symptoms is necessary for a diagnosis of GAD): Edginess or restlessness, easily fatigued, difficulty concentrating or mind going blank, irritability, muscle tension, sleep disturbance.

Practice Guidelines for the Treatment of GAD

Individuals can function with mild GAD and assume they are just worriers. Professional help is sought when symptoms increase, and they have a difficult time meeting the requirements of daily life or experience significant sleeping problems. The occurrence of several negative life events greatly increases the likelihood that GAD will develop into a chronic condition. The aim of management is to provide relief of psychological and somatic symptoms and minimize the impairment. These concerns can be addressed with pharmacotherapy and psychotherapy (Gautam et al., 2017; Powers et al., 2015).

Pharmacotherapy

First-line treatment usually consists of SSRIs or SNRIs such as duloxetine, escitalopram, paroxetine, or venlafaxine (Gautam et al., 2017; Powers et al., 2015). Second line treatment usually includes benzodiazepines such as diazepam, alprazolam, lorazepam, and clonazepam. Further treatments include buspirone and hydroxyzine. As with other psychiatric disorders, other medications from these categories are also used for GAD as an off-label treatment.

Adjunctive Treatment

Augmentation is achieved with antipsychotics such as olanzapine, risperidone, and quetiapine. Further treatments are pregabalin, tricyclic antidepressants, and beta-blockers (Gautam et al., 2017; Powers et al., 2015). Pregabalin is believed to have anxiolytic properties through its effects on calcium channels that reduces the release of glutamate, reduces the synthesis of excitatory synapses, and may block the trafficking of new voltage-gated calcium channels to the cell surface (Baldwin et al., 2013). Pregabalin is also effective at treating comorbid depression, somatic complaints, and sleep disturbance in those with GAD. Beta-blockers are often utilized to manage physical symptoms of anxiety such as an elevated heart rate and in this way reduce distress (Baldwin et al., 2013). A new FDA approved treatment for anxiety comorbid with depression is deep transcranial magnetic stimulation (Cohen et al., 2022).

Psychotherapy

The mainstay of psychotherapy is CBT that combines several different interventions: psychoeducation, worry exposure, relaxation, applied relaxation, problem solving, cognitive restructuring, and interpersonal psychotherapy. The most important ingredient is thought to be the exposure procedures (Powers et al., 2015). During exposure therapy the individual will incrementallybe introduced to stressors while applying coping and relaxation techniques. Applied relaxation teaches the patient a coping skill that will enable him or her to relax rapidly, to counteract and eventually abort the anxiety reactions better. Applied relaxation entails having people relax in actual anxiety-provoking situations. Acceptance and commitment therapy (ACT) and mindfulness are newer types of therapy, and initial studies are promising (Powers et al., 2015). These teach patients to focus on the present moment and follow actions guided by their values rather than by emotions and anxiety. Interpersonal psychotherapy and motivational interviewing have been evaluated for augmentation of CBT, with growing evidence of positive results.

Vocational Impact of GAD

Anxiety disorders can cause people to try to avoid situations that trigger or worsen their symptoms affecting job performance, schoolwork, and personal relationships. Having an anxiety disorder can have a major impact in the workplace. People may turn down a promotion or other opportunity because it involves travel or public speaking, make excuses to get out of office parties, staff lunches, and other events or meetings with coworkers, or be unable to meet deadlines (Anxiety and Depression Association of America [ADAA], 2022). In a national survey on anxiety in the workplace, people with anxiety disorders commonly cited these as difficult situations: dealing with problems, setting and meeting deadlines, maintaining personal relationships, managing staff, participating in meetings, and making presentations. Integrated mental healthcare and vocational rehabilitation programs demonstrate improved employment outcomes for many mental health disorders including GAD (Poulsen et al., 2017).

Reasonable Accommodations

As with other mental health disorders, the Americans with Disabilities Act of 1990 and the Amendments Act of 2008 protect against discrimination such that an employee may ask for reasonable accommodations if they satisfy the employer's requirements for the job (U.S. Equal Employment Opportunities Commission, 2008). An individual with GAD will work better in an environment that offers predictability, routine, time management, and breaks. Time management entails making to do lists and keeping a precise calendar of due dates. It is up to the individual to be aware of their symptoms and educate themselves on how to handle them at work. Allowing extra time and preparing in advance can significantly decrease symptoms of anxiety. Additionally, staying organized, planning enough sleep, exercise, and nutrition will all help with job performance for a person with GAD.

Costs of GAD

Recent data demonstrated that direct costs of anxiety disorders correspond to 2.08% of U.S. healthcare costs and 0.22% of GDP (Konnopka & König, 2020). These data are corroborated by an older study where the annual societal cost of anxiety disorders was estimated at $48.72 billion (Shirneshan, 2013). The annual overall direct medical costs associated with anxiety disorders was estimated at $1657.52 per person (SE: $238.83; $p < 0.001$), or $33.71 billion in total. Inpatient visits, prescription medications, and office-based visits together accounted for almost 93% of the overall cost. Regarding aspects of indirect cost or morbidity and mortality costs were estimated at $12.72 billion and $2.34 billion U.S. dollars in 2013, respectively. Generalized anxiety disorder and MDD frequently co-occur, which complicates disease diagnosis and treatment, increases health expenditures, and negatively impacts quality of life (Armbrecht et al., 2021). There is a high prevalence of comorbidity between the two disorders, and an estimated 62% of patients with GAD have an MDD episode in their lifetime. Treating this patient group requires a tailored approach, as patients with comorbid MDD and GAD have high rates of misdiagnosis and a higher percentage of treatment resistance than patients with either condition alone. Comorbid MDD and GAD is associated with greater healthcare resource use, elevated medical expenditures, and lower quality of life than either condition alone.

Obsessive-Compulsive Disorder (OCD)

Worry, doubts, and superstitious behavior are often a part of everyday experiences. Many people spend some time worrying, especially when psychosocial stressors are high. When worries become excessive or irrational or when certain actions are perceived as necessary to counteract these thoughts, then OCD is suspected. Important clinical features of OCD are that the thoughts and actions must be time consuming (greater than one hour per day), cause marked distress, and significantly impair everyday activities (APA, 2022).

Epidemiology and Course of Illness

OCD was once considered to be a rare disease by mental health professionals, however, in the United States, the 12-month prevalence rate is reported at 1.2% of the population (APA, 2022). People with OCD come from all ethnic backgrounds. There are slight gender differences, where men have higher rates during childhood and women have higher rates during adulthood. Generally, the onset of OCD is any age between preschool and adulthood. Most people develop OCD by the age of 40 years (March et al., 1997). Up to 50% of individuals with OCD report that their symptoms began during childhood. OCD often goes unrecognized even after an individual seeks treatment. It is estimated that the average person with OCD sees three to four different doctors and spends nine years seeking treatment before the correct diagnosis is made (March et al., 1997). Like other mental illnesses, OCD has genetic and physiological components. The symptoms are most likely due to an imbalance in neurotransmitters, as well as dysfunction in certain areas of the brain (APA, 2013; Denys et al., 2004; March et al., 1997). OCD symptoms are often chronic, although there may be periods of time when the symptoms are less severe.

Symptoms

The DSM-5-TR criteria for OCD includes the presence of obsessions, compulsions, or both. Obsessions are defined by recurrent and persistent thoughts, urges, or images that are experienced as intrusive and unwanted, and that in most individuals cause marked anxiety or distress. The individual attempts to ignore or suppress such thoughts, urges, or images, or to neutralize them with some other thought or action. Compulsions are defined by repetitive behaviors (e.g., hand washing, ordering, checking) or mental acts (e.g., praying, counting, repeating words silently) that the individual feels driven to perform in response to an obsession or according to rules that must be applied rigidly. The behaviors or mental acts are aimed at preventing or reducing anxiety or distress or preventing some dreaded event. The obsessions or compulsions are time consuming (more than one hour per day) or cause significant distress or impairment in functioning (APA, 2022).

Common obsessions are:

- Fear of contamination (e.g., by touching a doorknob or shaking hands)
- Repeated doubts (e.g., wondering if the stove was left on or if a check was signed)
- Symmetry (e.g., lining up shoes a certain way, positioning canned goods according to size, type)
- Forbidden or taboo thoughts (e.g., aggressive, sexual, and religious obsessions)
- Harm (e.g., fear of harm of oneself or others)

Common compulsions include the following (APA, 2022):

- Repetitive behaviors (e.g., hand washing, ordering, checking, touching)
- Repetitive mental acts (e.g., praying, counting, repeating words or phrases)

Practice Guidelines for the Treatment of OCD

Treatment of OCD includes both medications and psychotherapeutic interventions. Most people require the use of both modalities, as only 20% experience symptom remission with medications alone (APA, 2007, 2013; March et al., 1997). Treatment is divided into two phases: acute and maintenance. The respective treatment goals during the acute and maintenance phases are to end the current OCD episode and prevent future episodes. Most treatment occurs on an outpatient basis, as hospitalization is rarely necessary for the treatment of OCD. However, inpatient treatment may be an effective strategy for people with severe, chronic, treatment-resistant OCD (Boshen et al., 2008).

Pharmacotherapy

Antidepressants

SSRIs are the first-line pharmacologic treatment of OCD such as fluoxetine, fluvoxamine, paroxetine, and sertraline. Antidepressants that do not have serotonergic properties are typically not effective in the treatment of OCD (Pies, 1998). Most people will not have substantial improvement until they have been taking a SSRI for four to six weeks, and it may take as long as 10–12 weeks of treatment. If OCD symptoms do not diminish after an SSRI is initiated, it is recommended to increase the medication to the maximum tolerated dose within the approved dosage range (APA, 2007, 2013; Fenske & Petersen, 2015).

Adjunctive Treatment

If patients do not respond to conventional treatment, then another strategy is the use of adjunctive medications. Commonly used additional medications include clomipramine, antipsychotics (e.g., haloperidol, olanzapine, risperidone), and buspirone (an antianxiety agent) (APA, 2007, 2013; Fenske & Petersen, 2015). It is important to monitor for increased medication side effects or interactions when using multiple agents. Sedation is a common side effect of these medications, so it may be necessary to take them at bedtime. The FDA has approved transcranial magnetic stimulation for treatment-resistant OCD (Cohen et al., 2022).

Psychotherapeutic Interventions

Cognitive behavioral therapy is recommended for all individuals with OCD (APA, 2007, 2013; Fenske & Petersen, 2015). Cognitive behavioral therapy techniques utilized in the treatment of OCD include exposure and response or ritual prevention. Exposure consists of having the individual encounter a feared stimulus (e.g., dirty objects, shaking hands). The goal of this technique is to reduce anxiety with each exposure session. Response or ritual prevention is another key element to this process. This technique is defined as preventing the individual from any actions that are used to reduce anxiety when exposed to the feared stimulus, for example, not permitting the individual to wash her hands after touching something perceived as contaminated. Other CBT techniques used in OCD include thought stopping, distraction, and contingency management.

Individuals with OCD may also benefit from psychoeducation about the illness and ways to manage symptoms (APA, 2007, 2013; Fenske & Petersen, 2015). Also, support groups can be helpful because they provide an outlet for individuals to share experiences and receive peer support. OCD has a negative impact on an individual's interpersonal relationships, and significant others may become part of the destructive symptom cycle by enabling rituals. In these cases, it is especially important to include significant others in the treatment plan, including the use of marriage and family therapy.

Vocational Impact of OCD

OCD can have a devastating impact on vocational functioning. Commonly, individuals with OCD will work at a slow pace because of coping with obsessions and compulsions. An individual may feel compelled to check and recheck his/her work or a need to do certain rituals while working that make ordinary tasks take an extended period to complete. Individuals with OCD have a lower tolerance for stress. Everyday occurrences such as shaking someone's hand or counting money might induce obsessive thoughts and compulsive behaviors. Also, a stressful work environment can contribute to the severity and frequency of OCD symptoms. Distractibility can occur because the individual with OCD is often preoccupied with symptoms, detracting from the ability to concentrate and focus.

Reasonable Accommodations

An individual with OCD will work better in an environment that offers predictability and routine. This can help keep stress levels to a minimum and reduce the need to make decisions throughout the day, which may prove difficult, especially when symptoms are moderate to severe. It may be helpful to allow some flexibility in the setup of the workspace. Providing hourly goals may help establish pace of work. A workstation that is not near coworkers may decrease anxiety and distractibility. Last, flexible scheduling should be offered to accommodate medication management and CBT appointments.

Costs of OCD

In 1990, the total costs of OCD were estimated to be $8.4 billion, which was 5.7% of the estimated costs of all mental illnesses combined for that year, i.e., $147.8 billion (DuPont et al., 1995). Another study reports that the projected direct cost of OCD treatment is $5 billion per year (Hollander et al., 1997). Lost wages and underemployment are large contributors to the economic costs of OCD. More current research is needed about the economic impact of OCD.

Regarding quality of life, individuals with OCD have dysfunction in all areas (Macy et al., 2013). Those with OCD experience moderate to severe impairment in family and social relationships and ability to study or work. With treatment there is improvement in quality-of-life measures, but not to community norms.

Schizophrenia

In 1896, Emil Kraepelin provided the first descriptions of the disease known today as schizophrenia (Kendler, 2020). He used the term *dementia praecox* to describe individuals whose psychotic symptoms began early in life and continued a deteriorating course (Kendler, 2020). In 1911, Eugen Bleuler coined the term *schizophrenia* for the illness that Kraepelin called dementia praecox, because he thought it was a more fitting description of the illness. The word schizophrenia means a splitting (schizo) of the mind (phrenia), and not a split personality, which is a common public misperception about the illness (Kendler, 2020).

Early treatments for schizophrenia such as hypoglycemic coma, seizure therapy, and frontal lobotomies were typically unsuccessful and even harmful for the patient. Schizophrenia treatment was revolutionized in the early 1950s with the introduction of the first antipsychotic agent, chlorpromazine (Thorazine), allowing many patients to be treated in the community instead of in hospitals (Woo et al., 2017). In the early 1990s, pharmacotherapy entered another more promising phase with the introduction of the first atypical antipsychotic agent, clozapine. New antipsychotics continue to be developed, broadening the treatment options for schizophrenia.

Epidemiology and Course of Illness

The prevalence of schizophrenia and related psychotic disorders in the U.S. ranges between 0.25–0.64% (NIMH, 2022c). The incidence rate is similar across diverse geographical, cultural, and socioeconomic categories. The onset of schizophrenia can be gradual or sudden, but many individuals display signs that something is wrong (e.g., decreased sociality, withdrawal, anxiety, depression, unusual behavior, problems at school or work) before actual psychotic symptoms are apparent (Larson et al., 2010). The age of onset is typically adolescence to early adulthood, with men having an earlier onset than women. It is unusual to develop schizophrenia after the age of 40 (McEvoy et al., 1999). Earlier onset is associated with poorer outcomes, which may be attributed to the loss of age-appropriate milestones in the areas of education, interpersonal relationships, and employment (Lay et al., 2000). The course of schizophrenia is often chronic and disabling. Individuals may have periods of acute psychosis alternating with periods of symptom remission or a constant level of residual symptoms that can greatly impair functioning. Schizophrenia is one of the leading causes of disability worldwide and individuals with schizophrenia have an increased risk of premature mortality (NIMH, 2022c).

Schizophrenia is primarily a problem of brain functionality rather than brain structure. While the role of dopamine imbalance has been well documented, other neurotransmitters appear to be involved in schizophrenia as well, including serotonin, acetylcholine, norepinephrine, glutamate, and gamma-aminobutyric acid (GABA). The causes of schizophrenia are unknown but believed to be a combination of genetic predisposition and environmental factors that most likely occur *in utero* during the development of the brain. Trauma and psychosocial stressors such as living in an urban area and dysfunctional family communication also play a role in the development of schizophrenia (Tsuang, 2000).

Symptoms

The DSM-5-TR (2022) diagnostic criteria for schizophrenia are two or more of the following, each present during a one-month period: delusions, hallucinations, disorganized speech, grossly disorganized or catatonic behavior, or negative symptoms. At least one of the symptoms must be delusions, hallucinations, or disorganized speech, and continuous disturbance persists for at least six months. The main categories of symptoms in schizophrenia are *positive* referring to occurrences that are added to one's ordinary experience and *negative* referring to aspects of life that are taken away from one's ordinary experience.

Positive Symptoms

Positive symptoms include hallucinations, delusions, disorganized speech, and disorganized or catatonic behavior. Hallucinations can occur in all sensory modalities, but the most common are auditory. Auditory hallucinations are usually in the form of voices. A voice may provide a running commentary on a person's actions or thoughts; there may be two or more voices talking to each other or a single voice that commands a person to do things such as pray out loud or hide in the basement.

Delusions are false beliefs and may take on a bizarre quality such as believing one is from another planet or that one has two heads. Common categories of delusions include the following:

- Paranoid (believing one is being tracked by the CIA, is the victim of a communist plot, etc.)
- Grandiose (believing one is the president, a rock star, a religious prophet, etc.)
- Referential (believing that a song on the radio or popular novel is about oneself, etc.)
- Thought broadcasting (believing that one's thoughts are broadcasting out loud so that others can hear them)
- Somatic (believing one's teeth are soft or loose, that one's body is shrinking, etc.)

Negative Symptoms

Negative symptoms include flat affect (facial expressions of emotion are absent), alogia or poverty of speech (fluency and amount of speech are markedly reduced), avolition or lack of motivation or drive (decreased ability to initiate and continue goal-directed behaviors, little interest in any activity), anhedonia (loss of ability to feel pleasure, emptiness), anergia (lack of energy), and asociality (social isolation and withdrawal).

Associated Symptoms or Features

Other symptoms often found in schizophrenia include cognitive dysfunction (e.g., impaired memory, executive functioning, concentration, abstract thinking), inappropriate affect, dysphoric or depressed mood, anxiety, odd psychomotor activities (e.g., rocking, pacing), odd mannerisms or behaviors, lack of interest in eating and/or food refusal, and sleep disturbances (APA, 2022). Common comorbid conditions include substance abuse, depression, panic disorder, OCD, and PTSD (Buckley et al., 2009). It is important to note that treatment noncompliance is very common and further complicates the clinical picture of schizophrenia.

Practice Guidelines for the Treatment of Schizophrenia

There is no cure for schizophrenia, thus, treatment involves a broad range of interventions, both pharmacotherapy and psychosocial, designed to reduce the frequency and severity of symptoms and to improve functioning. The APA and the American Psychological Association have established treatment guidelines for schizophrenia (American Psychological Association, 2019; APA, 2021). The APA recommends that the guideline statement should be implemented in the context of a person-centered treatment plan that includes evidence-based nonpharmacological and pharmacological treatments for schizophrenia (APA, 2021).

The APA has conceptualized the treatment of schizophrenia into three phases: acute, stabilization, and stable (APA, 2009 2021). The acute phase is characterized by florid psychosis where patients are often unable to care for themselves and may be violent, homicidal, or suicidal. The goals of treatment during the acute phase are to reduce the acute symptoms and improve functioning. The stabilization phase typically lasts six months or more after the onset of the acute episode. Although the severity of the psychotic symptoms is reduced, symptoms and functioning are improved, but some impairment remains. Treatment goals during this phase include minimizing stress, minimizing the likelihood of relapse, improving community functioning, and continued reduction of symptoms. The stable phase is characterized by relatively stable symptoms that are less severe. Residual symptoms may be more nonpsychotic in nature, such as circumstantial thoughts or speech, overvalued ideas rather than delusions, and mild to moderate negative symptoms. Treatment goals during the stable phase include optimizing functioning and quality of life, minimizing the risk of relapse, and monitoring for medication side effects. Continuing antipsychotic treatment can reduce the relapse rate to less than 30% per year (APA, 2021).

Pharmacotherapy

The APA recommends that patients with schizophrenia be treated with an antipsychotic medication and monitored for effectiveness and side effects (APA, 2021). Patients with schizophrenia whose symptoms have improved with an antipsychotic medication should continue to be treated with an antipsychotic medication. Furthermore, for those whose symptoms have improved with an antipsychotic medication, they should continue to be treated with the same antipsychotic medication. Patients with treatment-resistant schizophrenia can be treated with clozapine, especially if the risk for suicide attempts or suicide remains substantial despite other treatments. Similarly, treatment with clozapine is recommended if the risk for aggressive behavior remains substantial despite other treatments. For those who have a history of poor or uncertain adherence they may receive treatment with a long-acting injectable antipsychotic medication. Many people with schizophrenia will have side effects from antipsychotics such as acute dystonia and this can be treated with an anticholinergic medication. Options for patients who have parkinsonism associated side effects with antipsychotic therapy are lowering the dosage of the antipsychotic medication, switching to another antipsychotic medication, or treating with an anticholinergic medication. Options for patients who have akathisia associated with antipsychotic therapy are lowering the dosage of the antipsychotic medication, switching to another antipsychotic medication, adding a benzodiazepine medication, or adding a beta-adrenergic blocking agent. For those patients who have moderate to severe or disabling tardive dyskinesia associated with antipsychotic therapy this side effect may be treated with a reversible inhibitor of the vesicular monoamine transporter 2 (VMAT2). Meta-analysis evaluation of decision-making competency in schizophrenia as analyzed by the MacCAT-CR scale demonstrates a difference in means of −4.43 (−5.76; −3.1, $p < 0.001$) for understanding, −1.17 (−1.49, −0.84, $p < 0.001$) for appreciation, −1.29 (−1.79, −0.79, $p < 0.001$) for reasoning, and −0.05 (−0.9, −0.01, $p = 0.022$) for expressing a choice (Hostiuc et al., 2018). Even though schizophrenia patients have a significantly decreased decision-making capacity, with reasonable accommodations they are capable of medical decision-making and vocational pursuits. Though schizophrenia patients have a significantly decreased decision-making capacity, they should be considered as competent unless very severe changes are identifiable during clinical examination. Enhanced informed consent forms decrease barriers to medical decision-making in schizophrenia patients and can be used when deciding on treatment for schizophrenia.

Antipsychotics

First generation or conventional antipsychotics include perphenazine, haloperidol, loxapine, and pimozide. Second generation or atypical antipsychotics include clozapine, olanzapine, risperidone, ziprasidone, quetiapine, aripiprazole, and lurasidone. Conventional antipsychotics are associated with troublesome and serious side effects such as tardive dyskinesia (abnormal, involuntary movements commonly of the mouth, face, or extremities) and extrapyramidal symptoms (restlessness, tremors, muscle contractions, and rigidity). Common side effects associated with the use of atypicals include drowsiness/sedation, dry mouth, constipation, dizziness, orthostatic hypotension, nausea, extrapyramidal symptoms (but reduced in comparison with conventional antipsychotics), weight gain, and metabolic effects. Since their introduction, atypical antipsychotics have been recommended over conventional antipsychotics due to their decreased risk of tardive dyskinesia and extrapyramidal symptoms. However, there has been some debate about this recommendation due to some evidence of comparable efficacy with conventional antipsychotics and the serious metabolic side effects that can occur with atypical antipsychotics (APA, 2009). The good news is that research continues into the development of effective antipsychotic treatment with tolerable side effects.

Adjunctive Medications

Commonly prescribed adjunctive medications in schizophrenia include anticonvulsants or mood stabilizers, antidepressants, benzodiazepines, and anticholinergics. Polypharmacy is common, where a second antipsychotic is added with the goal of a greater or more rapid therapeutic response. When polypharmacy is in use, it is increasingly important to regularly monitor clinical response, as well as side effects (Barnes & Paton, 2011).

Anticonvulsants/Mood Stabilizers

Commonly prescribed anticonvulsants/mood stabilizers include valproate, carbamazepine, and lithium. These agents have shown some evidence of augmenting antipsychotic response, improving mood, and reducing agitation, hostility, and irritability (Citrome et al., 2004; Sajatovic et al., 2008). Anticonvulsants are generally well-tolerated agents. Carbamazepine may interact with other drugs, including reducing the serum levels of antipsychotics and benzodiazepines. Common side effects of anticonvulsants include neurological symptoms (e.g., double vision, blurred vision, fatigue) and gastrointestinal distress (e.g., nausea, indigestion, vomiting, and diarrhea) (Woo et al., 2017).

Antidepressants

Depressive symptoms are common with schizophrenia and may expand the diagnosis to schizoaffective disorder (APA, 2022). Estimates of the prevalence of depression in this population range from 7% to 65% (Bartles & Drake, 1988; DeLisis, 1990). Antidepressants are indicated when the depressive symptoms are severe, causing significant distress, or are interfering with functioning (APA, 2021). SSRIs may increase the serum concentrations of certain antipsychotics (APA, 2010).

Benzodiazepines

Benzodiazepines (e.g., lorazepam, diazepam, clonazepam) are often implemented during acute psychosis and may be continued in the stabilization phase. Benzodiazepines are used to treat sleep disturbances, anxiety, agitation, and catatonia (APA, 2021). Additionally, patients with certain motor disturbances, such as akathisia, may show improvement with the use of benzodiazepines (Woo et al., 2017). Generally, benzodiazepines have few drug interactions and common side effects of benzodiazepines include sedation, drowsiness, and risk of dependence.

Anticholinergics

Anticholinergic medications (e.g., benztropine mesylate, trihexyphenidyl hydrochloride, amantadine) are used to prevent and treat extrapyramidal side effects. It is commonly necessary to use anticholinergics in individuals that are prescribed conventional agents. The use of these agents should be reconsidered whenever a change in the antipsychotic dosage is made, as lower dosages may have reduced side effects (APA, 2021). Anticholinergics generally do not interact with other drugs. Side effects of anticholinergics include dry mouth, dry eyes, urinary retention, constipation, and memory disturbances (APA, 2021).

Vesicular Monoamine Transporter Type 2 (VMAT2) Inhibitors

The vesicular monoamine transporter type 2 (VMAT2) inhibitors are agents that cause a depletion of neuroactive peptides such as dopamine in nerve terminals and are used to treat chorea due to neurodegenerative diseases such as Huntington's chorea or dyskinesias due to neuroleptic medications such as tardive dyskinesia (Tarakad & Jimenez-Shahed, 2018). As of 2019, three VMAT2 inhibitors have become available in the U.S. for management of dyskinesia syndromes, each with a somewhat different spectrum of approved indications: tetrabenazine, deutetrabenazine, and valbenazine. Clinical use is still limited but when tardive dyskinesia is disruptive to the individual these medications are recommended.

Psychosocial Interventions

The APA recommends that patients with schizophrenia who are experiencing a first episode of psychosis be treated in a coordinated specialty care program (APA, 2021). It is recommended that patients with schizophrenia are treated with supportive psychotherapy and cognitive behavioral therapy for psychosis (CBTp) (APA, 2021). An important part of treatment is psychoeducation about the illness to explain what is happening to the person. It is imperative that patients with schizophrenia receive supported employment services and assertive community treatment if there is a history of poor engagement with services leading to frequent relapse or social disruption (e.g., homelessness; legal difficulties, including imprisonment). Further interventions for patients with schizophrenia are aimed at developing self-management skills, enhancing person-oriented recovery, enabling cognitive remediation, and providing social skills training. Patients with schizophrenia who have ongoing contact with family are recommended to have family interventions.

Family and siblings of children and young people with a chronic illness are at increased risk of poor psychological functioning. Studies have attempted to implement and evaluate interventions targeting the psychological well-being of this at-risk group (McKenzie Smith et al., 2018; Vermaes et al., 2012). It is suggested that high well-being is positively related to good mental health and can be made up of the following ten components: competence, emotional stability, engagement, meaning, optimism, positive emotion, positive relationships, resilience, self-esteem, and vitality. Well-being interventions have been suggested to help improve psychological outcomes including anxiety, depression, stress, self-esteem, and coping of families and siblings of children and young people with a chronic illness. These interventions have taken various forms, including group interventions, sibling training, camps, and family-based support (McKenzie Smith et al., 2018).

Physical exercise may be valuable for patients with schizophrenia spectrum disorders as it may have a beneficial effect on clinical symptoms, quality of life, and cognition. Meta-analyses revealed that exercise was superior to control conditions in improving total symptom severity ($p < 0.001$), positive ($p < 0.01$), negative ($p < 0.001$), and general ($p < 0.05$) symptoms, quality of life ($p < 0.001$), global functioning ($p < 0.01$), and depressive symptoms ($p < 0.001$) (Dauwan et al., 2016). Yoga, specifically, improved the cognitive subdomain long-term memory ($p < 0.05$), while exercise in general or in any other form had no effect on cognition (Dauwan et al., 2016). These data demonstrate that physical exercise is a robust add-on treatment for improving clinical symptoms, quality of life, global functioning, and depressive symptoms in patients with schizophrenia.

Music therapy (MT) has been used in the treatment of schizophrenia for decades, and it is often used as adjunct therapy to medication. It can take the format of individual therapy, large group therapy, or a combination of individual and group therapy through either "passive listening" or "active participation." Every form of MT has an effect in schizophrenic patients to a certain extent. Treatment effects were significantly better in patients who received adjunct MT than in those who did not, in negative symptoms, mood symptoms, and positive symptoms (all $p < 0.05$) (Tseng et al., 2016). This significance did not change after dividing the patients into subgroups of different total duration of MT, amounts of sessions, or frequency of MT. The treatment effect on the general symptoms was significantly positively associated with the whole duration of illness, indicating that MT would be beneficial for schizophrenic patients with a chronic course. These findings provide evidence that clinicians should apply MT for schizophrenic patients to alleviate disease severity.

Treatment Refractory Schizophrenia

Treatment refractory schizophrenia remains a challenge to treat in the field of psychiatry. Approximately 10–30% of individuals diagnosed with schizophrenia have little to no response to antipsychotic treatment and up to 30% only have a partial response (APA, 2021). The criteria for treatment refractory schizophrenia are as follows: (1) persistent, moderately severe, positive symptoms; (2) at least a moderately severe illness overall; (3) poor social/occupational functioning during the last five years; and (4) drug refractory, that is, lack of improvement on at least two conventional antipsychotics (Kane et al., 1988). Treatment refractory individuals are often highly symptomatic, with higher rates of service use and rehospitalization. Strategies for treating refractory schizophrenia include a trial of clozapine, adjunctive medications, higher antipsychotic dosing, ECT, CBT, and cognitive remediation (APA, 2009; APA, 2021).

The lifetime risk of suicide and suicide attempt in patients with schizophrenia are 5% and 25–50%, respectively (Cassidy et al., 2018). A recent meta-analytic study aimed to determine risk factors associated with suicidality in subjects with schizophrenia (Cassidy et al., 2018). Depressive symptoms ($p < 0.0001$), Positive and Negative Symptom Scale general score ($p < 0.0001$), and number of psychiatric hospitalizations ($p < 0.0001$) were higher in patients with suicide ideation. History of alcohol use ($p = 0.0001$), family history of psychiatric illness ($p < 0.0001$), physical comorbidity ($p < 0.0001$), history of depression ($p < 0.0001$), family history of suicide ($p < 0.0001$), history of drug use ($p = 0.0024$), history of tobacco use ($p = 0.0034$), being white ($p = 0.0022$), and depressive symptoms ($p < 0.0001$) were the most consistent variables associated with suicide attempts. Being male ($p = 0.0005$), history of attempted suicide ($p < 0.0001$), younger age ($p = 0.0266$), higher intelligence quotient ($p < 0.0001$), poor adherence to treatment ($p < 0.0001$), and hopelessness ($p < 0.0001$) were the most consistently associated with suicide. These findings may help with future development of preventive strategies to combat suicide and treatment refractory schizophrenia.

Quality of life (QoL) has been linked to suicide risk among individuals with schizophrenia. QoL is a construct that evaluates functioning in the community (objective QoL) and perceived life satisfaction (subjective QoL). QoL has been increasingly recognized as a critical outcome in the evaluation of mental health service effectiveness among those with serious mental illness as an indicator of unmet need and vulnerability to suicide risk (Fulginiti & Brekke, 2019). A wide range of things can impact subjective and objective QoL over time, including clinical, psychosocial, and program-related factors. Disparity among suicide attempt survivors and non-attempters in QoL can potentially influence suicide risk disparity over time. Chronic disparity in subjective QoL was observed in work (b –0.51; 95% CI [–0.95, –0.06]), relationship (b –1.53; 95% CI [–2.68, –0.37]), and self-present life (b –2.04; 95% CI [–3.12, –0.95]) domains, with attempt survivors having lower QoL levels than non-attempters over time. Change disparity in objective QoL was observed in the relationship domain (b –0.23; 95% CI [–0.40, –0.07]), with attempt survivors having a lower rate of QoL change. Chronic and change disparities between attempt survivors and non-attempters suggests that QoL disparity could reflect a distinct clinical profile for attempt survivors over time, that service delivery efforts should account for attempt status to address enduring and emerging QoL gaps, and that suicide attempt status deserves more attention in schizophrenia treatment and research (Fulginiti & Brekke, 2019).

Patients diagnosed with schizophrenia often experience a relapse of their symptoms after successfully completing treatment. Patients are expected to be hospitalized several times within a few years of their first onset of a psychotic episode (Ji et al., 2018). Utilizing ratings of patients' level of schizophrenia symptoms and independent living skills at discharge are partially sufficient for deciding if they are ready for discharge without rehospitalization. Treatment providers in the community should attend to the patients' self-report of declining general mental health to prevent a rehospitalization. Findings that deterioration occurs during the period from six months to one year after discharge suggests that treatment providers should not assume that after six months the patient will remain stable and continue to monitor the patient (Ji et al., 2018).

Vocational Impact of Schizophrenia

Employment is a critical aspect of reintegration into the community. In recent years, the importance of employment among individuals with schizophrenia has received renewed interest, and more supported employment programs are available. However, most people with severe and persistent mental illness remain unemployed. The National Alliance on the Mentally Ill (NAMI) reports that the employment rates for people with mental illness dropped from 23% in 2003 to 17.8% in 2012 (NAMI, 2014). In fact, the literature indicates that employment rates for people with schizophrenia are much lower than in the general population, ranging between 14.5–17.2% in the United States, placing people with schizophrenia among those disability groups that are highly likely to be unemployed (Carmona et al., 2017). There are many factors that contribute to such low rates of employment, including residual positive and negative symptoms, interpersonal skills deficits, cognitive impairments, relapse, lack of appropriate vocational programs, and stigma. However, the benefits of paid employment are far-reaching, including an association with total symptom improvement, improvement in cognitive and negative symptoms, lower rates of hospitalization, and decreased rates of emotional discomfort (Bell et al., 1996; Bio & Gattaz, 2011). A study investigating the effects of paid work in individuals diagnosed with schizophrenia found improvements in QoL including increased motivation, sense of purpose, empathy, and decreased anhedonia (Bryson et al., 2002).

Access to employment plays a critical role in the recovery and functioning of people with schizophrenia. Vocational rehabilitation enhances employment outcomes for people with schizophrenia (Carmona et al., 2017). Engaging in a vocational intervention increases the likelihood of obtaining a competitive job (risk ratio (RR) = 2.31, 95% CI 1.85–2.88) and has a positive impact on hours worked in any job (standardized mean difference (SMD) = 0.42, 95% CI 0.16–0.68). Those receiving supported employment-based treatments show significantly better competitive job placement outcomes than those receiving other vocational treatments (RR = 2.49, 95% CI: 2.16– 2.88). There is no evidence of intervention efficacy regarding wages earned from competitive employment. Participation in rehabilitative vocational treatment is not sufficient to ensure work participation for people with schizophrenia. Comprehensive treatments are necessary to address functional deficits that hinder labor stability and job performance for people with schizophrenia (Carmona et al., 2017).

Reasonable Accommodations

Functional limitations will vary according to the individual based on differences in symptoms (both severity and domain) and effective coping strategies. Positive symptoms can make it difficult for clients to concentrate, handle stress, and interact with others. Negative symptoms can result in lack of motivation and energy, difficulty with initiating and completing a work task, and impaired social skills. Cognitive symptoms have a negative impact on concentration, attention, memory, and ability to problem solve or learn new information. Additionally, cognitive symptoms can cause difficulties in a client's ability to prioritize, filter out irrelevant information, and function socially.

Reasonable accommodations for clients with schizophrenia will vary according to individual needs and may change over time. Typically, accommodations are not costly, as they are not usually structural. Common reasonable accommodations for people with psychiatric disabilities include the following (MacDonald-Wilson et al., 2002):

- Flexible scheduling
- Job modification or restructuring
- Facilitating communication on the job
- Modifying employee training

- Providing training to staff or supervisors
- Modifying supervision
- Making policy changes
- Modifying the physical environment or providing special equipment
- Changing work procedures

Vocational Programs

Vocational program models include clubhouse programs, transitional employment, agency-sponsored or consumer-operated businesses, and supported employment. Supported employment has the most evidence as an effective employment strategy (Bond et al., 1997; Cook et al., 2005, 2008). Cook et al. (2008) found that people with schizophrenia who were enrolled in supportive employment had even better outcomes than people with other diagnoses in the control condition group. This is noteworthy given that at baseline, the schizophrenia group had more symptoms, more hospitalizations, lower education, earlier onsets, poorer work histories, and lower work motivation than the nonschizophrenia group. The basic tenet of supported employment is that any client can hold a job in the competitive workforce if provided the proper supports. Important features of supported employment include integration with treatment; client choice; ongoing, time-unlimited supports on or offsite; and integrated settings (Metcalfe et al., 2018).

Costs of Schizophrenia

The annual costs for schizophrenia are estimated to be in the range of $94 million to $102 billion, which translates into 0.02–5.46% of GDP of the U.S. (Chong et al., 2016). Improving medication adherence could reduce the economic burden of schizophrenia by decreasing the rates of symptom relapse, rehospitalization, and overall need for services. The Clinical Antipsychotic Trials of Intervention Effectiveness (CATIE) found that 74% of patients had discontinued their medication within 18 months due to efficacy, side effects, or other reasons (Lieberman et al., 2005).

A review of 22 studies found that in most cases, the atypical antipsychotics were at least cost-neutral and may be cost-effective when compared with conventional agents (Hudson et al., 2003). However, the CATIE trial found similar efficacy of a conventional antipsychotic (perphenazine) with several atypical antipsychotics (risperidone, ziprasidone, quetiapine) (Lieberman et al., 2005). In this study, one atypical antipsychotic (olanzapine) did have better outcomes in terms of efficacy than the conventional agent. Since these studies were published, several atypical antipsychotics are now available as generics, which significantly reduces their costs. A study investigating cost-effectiveness of one of the newer atypical antipsychotics (lurasidone) found lurasidone to be more cost-effective than generic risperidone due to less hospitalizations and minimal cardiometabolic effects (O'Day et al., 2013). Clearly, more investigation is needed to better quantify the cost-effectiveness, efficacy, and quality-of-life benefits of the atypical antipsychotics in comparison with each other and the older agents.

Mental Health in Children and Adolescence

Mental health is an ongoing aspiration for American youth as the rates of psychiatric disorders has steadily increased over the past years. In particular, the COVID-19 pandemic has caused increasing major depression and anxiety disorders in youth across the nation and worldwide. A meta-analysis of 29 studies including 80,879 youth globally, revealed the pooled prevalence estimates of clinically elevated child and adolescent depression and anxiety were 25.2% and 20.5%, respectively (Racine et al., 2021). The prevalence of depression and anxiety symptoms during COVID-19 doubled, compared with pre-pandemic estimates. Analyses revealed that prevalence rates were higher when collected later in the pandemic, in older adolescents, and in females. Much of the mental health burden is due to isolation, fear, family economic downturn, and the devastating morbidity and mortality from COVID-19 within families. When working with children and adolescents it is imperative to understand that this population has its own psychological needs, barriers, challenges, and FDA approved treatments. Thus, the life care planner must become familiar with standards of care for treating youth for mental health. Not all medications that are FDA approved for adults are approved for use in children. Furthermore, children may require increased supports and interventions to meet developmental milestones and mastery in school. There are also multiple adaptations for psychotherapeutic techniques used in children as well as child focused therapies. Examples are CBT that is adapted for children and various play therapy interventions (Landreth, 2012; Phifer et al., 2020). When working with children, parent or family work is vital for therapy to be successful (Novick & Novick, 2005). Individual and family therapy may supplement psychotherapeutic interventions in schools where there is both good access and efficacy (Yohannan & Carlson, 2019). Children have the resilience to make marked strides in mental health recovery, but the challenges that they face must be confronted head on (Yohannan & Carlson, 2019). Adverse childhood experiences are known to cause lifelong psychological and physical health complications and these adverse experiences are well defined (Centers for Disease Control and Prevention, 2022). Ultimately, life care plans for children and adolescents must encompass multidimensional treatment to be effective for psychological health.

The Impact of Mental Health Professionals on the Life Care Plan

Mental health professionals can help achieve recovery goals and while these specialties can vary by state, an overview includes psychiatrists, psychiatric nurse practitioners, psychologists, social workers, and counselors. The education and training are different for each of these paths. Psychiatrists are physicians that have earned a medical degree (MD) and specialize in psychiatry. Furthermore, psychiatric nurse practitioners have advanced level training in nursing and psychiatry (NP). Psychologists typically earn the degree of a Doctor of Psychology in clinical psychology (PsyD) or a Doctor of Philosophy in clinical psychology (PhD). Finally, a masters level education can be pursued to become a social worker or counselor.

These professionals assess, diagnose, and treat mental health, more broadly referred to as behavioral health. These professionals have some overlapping and varying contributions as providers of behavioral health. Overlap exists in the realm of diagnosis where these professionals utilize the *Diagnostic and Statistical Manual of Mental Disorders* 5th ed., Text Revision (APA, 2022) for diagnostic criteria. However, diagnosis may require input from more than one mental healthcare professional and is often done in the context of specialized care. There is further overlap in that these providers are all trained in psychotherapy so that they can treat symptoms and disorders with various psychotherapeutic techniques. Key differences between the mental healthcare providers are that psychiatrists prescribe medications and other medical interventions. Psychiatric nurse practitioners have prescribing authority as well, but often require physician oversight. The psychologist is trained in-depth on psychological and neuropsychological assessment; for example, Intelligence Quotient Tests, to determine intellectual potential. Social workers are trained to advocate for clients and connect them to community resources. A variety of mental health professionals provide comprehensive care in the field.

One or more mental health providers may be included on the multidisciplinary treatment team of the life care plan because chronic diseases and catastrophic injuries are strongly associated with psychiatric comorbidities (Missner & Cohen, 2019). Conditions commonly comorbid with illness are depressive disorders, anxiety disorders, trauma-based disorders, substance use disorders, impulse control disorders, dissociative disorders, somatic symptom disorders, sleep wake disorders, and neurocognitive disorders. The mental health provider's expertise allows the life care planner to create a solid foundation for the individual's mental healthcare needs that is based on medical and scientific evidence. Mental health providers often provide lifelong care to patients with mental health disorders who have sustained an injury or illness that results in permanent impairment and disability. The scope of topics these mental health professionals can address as a retained expert or consultant to the life care plan is summarized in Table 22.1.

Table 22.1 The Scope of Mental Healthcare Professionals in the Life Care Plan (Adapted from Missner & Cohen, 2019)

Preinjury psychiatric disorders	Did the individual have a premorbid mental health condition?
Psychiatric disorders related to the injury or chronic illness	Has a psychiatric disorder emerged or been exacerbated? Is there more than one psychiatric diagnosis?
Personality traits or disorders	Personality dimensions that are protective or risk factors for psychiatric morbidity.
Prognosis of psychiatric disorder	Will the condition be lifelong?
Psychosocial history and family dynamics	What supports does the individual have?
Psychosocial functioning and limitations	Individual's baseline premorbid and function currently?
Vocational functioning and limitations	Individual's baseline premorbid and function currently?
Psychological adjustment to disability	How is the individual adjusting to disability and how can the adjustment be improved?
Educational and vocational needs	Is educational or vocational rehabilitation recommended and what kind?
Attendant care or facility care	How much assistance is needed and in what setting?
Mental health treatment	Medications, psychotherapy, intensive outpatient treatment, hospitalization, and interventional psychiatry such electroconvulsive therapy, transcranial magnetic therapy, intravenous ketamine, intranasal ketamine.
Standard of care	Practice guidelines for illness.
Referrals to specialists	Neuropsychologists, specialized centers of care.
Costs of treatment	Brand versus generic medications, outpatient & inpatient programs.

The mental health professional employs the methodology that is normally used for creating evaluations: records analysis, examination of the evaluee, diagnostic testing, referrals, assessment, and long-term planning based on current scientific literature and published standards of practice (Missner & Cohen, 2019). Areas of particular concern in this population over the long-term are emotional responses to the new life situation; adjustment to disability; development of comorbid psychiatric disorders such as traumatic, mood, or neurocognitive disorders; exacerbation of prior psychiatric illness; and issues regarding malingering and secondary gain. Furthermore, the mental health specialist may provide recommendations related to education, employment, functional limitations, disability, need for attendant care, and costs related to psychiatric diagnoses. In addition, the mental health provider can determine if referrals are necessary for further evaluations as part of the multidisciplinary approach.

When the mental health professional prepares the recommendations for a LCP, all relevant modes of treatment should be considered (Missner & Cohen, 2019). Psychotherapy modalities include a range of therapies, such as supportive therapy, CBT, psychodynamic therapy, biofeedback, hypnotherapy, family therapy, and group therapy. Psychopharmacology is often recommended in patients with chronic or catastrophic illness and this falls under the purview of the psychiatrist or psychiatric nurse. Psychopharmacological interventions should be detailed and specific, including the rationale for the treatment approach and the predicted course of treatment. Side effects of psychotropic medications must be anticipated such as cognitive, attentional, sexual, and metabolic. Interventions to address these side effects must be elucidated. If it is likely that invasive treatments such as electroconvulsive therapy will be required, they should be included in the life care plan. The need for alternative interventional treatments, such as transcranial magnetic stimulation or ketamine infusions for medication resistant depression, should be addressed where relevant. As alternative treatments gain FDA approval, they may be added to the treatment plan where indicated. For example, new expensive medications may become available and preferable, or old drugs may develop new indications, such as with ketamine intravenous infusions or intranasal administration for treatment-resistant depression. The psychiatrist will advise the life care planner on frequency, duration, and the cost of these pharmacological treatments. Specific challenges that the mental health professional may face when creating recommendations for the life care plan include determination of long-term prognosis, developing enduring treatment plans, and detection of malingering. Psychologists can be referred to for neuropsychological testing and evaluation of malingering (Crighton et al., 2015; Zubera et al., 2015). Overall, mental health providers can play a key role in developing a holistic, individualized, and comprehensive life care plan.

Case Study

John is a 23-year-old single man who was diagnosed with schizophrenia at the age of 18. He has been hospitalized twice and attempted suicide at the age of 20. His experiences include auditory hallucinations, delusions, and negative symptoms. The voices he hears often instruct him to do things such as "Don't go outside!" or "Don't eat that food, it's poisoned!" His delusions are mostly of a paranoid nature. He believes that he is monitored by the Central Intelligence Agency through a chip implanted in his ear. When he walks down the street, he feels like others are staring at him. Sometimes he thinks that people are speaking in code about him at the supermarket. John also has a lack of motivation and drive. On a bad day, he stays on the couch for hours, barely moving. He sometimes has difficulty keeping up his hygiene. John often has trouble with his concentration and memory. To overcome this, he carries a small notebook with him everywhere he goes to remind him of things he needs to do such as appointments, grocery shopping, and laundry.

John takes numerous medications daily and requires the use of a medication organization box to keep track of them. Despite this, sometimes he still forgets his medication. John occasionally has delusions about his medications, believing that they are poisoned or hurting his body in some way. He sees his psychiatrist once a month for medication management. He also attends individual and group therapy once a week. John has received social skills training, psychoeducation, and vocational counseling in the past. He lives independently with a roommate, whereas previously he lived in a group home.

Although he had his first break at 18, John did complete high school. He has not had any other formal education. His work history is sporadic, with long periods of unemployment. He has worked as a grocery bagger, stocker, fast-food worker, pizza deliverer, and landscaper. He has morning sedation from his medications and is often late if he must be at work before 11:00 a.m. His chronic lateness resulted in several job terminations. John is currently unemployed but wants to work. He wants to try vocational counseling again because he is having a hard time finding a job on his own.

John receives Social Security Disability Insurance (SSDI) payments and has Medicare. His parents also contribute substantially to his living costs. John's parents want funds set up for when they are deceased, so that John will continue to receive appropriate treatment. They want to hire a life care planner to help them create these plans. Table 22.2 provides a sample life care plan for an individual with schizophrenia based on the format published in the *Life Care Planning and Case Management Handbook* (4th ed.) (Weed & Berens, 2018).

Conclusion

It is important to understand the complexity of mental illness when creating a life care plan. Factors to consider include the expected course of illness, chronicity of symptoms, response to treatment, and community integration. The costliest treatment modality is hospitalization. Individuals with a chronic, disabling course of illness may require multiple hospitalizations or longer-term stays. Treatment nonadherence is a major issue to consider, given that it is a widespread phenomenon and is associated with poorer outcomes and higher costs. While the goal of the life care plan is to prevent complications and to improve QoL, psychiatric disabilities are episodic in nature and thus, will likely involve periods of relapse that require intensive use of services (at intervals) and perhaps hospitalization.

Despite the differences among various mental illnesses in symptoms, treatment, and degree of disability, there are common areas to consider when creating a life care plan for this population. The checklists provided in Table 22.1 and Table 22.3 can help the life care planner cover the various areas required to create a plan for individuals with mental illness. Given the high price of mental illness in both direct costs and quality-of-life issues, life care planning for mental health is a necessary and overlooked resource.

Table 22.2 Example Entries for a Life Care Plan for an individual with Schizophrenia

Medications & Supplies	Time	Frequency	Purpose	Cost	Comment
Antipsychotic	2022–Life Expectancy (LE)	Per dosing recommendations	Treatment of delusions, hallucinations, disorganized speech, disorganized behavior, and negative symptoms	Generic: $15.00–$150.00/month Brand: $600.00–$2,407.00/month Option for Lab costs: $250.00–$500.00/unit monthly or four times a year	As prescribed by treating physicians
Anticonvulsant/Mood Stabilizer	2022–LE	Per dosing recommendations	Augment antipsychotic treatment	Generic: $15.00–$150.00/month Option for Lab costs: $250.00–$500.00/unit monthly or four times a year	As prescribed by treating physicians
Antidepressant	2022–LE	Per dosing recommendations	Treatment of depressive symptoms if present such as hopelessness, sadness, loss of motivation	Generic: $15.00–$150.00/month Brand: $350.00–$500.00/month	As prescribed by treating physicians
Benzodiazepine	2022–LE	Per dosing recommendations	Treatment of anxiety and agitation	Generic: $15.00–$75.00/month	As prescribed by treating physicians
Anticholinergic	2022–LE	Per dosing recommendations	In conjunction with conventional or atypical antipsychotic for side effects	Generic: $15.00–$30.00/month	As prescribed by treating physicians
Medication Organizer	2022–LE	Annually	To assist with pill organization	$5.00–$10.00	

(Continued)

Table 22.2 (Continued)   Example Entries for a Life Care Plan for an individual with Schizophrenia

Acute & Facility Care	Time	Frequency	Purpose	Cost	Comment
Hospitalization	2022–LE	For acute decompensation expect 1–2 weeks for stabilization; additional hospitalizations may be indicated in future	Inpatient treatment; indicated if individual is a threat to himself or others; initiate medications and provide stabilization	$1,250.00–$1,550.00/day	A 1:1 sitter may be needed for the first 24-36 hours.
Option 1 Residential Inpatient Treatment	2022–LE	Expect 1–6 months, depending on symptoms; additional residential treatment may be indicated in the future	Supervised housing and day treatment; indicated if individual is unable to complete activities of daily living (including taking medications as prescribed)	$783.33–$835.00/day	Self - pay rate.
Option 2 Residential living with an Outreach Counselor	2022–LE	This is a common scenario long-term	Live independently but in treatment center housing; includes twice daily visits by an outreach counselor for medication management and/or case management and/or supported employment	$200.00–$255.00/day	Self - pay rate.
Option 3 Residential Living with Limited Outreach	2022–LE	This is a common scenario long-term	Live independently but in treatment center housing; includes once weekly medication management and/or case management and/or supported employment	$125.00/day	Self - pay rate.
Option 4 Day Program	2022–LE	This is a long-term scenario for a person that wants structured activities a few times a week	Day treatment; does not include housing; indicated if individual needs increased daily structure	$150.00–$163.00/day	Self - pay rate.
Option 5 Group Home Supported Employment	2022–LE	Many individuals transition to living with one or two roommates without additional support services Biweekly over worklife expectancy	Living quarters; no treatment provided Support in job search, placement, and maintenance	$45.00 plus/day $100.00–$115.00/encounter	

* Costs are estimates and vary per location and plan (GoodRx, 2022; LuxuryRehab, 2022; Maryland Department of Health, 2018; Senior Living, 2022; Sheppard Pratt, 2022).

Table 22.3 Life Care Plan Checklist for Mental Health

- *Psychotherapeutic Interventions:* What types of therapy will be needed? Are there family or marriage issues that need to be addressed? How complex is the treatment plan? Will a case manager be needed to coordinate care? Are support groups available? Is substance abuse present? If so, what treatments will be needed?

- *Diagnostic Testing:* Often other illnesses need to be ruled out before a diagnosis of mental illness is made, especially in cases where symptoms might overlap with brain abnormalities (e.g., tumors). What tests are needed to rule out other illnesses? Will a psychological battery be needed? What level of education has the individual completed? Is separate educational testing needed as well?

- *Medication/Supply Needs:* Medication regimens can consist of multiple medications at various dosages. Some require blood serum monitoring, which will add to the overall cost. What medications are indicated (including daily dosages and how supplied)? Are they available in generic?

- *Routine Medical Care:* How often will the individual need to see a psychiatrist? In what kind of treatment setting will medication management take place? Will there be regular monitoring by other staff such as nurses? Comorbid conditions are common in people with mental illness. Will annual health checks be performed by medical personnel, including laboratory assessments?

- *Acute and Facility Care:* Is the illness at an acute stage where inpatient treatment is required? What is the expected course of illness? Are multiple hospitalizations likely? What impact do symptoms have on functioning? Is family present in the individual's life? Is the individual capable of independent living? If not, what level of support is required?

- *Vocational/Education Plan:* What is the individual's work history? What vocational services are offered in the geographical area? Has vocational potential been assessed? What are the costs of supported employment?

References

Akechi, T. (2012). Psychotherapy for depression among patients with advanced cancer. *Japanese Journal of Clinical Oncology, 42,* 1113–1119.

American College of Occupational and Environmental Medicine. (2003). ACOEM evidence-based statement. A screening program for depression. *Journal of Occupational and Environmental Medicine, 45*(4), 346–348.

American Psychiatric Association. (2007). *Practice guideline for the treatment of patients with obsessive-compulsive disorder.* Author. https://psychiatryonline.org/pb/assets/raw/sitewide/practice_guidelines/guidelines/ocd-1410197738287.pdf

American Psychiatric Association. (2004, February). *Practice guideline for the treatment of patients with schizophrenia, 2nd edition.* Author. https://psychiatryonline.org/pb/assets/raw/sitewide/practice_guidelines/guidelines/schizophrenia.pdf

American Psychiatric Association. (2009, September). *Guideline watch: Practice guideline for the treatment of patients with schizophrenia.* Author. https://psychiatryonline.org/pb/assets/raw/sitewide/practice_guidelines/guidelines/schizophrenia.pdf

American Psychiatric Association. (2010). *Practice guidelines for the treatment of patients with major depressive disorder.* Author. https://psychiatryonline.org/pb/assets/raw/sitewide/practice_guidelines/guidelines/mdd.pdf

American Psychiatric Association. (2013). *Guideline watch: Practice guideline for the treatment of patients with obsessive-compulsive disorder.* Author. https://psychiatryonline.org/pb/assets/raw/sitewide/practice_guidelines/guidelines/ocd-watch.pdf

American Psychiatric Association. (2021). *Treatment of patients with schizophrenia* (3rd ed.). Author. https://psychiatryonline.org/doi/pdf/10.1176/appi.books.9780890424841

American Psychiatric Association. (2022). *Diagnostic and statistical manual of mental disorders* (5th ed., Text Revision). Author.

American Psychological Association. (2019). *Clinical practice guidelines at a glance.* www.apa.org/monitor/2019/09/ce-corner-guidelines

Anxiety and Depression Association of America. (2022). *Anxiety and stress in the workplace.* https://adaa.org/managing-stress-anxiety-in-workplace/anxiety-disorders-in-workplace

Armbrecht, E., Shah, R., Poorman, G. W., Luo, L., Stephens, J. M., Li, B., Pappadopulos, E., Haider, S., & McIntyre, R. S. (2021). Economic and humanistic burden associated with depression and anxiety among adults with non-communicable chronic diseases (NCCDs) in the United States. *Journal of Multidisciplinary Healthcare, 14*, 887–896.

Baldwin, D. S., Ajel, K., Masdrakis, V. G., Nowak, M., & Rafiq, Z. (2013). Pregabalin for the treatment of generalized anxiety disorder: An update. *Neuropsychiatric Diseases and Treatment, 9*, 883–892.

Barnes, T. R., & Paton, C. (2011). Antipsychotic polypharmacy in schizophrenia: Benefits and risks. *CNS Drugs, 25*(5), 383–399.

Bartles, S. J., & Drake, R. E. (1988). Depressive symptoms in schizophrenia: Comprehensive differential diagnosis. *Comprehensive Psychiatry, 29*, 467–483.

Bell, M. D., Lysaker, P. H., & Milstein, R. M. (1996). Clinical benefits of paid work activity in schizophrenia. *Schizophrenia Bulletin, 22*, 51–67.

Benard, V., Vaiva, G., Masson, M., & Geoffroy, P. A. (2016). Lithium and suicide prevention in bipolar disorder. *Encephale, 42*(3), 234–241.

Bergeson, J. G., Jing, Y., & Forbes, R. A. (2012). Medical care costs and hospitalization in patients with bipolar disorder treated with atypical antipsychotics. *American Health Drug Benefits, 5*(6), 379–386.

Bio, D. S., & Gattaz, W. F. (2011). Vocational rehabilitation improves cognition and negative symptoms in schizophrenia. *Schizophrenia Research, 126*(1–3), 265–269.

Bond, G. R., Drake, R. E., Mueser, K. T., & Becker, D. R. (1997). An update on supported employment for people with severe mental illness. *Psychiatric Services, 48*, 335–346.

Boshen, M. J., Drummond, L. M., & Pillay, A. (2008). Treatment of severe, treatment-refractory obsessive-compulsive disorder. *CNS Spectrums, 13*(12), 1056–1065.

Bowden, C. L. (1996). Rapid cycling among bipolar patients. *Primary Psychiatry, 3*, 40.

British Association for Psychopharmacology. (2016). Evidence-based guidelines for treating bipolar disorder (3rd ed.). *Journal of Psychopharmacology, 30*(6), 495–553.

Bryson, G., Lysaker, P., & Bell, M. (2002). Quality of life benefits of paid work activity in schizophrenia. *Schizophrenia Bulletin, 28*, 249–257.

Buckley, P. F., Miller, B. J., Lehrer, D. S., & Castle, D. J. (2009). Psychiatric comorbidities and schizophrenia. *Schizophrenia Bulletin, 35*(2), 383–402.

Burcusa, S. L., & Iacono, W. G. (2007). Risk for recurrence in depression. *Clinical Psychology Review, 27*(8), 959–985.

Cade, J. F. (1999). Lithium salts in the treatment of psychotic excitement. *Australian and New England Journal of Psychiatry, 33*, 615–618.

Carmona, V. R., Gómez-Benito, J., Huedo-Medina, T. B., & Rojo, J. E. (2017). Employment outcomes for people with schizophrenia spectrum disorder: A meta-analysis of randomized trials. *International Journal of Occupational Medicine and Environmental Health, 30*(3), 345–366.

Cassidy, R. M., Kapczinki, F., & Passos, I. C. (2018). Risk factors of suicidality in patients with schizophrenia: A systematic review, meta-analysis, and meta-regression of 96 studies. *Schizophrenia Bulletin, 44*(4), 787–797.

Center for Behavioral Health Statistics and Quality. (2015). *Behavioral health trends in the United States: Results from the 2014 National Survey on Drug Use and Health* (HHS Publication No. SMA 15-4927, NSDUH Series H-20). www.samhsa.gov/data/

Centers for Disease Control and Prevention. (2022). *Adverse childhood experiences.* www.cdc.gov/violenceprevention/aces/index.html

Chong, H. Y., Teoh, S. L., Wu, B. C. D., Kotirum, S., Chiou, C. F., & Chaiyakunapruk, N. (2016). Global economic burden of schizophrenia: A systematic review. *Neuropsychiatric Disease Treatment*, *12*, 357–373.

Citrome, L., Casey, D. E., & Daniel, D. G. (2004). Adjunctive divalproex and hostility among patients with schizophrenia receiving olanzapine or risperidone. *Psychiatric Services*, *55*, 290–294.

Cloutier, M., Greene, M., Guerin, A., Touya, M., & Wu, E. (2018). The economic burden of bipolar I disorder in the United States in 2015. *Journal Affective Disorders*, *226*, 45–51.

Cohen, S. L., Bikson, M., Badran, B. W., & George, M. S. (2022). A visual and narrative timeline of US FDA milestones for Transcranial Magnetic Stimulation (TMS) devices. *Brain Stimulation*, *15*(1), 73–75.

Cook, J. A., Blyler, C. R., & Burke-Miller, J. K. (2008). Effectiveness of supported employment for individuals with schizophrenia: Results of a multi-site, randomized trial. *Clinical Schizophrenia & Related Psychosis*, *2*, 37–46.

Cook, J. A., Leff, H. S., & Blyler, C. R. (2005). Results of a multisite randomized trial of supported employment interventions for individuals with severe mental illness. *Archives of General Psychiatry*, *62*, 505–512.

Crighton, A., Wygant, D., Holt, K., & Granacher, R. (2015). Embedded effort scales in the repeatable battery for the assessment of neuropsychological status: do they detect neurocognitive malingering? *Archives of Clinical Neuropsychology*, *30*, 181–5.

Dauwan, M., Begemann, M. J. H., Heringa, S. M., & Sommer, I. E. (2016). Exercise improves clinical symptoms, quality of life, global functioning, and depression in schizophrenia: A systematic review and meta-analysis. *Schizophrenia Bulletin*, *42*(3), 588–599.

DeLisis, L. E. 1990. *Depression in schizophrenia*. American Psychiatric Press.

Denys, D., Zohar, J., & Westenberg, H. G. (2004). The role of dopamine in obsessive-compulsive disorder: Preclinical and clinical evidence. *Journal of Clinical Psychiatry*, *65*, 11–17.

Department of Veterans Affairs/Department of Defense. (2016). *Clinical practice guideline for the management of major depressive disorder*. Author. https://www.healthquality.va.gov/guidelines/MH/mdd/VADoDMDDCPGFINAL82916.pdf

Derry, S., & Moore, R. A. (2007). Atypical antipsychotics in bipolar disorder. A systematic review of randomised trials. *BMC Psychiatry*, *7*(40), 1–17.

Dilsaver, S. C. (2011). An estimate of the minimum economic burden of bipolar I and II disorders in the United States: 2009. *Journal Affective Disorders*, *129*(1–3), 79–83.

DuPont, R. L., Rice, D. P., Shiraki, S., & Rowland, C. R. (1995). Economic costs of obsessive-compulsive disorder. *Medicine Interface*, *8*, 102–109.

Edinoff, A., Ruoff, M. T., Ghaffar, Y. T., Rezayev, A., Jani, D., Kaye, A. M., Cornett, E. M., Kaye, A. D., Viswanath, O., & Urits, I. (2020). Cariprazine to treat schizophrenia and bipolar disorder in adults. *Psychopharmacology Bulletin*, *50*(4), 83–117.

Fenske, J. N., & Petersen, K. (2015). Obsessive-compulsive disorder: Diagnosis and management. *American Family Physician*, *92*(10), 896–903.

Ferrari, A. J., Charlson, F. J., & Norman, R. E. (2013). Burden of depressive disorders by country, sex, age, and year: Findings from the global burden of disease study 2010. *PLOS Medicine*, *10*(11), e1001547.

Fischler, G., & Booth, N. (1999). *Vocational impact of psychiatric disorders*. Aspen Publishers.

Fulginiti, A., & Brekke, J. S. (2019). Suicide attempt status and quality of life disparity among individuals with schizophrenia: A longitudinal analysis. *Journal for the Society for Social Work and Research*, *7*(2), 269–288.

Gautam, S., Jain, A., Gautam, M., Vahia, V. N., & Gautam A. (2017). Clinical practice guidelines for the management of generalised anxiety disorder (GAD) and panic disorder (PD). *Indian Journal of Psychiatry*, *59*(S1), S67–S73.

GoodRx. (2022). *Drug prices nationally*. www.GoodRx.com

Goodwin, F. K., & Jamison, K. R. (1990). *Manic-depressive illness*. Oxford University Press.

Greenberg, P. E., Fournier, A. A., Sisitsky, T., Simes, M., Berman, R., Koenigsberg, S. H., & Kessler, R. C. (2021). The economic burden of adults with major depressive disorder in the United States (2010 and 2018). *PharmacoEconomics*, *39*, 653–665.

Halcomb, E., Daly, J., Davidson, P., Elliott, D., & Griffiths, R. (2005). Life beyond severe traumatic injury: An integrative review of the literature. *Australian Critical Care*, *18*, 17–24.

Hama, S., Yamashita, H., Yamawaki, S., & Kurisu, K. (2011). Post-stroke depression and apathy: Interactions between functional recovery, lesion location, and emotional response. *Psychogeriatrics, 11*, 68–76.

Hilligoss, N. (2003). Life care planning for people with severe and persistent mental illness: An overlooked practice setting? *Journal of Life Care Planning, 2*, 56–72.

Hirschfeld, R. M., Lewis, L., & Vornik, L. A. (2003). Perceptions and impact of bipolar disorder: How far have we really come? Results of the National Depressive and Manic-Depressive Association 2000 survey of individuals with bipolar disorder. *Journal of Clinical Psychiatry, 64*, 161–174.

Hoffman, J. M., Bombardier, C. H., Graves, D. E., Kalpakjian, C. Z., & Krause, J. S. (2011). A longitudinal study of depression from 1 to 5 years after spinal cord injury. *Archives of Physical Medicine and Rehabilitation, 92*, 411–8.

Hollander, E., Stein, D. J., & Kwon, J. H. (1997). Psychosocial function and economic costs of obsessive-compulsive disorder. *CNS Spectrums, 3*(S1), 48–58.

Holmes, J. D., & House, A. O. (2000). Psychiatric illness in hip fractures. *Age and Aging, 29*, 537–546.

Horowitz, A., & Reinhardt, J. P. (2006). Adequacy of the mental health system in meeting the needs of adults who are visually impaired. *Journal of the Visually Impaired and Blind, 100*, 871–874.

Hostiuc, S., Rusu, M. C., Negoi, I., & Drima, E. (2018). Decision-making competence of schizophrenia patients in clinical trials: A meta-analysis and meta-regression. *BMC Psychiatry, 18*(2), 1–11.

Hudson, T. J., Sullivan, G., Feng, W., Owen, R. R., & Thrush, C. R. (2003). Economic evaluations of novel antipsychotic medications: A literature review. *Schizophrenia Research, 60*, 199–218.

Ji, P., Reynolds, J., Menditto, A., Beck, N., & Stuve, P. R. (2018). Differences in symptom severity and independent living skills between re-hospitalized and not re-hospitalized individuals with schizophrenia: A longitudinal study. *Community Mental Health Journal, 54*(7), 978–982.

Kamali, M., Krishnamurthy, V. B., Baweja, R., Saunders, E. F. H., & Gelenberg, A. J. (2017). Lithium. In A. F. Schatzberg & C. B. Nemeroff (Eds.), *Textbook of psychopharmacology* (5th ed., pp.889–922). American Psychiatric Association Publishing.

Kane, J. M., Honigfeld, G., Singer, J., & Meltzer, H. (1988). Clozapine for the treatment-resistant schizophrenic. *Archives of General Psychiatry, 45*, 789–796.

Keller, M. B., Trivedi, M. H., & Thase, M. E. (2007). The prevention of recurrent episodes of depression with venlafaxine for two years (PREVENT) study: Outcomes from the 2-year and combined maintenance phases. *Journal of Clinical Psychiatry, 8*, 1246–1256.

Kendler, K. S. (2020). The development of Kraepelin's concept of dementia praecox. A close reading of relevant texts. *JAMA Psychiatry, 77*(11), 1181–1187.

Kessler, R. C., Berglund, P., & Demler, O. (2005a). Lifetime prevalence and age-of-onset distributions of DSM-IV disorders in the national comorbidity survey replication. *Archives of General Psychiatry, 62*(6), 593–602.

Kessler, R. C., Chiu, W. T., Demler, O., & Walters, E. E. (2005b). Prevalence, severity, and comorbidity of 12-month DSM-IV disorders in the national comorbidity survey replication. *Archives of General Psychiatry, 62*, 617–627.

Konnopka, A., & König, H. (2020). Economic burden of anxiety disorders: A systematic review and meta-analysis. *Meta-Analysis Pharmacoeconomics, 38*(1), 25–37.

Landreth, G. L. (2012). *Play therapy: The art of the relationship* (3rd ed.). Routledge.

Larson, M. K., Walker, E. F., & Compton, M. T. (2010). Early signs, diagnosis, and therapeutics of the prodromal phase of schizophrenia and related psychotic disorders. *Expert Review of Neurotherapeutics, 10*(8), 1347–1359.

Lay, B., Blanz, B., Hartmann, M., & Schmidt, M. H. (2000). The psychosocial outcome of adolescent-onset schizophrenia: A 12-year follow up. *Schizophrenia Bulletin, 26*(4), 801–806.

Li, J., McCombs, J. S., & Stimmel, G. L. (2002). Cost of treating bipolar disorder in the California Medicaid (Medi-Cal) program. *Journal of Affective Disorders, 71*, 131–139.

Lieberman, J. A., Stroup, T. S., & McEvoy, J. P. (2005). Effectiveness of antipsychotic drugs in patients with chronic schizophrenia. *New England Journal of Medicine, 353*, 1209–1223.

LuxuryRehab. (2022). *Pricing*. https://luxuryrehabs.com/condition/depression/

MacDonald-Wilson, K. L., Rogers, E. S., Massaro, J. M., Lyass, A., & Crean, T. (2002). An investigation of reasonable workplace accommodations for people with psychiatric disabilities: Quantitative findings from a multi-site study. *Community Mental Health Journal, 38*(1), 35–50.

Macy, A. S., Theo, J. N., Kaufmann, S. C. C., Ghazzaoui, R. B., Pawlowski, P. A., Fakhry, H. I., Cassmassi, B. J., & IsHak, W. W. (2013). Quality of life in obsessive compulsive disorder. *CNS Spectrums, 18*(1), 21–33.

Manning, J. S., Haykal, R. F., Connor, P. D., & Akiskal, H. S. (1997). On the nature of depressive and anxious states in a family practice setting: The high prevalence of bipolar II and related disorders in a cohort followed longitudinally. *Comprehensive Psychiatry, 38*, 102–108.

Marangell, L. B., Dennehy, E. B., & Miyahara, S. (2009). The functional impact of subsyndromal depressive symptoms in bipolar disorder: Data from STEP-BD. *Journal of Affective Disorders, 114*(1–3), 58–67.

March, J. S., Frances, A., Carpenter, D., & Kahn, D. A. (1997). The expert consensus guidelines for the treatment of obsessive-compulsive disorder. *Journal of Clinical Psychiatry, 58*, 2–72.

Marwaha, S., Durrani, A., & Singh, S. (2013). Employment outcomes for people with bipolar disorder: A systematic review. *Acta Psychiatrica Scandinavica, 128*(3), 179–193.

Maryland Department of Health. (2018). Mental hygiene regulations. *Maryland Register, 45*(7), 357–393. https://health.maryland.gov/regs/Pages/10-21-25-Fee-Schedule-—-Mental-Health-Services-—-Community-Based-Programs-and-Individual-Practitioners-(BEHAVIORAL-HEALTH-A.aspx

Matsuoka, Y., Nishi, D., Nakajima, S., Kim, Y., Homma, M., & Otomo, Y. (2008). Incidence and prediction of psychiatric morbidity after a motor vehicle accident in Japan: The Tachikawa Cohort of Motor Vehicle Accident Study. *Critical Care Medicine, 36*, 74–80.

McEvoy, J. P., Scheifler, P. L., & Frances, A. (Eds.). (1999). The expert consensus guideline series: Treatment of schizophrenia. *Journal of Clinical Psychiatry, 60*, 3–80.

McKenzie Smith, M., Pinto Pereira, S., Chan, L., Rose, C., & Shafran, R. (2018). Impact of well-being interventions for siblings of children and young people with a chronic physical or mental health condition: A systematic review and meta-analysis. *Clinical Child & Family Psychology Review, 21*(2), 246–265.

Mental Health America. (2021). *The state of mental health in America*. Author. https://www.mhanational.org/research-reports/2021-state-mental-health-america

Metcalfe, J. D., Riley, J., McGurk, S., Hale, T., Drake, R. E., & Bond, G. R. (2018). Comparing the predictors of employment in Individual Placement and Support: A longitudinal analysis. *Psychiatry Research, 264*, 85–90.

Missner, S. C., & Cohen, Z. E. (2019). The impact of the psychiatrist on the life care plan. *The Journal of the American Academy of Psychiatry and the Law, 47*(2), 208–216.

Moltrecht, B., Deighton, J., Patalay, P., & Edbrooke-Childs, J. (2021). Effectiveness of current psychological interventions to improve emotion regulation in youth: A meta-analysis. *European Child & Adolescent Psychiatry, 30*(6), 829–848.

Morina, N., Stam, K., Pollet, T. V., & Priebe, S. (2018). Prevalence of depression and posttraumatic stress disorder in adult civilian survivors of war who stay in war afflicted regions: a systematic review and meta-analysis of epidemiological studies. *Journal of Affective Disorders, 239*, 328–38.

Mueller, T. I., Leon, A. C., & Keller, K. B. (1999). Recurrence after recovery from major depressive disorder during 15 years of observational follow-up. *American Journal of Psychiatry, 156*, 1000–1006.

National Alliance on the Mentally Ill. (2014). *Road to recovery: Employment and mental illness*. Author. https://www.nami.org/Support-Education/Publications-Reports/Public-Policy-Reports/RoadtoRecovery#:~:text=Acknowledgements%20and%20Gratitude,Katrina%20Gay%20and%20Jessica%20Hart.

National Institute for Health and Care and Excellence. (2014). *Bipolar disorder: Assessment and management clinical guideline*. Author. https://www.nice.org.uk/guidance/conditions-and-diseases/mental-health-behavioural-and-neurodevelopmental-conditions/bipolar-disorder

National Institute of Mental Health. (2022a). *Major depression*. www.nimh.nih.gov/health/statistics/major-depression

National Institute of Mental Health. (2022b). *Bipolar disorder*. www.nimh.nih.gov/health/statistics/bipolar-disorder

National Institute of Mental Health. (2022c). *Schizophrenia*. www.nimh.nih.gov/health/statistics/schizophrenia

Newton-John, T. R. (2014). Negotiating the maze: Risk factors for suicidal behavior in chronic pain patients. *Current Pain Headache Reports, 18*, 1–7.

Novick, K. K., & Novick, J. (2005). *Working with parents makes therapy work*. Rowman & Littlefield Publishers, Inc.

O'Day, K., Rajagopalan, K., Meyer, K., Pikalov, A., & Loebel, A. (2013). Long-term effectiveness of atypical antipsychotics in the treatment of adults with schizophrenia in the U.S. *Clinicoeconomics Outcomes Research, 5*, 459–470.

Oruch, R., Elderbi, M. A., Khattab, H. A., Pryme, I. F., & Lund, A. (2014). Lithium: A review of pharmacology, clinical uses, and toxicity. *European Journal of Pharmacology, 5*(740), 464–473.

Pagnin, D., Querioz, V., Pini, S., & Cassano, G. B. (2004). Efficacy of ECT in depression: A meta-analytic review. *Journal of ECT, 20*, 13–20.

Pan, Y., Knapp, M., & McCrone, P. (2012). Cost-effectiveness comparisons between antidepressant treatments in depression: Evidence from database analyses and prospective studies. *Journal of Affective Disorders, 139*, 113–125.

Papakostas, G. I., Shelton, R. C., & Smith, J. (2007). Augmentation of antidepressants with atypical antipsychotic medications for treatment-resistant major depressive disorder: A meta-analysis. *Journal of Clinical Psychiatry, 68*, 826–831.

Phifer, L. W., Crowder, A. K., Elsenraat, T., & Hull, R. (2020). *CBT toolbox for children & adolescents*. Pesi Publishing & Media.

Pies, R. W. (1998). *Handbook of essential psychopharmacology*. American Psychiatric Press.

Pollock, K., Dorstyn, D., Butt, L., & Prentice, S. (2017). Posttraumatic stress following spinal cord injury: A systematic review of risk and vulnerability factors. *Spinal Cord, 55*, 800–811.

Poulsen, R., Hoff, A., Fisker, J., Hjorthøj, C. & Eplov, L. F. (2017). Integrated mental health care and vocational rehabilitation to improve return to work rates for people on sick leave because of depression and anxiety (the Danish IBBIS trial): Study protocol for a randomized controlled trial. *Trials, 18*, 578.

Powers, M., Becker, E., Gorman, J., Kissen, D., & Smits, J. (2015). *GAD Clinical Practice Review Task Force Clinical practice review for GAD. Anxiety and Depression Association of America*. https://adaa.org/resources-professionals/practice-guidelines-gad

Price, L. H., Charney, D. S., & Heninger, G. R. (1986). Variability of response to lithium augmentation in refractory depression. *American Journal of Psychiatry, 143*, 1387–1392.

Racine, N., McArthur, B. A., Cooke, J. E., Eirich, R., Zhu, J., & Madigan, S. (2021). Global prevalence of depressive and anxiety symptoms in children and adolescents during COVID-19: A meta-analysis. *JAMA Pediatrics, 175*(11), 1142–1150.

Rao, M. D. (2002). Psychiatric aspects of traumatic brain injury. *Psychiatric Clinics of North America, 25*, 43–69.

Robins, L. N., & Reiger, D. A. (1991). *Psychiatric disorders in America: The epidemiologic catchment study*. Free Press.

Romera, I., Perez, V., & Ciudad, A. (2013). Residual symptoms and functioning in depression, does the type of residual symptoms matter? A post-hoc analysis. *BMC Psychiatry, 13*, 51.

Rush, A. J. (2003). Toward an understanding of bipolar disorder and its origin. *Journal of Clinical Psychiatry, 64*, 4–8.

Sajatovic, M., Coconcea, N., & Ignacio, R.V. (2008). Adjunct extended-release valproate semisodium in late life schizophrenia. *International Journal of Geriatric Psychiatry, 23*(2), 142–147.

Sanchez-Moreno, J., Martinez-Aran, A., & Taberes-Seisdedos, R. (2009). Functioning and disability in bipolar disorder: An extensive review. *Psychotherapy and Psychosomatics, 78*, 285–297.

Senior Living. (2022). *Nursing home costs*. www.seniorliving.org/nursing-homes/costs/

Shelton, R. C., Tollefson, G. D., & Stahl, S. (2001). A novel augmentation strategy for treating resistant major depression. *American Journal of Psychiatry, 158*, 131–134.

Sheppard Pratt. (2022). *Pricing and payment at The Retreat*. www.sheppardpratt.org/care-finder/the-retreat/pricing-payment/

Shirneshan, E. (2013). *Cost of illness study of anxiety disorders for the ambulatory adult population of the United States*. University of Tennessee Health Science Center. UTHSC Digital Commons.

Steadman, K., & Taskila, T. (2015). *Symptoms of depression and their effects on employment*. The Work Foundation. www.base-uk.org/sites/default/files/knowledge/Symptoms%20of%20depression%20and%20their%20effects%20on%20employment/382_symptoms_of_depression_final.pdf

Steigelmar, R., McKee, M. D., Waddell, J. P., & Schemitsch, E. H. (2001). Outcome of foot injuries in multiply injured patients. *Orthopedic Clinics of North America, 32*, 193–204.

Strassnig, M., Kotov, R., Fochtmann, L., Kalin, M., Bromet, E. J., & Harvey, P. D. (2018). Associations of independent living and labor force participation with impairment indicators in schizophrenia and bipolar disorder at 20-year follow-up. *Schizophrenia Research*, *197*, 150–155.

Suppes, T., Kroger, H., Pikalov, A., & Loebel, A. (2016). Lurasidone adjunctive with lithium or valproate for bipolar depression: A placebo-controlled trial utilizing prospective and retrospective enrolment cohorts. *Journal of Psychiatric Research*, *10*, 86–93.

Tarakad, A., & Jimenez-Shahed, J. (2018). VMAT2 Inhibitors in neuropsychiatric disorders. *CNS Drugs*, *32*(12), 1131–1144.

Trivedi, M. H., Fava, M., & Wisniewski, S. R. (2006). Medication augmentation after the failure of SSRIs for depression. *New England Journal of Medicine*, *354*, 1243–1252.

Tseng, P-T., Chen, Y-W., Lin, P-Y., Tu, K-Y., Wang, H-Y., Cheng, Y-S., Chang, Y-C., Chang, C-H., Chung, W., & Wu, C-K. (2016). Significant treatment effect of adjunct music therapy to standard treatment on the positive, negative, and mood symptoms of schizophrenic patients: A meta-analysis. *BMC Psychiatry*, *16*, 1–11.

Tsuang, M. (2000). Schizophrenia: Genes and environment. *Biological Psychiatry*, *47*(3), 210–220.

U.S. Burden of Disease Collaborators. (2013). The state of U.S. health, 1990–2010: Burden of diseases, injuries, and risk factors. *JAMA*, *310*(6), 591–606.

U.S. Equal Employment Opportunities Commission. (2008). *ADA Amendments Act of 2008*. www.eeoc.gov/statutes/ada-amendments-act-2008

Vallarino, M., Henry, C., & Etain, B. (2015). An evidence map of psychosocial interventions for the earliest stages of bipolar disorder. *Lancet Psychiatry*, *2*(6), 548–563.

Vasudev, K., Macritchie, K., Geddes, J., Watson, S., & Young, A. (2006). Topiramate for acute affective episodes in bipolar disorder. *Cochrane Database System Review*, *25*, CD003384.

Vermaes, I. P., van Susante, A. M., & van Bakel, H. J. (2012). Psychological functioning of siblings in families of children with chronic health conditions: A meta-analysis. *Journal of Pediatric Psychology*, *37*(2), 166–184.

Wang, P. W., Santosa, C., & Schumacher, M. (2002). Gabapentin augmentation therapy in bipolar depression. *Bipolar Disorder*, *4*, 296–301.

Weed, R., & Field, T. (2001). *The rehabilitation consultant's handbook* (3rd ed.). E&F Publications.

Weed, R., & Berens, D. E. (2018). *Life care planning and case management handbook* (4th ed.). Routledge.

Woo, T. U. W., Canuso, C. M., Wojcik, J. D., Noordsy, D., Brunette, M. F., & Green, A. I. (2017). Treatment of schizophrenia. In A. F. Schatzberg & C. B. Nemeroff (Eds.), *Textbook of psychopharmacology* (5th ed., pp.1241–1282). American Psychiatric Association Publishing.

Yohannan, J., & Carlson, J. S. (2019). A systematic review of school-based interventions and their outcomes for youth exposed to traumatic events. *Psychology in the Schools*, *56*(3), 447–464.

Zaretsky, A. E., Segal, S. V., & Gemar, M. (1999). Cognitive therapy for bipolar depression: A pilot study. *Canadian Journal of Psychiatry*, *44*, 491–494.

Zubera, A., Raza, M., Holaday, E., & Aggarwal, R. (2015). Screening for malingering in the emergency department. *Academy of Psychiatry*, *39*, 233–4.

Chapter 23

Life Care Planning for the Patient with Chronic Pain

Jarna R. Shah, Carrie Hyde, Gregory Lawson Smith,
Jaleesa Jackson, Chiedozie Uwandu, and
Johnathan H. Goree

The evaluation, management, and treatment of chronic pain is extremely challenging. There are a multitude of factors that contribute to this challenge. The first of which is the difficulty in evaluation. By its definition, pain is a personal subjective experience that cannot be divorced from innate biological, psychological, and/or social factors (Raja et al., 2020). Unlike hypertension, diabetes, or even physical injuries, objective assessment can only provide certain insights into the chronic pain patient's experience.

The second is the looming opioid epidemic. Since 1999, over 841,000 people in the United States have died from a drug overdose. Over 70% of those deaths have involved an opioid (Centers for Disease Control, 2020). Unfortunately, the statistics are not improving. It was estimated in 2021 that nearly 108,000 people died from overdoses (Centers for Disease Control, 2020). The Centers for Disease Control (CDC) has published guidelines to stem the tide (Dowell et al., 2016), but unfortunately, they have been ineffective and have offered little specific guidance on alternative treatment options. Also, some of the guidance seems arbitrary, leading to unnecessary weaning of opioids, increase in illicit drug use, and lack of acute and chronic pain treatment in primary care (Pergolizzi et al., 2019). The effects on public health, mental health, and access have been far reaching.

Cost is also a significant challenge. It has been estimated that 87% of patients suffer from low back pain at some point in their life (Deyo & Tsui-Wu, 1987). More specifically, the one year incidence of a first episode of low back pain ranges between 6.3–15.4% with a remission episode after one year at 54–90% (Hoy et al., 2010). In 2016, low back pain and neck pain were the most expensive diagnoses in the United States (Dieleman et al., 2020). An estimated $134.5 billion dollars were spent on patients in the United States with these conditions (Dieleman et al., 2020).

Another challenge is that surgical interventions are not always effective. In one study, the prevalence of post-spine surgery chronic pain was as high as 60% (Garcia et al., 2015). In the same study, the prevalence of residual post-surgical neuropathic pain was 89.9%. Post elective orthopedic procedures are also not encouraging. Up to 20% of total knee arthroscopy patients are dissatisfied due to pain and immobility (Pua et al., 2019).

Diagnostic Workup of Chronic Pain

A thorough history is a valuable tool when first beginning a patient workup. It provides the framework for building a differential diagnosis, which then guides treatment options. It includes the following and is not limited to:

- When did the pain begin and where is it located?
- Does it radiate in a specific direction?
- How is the pain described (i.e., sharp, dull, aching)?
- Is there associated numbness, tingling, and/or weakness?
- How is it rated on a scale from zero to ten?
- Does it impair functionality?
- Which inciting factors aggravate and alleviate the pain?
- Are there certain activities (i.e., standing, sitting, walking) that are associated with the pain symptoms?
- Are there any new changes in weakness, numbness, or strength?
- Does the patient have any bowel or bladder incontinence, and if so, for how long?
- What previous medications have been tried, and what were their degrees of effect?
- What prior treatment options/interventions have been trialed?

Other important history findings include medical comorbidities, psychiatric/psychological history, laboratory findings review, past surgeries, and social history. One must also consider if the patient is taking antiplatelet or anticoagulant therapy, and if they are currently on any medications for treating systemic infections, such as antibiotics.

For patients with cognitive impairments or disabilities, other important metrics include speaking with caregivers or family members to assess level of functionality. Is the patient sleeping well? Are they able to move around during the day without grimacing or wincing? Do they notice them favor a particular side when transferring between positions?

A full physical exam is integral to a proper workup for a patient with chronic pain. This includes an examination of the affected painful areas. One can assess the distribution of pain both subjectively and with objective physical examination maneuvers. Testing both sensory and motor strength of the upper and lower extremities is also important. Radiologic review may also be beneficial. This includes and it not limited to plain film x-rays, computed tomography (CT) scans, magnetic resonance imaging (MRI), myelograms, and nerve conduction velocity tests. An MRI is not appropriate for all patients (for example, in the presence of ferromagnetic foreign bodies or pacemakers). The American College of Radiology (ACR) is a good resource to determine whether further imaging is required or warranted in the presence of certain history and physical exam findings (American College of Radiology, n.d.).

While chronic pain assessment tools like Patient-Reported Outcomes Measurement Information System (PROMIS) scoring (Pope et al., 2021) and the Brief Pain Inventory (Chiarotto et al., 2019) provide some assistance, the visual analog scale and numeric rating scale are still the gold standard for pain assessments (Chiarotto et al., 2019).

Psychological Considerations of Pain

Pain is an incredibly complex phenomenon and difficult for physicians to control due to biological, psychological, and social factors and the heterogeneity in various treatments. In addition to decreased productivity, global disability, and uncontrolled persistent pain, chronic pain often co-occurs with behavioral health conditions, including mental and substance use disorders (Hooten, 2016). Suicidal ideation is also a common occurrence in persons with chronic pain.

The relationship between chronic pain (defined as pain longer than 3 months or longer than normal tissue healing) and depression/anxiety is bidirectional, as having either disorder increases the risk of developing the other condition (Bondesson, 2018). This relationship between pain and mental health disorders has been shown to share neural pathways, via functional imaging studies (Hooten, 2016). Pain is strongly associated with depression onset and relapse. A key factor that frequently complicates the diagnosis of depression is comorbid chronic pain, as patients presenting with pain are more likely to be investigated medically rather than as a broad biopsychosocial framework (Jaracz et al., 2016). Within this broad biopsychosocial model of pain, the fear-avoidance model explains the temporal relationship of chronic pain and behavioral response, which are important targets for treatment. First line non-drug interventions for a patient with chronic pain and concomitant depression include cognitive behavioral therapy (CBT), acceptance-based therapies, and multidisciplinary pain rehabilitation. Pharmacologic interventions should also be considered, and first line agents to consider include serotonin-norepinephrine reuptake inhibitors, tricyclic antidepressants, and anticonvulsants, which have indications for both pain and depression (Hooten, 2016). It is of paramount importance that clinicians pay attention to and treat both conditions to optimize pain outcomes.

The co-occurrence of post-traumatic stress disorder (PTSD) and chronic pain negatively impacts the course of both disorders and patients with both experience greater emotional distress, physical pain, and disability than those with either chronic pain or PTSD alone (Otis et al., 2003). There is evidence that suggests the interplay between PTSD and chronic pain has biologic/genetic and environmental factors. It is therefore important to screen for PTSD in patients with chronic pain to improve treatment outcomes and reduce long-term healthcare utilization (Gasperi et al., 2021).

Opioid Management

It is recommended that long-term opioids should not routinely be used for chronic pain. The clinical evidence does not support long-term (> 1 year) benefits to opioid therapy for chronic pain. Opioids should only be used when the benefits outweigh the risks, when there is low risk for substance abuse, and when other therapies (multi-modal non-pharmacologic treatments) have failed to provide adequate improvement in function. When initiating or titrating opioids, it is important to continue using medications and therapies in conjunction with the addition of opioids. Firstly, immediate release formulations should be used at the lowest effective dose. Extended release or long-acting opioids are reserved for persons who are considered to need long-term treatment for their pain. The latest CDC guidelines (Dowell et al., 2016) are to use caution with using more than 50 MME (morphine milliequivalent) per day due to the increased risk of addiction and overdose at doses greater than 50 MME. That being said, it is important to take each case and individualize it between the patient and their physician/prescriber. Generally speaking, after initiating opioids, it is imperative for close follow-up and reasonable to increase dosage by 50% until function improvement is achieved. If this is not achieved, it is reasonable to dose reduce and stop opioids. While all patients with non-cancer pain should be considered for dose reduction, a few of the populations who may not be good candidates for dose reductions are those with severe nociceptive pain (inflammatory arthritis, inflammatory bowel disease, sickle-cell related pain) and inflammatory or injury-related neuropathic pain (autoimmune demyelinating disorders, spinal cord injuries, complex regional pain syndrome, chemotherapy-induced neuropathy, and some phantom pain).

Complementary Medicine

Chinese Medicine

Acupuncture is defined by the Oxford Dictionary (2020) as "a system of integrative medicine that involves pricking the skin or tissues with needles, used to alleviate pain and to treat various physical, mental, and emotional conditions." The traditional Chinese medicine definition explains acupuncture as a technique for balancing the flow of energy or life force, known as Qi "chee," believed to flow through pathways (meridians) in your body. By inserting needles into specific points along these meridians, we believe that energy flow will re-balance. Studies have shown mixed results due to the difficulty with research, but acupuncture is very low risk and should be in the algorithm for adjuvant pain management. It is postulated that it is effective due to a strong placebo effect. It has been shown to have benefits in low back pain (Rubinstein et al., 2010), knee osteoarthritis (Berman et al., 2004), chronic headache/migraine (Linde et al., 2016), shoulder pain, and musculoskeletal pain.

Yoga

Yoga was developed in ancient India as a practice to unite the mind and body. There are many branches of yoga. All yoga styles can help balance your body, mind, and spirit, but they achieve it in various ways. Yoga therapy is defined as the application of Yogic principles to a particular person with the objective of achieving a particular spiritual, psychological, or physiologic goal. In a meta-analysis performed in 2012, looking at 16 trials, yoga slightly improved pain associated disability in pain conditions, including migraine, rheumatoid arthritis, and low back pain (Büssing et al., 2012). It can be recommended as a nonpharmacologic therapy option for low back pain.

Medical Cannabis

The use of cannabis and cannabinoids for chronic pain is controversial both legally and socially. Use of medical cannabis for pain is varied and dependent on several factors including state legalities, federal restrictions, and access to substances. Multiple trials and systemic reviews have reported mixed results on the efficacy for chronic pain. A 2017 report, *The Health Effects of Cannabis and Cannabinoids: The Current State of Evidence and Recommendations for Research*, found evidence of significant chronic pain reduction with use of cannabis or cannabinoids. In a 2018 meta-analysis of 47 randomized control trials of cannabis use for various types of chronic pain, there was moderate evidence that cannabis reduced pain by 30%, however adverse events were high (Stockings et al., 2018). Studies are difficult due to multiple available concentration strengths and methods of delivery. At the time of writing this book chapter, availability of cannabis and cannabinoids is increasing as more and more states are legalizing medical cannabis. It is highly likely that patients are going to seek approval or recommendations for the use of cannabidiol (CBD) or cannabis for use of their chronic pain or other medical conditions.

Axial/Non-Surgical Back Pain and Spinal Stenosis

Low back pain has a lifetime incidence of 51–84% and is a leading cause of disability globally (Hooten & Cohen, 2015). Low back pain is traditionally further classified as axial or radicular. Axial back pain is classified as non-radiating pain centered in the low back. Radicular back pain often radiates to the lower extremities in a dermatomal fashion (Hooten & Cohen, 2015). After an appropriate history, physical, and diagnostic workup is performed, the etiology of low back pain can be determined. Common causes of axial low back pain include:

1. Myofascial pain, evidenced by taut painful bands in muscle, fascia, or tendons
2. Facet-mediated pain, from osteoarthritis of the lumbar facet joints
3. Discogenic back pain from degeneration of intervertebral discs
4. Sacroiliitis from inflammation of the sacro-iliac joints
5. Spinal stenosis, a reduction in available space for neural elements due to degenerative changes

Management of Axial Low Back Pain

After an appropriate diagnosis has been made, management typically will begin with conservative measures. If pain persists even after a course of conservative treatment, interventions in the form of injections may be performed. Lumbar spinal stenosis is a very common condition in the elderly patient and has been found to be one of the most frequent reasons to perform spinal surgery in the elderly (Szpalski & Gunzburg, 2003).

Conservative Management/Physical Therapy

Pharmacologic management of axial back pain and spinal stenosis may include the use of acetaminophen, non-steroidal anti-inflammatory agents, gabapentin, pregabalin, and low dose opioids. Special consideration should be given to the use of these agents in the elderly population, due to cardiovascular, renal, and neurologic side effects (Lafian & Torralba, 2018). Due to the changes in physiology that occur with age, older adults may be more susceptible to adverse reactions and toxicities of these medications, particularly opioids (Brooks & Udoji, 2016). Physical therapy is widely used in the management of low back pain. Goals should be targeted to include core strengthening, posture correction, and increased stability (Lafian & Torralba, 2018).

Injection Therapy

Interventions can be quite helpful to alleviate pain while also avoiding the side effects of medications for pain. This is of great benefit to the elderly, as interventions may lead to a reduction of the use of oral medications, potentially decreasing side effects (Brooks & Udoji, 2016).

Lumbar epidural steroid injections

Lumbar epidural steroid injections (ESIs) are the most common intervention for pain worldwide (Cohen et al., 2013). They may be used for the treatment of pain from lumbar radiculitis, lumbar disc herniation, and spinal stenosis, among other diagnoses. A recent comprehensive review focused on reviewing the safety and efficacy of these injections found that there was a modest improvement

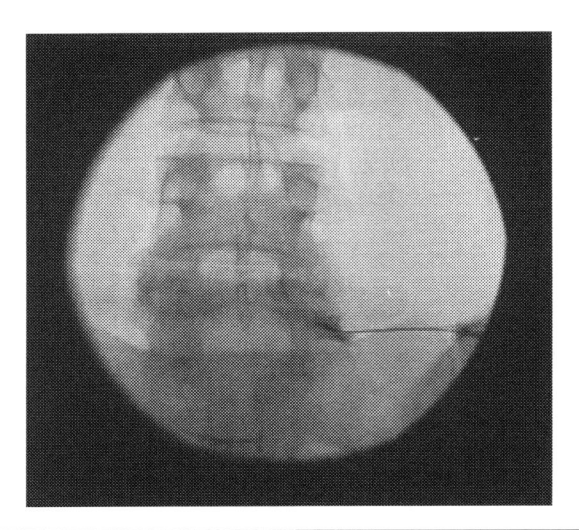

Figure 23.1 Transforaminal Epidural Steroid Injection

in pain lasting less than three months in appropriately selected individuals (Cohen et al., 2013). In this procedure, fluoroscopy is used to inject steroids with or without local anesthetic into the epidural space. Injection may be performed using an interlaminar, transforaminal, or caudal approach. There is no evidence for the ideal number of ESIs, thus the course of treatment should be tailored to each patient effects (Brooks & Udoji, 2016).

The sacroiliac joint (SIJ) is a diarthrodial joint at the junction of the sacrum and ilium effects (Brooks & Udoji, 2016). It is responsible for absorbing shock and transferring loads from the axial spine to the lower extremities (Rashbaum et al., 2016). Current literature has shown that SIJ pain may be the cause of low back pain in as much as 30% of patients (Rashbaum et al., 2016). If conservative therapy is not efficacious, sacroiliac joint injections can be performed. This injection is performed under fluoroscopy, using a small needle to access the joint. Local anesthetic steroid is then injected after confirmation of needle placement (Rashbaum et al., 2016). See Figure 23.2 for SIJ. Studies have been performed to determine the innervation of the SIJ. A recent cadaveric study found that innervation of the SIJ is supplied by the lateral branches of the posterior rami from L5–S4 (Roberts et al., 2014). Thus SIJ rhizotomy of these nerves can also be considered for longer term management of SIJ pain.

The lumbar facet joints are a common cause of axial back pain. In a study to determine the prevalence of lumbar facet joint pain among 100 adults, lumbar facet joint pain was prevalent in 30% of adults, and 52% in the elderly (Manchikanti et al., 2001). These joints serve to connect the vertebral arch of one vertebra to the adjacent vertebra. The joint contains synovial fluid, a cartilaginous surface, and a fibrous capsule (Cohen & Raja, 2007). Together with the intervertebral discs, these joints provide stability to the spine and serve to prevent injury (Cohen & Raja, 2007). Pain from the upper lumbar facets can refer to the thigh, hip and flank, while the lower lumbar facets can refer to the low back and, in some cases, the lateral leg. Injections can be performed directly into the facet joint using local anesthetic and/or steroid; however, the joint capsules are very small, and after injecting 1–2 cc of fluid, the capsules may rupture. See Figure 23.3 for lumbar facet injection.

Medial branch blocks are diagnostic blocks performed to determine whether facet joints are pain generators. This procedure is performed under fluoroscopy, during which the medial

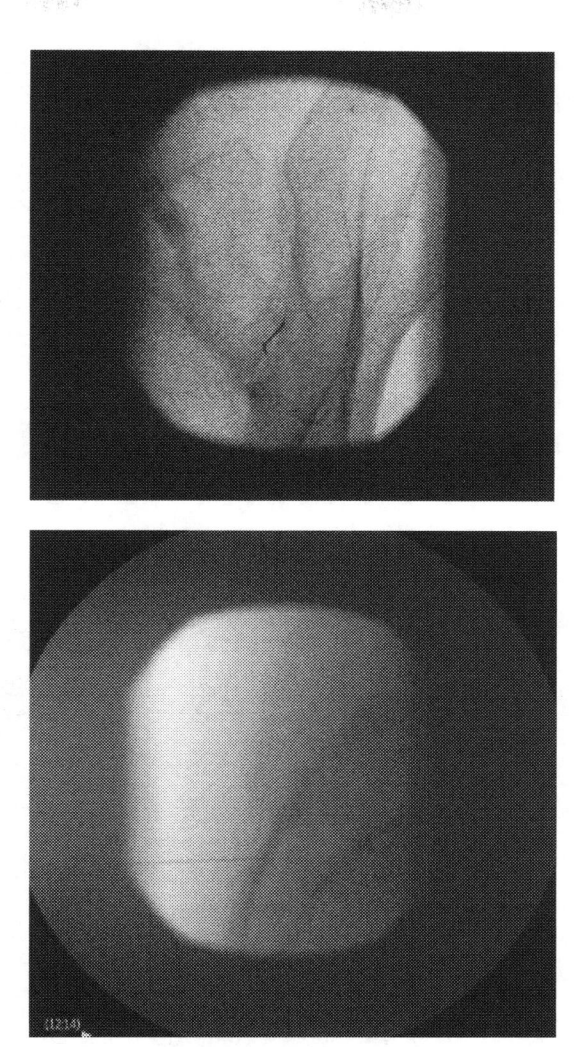

Figure 23.2 Sacroiliac Joint Injections

branch innervating the suspected facet joint(s) is anesthetized with a small amount of local anesthetic. If the pain generating lumbar facet is successfully anesthetized with the diagnostic block, a radiofrequency ablation of the medial branch nerves may be performed to provide longer lasting relief (Brooks & Udoji, 2016).

Traditionally, if conservative management options for spinal stenosis have been unsuccessful, surgical options including laminectomy, fusion, and discectomy were often the next step. However, there has been increased interest in the use of minimally invasive surgical approaches to minimize risks such as blood loss, tissue trauma, and improve recovery time. One such option is the minimally invasive lumbar decompression (MILD) procedure.

This procedure can be considered for patients with spinal stenosis and neurogenic claudication (i.e., low back or lower extremity pain that is worse with standing, ambulation, and improves with rest). The MILD procedure involves the decompression of stenosis by removing small amounts of

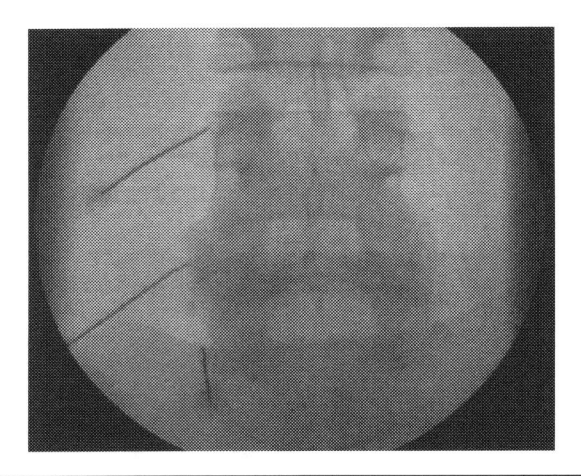

Figure 23.3 Lumbar Facet Injections

hypertrophic ligamentum flavum that contribute to stenosis (Mekhail et al., 2012). This leads to decreased intraspinal pressures and reduction of claudication symptoms. There should be radiologic evidence of lumbar spinal stenosis and ligamentum flavum hypertrophy greater than 2.5 mm prior to proceeding (Mekhail et al., 2012). This procedure can be done at multiple levels without increasing the risk of spinal instability. It is done through a small incision under fluoroscopic guidance. Patients are able to resume their usual activities within 24 hours. Procedure-related complications such as nerve injury, dural tear, infection, and bleeding have been assessed in multiple studies and found to be very low (Benyamin & Staats, 2016).

In patients with up to moderate lumbar spinal stenosis, indirect decompression via implantation of an interspinous spacer is a minimally invasive technique that can provide relief of pain associated with spinal stenosis and neurogenic claudication. The device acts as an extension blocker at the treatment level thus relieving compression of neural structures. It avoids the morbidity associated with open surgery (Benz et al., 2001). The implant that is currently mostly used is the Vertiflex Superion (Patel et al., 2015). The implant is percutaneously placed via a series of serial dilators also under fluoroscopic guidance.

Neuropathic Pain Syndromes

Neuropathic pain is not completely understood and is thought of more as a syndrome than a singular entity. It is defined by the International Association for the Study of Pain (IASP) as "pain caused by a lesion or disease of the somatosensory system" (Jensen et al., 2011, pp. 2204–2205). It manifests itself through different signs and symptoms which commonly include burning, pins and needles, tingling, and numbness (Abbott et al., 2011). The pain is more common in the extremities and lower back (Abbott et al., 2011; Szewczyk et al, 2022). It can be the result of trauma including spinal cord injuries. It can also be related to post-surgical outcomes, including: post laminectomy syndrome, failed back surgical syndrome, post amputation pain, or from a chronic disease process like diabetes, post herpetic neuralgia, multiple sclerosis, stroke, trigeminal neuralgia, chronic radiculopathy, HIV, etc. (Abbott et al., 2011; Jensen et al., 2011; Szewczyk et al., 2022). It is a syndrome that is diagnosed with increasing frequency as the general population ages (Szewczyk et al., 2022).

Neuropathic pain significantly alters a person's quality of life. The increase in perceived pain and fatigue lowers productivity, provokes disability/work absences, and affects the patients social, economic, and psychological well-being. (Abbott et al., 2011; Bates et al., 2019; Colloca et al., 2017; Szewczyk et al., 2022; Udall et al., 2019). The prevalence of neuropathic pain is most likely underestimated, though women ages 50–64 years tend to be affected more frequently (Mills et al., 2019; Steingrímsdóttir et al., 2017; Szewczyk et al., 2022). Low social status, unemployment, addiction history, family history, low education level, and poor physical activity are each risk factors for this and other chronic pain to develop (Mills et al., 2019; Steingrímsdóttir et al., 2017).

Pharmacologically, neuropathic pain is a challenge to treat and many patients with this type of pain respond only partially to treatment, are non-responders, or do not tolerate it due to side effects (Szewczyk et al., 2022). To complicate an already difficult to treat disease process, many patients will have nociceptive pain or other chronic pain in conjunction with their neuropathic pain (Szewczyk et al., 2022). Treatment for this debilitating syndrome can be broken down into two groups: conservative therapy and interventional therapy. This treatment will vary based upon patients' age and comorbidities. A comprehensive assessment including screening questionaries, thorough patient history/physical exam, and appropriate neurodiagnostic imaging such as MRI and testing like electroneuromyography (EMG) or a nerve stimulation study (NCS) should be performed before treatment is initiated (Bates et al., 2019).

Conservative Therapy

Multidisciplinary care is key when initiating neuropathic pain treatment. Psychology, physiotherapy, exercise therapy, and massage-based therapies should be utilized early on to address any psychologic issues (e.g., depression, anxiety) and functional issues such as sleep deprivation and deconditioning (Bates et al., 2019; Centre for Clinical Practice at NICE, 2013; Dworkin et al., 2010; Haanpää et al., 2009). The services by the above providers are invaluable in conjunction with the treatment of the managing physician to help the patient's mood and quality of life (Bates et al., 2019). It is recommended that a patient trial the above form of treatment for at least 6–8 weeks as the above care has been shown to decrease pain and improve mood and function (Shaygan et al., 2018).

Medications are the next line of treatment, in the form of tricyclic antidepressants (TCAs), serotonin-norepinephrine uptake inhibitors (SNRIs), gabapentinoids, lidocaine, capsaicin, and tramadol/tapentadol (Abbott et al., 2011; Bates et al., 2019; Centre for Clinical Practice at NICE, 2013; Dworkin et al., 2010; Haanpää et al., 2009; Jensen et al., 2011; Shaygan et al., 2018). These medications can be used alone or in conjunction with one another. Tricyclic antidepressants including nortriptyline and amitriptyline, SNRIs including venlafaxine and duloxetine, and gabapentinoids including gabapentin and pregabalin have been extensively studied for neuropathic pain and their use as a first line agent is supported across multiple guidelines (Bates et al., 2019; Centre for Clinical Practice at NICE, 2013; Dworkin et al., 2010; Finnerup et al., 2015; Haanpää et al., 2009; Sumitani et al., 2018). They should be trialed over 4–8 weeks (Dworkin et al., 2010). The side effect profile for TCAs, SNRIs, and gabapentinoids requires vigilant dosing, especially in the elderly as this patient population can have side effects even at the lowest doses (Bates et al., 2019). For TCAs and SNRIs, side effects include risk of falls, arrhythmia, urinary retention, orthostasis, and dry mouth; while for gabapentinoids side effects include somnolence, fatigue, dizziness, and edema (Bates et al., 2019; Wiffen et al.,

2017). Dose adjustments should occur if the patient fails the initial trial period or if they begin to have adverse effects.

In conjunction with the first line medications (TCAs, SNRIs, Gabapentinoids), topical medications are supported. Lidocaine patches and capsaicin are referred to most commonly. These medications are utilized for more focal neuropathic pain (post herpetic neuralgia) but have had limited success with post-surgical neuropathic pain or peripheral diabetic neuropathy with certain features (Bates et al., 2019). Lidocaine patches, creams as well as capsaicin cream are well-tolerated by the elderly and those who cannot take oral medications (Dworkin et al., 2010). Other topical agents such as ketamine, clonidine, and topical amitriptyline have limited evidence to support their use but may be helpful adjuncts (Dworkin et al., 2010).

After the above have failed tramadol or tapentadol should be considered. Most guidelines consider tramadol a second line treatment but can be included as a first line treatment in the face of acute neuropathic pain (Bates et al., 2019; Dworkin et al., 2010; Finnerup et al., 2015; Haanpää et al., 2009; Sumitani et al., 2018). Tapentadol is considered a third or fourth line treatment. It is more potent than tramadol (Bates et al., 2019). Tramadol has been proven to be effective in post herpetic neuralgia, diabetic neuropathy, and neuropathic cancer pain (Arbaiza & Vidal, 2007; Bates et al., 2019), while tapentadol may have some benefit for diabetic neuropathy (Bates et al., 2019; Schwartz et al., 2011). Only after the above medications have been trialed and interventional techniques been applied (will discuss in the next section) should low dose opioid management be attempted.

Interventional Therapy

When conservative therapy fails to provide adequate relief, or if the patient is having an acute flare up of their neuropathic pain, interventional techniques can be attempted. These therapies focus on specific structural targets that could be a source of a patient's neuropathic pain. These therapies include epidural injections, pulsed radiofrequency ablation, radiofrequency denervation, sympathetic blocks, and neuromodulation in the form of spinal cord stimulation (SCS) and dorsal root ganglion stimulation (DRGS).

Epidural injections provide a good starting place for patients suffering from neuropathic pain in a dermatomal distribution. It typically involves the use of a local anesthetic with or without the addition of a steroid to provide its analgesic effect. The American Pain Society and American Society for Interventional Pain Physicians, each gave recommendations that epidural therapy should be considered for neuropathic pain syndromes such as herpes zoster, persistent radiculopathies, and failed back surgical syndrome (Chou et al., 2015; Manchikanti et al., 2013). It is likely that these patients will need more than one epidural injection as the effects can be short lived.

There is limited evidence for the use of pulsed radiofrequency ablation or radiofrequency denervation. Pulsed radiofrequency ablation is a technique that attempts to change the synaptic transmission of a nerve via an electric field. Radiofrequency denervation is a technique in which the targeted structure is ablated using heat or cold. Most commonly the dorsal root ganglion of the desired nerve is the target. There is some support of pulsed RFA for post herpetic neuralgia and occipital neuralgia (Chang, 2018), but lack of evidence limits its use for trigeminal neuralgia or other peripheral neuropathies. Radiofrequency ablation of the DRG was also tested in the cervical and lumbar spine but ultimately performed no better than the sham treatment (van Kleef et al., 1996).

Neuromodulation in the form of SCS and DRGS has become increasingly popular for the treatment of many different pain syndromes including those with neuropathic pain components. The use of SCS and DRGS for post laminectomy syndrome, failed back surgical syndrome, and complex regional pain syndrome (CRPS) is well documented. As patients fail to respond to the above treatments, neuromodulation remains a viable choice even as patients age. Petersen et al. (2021) led a multicenter randomized clinical trial which compared conventional medical management (CMM) with SCS in the treatment of refractory painful diabetic neuropathy (PDN). The study concluded that SCS was superior to CMM for the treatment of PDN, with substantial pain relief and improved health and quality of life continuing at six months for patients with refractory PDN (Petersen et al., 2021). This lends credence that SCS and DRGS should be considered as a treatment for patients with neuropathic pain.

Neuropathic pain syndromes are challenging to treat. These diagnoses cause the patient physical, emotional, and spiritual pain and discomfort. As patients age, they are more likely to encounter this debilitating pain syndrome. As shown in this section, a multidisciplinary stepwise approach is needed to combat this pain process, reduce pain, and help each patient find balance and an acceptable quality of life.

Case Study/ Life Care Planning Needs

Patient is a 45 y/o female with chronic pain in her right leg status post an open reduction and internal fixation of the ankle after a motor vehicle accident three years ago. After the ankle surgery, the patient never improved. One year ago, she was diagnosed with CRPS. She currently has sensitivity to touch, swelling, intermittent color change, intermittent temperature change (coldness to touch), and lack of ankle mobility. She is able to ambulate about 40 feet with assistance of a cane but uses a knee scooter or wheelchair for longer distances. She is unable to drive. Previously, the patient worked as a construction worker. Since the injury, the patient has been unable to work due to pain and immobility. Patient has tried multiple medications including anti-neuropathic medications, antidepressants, opioids, non-steroidal anti-inflammatories, and others. Patient is currently taking oxycodone 15mg TID, gabapentin 800mg TID, nortriptyline 30mg daily, ibuprofen 600mg BID, and tizanidine 4mg BID. Patient rates her pain as eight on a 0–10 Numerical Rating Scale. She is currently being evaluated by a chronic pain physician.

The chronic pain physician suggests a sympathetic nerve block with extensive physical therapy. The plan is if that fails, then the patient will undergo neuromodulation, specifically DRGS targeting the L4 and S1 dermatomes to provide coverage for the ankle and foot.

Question:
Is this patient at their baseline? Are there other treatments that will be offered after the current plan?

Answer:
The patient is currently at her baseline if she does not move forward or does not improve with the current prescribed treatments because there is no other proven treatment that could be explored after SCS. We are hopeful that with these treatments, we will get symptomatic and functional improvement. We are also hopeful that we can reduce the medication burden of this patient, but if the patient fails these treatments, unfortunately, the patient will need to continue her current medication regimen for quality of life.

Question:
How often will the patient need visits over the next calendar year?

Answer:
The next year will be visit intensive. The patient will need 3–5 procedure visits for lumbar sympathetic injections with six weeks of extensive physical therapy up to three times per week. If this is ineffective, the patient will need a neuropsychological evaluation and an MRI for pre-surgical planning. Afterwards, the patient will need a neuromodulation trial visit and then if successful an implant visit. Post-surgical follow-up will conclude with a one week, six week, and 12 week follow-up. After which, if the patient is doing well, the patient will need to be seen every six months. If the patient refuses these treatments or does not improve with these treatments, the patient will need to be seen every 1–2 months for medication titration and monitoring of potentially addictive substances.

Question:
How often will this patient need to be seen subsequently?

Answer:
If stimulation and weaning of opioids is successful, the patient will only need follow-up every 3–6 months for routine maintenance of the device. Battery life of modern SCS products is 6–8 years, so she will need a battery replacement approximately every seven years. If the patient does not have success or refuses stimulation, she will need a visit every 1–2 months for life in order to maintain medication and potentially provide procedural intervention for temporary palliation. Patient will also probably have 1–2 emergency room visits per year due to severe pain exacerbations, falls, or depression associated with this disease.

Question:
What are the patient's permanent restrictions or limitations?

Answer:
We would suggest a functional capacity examination when the patient is stabilized from any effective procedural intervention. This will allow us to see the patient's functional limitations and capabilities to determine if based on her skill set and education, whether she has the opportunity to be gainfully employed. One of the challenges of CRPS is that it is the highest disease on the pain scale created by McGill University (Lee et al., 2014). Thus, acute exacerbations of chronic pain may be challenging for this patient to overcome leading to inability to focus on many tasks.

Question:
Is any equipment needed for this patient?

Answer:
If treatment is unsuccessful, the patient will need mobility equipment. She also may need modifications to her vehicle so that driving is possible without use of her right foot. She also may need modifications in the home to ensure that she is mobile and able to do her activities of daily living without worsening her condition or causing an acute exacerbation.

Conclusion

Chronic pain syndromes are challenging to treat. These diagnoses cause the patient physical, emotional, and spiritual pain and discomfort. As patients age, they are more likely to encounter this debilitating pain syndrome. Interventions and medications can offer improved quality of life for patients with many chronic pain conditions, when utilized appropriately. As shown in this chapter, a multidisciplinary stepwise approach is needed to combat this pain process, reduce pain, and help each patient find balance and an acceptable quality of life.

References

Abbott, C. A., Malik, R. A., Van Ross, E. R., Kulkarni, J., & Boulton, A. J. (2011). Prevalence and characteristics of painful diabetic neuropathy in a large community-based diabetic population in the UK. *Diabetes Care*, *34*(10), 2220–2224.

American College of Radiology. (n.d.). *ACR appropriateness criteria*. https://acsearch.acr.org/list

Arbaiza, D., & Vidal, O. (2007). Tramadol in the treatment of neuropathic cancer pain. *Clinical Drug Investigation*, *27*(1), 75–83.

Bates, D., Schultheis, B. C., Hanes, M. C., Jolly, S. M., Chakravarthy, K. V., Deer, T. R., Levy, R. M., & Hunter, C. W. (2019). A comprehensive algorithm for management of neuropathic pain. *Pain Medicine*, *20*(Supplement_1), S2–S12.

Benyamin, R. M., & Staats, P. S. (2016). MiDAS Encore Investigators. MILD® is an effective treatment for lumbar spinal stenosis with neurogenic claudication: MiDAS ENCORE randomized controlled trial. *Pain Physician*, *19*(4), 229–242.

Benz, R. J., Ibrahim, Z. G., Afshar, P., & Garfin, S. R. (2001). Predicting complications in elderly patients undergoing lumbar decompression. *Clinical Orthopaedics and Related Research (1976–2007)*, *384*, 116–121.

Berman, B. M., Lao, L., Langenberg, P., Lee, W. L., Gilpin, A. M., & Hochberg, M. C. (2004). Effectiveness of acupuncture as adjunctive therapy in osteoarthritis of the knee: A randomized, controlled trial. *Annals of Internal Medicine*, *141*(12), 901–910.

Bondesson, E., Larrosa Pardo, F., Stigmar, K., Ringqvist, Å., Petersson, I. F., Jöud, A., & Schelin, M. E. C. (2018). Comorbidity between pain and mental illness–evidence of a bidirectional relationship. *European Journal of Pain*, *22*(7), 1304–1311.

Brooks, A. K., & Udoji, M. A. (2016). Interventional techniques for management of pain in older adults. *Clinics in Geriatric Medicine*, *32*(4), 773–785.

Büssing, A., Ostermann, T., Lüdtke, R., & Michalsen, A. (2012). Effects of yoga interventions on pain and pain-associated disability: A meta-analysis. *The Journal of Pain*, *13*(1), 1–9.

Centers for Disease Control and Prevention. (2020). *Wide-ranging online data for epidemiologic research (WONDER)*. http://wonder.cdc.govb

Centre for Clinical Practice at NICE UK. (2013). *Neuropathic pain: The pharmacological management of neuropathic pain in adults in non-specialist settings*. www.nice.org.uk/guidance/cg173

Chang, M. C. (2018). Efficacy of pulsed radiofrequency stimulation in patients with peripheral neuropathic pain: A narrative review. *Pain Physician*, *21*(3), E225–E234.

Chiarotto, A., Maxwell, L. J., Ostelo, R. W., Boers, M., Tugwell, P., & Terwee, C. B. (2019). Measurement properties of visual analogue scale, numeric rating scale, and pain severity subscale of the brief pain inventory in patients with low back pain: A systematic review. *The Journal of Pain*, *20*(3), 245–263.

Chou, R., Turner, J. A., Devine, E. B., Hansen, R. N., Sullivan, S. D., Blazina, I., Dana, T., Bougatsos, C., & Deyo, R. A. (2015). The effectiveness and risks of long-term opioid therapy for chronic pain: A systematic review for a National Institutes of Health Pathways to Prevention Workshop. *Annals of Internal Medicine*, *162*(4), 276–286.

Cohen, S. P., & Raja, S. N. (2007). Pathogenesis, diagnosis, and treatment of lumbar zygapophysial (facet) joint pain. *The Journal of the American Society of Anesthesiologists*, *106*(3), 591–614.

Cohen, S. P., Bicket, M. C., Jamison, D., Wilkinson, I., & Rathmell, J. P. (2013). Epidural steroids: A comprehensive, evidence-based review. *Regional Anesthesia & Pain Medicine*, *38*(3), 175–200.

Colloca, L., Ludman, T., Bouhassira, D., Baron, R., Dickenson, A. H., Yarnitsky, D., Freeman, R., Truini, A., Attal, N., Finnerup, N. B., Eccleston, C., Kalso, E., Bennett, D. L., Dworkin, R. H., & Raja, S. N. (2017). Neuropathic pain. *Nature Reviews Disease Primers*, *3*(1), 1–19.

Deyo, R. A. & Tsui-Wu, J.Y. (1987). Descriptive epidemiology of low-back pain and its related medical care in the United States. *Spine (12),* 264–268.

Dieleman, J. L., Cao, J., Chapin, A., Chen, C., Li, Z., Liu, A., Horst, C., Kaldjian, A., Matyasz, T., Scott, K. W., Bui, A. L., Campbell, M., Duber, H. C., Dunn, A. C., Flaxman, A. D., Fitzmaurice, C., Maghavi, M., Sadat, N., Shieh, P., ... & Murray, C. J. (2020). US health care spending by payer and health condition, 1996–2016. *JAMA, 323*(9), 863–884.

Dowell, D., Haegerich, T. M., & Chou, R. (2016). CDC guideline for prescribing opioids for chronic pain—United States, 2016. *JAMA, 315*(15), 1624–1645.

Dworkin, R. H., O'Connor, A. B., Audette, J., Baron, R., Gourlay, G. K., Haanpää, M. L., Kent, J. L., Krane, E. J., LeBel, A. A., Levy, R. M., Mackey, S. C., Mayer, J., Miaskowski, C., Raja, S. N., Rice, A. S. C., Schmader, K. E., Stacey, B., Stanos, S., Treede, R.,... & Wells, C. D. (2010, March). Recommendations for the pharmacological management of neuropathic pain: An overview and literature update. *In Mayo Clinic Proceedings, 85*(3), S3–S14.

Finnerup, N. B., Attal, N., Haroutounian, S., McNicol, E., Baron, R., Dworkin, R. H., Gilron, I., Haanpää M., Hansson, P., Jensen, T. S., Kamerman, P. R., Lund, K., Moore, A., Raja, S. N., Rice, A. S. C., Rowbotham, M., Sena, E., Siddall, P., Smith, B. H., & Wallace, M. (2015). Pharmacotherapy for neuropathic pain in adults: A systematic review and meta-analysis. *The Lancet Neurology, 14*(2), 162–173.

Garcia, J. B. S., Rodrigues, D. P., Leite, D. R. B., do Nascimento Câmara, S., da Silva Martins, K., & de Moraes, É. B. (2015). Clinical evaluation of the post-laminectomy syndrome in public hospitals in the city of São Luís, Brazil. *BMC Research Notes, 8*(1), 1–7.

Gasperi, M., Panizzon, M., Goldberg, J., Buchwald, D., & Afari, N. (2021). Posttraumatic stress disorder and chronic pain conditions in men: A twin study. *Psychosomatic Medicine, 83*(2), 109–117.

Haanpää, M. L., Backonja, M. M., Bennett, M. I., Bouhassira, D., Cruccu, G., Hansson, P. T., Jensen, T. S., Kauppila, T., Rice, A. S. C., Smith, B. H., Treede, R., & Baron, R. (2009). Assessment of neuropathic pain in primary care. *The American Journal of Medicine, 122*(10), S13–S21.

Hooten, W. M. (2016, July). Chronic pain and mental health disorders: Shared neural mechanisms, epidemiology, and treatment. *In Mayo Clinic Proceedings, 91*(7), 955–970.

Hooten, W. M., & Cohen, S. P. (2015, December). Evaluation and treatment of low back pain: A clinically focused review for primary care specialists. *In Mayo Clinic Proceedings, 90*(12), 1699–1718.

Hoy, D., Brooks, P., Blyth, F., & Buchbinder, R. (2010). The epidemiology of low back pain. *Best Practice & Research Clinical Rheumatology, 24*(6), 769–781.

Jaracz, J., Gattner, K., Jaracz, K., & Górna, K. (2016). Unexplained painful physical symptoms in patients with major depressive disorder: Prevalence, pathophysiology and management. *CNS Drugs, 30*(4), 293–304.

Jensen, T. S., Baron, R., Haanpää, M., Kalso, E., Loeser, J. D., Rice, A. S., & Treede, R. D. (2011). A new definition of neuropathic pain. *Pain, 152*(10), 2204–2205.

Lafian, A. M., & Torralba, K. D. (2018). Lumbar spinal stenosis in older adults. *Rheumatic Disease Clinics, 44*(3), 501–512.

Lee, D. H., Noh, E. C., Kim, Y. C., Hwang, J. Y., Kim, S. N., Jang, J. H., Byun, M.S., & Kang, D. H. (2014). Risk factors for suicidal ideation among patients with complex regional pain syndrome. *Psychiatry Investigation, 11*(1), 32. https://doi.org/10.4306/pi.2014.11.1.32

Linde, K., Allais, G., Brinkhaus, B., Fei, Y., Mehring, M., Vertosick, E. A., Vickers A., & White, A. R. (2016). Acupuncture for the prevention of episodic migraine. *Cochrane Database of Systematic Reviews, 6.* https://pubmed.ncbi.nlm.nih.gov/27351677/

Manchikanti, L., Abdi, S., Atluri, S., Benyamin, R. M., Boswell, M. V., Buenaventura, R. M., Bryce, D. A., Burks, P. A., Caraway, D. L., Calodney, A. K., Cash, K. A., Christo, P. J., Cohen, S. P., Colson, J., Conn, A., Cordner, H., Coubarous, S., Datta, S., Deer, T. R., Diwan, S., Falco, F. J. E., Fellows, B., Geffer, S.... & Hirsch, J. A. (2013). An update of comprehensive evidence-based guidelines for interventional techniques in chronic spinal pain. Part II: Guidance and recommendations. *Pain Physician, 16*(2 Suppl), S49–S283.

Manchikanti, L., Pampati, V., Rivera, J., Fellows, B., Beyer, C., & Damron, K. (2001). Role of facet joints in chronic low back pain in the elderly: A controlled comparative prevalence study. *Pain Practice, 1*(4), 332–337.

Mekhail, N., Vallejo, R., Coleman, M. H., & Benyamin, R. M. (2012). Long-term results of percutaneous lumbar decompression mild® for spinal stenosis. *Pain Practice, 12*(3), 184–193.

Mills, S. E., Nicolson, K. P., & Smith, B. H. (2019). Chronic pain: A review of its epidemiology and associated factors in population-based studies. *British Journal of Anaesthesia, 123*(2), e273-e283.

Otis, J. D., Keane, T. M., & Kerns, R. D. (2003). An examination of the relationship between chronic pain and post-traumatic stress disorder. *Journal of Rehabilitation Research and Development, 40*(5–6), 397–406.

Oxford Leaners Dictionary. (20220). *Acupuncture*. Oxford University Press. www.oxfordlearnersdictionaries.com/us/definition/english/acupuncture

Patel, V. V., Whang, P. G., Haley, T. R., Bradley, W. D., Nunley, P. D., Davis, R. P., Miller, L. E., Block, J. E., & Geisler, F. H. (2015). Superion interspinous process spacer for intermittent neurogenic claudication secondary to moderate lumbar spinal stenosis: Two-year results from a randomized controlled FDA-IDE pivotal trial. *Spine, 40 (5),* 275–282.

Pergolizzi, J. V., Rosenblatt, M., & LeQuang, J. A. (2019). Three years down the road: The aftermath of the CDC guideline for prescribing opioids for chronic pain. *Advances in Therapy, 36*(6), 1235–1240.

Petersen, E. A., Stauss, T. G., Scowcroft, J. A., Brooks, E. S., White, J. L., Sills, S. M., Amirdelfan, K., Guiguis, M. N., Xu, J., Yu, C., Nairizi, A., Patterson, D. G., Tsoulfas, K. C., Creamer, M. J., Galan, V., Bundschu, R. H., Paul, C. A., Mehta, N. D., Choi, H., Sayed, D., Lad, S. P., DiBenedetto, D. J.... & Mekhail, N. A. (2021). Effect of high-frequency (10-kHz) spinal cord stimulation in patients with painful diabetic neuropathy: A randomized clinical trial. *JAMA Neurology, 78*(6), 687–698.

Pope, J. E., Fishman, M. A., Gunn, J. A., Cotten, B. M., Hill, M. M., & Deer, T. R. (2021). Cross-Validation of the Foundation Pain Index with PROMIS-29 in chronic pain patients. *Journal of Pain Research, 14,* 2677.

Pua, Y. H., Poon, C. L. L., Seah, F. J. T., Thumboo, J., Clark, R. A., Tan, M. H., Chong, H., Tan, J. W., Chew, E. S., & Yeo, S. J. (2019). Predicting individual knee range of motion, knee pain, and walking limitation outcomes following total knee arthroplasty. *Acta Orthopaedica, 90*(2), 179–186.

Raja, S. N., Carr, D. B., Cohen, M., Finnerup, N. B., Flor, H., Gibson, S., Keefe, F. J., Mogil, J. S., Ringkamp, M., Sluka, K. A., Song, X., Stevens, B., Sullivan, M. D., Tutelman, P. R., Ushida, T., & Vader, K. (2020). The revised IASP definition of pain: concepts, challenges, and compromises. *Pain, 161*(9), 1976.

Rashbaum, R. F., Ohnmeiss, D. D., Lindley, E. M., Kitchel, S. H., & Patel, V. V. (2016). Sacroiliac joint pain and its treatment. *Journal of Spinal Disorders and Techniques, 29*(2), 42–48.

Roberts, S. L., Burnham, R. S., Ravichandiran, K., Agur, A. M., & Loh, E. Y. (2014). Cadaveric study of sacroiliac joint innervation: Implications for diagnostic blocks and radiofrequency ablation. *Regional Anesthesia & Pain Medicine, 39*(6), 456–464.

Rubinstein, S. M., van Middelkoop, M., Kuijpers, T., Ostelo, R., Verhagen, A. P., de Boer, M. R., Koes, B. W., & van Tulder, M. W. (2010). A systematic review on the effectiveness of complementary and alternative medicine for chronic non-specific low-back pain. *European Spine Journal, 19*(8), 1213–1228.

Schwartz, S., Etropolski, M., Shapiro, D. Y., Okamoto, A., Lange, R., Haeussler, J., & Rauschkolb, C. (2011). Safety and efficacy of tapentadol ER in patients with painful diabetic peripheral neuropathy: Results of a randomized-withdrawal, placebo-controlled trial. *Current Medical Research and Opinion, 27*(1), 151–162.

Shaygan, M., Böger, A., & Kröner-Herwig, B. (2018). Predicting factors of outcome in multidisciplinary treatment of chronic neuropathic pain. *Journal of Pain Research, 11,* 2433.

Steingrímsdóttir, Ó. A., Landmark, T., Macfarlane, G. J., & Nielsen, C. S. (2017). Defining chronic pain in epidemiological studies: A systematic review and meta-analysis. *Pain, 158*(11), 2092–2107.

Stockings, E., Campbell, G., Hall, W. D., Nielsen, S., Zagic, D., Rahman, R., Farrell, M. B., Weier, M., & Degenhardt, L. (2018). Cannabis and cannabinoids for the treatment of people with chronic noncancer pain conditions: A systematic review and meta-analysis of controlled and observational studies. *Pain, 159*(10), 1932–1954.

Sumitani, M., Sakai, T., Matsuda, Y., Abe, H., Yamaguchi, S., Hosokawa, T., & Fukui, S. (2018). Executive summary of the clinical guidelines of pharmacotherapy for neuropathic pain: By the Japanese society of pain clinicians. *Journal of Anesthesia*, *32*(3), 463–478.

Szewczyk, A. K., Jamroz-Wiśniewska, A., Haratym, N., & Rejdak, K. (2022). Neuropathic pain and chronic pain as an underestimated interdisciplinary problem. *International Journal of Occupational Medicine and Environmental Health*, *35*(3), 1–16.

Szpalski, M., & Gunzburg, R. (2003). Lumbar spinal stenosis in the elderly: An overview. *European Spine Journal*, *12*(2), S170–S175.

Udall, M., Kudel, I., Cappelleri, J. C., Sadosky, A., King-Concialdi, K., Parsons, B., Hlavacek, P., Hopps, M., Arline Salomon, P., DiBonaventura, M., Clark, P., & Garcia, J. B. S. (2019). Epidemiology of physician-diagnosed neuropathic pain in Brazil. *Journal of Pain Research*, *12*, 243.

van Kleef, M., Liem, L., Lousberg, R., Barendse, G., Kessels, F., & Sluijter, M. E. (1996). Radiofrequency lesion adjacent to the dorsal root ganglion for cervicobrachial pain: A prospective double blind randomized study. *Neurosurgery*, *38*(6), 1127–1132.

Wiffen, P. J., Derry, S., Bell, R. F., Rice, A. S., Tolle, T. R., Phillips, T. & Moore, R. A. (2017). Gabapentin for chronic neuropathic pain in adults. *Cochrane Database Syst Rev*, *6*(6), CD007938.

Chapter 24

Life Care Planning for the Patient with Spinal Cord Injury

David Altman and Dan Bagwell

The spinal cord is the crucial conduit by which the brain communicates with the rest of the body. Injuries to the spinal cord, therefore, are among the most devastating of all neurological conditions, with profound, multidimensional consequences for both the individual and the family. Adults who have previously been independent are often devastated by their need for assistance with basic activities of daily living, such as feeding, bathing, grooming, and carrying out bowel and bladder functions. Consequently, a team approach is needed for the care, treatment, and rehabilitation of individuals with spinal cord injury (SCI), with contributions from medical and surgical specialties, nursing, multiple therapeutic disciplines, medical case managers, and other healthcare professionals. The rehabilitation process extends for years after the injury. Furthermore, the aging process compounds the effects of the SCI, necessitating proactive measures that include pharmacotherapy, physiotherapy, surgeries, counseling, environmental modifications, and an extensive array of adaptive devices, medical supplies, and durable medical equipment.

Epidemiology

Data from the 2021 SCI Data Sheet, National Spinal Cord Injury Statistical Center ([NSCISC], 2021b), indicate that there are approximately 17,900 individuals each year who sustain SCI, with an estimated 296,000 SCI survivors (from 252,000 to 373,000 persons) living in the United States. Males account for approximately 78% of new spinal cord injuries, but the average age at onset is currently 43 years, an increase from 29 years during the 1970s. Motor vehicle accidents (including motorcycle accidents) remain the leading cause of injury, accounting for 38.2%, followed by falls (32.3%), violence, primarily gunshot wounds, (14.3%), sports and recreation (7.8%), iatrogenic causes (4.1%), and other (3.3%). Furthermore, approximately 30% of persons with SCI are rehospitalized one or more times during any given year following injury, with diseases of the genitourinary system the leading cause of rehospitalization, followed by disease of the skin, while respiratory, digestive, circulatory, and musculoskeletal disease are also common causes.

Approximately 20% of spinal cord injuries occur in children and adolescents. Injuries before puberty are associated with a greater than 90% incidence of scoliosis. Children have a higher incidence of spinal cord injury without radiographic abnormality (SCIWORA) due to immaturity of the musculoskeletal system. Younger children with spinal cord injuries are more likely to be complete (Parent et al., 2011). Motor vehicle collisions are the leading cause of pediatric SCI, with falls and sports injuries (i.e., football, diving) thereafter (NSCISC, 2021b).

While life expectancies of SCI survivors improved substantially during the 1970s and well into the 1980s relative to just two decades preceding the 1970s, further gains were beginning to plateau as we entered the 1990s, with little gain seen through the first decade of the twenty-first century. This leveling of the improvement trend caught the attention of many who are involved in the care of those with SCI, as well as the spinal cord injured population generally. The average length of hospital stays in the acute care setting is currently less than half that of those who were injured in the 1970s, 11 days versus 24, and the average lengths of rehabilitation stay are currently just over one-third of those who received rehabilitation in the 1970s, 30 days versus 98 days (NSCISC, 2021). This compression of acute inpatient hospitalization has correspondingly limited the amount of time for individuals with newly acquired spinal cord injuries to develop adaptation and coping skills that are necessary for successful transition to the community.

Death rates remain much higher during the first year post-injury when compared with subsequent years, particularly for those who sustain greater levels of neurologic impairment. Multiple studies have also identified a number of socioeconomic risk factors that are believed to be associated with increased mortality rates among those with SCI (Krause et al., 2004; Krause & Saunders, 2010). Despite a leveling of the gains in life expectancies for those with SCI, long-term survival has improved immensely since the 1940s, when survival was estimated at just 18 months (Reyes & Morton, 2009). As a result of such gains, people with spinal cord injuries are living long enough to experience age-related health issues that are seen in the general population.

Data obtained from the 2021 NSCISC *Annual Report* indicate that diseases of the respiratory system remain the leading cause of death for those with SCI (21.4%), with 65.1% of these deaths due to pneumonia. The second leading cause of death was infective and parasitic disease (12.0%), of which 90.5% were the result of septicemia and usually associated with decubitus ulcers, urinary tract infections, or respiratory infections. Cancer (neoplasm) was the third leading cause of death in the SCI population (10.8%), followed closely by hypertensive and ischemic heart disease. Unintentional injuries were the sixth leading cause of death, followed by diseases of the digestive system, cerebral vascular disease, and suicide. It should be noted that while diseases of the genitourinary system represent the leading cause of rehospitalization, they constitute only 2.9% of overall deaths (NSCISC, 2021a).

During any given year, nearly one-third (30%) of patients with spinal cord injuries receiving care through the Spinal Cord Injury Model Systems of care are rehospitalized (NSCISC, 2021b). The average length of stay with rehospitalization is approximately 18 days. Far and away, the leading cause of rehospitalization within the first year continues to be diseases of the genitourinary system, at 30.0%. This is followed by diseases of the skin (11.4%) and diseases of the respiratory system (8.1%) for known or classified causes (NSCISC, 2021a). The incidences of rehospitalization for diseases of the skin and respiratory system increase substantially over time, accounting for up to 40.5% and 28.6% of rehospitalizations, respectively (NSCISC, 2020).

Spinal cord injuries usually occur during peak productivity years and survivors experience permanent disabilities that often impact employment opportunities. In fact, only 20.9% of SCI survivors in the United States are employed at five years post-injury and 26.5% at ten years post-injury (NSCISC, 2021a). Approximately 42% of these survivors have family household incomes that are less than $25,000 annually at post-injury year five, with only marginal changes from years 10–20 post-injury (NSCISC, 2021a).

Anatomy

The spinal cord is the crucial conduit between the brain and the body, and its small surface area contains millions of neurons and axons which innervate motor, sensory, and autonomic functions. Injuries to the spinal cord cause temporary or permanent changes in motor, sensory, and/or autonomic function. The resulting damage to the cord impairs physiologic transmission of signals to and from the brain below the level of the injury. Even small injuries to the spinal cord can result in profound functional loss, and the higher the level of involvement, the greater the degree of disability.

The human spinal cord is divided into 31 segments, and each segment projects a pair of mixed sensory and motor nerves, which combine before passing through spaces (foramina) between the vertebrae. The spinal cord generally terminates at the level of the first lumbar vertebra (L1), below which nerve roots within the vertebral column are referred to as the cauda equina (so named because the elongated nerve roots have the appearance of a horse's tail). The terminal spinal cord is referred to as the conus medullaris.

The spinal cord is surrounded and protected by 33 weight bearing bones, referred to as vertebrae, which are in turn separated by gelatinous disks which act as shock absorbers and supported by ligaments (Figures 24.1 and 24.2). There are seven cervical, 12 thoracic, five lumbar, five sacral and four fused coccygeal vertebrae. The cervical and lumbar portions of the vertebral column have a great deal of flexibility relative to the rigid thoracic vertebrae.

Each segment of the spinal cord is associated with a pair of dorsal ganglia, which are situated just outside the spinal cord, and which contain the cell bodies of sensory neurons (See Figure 24.3).

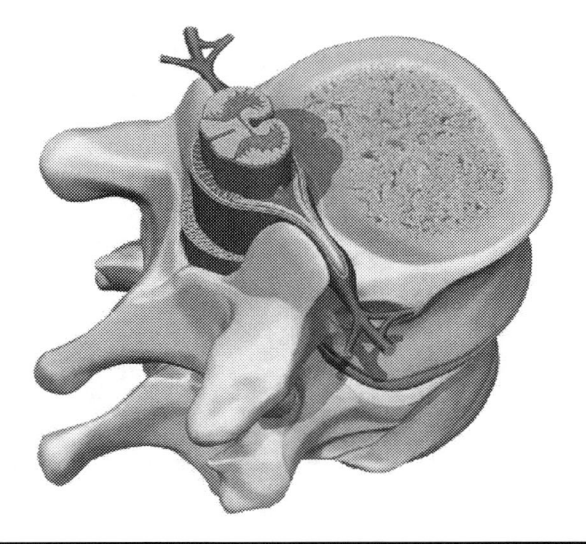

Figure 24.1 **Vertebrae Surrounding Spinal Cord and Other Neural Elements**

Source: Dreamstime L.L.C., Licensed Royalty Free June 09, 2016.

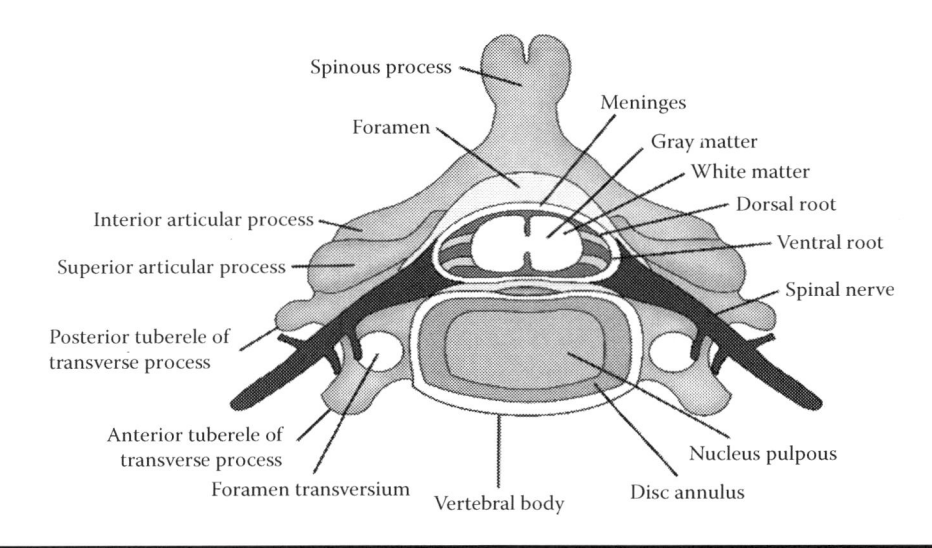

Figure 24.2 Cross Section of Vertebra Surrounding Spinal Cord and Other Neural Elements

Source: Dreamstime L.L.C., Licensed Royalty Free June 09, 2016.

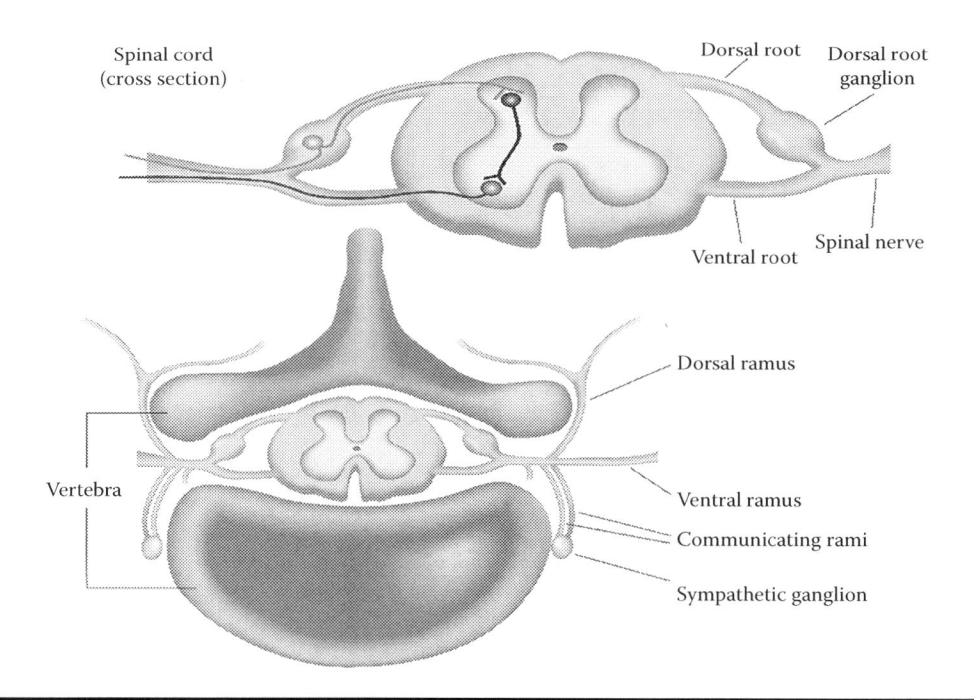

Figure 24.3 Cross Section of Spinal Cord

Source: Dreamstime L.L.C., Licensed Royalty Free June 09, 2016.

The spinal cord is organized somatotopically, such that the neurons that innervate muscles are located on its ventral portion, the fibers that carry proprioceptive and vibratory sensory modalities are positioned dorsally, and the nerve fibers that carry information for pain and temperature are located laterally. Understanding the somatotopic organization of the spinal cord can often allow for localization of lesions based upon relative involvement or preservation of these modalities.

Anatomically, the spinal cord is protected by three layers of tissue, referred to as the meninges. The outermost layer (dura mater) forms a tough protective coating. Between the dura mater and the surrounding bone of the vertebrae is the epidural space, which contains adipose tissue and an intricate network of blood vessels. The middle layer of the meninges is the arachnoid (spider) mater, which is separated from the innermost delicate (pial) layer by the subarachnoid space, which contains cerebrospinal fluid. The pial layer is extremely delicate and intimately associated with the surface of the spinal cord. The spinal cord is stabilized by the denticulate ligaments, which extend from the pia mater laterally between the dorsal and ventral roots.

Pediatric Spinal Cord Anatomy

Spinal column development begins by the sixth week of fetal growth. By birth, there are definable vertebral bodies as well as cartilaginous vertebral arches. Lamina and pedicles ossify during the first five years of life. Like adults, there are seven cervical, 12 thoracic, five lumbar, and five fused sacral/coccygeal vertebrae.

The infant spine (0–2 years) has increased mobility and elasticity. There is underdevelopment of the neck muscles and increased ligamentous laxity. The vertebral bodies are wedge shaped and incompletely ossified, with shallow, horizontally oriented facets. The relatively large size of the infant head with respect to the torso increases the likelihood of cervical spine injuries, especially between the skull and the first cervical vertebra.

Compared with adults, the pediatric spine exhibits increased mobility and elasticity. As a result, the spine can distract up to 2 inches, but the spinal cord can only distract 0.25 inches before being injured. These differences account for why the incidence of spinal column injuries is lower and the incidence of SCIWORA is higher.

Spinal cord injury without radiographic abnormality is a condition in which the spinal cord is damaged without obvious bony or ligamentous injury on plain radiographs or computed tomography. This pattern of injury is most common in children less than age five, and two-thirds of the time, the injury is identified only on MRI, where there is often rupture of the anterior or posterior longitudinal ligaments, cord disruption, and spinal cord edema (Altman, 2019).

Spinal Cord Injury Classification

The American Spinal Injury Association and the International Medical Society of Paraplegia have developed a worldwide nomenclature system which standardizes nomenclature and classification of spinal cord injuries, and which assists communication among clinicians, as well as clinical research and prognostic determinations. This system establishes a level of injury based upon the lowest neurological level that has intact sensory function and at least antigravity function. It is further classified through an A to E scale based upon the degree of preserved motor and sensory function below this level. These data are useful for the life care planner in projecting the type of medical and medically related goods and services that an individual with SCI will likely require, as well as providing a basis for projecting comorbidity and, where applicable, life expectancy.

Spinal cord injuries are classified using the American Spinal Injury Association (ASIA) Impairment Scale [AIS] developed by ASIA (2016), a modification of the Frankel Scale (See Figure 24.4). It has five levels from A to E that further define the extent of the injury. [AIS] "A" is a complete lesion, based on the absence of sensory or motor function in the S4 to S5 sacral segments; "B" is an incomplete lesion with sensation but no motor function below the neurological level. Sensation must be present in the S4 and S5 segments; "C" is an incomplete lesion with motor function present below the neurological level, and the majority of key muscles have a measured grade of strength less than three [five is normal strength]; "D" is an incomplete lesion with motor function present, and the majority of the key muscles below the neurological level has a muscle grade greater than or equal to three; and "E" represents preservation of normal sensory and motor function on neurological examination.

Often, the sensory and motor levels vary from side to side, and the sensory and motor levels can be different on the same side of the body. The physical examination should record the most caudal sensory and motor level on each side which results in the recording of four levels (sensory and motor from both right and left).

Muscle grades for testing motor power are as follows:

- Grade 0 – complete paralysis
- Grade 1 – flicker of contraction present
- Grade 2 – active movement with gravity eliminated
- Grade 3 – Active movement against gravity
- Grade 4 – Active movement against gravity and some resistance described as poor, fair, moderate strength.
- Grade 5 – Normal power

Preservation of Function by Neurologic Level of Injury

With each progressive level of neurologic lesion identified below, the gain in additional preservation of function is identified.

- C1–3: Preservation of tongue movement and swallowing, as well as neck extension flexion, rotation, and side bending. There is paralysis of all muscles of the trunk, upper extremities, and lower extremities. There is also loss of diaphragmatic function necessary for respiration.
- C4: Shoulder elevation (shoulder shrug). Under most circumstances, there is sufficient diaphragmatic function to breathe without a ventilator. Upper cervical paraspinals are also preserved.
- C5: Scapular adduction; shoulder abduction (partial), flexion, extension, and rotation; weak elbow flexion and forearm supination.
- C6: Full rotation and abduction of shoulder; scapular abduction and upward rotation; shoulder horizontal adduction; full elbow flexion; wrist extension and tenodesis grip (passive thumb adduction on the index finger during active wrist extension).
- C7: Shoulder internal rotation, adduction, and depression; elbow extension; forearm pronation; wrist flexion; finger and thumb extension; partial finger flexion.
- C8: Full wrist extension with abduction and adduction and wrist flexion; full finger flexion; thumb flexion, abduction, adduction, and opposition; flexion at the metacarpophalangeals with extension of the interphalangeals (incomplete lumbricals).

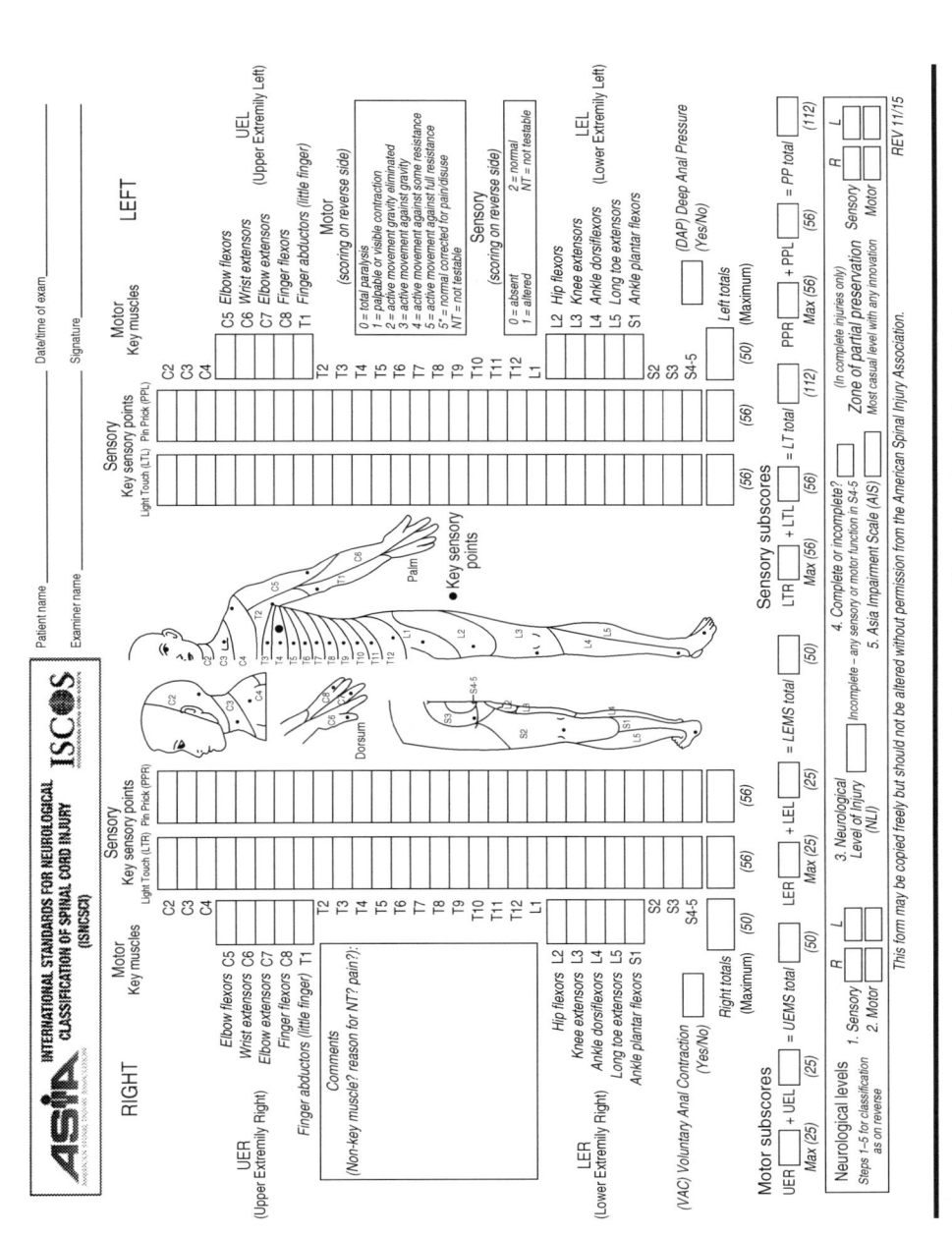

Figure 24.4 International Standards for Neurological Classification of Spinal Cord Injury

Source: American Spinal Cord Injury Association, 2016.

- T1–6: Complete innervation of lumbricals for flexion of the metacarpophalangeals and extension of the interphalangeals; finger abduction and adduction at the interphalangeals; extension of the thoracic spine; upper intercostals innervated.
- T7–12: Trunk flexion and rotation; some pelvic elevation.
- L1–2: Full pelvic elevation and hip flexion.
- L3–4: Lumbar extension; knee flexion and extension, hip adduction; ankle dorsiflexion (weak)

There are a number of incomplete spinal cord syndromes that are also important to recognize:

- Central cord syndrome: Central spinal cord swelling, or formation of a central syrinx (a fluid filled cavity) is often characterized by relative weakness in the upper extremities, a "floating" loss of temperature and pin prick sensation 1–2 levels below the level of the injury secondary to damage to the crossing spinothalamic tract fibers, and urinary retention.
- Brown-Sequard syndrome: Hemisection of the spinal cord results in ipsilateral weakness below the lesion (as a result of damage to the descending corticospinal tract) and contralateral sensory loss starting 1–2 levels below the lesion level (resulting from damage to the ascending and crossing spinothalamic tract fibers).
- Conus medullaris syndrome: Injury to the terminus of the spinal cord results in bowel and bladder dyscontrol, sexual dysfunction, and paraparesis.
- Cauda Equina Syndromes: Although not truly a spinal cord injury, lesions of the cauda equina result in loss of function to the lumbar plexus below the conus medullaris of the spinal cord. As such, it is a lower motor neuron lesion. These syndromes are characterized by sensory impairment in a saddle distribution, back pain, motor weakness of the lower extremities, neurogenic bowel and bladder, and sexual dysfunction.

Common Complications of Spinal Cord Injury

Spinal cord injuries result in numerous physiological changes that involve virtually every system of the body, which, in turn, can cause many complications. The life care planner must be familiar with these complications in order to project the need for medical interventions, equipment, supplies, and medications for anticipated treatment, symptom amelioration, or as possible, prevention.

Autonomic Dysfunction

The spinal cord is a critical component of the autonomic nervous system, and injury can often lead to changes in the quality of hair, skin, and nails, as well as the ability of the individual to respond to temperature changes (i.e., thermoregulation, including sweating). One of the most serious complications is autonomic dysreflexia, a syndrome associated with spinal cord lesions at or above the T6 level. Lesions above this level block the central nervous system's ability to regulate the outflow of the sympathetic ganglia that are located within the intermediolateral cell column. This condition is often provoked by noxious stimuli (i.e., urinary tract infections, urinary retention, constipation, ingrown toenails, labor and delivery, and decubitus ulcers), and is characterized by the following signs and symptoms:

- Severe headache
- Diaphoresis

- Piloerection
- Hypertension
- Tachycardia (occasionally bradycardia)
- General malaise
- Flushing or redness of the skin above the level of the spinal cord lesion

If unrecognized and untreated, autonomic dysreflexia can result in hypertensive cerebral hemorrhages, leading to severe disability and even death.

An opposite scenario is that of orthostatic hypotension, in which the individual with a spinal cord injury will experience sudden drops in blood pressure in response to position changes. This condition is characterized clinically by light headedness, dizziness, or even syncope. Proposed causes for orthostatic hypotension in the context of spinal cord injury include alterations in baroreflex receptor function, altered salt and water homeostasis, and impaired venous return from the lower extremities.

Poikilothermia is a condition that is defined by impaired thermoregulatory control. As individuals with spinal cord injuries are often unable to shiver, sweat or otherwise appropriately regulate peripheral blood vessels, they are at relatively high risk for becoming hypothermic or hyperthermic. As such, it is critical that they are able to closely monitor and regulate their environments with accurate and responsive thermostats. While outdoors, cooling vests offer some protection against hyperthermia in warmer climates.

Gastrointestinal Issues

Gastrointestinal problems occur in 27–62% of individuals with spinal cord injuries, and symptoms include incontinence, constipation, straining, diarrhea, distention, nausea, abdominal pain, rectal bleeding, hemorrhoids, and autonomic dysreflexia during bowel movements (Ebert, 2012; Hagen, 2015). The individual with SCI is at greater risk for gastritis as well as gastric ulcers, particularly if the level of injury is at or above the T6 level. Furthermore, spinal cord injury represents a threefold increased risk of developing gallstones. Possible explanations for this include gallbladder stasis with sludge formation and intestinal hypomotility that alters bile acid metabolism (Stinton & Shaffer, 2012). Complicating the situation is the fact that the clinical presentation of an acute abdomen is often subtle in this patient population, necessitating a low index of suspicion.

Neurogenic bowel dysfunction resulting in severe constipation and fecal incontinence is present in up to 85% of patients with SCI and has a marked impact on social and psychological well-being for patients with SCI (Smith & Decter, 2015; Valles et al., 2006). Neurogenic bowel can result from both upper (i.e., above the level of the conus medullaris) and lower motor neuron lesions (i.e., involving the conus medullaris and/or cauda equina). Most individuals with SCI experience an upper motor neuron syndrome, which is characterized by both the impaired sensation of rectal fullness as well as the inability to voluntarily relax the external anal sphincter. However, reflex bowel movements can still be triggered by intact nerve connections between the spinal cord, the colon, and the mesenteric plexus. In this scenario, fecal incontinence occurs suddenly and without warning as part of a mass reflex. Conversely, those with lower motor neuron lesions involving the distal conus medullaris and cauda equina have voluntary control of part or all of their abdominal muscles, but there is neither spinal cord-mediated peristalsis nor external anal sphincter control. This syndrome is generally characterized by constipation and requires that the rectum be kept empty by digital evacuation of stool.

For most individuals with neurogenic bowel, a complete bowel evacuation every other day is satisfactory. Less frequent bowel movements may result in fecal impaction. Some patients require daily evacuation to avoid incontinence between bowel programs. While most effective bowel evacuation programs take 30–60 minutes to complete, this may take up to two hours to complete and should be completed at a time that is convenient for both the patient and the caregiver. Stool softeners and bowel evacuants, along with digital stimulation are usually needed to obtain a reasonable degree of continence (absence of frequent bowel accidents).

Gastrointestinal motility can be further reduced by certain pharmacologic agents, such as narcotic analgesics and even some tricyclic agents. Where possible, these should be avoided. Broad-spectrum antibiotics may inadvertently alter gut flora and result in diarrhea. As patients with spinal cord injury often require these antibiotics, the bowel routine can be disrupted frequently, with need for replacement of normal gut flora with probiotic agents or other forms of lactobacillus, such as yogurt. The diet should also contain adequate amounts of water and fiber.

Most individuals with spinal cord injury experience constipation and an occasional fecal impaction. Younger individuals with SCI usually have fewer problems with chronic constipation than do older patients or individuals who are several years out from their injuries. Bowel programs generally evolve over time with changes in medication and the procedure used for bowel evacuation. However, most bowel regimens involve emphasizing the importance of adequate hydration and fiber intake to maintain proper stool consistency as well as bowel training, so that evacuation can occur at regular intervals. Other treatment options include the use of bisacodyl or saline enemas and oral medications such as cisapride, which facilitate the release of acetylcholine at the myenteric plexus (Badiali et al., 1991), sacral nerve stimulation (Gstaltner et al., 2008), non-invasive magnetic stimulation, and surgical placement of a colostomy or ileostomy (Branagan et al., 2003).

For those with refractory fecal incontinence who fail to achieve effective management of incontinence by the mainstay of oral medications, suppositories, and enemas, treatment of severe constipation or obstipation may be achieved with implementation of the antegrade continence enema (ACE) procedure. The ACE procedure allows a patient to administer an enema directly into the cecum by way of an easily accessible abdominal wall stoma. This has been shown to result in marked improvements in bowel programming for those with refractory fecal incontinence, and thus, significant improvements in overall quality of life (Smith & Decter, 2015).

Spasticity

Spasticity is defined as a velocity dependent increase in muscle tone resulting from hyperexcitability of the stretch reflex and is one of the hallmarks of spinal cord injury below the level of the lesion. The incidence of spasticity is reported to exceed 90% in the SCI population (Stampas et al., 2022). Clinical findings include hyperreflexia (often with clonus), muscle spasms, and clasp-knife responses. While mild spasticity in the lower extremities can assist with weight bearing and the reduction in venous stasis, markedly increased tone can interfere with or prevent the performance of functional activities, such as range of motion exercises. When more pronounced, it can result in painful spasms that can negatively impact an individual's quality of life (QoL).

It is important to treat spasticity to prevent the development of tendon shortening across a joint (i.e., contracture) and permanent loss of function. Stretching exercises, often performed by a therapist in the clinical setting and caregivers in the home setting, can help to reduce spasticity severity. Without periodic stretching and range of motion exercises, spastic extremities develop tendon shortening and permanent contractures.

Oral antispastic medications, such as baclofen and tizanidine, are commonly prescribed as first lines of therapy, along with benzodiazepine medications (i.e., diazepam, clonazepam), and occasionally dantrolene, which directly reduces the contractility of muscle tissue. For individuals who experience more severe spasticity, oral medications will often be insufficient for adequate management, or the dosing required of these agents may result in intolerable adverse effects, such as sedation, mental confusion, or elevated liver enzymes indicative of liver damage. Under these circumstances, neuromuscular blockade with botulinum toxin can be extremely effective, with effects lasting (in the authors' experience) for approximately three months between injections. Neuromuscular blockade can also be used adjunctively with orally administered antispastic agents.

Individuals with severe spasticity involving both upper and lower extremities may also benefit from the implantation of an intrathecal baclofen pump, a microprocessor controlled and programmable device that can administer miniscule quantities of medication through a catheter and into the intrathecal space, where spasticity can be greatly ameliorated with negligible systemic effects.

Respiratory Complications

With paralysis of the intercostal and abdominal muscles, normal respiratory function is impaired. Complications that develop following spinal cord injury are generally the result of impairments in ventilation and cough. The higher the level of the spinal cord lesion, the more likely and severe the respiratory complications will be. Cough is dramatically impaired in persons with cervical spine injuries from levels C4–C8. With chronic tetraplegia, a rapid and shallow breathing pattern is present. Over time and associated with age, late-onset ventilatory failure can develop due to diminution in vital capacity. These changes in ventilatory function lead to problems with atelectasis, pneumonia, and respiratory failure, resulting in a high incidence of morbidity and mortality from pulmonary complications. Respiratory failure is caused by either failure to ventilate, which is characterized by increased levels of carbon dioxide in the blood, or failure to oxygenate, in which there is reduced oxygen content within the blood. Global alveolar hypoventilation (GAH) is an insidious condition characterized by the gradual loss of pulmonary function as a result of reduced compliance from chronic hypoventilation. Its effects can be accentuated by comorbid scoliosis, kyphosis, and obesity. Individuals with vital capacities below 5–10 mL/kg are considered to be at highest risk for respiratory failure and may require assisted ventilation to support life. Other factors that can contribute to impaired respiratory status include pregnancy, scoliosis, spasticity, and syringomyelia.

The C3 through C5 nerve roots innervate the diaphragm through the phrenic nerves. Spinal cord injuries at or above these levels (particularly above C4) are usually associated with ventilator dependency. Ventilator dependency has significant implications for long-term post-injury survival and life expectancy. Older individuals and those with neurological lesions above T12 are most vulnerable to pulmonary problems associated with hypoventilation leading to a restrictive pattern of pulmonary disease because of intercostal muscle dysfunction.

Diseases of the respiratory system, particularly pneumonia, and septicemia as a consequence of pneumonia, continue to represent the leading cause of death for those with SCI (21.4%), while it is the third most common cause of rehospitalization for the SCI population overall (8.1%) (NSCISC, 2021a). For persons with tetraplegia, there is a much higher incidence of morbidity and rehospitalization due to diseases of the respiratory system, pneumonia in particular. As such, those with SCI should be given high priority for available flu, pneumococcal, and other vaccines that provide protection from respiratory infections. Optimal pulmonary management is critical for minimizing risk of serious, life-threatening pulmonary complications. All individuals with cervical or thoracic spinal cord injuries should undergo periodic clinical pulmonary assessments and pulmonary function testing and should receive recommended vaccinations in the absence of any contraindications. The need for periodic antimicrobial treatment for respiratory infections and bronchial inhalation therapies should be included as a probable need by the life care planner in the cervical and mid to high thoracic-level spinal cord injured individuals due to the reported infection occurrence rates and rehospitalization rate due to diseases of the respiratory system.

Chronic ventilation may become necessary to sustain life for those with global alveolar hypoventilation, particularly with vital capacities that are less than 5–10 mL/kg. There are a variety of devices that are employed to assist individuals with respiratory function. These include ventilation assist machines, such as continuous positive airway pressure (CPAP) and biphasic positive airway pressure (BiPAP), which can improve oxygenation and prevent hypercarbia. Phrenic nerve pacing (diaphragm pacing) is another option that electrically stimulates the diaphragm to produce more physiologic respirations. Phrenic nerve pacing provides many ventilator-dependent tetraplegics with freedom from total dependence upon mechanical ventilation. Even though many individuals with phrenic nerve pacing will still require periods of ventilator assistance throughout the day and night, the risk of death is diminished in the event of mechanical failure of the ventilator and affords time for back-up measures to be put into place.

In higher and complete cervical spine injuries (C1–4), ventilator assistance at some level is usually required and is administered through a tracheostomy tube. These individuals require 24-hour skilled nursing care to protect the airway, provide suctioning of secretions, pulmonary toilet, and management of the tracheostomy tube as well as to ensure accurate ventilator functioning.

Pain

Chronic pain occurs in 70–80% of individuals with spinal cord injury (Bryce et al., 2007; Cardenas & Felix, 2009). Approximately one-third of persons with SCI report chronic severe pain that interferes with activities of daily living and affects QoL. In one study, a survey of the spinal cord injured revealed that approximately one-third of individuals with chronic pain were willing to trade the possibility of recovery from SCI for pain relief (Nepomuceno et al., 1979).

Individuals with spinal cord injury often experience an array of nociceptive, visceral, and neuropathic type pain. Nociceptive pain is defined pathophysiologically by the transmission of pain impulses through the normal peripheral and central pathways. Examples of this type of pain would include the inflammatory pain from overuse of compensating joints or musculoskeletal tissue injury, such as rotator cuff syndrome. Visceral pain occurs in the abdomen or thorax and is generally described as a dull, aching, or cramping pain. It is most commonly associated with urinary tract infection, ureterolithiasis, cholelithiasis, or obstipation of the bowel with impaction. One of the particular challenges in caring for individuals with spinal cord injury is the often inchoate nature of their pain, which can mask serious underlying conditions, such as an acute appendicitis or nephrolithiasis. Neuropathic pain is caused by injury to the spinal cord or nerve roots and is believed to be the result of aberrant transmission of electrical impulses by damaged nerve pathways or by chronic electrochemical changes in the brain itself resulting from a spinal cord injury. It is therefore not at all unusual for individuals with spinal cord injury to experience pain in limbs that are insensate to external stimuli. While some individuals often describe this pain as "electrical," "stabbing," "shooting," or "burning," others may have difficulty articulating the specific nature of the pain. Another curious feature of neuropathic pain is the phenomenon of allodynia, in which a normally benign external stimulus (such as lightly stroking the skin) can be perceived as painful. Neuropathic pain itself can be further sub-divided into pain at the level of a spinal cord injury and pain below the level of the injury. It is important to recognize neuropathic pain and to treat it aggressively, since delayed treatment is believed to contribute to the chronicity and refractoriness of the pain.

In contrast to the use of nonsteroidal anti-inflammatory medications and prescriptive analgesics for the management of nociceptive pain, the treatment of neuropathic pain generally involves the use of anticonvulsant agents (i.e., gabapentin, pregabalin, lamotrigine), tricyclic antidepressants, and serotonin-norepinephrine reuptake inhibitors (i.e., duloxetine). For persons whose neuropathic pain responds suboptimally to oral agents, other treatment modalities include topical analgesics (i.e., lidocaine or compounded analgesics), electrical neurostimulation, and neuroablative techniques.

Many individuals with spinal cord injuries also experience secondary nociceptive pain caused by joint inflammation, tissue injury, and muscle spasms at some point in their lives. Approximately two-thirds of patients with upper extremity pain state that it interferes with their ability to transfer to and from a wheelchair, and rotator cuff tears are reported in 65% of those with chronic impingement syndrome with subacromial bursitis (Bagwell et al., 2010). Wrist pain is reported in 53–64% of persons with chronic SCI and this is attributed to compressive loading during transfers with the wrist in extension (Bagwell et al., 2010).

Joint pain can arise from either disuse or overuse of limbs, which can cause contractures in the former situation and tissue disruption in the latter. Rotator cuff tendinitis and tears as well as entrapment neuropathies of the ulnar and median nerves are common manifestations of overuse syndromes that occur in association with dependence upon the upper extremities to propel manual wheelchairs and perform frequent transfers. Interestingly, when no pain is present, QoL scores in SCI are similar to those of the general population. This highlights the potential for improved QoL post-injury, in line with population norms, if pain can be proactively managed and its impact reduced (Burke et al., 2018).

Genitourinary

To achieve urinary continence, the bladder must perform two functions: (1) store urine produced by the kidney; and (2) expel urine when appropriate. For success of both functions, neurological input is required from the cerebral cortex, spinal cord, and peripheral nervous system. Disruption anywhere along those neural pathways can lead to various degrees of bladder dysfunction (Lucas, 2019). Genitourinary dysfunction represents one of the most profound changes that occurs in spinal cord injury. For those with spinal cord injury, 70–84% have at least some degree of bladder dysfunction (Dorsher, 2012; Manack, 2011). Injuries that occur above the level of the conus medullaris (T12–L1) are associated with upper motor neuron dysfunction characterized by a spastic, hyperactive bladder, often with incoordination between the bladder musculature and the external sphincter, referred to as detrusor-external sphincter dyssynergia. If left untreated, this condition can result in renal injury from elevated pressures within the urinary tract.

Our understanding of how high, sustained intravesical pressures contribute to the development of chronic renal insufficiency and the consequent need to maintain low-pressure systems has been one of the greatest influences on improved survivals and life expectancies for those with SCI. In the 1960s, renal failure was a leading cause of death in the SCI population (Tribe, 1963). Deaths as a result of diseases of the genitourinary system in the SCI population as of 2021 were only 2.9%, representing the eleventh leading cause of death (NSCISC, 2021a). Renal failure in the general population is the tenth leading cause of death at 15.9 per 100,000 population (Centers for Disease Control, National Center for Health Statistics, National Vital Statistics System, 2021)

Spinal cord injuries below the level of T12–L1 (lower motor neuron bladder) are generally associated with a flaccid bladder that expands greatly, resulting in overflow incontinence as pressure from the distended bladder overwhelms the sphincter that is often incompetent. Intermittent catheterization represents the primary choice for urinary drainage in patients with neurogenic bladders. In most cases, this method reduces the incidence of recurrent urinary infection, urinary and ureteral reflux, and stone formation. Chronic indwelling catheterization is not generally recommended due to the increased risk for infection, bladder stones, and urethral trauma. Studies have also shown that bladder cancer risk and mortality are heightened in the spinal cord injured population compared with the general population and that chronic indwelling catheterization is a significant independent risk factor for the increased risk of and mortality caused by bladder cancer in the spinal cord injured population (Groah et al., 2002). However, this approach may be required when intermittent catheterization is not feasible to maintain a low-pressure system otherwise. This may occur when the individual is unable to perform clean intermittent catheterization independently while in a setting where competent assistance is not available to perform these procedures multiple times each day for the individual. Other factors may include difficult catheter insertion from a traumatized urethra or obstructive process. The surgical placement of a suprapubic catheter is another method of neurogenic bladder management; however, this procedure also contributes to increased risks for bacteremia and renal stone formation as well as significantly heightened risks for bladder cancer over time (Groah et al., 2002).

While deaths due to diseases of the genitourinary system in the spinal cord population have continued to decline since the 1960's with the understanding of proper urological management, these conditions continue to represent the leading cause of rehospitalization for every post-injury year by a large margin.

Proper urological management minimizes the risk of renal complications by reducing risk factors such as cystitis, pyelonephritis, vesicoureteral reflux, and trauma from the use of long-term indwelling catheters. The goals of treatment include establishment of a plan that maintains low detrusor pressures and allows complete bladder emptying. Continued urological follow-up is recommended to monitor for and reduce the risk of these renal, ureteral, and bladder complications.

Established protocols for follow-up and monitoring of the neurogenic bladder include the following:

The baseline urological evaluation (one time only):

- History and physical examination
- Urinalysis
- Urine culture & sensitivity
- 24-hour creatinine clearance or radionuclide scan
- Post void residual (when applicable)
- Renal scan and/or renal ultrasound
- Urodynamics
- CT urography or intravenous pyelogram (baseline assessment)

Subsequent Routine Follow-up:

- History and physical examination
- Urinalysis

- Urine culture & sensitivity
- Serum BUN and creatinine
- 24-hour creatinine clearance or radionuclide scan
- Kidney, ureter, bladder (KUB)
- Renal scan or renal ultrasound annually (Note: Some centers recommend renal scans annually as a preferred study to renal ultrasounds which are performed when the renal scan suggests concern for obstructive disease, such as renal/ureteral calculi. Other centers recommend ultrasound annually with intermittent renal scans otherwise.)
- Urodynamic evaluations performed at one year and as needed thereafter, usually every other year if the bladder appears to be stable

Post Void Residual When Applicable

- Urography: CT urography or intravenous pyelogram/cystourethrogram at approximately 3–5 year intervals
- Cystoscopy: Opinions on frequency vary greatly, but indications for cystoscopy include hematuria, recurrent symptomatic UTI, recurrent asymptomatic bacteremia with stone forming organism, i.e., Proteus mirabilis, episode of GU sepsis, eggshell calculus present with irrigating catheter, and management with long-term indwelling catheter

Diagnostic follow-up and treatment of neurogenic bladder is best performed by a urologist who is experienced with spinal cord injury and associated neurogenic bladder disorders. Improvements in the urological diagnostic investigation have reduced the incidence of progressive disease and death associated with end stage renal disease (ESRD) for the SCI population. While the risk of ESRD remains slightly higher due to inherent complications with urinary tract infection, obstruction, and reflux, the incidence rates continue to decline such that it is approaching those of the general population.

Metabolic Changes

While mortality rates for individuals with spinal cord injuries are declining for cancer, heart disease, arterial diseases, urinary diseases, digestive diseases, and suicide (NSCISC, 2020) these improvements are offset by increasing mortality rates for metabolic and endocrine diseases. Metabolic dysfunction following spinal cord injury is characterized by a high prevalence of lipid disorders, impaired glucose tolerance, and insulin resistance (Rankin et al., 2017). As a result of the reduced energy expenditure, most individuals with SCI experience weight gain that can further affect functional capabilities. For people with paraparesis, weight gain results in greater stress on upper extremity joints during transfers, increasing the risk for accelerated degenerative changes or overuse syndromes, such as rotator cuff injuries. The prevalence of obesity in this population is approximately 50% (Bloom et al., 2020). Weight gain also has negative implications for cardiovascular health. In addition, additional weight places more pressure on tissues during recumbence, substantially increasing the risk for decubiti.

The most common hormonal changes that accompany spinal cord injury include insulin resistance and reduced levels of growth hormone and testosterone. The incidence of diabetes mellitus is 2–3 times higher in individuals with SCI relative to the general population, with prevalence ranging from 13.66 to 20% compared with 5.91% in individuals without SCI (Cragg et al., 2013; LaVela et al., 2006). Low levels of growth hormone and testosterone have been associated with accelerated loss of lean muscle mass, impaired cellular repair mechanisms, and prolonged healing.

Heterotopic ossification (HO) refers to the formation of new bone in the peri-articular soft tissue. Clinically significant HO occurs in approximately 20% of individuals who have sustained spinal cord injuries (Kedlaya, 2018). The hips are commonly involved and those affected often present with impaired joint range of motion, associated with edema and warmth of the affected extremity. The diagnosis is typically made through the physical examination and x-rays, which clearly demonstrate the heterotopic bone formation.

Spinal cord injury results in profound bone demineralization caused by the lack of weight bearing. Approximately 16 months after a spinal cord injury, bone homeostasis occurs at a reduced rate, which can approach the fracture threshold. Osteopenia is thereafter facilitated by osteoclastic activity associated with the aging process. This leads to hypercalcemia and hypercalciuria, which likely contribute to the development of not only heterotopic ossification but also nephrolithiasis (kidney stones). Another consequence of demineralization is osteoporosis, with the attendant susceptibility to fractures, which can worsen overall disability. In fact, studies have reported that fractures occur in 21% of the SCI population and that the prevalence increases over time post-injury. The most common sites of fracture are the distal femur and proximal tibia (Bagwell et al., 2010). Common complications of these fractures include delayed union or non-union, pressure sores, and osteomyelitis. Individuals with SCI should undergo periodic monitoring (via DEXA scan) for the development of osteoporosis and should be maintained on vitamin D and calcium supplementation for prophylaxis. While some clinicians proactively prescribe bisphosphonates, recognizing the very high propensity toward long bone fractures, some studies have identified an association between the long-term use of this medication class with the development of osteonecrosis of the jaw (ONJ) (Blanchaert, 2021). Other options for prophylaxis include calcitonin and estrogen modulators (i.e., raloxifene).

Integumentary Issues

Spinal cord injury reduces or eliminates skin sensation in dermatomes below the injury site. Because individuals have either complete loss of sensation or impaired sensation, they may sit or lie for long periods of time on certain parts of their body. Due to associated muscle atrophy, the normal tissue padding that serves to cushion the skin is reduced. Normally, skin responds to pressure, mechanical stimulation, or inflammation with increased blood flow, but this reflex is blunted by SCI. Loss of this response not only adds to the vulnerability of the skin to pressure sores but reduces the ability of the skin to repair decubitus ulcers once formed.

Diseases of the skin represent a leading cause of first year post-SCI admissions, second only to disease of the genitourinary system, with increasing rates of rehospitalization with age and years post-injury (NSCISC, 2020). At any given time, approximately one-third of persons with SCI in the community have a decubitus ulcer and 15% have a stage 3 or 4 ulcer (NSCISC, 2020). Once a pressure sore is encountered, the scarred tissue upon healing is more fragile; therefore, the risk of recurrence is heightened. Approximately 35% of those who have sustained a spinal cord injury will experience three or more admissions for this condition over their lifetime (Bagwell et al., 2010). About 75% will admit in follow-up studies to having at least three ulcers at stage 3 or worse (Bagwell et al., 2010).

Decubitus ulcers are potentially life threatening, but progression of these wounds to advanced stages is largely preventable. Great care must be taken to prevent injury to the integument from pressure by shifting sitting positions and frequent turning. If sensory feedback is poor or nonexistent, many individuals use electronic devices such as watch alarms to provide timely cueing for lifting and repositioning. Special cushions for sitting and mattresses for extended recumbence have been developed to lessen the pressure upon bony prominences. Special seats that distribute the pressure are used in wheelchairs to prevent sacral decubiti. Vulnerable areas, such as the heels, must be padded. Seating devices must be maintained, and adjustments made to avoid shearing and contact with hard or abrasive surfaces due to impaired sensory feedback. Sheep skin and other materials are often used for heel and foot protection, as well as orthotic devices to fully offload pressure on the heels, a common site for decubiti. If a decubitus develops, all pressure must be removed, or the decubitus can progress to loss of skin and tissues to the point of exposing bone. The sores must be kept clean, or they can become infected. Extensive counseling and prevention education should be started early and continued in the years following the injury. Routine inspection by the patient, caregivers, and through periodic skilled nursing visits should usually identify the onset of these wounds in the earlier stages. Treatment of decubitus ulcers, once developed, requires extensive care, and may lead to costly hospitalizations with or without the need for plastic surgery intervention.

Cardiovascular Disease

One consequence of the reduced mortality from respiratory and renal complications is a relative increase in SCI deaths related to cardiovascular disease. Cardiovascular disease and associated complications are leading causes of long-term morbidity and mortality in individuals with spinal cord injury (Krassioukov et al., 2019). Contributing factors include reduced HDL cholesterol levels, higher incidences of obesity, and less exercise relative to the general population. Furthermore, individuals with SCI have smaller left ventricular volumes and mass, and altered systolic and diastolic function (Williams et al., 2019). Non-ambulatory individuals are also at risk for the development of phlebitis, deep venous thromboses, and pulmonary emboli, resulting from reduced sympathetic tone and diminished venous return. Therefore, it is critical that preventative measures be taken that include the frequent use of anti-embolic hose as well as frequent lower extremity exercises to reduce venous stasis. Individuals who are at particular risk for the development of deep venous thromboses may require chronic anticoagulation or even placement of devices within the inferior vena cava that can prevent clots from entering the pulmonary vasculature. Furthermore, the clinician should have a low threshold for ordering screening tests, such as Doppler ultrasonography to evaluate for the presence of clots that would necessitate more aggressive management.

Therefore, routine cardiac surveillance (i.e., periodic EKG's, echocardiography, Persantine stress test) should be instituted even in the younger SCI population, along with proactive recommendations that include aerobic exercise, weight control, and avoidance of tobacco products as well as other risk factors. Furthermore, those with spinal cord injury should anticipate the need for cholesterol lowering agents much earlier than the general population.

Individuals who are non-ambulatory are at substantially elevated risk for the development of various peripheral vascular complications, presumably secondary to the ineffective distribution of oxygenated blood and impaired venous return in the dependent regions of the body, especially the legs. One of the more common and serious conditions is the development of deep vein thrombosis (DVT). Studies on the incidence of DVT in this population are varied, ranging from as low as 7% to as high as 100% (Myers et al., 2007). Although the risk appears to be greatest during the first six months post-injury, DVT and thrombophlebitis remain lifelong concerns, particularly as the person ages. Risk factors include impaired mobility and reduced sympathetic tone, which contribute to venous pooling in the lower extremities. Once developed, DVT may continue to be problematic and require periods of prophylaxis and monitoring. With chronic changes in the peripheral venous system, the risk of venous pooling and thrombus formation again becomes a concern with aging.

Preventative measures include the use of anti-embolic hose to preserve the integrity of the peripheral venous system. Screening procedures include Doppler ultrasound, impedance plethysmography, and leg measurements. The definitive procedure for the diagnosis of DVT is venography, although this test is not without risk.

The most concerning risk of deep venous thrombosis is the development of a pulmonary embolism, which constitutes a significant cause of morbidity and mortality in the SCI population, with an incidence of approximately 5% in the first three months post-injury and 1–2% thereafter (Alabed et al., 2015). Pulmonary embolism may require diagnosis with the use of ventilation-perfusion (V/Q) scanning, although CT angiography of the pulmonary vasculature is today the most common diagnostic tool.

Infections

Infections of the respiratory and genitourinary tracts and the integument constitute the leading causes for hospital admissions for every post-injury year (NSCISC, 2021b). Urinary tract infections have consistently remained the leading cause of infection in patients with either traumatic or nontraumatic spinal cord injury, with an occurrence rate of 2.5 events per patient per year (Salameh et al., 2015). Most cases of septicemia in these patients can be attributed to the urinary tract, with a death rate of about 15% (Siroky, 2002). Infection rates are even higher in those who have chronic indwelling catheters. The increased risk of acquiring urinary tract infections in SCI is multifactorial, including reduced sensation of classical UTI symptoms, incomplete bladder emptying, frequent catheterizations, or chronic urinary tract catheters. Tofte (2017) stated:

> Due to the increased risk of acquiring recurrent or chronic UTIs and frequent antibiotic treatments, patients experience an increased risk of being infected with antibiotic-resistant bacteria like extended-spectrum β-lactamase-producing Escherichia coli or Klebsiella spp., but also bacteria like Pseudomonas aeruginosa inherently resistant to several antibiotics. Diagnosing the UTI can also be challenging, especially distinguishing harmless colonization from pathogenic infection.
> (Tofte et al., 2017, p. 385)

Of all individuals followed in model systems of care, urinary tract infections requiring antibiotic treatment have exceeded 50% in each 12-month period at post-injury year follow-up from years 1–40 (NSCISC, 2020). The number of UTIs requiring antibiotic treatment in the preceding 12-month period is delineated in Table 98 (p. 130) of the full public version of the NSCISC (2020) Annual Report for 1–2, 3–5, > 5 times per year, and unknown number of UTIs per year by post-injury year. As such, infections should be considered anticipated (i.e., probable) in the SCI population, not just potential complications. Individuals with higher level spinal cord injuries, particularly those with impaired respiratory function, are at substantially elevated risk for respiratory infections that can lead to sepsis. Other important risk factors for infection include the inability to weight bear and impaired mobility as well as the presence of bowel or bladder incontinence. Proactive measures, including pulmonary toilet, prevention of decubiti through frequent turning and skin surveillance, and the avoidance of chronic indwelling catheters can substantially reduce (but not eliminate) the incidence of infections.

The life care planner should project the need for periodic courses of both oral and intravenous antibiotics and recognize that with many years post-injury, the organisms become more resistant to conventional pharmacotherapy, necessitating the use of newer generation agents. Some patients with severe UTI recurrence may require chronic, prophylactic pharmacotherapies.

Overuse Syndromes

Overuse syndromes occur when individuals repeatedly perform the same movements, resulting in inflammation and damage to soft tissues (i.e., muscles, nerves, and tendons). These conditions are generally more prevalent in individuals with spinal cord injury who are living independently, without assistance (Heyward et al., 2017). Examples include the propulsion of wheelchairs, the use of canes, walkers as well as use of the arms for functional transfers. In one study (Curtis et al., 1999) 75% of subjects reported a history of shoulder pain since beginning wheelchair use. Such activities lead to accelerated degenerative changes, particularly in the shoulders but can also cause ulnar and median nerve entrapment syndromes at the elbow and wrist respectively, with wrist pain reported in up to 64% of persons with SCI (Dalyan et al., 1999). Diagnosis of shoulder injury (i.e., rotator cuff tear, bursitis, capsulitis) is usually made radiologically (i.e., MRI), while entrapment syndromes (i.e., the ulnar nerve at the cubital tunnel, the median nerve at the carpal tunnel) are definitively diagnosed by electrophysiological testing (i.e., EMG/NCV). Shoulder symptoms that prove refractory to conservative therapy or for which there is evidence of major structural pathology usually require arthroscopic surgery. Similarly, peripheral nerve entrapments that are not improved with orthotics and/or anti-inflammatory agents generally need decompression (i.e., ulnar nerve transposition, carpal tunnel release).

Sexual Function and Reproduction

Sexual function relies upon common neurologic pathways that innervate the bladder and bowel. Not surprisingly, spinal cord injuries that affect bowel and bladder function are likely to interfere with normal sexual function as well. Complete spinal cord injuries above the sacral segments produce a complete loss of psychogenic erectile function with relative preservation of reflex erectile functions. For males with erectile dysfunction caused by spinal cord injury, treatment modalities include the use of constriction bands, vacuum erection devices, oral pharmacologic agents (e.g., sildenafil, tadalafil, vardenafil, avanafil), prostaglandin penile injections, urethral suppository (MUSE/Alprostadil), and surgically implanted penile prosthesis. Testosterone levels should always be checked as well, as many men with spinal cord injuries experience deficiency of this hormone.

Females with spinal cord injury frequently experience disorders of genital sensation, arousal, and orgasm in addition to menstrual irregularities and even cessation of menstruation. Other comorbid conditions that impact sexual health include the presence of decubitus ulcers and bowel and bladder incontinence. The use of oral contraception for females with impaired mobility is relatively contraindicated secondary to the increased risk for deep venous thrombosis. Therefore, barrier contraception is generally recommended.

Spinal cord injury also impairs both male and female fertility and women who become pregnant have a higher incidence of premature and low birthweight neonates. Nonetheless, for couples who desire biological children, assisted reproduction techniques are available. For men, vibratory ejaculation and electrical stimulation allow for retrieval of sperm in the vast majority of cases. Testicular sperm extraction (TESE) and percutaneous epididymal sperm aspiration (PESA) are techniques that have a high success rate (Raviv et al., 2013). The cost for this, in the authors' experience, is reported to range from $3,000 to $12,000. Other assistive techniques include intravaginal insemination, intrauterine insemination, and *in vitro* fertilization.

Most individuals with SCI who experience sexual dysfunction and/or infertility benefit from counseling, not only to address the emotional sequelae, but also to learn about the spectrum of treatment options.

The life care planner must be aware of how both sexuality and fertility are affected by spinal cord injury and incorporate this knowledge into the interview and evaluation process. As each life care plan is individualized, it is important to consider age, relationship status, and desire for children, with an understanding that these are fluid.

Psychological Issues

Aside from physical disability, one of the most profound consequences of a spinal cord injury is the emotional impact upon the individual and their family, particularly after discharge from the hospital or rehabilitation facility. People with chronic disabilities, including spinal cord injury are at substantially greater risk for depression and anxiety as well as adjustment disorders. Not only can this result from the significant physical limitations, but also from the debilitating effects of secondary complications like pain, social isolation, and socioeconomic challenges that may limit access to adequate levels of healthcare.

While much of the literature references the greatest risk for depression occurring in the first months to one year following the onset of SCI, other longer-term follow-up studies have found ongoing problems with depression in SCI. For example, Anderson et al. (2007) reported depressive symptoms ranging from mild to severe in 27% of adults with childhood or adolescent onset of SCI, with 7% having suicidal thoughts in the prior two weeks, and 3% with symptoms consistent with probable major depressive disorder. It was concluded that depression is a significant problem among adults with pediatric-onset SCI and is associated with poorer outcomes and lower quality of life. Williams and Murray (2015) found the mean prevalence estimate of depression diagnosis after SCI was 22.2%, with a lower-bound estimate of 18.7% and an upper bound estimate of 26.3%. They concluded that the existing data on depression after SCI indicate that the prevalence of depression after SCI is substantially greater than that in the general medical population.

Family members are also subjected to social and psychological stress and may find themselves undergoing an adjustment process as they respond to changing roles and functions within the family unit. Depression and other psychological conditions are highly prevalent after SCI and counseling should be offered to address issues such as the acceptance of impairment and the impact of the disability upon the family, as well as sexual and vocational roles. A psychologist, counselor, or psychiatrist can assist other team members by clarifying the patient's behavior and recommending therapies that promote healthy adaptation. The judicious prescription of antidepressant medication is often appropriate in conjunction with adjustment counseling.

Home Modifications for Individuals with SCI

Those with SCI require modifications of most residential settings for accessibility and function commensurate with the level of their impairments. The residence will need to consider safe and unobstructed access from the location of vehicular storage (garage or carport), as well as routine and emergency ingress and egress for a wheelchair-dependent resident. Primary and emergency secondary egress ramping is recommended. Adequate storage space is required for supplies and the array of large and bulky durable medical equipment items, as well as sufficient space for living quarters and family circumstances for sleeping areas. Careful planning is required to construct a fully functional bathroom that is accessible by a roll-in shower chair and large enough to accommodate caregivers who may be required for assistance. The shower area will need to have sufficient interior space for transfers and turning in the shower chair, or gurney when applicable, and to enter and exit with the help of a caregiver when required. An area of the modified home will be required for home exercise programming, as well as a caregiver workstation. Standard doorways and hallways are usually too narrow to allow for ease of wheelchair access, or as may be required for maneuverability with other assistive devices. As such, personal injury, sheetrock, and baseboard trauma and damage to equipment can occur if this is not addressed during the planning phases. Proper architectural planning and construction consultation can alleviate many of these concerns and avoid unnecessary expense or potential injury to the wheelchair occupant or caregiver. Case management services can be most helpful to coordinate appropriate referrals for assistance with this process.

While the overall cost of medical care is generally higher for the individual with tetraplegia than the paraplegia, in the authors' experience, home modifications for the individual with paraplegia can be more involved, and thus, more costly than the requirements needed for most individuals with tetraplegia. This is because the individual with paraplegia has full use of the upper extremities and has greater functional independence than the individual with tetraplegia, if the home environment isandomizely modified. One example of this involves modifications of kitchens and laundry rooms. The individual with tetraplegia, especially those above C6, will have greater dependence upon others for meal preparation and kitchen clean-up, thus potentially negating the need for some of the more extensive modifications of cabinets. Under most circumstances, the individual with paraplegia can prepare meals and perform kitchen clean-up tasks, if necessary, items are located within reach at wheelchair level. This necessitates redesigning of cabinets, sinks, and counters, as well as acquisition and installation of ADA appliances that are accessible and functional at wheelchair level. Laundry rooms in most residential homes are, more often than not, smaller, and not accessible for those in wheelchairs. There are, however, washers and dryers that are designed for ADA compliance by a host of manufacturers with wide front-opening doors and eye level controls. Again, sinks and counter tops in the laundry room need to be at appropriate heights for accessibility and the space will need to be adequate for maneuverability in a wheelchair. As such, those with greater functional potential at wheelchair level will have needs for home modifications beyond those who have greater dependence upon others without disability for basic activities of daily living.

Another consideration in projecting the cost of home modifications is the location of the proposed project. Construction costs, particularly the costs for tradesmen and craftsmen, can vary widely from one region of the country to another. When deciding to modify an existing residence, the age of the residence is an important consideration and applicable construction codes. An older residence may be required to undergo complete updates of electrical and plumbing throughout the entire house to bring the structure current with applicable local codes, even if merely adding an addition to the home. This could be a game changer and should be investigated before incurring the cost of design, only to learn of this at the time of submitting plans for building permits.

The Department of Veterans Affairs provides Specially Adapted Housing Grants to help disabled Veterans and Service members to have access to wheelchair accessible homes. This can provide independent living that might not otherwise be possible. As of January 2022, the maximum grant amount is $101,754. It must be used for the purpose of constructing or modifying a home to meet adaptive needs. The maximum grant amount adjusts annually (www.benefits.va.gov/homeloans/adaptedhousing.asp). In the authors' opinion, this level of grant reflects a reasonable floor for estimating the basic needs for projected home modification expenses for those with SCI in the absence of an opportunity for formal architectural renderings and building proposals or when the disabled individual may be in temporary housing. Yet, few areas of cost projections in life care planning for the SCI will be as variable in cost ranges as home modifications due to the differences in specific living environments and the neurological level of injury. When in-home elevators are required, the cost is vastly greater. Load bearing walls, truss versus rafter roof construction, property setback restrictions, floor elevation requirements due to codes for flood risks (especially in coastal regions), and updating to local electrical and plumbing codes can all significantly impact the cost. When we have had the opportunity and benefit of consultation with architects and receive building proposals, it has not been uncommon to encounter cost projections ranging from $250,000 or more with some home modifications for those with spinal cord injury.

Vehicular Modifications for Individuals with SCI

A wide range of vehicular modifications exist for individuals with spinal cord injury. The level of injury and preservation of motor and sensory function are key factors in the determination of appropriate modifications for independence with vehicular transportation. Individuals with paraplegia who are young, otherwise healthy, and have lower thoracic or lumbar lesions may choose to opt for hand controls only. This will offer them the greatest selection of vehicles and styles that may be important to their self-esteem, although this requires the physical ability to lift, hoist, and maneuver their wheelchairs into the interior of the vehicle while sitting in the driver's seat or provide for an alternative way to secure the wheelchair within the vehicle during transit. Over time, the self-esteem derived from sports cars or trucks with lift kits usually gives way to the benefit of ease and efficiency of vehicular ingress and egress with comfort, convenience, and operational functionally, especially when inclement weather is a factor.

Independent vehicular operation is best accomplished with ramp vans. Well-known vehicular retrofitters, such as the Braun Corporation (BraunAbility: Rampvan, Companion Van, and Entervan) and Vantage Mobility International (VMI), provide safe and effective transportation. These vehicular adaptations provide for a ramp rather than an undercarriage power lift for entrance and egress. The vehicle can be raised or lowered hydraulically to reduce the angle of ascent or descent for ease of entrance and exit. Appropriate wheelchair securement is provided with multiple interior configurations available for driver and passenger location during transit. Modifications for vehicular operation may range from basic hand controls for the paraplegic to more sophisticated electronics with actuators, servo motors, touch screen controls, and joystick operation for the tetraplegic. There is now a vast array of vehicular choices from minivans and full-sized vans to several SUV models with either side or rear entry options. The cost for modifications for these vehicles, in the authors' experience, can range from $45,000 to more than $100,000, above and beyond the cost of the selected vehicle prior to modification. As one might expect, the sophisticated electronic control mechanisms needed for safe vehicular operation by individuals with lesions above C6 are at the higher end of the cost spectrum; however, being able to enter, exit, and operate a vehicle without assistance from others offers those with SCI a tremendous sense of freedom and autonomy.

A newer concept meeting the needs for individuals requiring vehicular modification is provided by Mobility Ventures. While the more established companies modify vans produced by major automotive manufacturers, Mobility Ventures has taken a "ground-up" approach to manufacture the entire vehicle, called the MV-1. This process also results in less overall costs for the total package of the vehicle and modifications. As such, individuals with disabilities now have an option for a sport utility vehicle. This is great news for many younger individuals who find it difficult to wrap their arms around the idea of driving a minivan.

The life care planner will need to consider that these modifications are required with each replacement vehicle purchased over time. In considering usual replacement cycles, it should be kept in mind that being stranded in a vehicle due to mechanical failure presents a very serious concern for individuals with paralysis relative to the able-bodied population.

Powered Robotic Exoskeletons in SCI

Prior to the development of robotic exoskeletons, individuals with SCI had few options for mobility aside from wheelchairs. Achieving the ability to walk again is without a doubt among the top priorities for individuals with SCI. The added benefits of improving overall physical, cardiovascular, and mental health further support the desire to return to walking. Powered robotic exoskeletons, first developed for use in the military, represent major technological advances toward the goal of functional ambulation for many with thoracic-level spinal cord injuries. These robotic exoskeletons are wearable orthoses that can be used as an assistive device to enable some individuals with SCI to walk or to augment rehabilitation. They can also increase activities of daily living, such as standing to cook or to reach objects and improve the ability to perform aerobic exercise to mitigate the risk of cardiometabolic syndrome (Kandilakis & Sasso-Lance, 2021).

On June 26, 2014, the FDA granted approval to Argo Medical Technologies (now marketed as ReWalk Robotics) for the sale of the ReWalk powered exoskeleton device for private use in the United States. With its initial release, the ReWalk was available in two versions, one for medical institutions for research and therapeutic applications under professional supervision, the ReWalk I, and another for personal use at home or in public, the ReWalk P. The newest iteration, the ReWalk Rehabilitation 6.0, features enhanced software for improved control and sizing options for taller individuals.

On March 10, 2016, the FDA granted Parker Hannifin permission to market and sell its Vanderbilt-designed Indego exoskeleton for clinical and personal use in the United States. The Indego Personal, at 29 pounds, is marketed to be considerably lighter and less bulky than the other exoskeletons under development. The Indego is reported to incorporate functional electrical stimulation and adjust robotic assistance automatically for users who have some preserved muscle function, allowing use of their own muscles while walking.

On April 4, 2016, the Ekso GT Robotic Exoskeleton (Ekso Bionics Holdings, Inc) was cleared by the FDA for use in the treatment of individuals with hemiplegia due to stroke, individuals with spinal cord injuries at levels T4 to L5, and individuals with spinal cord injuries at levels of T3 to C7 (ASIA D). The Ekso GT is the first exoskeleton cleared by the FDA for use with stroke patients. The EksoNR is the latest version of this technology and has also been approved for use in patients with acquired brain injuries.

Powered robotic exoskeletons can provide thoracic-level spinal cord injured individuals the ability to walk. They do require the use of a gait aid, such as forearm crutches, for support during walking. Individuals with lower thoracic lesions have greater preservation of truncal musculature, which helps with proficiency and speed of gait with less dependence upon their arms. Continued technological improvements will likely improve gait speed over time such that powered exoskeletal walking can be more efficiently used in the community and various terrains. The cost of these power robotic exoskeletons for personal use ranges from $75,000 to $80,000 for the device alone, although for devices such as the Esko, suitable for stroke and higher level SCI, it may reach $150,000 and is targeted for rehab centers for use by multiple patients (Lok, 2017). It should be noted that extensive training on the use of these devices is also required. The time required for such training is dependent upon a variety of factors, including the specific exoskeleton being used, comorbid conditions, and the user's functional goals.

Aging with Spinal Cord Injury and Personal Care Assistance Needs

Every person who lives long enough will eventually experience a decline in function. However, for people who have sustained a spinal cord injury, this process is accelerated and compounded by comorbidities, such as overuse syndromes, accelerated osteoarthritis, chronic pain, decubiti, infections, and recurrent hospitalizations (Hitzig et al., 2008). The individual with a spinal cord injury is typically younger at the time of their injury and experiences not only an immediate reduction in functional reserves but also in their financial resources. Since greater than 25% of all individuals with spinal cord injury are now more than 20 years post event (NSCISC, 2020), healthcare professionals must be aware of these changes and be proactive in implementing services that can mitigate this functional decline. Similarly, life care planning must consider the need for, and degree of personal care services based upon the age of the individual, the number of years since injury, the level of injury, the presence or absence of chronic pain, and other concomitant or comorbid medical conditions. Among the more age-specific problems that are unique to or more pronounced in this population are the following:

Spasticity That Contributes to Pain and Impaired Function

Overuse syndromes (i.e., rotator cuff injuries, tendinitis, and peripheral entrapment neuropathies) related to wheelchair mobility and transfers

Recurrent Decubiti from Hypomobility

The need for frequent courses of both oral and intravenous antibiotics with the subsequent development of highly resistant strains of bacteria

The vast majority of individuals with tetraplegia and many of those with paraplegia require personal care assistance (skilled nursing care if they are ventilator dependent and severe respiratory compromise otherwise) regardless of age. For most individuals with tetraplegia, living alone is not a viable option. While the younger person with a lower thoracic paraplegia may initially require little personal care assistance and only modest homemaking and household services, as they age, they will require increasing levels of personal care and homemaking assistance.

The Consortium for Spinal Cord Medicine develops and disseminates evidence-based clinical practice guidelines to professionals and consumers. Its membership consists of healthcare professional groups and payer and consumer organizations extensively involved with spinal cord injury. The Consortium publishes several clinical practice guidelines for health care professionals involved in the care and treatment of individuals with spinal cord injury. One such guideline is the Outcomes Following Traumatic Spinal Cord Injury (Paralyzed Veterans of America, 1999). This guideline is perhaps one of the most commonly used and cited guidelines for life care planners and case managers working with individuals with SCI. The guideline presents expectations of functional performance of SCI at one year post-injury and at each of eight levels of injury (C1–3, C4, C5, C6, C7–8, T1–9, T10–L1, and L2–S5).

The outcomes reflect a level of independence that can be expected of a person with motor complete SCI, given optimal circumstances. The categories presented reflect expected functional outcomes in the areas of mobility, activities of daily living, instrumental activities of daily living, and communication skills. The guidelines were based on consensus of clinical experts, available literature on functional outcomes, and data compiled from Uniform Data Systems (UDS) and the National Spinal Cord Injury Statistical Center (Paralyzed Veterans of America, 1999, p.11).

The panel participants of the Consortium of Spinal Cord Medicine identified a series of essential daily functions and activities, expected levels of functioning, and the equipment and attendant care likely to be needed to support the predicted level of independence at one year post-injury. The panel also emphasized that the expected functional outcomes "must be individualized to the unique characteristics, circumstances, and capabilities of each person with SCI" (Paralyzed Veterans of America, 1999, p.10).

The Functional Independence Measure (FIM) estimates are widely variable in several of the categories. It is unknown if those with SCI in the individual categories attained the expected functional outcomes for their specific level of injury or if there were mitigating circumstances such as age, obesity, or concomitant injuries, that would account for variability in assistance reported. An individualized assessment of needs is required in all cases.

While the guidelines published by the Consortium for Spinal Cord Medicine provide valuable information to serve as a basis point for planning and estimating levels of assistance required by neurological level of injury, life care planners, case managers, and other healthcare professionals should always recognize that the unique needs of each and every individual must be considered carefully when projecting the level and intensity of personal care assistance, rather than a "one size fits all" approach.

Life Expectancy of Individuals with SCI

The NSCISC publishes data from the Model Spinal Cord Injury System throughout the United States regarding life expectancies for the SCI population who are seen within these system programs. Since there is a substantially higher mortality within the first year post-injury, these survival data are included in a separate table. For individuals who have survived greater than one year post-injury, the data are sub-divided by age, level of injury, completeness of the injury (e.g., AIS A–D), and the need for ventilator assistance. Not surprisingly, those who have sustained higher levels of injury or who have complete spinal cord lesions experience reduced life expectancies, as they are at much greater risk for the development of decubiti, respiratory complications, and recurrent hospitalizations and surgeries. However, just as the need for personal care and skilled nursing services is highly dependent upon individual factors, it is critical that when estimating life expectancies, the life care planner also considers more than merely the statistical data. For example, an important limitation of these data is the fact that they do not consider the level of medical care that patients with SCI have received. Socioeconomic status can play an important role in access to care. Statistical data indicate that family income is less than $25,000.00 per year for 39.3–42.6% of individuals with SCI at years 1–25 post-injury (NSCISC, 2021a). Since proactive measures and careful clinical surveillance can prevent many of the common complications that are associated with morbidity and mortality, the data likely underestimate life expectancies for those who are vigilant with medical follow-up and have adequate resources to procure appropriate levels of medical and skilled nursing care. Other important considerations include comorbid medical conditions, as well as the degree and severity of complications that the individual has experienced since sustaining their injury. For example, a person who has already experienced multiple hospitalizations for serious respiratory infections and decubiti has greater risks of recurrence that can impact long-term survival and life expectancy relative to another person who is the same age and with the same level of injury who has been relatively free of such complications.

Case Study

John Smith, a 22.8 (23) year-old Hispanic male, sustained polytrauma in a motor vehicle collision on 08/25/20, including cervical and thoracic spinal fractures, multiple rib fractures, sternal fracture, and a posterior scalp laceration. He underwent spinal fusion surgeries and at greater than one year post-MVA, presents with a T6 AIS B neurologic level of function, with associated neurogenic bladder for which Mr. Smith self-catheterizes. He also endorses chronic thoracic pain, lower extremity spasms, depression, anxiety, insomnia, and erectile dysfunction.

The Life Care Cost Analysis is presented in specific categories designed to aid economic or financial experts with long-term financial planning and resource allocation. No adjustments have been made within the context of this plan for inflation, projected real rates of growth, or present value. The average residual life expectancy data are obtained from the National Vital Statistics Reports, Vol. 70, No. 19, March 22, 2022. Table 5. Life table for Hispanic males: United States, 2019 (Arias, 2022).

Table 24.1   Life Care Cost Analysis

TABLE I		
LIFE CARE COST ANALYSIS		
JOHN SMITH		
Date of Report: 01/28/22		Impressions:
Date of Birth: 04/14/99		MVA 08/25/20;
Current Age: 22.8 (23) Years		C Spine/T Spine Fractures;
Gender: Male		s/p C6-7 ACDF/C4-T8 Posterior Fusion;
Ethnicity: Hispanic		T6 AIS B; Neurogenic Bladder; ED; Spasticity;
Average Residual Life Expectancy: 57.9 (58) Years		Depression; Anxiety; Insomnia.
Projected Residual Life Expectancy: 45.2 (45) Years		

(Continued)

Table 24.1 (Continued) Life Care Cost Analysis

Service/Item	Begin At Age	Duration Years	Frequency per Year	Average Unit Cost	Annual Cost	Life Time Cost
Outpatient Physician Services						
PM&R/Neurology	23	45	2.5	$190.98	$477.44	$21,484.85
Psychiatrist	23	4	3.5	$228.11	$798.39	$3,193.55
Internist (Additional)	23	22	1.5	$157.67	$236.51	$5,203.22
Internist (Additional)	45	16	2.5	$157.67	$394.18	$6,306.94
Internist (Additional)	61	7	3.5	$157.67	$551.86	$3,863.00
Urologist (Neurogenic Bladder)	23	45	2	$190.98	$381.95	$17,187.88
Podiatrist	23	45	3.5	$58.94	$206.30	$9,283.58
Other Physician Consultation	23	22	1/3	$321.12	$107.04	$2,354.90
Other Physician Consultation	45	16	2/3	$321.12	$214.08	$3,425.31
Other Physician Consultation	61	7	1.5	$321.12	$481.68	$3,371.79
Therapeutic Services						
Physical Therapy Evaluation	23	45	1.5	$170.64	$255.96	$11,518.26
Occupational Therapy Evaluation	23	45	1.5	$193.63	$290.44	$13,069.95
Intermittent Physiotherapy	23	22	1/3	$4,010.50	$1,336.83	$29,410.37
Intermittent Physiotherapy	45	23	1/2	$4,010.50	$2,005.25	$46,120.80
Disability Adjustment Counseling	23	1	36	$176.24	$6,344.66	$6,344.66
Intermittent Supportive Counseling	24	3	1/3	$4,229.77	$1,409.92	$4,229.77
Medical Case Management	23	45	6	$805.50	$4,833.00	$217,485.00
Vocational Rehabilitation Evaluation	23	1	1	$1,067.50	$1,067.50	$1,067.50
Vocational Rehabilitation Counseling	23	2	1/2	$3,202.50	$1,601.25	$3,202.50
SCI Driver Evaluation	23	1	1	$510.67	$510.67	$510.67
SCI Driver Training Program	23	1	1	$1,253.33	$1,253.33	$1,253.33

(Continued)

Table 24.1 (Continued) Life Care Cost Analysis

Service/Item	Begin At Age	Duration Years	Frequency per Year	Average Unit Cost	Annual Cost	Life Time Cost
Medication						
Neuropathic Pain Agent	23	45	365	$5.93	$2,165.17	$97,432.55
Anti-Spasticity Agent	23	45	365	$2.04	$744.36	$33,496.16
Antidepressant	23	4	365	$4.89	$1,784.30	$7,137.19
Insomnia Agent	23	4	182	$4.86	$884.70	$3,538.78
Midodrine	23	45	365	$5.49	$2,002.21	$90,099.34
Prescriptive Analgesic	23	22	130	$2.17	$282.13	$6,206.82
Prescriptive Analgesic	45	23	182	$2.17	$394.98	$9,084.53
Prescriptive NSAID	45	23	182	$4.46	$811.13	$18,656.03
GI Prophylaxis	45	23	365	$3.32	$1,211.66	$27,868.21
Oral Antibiotics	23	22	2.5	$104.39	$260.97	$5,741.30
Oral Antibiotics	45	16	3.5	$104.39	$365.36	$5,845.69
Oral Antibiotics	61	7	4.5	$104.39	$469.74	$3,288.20
IV Antibiotics	23	22	1/5	$4,300.42	$860.08	$18,921.87
IV Antibiotics	45	16	1/3	$4,300.42	$1,433.47	$22,935.60
IV Antibiotics	61	7	1/2	$4,300.42	$2,150.21	$15,051.49
Topical Antibiotic/Antifungal	23	45	6	$43.46	$260.78	$11,735.10
Bladder Agent	23	45	365	$9.51	$3,471.15	$156,201.75
Calcium with D	23	45	365	$0.17	$61.06	$2,747.72
Erectile Dysfunction Agent	23	45	52	$42.98	$2,235.00	$100,575.19
Bowel Program						
Senna	23	45	365	$0.27	$99.10	$4,459.39

(*Continued*)

Table 24.1 (Continued) Life Care Cost Analysis

Service/Item	Begin At Age	Duration Years	Frequency per Year	Average Unit Cost	Annual Cost	Life Time Cost
Diagnostics						
Abdominal Flatplate	23	45	1	$119.36	$119.36	$5,371.21
Chest X-ray	23	22	1/2	$137.04	$68.52	$1,507.48
Chest X-ray	45	16	1.5	$137.04	$205.56	$3,289.04
Chest X-ray	61	7	2.5	$137.04	$342.61	$2,398.26
X-ray (Limbs, Hips)	23	45	1/3	$131.15	$43.72	$1,967.23
CT/MRI Spine	23	45	1/7	$1,648.94	$235.56	$10,600.33
CT/MRI Extremity	23	45	1/4	$1,514.99	$378.75	$17,043.65
Urodynamics	23	45	1/2	$2,531.32	$1,265.66	$56,954.73
Renal Ultrasound	23	45	1	$471.25	$471.25	$21,206.34
Renal Scan (Nuclear Medicine)	23	45	1/3	$802.81	$267.60	$12,042.12
Urography (IVP)	23	45	1/5	$425.28	$85.06	$3,827.49
Cystoscopy, In Office	23	45	1/3	$1,089.27	$363.09	$16,339.09
CBC (Additional)	23	22	1.5	$44.21	$66.31	$1,458.85
CBC (Additional)	45	16	2.5	$44.21	$110.52	$1,768.30
CBC (Additional)	61	7	3.5	$44.21	$154.73	$1,083.08
Metabolic Panel (Additional)	23	22	1.5	$58.35	$87.53	$1,925.68
Metabolic Panel (Additional)	45	16	2.5	$58.35	$145.88	$2,334.16
Metabolic Panel (Additional)	61	7	3.5	$58.35	$204.24	$1,429.67
Urinalysis (Additional)	23	22	1.5	$19.45	$29.18	$641.89
Urinalysis (Additional)	45	16	2.5	$19.45	$48.63	$778.05
Urinalysis (Additional)	61	7	3.5	$19.45	$68.08	$476.56
Urine C&S	23	22	2.5	$129.97	$324.93	$7,148.35
Urine C&S	45	16	3.5	$129.97	$454.90	$7,278.32
Urine C&S	61	7	4.5	$129.97	$584.87	$4,094.06
Cultures (Other)	23	22	1.5	$88.19	$132.29	$2,910.40
Cultures (Other)	45	16	2.5	$88.19	$220.48	$3,527.76
Cultures (Other)	61	7	3.5	$88.19	$308.68	$2,160.75
Sedimentation Rate	23	45	1.5	$22.99	$34.48	$1,551.68
Creatinine Clearance	23	45	2	$74.27	$148.54	$6,684.17
Bone Density Study	23	45	1/3	$360.73	$120.24	$5,411.00
Inpatient/Other Acute Care Services						
Problematic UTI	23	22	1/4	$42,581.37	$10,645.34	$234,197.55
Problematic UTI	45	16	1/3	$42,581.37	$14,193.79	$227,100.65
Problematic UTI	61	7	1/2	$42,581.37	$21,290.69	$149,034.80
Bacteremia, Urosepsis/Other	23	22	1/22	$159,909.17	$7,268.60	$159,909.17
Bacteremia, Urosepsis/Other	45	16	1/16	$159,909.17	$9,994.32	$159,909.17
Bacteremia, Urosepsis/Other	61	7	1/7	$159,909.17	$22,844.17	$159,909.17
Overuse Syndromes (Upper Ext.)	23	45	2/45	$17,691.67	$786.30	$35,383.35
Excision, Ingrown Nails	23	45	2/45	$418.20	$18.59	$836.41
Wound Care, Outpatient	23	45	1/4	$10,512.54	$2,628.14	$118,266.11
Decubiti (Non-operative)	23	45	1/15	$59,306.18	$3,953.75	$177,918.53
Decubitus (Surgical)	61	7	1/7	$157,102.46	$22,443.21	$157,102.46

(Continued)

Table 24.1 (Continued) Life Care Cost Analysis

Service/Item	Begin At Age	Duration Years	Frequency per Year	Average Unit Cost	Annual Cost	Life Time Cost
Home Health Care & Household Services						
CNA/HHA (4-8 Hrs/Day)	23	22	347	$96.00	$33,312.00	$732,864.00
CNA/HHA (12-16 Hrs/Day Illness/Other)	23	22	18	$224.00	$4,032.00	$88,704.00
Skilled Nursing Visits	23	22	18	$145.00	$2,610.00	$57,420.00
CNA/HHA (8-12 Hrs/Day)	45	16	335	$160.00	$53,600.00	$857,600.00
CNA/HHA (12-16 Hrs/Day Illness/Other)	45	16	30	$224.00	$6,720.00	$107,520.00
Skilled Nursing Visits	45	16	30	$145.00	$4,350.00	$69,600.00
CNA/HHA (16-24 Hrs/Day)	61	7	365	$320.00	$116,800.00	$817,600.00
Skilled Nursing Visits	61	7	45	$145.00	$6,525.00	$45,675.00
Household Services	23	45	52	$102.50	$5,330.00	$239,850.00
Supplies						
Wet Ones/Equivalent	23	45	365	$0.95	$346.99	$15,614.44
Skin Care Products	23	45	26	$44.50	$1,157.00	$52,065.00
Gloves Non Latex (Clean)	23	45	24	$7.87	$188.90	$8,500.68
Catheter Kits (4-6 Per Day)	23	45	365	$28.30	$10,329.50	$464,827.50
Antibacterial Soap	23	45	18	$2.39	$43.02	$1,935.90
Disinfectant Spray	23	45	18	$5.28	$95.04	$4,276.80
Heel Protectors	23	45	24	$8.25	$198.00	$8,910.00
Linen Protectors	23	45	365	$1.44	$524.83	$23,617.18
ADL Devices	23	45	1	$280.00	$280.00	$12,600.00
General Wound Care Supplies	23	45	12	$72.50	$870.00	$39,150.00
Equipment						
Electric Bed	23	45	1/10	$2,961.65	$296.16	$13,327.41
Specialty Mattress	23	45	1/8	$3,778.48	$472.31	$21,253.95
Powered Robotic Exoskeleton	25	43	1/8	$99,750.00	$12,468.75	$536,156.25
Software & Maintenance, Exoskeleton	25	43	1	$6,700.00	$6,700.00	$288,100.00
Training, Exoskeleton	25	43	1/5	$4,795.63	$959.13	$41,242.41
Manual Wheelchair & Custom Seating	23	45	1/5	$3,861.00	$772.20	$34,749.00
Power Assist Wheels	23	45	1/5	$8,385.58	$1,677.12	$75,470.23
Cushion, Jay/ROHO	23	45	1/3	$449.70	$149.90	$6,745.50
W/C Maintenance	23	45	1	$279.00	$279.00	$12,555.00
Portable Ramp	23	45	1/10	$452.00	$45.20	$2,034.00
Exercise Mat	23	45	1/3	$384.95	$128.32	$5,774.25
Easy Stand Evolv with Accessories	23	45	1/7	$6,190.63	$884.38	$39,796.91
Roll-in Shower Chair	23	45	1/5	$2,190.25	$438.05	$19,712.28
Travel Bath Bench	23	45	1/5	$259.00	$51.80	$2,331.00
Transfer Boards	23	45	3/5	$57.05	$34.23	$1,540.35
Clothing Adaptation	23	45	1	$675.00	$675.00	$30,375.00
Multi Podus Boots (Bilateral)	23	45	1/3	$301.00	$100.33	$4,515.00
Fleece Inserts (Pair)	23	45	1	$129.50	$129.50	$5,827.50

(Continued)

Table 24.1 (Continued) Life Care Cost Analysis

Service/Item	Begin At Age	Duration Years	Frequency per Year	Average Unit Cost	Annual Cost	Life Time Cost
Home & Vehicular Modifications						
Home Modifications	23	45	2/45	$112,896.00	$5,017.60	$225,792.00
Maintenance (Home Modification)	23	45	1/2	$625.00	$312.50	$14,062.50
Vehicular Modifications (Driver)	23	45	1/7	$49,035.20	$7,005.03	$315,226.29
Maintenance (Vehicular Modification)	23	45	1	$862.50	$862.50	$38,812.50
Potential Care Needs						
Deep Vein Thrombosis	23	45	1/45	$40,821.99	$907.16	$40,821.99
Bladder/Urinary Stones	23	45	1/45	$89,971.11	$1,999.36	$89,971.11
Fosamax/Boniva/Other	33	35	365	$2.78	$1,015.94	$35,557.94
Neurotoxin Injections for Spasticity						
Physician Administration	23	45	4	$820.49	$3,281.96	$147,688.42
Medication	23	45	4	$1,874.11	$7,496.42	$337,339.10
Spinal Fusion Extension	45	23	1/23	$216,926.29	$9,431.58	$216,926.29
Pre-Op Clearance	45	23	1/23	$481.86	$20.95	$481.86
Spine Surgeon (Pre/Post-Op, 4)	45	23	1/23	$763.91	$33.21	$763.91
X-Rays (Thoracic, Pre/Post-Op, 4)	45	23	1/23	$622.44	$27.06	$622.44

(Continued)

Table 24.1 (Continued) Life Care Cost Analysis

TABLE II

COST ANALYSIS SUMMARY

JOHN SMITH

SERVICE/ITEM	LIFE TIME COST TOTALS	PERCENT OF TOTAL
Outpatient Physician Services	$75,675.02	0.92%
Therapeutic Services	$334,212.81	4.06%
Medication	$641,022.89	7.79%
Diagnostics	$211,650.18	2.57%
Inpatient/Other Acute Care Services	$1,579,567.38	19.20%
Home Health Care & Household Services	$3,016,833.00	36.67%
Supplies	$631,497.50	7.68%
Equipment	$1,141,506.03	13.88%
Home & Vehicular Modifications	$593,893.29	7.22%
GRAND TOTAL	**$8,225,858.10**	**100.00%**
Potential Care Needs	$870,173.05	

References

Alabed, S., De Heredia, L. L., Naidoo, A., Belci, M., Hughes, R. J., & Meagher, T. M. (2015). Incidence of pulmonary embolism after the first 3 months of spinal cord injury. *Spinal Cord*, *53*(11), 835–837.

Altman, D. J. (2019). *Pediatric spinal cord injury* [Conference session]. International Academy of Life Care Planning and 25th Annual International Symposium of Life Care Planning Conference, Portland, OR, United States.

American Spinal Cord Injury Association. (2016). *International standards for neurological classification of spinal cord injury* (rev.). *Journal of Spinal Cord Medicine*, *39*(5), 504–512.

Anderson, C. J., Vogel, L. C., Chlan, K. M., Betz, R., & McDonald, C. M. (2007). Depression in adults who sustained spinal cord injuries as children or adolescents. *The Journal of Spinal Cord Medicine*, *30*(sup1), S76–S82.

Arias, E., & Xu, J. Q. (2022). United States life tables, 2019. *National Vital Statistics Reports*, *70*(19), 18. Hyattsville, MD: National Center for Health Statistics. 2022. https://dx.doi.org/10.15620/cdc:113096

Badiali, D., Corazziari, E., Habib, F. I., Bausano, G., Viscardi, A., Anzini, F., & Torsoli, A. (1991). A double-blind controlled trial on the effect of cisapride in the treatment of constipation in paraplegic patients. *Neurogastroenterology & Motility*, *3*(4), 263–267.

Bagwell, D., Winkler, T., & Reagles, K. (2010, September 13). *Long-term comorbidities in spinal cord injury: Consideration for anticipated versus potential complications with life care planning* [Conference session]. International Symposium on Life Care Planning, Orlando, FL, United States.

Blanchaert, R. H. (2021). *Bisphosphnate-related osteonecrosis of the jaw*. https://emedicine.medscape.com/article/1447355-overview

Bloom, O., Herman, P. E., & Spungen, A. M. (2020). Systemic inflammation in traumatic spinal cord injury. *Experimental Neurology*, *325*, 113143.

Branagan, G., Tromans, A., & Finnis, D. (2003). Effect of stoma formation on bowel care and quality of life in patients with spinal cord injury. *Spinal Cord*, *41*(12), 680–683.

Bryce, T. N., Ragnarsson, K. T., & Stein, A. B. (2007). Spinal cord injury. In R. L. Braddom (Ed.), *Physical medicine and rehabilitation* (3rd ed., pp.1285–1349). Saunders Elsevier.

Burke, D., Lennon, O., & Fullen, B. M. (2018). Quality of life after spinal cord injury: The impact of pain. *European Journal of Pain*, *22*(9), 1662–1672.

Cardenas, D. D., & Felix, E. R. (2009). Pain after spinal cord injury: A review of classification, treatment approaches, and treatment assessment. *PM&R*, *1*(12), 1077–1090.

Cragg, J. J., Noonan, V. K., Dvorak, M., Krassiouskov, A., Mancini, G. B. J., & Borisoff, J. F. (2013). Spinal cord injury and type 2 diabetes. *Neurology*, *81*(21), 1864–1868.

Curtis, K. A., Drysdale, G. A., Lanza, R. D., Kolber, M., Vitolo, R. S., & West, R. (1999). Shoulder pain in wheelchair users with tetraplegia and paraplegia. *Archives of Physical Medicine and Rehabilitation*, *80*(4), 453–457.

Dalyan, M., Cardenas, D. D., & Gerard, B. (1999). Upper extremity pain after spinal cord injury. *Spinal Cord*, *37*(3), 191–195.

Dorsher, P. T., & McIntosh, P. M. (2012). Neurogenic bladder. *Advances in Urology*, 816274. https://doi.org/10.1155/2012/816274

Dreamstime. (2016). [Photograph]. https://www.dreamstime.com/

Ebert, E. (2012). Gastrointestinal involvement in spinal cord injury: A clinical perspective. *Journal of Gastrointestinal & Liver Diseases*, *21*(1), 75–82.

Groah, S. L., Weitzenkamp, D. A., Lammertse, D. P., Whiteneck, G. G., Lezotte, D. C., & Hamman, R. F. (2002). Excess risk of bladder cancer in spinal cord injury: Evidence for an association between indwelling catheter use and bladder cancer. *Archives of Physical Medicine and Rehabilitation*, *83*(3), 346–351.

Gstaltner, K., Rosen, H., Hufgard, J., Märk, R., & Schrei, K. (2008). Sacral nerve stimulation as an option for the treatment of faecal incontinence in patients suffering from cauda equina syndrome. *Spinal Cord*, *46*(9), 644–647.

Hagen, E. M. (2015). Acute complications of spinal cord injuries. *World Journal of Orthopedics*, *6*(1), 17.

Heyward, O. W., Veger, R. J. K., de Groot, S., & van der Woude, L. H. V. (2017). Shoulder complaints in wheelchair athletes: A systematic review. *PloS ONE*, *12*(11), e0188410. https://doi.org/10.1371/journal.pone.0188410

Hitzig, S. L., Tonack, M., Campbell, K. A., McGillivray, C. F., Boschen, K. A., Richards, K., & Craven, B. C. (2008). Secondary health complications in an aging Canadian spinal cord injury sample. *American Journal of Physical Medicine & Rehabilitation, 87*(7), 545–555.

Kandilakis, C., Sasso-Lance, E (2021). Exoskeletons for personal use after spinal cord injury. *Archives of Physical Medicine and Rehabilitation, 102*(2), 331–337.

Kedlaya, D. (2018). *Heterotopic ossification in spinal cord injury.* https://emedicine.medscape.com/article/322003-overview

Krassioukov, A. V., Currie, K. D., Hubli, M., Nightingale, T. E., Alrashidi, A. A., Ramer, L., Eng, J. J., Martin Ginis, K. A., MacDonald, M. J., Hicks, A., Ditor, D., Oh, P., Verrier, M. C., & Craven, B. C. (2019). Effects of exercise interventions on cardiovascular health in individuals with chronic, motor complete spinal cord injury: Protocol for a andomized controlled trial (Cardiovascular Health/Outcomes: Improvements created by exercise and education in SCI (CHOICES) Study). *BMJ Open, 9*(1), e023540. https://doi.org/10.1136/bmjopen-2018-023540

Krause, J. S., DeVivo, M. J., & Jackson, A. B. (2004). Health status, community integration, and economic risk factors for mortality after spinal cord injury. *Archives of Physical Medicine and Rehabilitation, 85*(11), 1764–1773.

Krause, J. S., & Saunders, L. L. (2010). Life expectancy estimates in the life care plan: Accounting for economic factors. *Journal of Life Care Planning, 9*(2), 15.

LaVela, S. L., Weaver, F. M., Goldstien, B., Chen K., Miskevics, S., Rajan, S., & Gater, D. R. (2006). Diabetes mellitus in individuals with spinal cord injury or disorder. *Journal of Spinal Cord Medicine, 29*(4), 387–395.

Lok, C. (2017). *ReWalk, Ekso race to sell exoskeletons in tough rehab market.* https://xconomy.com/national/2017/12/04/rewalk-ekso-race-to-sell-exoskeletons-in-tough-rehab-market/

Lucas, E. (2019). Medical management of neurogenic bladder for children and adults: A review. *Topics in Spinal Cord Injury Rehabilitation, 25*(3), 195.

Manack, A., Motsko, S. P., Haag-Molkenteller, C., Dmochowski, R. R., Goehring Jr., E. L., Nguyen-Khoa, B. A., & Jones, J. K. (2011). Epidemiology and healthcare utilization of neurogenic bladder patients in a US claims database. *Neurourology and Urodynamics, 30*(3), 395–401.

Myers, J., Lee, M., & Kiratli, J. (2007). Cardiovascular disease in spinal cord injury: An overview of prevalence, risk, evaluation, and management. *American Journal of Physical Medicine & Rehabilitation, 86*(2), 142–152.

National Spinal Cord Injury Statistical Center, University of Alabama at Birmingham. (2020). *Annual report for the Spinal Cord Injury Model Systems.* Author. https://www.nscisc.uab.edu/public/AR2021_public%20version.pdf

National Spinal Cord Injury Statistical Center, University of Alabama at Birmingham. (2021a). *2021 Annual report for the Spinal Cord Injury Model Systems.* Author. https://www.nscisc.uab.edu/public/AR2021_public%20version.pdf

National Spinal Cord Injury Statistical Center, University of Alabama at Birmingham. (2021b). *Facts and figures at a glance.* https://medicine.umich.edu/sites/default/files/content/downloads/NSCISC%20SCI%20Facts%20and%20Figures%202021.pdf

Nepomuceno, C., Fine, P. R., & Richards, J. S. (1979). Pain inpatients with spinal cord injury. *Archives of Physical Medicine & Rehabilitation, 60,* 605–609.

Paralyzed Veterans of America. (1999). *Outcomes following traumatic spinal cord injury: Clinical Practice guidelines for health-care professionals.* https://pva.org/wp-content/uploads/2021/09/cpg_outcomes-following-traumatic-sci.pdf

Parent, S., Mac-Thiong, J. M., Roy-Beaudry, M., Sosa, J. F., & Labelle, H. (2011). Spinal cord injury in the pediatric population: A systematic review of the literature. *Journal of Neurotrauma, 28*(8), 1515–1524

Rankin, K. C., O'Brien, L. C., Segal, L., Khan, M. R., & Gorgey, A. S. (2017). Liver adiposity and metabolic profile in individuals with chronic spinal cord injury. *BioMed Research International,* 1364848. https://doi.org/10.1155/2017/1364818

Raviv, G., Madgar, I., Elizur, S., Zeilig, G., & Levron, J. (2013). Testicular sperm retrieval and intra cytoplasmic sperm injection provide favorable outcome in spinal cord injury patients, failing conservative reproductive treatment. *Spinal Cord, 51*(8), 642–644.

Reyes, R., & Molton, I. (2009). *Aging with a spinal cord injury*. Northwestern Regional Spinal Cord Injury System. https://sci.washington.edu/info/forums/reports/aging_6.09.asp

Salameh, A., Al Mohajer, M., & Daroucihe, R. O. (2015). Prevention of urinary tract infections in patients with spinal cord injury. *Canadian Medical Association Journal, 187*(11), 807–811.

Siroky, M. B. (2002). Pathogenesis of bacteriuria and infection in the spinal cord injured patient. *The American Journal of Medicine, 113*(1), 67–79.

Smith, P., & Decter, R. (2015). Antegrade continence enema procedure: Impact on quality of life in patients with spinal cord injury. *Spinal Cord, 53*, 213–215. https://doi.org/10.1038/sc.2014.223

Stampas, A., Hook, M., Korupolu, R., Jethani, L., Kaner, M. T., Pemberton, E., Sheng, L., & Francisco, G. E. (2022). Evidence of treating spasticity before it develops: A systematic review of spasticity outcomes in acute spinal cord injury interventional trials. *Therapeutic Advances in Neurological Disorders, 15*, 17562864211070657

Stinton, L. M., & Shaffer, E. A. (2012). Epidemiology of gallbladder disease: Cholelithiasis and cancer. *Gut Liver, 6*(2), 172–187. https://doi.org/10.5009/gnl.2012.6.2.172

Tofte, N., Nielsen, A. C., Trøstrup, H., Andersen, C. B., Von Linstow, M., Hansen, B., Biering-Sørensen, F., Høiby, N., & Moser, C. (2017). Chronic urinary tract infections in patients with spinal cord lesions–biofilm infection with need for long-term antibiotic treatment. *APMIS, Journal of Pathology, Microbiology, and Immunology, 5*(4), 385–391.

Tribe, C. R. (1963). Causes of death in the early and late stages of paraplegia. *Spinal Cord, 1*(1), 19–47. https://doi.org/10.1038/sc.1963.3

Valles, M., Vidal, J., Clav, P., & Mearin, F. (2006). Bowel dysfunction in patients with motor complete spinal cord injury: Clinical, neurological, and pathophysiological associations. *Official Journal of the American College of Gastroenterology, 101*(10), 2290–2299.

Williams, R., & Murray, A. (2015). Prevalence of depression after spinal cord injury: A meta-analysis. *Archives of Physical Medicine and Rehabilitation, 96*(1), 133–140.

Williams, A. M., Gee, C. M., Voss, C., & West, C. R. (2019). Cardiac consequences of spinal cord injury: Systematic review and meta-analysis. *Heart, 105*(3), 217–225.

Chapter 25

Life Care Planning for People with Visual Impairment

Christine Reid and Sandra Bullins

Life Care Planning for the Patient with Visual Impairment

The presence of a visual impairment or blindness in an individual's life impacts many aspects of that life—it significantly affects the personal, social, emotional, psychological, and vocational dimensions of life. Life care planners may need to develop plans for people whose visual impairment or blindness was caused by injury, such as anoxic brain injuries, industrial accidents, or misdiagnosed brain tumors. They could also work with people who had eye conditions exacerbated by injury, such as when someone's retinal tear becomes a detached retina in an automobile accident. Even if vision impairments are unrelated to the injury for which a life care plan is developed, they may interact with the injury that is the focus of the plan, affecting what recommendations should be made. Life care planners may encounter pre-existing eye conditions unrelated to the reason for developing a life care plan, but which affect how other recommendations in the life care plan can be carried out. For example, cataracts or macular degeneration could interfere with an individual's ability to read prescription labels, accurately dose insulin, etc. Some of those conditions might be progressive and expected to interact with how life care plan recommendations are implemented in the future. For example, a person with retinitis pigmentosa can expect a progressively decreasing visual field and the onset of night blindness, thus making it difficult, over time, to read sign language or drive an automobile. Additionally, life care planners should be aware of the fact that, as any disability interacts with the aging process, some degree of vision loss is expected for many people as they age (even if they do not yet have such a diagnosis), through mechanisms such as presbyopia, cataracts, macular degeneration, diabetic retinopathy, etc.

Understanding that visual impairment can be the focus of a life care plan or a consideration in developing a plan to address other disabilities, the goal of this chapter is to provide a foundation for understanding how blindness or visual impairments affect people over their lifespans and address implications for life care planning practice. As Weed and Wilkins (2018) stated in the fourth edition of this text, "The life care planner must have a thorough working knowledge of visual impairment, its effect and impact, and expertise regarding the types of equipment and technological advances for members of these populations" (p. 702).

Review of the Literature

To carefully and thoroughly develop a life care plan for an individual with a visual loss, the life care planner must understand the implications of visual impairment or blindness. How the life care plan is developed and documented must take into consideration the type of vision loss, the age of the individual at the time of onset, and how the visual impairment or blindness will progress over the individual's lifespan. The literature review that follows aims to address these issues and has been organized into categories, with headings to facilitate locating and reviewing essential information when it is needed.

Definitions and Prevalence

"Visual impairment" is often considered an umbrella term that describes the presence of a visual disability. This can encompass low vision, blindness, vision loss, and legal blindness. To assess visual acuity, a thorough eye exam is performed by an optometrist or ophthalmologist. The score for normal vision is referred to as 20/20. This means that an individual can clearly see at 20 feet away what a person with average, "normal" vision can see at that distance. In contrast, someone with 20/80 vision would need to be 20 feet away from something to see it as well as others with "normal" vision could see from 80 feet away. This is assessed separately for the right eye (O.D., *oculus dexter*) and the left eye (O.S., *oculus sinister*). It is important to differentiate between visual acuity that is aided (with eyeglasses or contact lenses) versus unaided. For example, if a person has 20/200 visual acuity in both eyes unaided, but their vision improves to better than 20/70 with eyeglasses, that person functions as legally blind unaided, but may be able to drive an automobile when wearing glasses.

In addition to visual acuity, the visual field is a key aspect of functional vision. Most people with "normal" vision are able to see a half-circle range (around 170–180°) around themselves when looking directly forward. With unimpaired peripheral vision, someone holding their arms straight out to their sides, perpendicular to their body, will not need to move those arms forward very much before the individual can see them. However, constricted peripheral vision ("tunnel vision") limits that visual field to just a center portion of the field; one's arms would have to move quite far from the side and to the front, in order to be seen. Reducing a visual field to around 40° is a significant visual impairment; reducing it to less than 20° satisfies the definition of legal blindness, regardless of the degree of visual acuity.

Blindness can be defined in several ways. One definition of blindness is the inability to see at all, or at best, to discern light from darkness. The National Federation of the Blind (2022a) uses a broader definition, which suggests blindness refers to sight that is bad enough, even with corrective lenses, that a person must use alternative methods to engage in any activity that people with normal vision would do using their eyes. Yet, the United States (U.S.) Bureau of Census question about "significant vision loss" includes both total or near-total blindness and "trouble seeing, even when wearing glasses or contact lenses." The definition of "legally blind" as used by the Social Security Administration (SSA) and various other agencies is that central visual acuity must be 20/200 or less in the better eye with the best possible correction, or that the visual field must be 20° or less (SSA, 2022). Visual acuity of 20/200 means that a person can only see at 20 feet away what a "normal" individual can see at a distance of 200 feet.

"Total blindness" is defined by some as having no light perception in either eye. Others will include in the definition of "total blindness" an individual who has some light perception, where they may be able to see vague patterns of light and shadows, recognize if it is daylight or dark, or identify if the lights are turned on in a room. In this case, the individual may also refer to themselves as blind with some light perception.

Vision loss and blindness are among the top ten disabilities in the United States (Kirtland et al., 2015). Flaxman et al. (2021) conducted a meta-analysis of studies on the prevalence of visual acuity loss or blindness in the United States. They defined blindness as vision that when corrected is 20/200 or worse in the better-seeing eye, and visual acuity loss as the best corrected visual acuity of 20/40 or worse in the better-seeing eye. Flaxman et al. estimated that just over 7 million people live with visual acuity loss, with just over 1 million of those living with blindness. They reported that although the majority of the individuals living with visual acuity loss were 40 years of age or older, over 1.6 million people with visual acuity loss were under the age of 40, and among those, about 141,000 are blind. Focusing on children, the American Foundation for the Blind (2022a) reported on results of the 2019 American Community Survey, stating that there were approximately 547,083 children under the age of 18 with "vision difficulty" in the United States at that time; 276,322 were males and 270,761 were females. The American Printing House for the Blind (APH) annually polls agencies in each state to discover how many legally blind children (through the age of 21 years) are eligible to receive free reading materials in Braille, large print, or audio format. They reported a total of 56,866 registered students in their most recent census (APH, 2021a).

The Centers for Disease Control and Prevention (CDC) (CDC, 2020a) reported that in the United States, approximately 6.8% of children under the age of 18 have a diagnosed eye and vision condition, and among children under the age of 18, nearly 3% are blind or visually impaired, even after correction with eyeglasses or contact lenses. The American Foundation for the Blind (2022b) reported findings from the 2019 American Community Survey that there were approximately 547,083 children with vision difficulties in the United States in 2018. Of that number, 276,322 were males and 270,761 were females. The children who were included in the survey results ranged in age from birth to 17 years old.

Looking beyond the United States, the Vision Loss Expert Group of the Global Burden of Disease Study (2020) estimated that an estimated 43.3 million people were blind worldwide, with 55% of them female. They predicted that by 2050, 61 million people will be blind, 474 million will have moderate or severe vision impairment, and 360 million will have mild vision impairment.

Etiology

According to Prevent Blindness America (2022), more than 50,000 Americans will lose part or all of their vision each year. The four leading causes of blindness in the United States are age-related macular degeneration, diabetic retinopathy, glaucoma, and cataracts (CDC, 2020b).

The National Institute for Occupational Safety and Health (n.d.) reported that thousands of people in the United States are blinded each year from work-related eye injuries. Life care plans may be developed because of such work-related injuries, as well as other injuries or medical mishaps. Swain and McGwin (2020) conducted a meta-analysis of studies on the prevalence of eye injuries and estimated that 24 million people in the United States have experienced eye injuries; among them, 1.5 million are visually impaired, 1.7 million are partially blind, and 147,000 are totally blind.

Zuckerman (2004) reported that blindness was caused by disease for nearly half of the population in the United States. The most commonly reported disease-related causes were diseases of the retina, diabetes, glaucoma, and cataracts. Accidents accounted for 15% of blindness in adults and 8% in children.

The most common causes of visual impairment among children are uncorrected refractive errors, amblyopia, corneal opacity, retinal disorders, and cataracts (Atowa et al., 2019). Some additional conditions have been identified by Helvin and Sutton (2011) as likely to be involved in the development of life care plans: cortical visual impairment and optic nerve anomalies (hypoplasia or atrophy). According to the World Health Organization (2019), the leading causes of vision impairment globally are uncorrected refractive errors, cataracts, age-related macular degeneration, glaucoma, diabetic retinopathy, corneal opacity, and trachomas (holes in the retina).

Life care planners should research the specific diagnoses of their evaluees' visual impairments because different diagnoses are associated with different prognoses, functional limitations, and treatment or rehabilitation options. Addressing every type of visual impairment is beyond the scope of this chapter, but here is an overview of some of the conditions a life care planner may encounter.

Refraction Errors

Refraction errors occur when the lens of the eye (which resides just behind the colored iris inside the eye) does not perfectly focus an image onto the retina at the back of the eye, causing blurry vision. Refraction errors could result in myopia (near-sightedness), hyperopia (far-sightedness), and/or astigmatism (uneven focusing errors from different sections of the lens). Refraction errors can often be corrected by wearing prescription glasses or contact lenses, or in some cases, through surgery. Refraction errors could be the same in both eyes, or the left and right eyes could have different refraction errors, such as when the lenses of the two eyes are shaped differently. When left untreated, especially if the refraction errors involve astigmatism or different refraction errors in each eye, amblyopia could result (Terbert. 2020).

Amblyopia

Amblyopia is a disorder in which the brain has difficulty reconciling different inputs from the two eyes, and essentially progressively ignores input from one of the eyes to reduce that dissonance. Basically, the brain and the problematic eye reduce communication, so the visual signal from that eye is reduced or lost. This disorder is commonly called "lazy eye," although it has nothing to do with laziness. If untreated in childhood (through correcting the underlying condition and/or through wearing an eye patch over the dominant eye), amblyopia can persist into adulthood and is one of the leading causes of monocular vision.

Monocular Vision

Monocular vision is vision using only one eye. It can result from untreated amblyopia, the need to cover one eye to stop diplopia (double vision), or from injury to or removal (enucleation) of one of the eyes. Monocular vision results in a decrease in the visual field (loss of about 30% of the periphery on the side without a functioning eye) and loss of depth perception (Hull University Teaching Hospitals, 2020). For the sole functioning eye, it is important to be vigilant about protecting and preserving vision.

Cataracts

Cataracts are cloudy opacities in the lens of the eye. They may be congenital or result from injury to the eye, but many of us develop them progressively over time, as we age. Minor cataracts result in reduced clarity of vision, but serious cataracts can result in complete loss of visual acuity. Treatment for cataracts typically involves replacing the opaque natural lens with an artificial lens.

Corneal Opacity

Corneal opacity is another type of opacity that interferes with light coming into the eye, but unlike a cataract, a corneal opacity is located on the front-most exterior part of the eye. Both the density of the opacity and the extent to which it covers the cornea affect the degree of vision loss. The greater the opacity, the greater the loss of acuity for the affected part of the visual field. The greater the surface of the cornea covered by that opacity, the greater the loss of visual field. Treatment for corneal opacity typically involves a transplant with a donor cornea.

Glaucoma

Glaucoma typically creates excessive pressure within the eyes, damaging the optic nerve, which transmits information from the retina to the brain. "Open-angle" glaucoma, the most common type, progresses slowly, and people may not notice that their vision is gradually decreasing until the disease is relatively well advanced. "Closed-angle" glaucoma usually involves pain and people suddenly noticing a problem with their vision. With either type, visual loss may start with a reduction of peripheral vision and the development of "blind spots." Untreated, it can progress to complete loss of vision (National Eye Institute, 2022a). Annually checking ocular pressures and having dilated eye exams are important for the early identification of glaucoma. Treatment for glaucoma typically involves medications (usually eye drops), laser treatment, or surgery.

Optic Nerve Disorders

Other include optic nerve hypoplasia and optic nerve atrophy. Optic nerve hypoplasia is insufficient development of the optic nerve(s) during pregnancy. Most people who have this condition exhibit nystagmus (rapid, abnormal involuntary eye movements). Their vision losses can range from mild impairments to total loss of light perception in one or two eyes. Optic nerve atrophy can have many different causes and different symptoms. Causes include insufficient blood flow, anoxia, pressure on the optic nerve (e.g., by a tumor), etc. Symptoms vary in type and intensity, including peripheral vision loss, blurred vision, reduction in sharpness, and color discrimination challenges. There are no known medical treatments for optic nerve hypoplasia or atrophy.

Cortical Visual Impairment

Cortical visual impairment is a neurological disorder in which the eyes themselves may be functioning normally, but the visual information is not interpreted correctly because of a disturbance in the visual neurological pathways or in the occipital lobe of the brain itself. This impairment can result in unique visual responses to people, educational materials, and the environment (Vermont Association for the Blind and Visually Impaired, 2022). Although there are no known medical treatments for cortical visual impairment, therapies focus on trying to reconnect the pathways between the eyes and the brain.

Retinal Diseases

Retinal diseases vary in their effects, depending on the areas of the retina they affect, and the ways they damage the retina. The retina is a multilayered network of neurons connected by synapses, featuring photoreceptor cells, attached at the posterior end of the interior of the eyeball. It receives light focused upon it by the lens inside the eye. The primary photoreceptor sensory cells are of two types: rods and cones. Cones are sensitive to color and are concentrated in the macula, the pigmented section near the center of the retina, while the rods are more sensitive to low-light conditions. At the center of the macula is the fovea, which is comprised entirely of cones and results in the sharpest, clearest part of the visual field, with the greatest visual acuity. If damage to the retina is due to its physical detachment from the interior wall of the eyeball, timely surgery to reattach it may be a feasible intervention to restore vision. Such detachment may occur with head injuries, such as those from automobile accidents or shaken baby syndrome. However, if the retinal injury causes death of the sensory cells within the retina, such as from ischemic injury, excessive ocular pressure, or anoxia, no medical interventions are available to restore vision. Similarly, vision loss is permanent for the following specific diseases affecting the retina.

Retinopathy of Prematurity

Retinopathy of prematurity is an eye disorder affecting premature infants. Various causes have been hypothesized, but regardless of causation, this disorder affects immature blood vessels of the retina and occurs just weeks after birth. A child is no longer a candidate for diagnosis with retinopathy of prematurity when the development of blood vessels is complete.

Albinism

Albinism refers to a group of inherited conditions characterized by the absence or reduction of pigment in the eyes, skin, or hair. This disorder results from genes that do not make normal amounts of the pigment melanin, which is required for the full development of the retina.

Colobomas

Colobomas are congenital holes or malformations resulting from irregularities in the development of parts of the eye tissue. Colobomas in the retina or the optic nerve are most likely to cause significant visual impairment.

Macular Degeneration

Macular degeneration, including age-related macular degeneration, is a retinal disease that negatively affects a person's central vision, including the part that offers the sharpest visual acuity. An individual's central vision is necessary for seeing objects clearly; it is needed to complete everyday tasks such as reading and driving. Age-related macular degeneration (AMD) can be categorized as "wet" or "dry." Wet AMD occurs when blood vessels behind the retina begin to grow abnormally under the macula, leading to the leaking of both blood and fluid. This leakage causes scarring of cells within the macula, which leads to a rapid loss of central vision. An early sign of wet AMD is when people with the condition look at a grid of straight lines, the lines appear wavy. Dry AMD occurs when there is a thinning of the macula over time, related to the aging process. An early sign of dry AMD is the blurring of the central vision (CDC, 2022a).

Diabetic Retinopathy

Diabetic retinopathy (DR) is the leading cause of blindness in working-age adults in the United States. Diabetic retinopathy is a progressive condition and is caused when there is damage to the blood vessels of the retina. Diabetic retinopathy typically affects both eyes and has four stages: mild, moderate, severe, and proliferative retinopathy (CDC, 2022a). Monitoring and maintaining appropriate blood glucose levels, maintaining healthy blood pressure, and prioritizing annual dilated eye exams focused on identifying signs of diabetic retinopathy can all contribute to minimizing the effects of diabetes on vision.

Retinitis Pigmentosa

Retinitis pigmentosa (RP) is a genetic eye condition that occurs when there is a breakdown of the cells in the retina. Retinitis pigmentosa is characterized by a loss of peripheral vision (tunnel vision) and trouble seeing at night (night blindness). Retinitis pigmentosa is a progressive condition and is relatively rare. Although prevalence rates vary in some geographic areas, especially those where Usher's Syndrome (involving both hearing loss and RP) is concentrated, it is estimated that overall, approximately 1 out of 4,000 individuals are affected by RP, both in the United States and worldwide (National Eye Institute, 2022b).

Non-24 Sleep Disorder

Non-24 sleep disorder is a relatively common circadian rhythm disorder among people who are blind. Lockley et al. (2015) reported the results of two consecutive placebo-controlled trials to assess the safety and efficacy of the drug tasimelteon to "entrain" blind people with non-24 syndrome into more effective sleep patterns. They reported that "Once-daily tasimelteon can entrain totally blind people with non-24; however, continued tasimelteon treatment is necessary to maintain these improvements" (p. 60031). Tasimelteon is available under the brand name Hetlioz; there is not yet a generic version available, in part due to patent protection in the early years of this drug's adoption. At the time this chapter was written, the monthly cost for Hetlioz was over $23,000 per month. For people who are blind and whose non-24 sleep disorders respond well to Hetlioz treatment, continued treatment with that medication is likely to be needed for the rest of their lives.

Expected Course of the Conditions

The projected course of a visual impairment depends on the etiology, as well as the timeliness of preventative interventions or treatments (if applicable). Some may be amenable to surgical interventions (such as cataracts, corneal opacity, and some retinal detachments), while others may not (such as optic nerve atrophy, albinism, or macular degeneration). For some, the condition will be stable (such as retinal colobomas, or enucleation of the eye), while for others it is likely to be progressive (such as retinitis pigmentosa, glaucoma, and diabetic retinopathy). Life care planners should be familiar with the expected courses of the particular types of eye diseases or injuries experienced by their evaluees, the treatments or interventions designed to limit the progression of those specific conditions (if applicable), functional implications of those types of visual losses, appropriate rehabilitation interventions to address the consequences of those conditions, and types of assistive technologies that can address the different limitations imposed by visual impairments caused by those etiologies.

Children and Youth

The presence of a visual impairment or blindness has an impact on many aspects of an individual's life. If the individual has grown and developed with a visual impairment since childhood, their adjustment is different from that of adults encountering vision loss (Farrell & Krahn, 2014). For children with visual impairment, the quality, quantity, and timeliness of appropriate interventions are important to help them function well within their environments, as they develop. Vervloed et al. (2020) emphasized the importance of early intervention, noting that the second year of life is a particularly vulnerable period for children with congenital blindness or visual impairment. They noted that important risk factors for setbacks in development for those children were the severity of visual impairment, neurological abnormalities, and social adversity. Atowa et al. (2019) noted that in general, loss of vision in childhood affects academic opportunities, career choices, and social life. They also separately examined the effects of different types of visual impairments, finding deficiencies in near vision influencing the ability to perform many tasks that require reading, and deficiencies in the visual field negatively affecting ambulation in challenging environments, as well as the use of peripheral vision. In their review of prevalence studies about visual impairment in school-aged children, Atowa et al. (2019) found that around 90% of children with visual impairments around the world are not receiving adequate education due to a lack of access to appropriate schools, discrimination, or stigmatization.

The American Printing House for the Blind (APH, 2021a) conducts an annual poll to see how many students with visual impairments (through age 21) in the United States qualify to receive free reading materials in alternate formats (large print, auditory, or Braille). In their most recent census, 84.5% of the students were reported by State Departments of Education, suggesting those students were mainstreamed into regular public or private schools. Students attending schools for the blind were 8% of the census; students participating in programs of rehabilitation agencies were 5.7%; and students attending programs focused on addressing multiple concurrent disabilities were 1.8% (APH, 2021a). Of the total 56,866 students registered with APH in 2021, 18% were "prereaders" and 30.7% were "symbolic readers or nonreaders" (illiterate). Among the literate students, 65% were visual readers (using large print, for example), 19% were auditory readers, and 16% were Braille readers. Literacy challenges for many of these students increase the difficulties inherent in achieving educational goals, and learning what they need to learn in order to become productive, engaged members of their communities in the future. These challenges may be complicated by additional co-occurring disabilities. For example, in a study reported by Zuckerman (2004), more than 40% of the children with visual impairments studied also had learning disabilities, and 20% had intellectual disabilities, although learning disabilities and intellectual disabilities were rare among the blind adults in that study.

Miyauchi (2020) identified some key elements for enhancing accessibility to school subjects for students with visual impairments, including having teachers possess effective pedagogical strategies, providing effective teaching-learning tools, and providing external support. Miyauchi and Paul (2020) looked at education from the students' perspectives and found three themes: barriers (physical environments of schools, accessibility, and social interactions), feelings of acceptance (homophily—seeking out people similar to themselves, and "fitting in"), and skills to be autonomous and assertive (for academic success and for initiating and building friendships).

The World Health Organization (2021) summarized the personal impact of vision impairment for those who experience it. Focusing on children who experience severe vision impairment at an early age, consequences can include delayed motor, language, emotional, social, and cognitive development, as well as lower levels of educational achievement. They noted that these effects have lifelong consequences.

Adults

Focusing on people who experience vision impairment for the first time in adulthood, the World Health Organization (2021) summarized how vision impairment severely impacts the quality of life. They pointed out lower rates of workforce participation and productivity (compared to populations without visual impairment), as well as higher rates of depression and anxiety. Looking more closely at the population of older adults with vision impairments, they noted problems with social isolation, difficulty walking, increased risk of falls and fractures, and a greater probability of entering nursing or care homes earlier than those without visual impairments.

For adult onset of visual impairment, there is a sudden impact on finances, identity, and sense of self-worth. The major effect on finances is that of employment. Employment statistics for the population of individuals who are visually impaired or blind have not changed much in several decades (McDonnall & Sui, 2019). According to the Bureau of Labor Statistics' (2022) Current Population Survey, the most recent employment rate for this group is 40%. Only four out of every ten individuals with a visual impairment or blindness between the ages of 16 and 64 are employed, an increase of only 10% from ten years ago (McDonnall et al., 2022; McDonnall & Sui, 2019).

Many things contribute to unemployment or underemployment of this population, including employer attitudes towards individuals with visual impairments or blindness, fear, and a lack of adequate transportation (Crudden, 2018; Crudden & Steverson, 2021). It is the latter that contributes to many issues that impact several areas of an individual's life. The lack of adequate and reliable transportation affects independence, health, and well-being, and contributes to feelings of isolation (Crudden et al., 2017). Although there have been some improvements in the availability of access to transportation, such as the availability of ride-share companies and public transportation in urban areas, those do not address the transportation challenge for rural areas (Crudden, 2018).

Stigmas and stereotypes that many employers hold is another contributing factor to the employment barriers faced by individuals with visual impairment or blindness (Fireison & Moore, 1998). Unger et al. (2005) studied charges of workplace discrimination filed with the United States Equal Employment Opportunity Commission by people with visual impairments. They found that people who had visual disabilities were more likely than other people filing disability discrimination complaints to receive settlement benefits from their employers, or to withdraw their complaints after receiving benefits without intercession from the Equal Employment Opportunity Commission. In an update to that study, Victor et al. (2017) found that, as evidenced by discrimination charges, individuals with visual impairments of each race and both genders perceived discrimination in all aspects of employment. For years, many individuals who had visual impairments or blindness were sent to work in sheltered workshops making rugs, brooms, or brushes, even though they had the skills and abilities needed to be employed elsewhere (Robert & Adele, 1999). The resistance of employers to hiring someone with a visual impairment may be related to fear of injury and subsequent costs for the employer, as well as the liability that the individual might get hurt. However, reasonable accommodations can make most work environments as safe for people with visual impairments as they are for sighted people.

Lack of or loss of employment leads to poverty. It has been suggested that the effects of having a visual impairment or blindness and being below the poverty level are both causes and consequences of each other. When an individual receives the diagnosis of vision loss, the effects are more than just physical. Loss of employment is a real concern, especially if the individual is the main source of household income. If the individual has assistive technology or the ability to return to an adaptive form of their former job, further education or training might be necessary to re-enter the workforce. Unemployment causes poverty, and poverty restricts access to needed services and technology essential for both employment and independent living in the community.

Functional Impact

Functional limitations associated with being partially sighted (low vision) differ from those associated with being blind (severe vision loss). People who have partial vision may try to act as if they do not have functional limitations, in hopes of appearing not to have a disability. In order to be accepted by society, they may struggle with not being able to see what they want to see, instead of using low vision aids (assistive devices) to read and take in information from the environment, or a cane to assist with orientation and mobility. This can result in anxiety, frustration, and even engaging in dangerous behaviors such as driving a motor vehicle when they do not have the level of vision required to do so legally (Falvo, 2019).

Key functional limitations for people who are blind focus on access to information in the environment, as well as barriers to orientation and mobility. Printed materials such as books or magazines, menus in restaurants, and labels on merchandise in stores, are inaccessible unless they are available in electronic form, or assistive devices are available to read them aloud. Another problem that people who are blind may face is limited awareness of the environment around them. For example, how would a person who is blind know if somebody is "lurking" outside their home or office, perhaps deciding whether or not to break into it? If the person who is blind lives or works in an environment where the norm may be to leave the doors unlocked, how would that person know when somebody has entered?

A significant barrier faced by almost all people who have visual impairments is transportation (Crudden et al. 2015; Crudden et al. 2016). Some people with visual impairments are able to drive automobiles, with appropriate eyewear or assistive devices; a list of driving restrictions for each state in the United States is provided by the American Academy of Ophthalmology (2020). However, the inability to drive and limited availability of public transportation are the two main factors making transportation the main barrier to employment and full community inclusion for most people with significant visual impairments or blindness. Furthermore, the lack of reliable transportation also impacts the health and well-being of an individual with a visual disability. Activities such as getting to medical appointments or to the grocery store are impeded by the inability to drive. Transportation is an important barrier to independent living and vocational success. In this area, technology may give reason for hope in the future. For example, if driverless car technology can advance to the point where it will be easily and safely available to people who have visual disabilities, this could reduce the significant transportation barrier.

Manduchi and Kurniawan (2013) described different functional limitations associated with different types of visual disabilities. For example, people with retinitis pigmentosa experience "tunnel vision," with a small spot in the center of the visual field visible and the periphery blurred or not visible. In contrast, macular degeneration results in some vision in the periphery, but reduced or missing vision in the center of the visual field, where vision for detail is normally the sharpest. Life care planners must understand the specific functional limitations associated with their evaluees' visual disabilities, as well as approaches those evaluees use or could use in the future if empowered with appropriate technology and training.

One common limitation experienced by people with visual impairments is fatigue. Schakel et al. (2019) conducted a systematic review and meta-analysis of studies of the relationship between visual impairment and fatigue and found "current moderate to high quality evidence" that people with visual impairments experience more severe fatigue symptoms than do people with normal sight (p. 399). Interestingly, they did not find a significant difference in fatigue severity between people with moderate visual impairment and people with severe visual impairment or blindness.

Jones et al. (2019) examined the impact of visual impairment on activities of daily living and vision-related quality of life for a population of adults. They found that people in their study who had visual impairments were more likely to be malnourished, and to report difficulty with shopping for, preparing, and eating food. They also reported poorer quality of life, compared to people without visual impairments. Jones et al. noted that there was a significant correlation between the level of visual impairment and reported difficulty with shopping for, preparing, and cooking meals.

Lockley et al. (2015) addressed sleep difficulties for people who are blind, noting that "most totally blind people have non-24-hour sleep-wake disorder (non-24), a rare circadian rhythm disorder caused by an inability of light to reset their circadian pacemaker" (p. 60031). Difficulty with sleep onset and with sleep latency, if not addressed, results in sleep deprivation. The effects of sleep deprivation on everyday functioning and productivity, as well as immune function and other health consequences, can be profound, and potentially life-threatening.

Focusing on the effect of visual impairment on employment, McKnight et al. (2021) found that age at disability onset interacted with time since disability onset in the prediction of whether or not a person with a visual impairment would be employed. Specifically, the odds of working after acquiring the visual impairment increased with time, but only for people who had their disability for at least four years. That makes sense because it takes some time to develop orientation and mobility skills, learn how to use new technology, and generally adjust to a new way of living after acquiring a vision loss. McKnight et al. (2021) also found that being female, receiving government benefits, and having multiple disabilities was associated with being less likely to work after disability onset while having sources of encouragement was associated with being more likely to work after disability onset.

Psychological Impact

The presence of a visual impairment or blindness affects many aspects of an individual's life. The coping and adjustment to a visual impairment or blindness is different than other chronic illnesses and disabilities based on the psychological impact it has on the individual (Moschos, 2014; Zapata, 2022). For many years, reference to Kubler-Ross' five stages of grief or loss was used to assist in understanding the emotions experienced by an individual with a diagnosis of visual impairment or blindness. The feelings of anger, bargaining, depression, acceptance, and denial were, and still are at times, valid emotional expressions felt (Moschos, 2014). The stages are fluid, and not necessarily experienced in a particular order.

Adjustment, acceptance, and identity development are influenced by several factors. The presence of support in the individual's life, such as family, friends, or other members of their inner circle, are a few of the initial factors. Other than close family and friends, that inner circle of support might include members of their church and clubs or organizations in which they might be a member or regular participant. The next layer of support might include the medical team including their physician, eye care professional, or any counselor or therapist that they might have an already established relationship with.

Another factor that contributes to adjustment and a level of acceptance is his or her development of personal identity (Gibson et al., 2018; Zapata, 2022). Zapata (2022) investigated how participating in a support group, focused on visual impairment or blindness, aided in more positive feelings and lowered feelings of anxiety and depression. The connection with other members of specific groups established a connection with individuals who had similar experiences, feelings, and struggles (Zapata, 2022).

People who have lost part or all of their vision often find that the loss has a tremendous impact on many aspects of their lives (Moschos, 2014; Stevelink & Fear, 2016; Stevelink et al., 2015). Some of the psychological issues faced by individuals who have a visual disability are a loss of self-sufficiency, being regarded as a burden, lack of privacy, a shift from independent to dependent, loss of financial security, and forced isolation (Moschos, 2014; Stevelink & Fear, 2016). Moschos (2014) conducted an intensive review of the literature and found three predominant responses to the loss of vision, which are acceptance, denial, and depression with anxiety. In Moschos' (2014) literature review, more than 90% of the subjects who were diagnosed with vision loss expressed feelings of depression, anxiety, and suicidal ideation. People who had only a partial loss of vision appeared to have a more difficult time adjusting to the vision loss than did people who experienced a total loss of their vision (Moschos, 2014). Gradual loss of vision can heighten and intensify feelings of isolation, inadequacy, and dependence (Moschos, 2014). Surakka et al. (2016) demonstrated the beneficial effects of regular exercises on the mental state of adults who were visually impaired or deafblind.

The development of posttraumatic stress disorder among people with visual impairments was addressed by van der Ham et al. (2021), who found that people with visual impairments may have a higher risk of exposure to traumatic events and limited or restricted access to situational information during those events may increase the stressfulness of those experiences. They also noted that visual impairment may shape the impact of traumatic events. In their systematic review of related studies, they found that posttraumatic stress disorder was prevalent in this population, with reported rates ranging from 4% to 50%.

Augestad (2017) conducted a systematic review of studies addressing self-concept and self-esteem among children and young adults with visual impairment, finding themes of independence in mobility, parenting style, social support, and friendships as important for enhancing self-concept and self-esteem among this population. Focusing on helping parents to cope with the stress of dealing with children who are blind so they could be more effective parents, Bahramfar and Ashori (2021) found stress inoculation training to be of benefit to when seeking to improve the emotional regulation and psychological problems of mothers of blind children.

Intersectionality

People who are members of intersecting marginalized communities often face increased barriers to employment and community inclusion. For example, someone who identifies as a biracial, transgender blind woman is likely to experience more situational and attitudinal barriers than someone who identifies as a white, cisgender blind man. It can be incredibly helpful for people to find ways to connect with the various communities with which they identify, despite the challenges of visual impairment or blindness.

Zuckerman (2004) noted that many blind adults also have other disabilities; for example, almost 1 in 5 have difficulty hearing, even with a hearing aid. As people age, the likelihood of developing hearing losses and/or visual losses increases. Reid and Bullins (2021) provided an overview of how vision and hearing losses interact, how hearing loss changes approaches upon which many people who are blind rely, and what kinds of services, assistive technologies, and rehabilitation interventions are important for people with dual sensory losses. The interaction between vision loss and hearing loss has more than just an additive effect; when vision is not available to supplement information reduced through hearing loss, the effect of the hearing loss is multiplied. Options such as cochlear implantation, which might not be considered necessary at a given level of hearing loss unless there is also a vision loss, become more important (Takano et al., 2016).

Vision loss can also interfere with the management of other kinds of disabilities or health conditions. For example, Giles et al. (2021) reported that people with visual impairments are known to be at an increased risk of experiencing medication errors, compared to those without visual impairments. Zhi-Han et al. (2017) studied a sample of this group and found that 89% of their respondents were unable to read their prescription labels, 75% did not know the expiration dates of their medications, 58% did not know the names of their medications, and 72% did not practice appropriate methods to store their medications.

Sometimes other disabilities can interfere with the identification of visual impairments. For example, Kroezen et al. (2020) found that although the prevalence of visual impairment and blindness is higher among people with intellectual disabilities than it is in the general population, visual impairment often goes undetected in people with intellectual disabilities. This result might be related to the problem of diagnostic overshadowing, in which behaviors that are associated with one disability (such as visual impairment) are incorrectly attributed to another disability (such as intellectual disability).

As visual impairments interact with the aging process, adaptations in approaches to literacy, orientation and mobility, etc. may be needed. Many adults, including those who are blind, develop diabetes and resulting peripheral neuropathy, which could reduce or preclude the use of Braille or other tactile ways of perceiving the world. Presbycusis (age-related hearing loss) can reduce the ability to use auditory input, upon which many people who are blind rely for their primary source of information. Arthritis may make physical movement challenging over time; cane navigation from a wheelchair is more difficult than from an upright, walking position. Life care planners should address these issues as potential complications for their evaluees with visual impairments, or if there is evidence that conditions such as these are more likely than not to occur as a particular evaluee ages, those conditions should be addressed in specific recommendations within that evaluee's life care planning tables.

Life Expectancy

Generally, conditions that cause blindness or visual impairments do not necessarily shorten life expectancy. Zuckerman (2004) noted that most blind adults are older than the general population; in that study of blind adults in America, the average age was 62, and one out of every three study participants was over the age of 75.

However, if appropriate rehabilitative services are not provided to help people who have visual impairments safely and competently navigate through the activities of their lives, risks to health and longevity can occur. Christ et al. (2014) conducted a longitudinal study to examine the relationships between visual acuity, daily functional status, and mortality. Although they did not find a direct effect between visual acuity and mortality, they did find an indirect effect, through instrumental activities of daily living. Basically, visual acuity loss adversely affected instrumental activities of daily living levels, which in turn affected mortality. They differentiated in their study between activities of daily living (ADL) which are necessary for fundamental daily function (such as bathing, dressing, and eating) versus instrumental activities of daily living (IADL) which relate to the degree to which an individual lives independently in the community (such as telephone use, shopping, and housework). Neither visual acuity loss nor ADL directly affected mortality, but IADL did. So, enhancing the extent to which an individual with a visual impairment or blindness can live independently in the community is likely to reduce the risk of premature death.

Medical Treatments

Some causes of blindness can be addressed through medical rehabilitation. Cataracts can often be surgically addressed by removing the clouded lens in the eye and replacing it with an artificial one. Clouded corneas can be replaced through a cornea transplant. Medications to treat glaucoma can halt or slow the progression of vision damage due to excess pressure within the eyes. Careful control of blood glucose levels can reduce the progression of diabetic retinopathy. However, many causes of blindness have no effective cure. Unfortunately, optical implants are not yet feasible for people who are blind. Conservation of residual vision, using assistive technology to accommodate vision loss, and developing alternative ways of approaching tasks without reliance on vision are necessary. Careful protection and monitoring of residual vision is important, even if that means having to find a way to get to a specialist far away from the local area, every 6–12 months.

Clinical Practice Guidelines

Clinical practice guidelines have been developed by the American Optometric Association (n.d.) for many different types of conditions causing visual impairments. They sort these guidelines into three different categories: Evidence-Based Clinical Practice Guidelines, Clinical Reports, and Consensus-Based Clinical Practice Guidelines. Keel et al. (2020) detailed plans for the World Health Organization to provide guidelines for treating the five most prominent causes of visual impairments. Cochrane Eyes and Vision, United States (2020) has a database of over 4,000 reviews, guidelines, and meta-analyses related to the eyes and various vision conditions. The quality of available clinical practice guidelines for addressing specific conditions is variable. Lingham et al. (2022) conducted a systematic review of clinical practice guidelines for childhood glaucoma, and based on their selection criteria, did not identify any high-quality clinical practice guidelines specifically targeted to this population. Chen et al. (2022) conducted a systematic review of clinical practice guidelines for myopic macular degeneration (MMD) and found that although high-quality clinical practice guidelines for MMD management were limited, intravitreal injection of anti-VEGF agents was recommended as an effective intervention for first-line treatment of one type of MMD.

Rehabilitation

Vision impairment and blindness caused by many major eye conditions (e.g., glaucoma and age-related macular degeneration) cannot be treated, and rehabilitation will be required. Rehabilitation aims to optimize the everyday functioning of those with vision impairment or blindness that cannot be treated in their environment, by maximizing the use of residual vision and providing practical adaptations to address the social, psychological, emotional, and economic consequences of vision impairment (World Health Organization, 2021).

Contrary to popular belief, losing vision does not "enhance" other senses. For example, Sorokowska et al. (2019) found examined whether blindness is associated with greater olfactory perception (sense of smell) and found no positive effects from visual impairment for any of the aspects of olfactory perception they studied: odor detection threshold, olfactory discrimination, or free and cued odor identification abilities. Instead of depending on the fictitious enhancement of other senses, people who are blind or visually impaired must learn how to better use and rely on their remaining senses; appropriate rehabilitative services are essential to this process.

Children who were born with or acquired a visual impairment soon after birth can begin learning basic skills from a Teacher for the Visually Impaired (TVI). A TVI can begin the instruction of Braille and basic mobility. This may be from an itinerant teacher working with the student who is mainstreamed in a regular local school, or in a specialized school for students who are blind or visually impaired. The schools for the blind do have a more focused and specific curriculum. The schools are not entirely residential; depending on the geographic location, there may be options for children to attend just during the day, as well as residential options. Mainstreamed children will need an Individualized Education Plan (IEP), developed with professionals who will take a role in the education of the child. For a child with a visual impairment or blindness, this might include an Orientation and Mobility Instructor who comes to the school to work with the child, an assistive technology professional familiar with devices and software that the child will use, and other professionals as the child might require. Life care planners should recognize that schools are only required to provide services that are educationally necessary through an IEP. Additional orientation and mobility services, independent living skills development, assistive technology, and other services may be necessary outside of the school setting to maximize the child's functional capacity despite the disability, and to minimize complications.

If adults who acquire vision loss are fully informed about what kinds of rehabilitative services may be helpful for improving their function and quality of life, they can discuss with life care planners what they perceive would be best suited for their individual needs and goals. Many states have rehabilitation centers for the blind, where an individual can learn skills to live independently, as well as develop vocational skills. There are several national centers where individuals can go to learn specific skills or receive training; many have the phrase "Lighthouse for the Blind" somewhere in the names of their programs. These centers commonly provide adjustment to blindness training/counseling, intensive Braille training, assistive technology assessments, and training for how to use technology recommended through those assessments, orientation and mobility skills training, independent living skills training, and depending on the facility, some types of vocational training. For example, World Services for the Blind (n.d.) in Arkansas provides all of these types of services and has a specialized training program designed to prepare their students to develop extensive skills with Microsoft Office programs, so they can become certified as Microsoft Office Specialists. Helen Keller National Center for DeafBlind Youths and Adults ([HKNC], 2022) with its main campus in New York and affiliates providing regional consultation and services around the country, serves people who have combined visual and hearing impairments. Life care planners should plan for more than one course of intensive training for their evaluees who are blind or visually impaired, such as those available from these centers. For people who experience vision loss or blindness as an adult, the most intensive services will be after the initial onset of the disability and should focus on orientation and mobility, adjustment to blindness/visual impairment, independent living skills training, assistive technology training, etc. However, as life circumstances or goals change, and as technology changes, additional training will be needed. Acquiring a new job, moving to a new area, and similar changes may require updated orientation and mobility training, assistive technology evaluation and training, etc. Other changes requiring additional training could be related to the interaction between disability and the aging process. For example, presbycusis (age-related hearing loss) may require shifting from a reliance on auditory input to more tactile ways of interacting with and receiving information from the environment.

Vision rehabilitation services allow people who are blind or have low vision to live independently and maintain quality of life. Certified Low Vision Therapists (CLVTs) instruct individuals in the use of residual vision with optical devices, non-optical devices, and assistive technology. Certified Low Vision Therapists also assist with helping to determine environmental modifications in the home, workplace, or school. Certified Vision Rehabilitation Therapists (CVRTs) teach adaptive independent living skills. Independent living skills enable adults who are blind or have low vision to confidently carry out a range of daily activities. Certified Orientation and Mobility Specialists (COMS or O&Ms) teach the skills and concepts that people who are blind or have low vision need in order to travel independently and safely in the home and in the community. They teach safe and independent indoor and outdoor travel skills, including the use of a white cane, electronic travel devices, public transportation, sighted guide (human guide), and pre-cane skills.

The specific assessments that are performed with an individual who is experiencing vision loss evaluate how much residual vision the individual has, what type of aids and assistance may be required, and individual function in regard to the activities of daily living (ADLs). Life care planners who are seeking professionals qualified to carry out such assessments could consult the Academy for Certification of Vision Rehabilitation and Education Professionals (ACVREP), which offers certification for Low Vision Therapists, Vision Rehabilitation Therapists, and Orientation and Mobility Specialists. The ACVREP provides a searchable database that will allow one to search by state.

Effective vocational evaluation is an important part of developing a vocational plan for a person who is blind or visually impaired. The vocational evaluator should be familiar with functional limitations and adaptations appropriate for the specific evaluee. Some tools, such as the McCarron-Dial Systems' (n.d.) Comprehensive Vocational Evaluation System (CVES) have been developed specifically to address some of the challenges of reliably and validly assessing the abilities of people who are blind or visually impaired. Life care planners should not make the erroneous assumption that a person who is blind or visually impaired cannot work and does not need a vocational plan. The importance of work or other productivity, and interventions to support those goals, were outlined by Reid and Riddick-Grisham (2015).

Braille literacy is important for people who are blind and cannot see printed materials, even with assistive technology to magnify or otherwise modify them. Braille uses a tactile code to translate letters and numbers, either directly (Grade I, uncontracted) or in an abbreviated form (Grade II, contracted). There is also a Nemeth code used to translate advanced mathematical concepts into Braille. People who use Braille can silently read materials, including their own notes, and can read Brailled markings in public places, such as on elevator buttons. It is estimated that fewer than 10% of school-age children with low vision or blindness can read or write braille (APH, 2021b). Those who learn to use Braille often start learning how to use it at a very early age from a TVI. Most people who lose their vision in adulthood choose to rely on auditory output instead of Braille, and for some adults, there are factors that make it more difficult for them to learn Braille. For example, if the adult also has diabetes and has peripheral neuropathy (nerve damage in the extremities), learning Braille may be more difficult due to reduced sensation in the fingertips.

Shahid and Wilkinson (2020) outlined recommendations for the rehabilitation of children with visual impairments. These recommendations included clinical low vision evaluations for all such children (regardless of the cause of their vision loss, their age, or the severity of their disabilities), to be provided by optometrists or ophthalmologists experienced with low vision rehabilitation care. They emphasized the need for collaboration between the eye care provider and the clinical low vision rehabilitation practitioner, in conjunction with teachers of students who are visually impaired, certified orientation and mobility specialists, the child's parents, and the children themselves as they mature.

Focusing on older adults, Natstasi (2020) found that group therapy, more hours of direct service over a shorter duration, and fitting older adults with low vision devices resulted in improvements in social participation outcomes. Smallfield and Kaldenberg (2020) provided an illustrative case study applying findings from the systematic review of occupational therapy for older adults with low vision, part of the American Occupational Therapy Association's evidence-based practice project.

Mobility and Travel

Certified Orientation and Mobility Specialists make recommendations based on assessments of an individual's goals, capabilities, and preferences. One of those assessments includes white cane skills. The basic white cane is still the most used mobility device, but there are now also white canes that have laser technology and canes equipped with global positioning systems (GPS) which uses speech technology in conjunction with smartphones. Orientation and mobility involve more than just learning how to use a white cane. It involves learning how to navigate around and avoid hazards in a particular environment, how to effectively use public transportation, etc. Life care planners should plan for periodic orientation and mobility evaluations and training, especially during times of transition (starting a new job, moving to a different home, etc.).

Orientation and mobility can also include working with a guide dog. A guide dog team is comprised of an individual with a visual impairment and a highly trained guide dog. An individual will travel to the guide dog school and stay for 21 to 26 days, learning commands, learning how to care for the specialized dog, and bonding with the guide dog. An individual with a visual impairment must have excellent independent travel skills before teaming with a guide dog and must have a daily routine that will allow the guide dog to work at least several hours per day. During training, the guide dog team must successfully complete multiple tasks to ensure the safety of both members of the team. After the guide dog team has worked together during the onsite stay, additional assistance may be required when they adjust to the specific routine in the home and work environments for the individual with a visual impairment. Several training facilities have recognized the need for a service dog to perform multiple tasks. Not only will the guide dog be a mobility tool; the training can address balance and/or stabilization, assistance with post-traumatic stress, and dealing with seizures or diabetic crises. A list of accredited guide dog schools can be found on the International Federation of Guide Dog Schools' website.

Assistive Technology

Advances in technology are constantly evolving (Madison et al., 2017; Mukamal, 2020). These advancements have been barrier-breaking for individuals with visual impairments or blindness (Madison et al., 2017) because, in the past, the lack of access to information has been a rather large obstacle and hindered the connection to the outside world. Assistive technology has two levels, those of basic or low-tech and the more advanced or high-tech. The life care planner who is working with an individual with visual impairment or blindness will most likely need to include both forms to enhance the basic independence and activities of daily living within the life care plan.

Any device or alteration to the environment is considered a form of assistive technology. When the term "basic" or "low-tech" is used, it typically refers to a simple modification. The use of bump dots, which are self-adhesive raised tactile dots or bumps, can be applied to household items such as microwaves, washers, dryers, dishwashers, stovetops, and ovens. Bump dots can also be placed on medications to assist in identification. Rubber bands can be utilized to help mark things such as shampoo and conditioner bottles, body washes, or other personal care items. For individuals with low vision, using contrasting colors for light switches, or even lighting the switch itself can assist in identifying the location of the switch to cut the lights off and on in a room. Many companies that market and sell independent living aids have a variety of computer keyboards that have altered keys. There are some keyboards that are predominantly black with white letters or symbols for contrast. There are also keyboards that have very large letters and symbols. The use of different strength or color light bulbs can assist someone with low vision, depending on their individual needs. Magnifiers or magnifying glasses can be useful in reading small print or labels.

One of the daily activities with which individuals with low vision or blindness may struggle is cooking. Basic tasks such as pouring a cup of hot coffee can cause fear of burning oneself. The acquisition of a liquid level indicator can ease that fear. The liquid level indicator is battery-powered and has two prongs that hang over the edge of a cup. When liquid is poured into the cup and it reaches the prongs, a tone or musical melody is played, letting the individual know that they are reaching the rim of the cup. The liquid level indicator typically leaves about an inch from the rim so that the cup will not overflow. Splatter guards for pots and pans can assist with keeping grease or other cooking oils from burning the individual while cooking. There are contrasting color measuring cups, gloves for cutting, silicon pads for placing hot pans, and even oven mitts made with silicon pads to prevent burns while taking things out of the oven or off of the stovetop. There are also talking food thermometers that assist individuals to test what they are cooking, so it may reach a safe temperature.

The management and identification of currency is another challenge faced by individuals with visual impairments or blindness. There are money organizers that allow for the placement of certain denominations, separated by liners. Another way to separate currency is to develop folding techniques that the individual feels comfortable doing. Many banking institutes will assist an individual organize their money during a visit to the bank.

Other helpful, inexpensive tools include writing guides and signature cards. Writing guides come in a variety of shapes, sizes, and purposes. There are letter-writing guides, guides for envelopes, and check-writing guides. Signature cards assist with signing credit card receipts or other documents that require a signature and are typically the size of a credit card and can easily fit in a person's wallet. Two popular companies with catalogs of such aids are Maxiaids and Independent Living Aids.

As the advancements in technology grow, so do the advancements in the technology used by individuals with disabilities (Mukamal, 2020). One high-tech advancement is that of smartphones. These devices allow for access to the internet, social media, texting, email, and a wide variety of applications (apps) that allow individuals with visual impairments or blindness to engage in daily activities with just taps on their screens (Madison et al., 2017; Mukamal, 2020).

As previously mentioned, diabetes is one of the leading causes of blindness in adults in the United States. Keeping tight control of blood glucose levels is key to minimizing health complications. Continuous Glucose Monitoring (CGM) systems have had a major impact on the management of diabetes in general but are especially helpful for individuals who are blind or have visual impairments. A small sensor and transmitter are placed on either the abdomen or back of the arm in adults, or the hip area for children. An app on one's smartphone will allow the individual to monitor blood glucose levels without the challenges of getting a small amount of blood into the right place on a small testing strip, to be inserted into a glucometer, without being able to clearly see those elements. Another app could be installed on the smartphone of a family member or caretaker, to allow them to also monitor the individual's blood glucose level. Alerts and alarms set within the app will let the individual, family member, and/or caretaker know when the blood glucose is over or below a certain range. This assists in preventing highs or dangerous lows. This app is especially beneficial for parents because even if the child is at school, the parent has access to the blood glucose readings at all times and will receive those alerts and alarms. This is also beneficial if children have experienced dangerous lows during the night. The parent's phone will sound an alarm and let the parent know what the blood glucose reading is so that the parent can act.

There are many free apps that assist with identifying colors, identifying money, or even playing games (Mukamal, 2020). The National Treasury has a free download for a money identifier that uses the camera on a smartphone. There are a variety of free downloadable apps to assist with identifying color. "Seeing AI" and "Tap See" are apps that allow an individual to snap a picture of an object. The app will then describe, in text, what is contained in the picture (Mukamal, 2020).

Kurzweil developed an application formerly called the KNFBReader Mobile. The title has recently been changed to the One Step Reader. The app uses Object Character Recognition software to optimize translating a print document into speech output. The app also has the capability to save files for future reference if needed. The app has many options, including various reading and language styles.

One of the most common text-to-speech software programs for use with a personal computer (PC) is Job Access With Speech (JAWS). It is compatible with most Microsoft products and can be purchased from Freedom Scientific. As with many assistive technologies, it does require some training for effective use. Apple products have an accessibility feature that comes with iPhones, iPads, and Macs, called VoiceOver. It uses the voice of Siri and can be accessed under the settings app. There are also some open-access software programs available for download, such as Non-Visual Desktop Access (NVDA).

Manduchi and Kurniawan (2013) addressed different types of technology that can help remove barriers in the workplace and the community for people who have visual disabilities. Examples include low-tech options such as lighted magnifying glasses and liquid level indicators, as well as high-tech solutions. Among the high-tech options are accessible global positioning systems, wayfinding devices, camera-based tools to access visual information, screen readers and tools to improve internet accessibility, and Digital Accessible Information System (DAISY) multimedia systems, as well as descriptive video services.

Determining which types of technology are most appropriate for an individual with a visual impairment requires understanding the technology options and how they interact with the individual's goals and preferences. Life care planners should plan for periodic assistive technology evaluations, purchase and updating of recommended hardware and software, and training for the individual to learn how to use that technology.

Transportation

Transportation is another very problematic barrier for people who are blind. Driving a vehicle can represent independence, as well as serve the function of facilitating employment and community engagement when public transportation options are limited or nonexistent. One of the top barriers to people with visual impairments or blindness feeling independent and not a burden is transportation (Crudden, 2018). Where the individual lives will determine how accessible public transportation is to them. Most large metropolitan areas have some public transportation. Although the cost of that public transportation is minimal, usually the cost of living in those areas is greater than the cost of similar homes or apartments in areas where public transportation is not available. Typically, the local public transportation system is partnered with paratransit. Paratransit is transportation accessible to people with disabilities and provides door-to-door services. However, the scheduling availability, timeliness, and reliability of paratransit services can be notoriously problematic.

Taxicab services are licensed by a governmental entity, requiring background checks as one of the conditions for securing those licenses. Taxi drivers are usually also required to go through training related to serving passengers who have disabilities. Ride-share companies (such as Uber or Lyft) offer popular alternatives to the cost of taxicab fare, but their drivers are not licensed by any governmental entity. There are risks involved in getting into the vehicle of a person who claims to be a driver for a ride-sharing company. For sighted people, there are apps available to provide a photo of the assigned driver, for visual comparison to the person who is driving a vehicle. However, such photos are of little use to someone with significant visual impairment. People who are blind or visually impaired may be willing to take on that extra risk if the ride-share service is more cost-effective than other alternatives, but that risk should be recognized.

When estimating transportation costs for evaluees who are blind or have visual impairments, life care planners can look at the average number of miles driven per year by a demographically similar individual who can see, calculate the cost of providing that amount of transportation through public transportation (if available), taxicabs, etc., and then subtract the average annual costs associated with purchasing and maintaining a vehicle to drive those miles. (Resources for estimating the average number of miles driven per year are available through websites such as the U.S. Department of Transportation's Federal Highway Administration page addressing average annual miles.) The difference between the cost of providing that transportation for the individual and the cost that individual would incur when driving if they were sighted is the cost of transportation that is attributable to the disability.

Life Care Planning with People Who Have Visual Impairments

Ensure the *accessibility* of your communications. Are your disclosure forms, checklists, forms you ask people to fill out, etc. accessible? Do they have any undescribed graphics? Are they text-based and readily available electronically? Are any PDF forms in a searchable format? If your documents are produced using Microsoft Word, are you using the headings function?

Understand the *functional* effects of visual impairment, as they affect daily life. What kinds of adaptations, services, or devices might help to address those functions? For example, what could take the place of a photo album, or a video tour of a building and the landscaping around it?

Consider how vision impairment *interacts* with other disabilities, both now and into the future as the evaluee ages. For example, if the evaluee is blind and has a hearing impairment, but does not quite reach the level of hearing loss designated as qualifying for a cochlear implant under traditional FDA guidelines, can anything be done?

Know what *team* you need. Like the wide range of differences in function and needs of individuals with visual disabilities, so is the need for varied specialists to contribute information for life care plan development, and to implement life care plans for this population. For example, ophthalmologists are usually the physicians who address the medical aspects of assessing and preserving the individual's vision. Neuro-ophthalmologists may be needed when the vision problem involves central processing (within the brain) or neural pathways. Optometrists assess visual acuity and determine what lenses may correct refraction errors, if applicable. Orientation and mobility (O&M) specialists provide assessments and training to increase the ability to safely travel and navigate in an environment. Teachers for the Visually Impaired (TVIs) assess and provide instruction for using Braille, as well as independent living skills. Counselors or psychologists help with adjustment to blindness, both for the individual with a vision impairment and for that person's family. They are essential for addressing the psychological and mental health needs, including feelings of isolation, depression, and anxiety that are experienced by many. Rehabilitation counselors help with identifying vocational goals, then developing and implementing plans to achieve those goals, with appropriate support as needed. Assistive technology specialists provide assessment of the technology needs of someone with a visual impairment, and training to use the technologies that may improve access and help that person more effectively pursue their goals. Social workers or case managers can assist with connecting people to much-needed resources and information. Providing effective services to address the needs of people experiencing blindness or vision impairment requires a coordinated, interdisciplinary approach.

Areas of Life Care Plan Recommendations

Below are several examples of areas to consider within each section of life care plan tables.

Medical Care

Is medical care needed to address conditions like insomnia or depression that commonly result from visual impairment? How often are visits to an ophthalmologist or neuro-ophthalmologist recommended? How will the visual impairment affect recommendations for medical treatment of other conditions the evaluee may have?

Procedures/Hospitalizations/Surgeries

Are any surgical interventions recommended, such as corneal transplant, cataract surgery, or laser surgery to reattach a detached retina?

Education

What kinds of education or training will this individual need to achieve desired life goals? For children, what kinds of educational support will be needed? For children and adults, what kinds of technology training, Braille training, orientation and mobility training, and independent living skills training are needed? For adults, and youths approaching transition to adulthood, what kinds of vocational training would be helpful?

Evaluations

What kinds of evaluations are needed because of the visual impairment? How often should low vision evaluations be conducted? When should technology evaluations occur? Who should conduct those evaluations?

Therapies

Is visual therapy recommended? What kinds of mental health counseling might be needed, and at what points in time? Would family counseling/education help the family to best provide an environment that empowers the person with a visual impairment?

Diagnostic Testing

Is diagnostic testing needed to guide educational placement and planning? Are assessments of visual acuity needed to prescribe appropriate eyeglasses or contact lenses? If so, how often, and by whom? Are modifications of diagnostic testing processes needed, such as for accurate monitoring of blood glucose levels?

Medications

Does the evaluee have sleep problems? If so, have they been evaluated for non-24 sleep-wake disorder, and has medication for this disorder been tried? Are medications needed for conditions such as glaucoma? How does visual impairment affect the administration of medications for other conditions?

Supplies

What kinds of consumable supplies are needed because of the visual impairment? Have you considered items such as Braille printer paper, 3D printer filaments, and earbud headphones?

Equipment

What kinds of technology is the evaluee using already? What else could address identified functional limitations? For example, might a 3D printer and Photo to Mesh software help to make two-dimensional photographs accessible? What has been recommended through assistive technology evaluation? What kinds of software are required to work with this equipment? What kinds of training are needed to use this equipment (which can be included in the Education section)?

Orthotics/Prosthetics

If one or both eyes are enucleated, would prosthetics improve the evaluee's appearance and confidence? Would wearing an eye patch help to treat a child's amblyopia?

Wheelchairs and Wheelchair Accessories/Maintenance

If the evaluee uses a wheelchair, or is expected to use one in the future for conditions unrelated to visual impairment, how does visual impairment affect the ability to use a wheelchair? What kinds of modifications would be needed in orientation and mobility techniques when using a wheelchair? Has technology progressed to the point where when you complete your evaluation, wheelchairs equipped with laser scanners and haptic robots are available?

Aids for Independent Living

What kind of annual allowance would be appropriate for various aids for independent living, such as liquid level indicators, talking thermometers, and a "pen friend" system for attaching to objects different labels that auditorily identify those items when the pen device is pointed at them? Is a guide dog planned? If so, what are the costs of caring for and maintaining the health of that canine companion?

Home Furnishings and Accessories

Is a security alarm system needed to alert the evaluee when someone is lurking around or trying to break into their home? Are storage units needed for things like 3D printouts? Unlike paper which can be easily stacked and put into a file cabinet, 3D printouts require organized shelving space to avoid chaos. Multiple shelving units provide the organized storage equivalent of one small filing cabinet for paper documents.

Home Care

Are there housekeeping, yard work, and home maintenance tasks that the evaluee cannot complete because of visual impairment, or that take more time because of the visual impairment? Would providing some assistance in this area help to free up time for some other tasks of daily living that require more time than would be needed for a sighted person?

Facility Care

Does the combination of visual impairment and other health conditions increase the likelihood that the evaluee will need assisted living services or placement in a skilled nursing facility at an earlier age than what would normally be expected? If so, what needs to happen for that facility to be accessible to people with visual impairments?

Case Management

Will case management services assist the evaluee or their family/caregiver to learn how to implement life care plan recommendations? If so, will the intensity of those services change over time?

Transportation

Are public transportation options available in this evaluee's area? If so, do they meet the individual's needs during the desired timeframes, with the needed degree of reliability? If not, what other transportation options are available? Have you deducted the average cost of owning and operating an automobile from those costs, to show the net increase in transportation costs that are due to the visual impairment?

Vocational Plan

What services can help this evaluee to achieve their vocational potential? Has a vocational evaluation been conducted? If so, what are the resulting recommendations? What are the evaluee's needs and vocational interests, and how do those relate to a vocational goal? Would career counseling and job placement services be helpful? Are supported employment or customized employment services needed? If so, for how long? If the person's combination of disabilities is so severe that employment is not a goal, what are plans for engaging in other types of productive activity in life? What kinds of services could help to attain those goals?

Health and Strength Maintenance

What can help this evaluee safely engage in physical and mental activities that will maintain their health and strength, despite limitations imposed by visual impairment? If membership in a gym would help, can personal training be provided to provide a hands-on orientation to the facility and equipment, as well as to monitor safe equipment use and technique? Are there ways to engage in outdoor activities with others, such as when riding a tandem bicycle? What kinds of hobbies interest the evaluee, and what might be needed to adapt equipment and processes so those hobbies can be enjoyed?

Architectural Renovations

Are the living and working spaces safe for people with visual impairments, or are there hazards such as platforms without railings? Will extra space be needed to hold bulky assistive technology devices, or to store things like 3D printouts?

Potential Complications

Potential complications are usually detailed in a life care plan report separately from the tables of recommendations and the projected costs of those recommendations. If there is evidence that something related to the disability is "more likely than not" to occur, it should be detailed within the life care plan itself, along with recommended services to address it. However, if the rate of occurrence is unknown or is lower than the level of "more likely than not," it should be listed as a potential complication. The purpose of listing potential complications is to provide information about what else *might* occur for the individual with that disability, given that it has been associated with the disability for some people in the past. Listing potential complications can also provide context for why some of the preventative recommendations are made, to minimize the risk of such complications. Examples of potential complications for people who are blind or visually impaired include:

- *Clinical depression or adjustment disorder.* Internalizing frustrations in adjustment to disability, if one isn't able to find healthy ways to cope with them, could lead to mental health crises. Including some mental health counseling services in the life care plan can help to minimize the risk of this complication.
- *Trip and fall injuries.* Not being able to see obstacles or uneven hazards in their paths, people with visual impairments are at increased risk for trip and fall accidents, which could result in broken bones, head injury, and other serious injuries. Interventions such as modifying the environment to minimize such hazards, and orientation and mobility training, should help to reduce the risk of these complications.
- *Cuts and bruises.* Without seeing (or seeing clearly) objects in their surroundings, people with visual impairments are at risk of "running into" them or hitting them with parts of their bodies. Providing a clear orientation to the environment and minimizing placement of hazardous objects directly in the areas surrounding where people with visual impairments live and work, can help reduce this risk.
- *Fire hazard.* People who are blind may have difficulty evacuating a burning building, especially if they are on an upper floor; they cannot see where the smoke or flames are originating and may not be sure which way to turn to avoid the hazard.
- *Deafblindness.* As people with visual impairments age, it is likely that they will lose some hearing. If they currently rely on hearing for much of their language and information reception but lose a great deal of hearing over time, they will experience significant challenges with dual-sensory loss. People with visual losses should monitor their hearing, and if they notice a decrease in hearing over time, seek intervention (hearing aids, cochlear implants, and/or rehabilitation services for people who have dual-sensory losses).
- *Pedestrian vs. traffic accidents.* People with visual impairments may not see automobiles approaching. When crossing a busy street intersection, they might not accurately identify where vehicles are located as they approach the intersection. This is especially challenging with quiet vehicles, such as electric cars. Orientation and mobility instruction, as well as environmental modifications such as crosswalks with traffic signals that provide auditory and tactile signals to pedestrians, can decrease this risk.
- *Violence or abuse.* Because people who are blind or visually impaired can appear vulnerable and not fully aware of their surroundings, they can risk seeming like "easy prey" for somebody seeking to victimize another human being. Tools such as home security systems can help to reduce this risk.

Assessment Questions to Ask

The following are examples of questions life care planners should ask as part of their evaluation process with an evaluee who has a visual impairment; they have been adapted from a protocol developed by the Helen Keller National Center:

1. How does this person describe their vision? What can they actually see? Does it vary under different circumstances?
2. If the person has any usable vision, what helps them to see best? What font type and size? What kind of lighting? Any assistive devices?
3. Orientation & Mobility: What kind of training has been accomplished and/or planned? How much? What works? Would more help? [Cane technique? Canine? Devices? Human guide? Other?]
4. Low Vision: What kind of evaluation has been done? What devices and techniques have been tried? What works? What could be improved? [Magnification, color, contrast? Portable devices? Closed Circuit Television (CCTV)?]
5. Braille: Has the evaluee tried it? What level? Is the evaluee interested in learning it, or improving their current Braille skills?
6. Safety/Security: How is this handled in the home? Outside the home?
7. Reading: How does this person read labels at home? Outside the home? Bills and correspondence? How do they generally read for information? For enjoyment?
8. Time: How much longer does it take, for activities of daily living (ADLs) and instrumental activities of daily living (IADLs) for interacting with the community)? For other tasks?
9. Assistance: What kinds of assistance are used now? Who provides the assistance, and how much?
10. Sleep: How well does the evaluee sleep each night? If there are problems, what kind of sleep problems are experienced?
11. Misses it: If the evaluee was sighted before but now has lost vision, what do they miss being able to do that they could do before?

Additional Resources

Low vision resources are available from the Foundation Fighting Blindness (2022) at https://www.fightingblindness.org/low-vision.

Three organizations of and for people who are blind include:

- American Council of the Blind (2022). Fostering voice, choice, and community. https://www.acb.org/
- American Foundation for the Blind (2022a). Moving forward. https://www.afb.org/
- National Federation of the Blind (2022b). Welcome to the movement. https://nfb.org/

Three examples of guide dog training programs are:

- Guide Dogs for the Blind (2022). Programs for the blind and visually impaired. https://www.guidedogs.com/get-a-guide-dog/programs-for-the-blind-and-visually-impaired
- Guide Dogs of America (2022). Our program overview. https://www.guidedogsofamerica.org/service-dog-information/
- Guiding Eyes for the Blind (2022). Who we are. https://www.guidingeyes.org/who-we-are/ https://www.guidingeyes.org/who-we-are/

Two other important resources for life care planners who work with people who are blind or visually impaired are a professional association and a research and training center. The Association for

Education and Rehabilitation of the Blind and Visually Impaired ([AER], n.d.) has many helpful resources, including the *Journal of Visual Impairment and Blindness*. The National Research and Training Center on Blindness and Low Vision (Mississippi State University, 2022) has resources for professionals, resources for families, research publications, training opportunities, and technical assistance services.

Case Study

When in high school, Betty Williams experienced chronic headaches and papilledema (swelling of the head of her optic nerves, where they attach to the retina) in both eyes before surgery was performed to remove a brain tumor. She experienced significant vision loss that did not improve with recovery from surgery; she was diagnosed as blind (with total loss of visual field in her left eye, and in her right eye nearly total loss which varied at times but was usually at the level of light perception only). At the time of her life care planning evaluation, she had engaged in significant rehabilitation services, including orientation and mobility training that enabled her to navigate using a white cane, independent living skills training, Braille training (reaching the advanced Grade 2—contracted Braille level, as well as Nemeth technique for using Braille in advanced mathematics), orientation to blindness training, etc. from a local Lighthouse for the Blind rehabilitation center. She graduated from high school, and at the time of the evaluation, she was a student in her junior year of college, living alone in an off-campus apartment. Her vocational goal was to run her own business in the hospitality industry; her college major was consistent with that goal. She also planned to start raising a family in about ten years, after first establishing her business. Supports at the time of her evaluation included services from the college's office of services for students with disabilities; a tuition waiver from her college; vocational counseling, assistive technology equipment, a stipend to assist with living expenses while in college, and other assistance from the vocational rehabilitation services department in her state; and transportation, shopping assistance, housekeeping assistance, and other supports from her family members.

During her interview with the life care planner, Ms. Williams reported symptoms of insomnia and depression. Oral administration of the Beck Depression Inventory II confirmed a serious level of depression, so a suicide risk assessment was included in the evaluation. Ms. Williams denied active suicidal ideation at that time but confirmed that she has previously considered ending her life. She said that her family members and her significant other help her get through the tough times, but it can be a challenge. Although Ms. Williams' general practitioner physician had prescribed Citalopram for depression and Trazodone for insomnia, both depression and insomnia remained significant problems despite medication. Later communication between the life care planner and Ms. Williams' physician confirmed that the physician said it "would be reasonable to explore" evaluation and treatment for non-24 sleep-wake disorder, but because such an evaluation had not been completed by the time the life care plan was due, recommendations for treatment of non-24 sleep-wake disorder were not included in the life care plan tables and cost calculations. A note for informational purposes was included in the life care plan narrative, detailing the projected costs for such treatment if, and only if, it is later recommended as a result of an evaluation by a qualified sleep disorders specialist who has experience working with people who are blind.

Ms. Williams' life care plan tables detailed services that were recommended going forward; they did not include services already provided in the past (such as Braille training, initial Orientation and Mobility Training, etc.).

Medical Care	Time	Frequency	Purpose	Cost	Comment
General Practitioner Physician	2022 – life	1x/year	Monitor medical treatment; address depression and insomnia.	$185 per visit	These visits are in addition to the annual visit recommended for everyone.
Ophthalmologist	2022 – life	2x/year	Monitor and treat the eye condition.	$245 per visit	Frequency recommended by the treating provider.

Education	Time	Frequency	Purpose	Cost	Comment
Adjustment to vision loss class	2023	Once, after completing her B.A. degree.	As she moves from a student role to that of an adult, adjusting to the effect blindness has on those changes.	$5,500 per class	Recommended by Lighthouse staff.
Orientation and Mobility (O & M) training, itinerant services	2023 2033 2063	10 days 4 days 4 days	In 2023, to increase her skill and confidence with navigating independently in the community, instead of relying on family members and friends to accompany her. Later, when she moves to a new residence, and much later, when challenges related to aging require O & M technique adjustments.	$700 per day	Each day listed assumes a full eight units of instruction are provided in that day. If the training is divided into partial days, the cost would increase because of additional transportation costs for the instructor.
Assistive Technology training, including itinerant services	2022 2023 2027 - life	5 days One class, after completing her degree. 5 days, every 5 years.	Training is needed as the combination of her needs and available technologies change over time.	$780 per day, or $5,500 per class.	Training as recommended after each assistive technology evaluation.

Figure 25.1 Example Life Care Planning Tables for Betty Williams

Evaluations	Time	Frequency	Purpose	Cost	Comment
Assistive Technology Evaluation	2022 – life	Once in 2022, once in 2023, then every 5 years.	Identify appropriate assistive technologies as the combination of needs and available tools evolve.	$2,500 per evaluation	Evaluations should occur before each round of assistive technology training.

Therapies	Time	Frequency	Purpose	Cost	Comment
Mental health counseling – 1st intensive course, and later two follow-up courses	2022 2032 2052	25 sessions 10 sessions 10 sessions	Treatment of current depression, and later adjustment challenges as blindness interacts with life events.	$80 - $190 per session.	Timing and actual number of the follow-up courses will vary.

Medications & Supplies	Time	Frequency	Purpose	Cost	Comment
Citalopram, 20 mg	2022 – life	Once per day	Treatment of depression.	$27 - $86 for 30 tablets.	Prescribed by her treating physician.
Trazodone, 50 mg	2022 – life	Once per day	Treatment of insomnia.	$17 - $26 for 30 tablets.	Prescribed by her treating physician.

Supplies	Time	Frequency	Purpose	Cost	Comment
Braille printer paper	2022 – life	1000 pages, 10 times per year.	Printing out Brailled text.	$35 - $48 per 1000 sheets.	Cost is for expenses above the average cost for regular paper.
Filaments for the 3D printer	2022 – life	2 spools per month.	Creation of three dimensional models and "photo mesh" textured images from two dimensional photographs.	$60 - $70 per spool.	Cost is for expenses above the average cost for regular printer toner.
Ear bud headphones	2022 – life	Three units every five months	For privacy and not interrupting others when listening to audio output on devices.	$8 - $17 per unit	Based on current use and replacement frequency.

Equipment	Time	Frequency	Purpose	Cost	Comment
Additional memory for	2022 – life	One unit every 5 years	Additional memory required to run memory-	$68 per unit	Cost of the entire laptop computer is not

Figure 25.1 (Continued) Example Life Care Planning Tables for Betty Williams

laptop computer			intensive screenreader programs.		included, because most people typically have laptop computers.
Perkins Brailler 2	2022 – life	One unit every 7 years	Print Brailled text.	$940 per unit	Cost for amount above cost of average regular printer.
Victor Reader Stream Portable	2022 – life	One unit every 5 years	For streaming audio materials	$460 per unit	Available from Humanware.
Talking scientific calculator	2022 – Working life	One unit every 5 years	For current courses future business use.	$290 per unit	Equipment included here is per Lighthouse recommendations.
Kurzweil 1000 scan-to-text and voice output software for laptop computer	2022 – life	Once every 5 years.	To make printed text materials accessible.	$1,200 per unit	Replacement schedule for software corresponds to replacement schedule for the laptop computer.
JAWS Pro screenreader software for laptop computer	2022 – life	Once every 5 years.	Voice output for text received on a computer.	$1,500 per unit	Replacement schedule corresponds to replacement schedule for the laptop computer.
Olympus digital voicerecorder	2022 – life	One unit every 5 years.	Recording notes, drafting messages, etc.	$230 per unit	Example of recommendation from the assistive technology evaluation.
Backpack for laptop computer	2022 – life	One unit every 5 years.	Backpack is needed to transport the laptop computer while leaving hands free for use of the white cane for mobility.	$40 - $55 per unit.	Frequency of replacement may be higher, depending on quality of the backpack and frequency of use.
TWAIN-compliant scanner that is compatible with the	2022 – life	One unit every 5 years.	Scanning printed text materials to prepare them for voice output.	$120 - $180 per unit	Smartphone scanning apps are not necessarily compatible with

Figure 25.1 (Continued) Example Life Care Planning Tables for Betty Williams

Kurzweil 1000 software					Kurzweil; a separate scanner is needed.
Phoenix Multi-Function Braille and Tactile Graphics System, 70PX000	2022 – life	One unit every 5 years.	Printing Brailled text and diagrams composed of raised dots.	$5600 - $6100	Also requires Duxbury software and Braille printer paper.
Extended warranty (3 years) for the Phoenix 70PX000	2022 – life	Once every 5 years.	Needed for the Phoenix system to be supported for five full years.	$1300 - $1400	Printer 5 year replacement schedule requires an extended warranty.
Peacemaker sound enclosure, 70PM0000	2022 – life	One unit every 5 years.	Reduces the VERY LOUD sound of Braille printing.	$1100 - $1200	Replacement schedule to coincide with printer replacement.
Duxbury Braille translation software	2022	Initial one-time purchase of one unit.	Translating electronic text into Braille code.	$690 - $980	After the first year, requires annual updates.
Annual updates for Duxbury software	2023 – life	Once per year, after the first year of software purchase.	Updates required to translate electronic text into Braille code.	$170 - $230	Charges start one year after initial software purchase.
Dual extruder 3D printer	2022 – life	One unit every 5 years.	Printing three-dimensional representations of environments, and textured "mesh" representations of photographs.	$4000 - $6000	Requires 3D scanner and storage space for a large footprint.
FARO Focus 3D X 130 scanner	2022 – work life.	One unit every 5 years.	Scanning of indoor and outdoor environments to create smaller-scale 3D (three dimensional) representations. This is important for Ms. Williams' planned business.	$59,000 per unit.	This can scan entire environments. Cost covers the scanner itself, tripod, batteries, and required training.
Photo to Mesh software	2022 – life	One unit every 5 years.	Improving the accessibility of flat images (such as photographs or drawings) by translating different	$50 per unit.	Available from Ransen software.

Figure 25.1 (Continued) Example Life Care Planning Tables for Betty Williams

			shades into varying textures.		
Aids for Independent Living	**Time**	**Frequency**	**Purpose**	**Cost**	**Comment**
Learning Ally membership renewal	2022 – life	Once per year.	Provides electronic access to printed books.	$135 per year	Available only to people with qualifying disabilities.
Ambutech graphite folding cane, marshmallow hook tip; rolling ball tip for the cane	2022 – life	One unit every 6 months.	Aid for orientation and mobility; visual signal to others that the user is blind.	$115	Replacement schedule based on prior history.
Trekker Breeze Plus handheld talking GPS system	2022 – life	One unit every 5 years.	Orientation and wayfinding assistance.	$800 - $900	Available from Humanware and other vendors.
Canine guide (service dog)	2022 – life	Multiple costs, summed to an annual total.	Orientation and mobility assistance.	$850 - $2200 per year.	No cost to the blind individual for acquiring the trained service dog; annual costs are for maintaining the dog's health.
Annual allowance for a variety of assistive devices to support independence	2022 – life	Cumulative costs summed into once per year.	Aids for independence, such as liquid level indicators, check-writing template guides, Braille labellers and adhesive labelling tape, Pen Friend recorder/reader and various labels to attach to objects so the pen can read aloud their identity when pointed toward those labels, tactile watch, weather alert radio, talking timers, etc.	$900 total per year.	Choice of assistive devices will vary from year to year, depending on needs at the time and personal preference.

Home Furnishings and Accessories	**Time**	**Frequency**	**Purpose**	**Cost**	**Comment**

Figure 25.1 (Continued) Example Life Care Planning Tables for Betty Williams

Oversize literature and mail sorting units for storing 3D printouts	2022 – life	Two units every 7 years.	3D printouts require organized shelving space to avoid chaos.	$1200 - $1600 per unit.	Replacement schedule based on IRS depreciation schedule for similar items.
Home security system and remote monitoring service	2022 – life	Ongoing, with monthly or annual charges.	Home safety when one cannot visually monitor the environment inside or outside of the home.	$300 - $700 per year.	Some systems also have initial equipment purchase costs, in addition to monthly ongoing charges.

Home Care	Time	Frequency	Purpose	Cost	Comment
Housekeeping support	2022 – 2031 2031 – life	25 weeks per year, for 10 years. 50 weeks per year.	Some housekeeping tasks cannot be completed by Ms. Williams at all, and other tasks may take considerably longer than they would take if she still had sight.	$150 - $180 per week.	Services are not expected for about two weeks per year, during times when Ms. Williams is traveling, such as on vacation with her family.
Personal assistance, including some driving and shopping assistance	2022 – life	Eight hours per week, 52 weeks per year.	Removing environmental barriers to instrumental activities of daily living (IADLs), engaging in the community.	$25 – 32 per hour	Time estimates for these tasks are based on Expectancy Data (2021) statistics.
Yardwork, including lawn care and shrub trimming	2032 – life	Once per week, 26 weeks per year.	After her projected move to a home with a yard in ten years, assistance with yardwork that requires vision is provided.	$170 - $260 per week.	Time estimates for these tasks are based on Expectancy Data (2021) statistics.

Case Management	Time	Frequency	Purpose	Cost	Comment
Case Management	2022 only 2031 only 2067 only	20 hours, one time 10 hours, one time 10 hours, one time	Limited case management services are included to assist with learning how to implement the life care plan.	$90 - $120 per hour.	After the first year, two other sets of limited case management assistance are provided at anticipated times of transition.

Figure 25.1 (Continued) Example Life Care Planning Tables for Betty Williams

Transportation	Time	Frequency	Purpose	Cost	Comment
Taxicab fare	2022 – life	Various times, with costs summed annually	Transportation, for the average amount that a female drives in the United States.	$26,000 - $29,000	Reduced by the average annual cost of owning and operating an automobile
Travel to and from the site where FARO provides training to use the 3D scanner.	2022	One time only	Travel for required training, for two.	$1400 - $2000	Travel for Ms. Williams and her assistant, who will also need to learn how to use the scanner.

Vocational Plan	Time	Frequency	Purpose	Cost	Comment
Career Counseling	2023	Ten sessions total, in one year.	Assistance with making the transition from student to employed worker, despite challenges faced because of blindness.	$90 - $250 per session.	Unemployment is associated with decreased quality of life and decreased life expectancy (Reid & Riddick-Grisham, 2015).
Job placement assistance	2023	80 total hours	Assistance with finding or entrepreneurially creating employment opportunities.	$70 - $120 per hour	Counteracts barriers to employment, including those of stigma, stereotypes, and reduced access to networks.

Health & Strength Maintenance	Time	Frequency	Purpose	Cost	Comment
Gym membership	2022 – life	12 months per year	Improving enjoyment of life, avoiding premature shortening of life due to reduced options for safe physical activity.	$40 - $60 per month	Fulfills dual goals of exercise and engaging with other people outside of her home.
Personal training	2022 only	40 sessions initially	Initial individual orientation to the facility; later personal training	$35 - $60 per session	Individual, hands-on assistance of a personal

Figure 25.1 (Continued) Example Life Care Planning Tables for Betty Williams

	2023-life	One session per month, after the first year	sessions once per month allow periodic monitoring for safety.		trainer is needed to ensure safe use of the equipment.
Tandem bicycle with sturdy frame for off-road use	2022 – life	Once every 10 years.	Outdoor exercise while engaging with another person.	$6,100 - $8,600	Tandem mountain bike. Replacement schedule is based on information from cyclingforums.com
Mountain bike helmets	2022 – life	Two helmets every 8 years	Helmets for safety of both bike riders.	$9.00 - $180.00 per helmet.	Replacement schedule per Helmets.org/replace.htm
Speedball Clay Boss Pottery Wheel	2022 – life	One unit every 7 years	Creative outlet for stress reduction and creating something useful	$610 - $720	Such productive activity could remain a hobby or even evolve into a potential source of second income.
Paragon Home Artist Kiln	2022 – life	One unit every 7 years	For firing ceramics creations (stress reduction, and benefits of productive activity)	$1,100 - $1,300	Ms. Williams stated that she enjoyed her ceramics classes in school but did not have the equipment at home needed to work with ceramics.

Architectural Renovations	Time	Frequency	Purpose	Cost	Comment
Additional space in Ms. Williams' home	2022 – life	Annually, if renting, OR Once every 13 years, if purchasing a home	Additional space is needed to accommodate assistive technology equipment and storage space for 3D printouts.	$1,800 per year if renting OR $24,000 per home purchase	Conservatively estimated, the increase in space needed in the home is at least 150 square feet.

Figure 25.1 (Continued)　Example Life Care Planning Tables for Betty Williams

Conclusion

Life care planners should not only understand the implications of blindness and visual impairments for people whose life care plans are developed because of such impairments; they should also understand how visual impairment interacts with other disabilities, either as a pre-existing condition or an additional disability that emerges as people age. Rehabilitation interventions such as orientation and mobility training, literacy enhancement (including Braille skills), independent living skills training, and assistive technology can be tremendously important. Preservation (and improvement, if applicable) of residual vision, monitoring (and enhancing, if needed) of hearing, addressing depression and other mental health challenges, and addressing sleep problems may require medical intervention or related therapies. Environmental modifications should include interventions such as moving obstacles that could become safety hazards, providing home security alert systems, and enabling easy access to public transportation or other transportation options. Combinations of rehabilitation, medical, and environmental interventions tailored to the needs of each individual who is blind or has a visual impairment can significantly improve functional outcomes and quality of life.

References

American Academy of Ophthalmology. (2020). *Driving restrictions per state*. https://eyewiki.aao.org/Driving_Restrictions_per_State

American Council of the Blind. (2022). *Fostering voice, choice, and community*. https://www.acb.org/

American Foundation for the Blind. (2022a). *Moving forward*. https://www.afb.org/

American Foundation for the Blind. (2022b). *Statistics on children*. https://www.afb.org/research-and-initiatives/statistics/statistics-blind-children

American Optometric Association. (n.d.). *Clinical practice guidelines*. https://www.aoa.org/practice/clinical-guidelines/clinical-practice-guidelines?sso=y

American Printing House for the Blind. (2021a). *Annual report, fiscal year 2021*. American Printing House, Inc. http://www.aph.org/annual-reports

American Printing House for the Blind. (2021b). *Vision rehabilitation services*. American Printing House, Inc. https://visionaware.org/everyday-living/essential-skills/vision-rehabilitation-services/

Association for Education and Rehabilitation of the Blind and Visually Impaired. (n.d.). https://aerbvi.org/

Atowa, U. C., Hansraj, R., & Wajuihian, S. O. (2019). Visual problems: a review of prevalence studies on visual impairment in school-age children. *International journal of ophthalmology*, 12(6), 1037–1043. https://doi.org/10.18240/ijo.2019.06.25

Augestad, L. V. (2017). Self-concept and self-esteem among children and young adults with visual impairment: A systematic review. *Cogent Psychology*, 4(1), 1–12. https://doi.org/10.1080/23311908.2017.1319652

Bahramfar E., & Ashori, M. (2021). The impact of stress inoculation training on cognitive emotion regulation and psychological problems of the mothers of blind children. *Journal of Child Mental Health*, 8(1), 27–42. http://childmentalhealth.ir/article-1-793-en.html

Bureau of Labor Statistics. (2022). Persons with a disability: Labor force characteristics summary-2021. https://www.bls.gov/news.release/disabl.nr0.htm

Centers for Disease Control and Prevention. (2020a). *Fast facts of common eye disorders*. Fast Facts of Common Eye Disorders | CDC

Centers for Disease Control and Prevention. (2020b). *Vision loss: A public health problem*. https://www.cdc.gov/visionhealth/basic_information/vision_loss.htm

Chen, Y., Han, X., Gordon, I., Safi, S., Lingham, G., Evans, J., Li, J., He, M., & Keel, S. (2022). A systematic review of clinical practice guidelines for myopic macular degeneration. *Journal of Global Health*, 12, 04026. https://jogh.org/2022/jogh-12-04026

Christ, S. L., Zheng, D. D., Swenor, B. K., Lam. B. L., West, S. K., Tannenbaum, S. L., Muñoz, B. E., & Lee, D. J. (2014). Longitudinal relationships among visual acuity, daily functional status, and mortality: The Salisbury Eye Evaluation Study. *JAMA Ophthalmology, 132*(12), 1400–1406. https://doi.org/10.1001/jamaophthalmol.2014.2847

Cochrane Eyes and Vision. (2020, September). CEV@US database of systematic reviews in eyes and vision [A database of systematic reviews and meta-analyses (SRMAs) across all eyes and vision conditions]. Retrieved August 5, 2022, from Cochrane Eyes and Vision.

Crudden, A. (2018). Transportation and vision loss: Where are we now? *Insight: The Journal of American Society of Ophthalmic Registered Nurses, 43*(2), 19–24.

Crudden, A., Antonelli, K., & O'Mally, J. (2016). Transportation self-efficacy and social problem-solving of persons who are blind or visually impaired. *Journal of Social Work in Disability and Rehabilitation, 15*(1), 52–61. https://doi.org/10.1080/1536710X.2016.1124254

Crudden, A., Cmar, J. L., & McDonnall, M. C. (2017). Stress associated with transportation: A survey of persons with visual impairment. *Journal of Visual Impairment & Blindness, 111*(3), 219–230.

Crudden, A., McDonnall, M. C., & Hierholzer, A. (2015). Transportation: An electronic survey of persons who are blind or have low vision. *Journal of Visual Impairment and Blindness, 109*(6), 445–456.

Crudden, A., & Steverson, A. C. (2021). Job retention and career advancement: A survey of persons who are blind or have low vision. *Journal of Rehabilitation, 87*(2), 28–35.

Falvo, D. R. (2019). *Medical and psychosocial aspects of chronic illness and disability.* Jones & Barnett Learning.

Farrell, A., & Krahn, G. (2014). Family life goes on: Disabilities in contemporary families. *Family Relations, 63*(1), 1–6.

Fireison, C., & Moore, J. (1998). Employment outcomes and educational backgrounds of legally blind adults employed in sheltered industrial settings. *Journal of Visual Impairment and Blindness, 92*(11). 740–747.

Flaxman, A. D., Wittenborn, J. S., Robalik, T., Gerzoff, R. B., Lundeen, E. A., Saaddine, J., & Rein, D. B. (2021). Prevalence of visual acuity loss or blindness in the US: A Bayesian Metameta-analysis. *JAMA Ophthalmology, 139*(7), 717–723. https://doi.org/10.1001/jamaophthalmol.2021.0527

Foundation Fighting Blindness. (2022). *Low vision resources.* https://www.fightingblindness.org/low-vision

Gibson, J., Pousson, J. M., & Laux, S. (2018). Disability identity development in people who have low vision or are blind. *Journal of Education and Human Development, 7*(3), 18–27. http://jehdnet.com/journals/jehd/Vol_7_No_3_September_2018/3.pdf

Giles, S. J., Panagioti, M., Riste, L, Cheraghi-Sohi, S., Lewis, P., Adeyemi, I., Davies, K., Morris, R., Phipps, D., Dickenson, C., Ashcroft, D., & Sanders, C. (2021). Visual impairment and medication safety: A protocol for a scoping review. *Systematic Reviews, 10*(1), 1–6. https://doi.org/10.1186/s13643-021-01800-8

Guide Dogs for the Blind. (2022). *Programs for the blind and visually impaired.* https://www.guidedogs.com/get-a-guide-dog/programs-for-the-blind-and-visually-impaired

Guide Dogs of America. (2022). *Our program overview.* https://www.guidedogsofamerica.org/service-dog-information/

Guiding Eyes for the Blind. (2022). Who we are. https://www.guidingeyes.org/who-we-are/https://www.guidingeyes.org/who-we-are/

Helen Keller National Center for DeafBlind Youths & Adults. (2022). *Helen Keller National Center for DeafBlind Youths & Adults.* https://www.helenkeller.org/hknc

Helvin, S. R., & Sutton, A. M. (2011). Life care planning for the visually impaired child. In S. Riddick-Grisham and & L. M. Deming (Eds.), *Pediatric life care planning and case management* (2nd ed.), pp. 696–714). CRC Press.

Hull University Teaching Hospitals. (2020). *Adapting to monocular vision (using the sight of one eye only).* https://www.hey.nhs.uk/patient-leaflet/adapting-to-monocular-vision-using-the-sight-from-one-eye-only/

Jones, N., Bartlett, H. E., & Cook, R. (2019). An analysis of the impact of visual impairment on activities of daily living and vision-related quality of life in a visually impaired adult population. *British Journal of Visual Impairment, 37*(1), 50–63. https://doi.org/10.1177/0264619618814071

Keel, S., Evans, J. R., Block, S., Bourne, R., Calonge, M., Chan, C., & Friedman, D. S. (2020). Strengthening the integration of eye care into the health system: Methodology for the development of the WHO package of eye care interventions. *BMJ Open Ophthalmology, 5,* e000533. https://bmjophth.bmj.com/content/5/1/e000533

Kirtland, K. A., Saaddine, J. B., & Geiss, Thompson, T. J., Cotch, M. F., & Lee, P. P. (2015, May 22). Geographic disparity of severe vision loss – United States, 2009–2013. *Morbidity and Mortality Weekly Report.* http://www.cdc.gov/mmwr/preview/mmwrhtml/mm6419a2.htm

Kroezen, M., van den Akker, N., van Genderen, M. M., & Wolkorte, R. (2020). Visual impairment and blindness in people with intellectual disabilities: A systematic review. *Optometry & Visual Performance, 8*(3), 109–121.

Lingham, G., Thakur, S., & Safi, S., Gordon, I., Evans, J. R., & Keel, S. (2022). A systematic review of clinical practice guidelines for childhood glaucoma. *BMJ open ophthalmology, 7*(1), e000933. https://doi.org/10.1136/bmjophth-2021-000933

Lockley, S. W., Dressman, M. A., Licamele, L., Xiao, C., Fisher, D. M., Flynn-Evans, E. E., Hull, J. T., Torres, R., Lavedan, C., & Polymeropoulos, M. H. (2015). Tasimelteon for non-24-hour sleep-wake disorder in totally blind people (SET and RESET): Two multicentre, randomised, double-masked, placebo-controlled phase 3 trials. *Lancet, 386*(10005),1754–1764. https://doi.org/10.1016/S0140-6736(15)60031-9

Madison, W., Bullins, S., & Wilkins, M. J. (2017). Assistive technology in the life care plan. *Journal of Life Care Planning, 15*(1), 9–12.

Manduchi, R., & Kurniawan, S. (2013). *Assistive technology for blindness and low vision.* CRC Press.

McCarron-Dial Systems. (n. d.). *CVES Comprehensive Vocational Evaluation System.* www.mccarrondial.com/CVESInfo.pdf

McDonnall, M. C., & Sui, Z. (2019). Employment and unemployment rates of people who are blind or visually impaired: Estimates from multiple sources. *Journal of Visual Impairment & Blindness, 113*(6), 481–492. https://doi.org/10.1177/0145482X19887620

McDonnall, M., Cmar, J., & McKnight, Z. S. (2022). Beyond employment rates; Full-time vs. part-time employment for people with visual impairments. *Journal of Visual Impairment and Blindness, 116*(1), 7–13. https://doi.org/10.1177/0145482X211072485

McKnight, Z. S., Crudden, A., & McDonnall, M. C. (2021). Personal characteristics associated with working after disability onset for people with visual impairments. *Journal of Visual Impairment and Blindness, 115*(2), 95–105. https://doi.org/10.1177/0145482X211000960

Mississippi State University. (2022). *National Research and Training Center on Blindness and Low Vision.* https://www.blind.msstate.edu/

Miyauchi, H. (2020). A systematic review on inclusive education of student with visual impairment. *Education Sciences, 10,* 1–15. https://doi.org/10.3390/educsci10110346

Miyauchi, H., & Paul, P. V. (2020). Perceptions of students with visual impairment on inclusive education: A narrative meta-analysis. *Human Research and Rehabilitation, 10*(2), 4–25. https://doi.org/10.21554/hrr.092001

Moschos, M. M. (2014). Physiology and psychology of vision and its disorders: A Review. *Medical Hypothesis, Discovery and Innovation Ophthalmology Journal, 3*(3), 83–90.

Mukamal, R. (2020). *Thirty apps, devices, and technology for people with vision impairments.* American Academy of Ophthalmology. https://www.aao.org/eye-health/tips-prevention/low-vision-impairment-apps-tech-assistive-devices

National Eye Institute. (2022a). *Glaucoma.* Eye conditions and diseases. https://www.nei.nih.gov/learn-about-eye-health/eye-conditions-and-diseases/glaucoma

National Eye Institute. (2022b). *Retinitis pigmentosa. eye conditions and diseases.* https://www.nei.nih.gov/learn-about-eye-health/eye-conditions-and-diseases/retinitis-pigmentosa

National Federation of the Blind. (2022a). *Blindness statistics.* https://nfb.org/blindness-statistics

National Federation of the Blind. (2022b). *Welcome to the movement.* https://nfb.org/

National Institute for Occupational Safety and Health. (n. d.). *Eye and face protection.* https://www.osha.gov/eye-face-protection

Natstasi, J. A. (2020). Occupational therapy interventions supporting leisure and social participation to older adults with low vision: A systematic review. *American Journal of Occupational Therapy, 74*(1), 1–9.

Prevent Blindness America. (2022). *Prevalence of vision loss.* https://preventblindness.org/prevalence-visual-acuity-loss-blindness-us

Reid, C. A., & Bullins, S. M. (2021). Sensory disabilities, functional limitations, and the role of technology. In Harley, D. A. & Flaherty, C. (Eds.), *Principles and practices of disability studies: An interdisciplinary approach* (pp. 325–346). Springer.

Reid, C., & Riddick-Grisham, S. (2015). The importance of work or productive activity in life care planning. *NeuroRehabilitation, 36*, 267–274.

Robert, H., & Adele, C. (1999). Innovative links to employment through industries for the blind. *Journal of Vocational Rehabilitation, 12*(1), 9-18.

Schakel, W., Bode, C., Elsman, E. B. M., van der Aa, H. P. A., de Vries, R., van Rens, G .H. M. B., & van Nispen, R. M. A. (2019). The association between visual impairment and fatigue: A systematic review and meta-analysis of observational studies. *Ophthalmic & Physiological Optics, 39*(6), 399–413.

Shahid, K. S., & Wilkinson, M. E. (2020). Evaluation and management consideration for children who are visually impaired. *Saudi Journal of Ophthalmology, 34*(2), 124–128. https://pubmed.ncbi.nlm.nih.gov/33575535/

Smallfield, S., & Kaldenberg, J. (2020). Occupational therapy interventions for older adults with low vision. *The American Journal of Occupational Therapy, 74*(2), 740239001p1-7402390010p5.

Social Security Administration. (2022). If you're blind or have low vision: How we can help. https://www.ssa.gov/pubs/EN-05-10052.pdf

Sorokowska, A., Sorokowski, P., Karwowski, M., Larsson, M., & Hummel, T. (2019). Olfactory perception and blindness: A systematic review and meta-analysis. *Psychological Research, 83*, 1595–1611. https://doi.org/10.1007/s00426-018-1035-2

Stevelink, S. A. M., & Fear, N. T. (2016). Psychosocial impact of visual impairment and coping strategies in female ex-service personnel. *Journal of the Royal Army Medical Corps, 162*(2), 129. https://doi.org/10.1136/jramc-2015-000518

Stevelink, S. A. M., Malcolm, E. M., & Fear, N. T. (2015). Visual impairment, coping strategies, and impact on daily life: A qualitative study among working-age UK ex-service personnel. *BMC Public Health, 15*, 1118. https://doi.org/10.1186/s12889-015-2455-1

Surakka, A., Venojarvi, M., & Pitkanen, K. (2016). Beneficial effects of regular exercises on mental state in visually impaired and deaf-blind adults. *Universal Journal of Psychology, 4*(1), 43–46. https://doi.org/10.13189/ujp.2016.040104

Swain, T., & McGwin, Jr., G. (2020). The prevalence of eye injury in the United States - Estimates from a meta-analysis. *Ophthalmic Epidemiology, 27*(3), 186–193.

Takano, K., Kaizaki, A., Saikawa, E., Konnno, A., Ogawawara, N., & Him, T. (2016). Outcomes of visually impaired patients who received cochlear implantations. *Auris Nasus Larynx, 43*(3), 242–246.

Terbert, D. (2020). Childhood eye diseases and conditions. American Academy of Ophthalmology. https://www.aao.org/eye-health/tips-prevention/common-childhood-diseases-conditions

Unger, D. D., Rumrill Jr., P. D., & Hennessey, M. L. (2005). Resolutions of the ADA Title I cases involving people who are visually impaired: A comparative analysis. *Journal of Visual Impairment & Blindness, 99*(8), 453–463.

Van der Ham, A. J., van der Aa, H. P. A., Brunes, A., Heir, T., de Vries, R., van Rens, G. H. M. B., & van Nispen, R. M. A. (2021). The development of posttraumatic stress disorder in individuals with visual impairment: A systematic search and review. *Ophthalmic & Physiological Optics, 41*(2), 331–341.

Vermont Association for the Blind and Visually Impaired. (2022). Five leading causes of visual impairments in children in the USA. https://www.vabvi.org/five-leading-causes-of-visual-impairments-in-children-in-the-usa

Vervloed, M. P. J., van den Broek, E. C. G., & van Eikden, A. J. P. M. (2020). Critical review of setback in development in young children with congenital blindness or visual impairment. *International Journal of Disability, Development & Education, 67*(3), 336–355.

Victor, C. M., Thacker, L. R., Gary, K. W., Pawluk, D. T. V., & Copollilo, A. (2017). Workplace discrimination and visual impairment: A comparison of Equal Employment Opportunity Commission charges and resolutions under the Americans with Disabilities Act and Americans with Disabilities Amendments Act. *Journal of Visual Impairment & Blindness, 111*(5), 475–482. https://doi.org/10.1177/0145482X1711100509

Vision Loss Expert Group of the Global Burden of Disease Study. (2020). Trends in prevalence of blindness and distance and near vision impairment over 30 years: An analysis for the Global Burden of Disease Study. *Lancet Global Health*, *9*(2), e130–e143. https://doi.org/10.1016/S2214-109X(20)30425-3

Weed, R. O., & Wilkins, R. (2018). Life care planning for the visually impaired. In R. O. Weed and & D. E. Berens (Eds.), *Life care planning and case management handbook* (4th ed., pp. 571–590). Routledge.

World Health Organization. (2019). *World report on vision*. Geneva, Author. www.who.int/publications/i/item/9789241516570

World Health Organization. (2021). *Blindness and vision impairment*. Geneva, Author. www.who.int/news-room/fact-sheets/detail/blindness-and-visual-impairment

World Services for the Blind. (n.d.). https://www.wsblind.org/

Yarali, M., Ozkan, J. B., Cinar, B., Merve, B., Arslan, F., Sennaroglu, G., Yucel, E., Atay, G., Bajin, D., & Sennaroglu, L. (2015). Bilateral sequential cochlear implantation in an adult with bilateral blindness. *Journal of International Advanced Otology*, *11*, 4.

Zapata, M. A. (2022). Group identity in blindness groups predicts life satisfaction and lower anxiety and depression. *Journal of Rehabilitation Psychology*, *67*(1), 42–52. https://doi.org/10.1037/rep0000432

Zhi-Han L., Hui-Yin Y., & Makmor-Bakry, M. (2017). Medication-handling challenges among visually impaired population. *Archives of Pharmacy Practice*, *8*(1), 8–14.

Zuckerman, D. M. (2004). *2004 blind adults in America: Their lives and challenges*. Washington, DC: National Center for Policy Research for Women & Families. https://www.center4research.org/blind-adults-america-lives-challenges/

Chapter 26

Life Care Planning for the Patient with a Brachial Plexus Injury

Scott H. Kozin and Mona Goldman Yudkoff

Life Care Planning for the Patient with a Brachial Plexus Injury

Neonatal brachial plexus palsy (a.k.a. obstetrical brachial plexus palsy) occurs with an incidence of 1–2 per 1,000 live births (Bager, 1997; Foad et al., 2008; Gilbert et al., 1999). In comparison, adult brachial plexus injuries have an annual incidence of 1–2 per 100,000 with an increased incidence in countries that rely on motorbikes or motorcycles for transportation (Cho et al., 2020). The incidence of neonatal brachial plexus palsy may be declining related to an increase in the rate of cesarean delivery and systemic changes in obstetric practice related to training/education (DeFrancesco et al., 2019; Draycott et al., 2008,). A considerable number of infants with brachial plexus palsy spontaneously recover in the first two months of life and subsequently progress to near-complete recovery of motion and strength (Greenwald et al., 1984; Sjoberg et al., 1988). However, those infants who do not have substantial recovery by three months of age will have a permanently limited range of motion, less strength, and a decrease in size and girth of the involved extremity. Currently, there continues to be debate about the timing and type of surgical intervention(s). The purpose of this chapter is to provide information regarding anatomy, epidemiology, diagnosis, classification schemes, and treatment options for neonatal brachial plexus palsy. This knowledge is necessary to formulate an appropriate life care plan.

Anatomy

The brachial plexus is formed by the C5–T1 (C5, C6, C7, C8, and T1) nerve roots and provides the basis for all sensibility (a.k.a. sensation) and function of the upper extremity (Kozin, 2014). The brachial plexus is subdivided into roots originating from their respective spinal level, trunks where the roots combine, divisions where the trunks divide into anterior and posterior parts, cords that

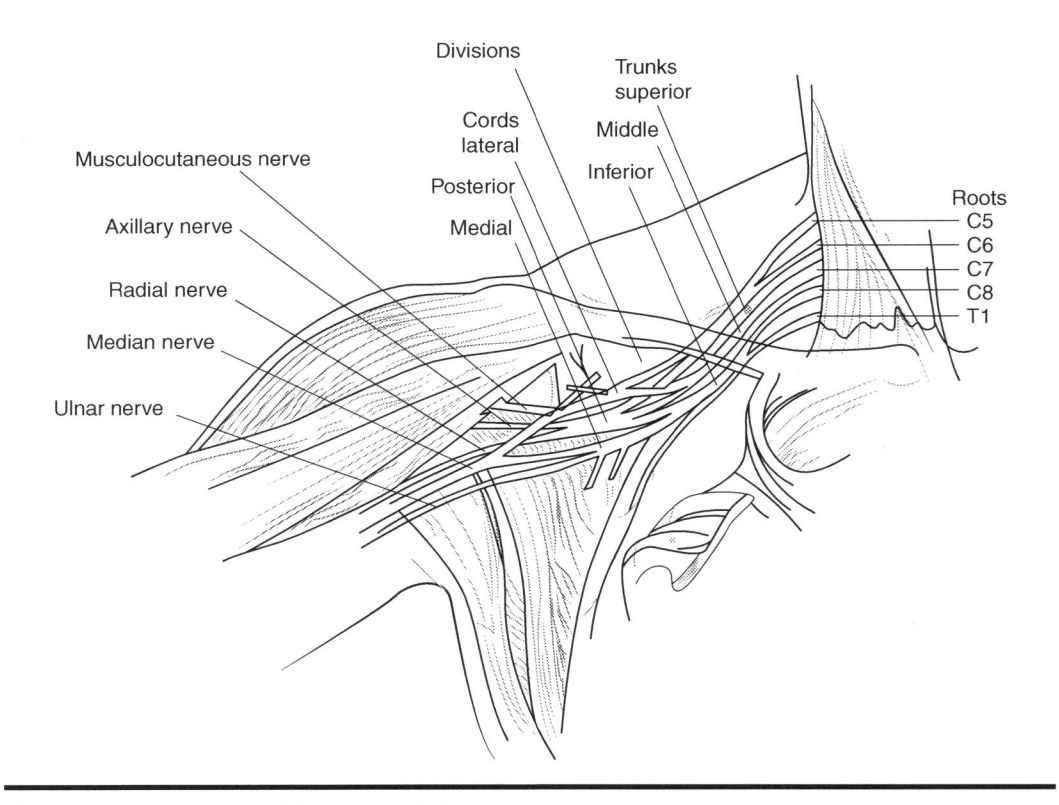

Figure 26.1 Anatomy of the Brachial Plexus

Source: (From Kozin, S. H. (2007). Injuries of the brachial plexus. In J. P. Iannotti & G. R. Williams, Eds., Disorders of the shoulder: Diagnosis and management (2nd ed., pp. 1087–1134). Lippincott Williams & Wilkins. With permission.)

represent combinations of the divisions, and last, branches that proceed into peripheral nerves. In addition, various peripheral nerve branches emanate along the way as the plexus proceeds from its nerve roots to its terminal peripheral nerves (Figure 26.1).

The C5 and C6 nerve roots combine to form the upper trunk, whereas the C8 and T1 nerve roots combine to form the lower trunk. The middle trunk is a continuation of C7. Subsequently, each trunk will divide into anterior and posterior divisions behind the clavicle. All three posterior divisions combine to form the posterior cord. The anterior divisions of the upper and middle trunk combine to form the lateral cord, whereas the anterior division of the lower trunk forms the medial cord.

The terminal branches form the major nerves to the upper extremity. Specifically, the ulnar nerve arises from the medial cord, the radial and axillary nerves arise from the posterior cord, the musculocutaneous nerve arises from the lateral cord, and the median nerve arises from a combination of the medial and lateral cords. Figure 26.1 shows the anatomy of the brachial plexus.

The phrenic nerve and the spinal accessory nerve are located in close proximity. The phrenic nerve receives innervation from the C3, C4, and C5 cervical roots. Injury to the phrenic nerve can occur during birth or at the time of surgery. Breathing and/or feeding difficulties may be present and require additional life care planning considerations. The spinal accessory nerve is cranial nerve XI and innervates the trapezius muscle yielding shoulder shrugging. This nerve is rarely injured during birth, but a portion of the nerve can be used during surgical reconstruction of the damaged plexus.

Epidemiology and Etiology

Birth-related brachial plexus palsies occur secondary to stretching of the nerve roots as they exit the spinal cord. In vertex deliveries, the stretching begins along the upper trunk (C5 and C6 nerve roots). A slight stretch will injure the myelin sheath that surrounds the nerve roots. This neurapraxia prohibits nerve conduction but the myelin will regenerate over six to eight weeks leading to complete recovery. A moderate stretch will cause myelin injury and additional damage to the axons within the upper trunk (axonotmesis). The axons can regenerate but at a slow rate of 1 mm/day or 1 inch/month). This slow process results in delayed recovery beginning between two and six months of age. This recovery is often incomplete with some residual loss of motion and permanent impairment. A severe stretch will tear the nerve (neurotmesis). The nerve can either tear in mid-substance (rupture) or pull directly from the spinal cord (avulsion). Complete tears will not recover and require surgical intervention. The ruptured nerve ends will fill with scarring (neuroma). Repair requires neuroma resection and nerve grafting to reconnect the nerve roots and distal nerve targets. Avulsions do not form neuromas and cannot be reconnected to the spinal cord. Reconstruction requires surgical reconnection to nerve roots that have been ruptured. For example, connecting a ruptured C5 nerve root to an avulsed lower trunk (C8 and T1 nerve roots) requires cortical neural plasticity as the C5 nerve will control hand function instead of shoulder function. This plasticity is readily available in the infant.

Major risk factors for brachial plexus birth palsies include fetal macrosomia, shoulder dystocia, and gestational diabetes. Additional risk factors include an instrumented delivery (vacuum or forceps), prolonged labor, and multiparity (Foad et al., 2008; Sibinski & Synder, 2007; Van Ouwekerk et al., 2000; Waters, 1997). Cesarean birth reduces the risk of brachial plexus palsy (100 fold) but does not eliminate it entirely (Sibinski & Synder, 2007). Fetal distress may contribute to relative hypotonia, making the infant and plexus more susceptible to stretch during delivery (Gurewitsch et al., 2006). These injuries tend to be transient without permanent sequelae.

Numerous etiologies of adult brachial plexus injuries exist (Kozin, 2014). The most common causes being vehicular trauma (especially motorcycle), athletic endeavors, domestic violence, and systemic disease. These etiologies can be divided into trauma (penetrating and nonpenetrating), entrapment, and infection (Table 26.1). There are other less common etiologies of brachial plexopathy related to tumors, neuropathies (e.g., Parsonage-Turner syndrome), and iatrogenic causes.

Patterns of Brachial Plexus Birth Palsies

The most common pattern (about 60%) of neonatal brachial plexus palsy involves the upper trunk (C5 and C6 nerve roots) and is known as an Erb's palsy (Tables 26.2 and 26.3) (Kozin, 2014). Additionally, the C7 root may also be involved, and this pattern is known as an extended Erb's palsy, which appears in approximately 20%–30% of cases Occasionally (~15%–20%), the entire plexus from C5 to T1 is injured, and this pattern is known as a pan-plexus, total, or global brachial plexus palsy. An isolated lower trunk injury to C8 and T1 nerve roots is extremely rare and is known as Klumpke palsy (Gilbert & Whitaker, 1991).

Table 26.1 Etiology of Brachial Plexus Injuries

Trauma
Nonpenetrating (traction)
Penetrating (knife, gunshot wound)
Nerve entrapment
Thoracic outlet syndrome
Infection
Viral plexopathy (Neuralgic amyotrophy or Parsonage-Turner syndrome)
Radiation
Fibrosis
Malignant degeneration after radiation
Tumors
Primary (schwannomas or neurofibromas)
Secondary (pulmonary apices)
Neuropathies
Iatrogenic
Axillary or scalene anesthesia
Surgical biopsy
Intraoperative positioning
Median sternotomy
Inadvertent traction

Table 26.2 Patterns of Brachial Plexus Injuries

Pattern	Nerve Roots Involved	Primary Deficiency
Erb–Duchenne lesion	C5 and C6	Shoulder abduction and external rotation
Upper brachial plexus		Elbow flexion
Extended Erb's lesion	C5 through C7	Above plus
Upper and middle plexus		Elbow and finger extension
Dejerine–Klumpke lesion	C8 and T1	Hand intrinsic muscles
Lower brachial plexus		Finger flexors
Total or global lesion	C5 through T1	Entire extremity
Entire brachial plexus		

Table 26.3 Practical Anatomy for Brachial Plexus Injury Pattern

Trunk (Roots)	Muscles	Sensation
Erb–Duchenne lesion Upper Trunk (C5 & C6)	Shoulder (rotator cuff and deltoid) Forearm supination (biceps & supinator) Elbow flexion (biceps & brachialis) Wrist extension (extensor carpi radialis longus)	Median nerve sensibility thumb & index finger
Extended Erb's lesion Middle Trunk (C7)	Elbow extension (triceps) Latissimus dorsi Forearm pronation (pronator teres) Wrist extension (extensor carpi radialis longus) Digital extension (MCP joints) Wrist flexion (flexor carpi radialis)	Median nerve sensibility long finger
Total or global lesion Lower Trunk (C8 & T1)	Forearm pronation (pronator quadratus) Extrinsic finger and thumb flexors (flexor digitorum profundus and flexor pollicis longus) Wrist flexion (flexor carpi ulnaris) Digital extension (IP joints) Intrinsic muscles	Ulnar nerve sensibility (ring and small fingers)

The prognosis following neonatal brachial plexus palsy is directly related to the number of roots injured. An isolated Erb's palsy has the best prognosis for spontaneous recovery and is associated with the least impairment. In contrast, a global palsy has the worst prognosis for spontaneous recovery and is associated with the greatest impairment. Children with global palsies require the most surgery, the largest amount of therapy, and the greatest assistance in their life care plan.

Diagnosis

The diagnosis of neonatal brachial plexus palsy is usually made shortly after birth by lack of arm movement. The physical examination of infants is more difficult because of their lack of cooperation and inability to follow commands. Extreme patience, diligence, and repeated examinations are required to obtain an adequate evaluation. Tactile stimulation is used to illicit movement. A variety of toys, props, and games are used to accomplish the examination (Figure 26.2). The goal is to determine the type and extent of injury. Practical anatomy is used to formulate the diagnosis regarding the number of nerve roots injured.

Primitive infant reflexes are often used to detect deficits in motion. For example, the Moro reflex is elicited by introducing a sudden extension of the neck, which subsequently causes abduction of the shoulders, extension of the elbows, and extension of the digits. An asymmetric response implies deficits in arm movement that may be related to a birth palsy. The palmar grasp reflex is also

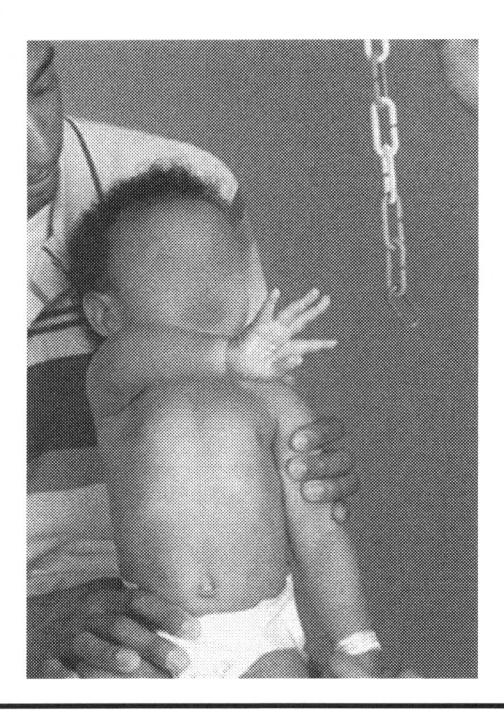

Figure 26.2 A Variety of Toys, Props, and Games Are Used to Examine Children

Source: (Courtesy of Shriners Hospital for Children, Philadelphia, PA.). Reprinted with permission.

useful. Placing a finger in the palm will provoke a reflexive palmar grasp reflex that lasts until about 5–6 months of age and is a reliable test for finger and thumb flexion indicative of a functioning lower trunk (C8 and T1 nerve roots).

The physician must assess for the presence or absence of Horner's syndrome (ptosis, meiosis, and anhidrosis), which indicates an avulsion injury to the lower roots (C8 and T1) and carries a poor prognosis (Gilbert & Whitaker, 1991; Michelow et al., 1994). Strength and sensibility assessments are impossible to determine in infants (and difficult in children) as they are unable to follow instructions for the assessment. Pain may be the only sensation that elicits a response.

The skilled therapist is very helpful during the initial examination as they have expertise in age-appropriate mobility and/or functional tasks coupled with consideration of developmental issues. The therapist can also administer an age-appropriate outcome measurement (e.g., Active Movement Scale, Toronto score, and Mallet classification) (Table 26.2 and Figure 26.3) (Abzug et al., 2010; Curtis et al., 2002). Last, the therapist can institute proper stretching exercises and provide an educational resource to the parents or caregivers (Figure 26.4).

Adolescents and adults with brachial plexus injuries are easier to examine. As long as the patient is compliant, specific manual muscle testing (MMT) can be performed and graded (Table 26.4) (Kozin, 2014). An inventory of the muscles innervated by the brachial plexus is imperative to accurately define the injury and provides a baseline to assess recovery. Sensibility is assessed using two-point discrimination or Semmes-Weinstein monofilament testing.

Modified mallet classification (grade I = no function, Grade V = normal function)						
	Grade I	Grade II	Grade III	Grade IV	Grade V
Global abduction	Not testable	No function	<30°	30° to 90°	>90°	Normal
Global external rotation	Not testable	No function	<0°	0° to 20°	>20°	Normal
Hand to neck	Not testable	No function	Not possible	Difficult	Easy	Normal
Hand on spine	Not testable	No function	Not possible	S1	T12	Normal
Hand to mouth	Not testable	No function	Marked trumpet sign	Partial trumpet sign	<40° of abduction	Normal
Internal rotation	Not testable	No function	Cannot touch	Can touch with wrist flexion	Palm on belly, no wrist flexion	

Figure 26.3 Modified Mallet Classification for Shoulder Motion

Source: (Adapted from Abzug, J. M. et al. (2009). Journal Pediatric Orthopaedics; Courtesy of Shriners Hospital for Children, Philadelphia, PA)

Early Rehabilitation of Brachial Plexus Injuries

Early intervention and therapy are medically necessary to maintain supple joint motion and to prevent the development of contractures. Therapy must be performed on a regular basis to avoid contractures about the shoulder, elbow, forearm, wrist, and digits. Conservative management is beneficial for preventing muscle tightness and subsequent joint contracture when further neurological recovery is anticipated. Intervention includes active and passive range of motion, strengthening, splinting, kinesiotaping, electrical stimulation, muscle/sensory re-education, and adaptive functional training.

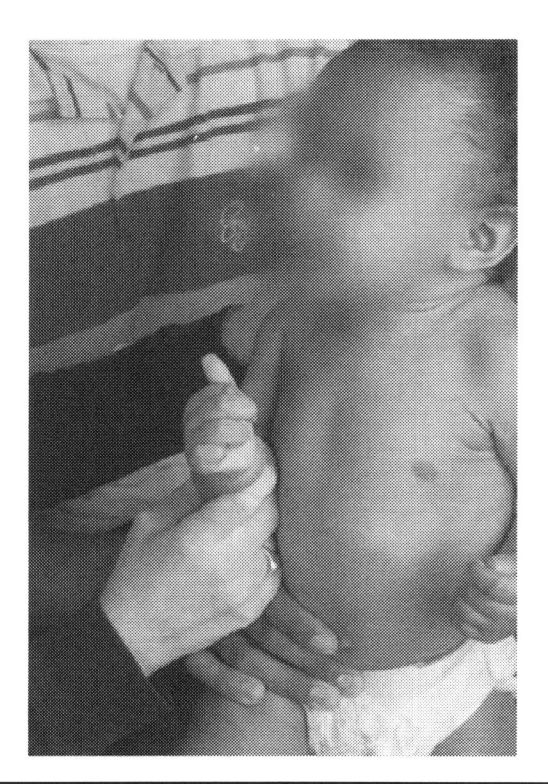

Figure 26.4 Proper Stretching Exercises Are Necessary to Prevent Joint Contracture

Source: (Courtesy of Shriners Hospital for Children, Philadelphia, PA.)

Table 26.4   Muscle Grading Chart

Muscle grade	Description
5, Normal	Full range of motion against gravity with full resistance
4, Good	Full range of motion against gravity with some resistance
3, Fair	Full range of motion against gravity
2, Poor	Full range of motion with gravity eliminated
1, Trace	Slight contraction without joint motion
0, Zero	No evidence of contraction

The use of electrical stimulation in the rehabilitation process is controversial. A variety of different forms of stimulation have been tried including neuromuscular stimulation (NMS), electrical muscle stimulation (EMS), and therapeutic electrical stimulation (TES). The theoretical goal is to stimulate nerves and muscles to produce analgesia, increase dormant motion, enhance bone growth, and improve circulation. However, the ability to obtain these goals is questionable. Currently, electrical stimulation is prescribed in certain centers and not used in other institutions.

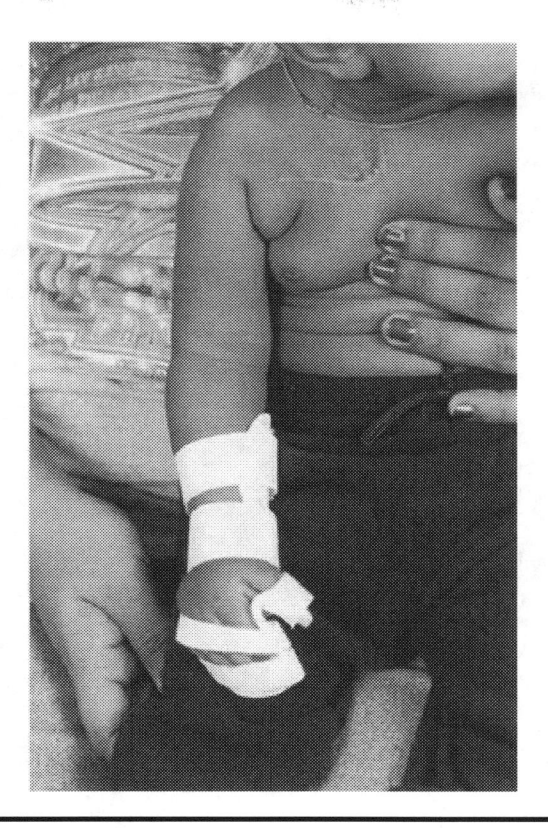

Figure 26.5A Fabricated Splint to Place the Arm Hand in a More Functional Position

The physician or therapists may recommend a splint for a variety of reasons. A splint may be requested to prevent or resolve a joint contracture. A splint may also place the arm/hand in a more functional position (Figure 26.5A). Lastly, the splint may be used as protection as a small percentage of children bite or self-mutilate their hands. The splint must be carefully fabricated for optimum fit without skin irritation or breakdown.

Ancillary Diagnostic Studies

Ancillary studies include X-rays of the affected limb to rule out a fracture causing a pseudo paralysis secondary to pain. Additional ancillary testing that may be helpful include imaging modalities and electrodiagnostic testing. Imaging studies include ultrasound, magnetic resonance imaging (MRI), and computerized tomography (CT) myelography. Ultrasound and MRI cannot discriminate between a neuroma-in-continuity (axonotmesis) that will recover versus a neuroma-in-discontinuity (neurotmesis) that will not recover. MRI or CT myelography may be useful in brachial plexus injuries, specifically for assessment of nerve root avulsion when the nerve root is pulled from the spinal cord. Following the nerve root avulsion, a meningeal pouch filled with cerebrospinal fluid (pseudomeningocele) forms outside the intervertebral foramen. CT myelography and MRI can visualize these pseudomeningoceles (Figure 26.5B). However, there are false-positive and false-negative results with both imaging modalities. More advanced techniques are under

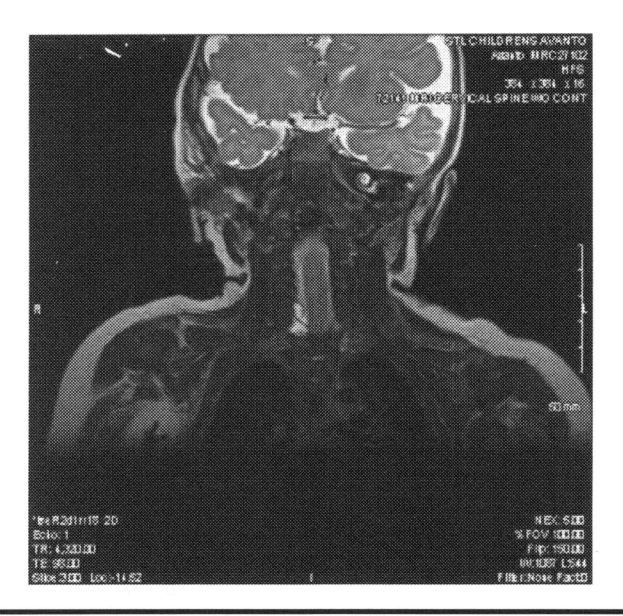

Figure 26.5B MRI with Meningeal Pouch Filled with Cerebrospinal Fluid (pseudomeningocele) outside the intervertebral foramen indicative of right sided nerve root avulsion

development to improve diagnostic accuracy, but their validity remains to be established. Magnetic resonance imaging currently offers the best evaluation of the brachial plexus trunks and cords with potential identification of a neuroma and/or nerve root avulsion (Kawai et al., 1989).

The use of electrodiagnostic studies including nerve conduction velocities and electromyography is also controversial. The lack of infant cooperation also confounds the interpretation. In general, electrodiagnostic studies tend to overestimate subsequent clinical recovery and should be interpreted with caution (Heise et al., 2007).

Electrodiagnostic studies are more useful in adolescents and adults with brachial plexus injury (Campion, 1996). Avulsion injuries separate the motor cell body in the spinal cord from its axons. In contrast, the sensory cell body is located in the dorsal root ganglion and remains connected to its axons. Therefore, the motor portion of the nerve undergoes wallerian degeneration, with degradation of the axons and myelin sheaths. In contrast, the sensory fibers are spared from wallerian degeneration but have been irrevocably detached from the spinal cord. The injury will cause clinical motor and sensory loss; however, electrodiagnostic studies will reveal abnormal motor findings with intact sensory conduction. In other words, the dorsal root is still functioning and is unaware that it is disconnected from the spinal cord. In addition, the adolescent or adult can comply with the electromyography (EMG) portion of the examination.

Potential Problems from Brachial Plexus Injury
Musculoskeletal

- Contractures can occur at the shoulder, elbow, and forearm due to overall muscle imbalance in the affected upper extremity.
- Joint subluxation of the humeral head can occur about the shoulder and of the radial head at the elbow.

Table 26.5 Active Movement Scale and Toronto Score

Active Movement Scale (AMS)			
Shoulder abduction	_____	*Gravity Eliminated*	*Score*
Shoulder adduction	_____	No contraction	0
Shoulder flexion	_____	Contraction, no motion	1
Shoulder external rotation	_____	<50% motion	2
Shoulder internal rotation	_____	>50% motion	3
Elbow flexion	_____	Full motion	4
Elbow extension	_____	*Against gravity*	5
Forearm supination	_____	<50% motion	6
Forearm pronation	_____	>50% motion	7
Wrist flexion	_____	Full motion	
Wrist extension	_____		
Finger flexion	_____		
Finger extension	_____		
Thumb flexion	_____		
Thumb extension	_____		
Total	_____		
Toronto Score			
Elbow flexion (0–2)		_____	
Elbow extension (0–2)		_____	
Wrist extension (0–2)		_____	
Finger extension (0–2)		_____	
Thumb extension (0–2)		_____	
Total			
Table for Scoring Toronto (All Movement Scored against Gravity)			
		Grade	Weight
No joint movement		0	0.0
Flicker		0+	0.3
<50% ROM		1–	0.6
=50%		1	1.0
>50% ROM		1+	1.3
Good but not full		2–	1.6
Full ROM		2	2.0

Source: Adapted from Curtis, C. et al., 2002, *Journal of Hand Surgery*, 27, 470.

- Compensatory winging of the scapula is usually observed due to altered kinematics of the glenohumeral joint and/or the weakness of the shoulder girdle musculature.
- Shortening of the affected arm is common and varies between 8% and 20%, proportional to the magnitude of the injury.

Sensory

- Self-mutilating or biting the arm (about 4%–5%) has been reported in children with brachial plexus injury.
- Persistent sensory deficits can occur in the arm or the hand, resulting in poor hand coordination and dexterity. The risk of injury is increased as some individuals are not able to feel pain when they are hurt (e.g., sustaining a burn on the hand).
- Persistent pain, relatively uncommon in brachial plexus birth palsy, affects 4%–5% of individuals.

Posture/Gait

- Awkward posturing of the affected arm occurs secondary to muscle imbalance and joint contracture.
- Altered swing phase during running occurs when the affected arm does not swing as much as the unaffected arm.

Psychological Issues

- Psychological problems are more than likely to emerge when the child starts to go to school and spends time with his or her age cohort. Even with good family support, a child can experience body image or self-concept problems (Louden et al., 2015).
- Psychological support services should be included in the life care plan.

Vocational Issues

- Individuals with physical deficits in the affected arm have vocational limitations.
- A vocational expert with experience in brachial plexus injuries is invaluable during the formation of a life care plan.
- A functional capacity can provide additional information on the adult patient population.

Surgical Intervention

Surgery is divided into two types: primary nerve surgery and secondary reconstructive procedures. The basic tenets will be discussed in this chapter, but the specific procedure is invariably dependent upon the child's injury pattern, surgeon philosophy, extent of recovery, and status of the underlying joints.

Clinical practice guidelines have been published using Canadian key opinion leaders (Coroneos et al., 2017). A modified Delphi approach was used to gain consensus from the opinion leaders. The guidelines discuss a variety of issues surrounding brachial plexus birth palsies. With reference to microsurgery, the guidelines state that microsurgery shoulder be offered for injuries consistent with root avulsion and for all injuries meeting center-defined operative criteria beginning at 3 months of age. There have not been similar guidelines formulated in the United States.

Life Care Planning for the Patient with a Brachial Plexus Injury ■ 749

Primary Nerve Surgery

Primary nerve surgery is performed on children who fail to considerably recover within the first few months of life. Generally, nerve reconstruction is performed between 3 and 8 months of age depending on the injury (Kozin, 2014). Earlier nerve surgery is performed for global injuries to allow ample time for nerve regeneration into the hand. A nerve torn outside the spinal cord is called an extraforaminal rupture or a postganglionic injury. This type of injury is usually reconstructed by first removing the scar (neuroma) that has formed between the nerve ends. The subsequent gap is bridged with nerve grafts harvested from the leg or legs depending upon the amount of graft needed (Figure 26.6).

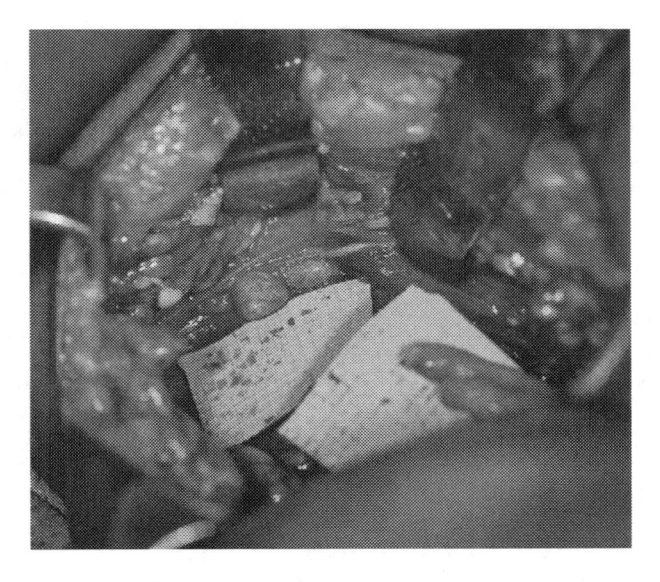

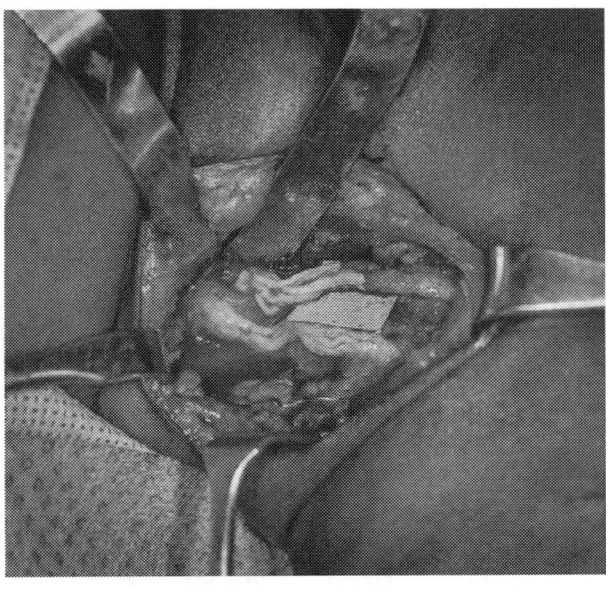

Figure 26.6 Five-Month-Old Female Child with Right Global Brachial Plexus Injury

A nerve torn directly from the spinal cord is known as an avulsion injury. Currently, there is no reliable technique to re-attach the nerve into the spinal cord. Therefore, alternative measures are necessary to reconstruct these damaged nerve segments. Nerve grafts can be placed from a ruptured segment to an avulsed nerve to provide nerve inflow. Another surgical option involves transferring part of a working nerve into the damaged segment (a.k.a. nerve transfer) (Figures 26.8 and 26.9) (Kozin, 2008). Examples include the spinal accessory nerve and/or the intercostal nerves. In extreme avulsion cases, nerves are passed from the uninjured contralateral brachial plexus (contralateral C7 nerve transfer) to the injured plexus (Vu et al., 2018).

Most primary surgeries use a combination of nerve grafting and nerve transfers to optimize outcome after nerve reconstruction. As stated earlier, the ultimate choice of nerve reconstruction is multifactorial and is often determined during the surgical procedure. Potential current procedural terminology (CPT) codes include microsurgical neurolysis (64713 and 64727), neuroma resection (64784), and nerve grafting and transfer (64885, 64886, 64901, and 64905).

Following primary surgery, the infant's head, neck, and limb are immobilized for between three and four weeks. Subsequently, therapy is gradually instituted to regain passive joint motion. Nerve regeneration occurs from the neck into the arm at a rate of only 1–2 mm/day. Therefore, no improvement in active limb movement is expected for ~6 months. Nerve regeneration occurs in proximal to distal direction. Motion should return in the shoulder before the arm and in the elbow before the hand. Maximum nerve recovery is obtained 2–3 years after primary surgery. Upper plexus (C5 and C6) injuries treated with neuroma resection and grafting produce encouraging results, with good recovery of shoulder function in 60%–80% and reliable return of biceps in ~80%–100% (Clarke et al., 1996; Gilbert, 1995; Hentz & Meyer, 1991; Kozin, 2014; Laurent et al., 1993; Waters, 1999). Unfortunately, global palsies have a more pessimistic outcome and more variable recovery (Kirjavainen et al., 2008).

Secondary Reconstructive Surgery

Secondary reconstructive procedures are performed in children with incomplete spontaneous recovery or persistent deficits after primary nerve surgery. Secondary reconstructions can involve the shoulder, elbow, forearm, wrist, and hand. Following any secondary reconstruction, there will be a period of immobilization (3–6 weeks) followed by an increase in therapy (2–3 months) to maximize surgical outcome. An occupational and/or physical therapist depending upon their comfort level rehabilitating brachial plexus injuries can administer the therapy.

Shoulder Involvement and Intervention

The shoulder is frequently impaired after a brachial plexus injury with loss of abduction and external rotation. The resultant muscle imbalance can cause an internal rotation contracture over time. An established internal rotation contracture (i.e., no external rotation) that does not respond to therapy and/or botulinum toxin injection requires surgical release as the shoulder joint will not develop normally. Arthroscopic or open capsular release is necessary to reposition and rebalance the ball within the socket (Bachy et al., 2022; Pearl et al., 2006, Pedowitz et al., 2007; Shahcheraghi et al., 2021, Waters & Bae, 2008). Following surgery, the postoperative cast immobilization is continued for 3–4 weeks. A splint is fabricated that replicates the casted position. The splint consists of a trunk portion and a posterior elbow splint with elbow flexion (Figure 26.7). The arm portion is

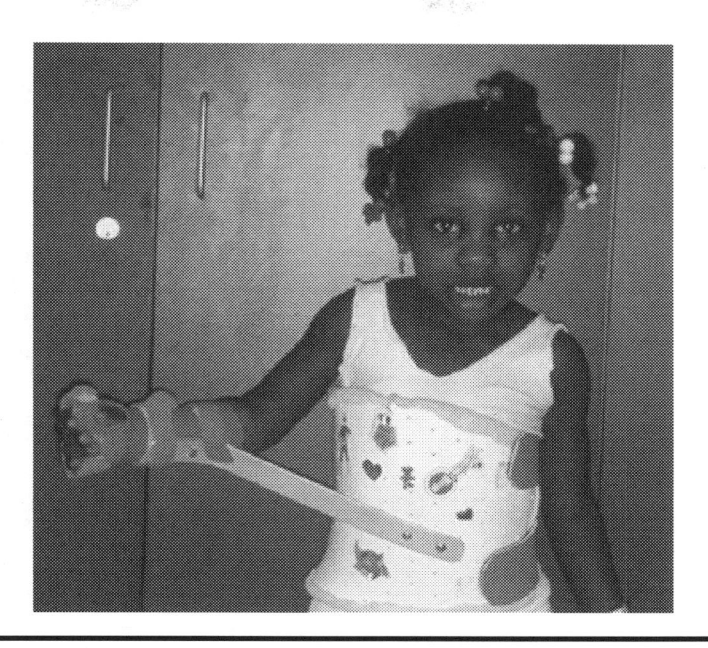

Figure 26.7 Fabricated Splint Consists of a Trunk Portion and a Posterior Elbow Splint With Elbow Flexion

Source: (Courtesy of Shriners Hospital for Children, Philadelphia, PA.)

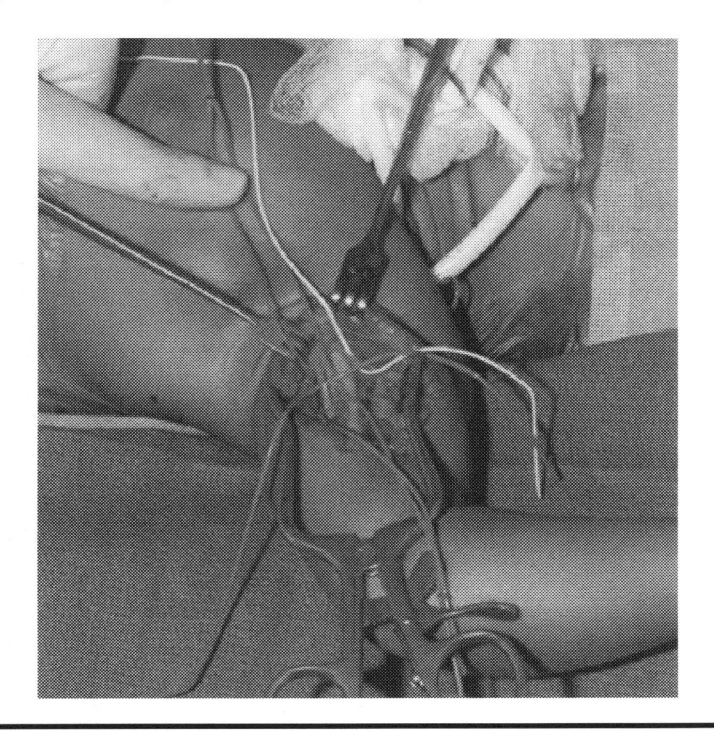

Figure 26.8 Nerve Transfer for Bicep's Function. Incision over the medial aspect of the arm to identify musculocutaneous and ulnar nerves

Source: (Courtesy of Shriners Hospital for Children, Philadelphia, PA.)

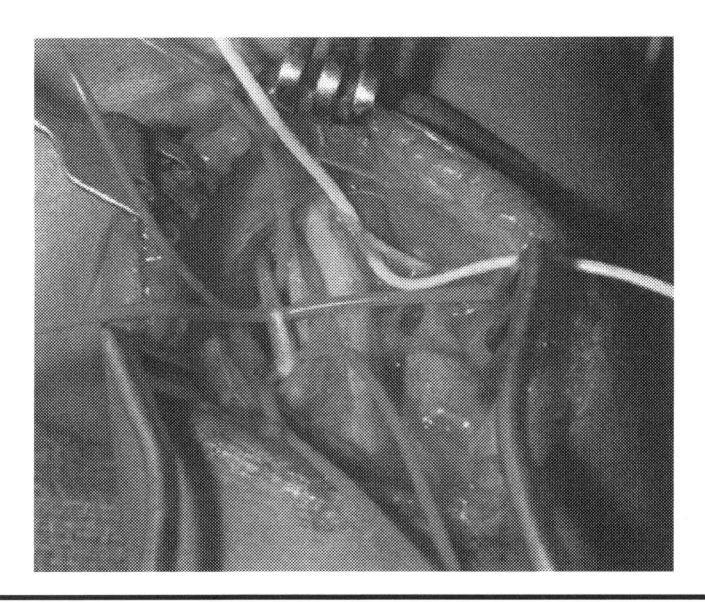

Figure 26.9 Isolation of a Group Fascicle from the Ulnar Nerve (left loop) for Transfer to the Musculocutaneous Branch to the Biceps Muscle (right loop)

Source: (Courtesy of Shriners Hospital for Children, Philadelphia, PA.)

securely attached to the trunk piece with the prescribed amount of abduction and external rotation. During the first 1–2 weeks, the splint is removed for bathing, therapy, and supervised play. Active range of motion exercises is started focusing on external rotation and shoulder elevation. Splint weaning is influenced by the presence of shoulder stiffness, active movement, and the patient's activity level. The splint is worn at night until 12 weeks after surgery. Caregiver education is a large component of early treatment to encourage carryover at home. Frequent practice of stretching, scar massage, and stabilizing techniques during therapy sessions increases confidence in the home program. Potential surgical CPT codes include shoulder arthroscopy (29806) and/or open reduction (23020). Spica cast application is also included (29055).

In children with persistent deficits in active abduction and/or external rotation, tendon transfers are performed to maximize motion (Abzug et al., 2022; Kozin et al., 2006; Pearl et al., 2006; Pedowitz et al., 2007, Shahcheraghi et al., 2021). The most common donors are the latissimus dorsi and teres major muscles (Kozin et al., 2006) (Figure 26.10). After four weeks of immobilization, a splint is fabricated to replicate the cast with the arm abducted and externally rotated. The splint is worn at night and weaned during the day for therapy, bathing, and supervised play. The splint is used at night until 12 weeks after surgery. Restrictions during the mobilization and light strengthening phases include avoiding passive internal rotation and shoulder adduction. Resistive and weight-bearing activities are also avoided. Potential CPT codes for tendon transfer are 23395 or 23397.

Older children with fixed deformity about the shoulder often lack external rotation. Changing the resting position of the arm can greatly improve activities requiring external rotation, such as hand to mouth and hand to neck (Abzug et al., 2010; Waters & Bae, 2006). A humeral osteotomy can improve an individual's function. Based on healing and patient-activity level, immobilization lasts for 4–6 weeks. Following dressing removal, a humeral fracture brace is fabricated to protect the healing bone (Figure 26.11). The splint is worn at all times, except bathing, until adequate

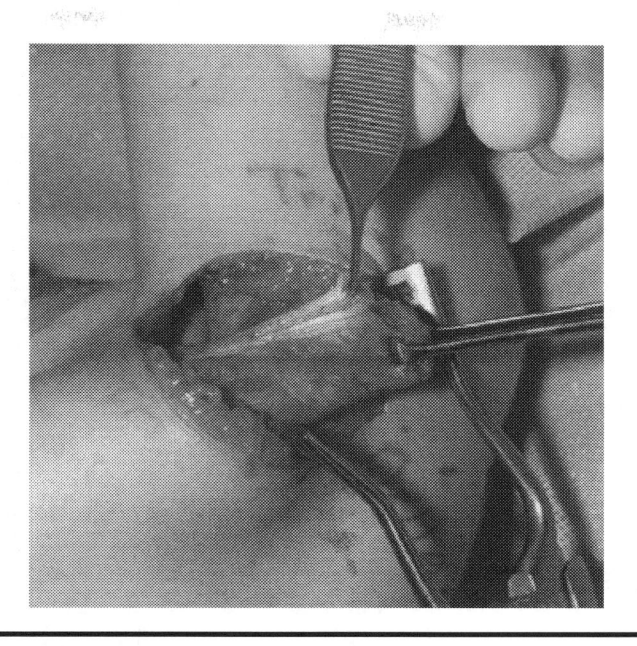

Figure 26.10 Tendon Transfer to Improve Shoulder Motion. Latissimus dorsi and teres major tendons transferred over triceps to posterior rotator cuff

Source: (Courtesy of Shriners Hospital for Children, Philadelphia, PA.)

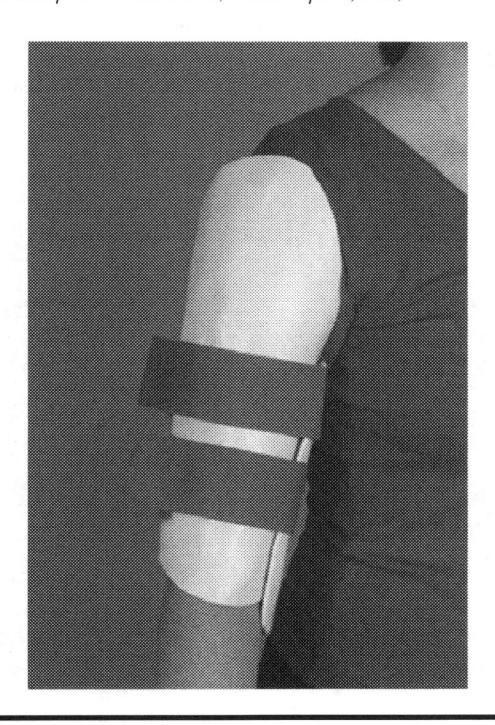

Figure 26.11 Humeral Fracture Brace to Protect Humeral Osteotomy and to Allow Elbow Motion

Source: (Courtesy of Shriners Hospital for Children, Philadelphia, PA.)

healing is noted. Resistive activities and passive range of motion are avoided until the bone healing is complete. Minimal therapy is needed, but rigorous activity is avoided for 3 months. The potential CPT code for humeral osteotomy is 24400.

Elbow Involvement and Intervention

In children who fail to regain elbow flexion, there is considerable impairment as hand-to-mouth function is impossible. A local muscle-tendon transfer may be required to regain elbow flexion and promote arm usage (Figure 26.12) (Kozin, 2014). Regardless of the muscle transferred for elbow flexion, the initial postoperative regimen is similar. The arm is splinted or casted in flexion for 4–6 weeks time dependent upon the status and effectiveness of the transfer sites. At the time of cast removal, a posterior long arm splint is fabricated with the elbow flexed at ~110°. The splint is primarily worn at night. The patient is also fitted with an adjustable elbow hinge brace that allows for locking flexion and extension range of motion. Initially, the extension hinge is locked to 110°, allowing further flexion and blocking extension beyond this point. During the early portion of mobilization, treatment focuses on muscle reeducation and scar management. When the patient can consistently recruit the tendon transfer, the range of motion can be progressed 15° each week. After achieving a 30° arc of motion (90°–120°), light resistive activities are initiated. This consists of against gravity active range of motion, hand-to-mouth activities, and more challenging tabletop activities. At ~10 weeks with sufficient tendon excursion, patients may begin formal strengthening. Passive elbow extension is not allowed for 3 months. Night splinting continues until 12 weeks from surgery. In children without local muscle-tendon donors, a free muscle may have to be removed from the leg and transferred into the arm. The muscle's nerve, artery, vein(s), and tendons need to be re-attached in the arm.

In children with spontaneous recovery of biceps and brachialis function, the elbow is prone to develop an elbow flexion contracture. The etiology is related to impaired muscle growth. The

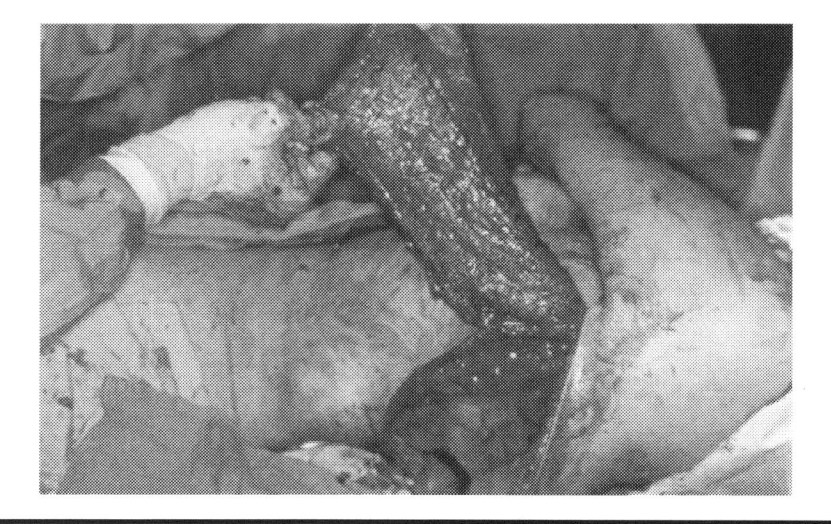

Figure 26.12 Tendon Transfer for Elbow Flexion. Bipolar Latissimus Dorsi Muscle Harvested from Flank for Elbow Flexorplasty

Source: (Courtesy of Shriners Hospital for Children, Philadelphia, PA.)

reinnervated biceps and brachialis fail to grow like normal muscle (Nikolaou et al., 2015). Hence, when the skeleton grows, the muscle tightens and causes an elbow flexion contracture. The contracture is more severe in children without triceps function. Therapy is often beneficial, especially if implemented early in the process. Splinting and serial casting are useful modalities. Botulinum toxin can be added in recalcitrant cases (CPT code 64614). Established contractures are difficult to treat, and capsular release has mediocre results with the inherent risk of losing pivotal elbow flexion. Therefore, an elbow release is rarely performed in patients with brachial plexus palsies.

A deficiency in elbow extension can result from a brachial plexus injury that involves the middle portion of the plexus (primarily C7 or the middle trunk). Surgical reconstruction is less commonly performed because elbow flexion is a greater priority and elbow extension can be accomplished by gravity (Jones et al., 1985). In certain cases, elbow flexion is adequate, and the lack of elbow extension is disabling. Deficient elbow extension will decrease the patient's available workspace and limits the ability to perform overhead tasks. In this case, a tendon transfer may be recommended to restore elbow extension (CPT code 24301).

Forearm Involvement and Intervention

An individual with brachial plexus birth palsy may lack supination, pronation, or both depending on the extent of the injury. Although supination is important for specific tasks such as accepting change, eating, receiving soap from a soap dispenser, and personal hygiene, these activities are unilateral and can be completed effectively with the unaffected arm. Pronation deficiency leads to difficulty with many more bimanual tasks such as keyboarding, writing, and tabletop activities (Figure 26.13). The decision to restore forearm movement requires careful consideration of the functional limitations and potential for gains and losses. Reconstructive options include a tendon transfer (CPT code 24301) or osteotomy of the radius and/or ulna (CPT code 25390 or 25365).

Wrist and Hand Involvement and Intervention

Wrist and hand impairment varies with the damage to the middle and lower plexus. Upper brachial plexus lesions have a minimal effect on hand use while global plexus injuries can severely hamper hand function. A definitive treatment algorithm is more difficult to formulate because of the variable clinical presentation. A detailed functional evaluation and manual muscle testing are the foundation for the development of a treatment paradigm. Individualized treatment is required, and tendon transfers may be necessary to maximize hand function.

The management of the hand follows the term "hierarchy of hand function." The most important movement is wrist extension, which aligns the finger flexors for maximum grip. In children without active grip, active wrist extension provides tenodesis for grip and for lateral pinch. The second most important task is lateral pinch, which affords the ability to perform numerous activities of daily living. Most activities that we perform every day can be accomplished with wrist extension combined with lateral pinch. The third essential motion is grasping, which allows us to hold objects. The fourth and last hierarchical movement is digital opening for object acquisition. The reason to place this function last on the ladder is that wrist flexion yields passive digital opening, which is often adequate for object procurement. In addition, synchronous digital opening is difficult to achieve via surgery as interphalangeal joint extension is primarily an intrinsic function and metacarpophalangeal joint extension is mainly an extrinsic function. Restoring both movements by tendon transfer(s) is a difficult task.

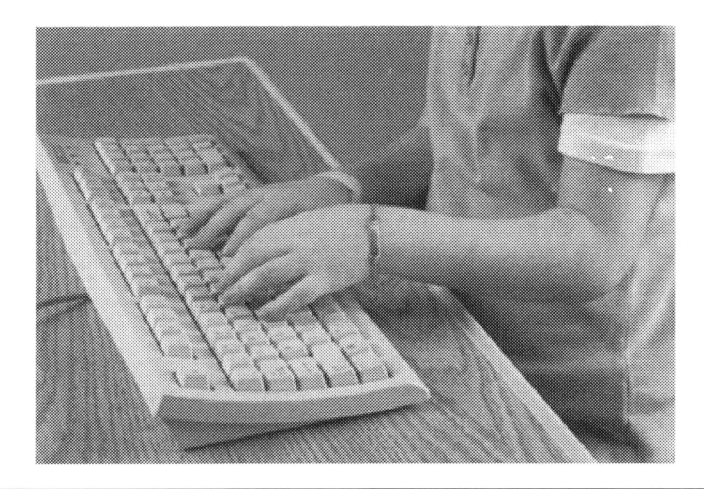

Figure 26.13 Pronation Deficiency Leads to Difficulty With Many More Bimanual Tasks Such As Keyboarding, Writing, and Tabletop Activities

Source: (Courtesy of Shriners Hospital for Children, Philadelphia, PA.)

The selection of available and appropriate donors for tendon transfer is crucial in children with residual brachial plexus palsy. We try to avoid using reinnervated muscles as donors because they tend to be weak and have limited excursion. Equally as important, we make every attempt to select a synergistic muscle as post-operative compliance in therapy is limited by age and cognition. Therefore, finger flexors are the preferred donors for wrist extension and wrist extensors are the favored choice for finger flexion. The principal donors are the flexor digitorum superficialis for wrist extension and extensor carpi radialis longus for finger flexion, respectively. When these tendons are unavailable, a search for alternative donors is based on the established principles of availability, expendability, synergy, and excursion.

General Principles of Rehabilitation Following Tendon Transfer

Following tendon transfer surgery, there are four main phases: immobilization, mobilization, light strengthening/functional training, and strengthening. Intervention during the immobilization phase focuses on edema management and the range of motion of the uninvolved joints. This phase typically lasts 3–4 weeks and will be determined by the type of tendon transfer, the quality of the tendons, and the strength of the suture repair.

The mobilization phase begins when the cast is removed and lasts until 6–8 weeks following surgery. Therapy is initiated with the fabrication of a protective splint that maintains a tension-free position of the tendon transfer. Resistive activities and active/passive movements that apply tension to the transfer are avoided. Treatment begins with muscle re-education of the tendon transfer. Cues to attempt the previous action of the transferred muscle in a protected position are useful for muscle re-education. Tapping and vibration can also facilitate recruitment. Biofeedback is a valuable modality for patients exhibiting difficulty with consistent recruitment of tendon transfers. Once consistent recruitment has been achieved with an active range of motion, functional activities should be incorporated into treatment. Incorporating play activities for children or identified functional goal activities can make sessions more meaningful to the patient. Scar management including scar massage and possible use of silicon products should be initiated as soon as incisions are healed (Widgerow et al., 2000).

The therapist should continually evaluate the patient for possible complications. A sudden or gradual lag in end-range movement may indicate weakness, deep scar formation, attenuation, or rupture of the tendon transfer. When weakness or scar formation is suspected, active-assisted range of motion or place-and-hold exercises can help build strength and promote tendon gliding. If limitations continue, neuromuscular electrical stimulation (NMES) may be beneficial to encourage gliding and strengthening. However, NMES should not be initiated until cleared by the surgeon, typically after 6 weeks following the procedure. In cases of suspected attenuation or rupture, the patient must be immediately evaluated by the surgeon. Mild attenuation may improve with healing and adaptive shortening of the muscle-tendon unit over time. However, substantial attenuation or rupture requires revision surgery to improve functional outcomes.

During the light-strengthening phase, the splint is worn only with sleep and for protection during highly resistive activities. Strengthening is initiated with light Thera-Bands and/or weights. The therapist must continue to monitor for complications. Muscle fatigue and undesired compensatory movement patterns should be avoided during the initiation of strengthening exercises. Passive motions that apply tension to the tendon transfer are avoided. Once cleared from restrictions (usually 12 weeks after surgery), splints are discontinued, and strengthening is progressed as tolerated.

Life Care Planning Considerations for the Patient with Brachial Plexus Injury

Brachial plexus injuries have a considerable impact on the patients with reference to avocational and vocational pursuits. There are many sections of the life care plan that should be considered when developing a life care plan for these patients. In addition to their orthopedic and equipment needs, the individual will likely have resulting impairment in activities of daily living and workspace limitations. These considerations should be identified throughout the individual's school and work life. A life care plan should consider these impairments and incorporate items/modifications to maximize independence and promote employability. Some of these considerations are discussed below.

Medical Surveillance

The brachial plexus specialist may be an orthopedic surgeon, physiatrist, neurologist, or neurosurgeon. Depending on the severity of the injury and the treatment recommendations, an interdisciplinary medical approach may be useful, especially in the early years.

The physician(s) specializing in the treatment of children with brachial plexus injuries will monitor musculoskeletal integrity and function. The therapy program will be directed, and decisions will be made regarding the role of surgical intervention, therapeutic modalities, splints and positioners, and adaptive devices.

Physician visits will generally be more frequent in early childhood. Once the child reaches skeletal maturity, the frequency of visits is likely to decrease. Follow-up in adulthood will focus on maintenance of function and crisis intervention.

The frequency of visits is likely to range from 2–6 per year in early childhood, 2–4 per year in adolescence, and then once every 1–3 years thereafter. The visit schedule will depend on the severity of the injury, the treatment plan, and other issues that may affect upper extremity function.

Diagnostic Studies

In addition to the physician's clinical evaluation, diagnostic studies may be used to define the extent of the injury and develop an appropriate treatment plan.

Imaging studies and electrodiagnostics are often used in early childhood. Plain X-rays and advanced imaging studies may be necessary. Infants have a high proportion of cartilage compared to bone. Magnetic resonance imaging (MRI) provides visualization of the cartilage and is frequently ordered to assess the glenohumeral joint (Kozin & Zlotolow, 2012). Ultrasound is also an imaging study that visualizes cartilage and can monitor the infant's shoulder for signs of humeral head subluxation (Bauer et al., 2017). The frequency of diagnostic testing is likely to be considerably reduced as the child grows into skeletal maturity. In general, women reach skeletal maturity at 14 years of age and men reach skeletal maturity at 16 years of age.

The cost of the study should include charges for both the professional and technical components of each test.

Therapeutic Modalities

The goals of therapy include maximizing function and preventing secondary disability by increasing the range of motion and strength. Therapy sessions are likely to include a combination of exercises, electrical stimulation, splinting, other modalities, and training in compensatory strategies for activities of daily living. The professional therapists will supervise these sessions and oversee the home-based exercise program.

Professional Therapy

The frequency of therapy is likely to vary from 2 to 12 times monthly. A combination of occupational and physical therapy is usually prescribed. Younger children may receive more frequent professional therapy sessions, while older children may be taught more home-based activities. Therapy frequency may be increased after surgery, during growth spurts, or during life transitions.

Therapy in the older adolescent and adult is likely to be episodic, focusing on the maintenance of function, crisis intervention, and adjustment to new life challenges.

When geographically available, therapy is usually best delivered at a center that treats many children/adolescents with brachial plexus injuries. School-based therapy is generally directed at facilitating the educational program and, in and of itself, may not provide sufficient attention to maximizing strength and range of motion. The life care plan should address the need for private therapy when school-based therapy cannot guarantee meeting the goals.

Home Exercise Program

Most children and adults with brachial plexus injury will benefit from a daily home exercise program, often supplemented with splinting. While exercise and splinting do not affect neurological recovery, they can prevent contractures, joint deformity, and loss of range of motion (ROM). The home exercise program will consist of all or some of the following elements:

- Passive ROM several times daily
- Tactile stimulation
- Weight-bearing activity to stimulate proprioception and muscle contraction
- Encouragement of bimanual activity

Splints/Positioners

The use of splints will depend on the extent of the injury:

- A resting hand splint is used to keep a flaccid hand and/or wrist in a functional position and prevent attenuation of tendons and/or injury to the nerves.
- A dorsal cock-up splint is used to increase grasp when wrist extension is limited.
- An elbow extension splint is used to reduce an elbow flexion contracture.
- A dynamic elbow flexion splint with rubber bands is used when the child has full elbow extension without elbow flexion.
- A "thumbs up" splint is used to reduce thumb adduction and maintain the thumb out of the palm.

Components of Surgical Costs

The cost of future surgical procedures should include the following:

- *Surgeon(s) fee*: Some procedures require more than one surgeon, either an assistant or a complimentary specialty. The physician charges should include the cost of each surgeon. It is helpful to have all of the appropriate CPT codes.
- *Facility fee*: The hospital charge will include the per diem, operating room charges, and ancillary costs. When obtaining costs from a particular facility, it is helpful to know the anticipated length of stay and expected time in the operating room. Some facilities also request CPT codes.
- *Anesthesiologist*: These charges are usually time-based. It is helpful to know the anticipated length of the procedure.
- *Postoperative rehabilitation*: Intensive physical and occupational therapy may be required. The life care plan should be careful not to duplicate therapy sessions that may have already been included in the plan. Only additional sessions, specific to the procedure, should be included in this section.

Pain Management

This is rarely an issue in birth injuries (4%–5% of children). However, acquired traumatic brachial plexus injuries, even in adolescents, can have a substantial component of pain. Some of these clients go on to manifest Reflex Sympathetic Dystrophy (RSD) or Complex Regional Pain Syndrome (CRPS) in the affected extremities. In these circumstances, pain management modalities can be a considerable cost factor.

Counseling/Psychological Support

Children with brachial plexus injuries will have to cope with differences and limitations through the various stages of normal development. They may have increased difficulty mastering the stages of independence. As they grow, self-image can be affected by the deformities in the arm and hand.

Professional counseling can facilitate a productive adjustment to disability. The family of the young child will benefit from strategies to cope with deviations in functional development and appearance. The adolescent must adjust to both his appearance and physical limitations. Young adults may face limited career opportunities and new physical demands as they pass through life stages.

Counseling is generally included in the life care plan in episodes lasting 3–6 months at various key transition stages (Alyanak et al., 2013).

Equipment/Home Modifications

Assistive devices and specially designed toys will facilitate function throughout childhood. The amount of equipment/home modification varies with the extent of brachial plexus injury. Grooming tools and other implements for activities of daily living and recreation may need adaptations for one-handed use. Storage of clothing, toys, and other personal belongings needs to be at shoulder height or lower when decreased shoulder motion is present. As the child grows, modifications in the kitchen and bathroom will be necessary to accommodate any limitation in reach.

During the school years, equipment to facilitate education may include book packs that can be opened easily with one arm, special holders to fix notebooks and papers to the desk for writing, other adaptive devices, and software to facilitate typing with one hand.

Depending on the severity of the injury, the young adult with a brachial plexus injury may need special adaptations to the steering wheel and dashboard to facilitate one-handed driving. A driving evaluation is usually part of the life care plan.

Examples of Assistive Devices

Assistive devices or adaptive equipment are recommended for individuals who are not able to fully participate in some aspects of their activities of daily living. These devices can assist with grooming, self-care, homemaking, leisure, and work activities:

- *Grooming*: one-handed nail clipper and nail brush.
- *Dressing*: buttonhook, zipper pull, elastic shoelaces, Velcro® fasteners, dressing stick, and a long-handled shoehorn.
- *Bathing*: long-handled brush, grab bars on the wall, and nonskid bathmat.
- *Homemaking*: enlarged or built-up handles for food preparation or cooking, right-angle rocker knife with a serrated edge, adapted cutting board, Dycem® to secure items on counter, and reacher.
- *Leisure*: adapted fishing reel, card shuffler, etc.
- *Work/school*: one-handed keyboard, voice recognition, and ergonomic workspace.

Driving Evaluation

A driving evaluation is routinely recommended for adolescents when they receive their driving permit. A certified therapist to ensure a safe driving experience performs this evaluation. In most cases, an automatic car is recommended. Additional recommendations include a spinner knob and modifications to the positions of the various controls for the turn signals, windshield wipers, etc.

Attendant Care/Replacement Services

Deficits in function will depend on the severity of the injury. Most adults with residual deficits from a brachial plexus injury will have limitations in performing tasks that require bimanual strength and dexterity. While many chores and activities of daily living can be successfully completed with one hand, those tasks that require climbing ladders, lifting heavy items, pulling, or pushing with both hands and two-handed dexterity may require outside assistance. Examples of tasks that are likely to present difficulties to the adult with a brachial plexus injury include

- Climbing ladders
- Carrying loads while ascending or descending stairs
- Styling hair and applying makeup
- Putting fitted sheets on a bed
- Running a vacuum cleaner
- Opening jars
- Cutting meat
- Lifting heavy pots of cooked food
- Tying shoes
- Fastening clothing
- Reaching into a back pocket
- Cutting nails
- Homemaking
- Leisure activities
- Working environment

The quantity of assistance in the life care plan should correlate with the functional deficits from the injury. A conversation between the treating physician and life care planner is always beneficial to ensure the formulation of a comprehensive plan.

Life Expectancy

Children with neonatal brachial plexus birth palsy have a normal life expectancy. Secondary overuse of the contralateral normal arm is a potential consequence in adulthood, however, there remains no evidence to support this sequela.

Conclusion

Children and adults who sustain a brachial plexus injury have varying degrees of permanent impairment based on the extent of the injury and the success of surgical/non-surgical intervention. There is ongoing research to improve nerve repair and nerve regeneration. As these techniques advance, persons with brachial plexus injury should have less impairment. Nonetheless, the future is now, and the formulation of a comprehensive life care plan is of utmost necessity to these patients and their families. The best life care plans are formulated with discussion between the treating physician, therapist, life care planner, and vocational expert.

References

Abzug, J. M., Chafetz, R. S., Gaughan, J. P., Ashworth, S., & Kozin, S. H. (2010). Shoulder function after medial approach and derotational humeral osteotomy in patients with brachial plexus birth palsy. *Journal of Pediatric Orthopaedics, 30,* 469–474.

Abzug, J. M., Miller, E., Case, A. L., Hogarth, D. A., Zlotolow, D. A., & Kozin, S. H. (2022). Single versus double tendon transfer to improve shoulder external rotation during the treatment of brachial plexus birth palsy. *Hand*, *17*, 55–59.

Alyanak, B., Kılınçaslan, A., Kutlu, L., Bozkurt, H., & Aydın, A. Psychological adjustment, maternal distress (2013), and family functioning in children with obstetrical brachial plexus palsy. *Journal of Hand Surgery-American*, *38*(1), 137–142.

Bachy, M., Lallemant, P., Grimberg, J., & Fitoussi, F. (2022). Palliative shoulder and elbow surgery in obstetrical brachial plexus birth palsy. *Hand Surgery & Rehabilitation*, *41S*, S63–S70.

Bager, B. (1997). Perinatally acquired brachial plexus palsy: A persisting challenge. *Acta Paediatrca*, *8*, 1214–1219.

Bauer, A. S., Lucas, J. F., Heyrani, N., Anderson, R. L., Kalish, L. A., & James, M. A. (2017). Ultrasound screening for posterior shoulder dislocation in infants with persistent brachial plexus birth palsy. *Journal of Bone Joint Surgery-American*, *99*(9), 778–783.

Campion, D. (1996). Electrodiagnostic testing in hand surgery. *The Journal of hand Surgery*, *21*(6), 947–956.

Cho, Á. B., Guerreiro, A. C., Ferreira, C., Kiyohara, L. Y., & Sorrenti, L. (2020). Epidemiological Study of Traumatic Brachial Plexus Injuries. *Acta ortopedica brasileira*, *28*(1), 16–18.

Clarke, H. M., Al-Qattan, M. M., Curtis, C. G., & Zuker, R. M. (1996). Obstetrical brachial plexus palsy: Results following neurolysis of conducting neuromas-in-continuity. *Plastic and Reconstructive Surgery*, *97*, 974–984.

Coroneos, C. J., Voineskos, S. H., Christakis, M. K., Thoma, A., Bain, J. R., Brouwers, M. C., & Canadian OBPI Working Group (2017). Obstetrical brachial plexus injury (OBPI): Canada's national clinical practice guideline. *BMJ open*, *7*(1), e014141. https://doi.org/10.1136/bmjopen-2016-014141

Curtis, C., Stephens, D., Clarke, H. M., & Andrews, D. (2002). The active movement scale: An evaluation tool for infants with obstetrical brachial plexus palsy. *Journal of Hand Surgery*, *27*, 470–478.

DeFrancesco, C. J., Shah, D. K., Rogers, B. H., & Shah, A. S. (2019). The epidemiology of brachial plexus birth palsy in the United States: Declining incidence and evolving risk factors. *Journal of Pediatric Orthopaedics*, *39*(2), e134–e140.

Draycott, T. J., Crofts, J. F., Ash, J. P., Wilson, L. V., Yard, E., Sibanda, T., & Whitelaw, A. (2008). Improving neonatal outcome through practical shoulder dystocia training. *Obstetrics & Gynecology*, *112*(1), 14–20.

Foad, S. L., Mehlman, C. T., & Ying, J. (2008). The epidemiology of neonatal brachial plexus palsy in the United States. *Journal of Bone & Joint Surgery-American*, *90*, 1258–1264.

Gilbert, A. (1995). Long-term evaluation of brachial plexus surgery in obstetrical palsy. *Hand Clinics*, *11*, 583–594.

Gilbert, A., & Whitaker, I. (1991). Obstetrical brachial plexus lesions. *The Journal of Hand Surgery: British & European Volume*, *16*, 489–491.

Gilbert, W. M., Nebitt, T. S., & Danielsen, B. (1999). Associated factors in 1611 cases of brachial plexus injury. *Obstetrics & Gynecology*, *93*(4), 536–540.

Greenwald, A. G., Schute, P. C., & Shiveley, J. L. (1984). Brachial plexus birth palsy: A 10 year report on the incidence and prognosis. *Journal of Pediatric Orthopaedics*, *4*, 689–692.

Gurewitsch, E. D., Johnson, E., Hamzehzadeh, S., & Allen, R. H. (2006). Risk factors for brachial plexus injury with and without shoulder dystocia. *American Journal of Obstetrics & Gynecology*, *194*(2), 486–492.

Heise, C. O., Siqueira, M. G., Martins, R. S., & Gherpelli, J. L. (2007). Clinical electromyography correlation in infants with obstetric brachial plexopathy. *Journal of Hand Surgery*, *32*, 999–1004.

Hentz, V. R., & Meyer, R. D. (1991). Brachial plexus microsurgery in children. *Microsurgery*, *12*, 175–185.

Jones, B. N., Manske, P. R., Schoenecker, P. L., & Dailey, L. (1985). Latissimus dorsi transfer to restore elbow extension in obstetrical palsy. *Journal of Pediatric Orthopaedics*, *5*, 287–289.

Kawai, H., Tsuyuguchi, Y., Masada, K., Heise, C. O., Siqueira, M. G., & Martins, R. S. (1989). Identification of the lesion in brachial plexus injuries with root avulsion: A comprehensive assessment by means of preoperative findings, myelography, surgical exploration and intraoperative diagnosis. *Neuro-Orthopedics*, *7*, 15–23.

Kirjavainen, M., Remes, V., Peltonen, J., Rautakorpi, S., Helenius, I., & Nietosvaara Y. (2008). The function of the hand after operations for obstetric injuries to the brachial plexus. *Journal of Bone & Joint Surgery British Volume, 90*(3), 349–355.

Kozin, S. H. (2014). Injuries of the brachial plexus. In J. P. Iannotti & G. R. Williams (Eds.), *Disorders of the shoulder: Diagnosis and management* (3rd ed., pp. 607–660). Lippincott Williams & White.

Kozin, S. H. (2008). Nerve transfers in brachial plexus birth palsies: Indications, techniques, and outcomes. *Hand Clinics, 24*, 363–376.

Kozin, S. H., Chafetz, R. S., Barus, D., & Filipone, L. (2006). Magnetic resonance imaging and clinical findings before and after tendon transfers about the shoulder in children with brachial plexus birth palsy. *Journal of Shoulder & Elbow Surgery, 15*, 554–561.

Kozin, S. H., & Zlotolow, D. A. (2012). Advanced imaging and arthroscopic management of shoulder contracture. *Hand Clinics Journal, 28*, 541–550.

Laurent, J. P., Lee, R., Shenaq, S., Parke, J. T., Solis, I. S., & Kowlik, L. (1993). Neurosurgical correction of upper brachial plexus birth injuries. *Journal of Neurosurgery, 79*, 197–203.

Louden, E., Allgier, A., Overton, M., Welge, J., & Mehlman, C. T. (2015). The impact of pediatric brachial plexus injury on families. *Journal of Hand Surgery-American, 40*, 1190–1195.

Michelow, B. J., Clarke, H. M., Curtis, C. G., Zuker, R. M., Seifu, Y., & Andrews, D. F. (1994). The natural history of obstetrical brachial plexus palsy. *Plastic & Reconstructive Surgery, 93*, 675–681.

Nikolaou, S., Hu, L., & Cornwall, R. (2015). Afferent innervation, muscle spindles, and contractures following neonatal brachial plexus injury in a mouse model. *Journal of Hand Surgery-American, 40*(10), 2007–2016.

Pearl, M. L., Edgerton, B. W., Kazimiroff, P. A., Burchette, R. J., & Wong, K. (2006). Arthroscopic release and latissimus dorsi transfer for shoulder internal rotation contractures and glenohumeral deformity secondary to brachial plexus birth palsy. *Journal of Bone & Joint Surgery-American, 88*, 564–574.

Pedowitz, D. I., Gibson, B., Williams, G. R., & Kozin, S. H. (2007). Arthroscopic treatment of posterior glenohumeral joint subluxation resulting from brachial plexus birth palsy. *Journal of Shoulder & Elbow Surgery, 16*, 6–13.

Shahcheraghi, G. H., Javid, M., & Zamir-Azad, M. (2021). The outcome of soft-tissue release and tendon transfer in shoulders with brachial plexus birth palsy. *Journal of Shoulder and Elbow Surgery International, 3*(5), 905–911.

Sibinski, M. & Synder, M. (2007). Obstetric brachial plexus palsy: Risk factors and predictors. *Journal of Orthopaedics, Traumatology & Rehabilitation, 9*, 569–576.

Sjoberg, K., Erichs, K., & Bjerre, I. (1988). Cause and effect of obstetric (neonatal) brachial plexus palsy. *Acta Paediatrica, Scandinavia, 77*, 357–364.

Van Ouwekerk, W. J., van der Sluijs, J. A., Nollet, F., Barkhof, F., & Slooff, A. C. (2000). Management of obstetric brachial plexus lesions: State of the art and future developments. *Child's Nervous System, 16*, 638–644.

Vu, A. T., Sparkman, D. M., van Belle, C. J., Yakuboff, K. P., & Schwentker, A. R. (2018). Retropharyngeal contralateral C7 nerve transfer to the lower trunk for brachial plexus birth injury: Technique and results. *Journal of Hand Surgery-American, 43*(5), 417–424.

Waters, P. M. (1997). Obstetric brachial plexus injuries: Evaluation and management. *Journal of the American Academy of Orthopedic Surgeons, 5*, 205–214.

Waters, P. M. (1999). Comparison of the natural history, the outcome of microsurgical repair, and the outcome of operative reconstruction in brachial plexus birth palsy. *Journal of Bone & Joint Surgery-American, 81*(5), 649–659.

Waters, P. M., & Bae, D. S. (2006). The effect of derotational humeral osteotomy on global shoulder function in brachial plexus birth palsy. *Journal of Bone & Joint Surgery-American, 88*(5), 1035–1042.

Waters, P. M., & Bae, D. S. (2008). The early effects of tendon transfers and open capsulorrhaphy on glenohumeral deformity in brachial plexus birth palsy. *Journal of Bone & Joint Surgery-American, 90*(10), 2171–2179.

Widgerow, A. D., Chait, L. A., Stahls, R., & Stahls, P. (2000). New innovations in scar management. *Aesthetic Plastic Surgery, 24*(3), 227–234.

Chapter 27

Forensic Issues in Life Care Planning

Rick H. Robinson

Forensic Issues in Life Care Planning

The process of building a life care plan within the context of a litigated matter can be effectively conceptualized and compared to the process of connecting individual links to construct a chain that ultimately bears the weight of the life care planner's opinions and conclusions. A chain is best described as a series of links, connected one after another, to form a flexible yet high-strength apparatus for connecting elements together, holding elements down, and pulling things along. Regardless of the application, each link in the chain contributes to the overall strength and effectiveness of the apparatus as a whole. The overall strength of the chain, in sum, is only as strong as its weakest link. This is also the case for life care planning within a forensic application. This chapter will provide a brief overview of the American legal system and how the specialty practice of life care planning is performed within this legal system.

Structure of the American Legal System

English Common Law

American law is derived in large part from English common law dating back to the eleventh century (Scheb & Sharma, 2020). Very early, English common law drew a distinction between civil law and criminal law. Where criminal law sought to punish persons committing offenses against the Crown or that could be seen as harming society, civil law addressed offenses against private parties, versus society in general (Scheb & Sharma, 2020). The focus of this chapter will be toward matters involving civil wrongs against individuals or private parties. In English common law, the aggrieved party was referred to as the plaintiff, while the party accused of wrongdoing was referred to as the defendant (Scheb & Sharma, 2020). The common law system forms the typical legal structure of most English-speaking countries (Dunn, 2014).

Predating English common law, trials took the form of what Scheb and Sharma (2020) referred to as irrational modes, such as trial by combat or trial by ordeal. In trial by combat, the parties in dispute would engage in combat or hire others to fight on their behalf. In trial by ordeal, "the defendant was tortured by fire or water. If a defendant survived the ordeal, it was said that God had intervened to prove the defendant's innocence before the law" (Scheb & Sharma, 2020, p. 15). With the widespread success of English common law, came also the process of a jury trial. By the fourteenth century, the jury system in England had become well established, with two types of recognized juries. The grand jury, decided whether an individual accused of a crime should be indicted for said crime, while a petit jury came to serve as the finder of facts in both civil and criminal cases (Scheb & Sharma, 2020).

Trial by jury became the standard means of resolving both criminal and civil matters. The jury would hear the evidence and ultimately decide the factual issues of greatest importance in the matter. The judge presided over the trial and ruled on questions of law (Scheb & Sharma, 2020). The law, as it is applied in the modern world, provides a framework for resolving conflicts between individuals, groups, families, corporations, and governments. This framework developed into an adversarial system of justice where opposing parties argue each side's position to try to achieve a favorable outcome for their particular side. Scheb and Sharma (2020, p. 16) provided great insight into this process, stating:

> the adversarial system of justice assumes that truth and justice are most likely to emerge from the clash of opposing factual and legal claims. In general, this may be true—but there is no assurance that competition in the courtroom always will produce truth or justice.

Common Law in America

As the dust of the American Revolution settled, it became obvious that English common law would need to be Americanized. The colonies would need to choose what parts of English common law to keep and which to disregard (Friedman, 2019). This period in American history was necessarily an age of "innovation in fundamental law" (Friedman, 2019, p. 86). American states and the national government began to draft written constitutions that set out the structure of government and the individual rights of its citizens.

The Constitution of 1787 created a new system of federal courts in the United States (U.S.). This new federal system of courts was limited to matters of federal law or citizens of different states. Unless the issue in question was clearly related to "a real federal question" (Friedman, 2019, p. 110), the final word on the issue was decided in state courts. Accordingly, very early after the birth of the nation, federal and state courts began to resolve matters of conflict within their respective jurisdictions, thus creating the very foundations of American case law—albeit not well documented. Friedman (2019, p.61), wrote:

> Case law—court decisions—did not easily pass from colony to colony. There were no printed reports at all, though in the eighteenth century some manuscript materials did circulate among lawyers. These could hardly have been very influential. No doubt custom and case law slowly seeped from colony to colony. Travelers and word of mouth must have spread some knowledge of living law.

Because of the evolving requirement for courts to resolve successive similar issues or questions in the same or similar manner to previous proceedings, case law became an essential foundation for the legal process. The legal doctrine of stare decisis states that courts will adhere to precedent in making their decisions (Cornell School of Law, n.d., stare decisis). In considering the weight of a particular court decision, it is important to appreciate that case law within the jurisdiction where a matter is being heard, has the greatest degree of weight; wherein case law from other jurisdictions has little to no persuasive weight (Dunn, 2014). Consistent with the doctrine of stare decisis, lawyers must prepare extensive research on *case law*, or previous decisions from courts in the relevant jurisdiction, to form an argument supporting their client's claim or defense (Dunn, 2014). The rare exception to this doctrine is when a court is hearing a case of first impression which is a case that presents a legal issue that has never been decided by the governing jurisdiction (Cornell School of Law, n.d., case of first impression). In such a case, legal decisions from other jurisdictions may be argued and considered by the court in arriving at a common law rule that the jurisdiction will follow in subsequent similar cases (Dunn, 2014).

While common law clearly carries great weight within the jurisdiction having decided an issue, it is subordinate to both constitutional and statutory bodies of law (Dunn, 2014). The area of constitutional law refers to rights articulated in both federal and state constitutions. Most of this body of law has evolved from state and federal Supreme Court rulings, which interpret their respective constitutions and ensure that the laws passed by their respective legislatures do not violate constitutional limits (Roger Williams University School of Law, 2022, Constitutional Law). The area of statutory law encompasses a body of written laws, usually enacted by a legislative entity. Statutory laws can range from regulatory and administrative laws passed by executive agencies, to common law, or law created by prior court decisions. Unlike common law, however, which is subject to interpretation in its application by the court, statutory laws are generally strictly construed by courts. Statutory law is proposed, debated, and created by democratically elected representatives of federal, state, and local governments (Dunn, 2014).

In describing the complexity of this multitiered system of lawmaking and dispute resolution, Dunn (2014, p. 240) offered the following commentary "the total amount of case law, statutory law, and regulatory law has become quite immense. Further complicating the matter is the lack of uniformity that can come from differences between state jurisdictions in the interpretation of the law."

The Structure of Courts in the United States

The United States Constitution is the supreme law of the land in the United States. The Constitution creates a federal system of government in which power is shared between the federal government and state governments (United States Courts, 2022). Both the federal government and each of the state governments have their own court systems.

The Federal Court System

Article III of the United States Constitution states "The judicial Power of the United States, shall be vested in one supreme Court, and in such inferior Courts as the Congress may from time to time ordain and establish" (National Constitution Center, 2022). This article invests the judicial power of the United States in the federal court system and specifically creates the U.S. Supreme Court and gives Congress the authority to create the lower federal courts (United States Courts, 2022). This constitutional power has been utilized by the United States Congress to establish a judicial system of 13 Federal Courts of Appeals, 94 Federal District Courts, the U.S. Court of Claims, and the U.S. Court of International Trade (United States Courts, 2022). A party who is dissatisfied with the ruling of a district court may appeal to one of the U.S. Court of Appeals (United States Courts, 2022). A party who is dissatisfied with a decision of the U.S. Court of

Appeals may request the U.S. Supreme Court to review the decision. However, the Supreme Court usually is under no obligation to do so unless there is a constitutional question—for which the U.S. Supreme Court is the final arbiter (United States Courts, 2022). Federal courts typically hear cases dealing with the constitutionality of a law; cases involving ambassadors and public ministers; disputes between two or more states; admiralty law; bankruptcy; and issues related to habeas corpus (United States Courts, 2022).

The U.S. Constitution requires that federal judges be nominated by the President of the United States and confirmed by the U.S. Senate. Federal judges hold office during good behavior, typically, for life, and can only be removed through impeachment for misbehavior (United States Courts, 2022).

The State Court Systems

Whereas the U.S. Constitution grants power to the federal court system, at the state level, it is the Constitution and laws of each state that establish the state courts (United States Courts, 2022). State courts typically hear cases related to criminal matters; probate (involving wills and estates); contract cases, tort cases (personal injuries), family law (marriages, divorces, adoptions), etc. (United States Courts, 2022). State-level courts vary from state to state in their structure, but in most cases, there are three levels of courts: the trial court, the appeals court, and the Supreme Court (Dunn, 2014).

The lowest level of court is the trial court, where the issue in dispute is initially decided. Trial courts in various states may be referred to by different names, such as general sessions courts, chancery courts, court of claims, etc. (Dunn, 2014). In these trial courts, attorneys bring and defend actions from all areas of the law. In this setting, legal arguments are presented to the court along with evidence in support of the plaintiff's argument or in opposition to the plaintiff's arguments. Through this process, the trial court's primary purpose of making an initial determination of a matter is fulfilled through the gathering of relevant facts, and application of relevant law (Dunn, 2014).

Once a trial court has decided the outcome of a matter, a dissatisfied party may attempt to appeal the decision of the court. To pursue an appeal, there must be a basis for questioning the findings of the trial court, such as with the admission of a piece of evidence or the perceived misapplication of a particular element of the law (Dunn, 2014). Upon evaluating the merits of the appeal, the Court of Appeals may agree to hear the appeal or reject the request. It is important to understand that it is not the role of the Court of Appeals to retry the case. In fact, at this level, the Court of Appeals does not collect new evidence, but instead engages only in a review of the merits of the case (Dunn, 2014).

At the state court level, a court of last resort, often known as a Supreme Court, usually is the highest court (United States Courts, 2022). Similar to the lower Court of Appeals, not all cases referred to the state Supreme Court will be heard. The state Supreme Court will consider the merits of the appeal, and if accepted, will grant a writ of certiorari to the petitioning party (Dunn, 2014). State courts are the final arbiters of state law and their respective state constitutions. Upon a state Supreme Court deciding an issue, the decision is final as to action within the state court (Dunn, 2014). Beyond the state Supreme Court, the remaining means of appeal would be to the Supreme Court of the United States, usually on the basis of some violation of Constitutional law (Dunn, 2014).

Within the state court system, judges are selected in a number of different ways depending on the state's constitution and laws. At the state level, judges may be selected by election; by appointment for a specific number of years or even to life; or by combinations of these methods (United States Courts, 2022).

Rules of Civil Procedure

As a point of general discussion, the Federal Rules of Civil Procedure (The Committee of the Judiciary, 2020b) will be the focus of this section. Each state has adopted, through its legislature and courts, rules that apply specifically to that state's court system in terms of process and procedure to be followed within that jurisdiction. While most state rules of civil procedure may be similar to the Federal rules, they are not the same and may materially vary—such variance is beyond the scope and purpose of this chapter. Readers are referred to the Cornell Law School Legal Information Institute for links to the Rules of Civil Procedure by state, which are provided at www.law.cornell.edu/wex/table_civil_procedure.

The *Federal Rules of Civil Procedure* govern civil proceedings in United States district courts. The stated purpose of the rules is "to secure the just, speedy, and inexpensive determination of every action and proceeding" (The Committee of the Judiciary, 2020b, p. 1). The set of rules were adopted by order of the Supreme Court on December 20, 1937, and became effective on September 16, 1938. The most recent revision of the rules became effective on December 1, 2020 (The Committee of the Judiciary, 2020b).

According to Dunn (2014), various forms of legal remedies may be pursued through a civil action, but the remedies can generally be separated into two broad categories: "*legal remedies* (payment of money to make the injured party 'whole') and *equitable remedies* (injunctions or orders by the court to force a party to take an action or to cease and desist from some action)" (p. 247). In 2010, the Congressional Committee on the Judiciary merged courts of law and equity within the Federal Rules of Civil Procedure by recognizing that cases brought before a federal court were brought not as a separate law or equity action, but more broadly as a civil action (Dunn, 2014). In a civil action, a plaintiff pursues some form of civil remedy from a defendant who has, could, or is causing injury to the plaintiff in some way. This claim of injury forms the rationale for pursuing damages wherein the plaintiff will demonstrate the defendant is liable for injuries and should pay an amount in damages (Dunn, 2014). The process by which the plaintiff will pursue alleged damages are detailed in the Rules of Civil Procedure.

The Complaint

A civil action is commenced by filing a complaint with the court (The Committee of the Judiciary, 2020b). The complaint must include at least three elements by rule that include: (1) a short and plain statement of the grounds for the court's jurisdiction, unless the court already has jurisdiction and the claim needs no new jurisdictional support; (2) a short and plain statement of the claim(s) against the defendant showing that the plaintiff is entitled to relief; and (3) a demand for the type of remedy or relief being sought (The Committee of the Judiciary, 2020b, § 8(a)(1–3)). Upon receipt of the complaint by the Defendant, they must respond with an answer to claims detailed in the complaint (Cornell School of Law, n.d., complaint). Until relatively recently, complaints did not need to specify the alleged facts the plaintiff intends to prove. In 2007, the U.S. Supreme Court introduced a heightened standard in the decision of *Bell Atlantic v. Twombly*, wherein it was determined that a complaint must allege "enough facts to state a claim to relief that is plausible on its face" (Bell Atlantic v. Twombly, 2007, p. 4).

Service

Upon filing a complaint with the court, the complaint must then be served on the defendant. According to Dunn (2014, p. 249):

> Service implicates Constitutional issues of due process because the defendant is threatened with a deprivation of property in a civil case, and the manner of service must be calculated to actually inform the individual of the civil action and provide them with a right to be heard in a court.

The service document, referred to as a summons, must include: the name of the court and the parties; be directed to the defendant(s); state the name and address of the plaintiff's attorney or—if unrepresented—of the plaintiff; state the time within which the defendant must appear and defend; notification to the defendant that a failure to appear and defend will result in a default judgment against the defendant for the relief demanded in the complaint; be signed by the clerk; and bear the court's seal (The Committee of the Judiciary, 2020b, § 4(1)).

Pre-answer Motions and the Answer

Having been appropriately served, the defendant may choose to file a motion to the court requesting the complaint be dismissed. There are a number of defenses that may be asserted by motion to the court, such as: lack of subject matter jurisdiction; lack of personal jurisdiction; improper venue; insufficient process; insufficient service of process; failure to state a claim upon which relief can be granted; or failure to join a party to the complaint (The Committee of the Judiciary, 2020b, § 12(b)).

If the pre-answer motions fail to result in the complaint being dismissed by the court, the defendant then must provide an answer to the complaint (Dunn, 2014). In providing a formal response to the complaint, the defendant must respond to each factual allegation made by the plaintiff by denying, admitting, stating additional facts, or claiming affirmative defenses to the defendant's actions (Dunn, 2014). In a tort action, there are a number of potential affirmative defenses that can be raised, which, if found to be credible, will negate liability even if it is proven that the defendant committed the alleged acts (Cornell School of Law, n.d., affirmative defense).

A defendant's written response may also counter the plaintiff's facts with their own facts that may absolve the defendant of liability or include counterclaims against the plaintiff. A plaintiff who faces a counterclaim then stands in the role of both plaintiff and defendant. After the answer has been provided to the Plaintiff, either party may move for a judgment. Such a judgment may be granted by the court if either side can demonstrate circumstances that will cause either the specified relief to be granted or the case to be dismissed (Dunn, 2014). If such a motion is made and denied by the court, the civil action now moves forward toward joinder and discovery.

Joinder of Claims and Parties

Joinder involves bringing additional parties or claims into the lawsuit (Cornell School of Law, n.d., joinder). The most common type of claims under joinder are counterclaims and crossclaims (Dunn, 2014). A counterclaim is a claim for relief filed against an opposing party after the original claim is filed—most commonly, a claim by the defendant against the plaintiff (Cornell School of Law, n.d., counterclaim). A cross-claim, on the other hand, is a claim brought by a plaintiff against a co-plaintiff, or by a defendant against a co-defendant. A crossclaim will not be allowed unless the subject matter relates closely to the original cause of action (Cornell School of Law, n.d., cross-claim).

Disclosures

Disclosures and Discovery are legal processes for obtaining evidence in support of a cause of action or in defense of a legal action. Disclosures and discovery can come in multiple forms—physical documents, electronic information, objects, first-hand observation by witnesses, and the opinions of experts (Dunn, 2014). Disclosure involves the production of documents, items, or related materials that have relevance to the case, whereas discovery is the act of obtaining new evidence or expanding upon what is already known to a party through disclosure (Dunn, 2014).

Initial Disclosures

In general, initial disclosures begin with the parties providing known and relevant information concerning the matter in controversy to other parties in the action (Dunn, 2014). During the initial disclosure phase, unless otherwise stipulated or ordered by the court, a party must, without awaiting a discovery request, provide to the other parties certain information:

1. The name and, if known, the address and telephone number of each individual likely to have discoverable information—along with the subjects of that information—that the disclosing party may use to support its claims or defenses, unless the use would be solely for impeachment.
2. A copy or a description by category and location of all documents, electronically stored information, and tangible things that the disclosing party has in its possession, custody, or control and may use to support its claims or defenses, unless the use would be solely for impeachment.
3. A computation of each category of damages claimed by the disclosing party who must also make available for inspection and copying the documents or other evidentiary material, unless privileged or protected from disclosure, on which each computation is based, including materials bearing on the nature and extent of injuries suffered.
4. Any insurance agreements under which an insurance business may be liable to satisfy all or part of a possible judgment in the action or to indemnify or reimburse for payments made to satisfy the judgment (The Committee of the Judiciary, 2020b, § 26(a)(1)(A)).

Parties are expected to make these initial disclosures quickly and cannot claim excuses such as failure to properly investigate or a failure of other parties to fully disclose (Dunn, 2014). For initial disclosures, a party must make the required disclosures at or within 14 days following the discovery, planning conference unless a different time is set by stipulation or court order, or unless a party objects during the conference that initial disclosures are not appropriate in this action and states the objection in the proposed discovery plan (The Committee of the Judiciary, 2020b, § 26(a)(1)(C)). For parties who were served or joined after the discovery planning conference, they are required to make their initial disclosures within 30 days after being served or joined, unless a different time frame is set by stipulation or court order (The Committee of the The Committee of the Judiciary, 2020b, § 26(a)(1)(D)).

The rules of civil procedure, require that a party make its initial disclosures based on the information that is reasonably available. A party is not excused from making its disclosures because of a claim it has not fully investigated the case or because it challenges the sufficiency of another party's disclosures or because another party has not made its disclosures (The Committee of the Judiciary, 2020b, § 26(a)(1)(E)).

Expert Disclosures

Disclosure of expert witness testimony is guided by a separate set of disclosure rules. In addition to the initial disclosures, a party must also disclose to the other parties the identity of any witness it may use at trial to present evidence under the Federal Rules of Evidence (The Committee on the Judiciary, 2020a), rules 702, 703, or 705 (The Committee of the Judiciary, 2020b, § 26(a)(2)(A)). Unless otherwise stipulated or ordered by the court, this disclosure must be accompanied by a written report prepared and signed by the witness, provided the witness has been retained or specially employed to provide expert testimony in the case or one whose duties regularly involve providing expert testimony (The Committee of the Judiciary, 2020b, § 26(a)(2)(B)). Disclosure of an expert report must contain the following:

1. A complete statement of all opinions the witness will express and the basis and reasons for them;
2. The facts or data considered by the witness in forming their opinions;
3. Any exhibits that will be used to summarize or support their opinions;
4. The witness's qualifications, including a list of all publications authored in the previous 10 years;
5. A list of all other cases in which, during the previous 4 years, the witness testified as an expert at trial or by deposition; and
6. A statement of the compensation to be paid for the study and testimony in the case (The Committee of the Judiciary, 2020b, § 26(a)(2)(B).

For a life care planner, much of the information required to be produced as part of the expert disclosures can be satisfied by the production of the life care plan and accompanying narrative report; attachment of the life care planner's billing statement or invoice; and attachment of the life care planner's current curriculum vita.

Pre-Trial Disclosures

In addition to the initial and expert disclosures, parties are also required to provide pre-trial disclosures at least 30 days prior to trial (The Committee of the Judiciary, 2020b, § 26(a)(3)(B)). Pre-trial disclosures require the parties to disclose evidence they may present at trial other than solely for impeachment. Pre-trial disclosure must contain the following:

1. The name and, if not previously provided, the address and telephone number of each witness—separately identifying those the party expects to present and those it may call if the need arises;
2. The designation of those witnesses whose testimony the party expects to present by deposition and, if not taken stenographically, a transcript of the pertinent parts of the deposition; and
3. An identification of each document or other exhibit, including summaries of other evidence—separately identifying those items the party expects to offer and those it may offer if the need arises (The Committee of the Judiciary, 2020b, § 26(a)(3)(A)).

Discovery

Before the Federal Rules of Civil Procedure were adopted in 1938, a plaintiff was essentially required to "prove their case" before filing a civil suit (Cornell School of Law, n.d., discovery). However, the adoption of the Federal Rules of Civil Procedure changed this requirement. Under the current rules, plaintiffs who strongly suspect they were wronged can file a lawsuit, even if they do not have solid evidence (Cornell School of Law, n.d., discovery). During discovery, a plaintiff can force the defendant to disclose to them evidence that can be used to build their case, essentially using the pre-trial discovery process to gather information in preparation for trial (Cornell School of Law, n.d., discovery).

The process of discovery seeks to expand upon previously disclosed information or identify new relevant information of value to the plaintiff in pushing forward a claim or assisting the defendant in defending a claim (Dunn, 2014). The parties involved meet to discuss the need for and rationale for discovery and develop a proposed discovery plan (The Committee of the Judiciary, 2020b, § 26(f)(2)). Despite the usually broad manner in which discovery is pursued, some information is excluded from being discoverable as it is privileged. Information deemed privileged cannot be inquired into in any way (Cornell School of Law, n.d., privilege) as it cannot be asked about in testimony. Information considered privileged includes confidential conversations between an attorney and their client, such as the attorney's thoughts on case strategy, theory, and trial preparation tactics (Dunn, 2014). A second exception to the discovery process is information covered under the work product doctrine (Dunn, 2014). Attorney work product doctrine is a form of privilege that permits attorneys to withhold documents or other tangible materials prepared in anticipation of litigation by or for another party or its representative (The Committee of the Judiciary, 2020b, § 26(b)(3)). As with attorney-client privilege, work product privilege does not protect the underlying facts of a case, and in fact, work product privilege may be overcome if there is a substantial need for materials to prepare the case and the opposing party cannot reasonably obtain their substantial equivalent materials by any other means (Cornell School of Law, n.d., attorney work product privilege). As an example, a life care planner may be asked to review an opposing life care plan and to prepare a report or memorandum in preparation for a pending trial, rather than for use at trial. In such a case, the life care planning expert may not be disclosed to the court and their opinions thus are not discoverable nor usable at trial. In some circumstances, a party to the discovery process may believe that a request for information is inappropriate due to privilege. In such cases, the party claiming privilege can request the court grant a protective order that prevents the discovery of all, or part of the information requested (Dunn, 2014). However, such a request for a protective order may be denied by the court and in such an instance, compel the party to comply with the discovery request (Dunn, 2014).

The process by which discovery proceeds may take many different forms. One of the most common discovery tools is the deposition (Dunn, 2014). A deposition is a witness's sworn out-of-court testimony used to "discover" information and in some circumstances may be used at trial (Cornell School of Law, n.d., deposition). The witness whose sworn testimony is the subject of the deposition is referred to as the deponent (Cornell School of Law, n.d., deposition). Generally, depositions do not directly involve the court but are instead initiated and supervised by parties representing the plaintiff and defense in a matter. Generally, the only persons present at a deposition are the deponent, attorneys for all interested parties, a person qualified to administer oaths, and in most cases a stenographer to document the testimony (Cornell School of Law, n.d., deposition). Deposition testimony is usually considered to be hearsay and is thus generally inadmissible at trial with three exceptions (Cornell School of Law, n.d., deposition): (1) when a party admits something in a deposition that is against their interest; (2) when a witness's testimony at trial contradicts their deposition testimony; (3) when a witness is unavailable to provide live testimony at trial (The Committee of the Judiciary, 2020b, § 32).

In completing a deposition, the deponent is placed under oath and provides testimony under penalty of perjury (Dunn, 2014). Questions posed to the deponent may be objected to by a party, but the deponent must answer the question (unless directed not to answer due to an issue related to legal privilege). If necessary, the court will later consider any objections posed during the deposition, and if necessary, redact any witness answers to which the objection is sustained by the court (The Committee of the Judiciary, 2020b § 30(c)(2)).

Following completion of a deposition, the deponent will be given the opportunity to either read and make corrections to their testimony or waive this right. In its simplest function, the deposition gives the opposing party the opportunity to explore and memorialize in writing, the life care planner's opinions and thoughts as they relate to the scope of expert disclosure in a matter. If a case is not resolved prior to the scheduled trial, the life care planner may very likely be called to testify at trial. In this circumstance, it is imperative that the life care planner not deviate from testimony elicited through deposition testimony. Such deviation at trial from deposition testimony opens the witness up to potential impeachment, thus compromising the witness's credibility to the court. If the deponent is expected to produce documents as part of the deposition, the deponent will be served with a subpoena duces tecum, that lists the scope of documents to be produced by the deponent (The Committee of the Judiciary, 2020b § 30(b)(2)).

Pre-Trial Conferences and Dismissals

By the conclusion of the disclosure and discovery process, pertinent issues related to the points of contention should be well-defined for the court (Dunn, 2014). In any action, the court is likely to compel the attorneys and any unrepresented parties to attend a pre-trial conference to discuss a broad range of issues for such purposes as: (1) expediting disposition of the action; (2) establishing early and continuing control so the case will not be protracted because of lack of management; (3) discouraging wasteful pre-trial activities; (4) improving the quality of the trial through more thorough preparation; and (5) facilitating settlement (The Committee of the Judiciary, 2020b § 16(a)).

In lieu of proceeding to trial, multiple alternative resolution mechanisms exist. One or the other party may file a motion to dismiss the case entirely (The Committee of the Judiciary, 2020b § 12(b)) by filing a motion for judgment on the pleadings, a motion for default judgment, a motion for voluntary or involuntary dismissal, or settlement (Dunn, 2014). If, after all, other methods of having the matter dismissed are unsuccessful, the one final alternative to achieve case resolution prior to going to trial, is a motion for summary judgment (Dunn, 2014). A motion for summary judgment is a motion asking the court to rule on at least one claim comprising the issues in contention. A party may move for summary judgment, identifying each claim or defense—or the part of each claim or defense—on which summary judgment is sought (The Committee of the Judiciary, 2020b § 56(a)). If the motion is granted by the court, a decision is made on at least one element of the claim without holding a trial. Typically, the motion must show that no genuine issue of material fact exists, and that the opposing party loses on that claim even if all its allegations are accepted as true (Cornell School of Law, n.d., motion for summary judgment).

The Trial

Once a matter or claim(s) has been found to have merit, it proceeds to trial. Civil trials must be by jury unless: (1) the parties or their attorneys file a stipulation to a nonjury trial or so stipulate on the record; or (2) the court, on motion or on its own, finds that on some or all of the issues, there is no federal right to a jury trial (The Committee of the Judiciary, 2020b § 39(a)(1-2)). The trial process begins with the selection of a jury from a potential jury pool that has been randomly selected from the community where the trial will occur. Jury selection involves summoning, questioning, and selecting jurors to serve on a jury for a particular trial (Cornell School of Law, n.d., jury selection). The jury pool is then randomly divided into smaller jury panels and assigned to different courtrooms to potentially serve on juries for trials beginning that week. Before potential jurors begin to be questioned, the judge presiding over the trial will introduce to the panel the type of case to be tried (Cornell School of Law, n.d., jury selection). Prospective jurors are placed under oath and questioned and challenged by judges and lawyers on both sides of the case to determine if they can decide the case impartially. This process of questioning is called voir dire, meaning to speak the truth (Cornell School of Law, n.d., jury selection). Questions concerning the suitability of jurors typically involve inquiry as to whether they have any information about the case, if they are related to a party in the trial, or whether their prior experiences might make them prejudiced (Cornell School of Law, n.d., jury selection). A prospective juror will be excluded if a lawyer can show to the judge that they may act unfairly or in a prejudicial manner at trial. Parties have a limited number of peremptory challenges that result in the exclusion of a potential juror without the need to provide a reason or explanation—unless the opposing party can demonstrate the challenge was used to discriminate on the basis of race, ethnicity, or sex (Cornell School of Law, n.d., peremptory challenge). Once jurors to be seated in a trial have been decided, the jury panel is sworn in to try the case, while those not selected to serve on the jury are sent home (Cornell School of Law, n.d., peremptory challenge). In Federal cases, a jury must be comprised of at least six members, but no more than twelve members (The Committee of the Judiciary, 2020b § 48(a)).

Once seated, the jury determines the answers to questions of fact presented in the trial—the jury become the *triers of fact* (Cornell School of Law, n.d.ee, trier of fact). Evidence presented in a trial is done so in accordance with the Federal Rules of Evidence, with the credibility, weight, and impact of the evidence solely up to the discretion of the jury (Dunn, 2014). Judges, on the other hand, make determinations on the admissibility of evidence and manage the trial from beginning to end (Dunn, 2014). The trial then proceeds through a standard process with the presentation of the plaintiff's case, followed by the presentation of the defendant's defenses (Dunn, 2014). The plaintiff will begin the trial with an opening statement, which is their first opportunity to address the jury directly (Cornell School of Law, n.d., opening statement). The opening statement is not evidence itself (Dunn, 2014), but is intended to provide jurors a preview of the case by describing the nature of the issue(s) in dispute, providing an overview of the facts and evidence, and providing context to frame the evidence in a light that is favorable to their client's case (Cornell School of Law, n.d., opening statement). The defendant may also make an opening statement after the plaintiff but may also choose to wait until the beginning of the presentation of their case (Dunn, 2014). Following opening statements by the parties, the plaintiff begins presenting the evidence that will serve as proof of their claim. The introduction of evidence is generally accomplished through the examination of witnesses who have been disclosed during pre-trial discovery (Dunn, 2014). The initial examination of plaintiff witnesses is referred to as direct examination, which is then followed by cross-examination by the opposing party. The process of direct and cross then repeats sequentially until the parties have no additional questions. According to Dunn (2014, p. 257):

> Cross-examinations are limited to those matters raised as part of the direct examination. Redirect and Recross examinations are limited to the matters raised in subsequent

rounds of questioning, narrowing the scope of the examination until eventually the potential avenues of questioning by both parties is exhausted.

Following the completion of the plaintiff's case, the defendants may immediately move for a directed verdict (Dunn, 2014). A directed verdict is a ruling issued by the trial judge on an issue where the court finds that a reasonable jury would not have a legally sufficient evidentiary basis to find for the plaintiff on that issue (The Committee of the The Committee of the Judiciary, 2020b § 50(1)). In the case of a directed verdict, the court may resolve the issue against the party; and grant the motion for judgment as a matter of law against the party on a claim or defense that, under the controlling law, can be maintained or defeated only with a favorable finding on that issue (The Committee of the Judiciary, 2020b § 50(a-b)). A directed verdict may be granted at any time but usually occurs after at least one party has fully presented their case to the jury (Cornell School of Law, n.d.o, directed verdict). When all evidence has been presented by the parties, and motions for directed verdicts denied, the process moves on to closing arguments (Dunn, 2014). Closing arguments occur after all evidence has been presented and both sides have rested their cases. Closing arguments can be very impactful since it is the last thing the jury will hear. The closing argument is each party's final opportunity to tell the judge and/or jury why they should prevail in the case. The parties explain how the evidence supports the theory of their case and clarifies for the jury the issues they must resolve to ultimately render a verdict (Cornell School of Law, n.d.i, closing argument). During closing arguments, the parties may comment on the evidence that has been presented, but they are not allowed to submit new information as part of the closing argument. Upon completion of closing arguments, the judge will then charge the jury and have them *retire* to consider the composite of the evidence and arrive ultimately at a verdict on the issues in dispute (Dunn, 2014).

It is also the judge's role to provide instructions to the jury on the definition and/or meaning of laws influencing the matter at hand and ultimately, the jury's ability to interpret and find meaning from the evidence presented. At the conclusion of the trial, the parties will propose to the judge a set of jury instructions, often seeking specific phrasing that is advantageous to their client (Cornell School of Law, n.d., jury instructions). Ultimately, the judge will formulate a set of literal written instructions for jury deliberation (Cornell School of Law, n.d., jury instructions). Jury instructions are the only guidance that the jury should receive when deliberating and are meant to keep the jury on track regarding the basic procedure of the deliberation and the substance of the law on which their decision must be based (Cornell School of Law, n.d., jury instructions). Jury instructions should ideally be brief, concise, nonrepetitive, relevant to the details of the case, understandable to the average juror, and should correctly state the law without misleading the jury or inviting unnecessary speculation (Cornell School of Law, n.d., jury instructions).

Verdict and Judgment

A jury's findings or conclusions on the factual issues presented in a matter are referred to as a verdict (Cornell School of Law, n.d., verdict). Based upon the jury's verdict, a judgment then is a court order that determines each party's rights and obligations with respect to the issues in dispute (Cornell School of Law, n.d., judgment). Whether an order counts as a judgment often determines whether it can be immediately appealed to a higher court. In formulating a judgment, the judge may request the jury provide either a general verdict or a special verdict (Dunn, 2014). For a general verdict, the court may submit to the jury forms, together with written questions on one or more issues of fact that the jury must decide. The court must be given the instructions and explanations necessary to enable the jury to render a general verdict and answer the questions in writing (The

Committee of the The Committee of the Judiciary, 2020b § 49(b)). In a special verdict, the court may require a jury to return only a special verdict in the form of a special written finding on each issue of fact (The Committee of the Judiciary, 2020b § 49(a)). The court may do so by:

> Submitting written questions susceptible of a categorical or other brief answer; by submitting written forms of the special findings that might properly be made under the pleadings and evidence; or by using any other method that the court considers appropriate" (The Committee of the Judiciary, 2020b §49(a)(1)(a-c)).

Once the special verdict is known, the judge then decides the questions the jury should answer, and the judge draws legal implications from the jury's answers (Cornell School of Law, n.d., special verdict). In the process of deliberating, the jury must find that one party or the other is more likely to be correct in their case theory and assertions by considering the preponderance of the evidence (Dunn, 2014). According to Dunn (2014, p. 257):

> Preponderance of the evidence may be thought of as finding one party to be more than fifty percent likely to have the more valid claim. Some actions in court require a higher standard, clear and convincing evidence, which means that a party's cause is not merely more than likely, but probable. The highest standard, beyond a reasonable doubt, is preserved for criminal causes of action.

In Federal court, jury verdicts must be unanimous, which is a significant element of deviation from some state court systems which permit majority verdicts rather than unanimous verdicts in some settings (Dunn, 2014).

Even after the reading of the judgment by the jury, the parties still have the right to once again introduce a motion for a new trial as a matter of law (Dunn, 2014). Dunn (2014, p. 257) stated:

> The judge in the case, on considering the matter, may grant such relief when, in their judgment, no reasonable jury could have reached the conclusions that they did. The judge may also grant a dismissal and order a new trial on the issue. In this role, the judge is sometimes referred to as a "13th juror," with a veto power over the jury in a civil action.

On occasion, a trial court will issue an order in response to an excessive damage award by the jury. Such an order, referred to as a remittitur, gives the plaintiff the option to accept a reduced damage award or the court may order a new trial (Cornell School of Law, n.d., remittitur). The purpose of a remittitur is to give a trial court the ability, with the plaintiff's consent, to correct an inequitable damage award or verdict without having to order a new trial. Prior to granting a remittitur, specific criteria must be met that include: (1) unliquidated damages are assessed by a jury; (2) the verdict is not influenced by passion or prejudice; (3) the award is excessive; and (4) the plaintiff agrees to the reduction in damages (Cornell School of Law, n.d., remittitur).

Relief and Appeals

Following the court entering a judgment following trial, in certain circumstances, a party may seek relief from the court (Dunn, 2014). Requests for relief from judgment must be made within a reasonable time, but not more than one year after the entry of the judgment or order or the date of the proceeding (The Committee of the Judiciary, 2020b, § 60(c)(1)). Once a judgment is entered by the court, the court must next enforce its order of judgment by permitting the plaintiff to acquire property they are due from the defendant (Dunn, 2014). There are primarily four ways the court may satisfy a judgment that include attachment, garnishment, replevin, and sequestration (Dunn, 2014). An attachment is an order by the court seizing specific property and is used both as a pre-trial provisional remedy and to enforce a final judgment and prevent it from being otherwise disposed of (Cornell School of Law, n.d., attachment). Garnishment is a legal process that allows a third party to seize the assets of a debtor, such as acquiring the wages of a debtor through the debtor's employer (Cornell School of Law, n.d., garnish). Replevin is an action seeking to return the personal property of the plaintiff that was wrongfully taken or held by the defendant. For example, a bank may file a replevin action against a borrower to repossess a car after he/she missed too many payments on (Cornell School of Law, n.d., replevin). Last, sequestration involves the process of removing property from its possessor, pending the outcome of a judicial dispute between multiple parties who claim ownership of the same property (Cornell School of Law, n.d., sequestration).

An appeal is a challenge to a previous legal determination and is generally directed towards a legal power that is higher than the court making the challenged determination. In most states and in the federal system, trial court determinations can be appealed in an appellate court. An appellate court is a higher court that reviews the decision of a lower court when a losing party files an appeal (Cornell School of Law, n.d., appellate court). The rulings of appellate courts may be reviewed by a court of last resort, which in the federal court system, is the United States Supreme Court. The party or person pursuing an appeal is called an appellant, while the party or person defending the lower court's ruling is the appellee or respondent (Cornell School of Law, n.d., appeal). Courts of appeals do not gather new evidence in a matter but review the record of the trial court in determining whether a matter should be reconsidered (Dunn, 2014). The appellate court may apply one of three standards in conducting their review (Dunn, 2014). First is a *de novo* review, wherein the court is deciding the issues without reference to any legal conclusion or assumption made by the previous court to hear the case (Cornell School of Law, n.d., de novo). An appellate court hearing a case *de novo* may refer to the lower court's record to determine the facts, but will rule on the evidence and matters of law without deferring to that court's findings (Cornell School of Law, n.d., de novo). The next type of appellate review is a review for clear error and is the standard of review in civil appellate proceedings when a finding is "clearly erroneous" and there is evidence to support the error (Cornell School of Law, n.d., clearly erroneous). Lastly, an appellate court may review a decision for a judicial abuse of discretion (Dunn, 2014). An abuse of discretion standard is used when a lower court has made a discretionary ruling, and if challenged on appeal, the appellate court will use the abuse of discretion standard to review the ruling to determine if an error was made (Cornell School of Law, n.d., abuse of discretion). An abuse of discretion standard is considered when a judge has properly applied the law, but when there may be no rational basis for the decision that was made by the lower court (Dunn, 2014). For the majority of cases, an appeal to the appellate level will be the end of the appeals process, unless it is accepted by the Supreme Court (Dunn, 2014).

Types of Experts in Life Care Planning

Within the legal environment, experts occupy a unique position and role. As expert life care planners, we serve as tutors and/or educators in the life care planning process to evaluate the existing evidence, develop new evidence related to future care needs, and develop opinions related to these analyses (Field, 2013). There are generally three types of experts which include consulting experts, testifying experts, and court-appointed experts (Sunday & Kennedy Arnold, 2011). During the initial contact with the retaining attorney, it is vital that the life care planner clearly determine which of these expert roles they will be expected to fulfill in the course of their engagement. In the role of a consulting expert, the life care planner may not be disclosed to the opposing parties. In this role, the life care planner may be retained to educate the attorney on pre-suit life care planning issues and expectations or to critique the work of other life care planning experts, if such work has already been produced. Generally, the existence of the non-disclosed consulting life care planner and any of the work product produced, will not be known by the court or the opposing attorney—this is purely a behind-the-scenes role (Heitzman et al., 2014). Non-disclosed consulting experts render their opinions only to those who hire them. Life care planners may also be retained as disclosed or testifying experts by a party engaged in the litigation to develop independent opinions and provide sworn testimony at a deposition and/or trial (Sunday & Kennedy Arnold, 2011). Occasionally, a judge presiding over a matter may retain a life care planner as a neutral, court-appointed expert on issues related to life care planning (Sunday & Kennedy Arnold, 2011).

As a discipline, life care planning is a transdisciplinary specialty practice (Mauk, 2019; Weed & Berens, 2018). To even be considered for certification as a life care planner, a practitioner should meet the basic professional qualifications of at least one of just a few credentialing bodies. The International Commission on Healthcare Certification (ICHCC™) states "Qualifying for the Certified Life Care Planner credential is based upon two factors; 1) meeting the definition of a "Qualified Healthcare Provider, and 2) the applicant's education and training" (ICHCC™, n.d.). According to the ICHCC (2021), this designation of qualified healthcare professional is based on a background of education, training, and practice qualifications. A background of only experience and/or designated job title is not accepted as defining a qualified healthcare professional. Completion of training in the respective credential's focus area, experience, or being qualified in the court system as an expert witness do not necessarily meet the definition of a qualified healthcare professional under the ICHCC™ standards. This definition can only be met when all educational, training, and practice qualification components are reviewed and met (p. 11).

Other certification boards have evolved to offer life care planning certification to specific professional specialties within the healthcare field, such as the Certified Nurse Life Care Planner (CNLCP®) provided through the Certified Nurse Life Care Planner Certification Board. For certification as a CNLCP®, the board requires the following:

> Provision of proof of valid Registered Nurse licensure or its equivalent in other countries, for at least the prior three (3) years immediately preceding application. The license must be active, without any restrictions, and a current copy of the license must be submitted with the Candidate's application (Certified Nurse Life Care Planner Certification Board, n.d., para. 3).

Most recently, the credential of Certified Physician Life Care Planner (CPLCP™) has been offered through the Certified Physician Life Care Planner Certification Board. The basic qualification requirements to qualify to take the CPLCP™ certification examination include the following:

1. Be licensed as a Medical Doctor (MD), or Doctor of Osteopathic Medicine (DO) in the United States, or the equivalent in other countries, for at least 3 years following the completion of residency. Any license must be currently active, without any restrictions;

2. Be Board Certified in Physical Medicine & Rehabilitation (Physiatry) as designated by the American Board of Physical Medicine & Rehabilitation (ABPMR), or by the American Osteopathic Board of Physical Medicine & Rehabilitation (AOBPMR);
3. Be a Certified Life Care Planner (CLCP™), as designated by the International Commission on Health Care Certification (ICHCC™) (Certified Physician Life Care Planner Certification Board, n.d., para. 3).

For the past 30 years, approximately every decade, Neulicht has conducted life care planning surveys to evaluate processes, methods, and protocols utilized in the area of life care planning (Neulicht et al., 2010). The most recent survey, completed in 2009, found that approximately 47% of survey respondents identified nursing as their primary healthcare profession, while an additional approximately 37% identified rehabilitation counseling as their primary healthcare profession (Neulicht et al., 2010). Neulicht et al. are currently in the process of updating the life care planning survey, with the results likely to be released in 2023. It is likely that this updated survey will reflect a much broader range of healthcare disciplines prominently represented in the life care planning community including occupational therapists, physical therapists, speech-language therapists, psychologists, and physicians. Regardless of professional discipline, life care planners work within their specific standards and scope of professional practice for their discipline to ensure accountability, responsibility, and professional standards for which they are accountable (Johnson & Weed, 2013; Mauk, 2019). For further discussion of the scope of practice for life care planners from various professional disciplines, the reader is referred to Issue 17(1) of the *Journal of Life Care Planning*—a special edition dedicated to this topic.

Qualifications

The scope of practice for each individual life care planner rests upon the individual's knowledge, educational, and work-related experience stemming not only from their training in the field of life care planning but, more importantly, within the field that qualifies them as a healthcare practitioner (Sunday & Kennedy-Arnold, 2011). Presently, life care planners are not required to be licensed as a life care planner, however, are required to hold a professional license or board certification in the primary practice area that qualifies the individual as a qualified healthcare professional (Sunday & Kennedy-Arnold, 2011). No one specific healthcare discipline qualifies a life care planner to render recommendations across the entire healthcare or rehabilitation continuum of care. Because the specialty practice of life care planning is truly transdisciplinary, it necessarily draws upon the collective expertise of professionals from many healthcare and related supportive disciplines.

While it is important that a life care planner be knowledgeable of various healthcare systems, including billing and coding systems, it is even more important for the life care planner to be familiar with the role and function of the various healthcare professionals within the healthcare and rehabilitation systems. Consultation with other healthcare professionals involved in the evaluee's care and treatment is necessary when developing a life care plan that includes recommendations that are outside the professional scope of practice of the retained life care planner. Further, while consultation with other healthcare professionals is a necessary element in a transdisciplinary life care planning process, the life care planners' qualifications, and professional experience also serve to define the types of cases, a life care planner may choose to accept. Life care planners must consider their own individual qualifications and experiences to effectively evaluate their personal competency to appreciate the unique elements of a particular life care planning case (Sunday & Kennedy-Arnold, 2011).

Retention: Expert versus Clinical Practice

Nearly 30 years ago, Blackwell et al. (1994) dispelled the notion that experts are advocates in the role they fulfill within the legal system—instead, acknowledging that the attorney's engaging the services of an expert are the advocates within a legal setting. Blackwell et al. (1994, p. 103) opined that retained experts are "advocates for their knowledge. Objectivity and independence are never static. These qualities evolve with the constant assessment of [the evaluees'] needs and public responsibility." This expectation of neutrality often places the life care planner at odds with a legal system that expects and challenges the retained expert to carry favor toward the party retaining him/her and ultimately paying the bill for services (Barros-Bailey & Carlisle, 2014). Given this often unspoken expectation of retaining attorneys, an inexperienced expert may be placed into the unenviable position of feeling pressured or tempted to alter their professional methodology to ultimately support a favorable conclusion for the retaining attorney—thus demonstrating significant role confusion by the expert. Although specifically addressing vocational issues, the same concerns offered by Woodrich and Patterson (2003) are applicable to life care planners. Woodrich and Patterson (2003) opined that role confusion can result in compromised ethical behavior, such as the temptation to be pulled away from a position of a neutral educator and more toward a biased advocate.

The expectation that a retained expert will be partial to the retaining party extends beyond the expert. Rule 3.4(b) of the Model Rules of Professional Conduct (2019)—published by the American Bar Association (ABA—states "A lawyer shall not ... falsify evidence, counsel or assist a witness to testify falsely, or offer an inducement to a witness that is prohibited by law." Clearly, the ABA expects that attorneys will not exert influence over witnesses through inducements to promote false or misleading testimony on behalf of the clients. Objectivity and impartiality of retained experts, including life care planners, have been expected in the code of ethics and rules of professional conduct for healthcare professionals and attorneys alike for some time (Barros-Bailey & Carlisle, 2014). Ultimately, this theme in forensic applications addresses the common ethical principle of justice and clearly is equally expected of the retained expert and the attorney hiring the expert (Barros-Bailey & Carlisle, 2014).

Methodology: The Standard for Opinions

In developing opinions, whether as a disclosed testifying life care planner or as an undisclosed consulting life care planner, it is vital that the life care planner follow published and generally accepted life care planning methodology. Deviation from accepted life care planning methodology can ultimately result in the life care planner's testimony being limited or altogether excluded. Any deviations from accepted life care planning methodology need to have a clear rationale and be well documented but even then, such deviations may become the subject of opposing counsel's motion to limit or exclude (Sunday & Kennedy-Arnold, 2011).

Rule 702 of the current (2020) Federal Rules of Evidence clearly articulates the evidentiary bar by which an expert witness's testimony is measured and evaluated. Any witness presented as serving in the role of an expert by way of knowledge, skill, experience, training, or education may testify in the form of an opinion or otherwise, if four prongs are satisfied. First, the expert's scientific, technical, or other specialized knowledge will help the trier of fact to understand the evidence or to determine a fact in issue (Rule 702(a)). This is the educational role wherein the life care planner is expected to assist the trier of fact (either a judge or jury or both) to understand the life care planning issues relevant to the case. Second, the expert's testimony is based on sufficient facts or data (Rule

702(b)). For the second prong of the admissibility test, the court is evaluating the foundation of facts and data considered by the life care planner in arriving at their ultimate opinions. For example, a life care plan recommending regular opiate monitoring in a case where opiate medication is not recommended would likely be questioned because of insufficient facts and/or data. For the third prong of the admissibility test, the court is evaluating whether the testimony is the product of reliable principles and methods (Rule 702(c)). This prong requires that the life care planner adhere to the generally accepted principles and methods of their healthcare discipline and of the specialty practice area of life care planning. Earlier, the importance of the life care planner clearly documenting the need and rationale for any deviations from generally accepted life care planning principles and methods was discussed. Even documenting a clear rationale for deviating from accepted principles and methods does not ensure that the life care planner will prevail should a motion to limit or exclude their testimony be introduced to the court. Lastly, the fourth prong of the admissibility test examines whether the expert has reliably applied the principles and methods to the facts of the case (Rule 702(d)). This prong is examining facts evaluated in the second prong as being reliably applied within the methods described in the third prong of admissibility. As an example, if a life care planner failed to consult with other medical experts for the foundation of life care plan recommendations, and personally provided all recommendations within the plan (across multiple professional disciplines), then they have likely failed to apply one of the most basic tenets of life care planning which is to consult with necessary allied healthcare providers in a transdisciplinary manner.

Often, deviation from the accepted methodology is outside of the control of the life care planner. A common example is when one party denies permission for the opposing party to meet with the plaintiff to discuss their injuries and treatments. In such deviations, the life care planner should document such positions in the case file in the event the same counsel who prevented an in-person meeting, also attempts to exclude the expert for deviating from the generally accepted methodology.

Currently, there is a movement within the federal judiciary's Advisory Committee on Evidence Rules to amend Rule 702 of the Federal Rules of Evidence as described above. As of February 2022, the comment period for the amendment to the Federal Rules of Evidence on expert testimony closed, and it is expected that the changes will be approved by the Supreme Court and take effect in December 2023 (Bernard, 2022). The proposed changes will clarify and emphasize that ultimate admissibility as set forth in the rule must be established to the court by a "preponderance of the evidence" (Behrens & Jackson, 2021). Currently, Rule 702 (which has been in effect since 2000) does not explicitly include the preponderance of the evidence standard. The Advisory Committee noted that, since 2000, when the current rules were published, "the admissibility of all expert testimony is governed by the principles of Rule 104(a)," under which "the proponent has the burden of establishing that the pertinent admissibility requirements are met by a preponderance of the evidence" (Behrens & Jackson, 2021, para. 2). Drawing from this rule, the Advisory Committee concluded "many courts" have incorrectly applied both Rule 702 and 104(a) by interpreting that "the critical questions of the sufficiency of an expert's basis, and the application of the expert's methodology, are questions of weight and not admissibility" (Behrens & Jackson, 2021, para. 2). The proposed changes to Rule 702 requires the proponent of the expert testimony to show admissibility by a preponderance of the evidence, and further to show the expert's opinion is reliable in light of the facts and applicable principles or methodology (Bernard, 2022).

Report Writing: Consensus Statement and Standards

In documenting life care planning opinions and/or developing the life care plan or narrative report, it is important for the life care planner to be cognizant of the evidentiary demands described in the

Federal Rules of Evidence as described in the previous section. The current rules for the admissibility of expert witness testimony grew in part from the 1993 hallmark case of *Daubert v. Merrell Dow Pharmaceuticals*, otherwise referred to by many experts as the *Daubert* decision (Weed, 2018b). This Federal ruling inferred that any testimony in a Federal court offered by a scientific expert must be founded on a methodology or underlying scientific reasoning that is scientifically valid and can be properly applied to the facts of the case at hand (Field, 2018). The criteria for admission of expert witness testimony in Federal cases have been highly influenced not only by the *Daubert* decision, but also through the subsequent decisions of *General Electric Co. v. Joiner* in 1996, and *Kuhmo Tire Co. v. Carmichael* in 1999. This trio of U.S. Supreme Court decisions regarding the admissibility of expert witness testimony are jointly referred to as the "*Daubert* Trilogy" (Field, 2018, p. 820) and have jointly made a significant impact on the parameters within which expert testimony, opinions, and conclusions must comport.

As a life care planner develops a life care plan, it is paramount they remember that the plan is, first and foremost, a dynamic multidisciplinary case management tool that is based upon the actual needs of the individual who is the focus of the plan (Pomeranz & Shaw, 2006). A plan that fails to satisfy this most basic element, such as not being transdisciplinary, or representing needs that are improbable or just possible as being necessary, will likely be met with abundant critique within a forensic venue. A well-designed life care plan can best be viewed as a "roadmap" for a case manager, family member, or even the evaluee to be able to implement the recommendations of the plan over the person's life expectancy (Pomeranz & Shaw, 2006). To achieve this goal, the life care planner should utilize a systematic and coordinated approach that maximizes the evaluee's potential, attempts to prevent future complications, and sustains or enhances the evaluee's quality of life (Pomeranz et al., 2014).

In the course of developing the life care plan, it is paramount that the life care planner works collaboratively with other professionals involved in the evaluee's care and treatment, as well as the evaluee, and their family members, as necessary. Other professionals involved in contributing recommendations to a life care plan will vary by the nature and needs of each case. Other involved healthcare professionals often include physicians, nurses, psychologists, physical therapists, occupational therapists, and vocational rehabilitation counselors. Pomeranz et al., 2014, p. 393) opined that "Collaboration between the life care planner and these allied health care professionals is a hallmark feature of a comprehensive LCP." Regardless of the discipline from which the life care planner comes (e.g., rehabilitation counseling, nursing, medicine), it is critical that they recognize that because the life care plan is, by definition, transdisciplinary, many sections of the plan are likely to be outside of their scope of practice or professional expertise (Pomeranz et al., 2014). It is in these areas, where the life care planner is most susceptible to critique if they fail to appropriately consult with allied health care professionals.

Despite the high degree of variability of the types of cases a life care planner is typically involved in, the process and methodology undertaken must be consistent within the generally accepted principles and methods utilized in the field of life care planning. Over time, what is generally accepted evolves, so it is critical that the life care planner evolve with the literature and case law within the jurisdiction where they practice. A good example of this evolution of methodology is presented by the current state of the Collateral Source Rule. The Collateral Source Rule is a long-standing legal doctrine that holds that if an injured party receives compensation for injuries incurred from a source independent of the person responsible for the injuries, those payments are not deducted from the damage award (Stern & Owen, 2022). Recently, this doctrine has begun to be challenged across the country leading to significant variability in how this doctrine is applied from state to state (Stern & Owen, 2022). To sufficiently address this issue, Stern and

Owen (2022, p. 35) made specific recommendations regarding how the life care planner can best address these evolving issues, which included consulting life care planning guiding documents such as standards of practice (International Academy of Life Care Planners, 2022); reading previously published materials on the Collateral Source Rule (Field et al., 2015) using usual, customary and reasonable pricing; inquiring about previous court decisions related to life care planning issues; and understanding the individual approach of the court where each life care plan is prepared.

It is likely that since this issue remains unsettled, variations in how courts address the Collateral Source Rule will likely influence how a life care planner's testimony is received by the courts. While staying abreast of these types of evolving issues within the field of life care planning is crucial, it is just as critical that in these gray areas, unless the courts have clearly provided direction, the life care planner remains in alignment with the life care planning literature, on issues, such as costing, where the consensus of life care planners has been to use "Non-discounted/market rate prices" (Johnson et al., 2018, p. 17).

Similar guidance on a range of issues related to the specialty practice of life care planning is provided in Consensus and Majority Statements (Johnson et al., 2018) derived from nine separate life care planning summits held between 2000 and 2017 and updated in 2018. The most recent summit was held in 2022, but the results have not yet reached publication as of the date of this writing. To date, these summits have produced 96 unique consensus statements focused specifically on the specialty practice of life care planning that are relevant and applicable to all life care planners (Johnson et al., 2018, p. 17). Likewise, the International Academy of Life Care Planners (2022) has published the *Standards of Practice for Life Care Planners*. These standards reflect the progress of life care planning and how the practice has become more objective and research-based over time (International Academy of Life Care Planners, 2022). The standards provide measurable criteria for evaluating the consistency between actual life care planning practice and what is considered within the field to be the standard of practice (International Academy of Life Care Planners, 2022). Additional life care planning Standards of Practice have been published by the American Association of Nurse Life Care Planners (AANLCP®) and the International Commission on Health Care Certifications™ (ICHCC™). Whether the life care planner is new or highly experienced, consistency between published Majority and Consensus Statements and Standards of Practice will place the life care planner in the best position to minimize the potential for their work to be excluded or limited as the legal process evolves.

Having gained a complete and thorough understanding of a particular case, the life care planner is ready to prepare a narrative report and life care plan document. The narrative report details the life care planner's findings in interviews, records reviews, and consultations with other allied providers, and essentially helps build the initial foundation of elements and data that the actual life care plan will be built upon and evaluated against. The narrative report should be comprehensive and clearly articulate the unique aspects of the particular case—not simply reflect a basic template that is generic to all of the life care planners' work. The typical categories detailed in the life care plan are well established within the life care planning literature and include the following:

- Future Medical Care—Routine
- Future Medical Care—Surgical Interventions or Aggressive Treatment
- Projected Evaluations
- Projected Therapeutic Modalities
- Health and Strength Maintenance
- Diagnostic Testing/Educational Assessment
- Orthopedic Equipment Needs

- Wheelchair Needs
- Wheelchair Accessories and Maintenance
- Aids for Independent Function
- Orthotics and Prosthetics
- Home Furnishing and Accessories
- Drug and Supply Needs
- Transportation
- Architectural Considerations
- Vocational/Educational Plan
- Home Care/Facility Care
- Potential Complications (Deutsch & Sawyer, 1985; Weed & Field, 2001).

Not every life care plan will address every category of need as described above. To remain consistent with the life care planning literature, the life care planner should make use of those categories of need that are clearly necessary, consider those that may be necessary, and disregard those that have no bearing on the specific case. For consistency of methodology, the life care planner should be consistent from case to case in how categories are considered and applied in your life care planning report preparation.

Establishing and Maintaining Files

It is worth noting the life care planner's file will serve as an essential tool throughout the life of the consultant's involvement in a case. The file may contain both digital and hardcopy materials, but in either form, serve as the central storage point for data in support of life care planning recommendations. The file should contain any written reports, backup documentation, billing materials, etc. When the life care planner is initially setting up their file, they should assume the file will be used as a reference during testimony, therefore it is subject to discovery. The life care planning professional should be careful to keep all notes and memorandum objective and on point. The file should not include extraneous materials, such as informal notes or doodles in the margins (Sunday & Kennedy Arnold, 2011).

With respect to the maintenance of life care planning files after case closure, that will generally be guided by the rules and regulations of each individual state. A general rule of thumb is seven years.

Work Product Rules

In the normal course of healthcare delivery, an appropriately executed medical release will likely yield any medical records in a provider's possession. These same rules do not necessarily apply within the legal system. In the normal course of litigation, certain materials, referred to as work product, and prepared by an attorney who is acting on behalf of their client in preparation for litigation, are privileged from disclosure to the opposing party. The work product rule is an exception to the usual sharing of information. The rule can include a wide range of materials, such as research, records, correspondence, reports, or memoranda to the extent they contain the opinions, theories, strategies, mental impressions, or conclusions of the client, the attorney, or persons participating in the case with the attorney.

Mediation and Arbitration

Two commonly used conflict resolution mechanisms are mediation and arbitration. In mediation, an impartial third party, or mediator, assists the disputing parties resolve their conflict through a structured process of communication and negotiation (Florida Courts, n.d.). The life care planner's role is to educate all parties involved, including the attorney, an economist, a structured settlement specialist, a mediator, and any other interested parties (Sunday & Kennedy Arnold, 2011). In this setting, the mediator is not allowed to dispense legal advice, decide who is right or wrong, or express how the parties should resolve their dispute. While the goal of mediation is certainly dispute resolution, the parties involved may decide, in the end, that resolution or settlement of the dispute is not in their best interest and fail to resolve the issue at mediation.

A second, commonly utilized, conflict resolution mechanism is arbitration. Arbitration makes use of a neutral third party, called an arbitrator, to ultimately resolve a dispute outside of the courtroom environment. However, unlike a mediator, the arbitrator serves as a form of private judge or Special Master to listen to the evidence, and ultimately make a ruling on the outcome of the issues in dispute. The decision by the judge or Special Master is binding and no trial will follow (Sunday & Kennedy Arnold, 2011) As in mediation, the life care planner's role is to educate the parties involved, including the attorney, an economist, structured settlement specialist, judge or Special Master, and any other interested parties (Sunday & Kennedy Arnold, 2011).

Testimony: Deposition

One of the best litmus tests of the quality of your expert report and of your value to the litigation process is your ability to provide deposition testimony. Your life care plan report and your subsequent deposition testimony during discovery are keystones to your later acceptance by the court. During discovery when opposing counsel is taking sworn testimony from the experts, you will not be an exception. Most often, you will receive a subpoena for deposition testimony. In most cases, the attorneys will coordinate the deposition with your schedule, but if this does not happen, then you have the right to schedule the deposition consistent with your availability, provided your availability does not breach any court-imposed discovery deadlines. If you are not able to keep to the schedule described in the deposition, you must notify the attorneys accordingly, so it may be rescheduled at a mutually agreeable time and place.

In a deposition, one of the attorneys will usually question the expert or lay witness named by the other side of the matter (Sunday & Kennedy Arnold, 2011). Depositions are normally taken orally, although they can be taken in writing. Prior to giving deposition testimony, the witness is sworn in by an officer of the court who also serves as the court reporter to document both questions and answers verbatim. Some states limit the number of hours a deposition can last in one day. Because of the complexity often involved in putting a life care plan together, you would do well to anticipate a full-day commitment, due to travel, pre-deposition conference with the retaining attorney, the actual deposition time, and any post-deposition discussion the retaining attorney may desire (Sunday & Kennedy Arnold, 2011).

The notice of intent to take deposition will include the name of the party filing the notice, which is generally the opposing party, the date, time, and location of the deposition, and if applicable, information regarding the recording of the deposition (Sunday & Kennedy Arnold, 2011).

On the day of the deposition, it is worth looking at the process as a form of dress rehearsal. The attorney taking the deposition has the opportunity to see what to expect from each witness being offered to the court for testimony by the opposing party. However, for you as a life care planner, it provides insight into what issues to expect during cross-examination at trial.

The life care planner will likely also receive a subpoena duces tecum, which includes a list of documents or items they should bring with them to the deposition. Such items often include an up-to-date curriculum vitae, a list of cases the life care planner has testified in, and the complete case file including written reports, billing, notes, research, etc. One keynote here is that unless a list or single item requested in the subpoena duces tecum has previously been prepared or drafted, production of such documents in arrears is not expected or required.

In some cases, the variable of time works against the life care planner. In other words, a significant amount of time passes between the time the written report is published and the date when the deposition is taken. Examples would be outdated reference sources, outdated treatment recommendations, and aging. In these circumstances, the life care planner would do well to update the life care plan and re-submit the document as far in advance of the deposition as possible.

It is not at all uncommon for the life care planner and the retaining attorney to meet in advance of the deposition. Such a preparatory meeting can last as little as 30 minutes and as long as several hours depending upon the complexity of the case and the experience of the life care planner and attorney (Sunday & Kennedy Arnold, 2011). An important issue to remember is the life care planner should never discuss any case-related details with anyone other than the retaining attorney.

The life care planner should be well prepared for the deposition, dressed in a dark suit, with a plain blouse or shirt and minimal jewelry (Sunday & Kennedy Arnold, 2011). The same cautions that bear out in trial testimony also are applicable to deposition testimony. Because deposition testimony is taken under oath, the life care planner is obligated to answer questions truthfully or run the risk of being charged with perjury. The typical deposition follows a rather predictable course that includes a discussion of educational credentials and qualifications; the life care planner's past and current employment, duties, and responsibilities; and the life care planner's assumptions and methodology as it relates to the current and other life care plans (Sunday & Kennedy Arnold, 2011). It is important to remember that when it comes to deposition testimony, the minimal possible answer is best. If a question can be addressed adequately with a simple "yes" or "no," then you should answer in this way to help minimize the potential for offering unintentional information to the opposing party. However, in some cases, the question is focused on a hypothetical question that has no obvious relationship to the facts of the case at hand. In these circumstances, be cautious of intent (although intent may not be obvious), and do not simply agree with the opposing attorney. Rather, remain calm, confident, and above all credible (Sunday & Kennedy Arnold, 2011).

During the deposition, the retaining attorney may "object" to a question, or the form of a question asked by the opposing attorney. In these circumstances, it is usually a technical objection, and it rarely results in the life care planner ultimately not answering the question. Once the opposing attorney has completed their line of questioning, the retaining attorney will have the opportunity to clarify any points that were not clear in the testimony. Once both sides have rested from questions, the deposition will conclude. The court reporter will generally ask the witness if they would like to read their deposition testimony or do they waive that right. If you choose to read the transcript, then the court reporter will send the life care planner a copy of the transcript to review and make any necessary edits. The corrected and signed copy will then be distributed to all of the attorneys and other witnesses. The life care planner should also retain their own copy of the deposition transcript for review prior to providing trial testimony.

Testimony: Trial

Only a very small number of personal injury and medical malpractice cases actually go to trial, as most are successfully resolved through mediation (Sunday & Kennedy Arnold, 2011). When a case ultimately proceeds to trial, the life care planner must become prepared with all of their case materials for trial testimony. In most states, all testifying witnesses are typically excluded from the courtroom except when they testify (Sunday & Kennedy Arnold, 2011). Up to this point in the litigation process, the only party likely who has performed a full examination of the life care planner is the opposing counsel in a deposition. However, at trial, the retaining party will perform their full examination with cross-examination then being provided by the opposing counsel. However, regardless of which attorney's side has retained the life care planner, their role remains to educate the judge and jury about the plaintiff's impairments and treatment costs associated with ongoing management of their newly acquired disabilities (Sunday & Kennedy Arnold, 2011). The time for testimony at trial is condensed compared to deposition. Additionally, it is not uncommon for the retaining attorney to have exhibits, demonstrations, and visual aids prepared to help guide the life care planner's trial testimony. Once the trial testimony is complete, the life care planner should immediately prepare an invoice to the retaining attorney that outlines accumulated costs in an effort to expedite payment.

Conclusion

Developing a process that guides your work from initial retention through to file closure is a vital element towards providing life care planning services within the legal-forensic setting. It is through this process that the life care planner learns to consistently engage a case in a manner that is aligned with your education, professional credentials, and experience. By repeatedly carrying out this evolved process, you will, through repeated exposure, learn to fluidly execute and describe the process from beginning to end.

References

American Bar Association. (2019). *Text of the model rules of professional conduct, ABA.* www.americanbar.org/groups/professional_responsibility/publications/model_rules_of_professional_conduct/rule_3_4_fairness_to_opposing_party_counsel/

Barros-Bailey, M., & Carlisle, J. (2014). Professional identity, standards, and ethical issues. In R. Robinson (Ed.), *Foundations of forensic vocational rehabilitation* (pp. 443–465). Springer.

Bell Atlantic v. Twombly et al., 550 U.S. 544 (2007).

Behrens, M. A., & Jackson, K. R. (2021). *Federal judiciary advisory committee proposes amendments to expert testimony rule.* The Federalist Society. https://fedsoc.org/commentary/fedsoc-blog/federal-judiciary-advisory-committee-proposes-amendments-to-expert-testimony-rule

Bernard, E. (2022). *Analysis: Say goodbye to "Daubert motion," hello to new rule 702(1).* Bloomberg Law. https://news.bloomberglaw.com/bloomberg-law-analysis/analysis-say-goodbye-to-daubert-motion-hello-to-new-rule-702

Blackwell, T. L., Martin, W. E., & Scalia, V. A. (1994). *Ethics in rehabilitation: A guide for rehabilitation professionals.* Elliott & Fitzpatrick.

Certified Nurse Life Care Planner Certification Board. (n.d.). Certification by examination. https://cnlcp.org/certification-by-examination

Certified Physician Life Care Planner Certification Board. (n.d.). The Pinnacle of Life Care Planning. Certified Physician Life Care Planner (CPLCP™) Certification. https://cplcp.org/Certification.aspx

Cornell School of Law. (n.d.a). *Abuse of discretion*. In Legal Information Institute. www.law.cornell.edu/wex/abuse_of_discretion

Cornell School of Law. (n.d.b). *Affirmative defense*. In Legal Information Institute. www.law.cornell.edu/wex/affirmative_defense

Cornell School of Law. (n.d.c). *Appeal*. In Legal Information Institute. www.law.cornell.edu/wex/appeal

Cornell School of Law. (n.d.d). *Appellate court*. In Legal Information Institute. www.law.cornell.edu/wex/appellate_court

Cornell School of Law. (n.d.e). *Attachment*. In Legal Information Institute. www.law.cornell.edu/wex/attachment

Cornell School of Law. (n.d.f). *Attorney work product privilege*. In Legal Information Institute. www.law.cornell.edu/wex/attorney_work_product_privilege

Cornell School of Law. (n.d.g). *Case of first impression*. In Legal Information Institute. www.law.cornell.edu/wex/case_of_first_impression

Cornell School of Law. (n.d.h). *Clearly erroneous*. In Legal Information Institute. www.law.cornell.edu/wex/clearly_erroneous

Cornell School of Law. (n.d.i). *Closing argument*. In Legal Information Institute. www.law.cornell.edu/wex/closing_argument

Cornell School of Law. (n.d.j). *Complaint*. In Legal Information Institute. www.law.cornell.edu/wex/complaint

Cornell School of Law. (n.d.k). *Counterclaim*. In Legal Information Institute. www.law.cornell.edu/wex/counterclaim

Cornell School of Law. (n.d.l). *Cross-claim*. In Legal Information Institute. www.law.cornell.edu/wex/cross-claim

Cornell School of Law. (n.d.m). *De novo*. In Legal Information Institute. www.law.cornell.edu/wex/de_novo

Cornell School of Law. (n.d.n). *Deposition*. In Legal Information Institute. www.law.cornell.edu/wex/deposition

Cornell School of Law. (n.d.o). *Directed verdict*. In Legal Information Institute. www.law.cornell.edu/wex/directed_verdict

Cornell School of Law. (n.d.p). *Discovery*. In Legal Information Institute. www.law.cornell.edu/wex/discovery

Cornell School of Law. (n.d.q). *Garnish*. In Legal Information Institute. www.law.cornell.edu/wex/garnish

Cornell School of Law. (n.d.r). *Joinder*. In Legal Information Institute. www.law.cornell.edu/wex/joinder

Cornell School of Law. (n.d.s). *Judgement*. In Legal Information Institute. www.law.cornell.edu/wex/judgment

Cornell School of Law. (n.d.t). *Jury instructions*. In Legal Information Institute. www.law.cornell.edu/wex/jury_instructions

Cornell School of Law. (n.d.u). *Jury selection*. In Legal Information Institute. www.law.cornell.edu/wex/jury_selection

Cornell School of Law. (n.d.v). *Motion for summary judgement*. In Legal Information Institute. www.law.cornell.edu/wex/motion_for_summary_judgment

Cornell School of Law. (n.d.w). *Opening statement*. In Legal Information Institute. www.law.cornell.edu/wex/opening_statement

Cornell School of Law. (n.d.x). *Peremptory challenge*. In Legal Information Institute. www.law.cornell.edu/wex/peremptory_challenge

Cornell School of Law. (n.d.y). *Privilege*. In Legal Information Institute. www.law.cornell.edu/wex/privilege

Cornell School of Law. (n.d.z). *Remittitur*. In Legal Information Institute. www.law.cornell.edu/wex/remittitur

Cornell School of Law. (n.d.aa). *Replevin*. In Legal Information Institute. www.law.cornell.edu/wex/replevin

Cornell School of Law. (n.d.bb). *Sequestration*. In Legal Information Institute. www.law.cornell.edu/wex/sequestration

Cornell School of Law. (n.d.cc). *Special verdict*. In Legal Information Institute. www.law.cornell.edu/wex/special_verdict

Cornell School of Law. (n.d.dd). *Stare decisis*. In Legal Information Institute. www.law.cornell.edu/wex/stare_decisis

Cornell School of Law. (n.d.ee). *Trier of fact*. In Legal Information Institute. www.law.cornell.edu/wex/trier_of_fact
Cornell School of Law. (n.d.ff). *Verdict*. In Legal Information Institute. www.law.cornell.edu/wex/verdict
Daubert v. Merrell Dow Pharmaceuticals, 509 U.S. 579 (1993)
Deutsch, P., & Sawyer, H. (1985). *Guide to rehabilitation*. AHAB Press.
Dunn, P. (2014). Introduction to the American legal system and rules of civil procedure: A primer for vocational experts. In R. Robinson (Ed.), *Foundations of forensic vocational rehabilitation* (pp. 239–260). Springer.
Field, D. L. (2013). *The expert*. Iuniverse.
Field, T. F. (2018). Admissibility considerations in life care planning. In R. Weed & D. Berens (Eds.), *Life care planning and case management handbook* (4th ed., pp. 819–832). Routledge.
Field, T., Johnson, C. B., Choppa, A. J., & Fountaine, J. D. (2015). The collateral source rule and the Affordable Care Act: Implications for life care planning and economic damages. *Journal of Life Care Planning, 13*(3), 3–16.
Florida Courts. (n.d.). Mediation in Florida. www.flcourts.org/Resources-Services/Alternative-Dispute-Resolution/Mediation-in-Florida
Friedman, L. M. (2019). *A history of American law* (4th ed.). Oxford University Press.
General Electric Company v. Joiner, 522 U.S. 136 (1997).
Heitzman, A. M., Amundsen, C., Gann, C., & Christensen, D. R. (2014). Consultation in employment law. In R. Robinson (Ed.), *Foundations of forensic vocational rehabilitation* (pp. 363–378). Springer.
International Academy of Life Care Planners. (2022). *Standards of practice for life care planners* (4th ed.). https://cdn.ymaws.com/rehabpro.org/resource/collection/D5B16132-B4BE-4918-BA5A-1BABE8C2E1A4/SOP4_101122.pdf
International Commission on Health Care Certification. (2021). *Practice standards and guidelines*. https://ichcc.org/images/PDFs/Standards_and_Guidelines.pdf
International Commission on Health Care Certification. (n.d.). Certified Life Care Planner. www.ichcc.org/certified-life-care-planner-clcp.html
Johnson, C., Pomeranz, J., & Stetten, N. (2018). Consensus and majority statements derived from life care planning summits held in 2000, 2002, 2004, 2006, 2008, 2010, 2012, 2015 and 2017 and updated via delphi study in 2018. *Journal of Life Care Planning, 16*(4), 15–18.
Johnson, C., & Weed, R. (2013). The life care planning process. *Physical Medicine and Rehabilitation Clinics of North America, 24*(3), 403–417.
Kuhmo Tire Company v. Carmichael, 526 U.S. 137 (1999)
Mauk, K. L. (2019). Revisiting the concept of transdisciplinary life care planning. *Journal of Life Care Planning, 17*(1), 5–6.
National Constitution Center. (2022, April 29). *Article III*. Judicial Branch. https://constitutioncenter.org/interactive-constitution/article/article-iii
Neulicht, A. T., Riddick-Grisham, S., & Goodrich, W. R. (2010). Life care plan survey 2009: Process, methods and protocols. *Journal of Life Care Planning, 9*(4), 129–214.
Pomeranz, J. L., & Shaw, L. R. (2006) International Classification of Functioning, Disability and Health: A model for life care planners. *Journal of Life Care Planning, 6*(12), 15–24.
Pomeranz, J., Yu, N., & Robinson, R. H. (2014). Introduction to life care planning In R. Robinson (Ed.), *Foundations of forensic vocational rehabilitation* (pp. 391–399). Springer.
Roger Williams University School of Law. (2022, April 29). Constitutional Law. https://law.rwu.edu/academics/msl-program/constitutional-law
Scheb, J. M., & Sharma, H. (2020). *An introduction to the American Legal System* (5th ed.). Aspen Publishing.
Stern, B., & Owen, T. (2022). Collateral source rule approaches and its implications for usual, customary and reasonable pricing. *Journal of Life Care Planning, 20*(1), 27–42.
Sunday, C., & Kennedy Arnold, T. (2011). Use of the life care planning expert in legal cases. In S. Riddick-Grisham & L. M. Deming (Eds.), *Pediatric life care planning and case management* (2nd ed., pp. 839–853). CRC Press.
The Committee on the Judiciary—House of Representatives. (2020a). *Federal rules of evidence*. U.S. Government Pricing Office.

The Committee on the Judiciary—House of Representatives. (2020b). *Federal rules of civil procedure*. U.S. Government Pricing Office.

U.S. Courts. (2022, April 29). *About federal courts*. Comparing Federal & State Courts. www.uscourts.gov/about-federal-courts/court-role-and-structure/comparing-federal-state-courts

Weed, R. (2018a). Life care planning: Past, present, and future. In R. Weed & D. Berens (Eds.), *Life care planning and case management handbook* (4th ed., pp. 3–20). Routledge.

Weed, R. (2018b). Forensic issues for life care planners. In R. Weed & D. Berens (Eds.), *Life care planning and case management handbook* (4th ed., pp. 609–629). Routledge.

Weed, R., & Field, T. (2001). *The rehabilitation consultant's handbook*. Elliott & Fitzpatrick.

Woodrich, F., & Patterson, J. B. (2003). Ethical objectivity in forensic rehabilitation. *The Rehabilitation Professional, 11*(3), 41–47.

Chapter 28

Admissibility Considerations in Life Care Planning

Timothy F. Field

Admissibility Considerations in Life Care Planning

The admissibility of expert testimony in federal and state courts has evolved into a major issue related to civil cases of personal injury and life care planning (Elliott, 2010; Gunn, 2010). *In limine* motions to strike testimony are not uncommon and are usually directed toward the expert's credentials and/or methodologies relied upon in developing conclusions and opinions for presentation and trial (*Crouch v. John Jewel Aircraft*, 2016; Elliott, 2010; Gunn, 2010). This chapter discusses the history and development of rules and regulations which govern the testimony of an expert and clarifies some issues and confusion regarding the intent and meaning of recent court cases on this issue.

The Daubert *Trilogy*

Three US Supreme court cases are referred to as the *Daubert* trilogy (*Daubert v. Merrill Dow Pharmaceutical*, 92-102, US Sp Ct, 1993a; (hereafter *Daubert*) *General Electric Co. v. Joiner (*hereafter *Joiner)*96-188, US Sp Ct, 1997; and *Kumho Tire Co. v. Carmichael* (hereafter *Kumho*) 526 137, US Sp Ct, 1999). All three cases and the related U.S. District Court and U.S. Court of Appeals decisions leading up to the final rulings were meant to clarify and refine the guidelines for the admissibility of expert testimony in federal courts. The *Daubert* decision was a departure from the long-held decision of *Frye v. United States* (1923) and further emphasized the substantial importance of Rule 702 of the Federal Rules of Evidence 702 (FRE 702 was subsequently amended in 2000). The *Daubert* trilogy has had a significant impact on the parameters and meaning of such concepts as: What has changed from *Frye;* what are the criteria for admissibility that apply in any or all federal cases and in particular, for the rehabilitation and life care planning community, what is acceptable methodology and testimony—especially in light of the *Daubert* criteria for admissibility? This chapter will review the various federal rulings to examine how the rules apply to life care planning and rehabilitation experts. An analysis of several tort cases will be presented to illustrate how the courts have decided on issues of admissibility.

Frye v. United States

Frye involved the case of a defendant who was convicted of the crime of second-degree murder. During the course of appeal, the defendant offered an expert who used a "deception test" based on the theory that "truth comes without conscious effort, while the utterance of a falsehood requires a conscious effort, which is reflected in the [systolic] blood pressure" (p. 1). The government objected to the presentation of the expert who conducted the test prior to trial, and the objection was sustained by the court. Given the fact that this "deception test" was relatively new to the scientific community, the court stated that:

> the principle must be recognized, and while courts will go a long way in admitting expert testimony deduced from a well-recognized scientific principle or discovery, the thing from which the deduction is made must be sufficiently established to have gained general acceptance in the particular field in which it belongs (p. 1).

Thus, the principle of "general acceptance" became the standard for admissibility of testimony from 1923 until *Daubert* was decided in 1993. However, as will become apparent, the *Daubert* ruling did not fully clarify the issue of admissibility, as approximately one-half of the states still rely on *Frye* as their standard for admissibility in their respective state courts.

Feinman (2011) raised the question of who decides the admissibility of a generally accepted principle or technique; and who decides who constitutes the relevant scientific community? Feinman suggests that issues of science should be determined by adequately defined scientific research with controlled and randomized studies. The "opinions of respected authorities, based on clinical experience, descriptive studies, or reports of experts committees" (p. 4) should be the least likely path to establishing general acceptance. In the area of the soft sciences, such as life care planning, the same two questions apply: What is the agreed upon methodology, and is general acceptance by collegial experts sufficient for admissibility?

Daubert v. Merrill Dow Pharmaceuticals

Jason Daubert (and Eric Schuller) were born with deformities after their mothers ingested the drug Bendectin during pregnancy. The issue before the court was whether Bendectin caused those deformities. The respondent, Merrill Dow Pharmaceuticals, was granted a summary judgment by the U.S. District Court (1989) which was affirmed by the U.S. Court of Appeals, 9th Circuit (1991). A summary of the District Court's ruling follows:

> The summary judgment based on a well-credentialed expert's affidavit concluding, upon reviewing the extensive published scientific literature on the subject, the material use of Bendectin has not been shown to be a risk factor for human birth defects. Although petitioners had responded with the testimony of eight other well-credentialed experts, who based their conclusion that Bendectin can cause birth defects on animal studies, chemical structural analyses, and the unpublished "reanalysis" of previously published human statistical studies, the court determined that the evidence did not meet the applicable "general acceptance" standard for the admission of testimony. The Court of Appeals agreed and affirmed, citing *Frye v. United States*, for the rule that expert

opinion based on scientific technique is inadmissible unless the technique is "generally accepted" as reliable in the relevant scientific community (*Daubert v. Merrill Dow Pharmaceuticals Syllabus*, 1993a, p. 1).

In *Daubert* (1993b), the U.S. Supreme Court summarized the expert testimony of both the petitioners and the defense. Steven Lamm, a physician and epidemiologist testified that he had reviewed over 30 published research studies involving over 130,000 patients and had concluded that Bendectin "during the first trimester of pregnancy has not been shown to be a risk factor for human birth defects" (p. 1). The petitioners, on the other hand, presented eight experts who had "concluded that Bendectin can cause birth defects" (p. 1) based on animal studies that did find a link between Bendectin and malformations. The Court noted that the District Court (1993, p. 1) had relied upon the *Frye* rule and found that the petitioner's evidence was not "sufficiently established to have general acceptance in the field to which it belongs." The U.S. Court of Appeals (1991) essentially reached the same conclusion that the petitioner's evidence did not reach the level of general acceptance. The Appeals Court affirmed the District Court's decision by rejecting the "petitioners' reanalysis as unpublished, not subjected to the normal peer review process, and generated solely for use in litigation" (p. 2). The Supreme Court (1993) took the next step to address the issue by contending that the Federal Rules of Evidence (FRE) (i.e., FRE 401, FRE 402, and FRE 702) superseded the *Frye* test of 1923. FRE 402 (p. 3) established a baseline:

> All relevant evidence is admissible, except as otherwise provided by the Constitution of the United States, by Act of Congress, by these rules, or by other rules prescribed by the Supreme Court pursuant to statutory authority. Evidence which is not relevant is not admissible.

FRE 401 (p. 3) defines the meaning of relevance:

> Relevant evidence is defined as that which has any tendency to make the existence of any fact that is of consequence to the determination of the action more probable or less probable than it would be without the evidence.

The Supreme Court further noted that the FRE 702 governed expert testimony, and in doing so, that there was nothing in the rule that "established general acceptance as an absolute prerequisite to admissibility." In 1993, FRE 702 (p. 3) defined the role of the expert as follows:

> If scientific, technical, or other specialized knowledge will assist the trier of fact to understand the evidence or to determine a fact in issue, a witness qualified as an expert by knowledge, skill, experience, training, or education, may testify thereto in the form of an opinion or otherwise.

The amended FRE 702 (2000 p. 1), in addition to the above, added the following narrative at the end of the above definition:

> … if (1) the testimony is based upon sufficient facts or data, (2) the testimony is the product of reliable principles and methods, and (3) the witness has applied the principles and methods reliably to the facts of the case.

In 2022, the federal's judiciary's *Advisory Committee on Evidence Rules* has proposed a second amendment to FRE 702 which would be added to the end of the current definition of FRE 702 (if approved by the U.S. Supreme Court). The new language would be as follows:

> …the court finds that the proponent has demonstrated by a preponderance of the evidence that the expert's opinion reflects a reliable application of the principles and methods to the facts of the case (Behrens & Jackson, 2021, p. 2).

At issue with this most recent development of the proposed 2022 Amendment to FRE 702, is a greater role by the gatekeeper in determining a proper admissibility of an expert. This amendment will require that the gatekeeper finds the "proponent has demonstrated by a preponderance of the evidence" and that the "expert's opinion reflects a reliable application of the principles and methods to the facts of the case" (Ward, 2021, p. 1).

As a consequence of these rule developments, the Supreme Court noted that a rigid general acceptance requirement (i.e *Frye*) would be at odds with the liberal thrust of the FRE the [rules] general approach to relaxing the traditional barriers to opinion testimony. The standard of "general acceptance" for admitting testimony became incompatible with the FRE. The Court emphasized, however, that testimony or evidence must be both *rele*vant and *reliable*. The court then took the next step to examine the issue of "knowledge" which is contained in FRE 702. Noting that knowledge can exist within three domains (scientific, technical, or other specialized) the Court argued that the "adjective scientific implies a grounding in the methods and procedure of science" (p. 4). As will become evident when the *Kumho* ruling is reviewed, technical and other specialized knowledge clearly differs from scientific knowledge, requiring a different approaching to evaluating a relevant and reliable methodology. The Court, in *Daubert*, a legal case involving an issue of science (i.e., scientific knowledge) suggested that:

Many factors will bear on the inquiry, and we do not presume to set out a definitive checklist or test. But some general observations are appropriate.

1. Scientific knowledge today is based on generating hypotheses and testing them to see if they can be falsified.
2. Another pertinent consideration is whether the theory or technique has been subjected to peer review.
3. In the case of a particular scientific techniques, the court ordinarily should consider the known or potential rate of error.
4. Finally, 'general acceptance' can yet have a bearing on the inquiry. The inquiry envisioned by FRE 702 is, we emphasize, a flexible one (p. 5).

In an Endnote (#8) on the *Daubert* case (1993a), the Court observed that " Rule 702 also applies to 'technical, or other specialized knowledge.' Our discussion is limited to the scientific context because that is the nature of the expertise offered here" (p. 9).

General Electric Co. v. Joiner

Robert Joiner was working as a maintenance electrician on the city's Water and Light Department in Thomasville, Georgia. He was exposed to a mineral-based dielectric fluida contaminate fluid with polychlorinated byphenyls (PCBs). Subsequently, Joiner was diagnosed with small cell lung cancer. The District Court granted a summary judgment to the petitioners (GE) for the following reasons:

(1) there was no genuine issue as to whether Joiner had been exposed to furans and dioxins, and (2) the testimony of Joiner's experts had failed to show that there was a link between exposure to PBCs and small cell lung cancer. The court believed that the testimony of the respondent's experts to the contrary did not rise above 'subjective belief or unsupported speculation. Their testimony was therefore inadmissible (p. 2).

The Court of Appeals for the 11th Circuit held that the District Court "had erred in excluding the testimony of Joiner's expert witnesses" (p. 3) and reversed for two reasons. First, the Court concluded, the jury should decide the correctness of an expert's testimony. Second, there was a genuine issue of the question of furans and dioxins. The US Supreme Court (1997) disagreed and reversed, holding that the Appeals Court held a view of testimony that was too stringent and that under the FRE, which now superseded *Frye*, the District Court was allowed to admit a much broader view of evidence. The gatekeeper role of the district judge had considerable discretion and latitude in admitting evidence at trial. The *GE-Joiner* decision is often referred to as the "discretion rule." The following paragraph best describes the essence of the Joiner decision:

Most significant to experts was the Supreme Court's finding that the trial court properly excluded the plaintiff's expert's testimony because there was "simply too great an analytical gap between the data and the opinion proffered" (Pearson, 2014, p. 6). In other words, the Court found the expert's opinion to be speculative because it could not be supported by the underlying methodology, even when the methodology itself is reliable. Furthermore, the Court noted that an expert cannot rely solely on his or her qualifications as validation that an expert opinion is reliable.

Kumho Tire Co. v. Carmichael

After a period of confusion by many as to what the Supreme Court actually meant and intended with regard to admissible testimony, the *Kumho Tire Co. v. Carmichael* (1999) case was selected as a means to clarify and expand on this issue. Patrick Carmichael purchased a used minivan with a significant amount of wear on the tires. While driving the van in 1993, a rear tire blew out causing a serious accident which resulted in one death and several injured. Carmichael sued *Kumho Tire* claiming that the tire was defective. Dennis Carlson, a tire construction expert, testified for the petitioner and concluded that a defective tire caused the accident when the tread separated from the carcass of the tire. The essence of this presentation to the court was a four-part criteria which he used in evaluating the tire that included "(a) tread wear on the tire's shoulder that is greater that the tread wear along the tire's center; (b) signs of a bead grove where the beads have been pushed too hard against the bead seat on the inside of the tire's rim; (c) sidewalls of the tire with physical signs of deterioration such as discoloration; and (d) marks on the tire's rim flange" (p. 2). Note that the four-point *Daubert* criteria were not used in Carlson's analysis. With his own criteria, conclusions from two criteria of which were observations Carlson concluded that a defect must have caused the separation. The District Court (*Carmichael v. Samyang Tires, Inc.*, 1996) found that Carlson's credentials were not at issue but his methodology was relevant when evaluated in light of the *Daubert* factors. The District Court "found that all those factors argued against the reliability of Carlson's methods and it granted a [defendant's] motion to exclude the testimony. The plaintiffs, arguing that the court's application of the *Daubert* factors was too "inflexible" (p. 3) and asked for reconsideration. Observing that the method employed by Carlson used a visual inspection (observation) of the tire, the District Court again affirmed its earlier decision and found for the defendant in rejecting Carlson's methodology.

The US Court of Appeals for the 11th Circuit (*Carmichael v. Samyang Tires, Inc.*, 1997) reversed the court's decision for applying *Daubert* factors as a means to establish reliability of a methodology. The Appeals Court was clear in their clarification of interpretation of the *Daubert* factors:

> The Supreme Court in *Daubert* explicitly limited its holding to cover only the scientific context, adding that 'a *Daubert* analysis' applies only where the expert relies on 'the application of scientific principles' rather than 'on-skill or experienced-based observation.' [The court] concluded that Carlson's testimony, which it viewed as relying on experience, falls outside the scope of *Daubert,* that the district court erred as a matter of law by applying *Daubert* in this case, and that the case must be remanded for further (non-*Daubert*-type) consideration under FRE 702 (p. 3).

With the *Kumho* ruling, the Supreme Court took into consideration the following factors. First, *Daubert* does still apply with an emphasis on reliable methods in evaluating scientific, technical or other specialized knowledge. Next, a consideration must be made related to the proper manner in which a methodology is evaluated. There are several considerations to be made in this evaluation process. The FRE 702 rule imposes a special consideration regarding both the relevance and reliability of evidence. In fact, FRE 702 is so central to the issue of admissibility that the U.S. Supreme Court basically predicated the decisions of the *Daubert* trilogy on this rule. The role of the expert begins with this rule and all else follows, i.e., credentials, the type of knowledge, and emphasis on a reliable methodology. Next, a consideration must be made regarding the type of knowledge that is required in establishing a measure of evidentiary reliability. Not all knowledge is scientific (requiring an evaluation with the application of the four *Daubert* factors); some knowledge is technical or specialized (requiring relevant factors that fairly evaluate the nature of the knowledge and reliable methods relative to the facts of the case). The Court made it abundantly clear that the trial judge "may consider several more specific factors" (p. 5) other than the *Daubert* factors which, by way of emphasis, is within the domain of the gatekeeping role of the trial judge allowing (i.e., discretion). The Supreme Court concluded "that we can neither rule out or rule in for all cases and for all time the applicability of the factors mentioned in *Daubert,* nor can we now do so for subsets of cases categorized by category of expert or by kind of evidence" (p. 5). Furthermore, "whether *Daubert*'s specific factors are or are no reasonable measures of reliability in a particular case is a matter that the law grants the trial judge broad latitude to determine" (p. 7). And "the relevant reliability inquiry should be 'a flexible one,' that its 'over-arching subject should be validity and reliability,' and that *Daubert* was intended neither to be exhaustive nor to apply in every case" (p. 8).

Kumho, therefore, emphasized several factors that are the essence of admissibility including FRE 702, the type of knowledge relative to the facts of the case, *Daubert's* requirement of relevance and reliability, gatekeeping discretion on the part of the trial judge with considerable leeway in contemplating other factors (other than *Daubert*) in evaluating the reliability of a methodology. Taken collectively, all of these considerations provide ample opportunity for rehabilitation experts and life care planners to develop appropriate testimony without the threat of being disallowed in district courts. However, being able to side-step the *Daubert* criteria in no way alleviates the expert from due diligence in opinion development for depositions and trials. The *latitude* provided by *Kumho* offers much more flexibility for the gatekeeper role of the trial judge and *may* involve different criteria in establishing reliability of a methodology use in evaluating the facts of the case. Note: The two words *latitude* and *may* were italicized for emphasis in the Supreme Court's summary of *Kumho*. This flexibility, however, can also serve as an unwanted pitfall for those who fail to take the admissibility requirements seriously. Assuming that the U.S. Supreme Court affirms the proposed amendment to FRE 702 with an emphasis on a gatekeeper evaluating a preponderance of the evidence proffered by an expert the vocational expert and/or life care planner should be cautioned to use a reliable methodology in developing an opinion based on the facts of the case. In order to further clarify this issue for rehabilitation consultants offering technical or specialized testimony, a review of select cases are discussed to illustrate how some cases were adjudicated in this area.

Practical Implications of the 702 Amendment for the Life Care Planner

The proposed (Amaru, 2022) Amendment to FRE 702 will impact litigation when expert witnesses are used in civil cases and will likely result in more challenges on the reliability of the principles and methods utilized in forming an opinion. Most notably, the expert should be prepared to respond to an examination of the "preponderance of evidence" issue as qualifying for admissibility of opinion. While credentials will continue to be an important area of concern, the expert will be examined more carefully based upon their opinion (evidence) and will need be prepared to explain how they reached their conclusion by utilizing the discipline's principles and methodologies. Leading up to a deposition or trial, the various players in the litigation process, including the life care planner or legal representatives, should consider the following six points of preparation and strategy in opinion development (*Amaru et al.*, 2022, p. 4).

1. Contacting experts sooner to provide more time for foundational development of expert reports and testimony;
2. Selecting qualified and experienced experts and ensuring an adequate foundation is laid for expert testimony;
3. Seeking modification of litigation timelines to allow more time for experts to complete merits and rebuttal reports;
4. Closely scrutinizing the methods utilized by experts in developing their opinions to first determine their reliability, and second to ensure the opinion is an accurate output of such methodology.
5. Anticipating more aggressive challenges to expert opinions during discovery rather than deferring such challenges until trial; and
6. Anticipating possible changes in strategy regarding expert report submissions and filing motions to exclude expert opinion knowing that courts will be closely examining the admissibility of both.

Life care planners are cautioned to be aware of the potential strategies by opposing legal counsel.

Case Discussion

This section includes selected cases to illustrate some of the issues life care planners may encounter in the role of a forensic and life care planning expert, including admissibility, credentials, evidence, methodology, and the impact of the federal rulings (*Daubert, Kumho, and Joiner*) and the FRE. The following is a discussion of various motions to exclude a life care planning expert from testifying in trial for whatever reason. All of these cases reference FRE 702 as the basis for a decision on a challenge on expert admissibility, and a few specifically reference the *Daubert* decision in a secondary manner.

The *Daubert* Challenge: Credentials and Evidence

The *Daubert* challenge is an *in limine motion to exclude* by either the plaintiff or defense usually directed toward an expert regarding the expert's credentials, attention to procedure, or methodology issues (including a review of the preponderance of the evidence of the case). The context of the importance of a *motion to exclude* is illustrated by the abstract from a case that was adjudicated (*M.D.P. v. Middleton*, 2013) which is typical of nearly all challenges in federal courts. For a more detailed discussion of the importance of FRE 702, the reader is directed to Field (2011).

> The admissibility of expert testimony is governed by FRE 702 which provides:
>
>> A witness who is qualified as an expert by knowledge, skill, experience, training, or education may testify in the form of an opinion or otherwise if: (a) the expert's scientific, technical, or other specialized knowledge will help the trier of fact to understand the evidence or to determine the fact at issue; (b) the testimony is based on sufficient facts or data; (c) the testimony is the product of reliable principles and methods; and (d) the expert has reliably applied the principles and methods to the facts of the case (p. 7).
>
> As noted in *M.D.P. v. Middleton* (2013):
>
>> [I]n determining the admissibility of expert testimony under FRE 702, and the trial court must conduct a rigorous three-part inquiry considering whether: (1) the expert is qualified to testify competently regarding the matter he intends to address; (2) the methodology by which the expert reaches his conclusions is sufficiently reliable as determined by the sort of inquiry mandated in *Daubert*; and (3) the testimony assists the trier of fact through the application of scientific, technical, or specialized expertise to understand the evidence or to determine a fact at issue" (p. 2).

Motions *in limine to exclude* should always be addressed with some caution and concern. In *Marten v. State of Montana* (2019), the court was confronted with a total of six motions with two being forwarded by the plaintiff and four by the defense. The motions once decided resulted in a total of nineteen separate motions of which six were denied and 13 were granted. In *Perez v. United States of America* (2018), a total of 12 motions of *in limine to exclude* were advanced to reject or limit the testimony of several experts (ten motions were denied; two were allowed). Relevance to rehabilitation experts who offer testimony on economic issues is the use of foundation information and data in offering an opinion of loss of earning capacity. While the court ruled that the expert was qualified on credentials. The challenge was directed at the improper use of certain economic data under California law. The court allowed the testimony and suggested that the correctness of the expert calculation can be challenged under cross-examination. In *McGee v. Target Corp.* (2022), a similar argument for the exclusion of economic testimony be disallowed; the court noted that such testimony could be examined under cross-examination.

Ngatuval v. Lifetime Fitness (2020)

Ngatuval v. Lifetime Fitness (2020) illustrates the potential pitfalls of an expert's credentials or testimony to be challenged by a total of five motions *in limine to exclude* both the expert's credentials and the expert's testimony. The court ruled that the expert was qualified to testify, but part of the expert's report was predicated on a report by another expert's report that was brought into question. Consequently, part of the expert's report was not allowed.

Beavers v. Victorian (2014)

In *Beavers v. Victorian* (2014), the defendant challenged both the qualifications (related to a specific opinion) and the reliability of a portion of the expert's life care plan. The defendant's "challenge only [the life care planner's] expertise regarding the effects of plaintiff's traumatic brain injuries" and further arguing that the [life care planner] "makes a 'speculative leap' between the [doctor's] findings and a need for assisted living services beginning at age 70 and through life expectancy" (p. 2). The Court rejected both the challenge to the expert's credentials and determined that the expert relied on the medical opinions expressed, making the expert's opinions sufficiently reliable to be admissible.

Worley & Worley v. State Farm Mutual Automobile Insurance Co. (2013)

In *Worley & Worley v. State Farm Mutual Automobile Insurance Co.* (2013), a defendant's motion was presented to exclude or limit the testimony of a life care planner. The Court summarily determined that the expert was qualified to offer testimony. The defendant next challenged the expert's opinions as unreliable because the expert relied on a standard reference for costs of certain future medical costs. The Court "must insure that speculative, unreliable expert testimony does not reach the jury."(p. 5). This decision by the court is a good example of the latitude the judge has in determining the admissibility of evidence (i.e., *General Electric v. Joiner,* 1997).

Mettias v. United States of America (2015)

In *Mettias v. United States of America* (2015), the defendant's motion to exclude the testimony of a life care planner on the issues of qualifications and methodology was denied. The court ruled that the expert was qualified stated:

> [expert's] testimony was highly relevant to the issue of [plaintiff's] future costs. Relying on FRE 702, the court addressed the issue of reliability with regard to the expert's] , methodology in preparing a life care plan. The challenge centered on the argument that the [expert] had no expertise in the area of assessing the needs of a person disabled by gastric bypass surgery, that he conducted no independent research of the future needs of [plaintiff], and that he relied entirely on the opinions of [doctor]. In relying on the requirements inherent in FRE 702 the court ruled "that the [expert] does not have specific experience with assessing the needs of a person disabled with gastric bypass surgery in particular does not make him unqualified as an expert (p. 6).

The expert stated that he:

> followed the accepted methodology and standards of practice in the field by looking to the medical providers to define the nature and extent of impairments and then translated those limitations and recommendations to the world of work, independent living, coordination of future medical and rehabilitation services and the associated costs (p. 6). The motion to exclude was denied.

Ancar & Ancar v. Brown & TNE Trucking (2014)

In *Ancar & & Ancar v. Brown & TNE Trucking* (2014), as is sometimes the case, a challenge to the expert testimony is sometimes allowed, in whole or in part. The expert in this case made recommendations regarding medication (allowed), physical therapy (allowed), weight-loss and home-exercise program (not allowed), and epidural steroid injections (allowed), but the expert was subjected to a vigorous cross-examination as suggested in the *Daubert* ruling (509 U.S. at 596) noting that "vigorous cross-examination and other traditional safeguards are appropriate means of attacking shaky but admissible evidence" (p. 4).

Crouch v. John Jewell Aircraft (2016)

Finally, in *Crouch v. John Jewell Aircraft* (2016), the Court, beginning with a reference to FRE 702, addressed the issues related to the plaintiff's testimony: (a) failure by the expert to fully disclose information (violations cited with reference to FRCP 26 & 37) e.g., rules that outlined requirements for disclosure of a statement of opinions, (b) facts and data considered by the experts in each case, exhibits, (c) expert qualifications (including publications over the last ten years), (d) a list of cases over the last four years, and (e) whether or not the omissions were harmless to the current case. The defendant argued that the expert did not fully comply with the requirements of FRCP 26, and when given the opportunity to supplement his testimony post-deposition, the expert failed to comply. There was also some confusion by the expert about which reports were used in forming his opinion. The Court found "that this [expert's] reports were plagued with deficiencies" and the "most egregious is his failure to include the source(s) of the information used to formulate the costs utilized in the life care plan [for defendant]" (p. 3). Further, the expert "testified that he had a conversation with [physician], a rehabilitation medicine specialist, who suggested changes in Crouch's life care plan" (p. 3), which was not disclosed in the expert's report. The court determined that the [expert's] reports were stricken and was prohibited from testifying at trial. This case illustrates the need for an expert to carefully prepare any testimony consistent with the rules related to admissibility. This being a federal court case the FRE (amended 2000) and the Federal Rules of Civil Procedure (FRCP 26 & 37) applied. In state courts, the appropriate state rules would apply.

Foundation and Methodology

Aside from the credentials that an expert needs to qualify as a life care planner, using proper foundation to develop a plan that will withstand a challenge and cross-examination during trial is essential (Weed & Johnson, 2006). Proper, relevant, and reliable methodologies are emphasized in *Kumho v. Carmichael* (1999) and FRE 702 (2000). In reviewing several legal cases (illustrated below), the second most common basis for a *motion to exclude* testimony is related directly to the expert methodology for forming an opinion (the first motion is usually related to the expert's credentials' as previously discussed). As noted above, a frequent mistake made by an expert is the failure to rely on a proper foundation as the basis for a life care plan.

In *Tucker v. Cascade General* (2014), the life care planning expert consulted with the plaintiff's physicians and medical providers who provided needed information regarding future medical care.

Based on these discussions, [expert] "determined the need for future medical care and treatment and its cost, in multiple disciplines for the remainder of his life. [The plan] included necessary medical services as well as other vocational and domestic assistance, and the costs of prescription medications" (p. 20).

The primary treating physician "reviewed the [expert's] life care plan and agreed the services were necessary" (p. 25). This case is an excellent example of the proper approach a life care planner should take in developing a life care plan. Following a review of all the relevant reports and documents, the expert proceeded to develop a plan based on the medical evidence, and ultimately had the plan reviewed by the physician. The methodology was sound and in keeping with the guidelines for plan development by the *Standards of Practice for Life Care Planners* (International Academy of Life Care Planners, 2022, pp. 5–20).

In *Riha v. Offshore Service Vessels* (2021), part of the testimony of a rehabilitation expert was disallowed because there was lacking information from a report provided by an economic expert. Without proper foundation information, the rehabilitation expert was not allowed to testify on the plaintiff's future lost earning capacity. In a related case (*Bergeron v. Great Lakes Dredge and Dock Co.*, 2019) on the issue of admissibility of testimony by the plaintiff's life care planning expert, the court denied a motion to dismiss the expert's testimony because the expert clearly relied on medical foundation information in recommending long term pharmaceutical care for the plaintiff.

The defendant, in *Sandretto v. Payson Healthcare Management, Inc.* (2014) argued, on appeal, that the life care planner's testimony for the plaintiff was allowed when it should have been denied, an error in discretion by the lower court. The specific complaint by the defendant was that the life care planning expert "did not provide proper foundation to testify about the cost of [plaintiff's] future medical care" (p. 6). Citing Arizona's *Rule of Evidence 703*, the court noted that "facts or data in the case that the expert has been made aware of or personally observed" (p. 6) serves as proper sources of information for expert opinions. Given the importance of relying upon a proper foundation for plan development, the following is a summary of the [expert's] own explanation to the court on her approach and cognizance of the foundation issue:

> [Expert] testified that she relied on her own observations and experience as well as input from medical doctors and readily available pricing information for procedures, medications, and other line items. [Expert] also met with the plaintiff and the treating physician (on two occasions) and typically relied on physicians to provide medical justification for individual line items in the life care plan, and then she would determine the costs of the plan. [Expert] testified her expertise includes the calculation of the costs of the plan, but the doctors determined whether a particular line item was appropriate (pp. 6–7).

The defendant continued to argue that the "[expert] was not candid in the preparation of her life care plan" (p. 7), but the trial court determined that this issue went to the weight of the evidence, not the issue of admissibility. On the issue of abuse of discretion by the trial court the appeals court ruled that the "trial court did not err in admitting the [life care planner's] testimony the life care plan" (p. 7) the motion for a new trial was denied.

In *Cuevas v. Contra Costa County* (2017), the defendant did not contest the findings of liability of the plaintiff life care plan, but rather, challenged the damages as presented by the plaintiff's expert. At issue was the projected costs of the life care plan. The plaintiff's expert relied on a national database that reflected the average costs for each type of service recommended for the plaintiff. The defendant's life care planning expert illustrated the discounted costs of a life care plan by suggesting that the *Affordable Care Act* (ACA, 2010) could offset the cost of some of the damages. In addition, the defendant's expert illustrated how the damage costs could be further reduced by comparing the plaintiff's recommendation on costs to the lower costs for the same services provided by the Medi-Cal program. The court remanded a new trial of the issue on the plaintiff's future medical damages. This case illustrates the importance of proper reliable methodology and the use of resources utilized in developing an opinion.

The case of *Brown v. USA Truck, Inc. and Watkins* (2013) presents a situation involving differing medical opinions relied upon by the plaintiff's ife care planner. As noted previously and as illustrated in the Sandretto case (2014), proper medical foundation is essential in developing life care plans. While no fault resided with the life care planner, the court determined that the "preponderance of the evidence …is not sufficient to establish" (p. 3) the inability of the plaintiff to be employed in the future. Consequently, the court ruled that the plaintiff is not "entitled to recover damages based on future lost income, a decision that negated the need for the plaintiff's life care plan" (p. 3).

In *Taylor v. Speedway Motorsports, Inc.* (2003) a case where the testimony of a life care planner was excluded the issue of "foundation" for her testimony was the central focus. The life care planner was excluded because the court found that "the witness wishes to express an opinion or numerous opinions without proper foundation" (p. 33). The court found the life care planner's opinions "entirely speculative" (p. 33). Relying on the federal rulings of both *Daubert* and *Kumho* that the "proffered testimony is unreliable and is not relevant … and would not be helpful and will not assist the jury in understanding the evidence or determining the facts in issue" (p. 34). Adopting language from FRE 403, the court held that "such testimony is substantially outweighed by the danger of unfair prejudice, misleading the jury and a waste of time" (p. 34).

The decision by the court in this case seems harsh and the decision clearly was a firm rejection of the life care plan. However, this early case established a precedent that life care plans must be without speculation and developed with a proper foundation of relevant and reliable data and information. Preparation, or the lack thereof, was illustrated as well in a recent case (*CSC v. USA*, 2013) where the life care plan for the defendant was found to be deficient. The court determined that the life care planner never met the plaintiff, or the child's parents, was not a certified life care planner, and relied only on the viability of the *Affordable Care Act* as too speculative as a funding source.

In *John v. Friesen* (2022), a certified life care planner provided "a life care plan and a written report concerning the plaintiff's current condition, future treatment, future care and life adjustments, and any disability or work restrictions." (p. 1). The defense asserted that the expert's report "provides no information on what methodology he employed to arrive at his conclusion" (p. 2). Following a review of FRE 702 and the admissibility requirements under this rule, the Court agreed that the [report] provides no information on how {expert} arrived at his conclusion … his report provides no basis to conclude this statement resulted from 'reliable principles and methods' as required by FRE 702" (p. 2).

Standards of Practice

The *Daubert* trilogy rulings made it very clear that a relevant and reliable methodology was critical to the admissibility of opinion and testimony in federal courts (similar requirements also apply in state courts). The foundation for expert testimony is Federal Rule 702 which emphasized the three essential factors for the court to consider in determining admissibility:

> (1) the testimony is based upon sufficient facts or data, (2) the testimony is the product of reliable principles and methods (3) the witness has applied the principles and methods reliably to the facts of the case.

For the life care planner and testifying expert, in addition possessing proper credentials, methodology is central to the development of a life care plan. Membership and participation in relevant life care planning professional associations can further enhance and clarify the work of the life care planner by providing guidance for the expert. The advantage of membership in such associations are the ongoing educational opportunities through regional and national conferences, and the many opportunities for networking and/or collaborating with other professionals, including participation in professional listservs and webinars. However, one of the most valuable sources of information is the "standards of practice" – a document which has been developed over time by the very professionals who are members of the professional associations. For example, the *Standards of Practice for Life Care Planners* (2022) was most recently revised in 2022 by an advisory group and a revision committee (a total of 48 professionals), all of whom have been active life care planners for many years. These professionals have all earned degrees in academic fields such as rehabilitation counseling, case management, and nursing; several have earned doctorates. In addition, many of the professionals have years of experience as life care planners, have been leaders and resource people at conferences, and possess a number of professional certifications in various practice areas related to rehabilitation and life care planning. Other life care planning standards were developed specifically for nurse and physician life care planners. The American Association of Nurse Life Care Planners Scope and Standards of Practice (1st edition) (AANLCP®2016) was published by the American Association of Nurse Life Care Planners. Additionally, for physician life care planners, the American Academy of Physician Life Care Planners published Standards of Practice (2014–2022). For a more complete discussion of standards for the life care planner, the reader is referred to the chapter in this text titled *Methodology, Scope of Practice, Standards of Practic, and Consensus in Life Care Planning*.

Professional standards of practice provide important guidelines for life care planners. These standards serve as a basis for a consistent and comprehensive methodological approach which contributes significantly to reaching the needed levels of relevance and reliability for admissibility of testimony in state and federal courts.

However, a note of caution, in *Adams v. Laboratory Corp. of America* (2014), the court addressed the issue of the extent to which a testifying expert could or should rely on a professional association *Standards* in the preparation of a work product. The court noted that standards could be self-serving, are not objective findings, and that the district court reliance on the standards by permitting them as evidence for admissibility was an abuse of discretion. The court further noted the following:

> neither *Daubert* or *Kumho* permits a scientific or medical community to define a litigation standard that applied when its members are sued … but may consider the degree of acceptance of a scientific technique or theory in the relevant scientific community (p. 2).

It can be assumed that the same general admissibility standard would apply in cases involving "specialized or other technical knowledge" (i.e., FRE 702) such as would be present with life care plans. This ruling suggests that the *Standards of Practice for Life Care Planners* should serve as a guideline for both practice and the development of opinion and testimony in state and federal courts. The *Standards* should not be construed as the basis for admissibility, however. An excellent example of how this issue on *Standards* was considered for admissibility can be found in *Roach & Roach v. Hughes, Chicot, Chicot Sales, & Wheels* (2015) which included a *motion to exclude* the opinion of the life care planner in this case. The motion was denied and the court determined that the life care planning expert

> … followed the standards of the [professional association] in developing the life care plan and based her opinions on sufficient facts and data, including medical records,

the opinions and recommendations of multiple medical providers, consulting with [plaintiff], and her own research. The court finds that the principles and methodology utilized in the life care planning field are reasonable measures of reliability of [expert's] methodology and opinions (p. 3).

On the other hand, in *Vaughn v. Hobby Lobby Stores, Inc.* (2021), the court found that a life care planner's testimony:

> failed to carry the burden that [expert's] testimony [was] based upon sufficient facts and data, or that [expert's] testimony [was] the product of reliable principles and methods, or that the [expert] applied the principles and method reliably to the facts of the case (p. 12).

Life care planning experts will need to take note and be prepared to develop and adjust their testimony accordingly.

Table 28.1 Admissibility Related Topics Checklist

• Do you have appropriate life care planning related specialized education, training, experience, and credentials?
• Do you have life care planning relevant specialized training?
• Are you certified as a life care planner?
• Do you belong to and, even better, are you active in appropriate organizations that have life care planning education as part of its mission?
• Do you develop life care plans according to established and accepted standards of practice, ethics and published methodologies?
• Do you make sure that life care plans include proper foundation (including medical)?
• Do you stay current with the parameters of the profession?
• Are you familiar with relevant life care planning literature?
• Are you intimately familiar with life care planning related Standards of Practice?
• Are you familiar with the rules of the jurisdictions in which you practice?
• Are you knowledgeable about applicable Federal Rules of Evidence when testifying in personal injury litigation?
• Is your report written to meet FRCP 26 requirements? And do you have a list of all publications authored within the preceding ten years and a listing of any other cases in which you have testified as an expert at trial or by deposition within the preceding four years?
• When you author a life care plan, are you an active participant/collaborator? (Rather than a "secretary" simply writing down whatever someone else recommends, or a "know-it-all" who believes he/she needs no participation from others.)
• Are you mindful about staying within one's area of expertise or scope of practice?
• Are you knowledgeable about the disability/disabilities for which life care plans are developed?

Conclusion

Professionals who are involved in the practice and development of life care plans should be familiar with and have a working knowledge of the following important areas of information:

1. The *Frye, Daubert, Kumho,* and *Joiner* federal rulings on admissibility.
2. The FRE (i.e., FRE 401, FRE 402, FRE 403, and FRE 702) and the FRCP (i.e., FRCP 26). The proposed amendment to FRE 702 (2022).
3. *Standards of Practice.*
4. Following current case law developments.
5. Following these suggestions, the reader is referred to Table 28.1, which can serve as a checklist or guide in development of a life care plan.

In addition, being active in one's respective professional association through such activities as attending conferences (for continuing education, certification credit, and networking), participating in leadership roles (committee memberships, presenting on topics, and representing the profession), and engaging in knowledge development (i.e., authoring for journals) will assist the professional with establishing a substantial foundation of knowledge upon which to rely.

References

Adams v. Laboratory Corp. of America, No. 13-10425, US Ct of Appl, 11th Cir (2014).
Amaru, S., Elliott, M., & Huang, R. L. (2022). *White paper: Consideration for vocational experts to be accepted by the Social Security Administration.* International Association of Rehabilitation Professionals.
American Association of Nurse Life Care Planners (2015). *Scope and standards of practice* (1st ed.). American Association of Nurse Life Care Planners.
American Academy of Physician Life Care Planners (2014–2023). Standards of practice. https://aaplcp.org/About/PracticeStandarts.aspx
Ancar & Ancar v. Brown & TNE Trucking, No. 3:11-ev-595-DPJ-FKB, US Dist Ct for the So Dist of MA, No Div (2014). https://casetext.com/case/ancar-v-brown-1
Beavers v. Victorian, No. CIV-11-1442-D, US Dist Ct for the W Dist of OK (2014). https://casetext.com/case/beavers-v-victorian-6
Behrens, M., & Jackson, K. (September 20, 2021). *The federalist society.* https://fedsoc.org/
Bergeron v. Great Lakes Dredge and Dock Co., No. 17-0002, US Dist Ct, W.D. Louisiana, 2019.
Brown v. USA Truck, Inc. and Watkins, No. CIV-11-856-D, US Dist Ct for the W Dust of OK (2013). https://casetext.com/case/brown-v-usa-truck
Carmichael v. Samyang Tires, Inc., US Dist Ct, 923 F. Supp. 1514, 1521–1522, SD Ala. (1996). https://law.justia.com/cases/federal/district-courts/FSupp/923/1514/1946875/
Carmichael v. Samyang Tires, Inc., US 11th Cir Ct, 131 F 3d 1433 (1997). https://casetext.com/case/carmichael-v-samyang-tire-inc
Compilation of Patient Protection and Affordable Care Act, Public Law 111-148, 111th US Congress, May, 2010.
Crouch v. John Jewell Aircraft, Inc., No. 3:07-CV-638-DJH, US Dist Ct for the W Dist of KY, Louisville Div (2016). https://casetext.com/case/crouch-v-john-jewell-aircraft-inc-5
Cuevas v. Contra Costa County, 11 Cal. App. 5th 163 (2017).
CSC, a minor, and Bryant and Cobbs v. United States of America, No. 10-910-DRH, US Dist Ct for the S Dist of IL (2013). https://casetext.com/case/csc-v-united-states-1
Daubert v. Merrell Dow Pharmaceutical, 727 F. Supp. 570, 572 SD Cal. (1989). https://law.justia.com/cases/federal/district-courts/FSupp/727/570/1461114/

Daubert v. Merrell Dow Pharmaceuticals Syllabus, 92-102, US Sp Ct. (1993a). www.law.cornell.edu/supct/html/92-102.ZS.html

Daubert v. Merrell Dow Pharmaceuticals, 92-102, US Sp Ct. (1993b). https://supreme.justia.com/cases/federal/us/509/579/

Daubert v. Merrell Dow Pharmaceuticals, 951 F. 2d 1128, US Ct of Appl, 9th Cir. (1991). https://casetext.com/case/daubert-v-merrell-dow-pharmaceuticals-inc-3

Elliott, T. (2010). A plaintiff's attorney's perspective on life care planning. In R. O. Weed & D. E., Berens (Eds.), *Life care planning and case management handbook* (3rd ed., pp. 761–782). Routledge.

Federal Rules of Civil Procedure. www.law.cornell.edu/rules/frcp

Federal Rules of Evidence (Amended 2000). www.law.cornell.edu/rules/fre

Federal Rules of Evidence: Notes of Advisory Committee on Rules. (2000). www.uscourts.gov/rules-policies/archives/committee-reports/advisory-committee-evidence-rules-may-2022

Feinman, R. (2011). *Evidence-based medicine: Who decides admissibility? The* Frye *standard.* http://rdfeinman.wordpress.com/2011/05/06/evidence-based-medicine

Field, T. (2011). *Federal rule 702 in light of the* Daubert, Kumho *and* Joiner *rulings on the admissibility of expert testimony.* Elliott & Fitzpatrick.

Frye v. United States, 3968, 293 F 1013 DC Cir, (1923). https://casetext.com/case/frye-v-united-states-7

General Electric Co. v. Joiner Syllabus, 96-188, US Sp Ct. (1997). https://supreme.justia.com/cases/federal/us/522/136/

General Electric Co. v. Joiner, 96-188, US Sp Ct. (1997). https://supreme.justia.com/cases/federal/us/522/136/#tab-opinion-1960211

Gunn, R. (2010). A defense attorney's perspective on life care planning. In R. O. Weed & D. E., Berens (Eds.), *Life care planning and case management handbook* (3rd ed., pp. 783–797). Routledge.

International Academy of Life Care Planners. (2022). Standards of practice for life care planners, 4th edition. *Journal of Life Care Planning, 20*(3), 5–25.

Johnson, J. T. v. Friesen, J. R. No. 8-19-CV-322. US Dist Ct, NE, (2022).

Kumho Tire Co. v. Carmichael, 97-1709, 526-137, US Sp Ct. (1999). https://supreme.justia.com/cases/federal/us/526/137/

Martin v. State of Montana, No. CV 17-31-H-CCI, US Dist Ct, D Montana, Helena Div. (2019).

McGee v. Target Corp. et al., No. 2:20-cv-00345-KJD-DJA, US Dist Ct, D, Nevada, (2022).

M.D.P. v. Middleton, No. 1:11cv461-WHA (wo), US Dist Ct for the Middle Dist of AL, So Div. (2013). https://casetext.com/case/mdp-v-middleton-1

Mettias v. United States, Civ. No. 12-00527 ACK-KSC, US Dist Ct for the Dist of HI (2015). https://casetext.com/case/mettias-v-united-states-2

Neulicht, A., Riddick-Grisham, S, Hinton, L., Costantini, P., Thomas, R., & Goodrich, B. (2002). Life care planning survey 2001: Process, methods, and protocols. *Journal of Life Care Planning, 1*(2), 97–148.

Ngatuval v. Lifetime Fitness, No. 2:16-cv-39-JNP-DBP, US Dist Ct, D, Utah (2020).

Pearson, W. (2014). *What to expect when you're an expert: Admissibility of expert testimony.* www.ims-expertservices.com/admissibility

Perez v. United States, No. 16cv01911 JAH-MDD, US Dist Ct, S.D. California, 2018.

RIHA v. Offshore Service Vessels, No. 20-2234, US Dist Ct, E.D. Louisiana, 2021.

Roach & Roach v. Hughes, Chicot, Chicot Sales, & Wheels, No. 4:13-CV-00136-JHM, US Dist Ct for the W Dist of KY, Owensboro Div. (2015).

Sandretto v. Payson Healthcare Management, Inc., No. 2 CA-CV 2013-0044, Court of Appeals of Arizona, Div Two (2014). https://casetext.com/case/sandretto-v-payson-healthcare-mgmt

Taylor v. Speedway Motorsports, Inc., 01-CVS-12107, Mecklenburg Cty Sup Ct, NC (2003).

Tucker v. Cascade General, 3:09-cv-1491-AC, US Dist Ct for the Dist of OR, Portland Div. (2014). https://casetext.com/case/tucker-v-cascade-gen-inc-2

Vaughn v. Hobby Lobby Stores, Inc., US Dist Ct, W Div of Louisiana, No. 6:19-cv-00293 (2021). https://casetext.com/case/vaughn-v-hobby-lobby-stores-3

Ward, F. (2021). *Will the proposed amendments to FRE 702 curb unreliable expert testimony.* www.franzward.com/news-willtheproposedamendments

Weed, R., & Johnson, C. (2006). *Life care planning in light of* Daubert *and* Kumho. Elliott & Fitzpatrick.

Worley & Worley v. State Farm Automotive Ins., US Dist Ct, Middle Dist of FL, Jacksonville Div., 3-12-cv-1041-J-MCR (2013).

Chapter 29

A Plaintiff's Attorney's Perspective on Life Care Planning

Bruce H. Stern

Note: Some material in this chapter is excerpted from Stern & Owen (2022), Collateral source rule approaches and its implications for usual, customary, and reasonable pricing. *Journal of Life Care Planning*, 20(1), pp. 5–20. Reprinted with permission.

This chapter is adapted from Stern, B. (2011). Use of a life care plan in a lawsuit involving a child. In Riddick-Grisham, S. & Deming, L. M. (Eds.), Pediatric life care planning and case management (2nd ed., p. 805–817). CRC Press.

A Plaintiff's Attorney's Perspective on Life Care Planning

Many individuals with disabilities require a lifetime of medical care and support. They may require ongoing medication, a variety of supplies, and specialized medical equipment, such as wheelchairs. Because the individual's enjoyment of and participation in past activities (once taken for granted) may be greatly curtailed or eliminated, an injury's effect on an individual and their family will be immense.

When a person's disability has been caused by another's negligence, they may recover damages from the other person for all past, present and prospective harm (*Singh v. Larry Fowler Trucking, Inc.*,[1] 2012). The measure of damages generally recoverable is the amount which will compensate for all the harm, losses, and damages proximately caused by the tort. In this recovery process, a plaintiff may recover two types of damages: economic (or pecuniary) damages and non-economic (or personal) damages (*Golden Eagle Archery v. Jackson*, 116 S.W. 3d 757, 763 (Tx. 2003).

Damages

Non-economic Damages

Non-economic damages are subjective, non-monetary losses suffered by the plaintiff. Non-economic damages include compensation for pain, suffering, mental anguish, and disfigurement. Hedonic damages are another type of non-economic damages and compensate for loss of enjoyment of life (Golden Eagle Archery, Id. at 763). "Hedonic losses include the inability to perform the plaintiff's usual specific activities which had given pleasure to this particular plaintiff, such as playing golf, dancing, bowling, playing musical instruments, and engaging in specific outdoor sports," which must be distinguished from "[b]asic losses" or "disability losses" that "include the inability to perform the basic mechanical body movements of walking, climbing stairs, feeding oneself, and driving a car" *Ramos*[2] *(1992*, p. 43).

In litigation today, compensation for non-economic damages comes under daily attack by those who seek to avoid responsibility and accountability. Currently, eleven states cap non-economic damages in general tort or personal injury cases, including Alaska, Colorado, Hawaii, Idaho, Kansas, Maryland, Mississippi, Ohio, Oklahoma, Oregon, and Tennessee.[3] Twenty-nine states have caps on non-economic damages in medical malpractice cases.

Economic Damages

Economic damages include past medical expenses, future medical expenses, lost wages, and lost earning potential. Included in the prospective harm for which damages may be recovered is the reasonable cost of the medical services that will likely be incurred because of the lingering effects of the injuries caused by the negligent person (*Singh v. Larry Fowler Trucking, Inc.*, 2012).

> A person who is injured by another's negligence may recover damages from the other person for all past, present, and prospective harm. Included in the prospective harm for which damages[1] may be recovered is the reasonable cost of the medical services that will probably be incurred because of the lingering effects of the injuries caused by the negligent person. To remove awards for future medical expenses from the realm of speculation, persons seeking future medical expenses must present evidence (1) that additional medical treatment is reasonably certain to be required in the future and (2) that will enable the trier-or-fact to reasonably estimate the cost of the expected treatment (*Henley v. Amacher*, 2002 WL 100402 (Tenn. Ct. App. Jan 28, 20002), cited with approval (*Singh v. Larry Fowler Trucking, Inc.*, 2012, p. 287).

Anchoring Economic Damages

The plaintiff counsel's ability to present concrete economic losses to a jury has become ever more important. As David Ball (2005, p. 175) explains: Jurors often base their intangibles (non-economic damages) on the tangible (economic) amount.

> Jurors use the economic losses as a benchmark for measuring non-economic losses … the higher, the more concrete, and the more persuasive your tangible figure is, the more money you are likely to get for intangible damages as well.[4]

This is a heuristic known as anchoring bias (Tversky & Kahneman, 1974)[5]

> The anchoring effect refers to the cognitive bias in which human beings rely too much on the first piece of information encountered, or other (even possibly irrelevant) information in their consciousness, when making decisions. Its power in affecting human decision-making is well-established in the literature of psychology.[6]

For instance, Tversky and Kahneman (1974) found that even arbitrary numbers could lead participants to make incorrect estimates. In one example, participants spun a wheel to select a number between 0 and 100. The volunteers were then asked to adjust that number up or down to indicate how many African countries were in the United Nations. Those who spun a high number gave higher estimates while those who spun a low number gave lower estimates. In each case, the participants were using that initial number as their anchor point to base their decision[7] (Cherry, 2019).

This anchoring bias applies to litigation as well.[8] Hastie et al. (1999) demonstrated that jurors will award more money in compensation, the more money plaintiff's attorney requests. Raclinski et al. (2006) observed this same behavior pattern in judges.[9] The cost of the plaintiff's future healthcare needs can also serve as an anchor, especially in states where attorneys are prohibited from asking the jury for a specific figure for non-economic damages. Recognizing this bias, a life care plan should only be used where the cost projection of future medical needs is sufficiently high. A projection that is too low may have a negative effect and result in a lower jury award. (Ball, 2013, p.189).[10] With low economic damages, an economic-damages anchor can work against you. Low economic figures lead to low economic figures."

Hiring a Life Care Planning Expert

Plaintiff's attorneys have traditionally obtained reports on the need for future medical care from their client's treating or examining physicians. Although this may lay the foundation for the life care planner's later testimony, most physicians are limited to providing acute medical care. Long-term rehabilitative care is not something the treating neurosurgeon, for example, routinely provides after the catastrophically injured individual is through the acute life-threatening episode. Neurosurgeons generally discharge and refer the patient to the care of rehabilitative specialists. Very few physicians have the training or expertise to evaluate and prepare a comprehensive long-term life care plan that involves the coordination of multidisciplinary professionals. In today's age of managed health care, physicians rarely know the reasonable or acceptable reimbursement rate for the treatment they, themselves, provide, let alone the reimbursement rate for treatment by other specialists. This is one of the very reasons that life care planning has evolved as a profession.

When representing an injured plaintiff and their family, the plaintiff's trial counsel must retain a well-qualified life care planner who can properly quantify the costs of future medical care and provide the necessary support to replace services that can no longer be performed. It is critical that the life care planner provide thoughtful input into the long-term medical, educational, rehabilitative, social-emotional, leisure, and vocational needs that will arise throughout the individual's lifetime[11] (Sellars, 1996).

The need for periodic appointments and treatments, the monitoring and future costs of medication, and the potential need for and costs of supportive care loom large; however, for many individuals with catastrophic injuries, their greatest losses reside in their inability to perform or experience activities once an integral part of life. Therefore, in addition to identifying health-related services, the life care planner should also address quality-of-life and psychosocial and behavioral needs, and educational, vocational, recreational, home, and community support systems.

Retaining the best-qualified life care planner is essential. Under the *Federal Rules of Evidence* 702 and evidence rules in most state courts, a witness will qualify as an expert based on knowledge, skill, experience, training, and/or education.[12] The life care planner retained should be academically, clinically, and socially qualified (Sellars, 1996). The life care planner should be familiar with clinical management and long-term planning. In this day of specialization, some life care planners, for example, work exclusively with individuals with certain disabilities (e.g., brain injuries and spinal cord injuries).

In 1996, the International Commission on Health Care Certification[13] offered the first certification examination for life care planners. One cannot, however, assume that certified life care planners have demonstrated basic competency in the field. The plaintiff's attorney should therefore be advised to look beyond simple certification and investigate the life care planner's academic training and work-related experience. The attorney should question whether the candidate has a broad breadth of experience in the rehabilitation field and attends continuing education to maintain and upgrade life care knowledge. It is critical that the life care planner also read relevant literature as healthcare, disability policies, and healthcare costing are constantly changing.

Life care plans are by their very nature educational documents. Therefore, another major consideration when hiring a life care planner is whether the life care planner can present the life care plan in the courtroom setting or in a deposition to educate interested parties. Because direct examination is about persuasion and communication, the life care planner must be able to communicate complex issues in the life care plan, appear credible, and persuade the jurors they should agree with the planner's opinions. Cross-examination is one of the most difficult and challenging aspects of being a life care plan expert. Opposing counsel will work to lessen the expert's credibility by seeking to expose bias; impeaching the expert with prior statements or writings; and challenging the expert's opinions, methodology, facts, and data.[14]

Working with the Life Care Planner

Although preparing a long-term care plan may be premature at the outset, ideally the life care planner will be retained shortly after the attorney is retained, so the life care planner can work with the plaintiff's doctors and medical providers to help establish a workable plan for both acute and long-term care. The life care planner can also interact with medical insurance company adjusters and representatives to help avoid the common delays in medical treatment that patients and families encounter when dealing with insurance representatives. Because a life care plan is an evolving, dynamic document, early retention of a life care planner can facilitate the development of an effective and well-considered plan for the plaintiff.

It is imperative that the life care planner personally interview the injured individual and family and observe the person in the home environment. Using only a "record review" to prepare a life care plan subjects the life care planner to intense cross-examination.[15] The plaintiff's attorney needs to obtain all of the injured individual's medical and employment records to properly assist the life care planner in formulating a life care plan. The plaintiff's attorney should also obtain a prognosis from each of the patient's physicians that includes their expectations for the care the person will need.

The need for expert medical opinion upon which the life care planner relies is well illustrated by *First National Bank of Fort Smith v. The Kansas City Southern Railway Co.*[16] While the Court found the plaintiff's life care planner to be qualified, the Court concluded that the life care planner's opinion that the plaintiff would become a paraplegic or confined to a wheelchair should have been excluded as no doctor or other qualified medical expert testified as such.

Conversely, after the life care planner prepares the life care plan, the plaintiff's attorney should review it to ensure that each of the recommended treatments has proper foundational support. Anything that seems unnecessary or frivolous should be omitted, as such items will undermine the credibility of the plan and destroy the jurors' confidence in the validity and necessity of every part of the plan (Ball, 2005).

A life care plan is a dynamic document that may require modifications as time goes on. Therefore, medical reports that post-date the life care plan must be sent to the life care planner for consideration and the plan should be modified as required. It is inexcusable for an attorney to present a life care planner who was not furnished with the client's medical records when such a review could easily have been accomplished.

In preparing the plan, the life care planner must address what effect the injuries have had not only on the catastrophically injured person but also on the person's family. The emotional turmoil suffered by caregivers cannot be discounted or ignored.[17] Families who have sustained a relative's traumatic injury often suffer from isolation, depression, anxiety, stress, and fatigue (McDaniel et al. (2012); Qadeer et al., 2017).[18] [19] Thus, it is necessary that the life care planner assess whether family members will also require related medical care, such as family or individual counseling.

Finally, because the life care plan will document the need for future care over the individual's entire life, it must be presented in today's dollars. Because most life care planners lack the qualifications and the expertise to perform the economic analysis necessary required to present the cost in today's dollars, it will be necessary to retain an economic expert to make this calculation. For a discussion of the role of the economist, see Chapter 18 "The Role of the Economist in Life Care Planning."

Defense Attack of Life Care Planners

The object of the life care plan is to fully and fairly compensate the injured person and enhance the quality of life to the greatest extent. Defense counsel in personal injury actions has the duty to advocate for their client. To that end, the role of defense counsel is to minimize, or contain, the cost or recovery. One can expect the defense attorney and the insurance carrier to mount an all-out attack against the plaintiff's life care planner. These attacks are commonly centered on the life care planner's credentials and qualifications, the methodology used in preparing the life care plan, and ultimately the plan itself.

Daubert and the Admissibility of Expert Life Care Planner Testimony

In *Daubert v. Merrill Dow Pharmaceuticals*, (1993)[20] the United States Supreme Court held that trial judges were to act as gatekeepers for the admissibility of expert testimony. The Court enunciated five factors to be considered:[21]

> (1) whether the expert's technique or theory can be or has been tested—that is, whether the expert's theory can be challenged in some objective sense, or whether it is instead simply a subjective, conclusory approach that cannot reasonably be assessed for reliability;

(2) whether the technique or theory has been subject to peer review and publication;
(3) the known or potential rate of error of the technique or theory when applied;
(4) the existence and maintenance of standards and controls; and
(5) whether the technique or theory has been generally accepted in the scientific community.

In 2000, the Daubert holding was codified under Federal Rules of Evidence 702. Committee Notes to the 2000 Amendment explained:

> The amendment affirms the trial court's role as gatekeeper and provides some general standards that the trial court must use to assess the reliability and helpfulness of proffered expert testimony. Consistently with *Kumho*, the Rule as amended provides that all types of expert testimony present questions of admissibility for the trial court in deciding whether the evidence is reliable and helpful. Consequently, the admissibility of all expert testimony is governed by the principles of Rule 104(a). Under that Rule, the proponent has the burden of establishing that the pertinent admissibility requirements are met by a preponderance of the evidence. *See Bourjaily v. United States*, 483 U.S. 171 (1987).

Presently the Advisory Committee on Evidence Rules has recommended two amendments to Rule 702. These changes will take place in December 2023. First, the proposed rule would be amended to clarify and emphasize that the admissibility requirements set forth in the rule must be established to the court by a preponderance of the evidence. The Committee noted:

> There is no intent to raise any negative inference regarding the applicability of the Rule 104(a) standard of proof for other rules. The Committee concluded that emphasizing the preponderance standard in Rule 702 specifically was made necessary by the courts that have failed to apply correctly the reliability requirements of that rule. Nor does the rule require that the court make a finding of reliability in the absence of objection.
>
> The amendment clarifies that the preponderance standard applies to the three reliability-based requirements added in 2000—requirements that many courts have incorrectly determined to be governed by the more permissive Rule 104(b) standard. But it remains the case that other admissibility requirements in the rule (such as that the expert must be qualified and the expert's testimony must help the trier of fact) are governed by the Rule 104(a) standard as well. Some challenges to expert testimony will raise matters of weight rather than admissibility even under the Rule 104(a) standard. For example, if the court finds it more likely than not that an expert has a sufficient basis to support an opinion, the fact that the expert has not read every single study that exists may raise a question of weight and not admissibility. But this does not mean, as certain courts have held, that arguments about the sufficiency of an expert's basis always go to weight and not admissibility. Rather it means that once the court has found it more likely than not that the admissibility requirement has been met, any attack by the opponent will go only to the weight of the evidence. It will often occur that experts come to different conclusions based on contested sets of facts. Where that is so, the Rule 104(a) standard does not necessarily require exclusion of either side's experts. Rather, by deciding the disputed facts, the jury can decide which side's experts to credit. "[P]roponents 'do not have to demonstrate to the judge by a preponderance of the evidence that the assessments of their experts are correct, they only have to demonstrate by

a preponderance of evidence that their opinions are reliable .... The evidentiary requirement of reliability is lower than the merits standard of correctness.'"[22]

The second proposal would emphasize that a trial judge must exercise gatekeeping authority with respect to the opinion ultimately expressed by a testifying expert. The Committee noted:

> (2) Rule 702(d) has also been amended to emphasize that each expert opinion must stay within the bounds of what can be concluded from a reliable application of the expert's basis and methodology. Judicial gatekeeping is essential because just as jurors may be unable, due to lack of specialized knowledge, to evaluate meaningfully the reliability of scientific and other methods underlying expert opinion, jurors may also lack the specialized knowledge to determine whether the conclusions of an expert go beyond what the expert's basis and methodology may reliably support.
>
> The amendment is especially pertinent to the testimony of forensic experts in both criminal and civil cases. Forensic experts should avoid assertions of absolute or one hundred percent certainty—or to a reasonable degree of scientific certainty—if the methodology is subjective and thus potentially subject to error. In deciding whether to admit forensic expert testimony, the judge should (where possible) receive an estimate of the known or potential rate of error of the methodology employed, based (where appropriate) on studies that reflect how often the method produces accurate results. Expert opinion testimony regarding the weight of feature comparison evidence (i.e., evidence that a set of features corresponds between two examined items) must be limited to those inferences that can reasonably be drawn from a reliable application of the principles and methods. This amendment does not, however, bar testimony that comports with substantive law requiring opinions to a particular degree of certainty.[23]

Since the United States Supreme Court's landmark decision in *Daubert v. Merrill Dow Pharmaceuticals, Inc.* (1993), and its codification in the Federal Rules of Evidence, federal and state court trial judges have scrutinized the opinions and methodologies used by all experts called to testify on behalf of the parties. Experts who previously had no difficulty qualifying and giving expert opinions are finding their testimony barred and their opinions excluded when they cannot demonstrate that they have followed an accepted methodology or standards of practice. Life care planners are no exception (*Sandretto v. Payson Healthcare*, 2014).[24] [25]

Common Defense Arguments Against Life Care Planners

A life care planner's testimony is admissible, but before a life care planner may testify, the adversary attorney and trial court will scrutinize the plan's methodology. One attack against a life care planner may focus on the recommendations included in the life care plan that did not come from a physician. Second, the life care planner's testimony may be attacked and a motion to strike may be filed to argue that the proposed testimony and opinions are outside of the scope of the life care planner's expertise because a life care planner is not a medical doctor. This latter argument recalls the misguided belief that only physicians are qualified to give medical opinions about future medical care needs. For additional information about the scope of practice for life care planners from various professional disciplines, the reader is referred to the *Journal of Life Care Planning*, *17*(1). While courts historically did not permit non-physicians to give medical opinions including diagnosis, causation, and prognosis, that has changed in most states recognizing the ability of a non-physician expert, who has the requisite knowledge, skill, experience, training, and/or education in the particular field, to provide such opinions.

In presenting the life care planner as an expert, it is important not only to provide the court with an outline or summary of the expert's education, training, and experience but also to educate the court about the functions of the life care planner and clarify for whom the life care planner provides reports. While used in litigation, it should be noted that the insurance industry and the federal government use life care plans. Insurance companies set reserves regarding the costs of future medical care, as does the government in funding Social Security, or Medicare payments, the Vaccine Injury Compensation Board, and the Veterans Administration. To make such assessments, the insurance industry and federal government often retain life care planners to make these calculations, frequently without the assistance or intervention of any medical personnel.

The argument that no qualified physician has offered foundational testimony about the need for, and type of future medical care is a central attack designed to undermine the entire specialty practice of life care planning as a profession. This long-standing defense argument attempts to reduce the life care planner to nothing more than a clerical staff member whose only responsibility is to quantify the costs of future medical care prescribed or recommended by a physician. The assault will further contend that, to prepare a life care plan, the life care planner must consult with a treatment team who will recommend a list of medical treatments for the person's future health care.

In negating this argument, the plaintiff's attorney must retain a life care planner with experience in preparing life care plans and, more importantly, one who has experience in treating patients who have sustained traumatic injuries or who have chronic health conditions. It also is important for the attorney to understand life care planning and to establish that a particular life care planner's methodology is both appropriate and acceptable.

A good example of a life care planner having her testimony stricken is *Vaughn v. Hobby Lobby Stores* (2021),[26] where the federal court barred the testimony of the plaintiff's life care planner, finding the life care planner failed to demonstrate her plan was based upon sufficient facts or data. Specifically, the court found the life care planner failed to cite with sufficient specificity any written report, medical record, or deposition testimony that [plaintiff] will more probably than not need the treatment recommended. The Court found that the proposed testimony was not predicated upon the testimony of treating physicians (other than herself), as to the reasonable need for future care. "Her own diagnosis of any disorder or condition or the future medical costs related thereto is not sufficient"(p.13).

Trial courts have upheld life care planners' qualifications when education, training, and experience in preparing life care plans are established, as in *Coleman v. United States of America and Touchette*[27] (2003). Conversely, in *Fairchild v. United States*[28] (1991), a Louisiana federal court rejected the qualifications of a life care planner who had taken only two seminars in life care planning and had compiled only 25 life care plans.

Will the life care planner be permitted to present expert opinion detailing what medical care will be needed, or will the testimony be limited solely to providing testimony regarding the costs of that care? In *Kent Village Associates Joint Venture v. Smith*[29] (1995), that issue was presented to the Court of Special Appeals of Maryland. The case involved a tragic accident in which the plaintiff sustained paraplegia. The plaintiff produced the expert testimony of a life care planner who held a doctorate in rehabilitation counseling and was certified as a national rehabilitation counselor and in her state. Her expertise as a rehabilitation counselor was not contested by defense counsel. Instead, the principal attack on the life care planner's testimony was that there was "no medical evidence from qualified medical experts sufficient to support" her opinion (pp. 523–524). The court rejected this defense, finding:

> We are satisfied, having reviewed her testimony and the exhibit prepared by her, that her opinions were adequately supported by medical evidence, where that kind of support was required, or by other facts that it was reasonable for [life care planner] to consider (*Kent Village Associates Joint Venture v. Smith*, 1995, p. 524).

Conversely, in *Norwest Bank v. Kmart Corp.*[30] (1997), the court granted defendant Kmart's motion to exclude the testimony of the plaintiff's life care planner because, after reviewing the life care planner's qualifications, the District Court found that, although the life care planner had the necessary qualifications and experience to be qualified as an expert, the witness testimony must still "fit the witness's expertise."(p.2). The court was of the antiquated opinion that the projected need for future medical care called for a medical opinion, for which the life care planner was not qualified to provide. Accepting this rationale, virtually every life care planner in the country today would not be qualified to provide expert testimony regarding the life care needs of an individual, rendering the field of forensic life care planning extinct.[31] The court barred this testimony.

In looking back at the *Norwest* decision, this case was decided before the U.S. Supreme Court's decision in *Kumho Tire Co. v. Carmichael* (1999).[32] There, the U.S. Supreme Court clarified that the factors referenced in *Daubert v. Merrill Dow Pharmaceuticals, Inc.* (1993) were neither exclusive nor all-inclusive and that the trial court appeared to have employed an improper analysis. The issue for any trial court is to determine whether a specific expert's methodology is scientifically valid. To make that determination, the trial court must look to see whether that methodology is accepted and used in the specific scientific community. The court was critical because the life care planner could provide no literature to support his specific methodology. The court stated in *Norwest*:

> His opinion appears to have been based on his years of experience in the field, for which consumers in the market pay him. But under 'the higher standard for the admissibility of expert witness testimony' that has emerged in the wake of *Daubert*, the court must assure that opinion testimony is linked to scientific principal as well as to individual expertise (p.5).

In strictly applying the *Daubert v. Merrill Dow Pharmaceutical, Inc.* (1993) criteria or factors, one quickly understands that the specific factors, such as error rate, for example, simply do not apply to life care planning. *SeaRiver Maritime, Inc. v. Pike*[33] (2006) illustrates well the adjustment necessary to obtain the admissibility of one's life care planner. In this case, the plaintiff retained the same life care expert whose methodology was questioned in *Norwest Bank v. Kmart Corp.* (1997). Here, the defendants appealed a plaintiff's verdict complaining that the trial court erred by failing to exclude the entire testimony of the plaintiff's life care planner. Defendants asserted that the life care planner was not qualified, and his testimony was irrelevant and unreliable. Defendants argued that the plaintiff's expert should not have been permitted to testify as to the need for future care, as he was not a medical doctor. In making their argument, the defendants relied upon *Norwest v. Kmart Corp.* (1997).

On appeal, the Texas Appellate Court rejected the defendant's arguments. First, the court found that the expert was qualified to testify based on his "work in the field of life care planning for over 20 years and his 30 years of experience in health care management for people with disabilities" (*Norwest v. Kmart Corp.*, 1997, para. 2) In deciding, the court also relied upon the expert having operated his own facility for rehabilitation, particularly for patients with neurologic impairments, his master's degree in rehabilitation counseling, and his doctorate degree in counseling.

Regarding the defendants' *Norwest* argument, the appellate court distinguished that case from the facts and testimony presented here. The court stated:

> *Norwest* is plainly distinguishable. As we read [the expert's] testimony, his approach in this case avoided the mistakes in *Norwest*. He based much of his cost evaluation upon the records and recommendation[s] of the treating physicians. Unlike *Norwest,* other qualified health care providers testified and related many of the components of the health care plan. Further, unlike *Norwest, SeaRiver* also provided health care evidence through its own life care expert (*Sea River Maritime, Inc. v. Pike,* 2006).

Finally, the defendants argued that the opinions were unreliable, selectively choosing three items of cross-examination where the expert admitted there was no doctor recommendation for the stated therapy. The court noted that, while no specific objections had been lodged to that testimony, the court went further, finding that the expert life care planner had considerable expertise to assess actual medical costs and had consulted and confirmed with the treating doctors their opinions on both the need for and cost of ongoing treatment. The court found that under the circumstances, it could not say that the trial court abused its discretion in admitting the testimony.

Two additional cases, *Oram v. DeCholnoky* (2008) and *Marcano v. Turabo Medical Center Partnership* (2005) have also rejected that a life care planner, to be admitted as an expert, must be a physician or that the life care planner's opinions must be based upon the testimony of a medical physician regarding the need for future medical care. In *Oram v. DeCholnoky*[34] (2008), the testimony of a life care planner was deemed admissible although the life care planner was not a medical doctor, because the planner had years of experience, was certified, was a fellow of the International Academy of Life Care Planners and was also certified as a disability analyst and vocational evaluator. The court rejected the defendant's argument that the expert's testimony was inadmissible because he was not a medical doctor.

Similarly, in *Marcano v. Turabo Medical Center Partnership*[35] (2005), the 1st Circuit upheld the U.S. District Court for the District of Puerto Rico's denial of a motion to strike a life care planner as an expert. The life care planner was allowed to testify as an expert wherein he had sufficient education and professional credentials, had been admitted as an expert on rehabilitation and life care planning in numerous state and federal courts, and his proposed plan was based on a review of records from an agency providing the child with skilled medical care, a letter from the child's physician, and an interview of the child's family and caregiver. The court stated, "although [the expert's] report might have benefitted from a physician's review of the projections regarding [the child's] future needs, the court did not abuse its discretion in determining that [the planner's] methodology was sufficiently reliable for admissibility" (*Marcano v. Turabo Medical Center Partnership,* 2005, p. 171).

Remembering that the defense attorney's mission is cost containment and damage control, it is logical that the defense will next attack the assumptions made and the opinions rendered by the plaintiff's life care planner. From the perspective of a plaintiff's life care planner, the life care plan is based on assessing real costs, highlighting necessary care, and developing a plan that creates the least restrictive environment for the injured person. Defendants often attempt to place the injured person in the least costly environment, arguing that the person's spouse should provide needed care or recommend placement in a restricted environment, based solely on cost. However, it is not only unfair but also wrong to reject needed care and, instead, place that burden of care on the injured plaintiff's spouse because the defendant caused the injury that resulted in the need for care and should be held responsible for the entire harm caused.

Defendant Retained Life Care Planners

Defendants will sometimes hire their own life care planner to counter the plan that the plaintiff's life care planner submits. Most defendants will not do so, however, because they fear setting a monetary floor at which the jury will begin when determining an appropriate figure for future care. The common purposes for presenting the defense life care planner are cost containment and damage control. The defense life care planner may eliminate as much of the proposed care as possible and may shift the burden of care from trained professionals to an individual's family members. It is also not uncommon to see defense life care planners claiming a reduced life expectancy for the injured individual.

More recently, defendants have retained life care plan experts as expert witnesses to attack the qualifications or methodology used by the plaintiff's experts. In these circumstances, the defendants' expert does not prepare their own life care plan but rather attacks the qualifications, methodology, or projections provided by the plaintiff's expert.

To defeat this approach, it is important for the plaintiff's counsel to take the deposition of the defendant's life care planning expert and walk that expert through the plaintiff's own life care plan getting the defense expert to agree or disagree as to the need for every component of the plaintiff's life care plan. When successfully done, the plaintiff's counsel can compel the defendant's expert to essentially prepare a life care plan at the deposition and compel the defendants to concede the cost of much of the plaintiff's expert's report.

The case of *Cogg v. Dawson*[36] (2007) provides an interesting attack by the plaintiff's counsel on such a defense expert who was hired not to project her own life care plan but to attack the methodology used by the plaintiff's expert. There, the plaintiff sought to exclude the expert testimony of the defendants' life care planner regarding the details of the life care plan created by the plaintiff's retained expert. The plaintiff did not challenge the defense expert's qualifications to testify competently, and the court found no reason to doubt her expertise, finding that her experience as a counselor with an advanced degree in rehabilitation counseling, a quarter-century's worth of experience, and that she had prepared over 20 life care plans satisfied the court she was qualified to testify.

Having determined the defendant's expert was qualified to testify, the court then needed to determine the reliability of the testimony. The plaintiff argued before trial that the plaintiff's expert could not challenge the "specifics of one plan without possessing the knowledge to create her own." (p.4).

The defendant conceded that no "reliability argument" could be made regarding her own life care plan and, at most, "it would appear that [the defendant's expert] can testify as to how to make a life care plan and what steps are involved in its creation." (p. 5). However, the court held that the defendant's expert could not testify specifically regarding the need of the injured plaintiff as the defendant's expert had not tried to educate herself regarding the specific needs of the plaintiff. The court held that all the defendant's expert could do was criticize the plaintiff's expert's methodology but not his findings, and the defendant's expert could not dispute the facts the plaintiff's expert used in creating his plan.

Role of Medical Providers in Life Care Planning

As most life care planners are not physicians, some states require the life care planner to base the life care plan on the recommendations and opinions of medical physicians, whose opinions are based on a reasonable degree of medical probability. In preparing a life care plan, the life care planner will normally interview the injured plaintiff and members of their family, review medical records, and often speak with or submit questionnaires to physicians regarding the need for future medical care.[37] This has often resulted in defendants objecting to the life care planner testifying, asserting the life care planner's opinions are based on hearsay. The *Federal Rule of Evidence* 703[38] states:

> An expert may base an opinion on facts or data in the case that the expert has been made aware of or personally observed. If experts in the particular field would reasonably rely on those kinds of facts or data in forming an opinion on the subject, they need not be admissible for the opinion to be admitted. But if the facts or data would otherwise be inadmissible, the proponent of the opinion may disclose them to the jury only if their probative value in helping the jury evaluate the opinion substantially outweighs their prejudicial effect.

Morales-Hurtado v. Reinoso[39] (2020) provides an illustrative example. Juan Morales-Hurtado was injured in a motor vehicle crash. He sustained neck and back injuries, which after conservative treatment, underwent a lumbar fusion. Plaintiff claimed his injuries were permanent. Plaintiff's attorney retained a life care planner who met with the plaintiff and his wife at their home and reviewed numerous medical records. Following her consideration of the medical records, the life care planner followed up with the medical offices, either by talking to staff or sending comprehensive questionnaires. She also sent a summary letter to a doctor confirming the information she received. The doctor would indicate approval by signing the summary.

Although the court found the expert qualified to render an opinion in the field of life care planning, and though the expert testified the medical records and questionnaires she relied upon were of the type reasonably relied upon by experts in her field, the trial court nonetheless precluded her from testifying. In doing so, it appears the court believed that if the underlying data and records were inadmissible, the expert's opinion must be barred.[40]

On appeal, the New Jersey appellate court, reversed the decision, finding:

> Experts are permitted to "apprise the trier of fact of the bases for [their] opinion, including the opinions of other experts," but are not entitled "to introduce an out-of-court expert's report for its 'truth', where it is critical to the primary issue in the case and the adversary objects." … Exclusion of the information or data an expert has relied upon does not require exclusion of the expert's opinion.
>
> The court appears to have made the same mistake concerning the expert's interview with [the] plaintiff's wife. The court noted plaintiff's spouse had not been named as a witness and could not testify at trial. Nonetheless, the expert had the right to apprise the jury she relied on, among other things, interviews with plaintiff and his wife. Of course, a trial court should provide a limiting instruction to the jury in situations where a testifying expert identifies or alludes to the sources upon which he or she has professionally relied'(citation omitted) (p.1006).

Defendant appealed to the New Jersey Supreme Court. There, the Supreme Court, relying on N.J.R.E. 703, which provides an expert may rely on "facts or data in the particular case," which "may be those perceived by or made known to the expert at or before the hearing," and that such facts or data need not be admissible in evidence "[i]f of a type reasonably relied upon by experts in the particular field in forming opinions or inferences upon the subject."[41] (p. 243). The Supreme Court noted:

> That principle, however, does not obviate the need to demonstrate that the treating physician on whom the life care expert relies actually holds the opinion attributed to him or her, which can be accomplished by means of a report by the treating physician, his or her trial testimony, or other competent evidence. [42] (p.243).

In a footnote the Court upheld the use of a questionnaire, advising:

> A questionnaire may be an appropriate device for a life care expert to use in the collection of facts or data relevant to his or her opinion. We address only the expert's use of questionnaires in this case to elicit the opinions of treating physicians as to plaintiff's future need for medical care. (p.243).

A similar decision was announced in *Hale v. Gannon* (2012).[43] In this case, the defendant moved to bar the introduction of a life care planner, who also relied on physician questionnaires. In upholding this practice, the District Court explained in a footnote:

> The Defendants also object to [life care planner's] testimony because, they assert, she may not rely on inadmissible questionnaires as a basis for including certain treatment in her life care plan. However, the Defendants conflate the standard for evidence on which the *jury* may rely to find that certain treatment is necessary with the standard for evidence on which a *life care planner* may rely to include in her life care plan. Federal Rule of Evidence 703 provides: "An expert may base an opinion on facts or data in the case that the expert has been made aware of .... If experts in the particular field would reasonably rely on those kinds of facts or data in forming an opinion on the subject, they need not be admissible for the opinion to be admitted." [Life care planner] testified that one of the step-by-step procedures outlined in the life care planning handbook for following-up with treating physicians is composing a letter outlining the "right" questions to assure that the planner is soliciting the needed information. Furthermore, all parties agree [life care planner] may not render medical treatment opinions herself. Therefore, the Court finds that submitting questionnaires to treating physicians requesting additional information is a reasonable practice (p.5–6).[44]

What these cases teach, is that the opinions of life care planners should incorporate the opinions of a plaintiff's doctors, when possible and not solely the life care planner's own opinions and recommendations. While it may not be necessary for the plaintiff's counsel to call each and every physician whose opinion is relied upon to form the basis for the life care plan, where practical, the attorney may strongly consider doing so, to avoid this hearsay objection.[45]

Presenting the Life Care Planner in Court

Economic damages are often the benchmark or jumping-off point for jurors when they deliberate to award non-economic damages. Remember that none of the funds sought for the life care plan will ultimately go to the plaintiff, but will pay for future medical, support, or replacement care. As

Ball (2001) cautions, economic testimony is important because the jurors should know the purpose each item serves, to which specific injury the item relates, and what will happen if the item is not provided. He states further:

> Some attorneys tend to rush testimony about the life-care plan because it seems tedious. It is quick and easy to describe a few representative examples of the items on the life-care plan, and then give a grand total. But that is what the defense hopes you will do. The defense does not want you to present your life-care plan carefully and concretely. The defense prefers you to leave the jury with only a vague idea of the life-care plan's content(Ball, 2001, p. 176).

In presenting the testimony of the life care planner, Ball (2012) recommends:[46]

1. The life care planner is responsible for teaching the attorney the questions to ask;
2. Explain the steps the life care planner takes to arrive at his/her opinion;
3. Demonstrate not only that the adversary's life care plan is wrong, but show where the other side's life care planner did not follow the rules of their profession;
4. Explain what will happen to the plaintiff if the plaintiff is not awarded the full amount of the life care plan;
5. Show how the items in the life care plan will help the plaintiff maintain his/her self-respect, [and] mobility and avoid isolation.

Rarely will the defense be able to attack every item. Rather, defense counsel will pick a few specific items to discredit the entire report and will attack the plan either through cross-examining the plaintiff's life care planner or through the direct testimony of its own life care planner. If the life care planner has omitted those controversial items, the plan is more difficult to attack. However, the defense will always argue that certain items are unnecessary. If the life care planner has presented every item, it is then easy for the plaintiff's counsel, in summation, to tell the jury to eliminate those items in dispute, which will leave much of the life care plan intact and still present a formidable damage amount.

A Case Illustration: United Planters Bank v. United States

On July 18, 1998, Kimberly Coleman presented to Touchette Regional Hospital in labor. Because her regular obstetrician was unavailable, she was assigned to the obstetrician on call. Due to that obstetrician's negligence, as determined by the court sitting without a jury, the infant plaintiff, Javan Coleman, was born profoundly impaired with an approximate IQ of 20. He was born with hypotonic ataxic cerebral palsy. He has difficulty with gross motor skills and trouble swallowing, cannot chew food, and has visual impairments. The court found the multiple impairments to be significant. The plaintiff's counsel retained the services of a rehabilitation professional life care planner, whom the court found was a "very impressive witness, who presented with a tremendous background of academia and practical experience" (p. 5).[47] The court also found his testimony was "highly credible and carried great weight" (p.5).

In awarding damages, the court found that the plaintiff's life care plan was a very "detailed one," and considered as many of Javan's needs as contemplated. The plaintiff's life care planner considered "doctors, facilities, personal care items, and seemingly every conceivable need within a reasonable degree of contemplation by a life care planner" (p. 6). The defense, on the other hand, retained a board-certified physician who rendered the opinion that the infant should be admitted to a nursing home where he should be "sufficiently medicated to allow the relatively non-professional nursing home staff to manage him" (p.6). He also rendered the opinion after considering "every known article on the subject" of life expectancy that Javan's ailments and disabilities would reduce his life expectancy to 40 years of age (p. 6).

The court rejected the opinions offered by the defendant's physician, for the plan submitted by the plaintiff's life care planner. The court found that the defendant's expert's testimony was much less impressive and internally inconsistent. The court found that the defense plan was not in the child's best interest, but it favored the defendant. The court rejected the opinion that the infant's life expectancy would be shortened because of the disabilities and impairments, which resulted from the defendant's medical negligence. Finally, the court rejected outright the suggestion by the defendant's life care planner that any nursing home would do for the child's care.

This case illustrates many issues addressed in this chapter: the court found for the life care plan prepared by the plaintiff's life care planner, a non-physician professional, over that of a board-certified physician. Similarly, the court dismissed the defendant's argument that the plaintiffs could be substituted as caregivers over professional staffing and that the infant plaintiff should be institutionalized in a nursing home to help contain the cost of future medical care. Finally, the court rejected the government's use of the Strauss and Shavelle (2008) life expectancy studies[48] often relied upon by defense attorneys and their life care planners.

Economic Valuations of Life Care Plans

Because life care plans project medical care costs over the plaintiff's lifespan, in most states, if not all, the plan must be presented in today's dollars. This is called discounting. Because the plaintiff will receive the cost of the life care plan today for medical care needed, the plaintiff can invest those monies and earn interest. It is necessary to consider the effect of inflation on the value of money. Where interest earned outpaces inflation, the life care plan must be reduced to reflect its present value. But if the effect of inflation on the cost of medical care is greater than the interest that can be earned on that investment, the present value of the life care plan must be increased. This is called a net negative discount effect. Where the interest rate and the inflationary rate are equal, this is called a total offset. Some states as a matter of law mandate the total offset method, thus eliminating the need to present evidence of present value, the majority leave it to the parties to present expert testimony.

It is not recommended that the life care planner calculate the present value of the life care plan. Rather, it is recommended that the plaintiff retain an economist to perform the calculation. Inflationary trends and discount rates are not traditionally in the life care planner's qualifications and it is simpler and less confusing to the jury to let different professionals explain the costs of future medical needs and the costs in today's dollars.

Defendants will often retain an economist who will use an inappropriate discount rate, which will have the effect of severely reducing the present value of the life care plan, providing inadequate funds to care for the plaintiff over their lifetime. To appreciate the significance of the discount rate used, consider this example: Johnnie Smith is a three-year-old male child who sustained a traumatic brain injury in a car crash. The child will likely require future medical care and some assistance in terms of living independently. He is expected to have a normal life expectancy. The economist calculated the present value of the cost of the life care plan to be $3,646,562, using the total offset methodology to arrive at the present value of the loss. Another economist, employing a one percent net discount rate, opined that the cost was $2,403,015, a reduction of over one million dollars. A third economist used a two-percent net discount rate, resulting in a present value cost of $1,619,559, a reduction of over two million dollars. An economist who used a net negative discount rate, i.e., the rate of medical inflation outpaced the interest rate, would have to increase the value over the $3,646,562 million figure used by the economist who used a total offset.

Finally, in a continuing effort at cost containment, defendants will retain or make use of an annuity expert who can minimize or reduce the cost of the life care plan by proffering that an insurance annuity purchased at a far cheaper cost can fund the specific life care plan and provide an income stream for the plaintiff's future medical needs. From a legal standpoint, this is flawed because no state requires an injured plaintiff to purchase an annuity with the proceeds of a personal injury award. The cost of the annuity is based on the risk assumed by the issuing insurance carrier, and the purchase of such an annuity establishes a fixed rate of return. The question then arises as to why the defendant who caused the harm should make these determinations. The plaintiff should decide how the settlement funds or jury's verdict should be invested for their future medical needs.

The cost of an insurance annuity is not based solely on projecting the present value of the projected future cost of the medical needs. Rather, in pricing an insurance annuity, the insurance carrier considers its own determination of the child's life expectancy, future inflation, rate of return, overhead costs and expenses, investment risk, market strategy, and profit level (Langerman, 2001).[49] Such testimony is inadmissible, despite continued attempts by defendants to introduce it. In *Hinsdale v. N.Y., NHHRR Co.*[50] (1903), the trial court excluded this testimony, ruling:

> We do not think that evidence of the cost of an annuity should be admitted, as it is calculated to distract the attention of the jury from the real duty … to fix what they deem a fair and just compensation. (p. 621).

The Tennessee Supreme Court in *Mercer v. Vanderbilt University, Inc.* (2004) upheld a trial court ruling, excluding the testimony of the defendant's structural annuity specialist.[51] Defendant's offer of proof indicated that its expert would have testified about the cost of an annuity policy that could have been purchased to ensure a stream of cash payments to cover Qualls's future medical expenses. The trial court ruled that this evidence was "too speculative." The Tennessee Supreme Court ruled:

> We conclude that the trial court did not abuse its discretion by excluding this testimony. Many changing variables affect the quote that an annuitist delivers to the jury. For instance, time limits and market factors both impact annuity rates. Moreover, an insurance company is in no way bound to the quoted rate or to its initial underwriting decision. These factors not only make the testimony as to the cost of an annuity speculative, but they also raise questions about its potential to mislead the jury. Furthermore, such testimony invites the jury to depart from its legal duty to award present cash value. (p.133–4).

By contrast in *Diede v. Burlington Northern Railroad Co.*,[52] (1983) the U.S. District Court ruled on the admissibility of annuity testimony:

> On the issue of damages, the district court permitted the railroad's witness to testify extensively about the cost of an annuity that would provide a stream of payments to replace Diede's future income. But the court would not permit the witness to testify about the non-taxability of the annuity payments if the railroad purchased the annuity for Diede. Nor would the court admit into evidence the railroad's proposed stipulation

to purchase an annuity. The railroad argues that the failure to admit both the testimony about non-taxability and the proposed stipulation to purchase an annuity resulted in an inflated verdict (p. 594).

On appeal the appellate court upheld the trial court's decision, finding its probative weight was outweighed by the danger it would confuse the issues. The appellate court also noted there were significant constructive receipt problems (p.596–7).

Reasonable and Necessary Future Medical Costs

In most states, an injured person may seek reimbursement for all reasonable and necessary future medical costs causally related to the traumatic event. One currently debated issue centers on whether the proposed care is both reasonable and medically necessary. Some life care planners may be tempted to follow or adopt an insurance reimbursement model based on medical problems, failing to take into account quality of life and only looking for the least expensive treatment. According to Voogt[53] (1996, p. 1), however, "quality of life is generally not an issue that is addressed under this model." Some defendant-retained life care planners look to the least expensive treatment or prepare a plan that attempts to make use of free governmental services. Sometimes a defendant-retained life care planner will argue that the individual's family members should provide care, thereby reducing the need for outside providers and lowering the costs of the life care plan. Unfortunately, such plans fail to compensate fully the injured plaintiff and do not return the individual and family to their position before the traumatic event. It behooves the life care planner to be familiar with the body of literature addressing the physical, psychological, and financial impact of caregiving when providing care for a family member.

Reasonableness of Costs

To sustain an award of future medical expenses, the claimant must present evidence to show there is a reasonable probability that the medical expenses will be incurred; they must also show the reasonable costs of such care (*Columbia Medical Center of Las Colinas v. Bush*,[54] 2003; *Ibrahim v. Young*,[55] 2008). Medical expenses include the costs of doctors' services, hospital services, medicines, medical supplies, medical tests, and any other charges for medical services. The payment is the fair and reasonable value of such medical expenses.

Usual, Customary, and Reasonable[56]

For decades in the United States, the reasonableness of medical costs was rarely disputed in litigation. Life care planners involved in litigation may have had different opinions about what was contained in the plan, but the reasonableness of the cost was typically not discussed. A review of 13 years of *The Neurolaw Letter* (HDI Publishers, 1991–2003), a monthly publication devoted to attorneys and professionals who provide services to survivors of brain injury and spinal cord injury, found fewer than a dozen articles discussing life care planning in general and no articles discussing the usual, customary, or reasonableness of medical costs. In fact, in 1999, life care planner Robert Voogt wrote "A dollar amount can easily be assigned to physician visits, in-home healthcare, medication, therapy, equipment and surgeries" (Voogt[57], 1999, p. 5), implying that assignment of cost could be easily performed.

Collateral Source Rule

In the late 1980s and 1990s, a major piece of the tort reform movement centered on attacking the Collateral Source Rule defendants, manufacturers, and insurance companies argued that plaintiffs should not recover for incurred or to be incurred medical expenses covered by third parties such as private insurance or Medicare/Medicaid. The issue centers on who should benefit from the injured person's own insurance policy. From the injured plaintiff's perspective, a culpable tortfeasor has no right to obtain the advantage of a policy whose premiums were paid for by the plaintiff or obtained as an employee benefit. Defendants, manufacturers, and the insurance industry argue, however, that an injured plaintiff whose medical expenses or lost wages have been paid by private health insurance or reimbursed by a disability carrier receives a double recovery through reimbursement for expenses paid by a third party.

At common law, the law favored the innocent injured plaintiff, finding that a culpable defendant should not reap the windfall because of the fortuitous happenstance that the plaintiff had their own insurance coverage. However, during the past 15 years of tort reform battles, the defense industry has argued there would be greater availability, at less cost, if defendants were not responsible for payment of medical expenses or wage benefits already reimbursed or were reimbursable, by a third-party entity.

Starting in the late 1980s-early 1990s, states began enacting legislation to eliminate recovery for medical expenses paid or payable by private insurance[58] (NJ Rev Stat § 2A:15-97, 2013). By 2007, it was noted that 44 of the 50 states had taken legislative steps to limit the collateral source rule[59] (Zorogastua, 2007). In 2011, the California Supreme Court decided the case of *Howell v. Hamilton Meats & Provisions, Inc.*[60] In *Howell* (2011) the California Supreme Court wrote, "The collateral source rule precludes certain deductions against otherwise recoverable damages but does not expand the scope of economic damages to include expenses the plaintiff never incurred" (p. 548).

Current Status of Collateral Source Rule

As of 2021, there is no consensus among state courts as to the collateral source rule. State courts have essentially taken four approaches of[to] whether to admit undiscounted medical bills into evidence when the bills have been satisfied for less. These are (1) the "actual amount paid" approach, which allows into evidence only the actual amount paid for medical care; (2) the "benefit of the bargain" approach, which allows the undiscounted medical bills into evidence if the plaintiff paid meaningful consideration for the insurance or other collateral source from which payment was made; (3) the "reasonable value" approach, which allows admission of undiscounted medical bills without restriction as at least evidence of the medical services' value (*Dedmon v. Steelman*,[61] 2017; *Weston v. AKHappyTime, LLC*[62], 2019); and (4) a hybrid approach. However, the vast majority of states adhere to the "reasonable value" approach.

The "Actual Amount Paid" Approach

Howell v. Hamilton Meats & Provisions, Inc. (2011) provides an excellent example of the actual amount paid approach. In *Howell*, the issue presented was whether an injured plaintiff whose medical expenses were paid through private health insurance could recover as economic damages the amount billed by the medical provider, or were they limited to the actual amount paid by the insurer. The California Supreme Court ruled a plaintiff could not recover as economic damages more than the discounted amount paid by the private insurer. The Court reasoned:

Because they do not represent an economic loss for the plaintiff, they are not recoverable in the first instance. The collateral source rule precludes certain deductions against otherwise recoverable damages but does not expand the scope of economic damages to include expenses the plaintiff never incurred. (p.549).

...The rule that a plaintiff's expenses, to be recoverable, must be both incurred *and* reasonable accords, as well, with our damages statutes. 'Damages must, in all cases, be reasonable (Civil Code, § 3359)....' But if the plaintiff negotiates a discount and thereby receives services for less than might reasonably be charged, the plaintiff has not suffered a pecuniary loss or other detriment in the greater amount and therefore cannot recover damages for that amount (Civil Code, §§ 3281, 3282). The same rule applies when a collateral source, such as the plaintiff's health insurer, has obtained a discount for its payments on the plaintiff's behalf. (p.556)

The Court concluded that the plaintiff's recovery was limited to the discounted value of the medical expenses. The Court did acknowledge that a tortfeasor who injured an individual insured under a managed care insurance policy would pay less than if the injured person was uninsured. As of the writing of this chapter, it is noted that six states have adopted the actual amount paid approach: California, Idaho, Michigan, New York, Pennsylvania, and Texas.

The "Benefit of the Bargain" Approach

A few states have adopted an alternative sometimes called the "benefit of the bargain" approach. Under the benefit of the bargain approach, the plaintiff who has purchased insurance is assumed to have paid for the negotiated rate differential as much as for the actual cash payments made by the insurer to medical care providers. However, plaintiffs who did not pay for the benefit of discounted rates and write-offs (e.g., beneficiaries of Medicare and Medicaid) may not introduce their undiscounted billings. In these cases, the court "treat[s] the amount paid by Medicare [or Medicaid] as dispositive of the reasonable value of healthcare provider services" (*Weston v. AKhappyTime*, 2019 p. 1026). See also (*Bozeman v. State*[63], 2004; *Stayton v. Delaware Health Corp.*,[64] 2015). As of the writing of this chapter, two states have adopted the benefit of the bargain approach: Delaware and Louisiana.

The "Reasonable Value" Approach

The reasonable value approach allows the admission of undiscounted medical bills without restriction, as evidence of medical services' value. Courts following this approach "adhere to the traditional collateral source rule, as outlined in the Restatement (Second) of Torts § 920A. that tortfeasors should be responsible for all the damage they cause and that plaintiffs, not tortfeasors, should benefit from any negotiated discount" (Weston, 2019, p. 1026).

Some of these courts emphasize that because the value of medical services is a fact-intensive question, juries should receive all relevant evidence, including undiscounted medical bills. An example is *Arthur v. Catour*,[65] 2005. In this case, all of the plaintiff's bills were paid by health insurance. Defendant moved for partial summary judgment, seeking to limit the plaintiff's claim for medical expenses to the amount paid rather than the amount billed. The Illinois Supreme Court rejected the defendant's argument, upheld the collateral source rule, and determined plaintiff could present to the jury the amount that her healthcare providers initially billed for services rendered.

The Tennessee Supreme Court decision in *Dedmon v. Steelman* (2017) is illustrative of this approach. In this case, the defendants filed a motion to limit the plaintiff's recovery for past medical expenses to those amounts actually accepted by medical providers. The Tennessee Supreme Court reviewed the approaches taken by courts throughout the United States and rejected abrogating the collateral source rule, holding:

> All of the alternative common-law approaches have the effect of undermining the collateral source rule and the significant public policies it continues to serve. A decision to depart from the established precedent of the collateral source rule would have to be supported by the firm belief that justice dictates a different path. None of the common-law alternatives to the collateral source rule give us such a firm belief.
>
> Importantly, we have no assurance that adoption of any of the alternative approaches would result in a more just and accurate assessment of the reasonable value of medical services received by plaintiffs in personal injury cases. The discounted amount of medical services does not necessarily, and in fact probably does not, reflect the true value of services rendered … A discounted rate, however, generally reflects the third-party payor's negotiating power and the fact that providers enjoy prompt payment, assured collectability … . (p. 465).
>
> We also decline to alter existing law in Tennessee regarding the collateral source rule. Consequently, the Plaintiffs may submit evidence of Mrs. Dedmon's full, undiscounted medical bills as proof of her "reasonable medical expenses," and the Defendants are precluded from submitting evidence of discounted rates for medical services accepted by medical providers as a result of Mrs. Dedmon's insurance. The Defendants remain free to submit any other competent evidence to rebut the Plaintiffs' proof on the reasonableness of Mrs. Dedmon's medical expenses, so long as the Defendants' proof does not contravene the collateral source rule. (p.467).

In essence, the Dedmon Court decision reaffirmed the reasonable value approach whereby a plaintiff may recover the amount of the full (undiscounted) medical bill. In deciding the case, the Dedmon Court acknowledged the increasing complexity of healthcare pricing, stating:

During this same period since [the] adoption of the rule, the pricing, payment, and reimbursement system for healthcare providers has become exponentially more complex. The rise of managed care organizations has distorted pricing for health care services, as the deep discounts demanded by the MCOs require providers to offset those discounts by charging higher prices to other patients. As observed by the Court of Appeals below, all of these developments have caused:

> the issue of what constitutes a reasonable medical charge or expense [to become] the subject of increased litigation due to the increased involvement of government payors, the complexity of health care reimbursement provisions, financial pressures on hospitals, and the significance of medical expense recovery in personal injury litigation" Dedmon p. 452).

As of the writing of this chapter, it is noted that 18 states continue to follow the reasonable value approach: Alaska, Arizona, Arkansas, Colorado, Hawaii, Illinois, Kansas, Kentucky, Maine, Maryland, Massachusetts, Montana, Oregon, South Dakota, Tennessee, Virginia, West Virginia, and Wisconsin.

Collateral Source Rule and Life Care Planning

The collateral source rule has a significant impact regarding life care plans and a plaintiff's ability, or inability, to obtain compensation for future needs. In those no-fault states or states with the collateral source rule, a life care plan that exclusively outlines expenses for future medical treatment will be of limited use to a plaintiff as the cost of that treatment will not be admissible. While it will be helpful for the jury to understand the plaintiff's future medical treatment needs, the significant impact of introducing a real economic loss and need is eliminated. From a plaintiff's perspective, plaintiffs are advised to retain a life care planner who does not follow the strict insurance medical reimbursement model; while in collateral-rule states, the plaintiff should retain a life care planner who properly quantifies the economic cost for replacement services. Because these expenses are not for medical treatment and are not reimbursable under most medical insurance policies, the collateral source rule is inapplicable.

Day In the Life Video

A day-in-the-life video is a snapshot of a plaintiff's life following an injury. It is very effective in demonstrating the disability, impairments, and limitations the losses and harms caused by the defendant have imposed upon the injured plaintiff and family members. It is also effective in highlighting the need for the proposed life care plan. Often because the injured plaintiff and family lack resources to obtain all the care recommended in the life care plan, a day-in-the-life video can highlight not only what the plaintiff endures on a daily basis but how the plaintiff's life can be enhanced with the recommended life care plan.

Conclusion

In every case in which the plaintiff's counsel represents a person with significant injury, a life care plan is essential. Even cases involving a mild brain injury can prevent the person from performing certain activities for which replacement support care will be needed. Remember, only a small part of the life care plan involves future medical care to treat physical residuals. A person with a significant traumatic injury will have suffered intangible losses for which a life care plan can establish economic value. Omitting a life care plan will undermine the plaintiff's case and prevent the plaintiff from obtaining true compensation for all that has been lost. Compensation, the principle upon which our civil justice system is based, is the provision of balance. Justice balances harm with proper compensation. Cost containment and damage control may be the principles the defense must ensure, but they are not the principles upon which a life care plan should be based.

Notes

1. Singh v. Larry Fowler Trucking, Inc., 390 S.W.3d 280 (Tenn. 2012) https://casetext.com/case/singh-v-larry-fowler-trucking
2. Ramos v. Kuzas, 65 Ohio St.3d 42, 600 N.E.2d 241, 243 (1992)
3. (Expert Institute https://www.expertinstitute.com/resources/insights/state-state-damage-caps/#:~:text=Connect%20with%20industry%20professionals%20whose%20credentials%20meet%20all%20your%20requirements.&text=Currently%2C%20eleven%20states%20cap%20non,Oklahoma%2C%20Oregon%2C%20and%20Tennessee.)

4. Ball, D. (2005). *David Ball on damages: A plaintiff's attorney's guide for personal injury in wrongful death cases* (2nd ed., rev. and expanded). National Institute for Trial Advocacy.
5. Tversky, A., & Kahneman, D. (1974). Judgment under uncertainty: Heuristics and biases. *Science 185*(4157), 1124–31.
6. Chang, Y-C., Chen, K-P., & Lin, C-C. (2016). Anchoring effect in real litigation: An empirical study. *Coase-Sandor Working Paper Series in Law and Economics, 744*, 4. https://chicagounbound.uchicago.edu/cgi/viewcontent.cgi?article=2489&context=law_and_economics
7. Cherry, K. (2020, April 30). *How anchoring bias psychology affects decision making*. https://www.verywellmind.com/what-is-the-anchoring-bias-2795029
8. Hastie, R., Schkade, D. A., & Payne, J. W. (1999). Juror judgments in civil cases: Effects of plaintiff's requests and plaintiff's identity on punitive damage awards. *Law and Human Behavior, 23*, 445–470. https://doi.org/10.1023/A:1022312115561
9. Rachlinski, J. J., Guthrie, C., & Wistrich, A. J. (2006*).* Inside the bankruptcy judge's mind. *Boston University Law Review 86*(5), 1227–1265.
10. Rachlinski, J. J., Guthrie, C., & Wistrich, A. J. (2007). Heuristics and biases in bankruptcy judges. *Journal of Institutional and Theoretical Economics, 163*(1),167–186.
11. Sellars, C. W. (1996). Life care planning for young children with brain injuries. *Neurolaw Letter, 6*(4), 106–107.
12. The National Court Rules Committee. (2022). *The federal rules of evidence, Rule 702*. https://www.rulesofevidence.org/
13. International Commission on Health Care Certification. (2022). *Certified life care planner™*. https://ichcc.org/certified-life-care-planner-clcp.html
14. Keller, J. (n.d.). *Cutting it down to size: Strategies for handling like care plans.* Deutsch Kerrigan. https://trial.com/wp-content/uploads/2020/01/18-Keller.pdf
15. International Academy of Life Care Planners. (2022). *Standards of practice for life care planners* (4th ed.). International Association of Rehabilitation Professionals.
16. First National Bank of Fort Smith v. The Kansas City Southern Railway Company., 865 S.W. 2d 719 (Mo. Ct. App. 1993).
17. Brain Injury Association of New York State. (2022). https://bianys.org/resources/caregivers/
18. Qadeer, A., Khalid, U., Amin, M., Murtaza, S., Khaliq, M. F., & Shoaib, M. (2017). Caregiver's burden of the patients with traumatic brain injury. *Cureus, 9*(8), e1590. https://doi.org/10.7759/cureus.1590
19. McDaniel, K. R., & Allen, D. G. (2012). Working and Care-giving: The Impact on Caregiver Stress, Family-Work Conflict, and Burnout. *Journal of Life Care Planning, 10*(4), 21-32.
20. Daubert v. Merrill Dow Pharmaceuticals, Inc., 509 U.S. 579 (1993)
21. Daubert v. Merrill Dow Pharmaceuticals, Inc., 509 U.S. 579 (1993)
22. Advisory comments to the Proposed amendment to Federal Rule of Evidence 702, Committee on Rules of Practice and Procedure, June 7, 2022, pages 892-4
23. Advisory comments to the Proposed amendment to Federal Rule of Evidence 702, Committee on Rules of Practice and Procedure, June 7, 2022, pages 894-895
24. Sandretto v. Payson Healthcare Management, Inc., 322 P. 3rd 168, 234 Ariz. 351 (Ct. App. 2014)
25. Gurley v. Nebraska Methodist Health System, Inc., 663 N.W. 2d 43, 265 Neb. 918 (Neb. 2003)
26. Vaughn v. Hobby Lobby Stores, Civ. # 6:19-cv-00293 (USDC W.D. LA March 5, 2021)
27. Union Planters Bank, No. 01-CV-0314-DRH U.D.D.C. (S.D. Il. July 15, 2003)
28. Fairchild v. United States, 769 F Supp. 964, 968 (WD La. 1991)
29. Kent Village Associates Joint Venture v. Smith, 657 a.2d 330, 104 Md. App. 507 (Ct. of Special App. Md. 1995)
30. Norwest Bank v. Kmart Corp., 1997 U.S. Dis. Lexis 3426 (USDC NDIN, January 29, 1997)
31. May III, V. R., & MoradiRekabdarkolaee, H. (2020). The International Commission on Health Care Certification Life Care Planner Role and Function Investigation. *Journal of Life Care Planning, 18*(2).
32. Kumho Tire Co. v. Carmichael, 526 U.S. 137 (1999)
33. SeaRiver Maritime, Inc. v. Pike, Wl1553264 (Tex. App. - Corpus Christie, 2006)
34. Oram v. DeCholnoky, Wl 4984752 (Conn. Sup. 2008)
35. Marcano v. Turabo Medical Center Partnership, 415 F.3d. 162, 171 (1st Cir. 2005)

36. Cogg v. Dawson, WL 4373255, U.S. Dist. Lexis 91177 (M.D. Ga. 2007)
37. International Academy of Life Care Planners. (2022). *Standards of practice for life care planners* (4th edition). International Association of Rehabilitation Professionals.
38. The National Court Rules Committee. (2022). *The federal rules of evidence, Rule 703*. https://www.rulesofevidence.org/
39. Morales-Hurtado v. Reinoso, 230 A.3d 241, 241 N.J. 590 (NJ 2020)
40. Morales-Hurtado v. Reinoso, 198 A.3d 987, 1006, 457 N.J. Super. 170 (N.J. App. Div. 2018)
41. NJRE 703
42. Morales-Hurtado v. Reinoso, 230 A.3d 241, 243, 241 N.J. 590 (NJ 2020)
43. Hale v. Gannon, Cause No. 1:11-cv-277-WTL-DKL (U.S.D.C IN (2012). https://casetext.com/case/hale-v-gannon-3
44. Mertes, A. P., & Albee, T. (2020). The effects of post-Sanchez hearsay in life care planning. *Journal of Life Care Planning, 18*(2), 81-89.
45. New Jersey Rules of Evidence 808. https://www.njcourts.gov/attorneys/evidence.html
46. Ball, D. Transcript of David Ball, Trial Consultant 2012 International Symposium on Life Care Planning-Persuasive Life Care Planner Testimony-Serving the Injured client. *Journal of Life Care Planning, 11*(4), 7-18.
47. Union Planters Banks. V. United States, No. 01-CV-0314-DRH, (U.S.D S.D. Ill. 2003).
48. Strauss, D., Brooks. J., Rosenbloom, L., & Shavelle R. (2008). Life expectancy in cerebral palsy: An update. *Developmental Medicine & Child Neurology, 50*, 487–93. doi:10.1111/j.1469-8749.2008.03000
49. Langerman, A. G. (2001). *Defendant's annuity witness* [Conference paper]. American Trial Lawyers of America Conference, Atlanta, GA.
50. Hinsdale v. N.Y., NHHRR Co., 81 N.Y.S. (356, 81 N.Y. Supp. 356 (1903)
51. Mercer v. Vanderbilt University, Inc., 134 SW 3d 121, 134 (Tenn. 2004)
52. Diede v. Burlington Northern Railroad. Co., 772 F.2d 593 (9th Cir. 1983)
53. Voogt, R. D. (1996). What are we going to be when we grow up and become an industry? *Viewpoints, 34*, 1.
54. Columbia Medical Center of Las Colinas v. Bush, 122 S.W. 3d 835,862-63 (Tex. App.-Fort Worth 2003, pet. denied) https://case-law.vlex.com/vid/columbia-medical-center-v-889085096
55. Ibrahim v. Young, 253 S.W.3d 790 (Tex. App. 2008). https://casetext.com/case/ibrahim-v-young
56. The discussion on usual, customary, and reasonable is excerpted from Stern, B. & Owen, T. R. (2022). Collateral Source Rule approaches and its implications for usual, customary, and reasonable pricing. *Journal of Life care Planning, 20*(1), 5-20.
57. Voogt, R. D. (1999). Brain injury litigation: What is the missing link in defining damages? *The Neurolaw Letter 9*(1), 4.
58. NJ Rev Stat § 2A:15-97, 2013
59. Zorogastua, G. G. (2007). Improperly divorced from its roots: The rationales of the Collateral Source Rule and their implications for Medicare and Medicaid write-offs. *Kansas Law Review, 55*(2), 464-500.
60. Howell v. Hamilton Meats & Provisions, Inc., 52 Cal. 4th 541, 129 Cal. Rptr. 3d 325, 257 P.3d 1130, 1135-46 (Cal. 2011). https://casetext.com/case/howell-v-hamilton-meats-provisions-inc-2\
61. Dedmon v. Steelman, 535 S.W.3d 431, 457 (Tenn. 2017). https://casetext.com/case/dedmon-v-steelman-2
62. Weston v. AKHappyTime LLC, 445 P.3d 1015 (Ak. 2019)
63. Bozeman v. State, 879 So. 2d 692, 705 (La. 2004)
64. Stayton v. Delaware Health Corp., 117 A.3d 521, 531 (Del. 2015)
65. Arthur v. Catour, 833 N.E. 2d 847 (Ill. 2005)

Chapter 30

A Defense Attorney's Perspective on Life Care Planning

Aubrey Lyon and Simão Ávila

A Defense Attorney's Perspective on Life Care Planning

The basic purpose of a life care plan in personal injury cases is to assist in proving the future cost of the plaintiff's needs. The life care plan is an efficient method for presenting this evidence as it consolidates future care needs into a singular report. The plan is presented and explained to the jury by the life care planner as a qualified expert. The explanation of each feature of the plan allows the life care planner an opportunity to reinforce the extent of the injury and associated impacts on the plaintiff's life.

The defense may be at a disadvantage if it is not properly prepared to present a more compelling case to the jury. Therefore, the defense must prepare to oppose the plaintiff's plan by evaluating the credentials of the life care planner, the foundational requirements of necessity and reasonableness for each plan element, and the scope of the plan for inclusion of only legally recoverable damages. Effective arguments against the admissibility of the plan, or parts of the plan, may be necessary. Proper cross-examination may demonstrate a lack of foundation for essential elements of the plan and show overreach by the plaintiff. In some cases, presentation of the defense's own life care plan may be appropriate—or even required—as will be discussed in this chapter.

The Scope of a Life Care Planner's Role in Litigation

Life care planners have an important role in litigation, as well as in mediation or negotiation,[1] when the parties need an expert to assist them or the trier of fact[2] to understand the evidence or to determine a fact at issue in a case. As a witness, qualified as an expert, the life care planner may testify about the facts and provide opinions if (1) the testimony is based upon sufficient facts or data,

(2) the testimony is the product of reliable principles and methods, and (3) the witness has applied the principles and methods reliably to the facts of the case.[3]

The specific role that a life care planner may play will depend, in part, on the knowledge, skill, experience, training, or education of the individual. Life care planners have different and varied professional backgrounds, including healthcare, vocational rehabilitation, counseling, education, psychology, and mental health. It is essential to consider the diversity of these backgrounds to be able to evaluate the appropriateness of the role of a life care planner in a specific case. These backgrounds will guide the bases for an individual's expertise. Defense counsel must determine, for example, whether the individual has sufficient experience to qualify as an expert witness in the field of life care planning. Ultimately, a judge will determine whether there is sufficient evidentiary foundation to support the facts and opinions emanating from the plan and the reliability of underlying assumptions leading to those opinions.

Anatomy of a Case

Life care planners' expertise is often sought in personal injury or professional negligence actions. In most jurisdictions, the cause of action that a plaintiff must prove to be entitled to recovery in those cases is a version of "negligence." A negligence cause of action commonly has four elements that the plaintiff must prove: duty, breach, causation, and damages.[4] The elements of duty, breach, and causation are sometimes referred to as the "liability" portion of a negligence case. In lay terms, the elements of a negligence case require the plaintiff to show that the defendant did something wrong and that the wrongful conduct caused the plaintiff some form of harm. The life care plan, and the life care planner's testimony, are almost always used for the damages element of a negligence case.

Standards for Admitting Expert Testimony

In this chapter, we refer to the Federal Rules of Evidence (FRE) and decisions interpreting those rules. Generally, these authorities apply only in federal courts, and different requirements may apply in state courts and other jurisdictions. However, many states have patterned their rules of evidence after the federal rules and have adopted certain case law interpreting the federal rules as persuasive in their respective jurisdictions. As such, and because of the burden of separately considering the specific evidentiary standards of every potential jurisdiction where a life care planner's opinions may be offered, the discussion of the admissibility of life care plans and the standard for qualification of the life care planner as an expert witness in this chapter will focus on federal evidentiary standards.[5]

The Frye *Standard: General Acceptance Test*

The admissibility of expert testimony before 1993 was generally based on "the *Frye* Standard." That standard originated from a District of Columbia case in 1923, which rejected the scientific validity of the precursor to the polygraph machine as a lie detector. In *Frye v. United States*,[6] the District of Columbia court established the following for determining the admissibility of scientific examinations:

> Just when a scientific principle or discovery crosses the line between the experimental and demonstrable stages is difficult to define. Somewhere in this twilight zone the

evidential force of the principle must be recognized, and while the courts will go a long way in admitting experimental testimony deduced from a well-recognized scientific principle or discovery, the thing from which the deduction is made must be *sufficiently established to have gained general acceptance in the particular field in which it belongs.*

Id. at p. 1014 (emphasis added by authors)[7]

This standard prevailed in many states and in federal courts for many years. It is still applicable today in a few states. Accordingly, courts had to decide if the procedure, technique, or principles in question were generally accepted by a meaningful proportion of the relevant scientific community.

The Daubert *Standard*

In 1993, the United States Supreme Court had an opportunity to revisit evidentiary standards, given that there were vigorous debates about the merits of the *Frye* Standard and because of a conflict in the interpretation of that test among Federal Courts of Appeal. In *Daubert v. Merrell Dow Pharmaceuticals, Inc.*,[8] the United States Supreme Court held that the FRE—specifically Rule 702, which postdated the *Frye* decision by many years—superseded *Frye*'s narrow "general acceptance" test. The Supreme Court explained that, under the FRE, the trial judges are the final decision-makers or "gatekeepers" on the admissibility of relevant evidence and the acceptance of a witness who may testify as an expert within their own courtrooms. The court noted that Rule 702 of the FRE provided a more expansive standard than the *Frye* test. Thus, in deciding if the science and the expert in question should be permitted, judges should consider the following questions:

- What is the basic theory, and can it be or has it been tested?
- Has the theory or technique been subjected to peer review and publication?
- What is the known or potential error rate?
- Are there standards controlling the technique?
- Is there general acceptance of the theory?[9]
- Has the expert adequately accounted for alternative explanations?
- Has the expert unjustifiably extrapolated from an accepted premise to an unfounded conclusion?

Responding to arguments that having a broader standard would open the floodgates and result in a "free-for-all" in which befuddled juries are confounded by all kinds of evidence presented at trial, the Supreme Court noted that the FRE place limits on the admissibility of purportedly scientific evidence. Thus, trial judges must ensure that any and all scientific testimony or evidence admitted is both relevant and reliable. Concerns about questionable evidence and its admissibility also could be scrutinized. Defense counsel could vigorously cross-examine the expert, present contrary evidence to that proffered by the expert, and seek careful instructions to a jury on the burden of proof.[10]

Four years after the *Daubert* decision, the Supreme Court further expanded on its ruling and reasoning. In *General Electric Co. v. Joiner*,[11] the Supreme Court clarified that when determining admissibility, the focus of inquiry should be the expert's methodology in addition to the ability to reach an accurate conclusion. In other words, there must be a correlation between supportive data and the conclusion reached for the evidence to be admissible.

In another decision shortly after *General Electric*, the Supreme Court extended once more the reach of *Daubert*. In *Kumho Tire Co. v. Charmichael*,[12] in a fatal tire blowout case, the court extended the *Daubert* Standard beyond scientific techniques. It ruled that the standard should also apply in fields of "technical" and other "specialized knowledge." With this case, it is now clear that the *Daubert* Standard is appropriate to determine the admissibility of evidence in other disciplines or expertise, such as economics, psychology, and "soft sciences."

Scientific, technical, and specialized knowledge expert testimony is now subject exclusively to the *Daubert* Standard in federal courts and also in many states that follow that rule and its premises. However, some states use a modified *Daubert* Standard, and some even continue to use the *Frye* Standard or a modified version of it. Attorneys should familiarize themselves with the applicable standard in the jurisdiction where the matter is heard, as should the life care planner.

Federal Evidence Rule 702: New Amendments

In 2021, the Advisory Committee on Rules of Practice and Procedure—Judicial Conference of the United States unanimously approved a proposal to amend FRE 702. After a hearing and a comment period, which ended in February 2022, the amendments to FRE 702 will likely be approved by the U.S. Supreme Court and take effect on December 1, 2023. As a consequence, the amendments will have to be followed in all federal courts. Similarly, the states that follow the FRE will also likely adopt this new and more precise standard.

The two new changes to the text of FRE 702[13] will establish that:

(1) the proponent of the expert testimony must show admissibility by a *preponderance of the evidence*;[14] and
(2) the expert's opinion must reflect a reliable application of the principles and methods applicable to the facts of the case.

These changes will further clarify the applicable standards for the admissibility of expert testimony in Federal court litigation that involves scientific, technical, or other specialized theories and where experts are necessary to assist the trier of fact to make a determination in the case.

One hopes the new amendments will establish the trial courts as the gatekeepers instead of allowing the juries to hear the evidence and decide what weight to give it in deliberations before reaching their decision. The Committee's note specifies that:

> Rule 702(d) has also been amended to emphasize that the trial judge must exercise gatekeeping authority with respect to the opinion ultimately expressed by a testifying expert. A testifying expert must stay within the bounds of what can be concluded by a reliable application of the expert's basis and methodology (p. 310).[15]

Similarly, for *forensic* experts, the Committee's note specifies that:

> the judge should (where possible) receive an estimate of the known or potential rate of error of the methodology employed, based (where appropriate) on studies that reflect how often the method produces accurate results. Expert opinion testimony regarding the weight of feature comparison evidence (i.e., evidence that a set of features corresponds between two examined items) must be limited to those inferences that can reasonably be drawn from a reliable application of the principles and methods (p. 311).[16]

A few other comments from the Committee's note, itemized here, may be helpful to defense counsel, both in the preparation to question the admissibility of a life care plan or to prepare to cross-examine the plaintiff's experts. The following are some of the other reasons for the Committee's amendments:

- Many courts have held that the critical questions of the sufficiency of an expert's basis, and the application of the expert's methodology, are questions of what "weight" to give the evidence. This is an incorrect application of the rule. The amendment, requiring the proponent of the evidence to establish admissibility by the preponderance of the evidence, will correct this problem.
- The preponderance of the evidence standard will apply to all three reliability-based requirements itemized in the rule.[17]
- Once the court has found the admissibility requirement to be met, by a preponderance of the evidence, any attack by the opponent will go only to the weight of the evidence.
- Experts may come to different conclusions based on contested sets of facts. The preponderance of the evidence standard does not necessarily require the exclusion of either side's experts. Rather, by deciding the disputed facts, the jury can determine which side's experts to credit.

Exploring the Plaintiff's Life Care Planner's Qualifications

The attorney's role in responding to an opposing party's expert witnesses is to challenge the basis of opinions, question the expert's conclusions, and expose inaccuracies for the finder of fact. Every case and every expert is unique, and challenging an opposing party's expert witness can range from seeking the total exclusion of the expert's testimony to pointing out weaknesses on cross-examination. A life care planner's testimony and plan are presented in litigation as expert opinions, and therefore a defense attorney will approach an opposing expert with this range of goals in mind.

Expert opinion testimony is subject to specific rules for admissibility. Lay witnesses may not testify in the form of an opinion, subject to certain exceptions.[18] A witness who is qualified as an expert, however, may testify in the form of an opinion, though again, subject to certain limitations.[19] In order to qualify as an expert, a witness must have specialized "knowledge, skill, experience, training, or education."[20]

Even if a witness qualifies as an expert, the scope of an expert's opinions have specific boundaries:

- an expert may testify in the form of an opinion only to the extent the opinion will help the finder of fact understand the evidence or determine a fact in issue
- is based on sufficient facts and data
- is the product of reliable principles and methods, and
- is the product of the expert reliably applying the principles and methods to the facts of the case.[21]

Whether a witness qualifies as an expert and whether an expert's opinions are admissible are questions of law and are therefore determined by a judge.[22] This is sometimes referred to as the "gate-keeping function of the trial judge."[23] This determination is left to the sound discretion of the trial court and will not be reversed on appeal absent an abuse of that discretion.[24]

With this structure in mind, a good place to start in determining how to challenge a life care planner's opinions is to evaluate the life care planner's qualifications. That is, does the life care planner have specialized knowledge, skill, experience, training, or education that will assist the trier of fact in understanding the evidence or determining a fact in issue? A successful attack on a life care planner's qualifications can exclude the life care planner and associated opinions from the jury's consideration.

A life care planner must have two levels of qualifications. First, the expert must be qualified generally in the area of life care planning. Second, the life care planner must have specific expertise in each substantive element of the plan, to the extent required by the jurisdiction's substantive law, or rely on the opinion of a separate qualified expert.

Qualifications as a Life Care Planning Expert Generally

As with any testifying expert witness, a life care planner must be recognized by the court as an expert before being allowed to offer expert opinions. To qualify as an expert, a witness must have specialized knowledge, skill, experience, training, or education.[25] A witness need only have one of those five qualities to potentially be admitted as an expert.[26] Thus, a properly qualified expert may have no practical experience in the particular area about which the expert testifies.[27] Similarly, a witness may qualify as an expert in a field in which the expert has no formal training, education, degree, or certification. Certain items in a life care plan may be appropriate even without being based on a recommendation by a physician; a particular plaintiff may need certain items and services that are not within a physician's expertise and, rather, may be within a non-physician life care planner's area of expertise.[28]

Expert testimony is generally proper in any scientific field that has reached a level of general acceptance. Life care planners and their plans can generally be expected in catastrophic injury cases.[29]

Qualification to Present the Particular Life Care Plan

Often challenging an opposing party's life care planner's qualifications to opine as to each element of the plan has more bountiful opportunities than challenging the qualifications of the witness as an expert in general. Even if a life care planner is accepted as an expert witness, the party offering the life care planner's testimony must still establish that the life care planner's opinions in that case are based on sufficient facts and data, are the product of reliable principles and methods, and are the product of the expert reliably applying the principles and methods.[30]

For example, in cases involving claims of personal injury, courts around the country generally hold that expert testimony is required on the issue of whether treatment claimed as damages is medically necessary. Under this rule, many elements of a life care plan may require qualified medical expert testimony to be properly presented to the jury as a claimed element of damages. Often, this foundation requires the testimony of a physician.[31] Therefore, defense counsel should analyze the necessity of each item in a life care plan with an eye toward the foundational basis for each item and whether the proponent of each item of a plan has the qualifications to recommend that care. Where an item in a plan is recommended by someone who lacks the expertise to recommend such care, whether that be a physician or non-physician life care planner, that element of the plan should be challenged. Depending on the individual qualifications of the plaintiff's life care planner, the defense should consider taking the position that each element of the life care plan must also be independently supported by a separately qualified expert's testimony as to that element's reasonableness and necessity in the given case.

Failure by the plaintiff to properly limit the scope of the life care planner's proposed expertise may result in the entire plan and the planner's entire testimony being precluded or stricken.[32] Life care planners must, therefore, ensure that not only are they qualified to testify as life care planners generally, but also that they are qualified to testify concerning the necessity of each individual element of the plan not independently supported by appropriate medical or other expert testimony. In many cases, the plaintiff's life care planner can best serve the client by enlisting the services of the proper medical and rehabilitation experts, rather than by attempting to support the plan based on the life care planner's testimony alone.[33] It is common for a medical expert, especially a non-retained treating provider, not to provide all the foundational detail needed for an element of a plan, such as length of treatment or appropriateness of alternative, less expensive medications. In such situations, particularly where the non-retained treating provider is not easily accessible to the life care planner, it can be tempting for the life care planner to fill in the gaps, and the defense attorney should be on the lookout for such opportunities to exclude an element of a plan. A defendant's own life care planning consultant can be of great assistance in helping defense counsel to identify any weaknesses in the plaintiff's proposed expert's qualifications to testify regarding the need for any given treatment element in the plan.

In general, a rehabilitation or habilitation expert will attempt to translate the physical or mental impairment into a disability in order to assess the effect upon the injured party's ability to participate in activities of daily living or instrumental activities of daily living. It is the role of the qualified healthcare provider to establish the existence of a physical or mental impairment, and it is inappropriate for a life care planner, without appropriate qualifications, to present opinion testimony as to the existence of a medical condition or its likely progression. Rather, the foundation for the impairment must be laid by a qualified healthcare provider, including any expected complications or progression. This medical opinion can then be translated by the life care planner into the disabling effects of the condition and its impacts on the activities of daily living and instrumental activities of daily living.

Types of Expert Roles

In a civil case, a retained expert can generally be used for one of two roles: as an expert expected to testify at trial or as a non-testifying consulting expert.[34] The scope of permissible discovery into an expert's opinions differs greatly depending on which role the expert plays. A party is entitled to broad, in-depth discovery of the opinions and bases of opinions of an opposing party's retained expert who is expected to testify at trial.[35] In order to offer an expert's opinion testimony at trial, the opinions and basis of those opinions must be timely and fully disclosed to the opposing party.[36] The conversations between an attorney and a testifying expert that the attorney has retained for the trial are not protected by the attorney-client privilege or the full work product doctrine.[37] However, the opposing party is entitled to almost no discovery of an opposing party's non-testifying consulting expert.[38]

It is not uncommon for a defendant in a civil case to retain a life care planner as a non-testifying consulting expert who is charged with analyzing the plaintiff's life care plan and recommending areas for objections and cross-examination. The benefits of this approach are that the opinions (and even the identity of) the consulting expert are nearly impossible for the plaintiff to obtain during discovery and that the defendant is not placed in a position of presenting the defense's own life care plan, which may implicitly suggest to the jury that the defendant may be liable.

This approach should be used cautiously, though. In some cases, especially cases with catastrophic damages or a complex life care plan, the defense may lose an important opportunity to present a reasonable plan to the jury if the defense life care planner has not been disclosed as an expert expected to testify at trial.

A cautious defense counsel will retain a life care planning expert early in a case with the thought that the expert may be disclosed or not, depending on how discovery develops. Expert disclosures are often a time-pressured period in the course of litigation, and waiting until the plaintiff's life care plan is in hand to determine whether a defense life care planner is needed can be too late. Also, just because a life care planner has been disclosed to the opposing party does not mean that the disclosing party needs to actually have the life care planner testify at trial. If, by the time the trial begins, the defense has determined that it is tactically beneficial not to put on its own life care planning expert, the defense can decline to call that witness, and the jury never is the wiser. As with any expert, prior to disclosing a life care planner, attorneys should consider whether the expert has to discuss opinions that are damaging to their client's case.

Considering the variability in roles of a defense life care planner, life care planners might consider asking the following questions of defense counsel at the outset of the retention:

- Does counsel expect the life care planner to be in a consulting or testifying expert role?
- Does counsel expect the life care planner to critique someone else's plan, prepare an original life care plan, or both?
- Does counsel expect the life care planner to perform any roles beyond the life care plan such as developing vocational rehabilitation opinions?
- Will the life care planner have access to the injured party's treatment team?
- What kind of medical experts has the defense retained who the life care planner can consult with in preparation of the life care plan?
- Does the jurisdiction have any specific requirements regarding the scope of opinions allowed by a life care planner?

Foundational Objections, the *Daubert* Standard, and Other Preclusions

Beyond challenges to the general and specific qualifications of a plaintiff's life care planner expert, other grounds for excluding the expert's testimony may exist. Common grounds for seeking the exclusion of a witness's testimony include:

- failure to timely disclose the expert or the expert's report;[39]
- failure to timely disclose a specific opinion;
- failure to disclose the methodology the expert applied to reach the expert's opinion;
- failure to disclose the facts and data the expert used in reaching an opinion;[40]
- speculative opinions; and
- inappropriately opines on causation.

Some of these grounds are discussed in more detail below. Potential for objections based on speculation or lack of factual support may arise where, for example, the life care planner intends to testify regarding the cost of certain treatment, but no medical evidence has been proffered to indicate that such treatment is reasonable, necessary, or caused by the relevant accident.

The legal element of "causation" to establish a cause of action in the lawsuit is another common ground for objection in many life care plan opinions. The life care plan itself is not an appropriate vehicle to argue the legal cause of the injury at issue. Rather, the life care plan should adopt a cause as the basis for the plan and provide conclusions with that cause as one factor in the plan. Being qualified to prepare and opine on a life care plan is not the same as being qualified to offer opinions on causation. A defense attorney who encounters a life care plan that contains causation opinions, unsupported by a qualified expert, should seek to exclude those opinions or the entire plan.

A plan may also be objectionable as speculative, where it relies on new or experimental treatments. As discussed above, each element must meet the *Daubert* Standard or other applicable standard for admissibility. The defense should evaluate the plan for the inclusion of therapeutic modalities which are not generally accepted as "necessary" for the treatment. For example, the use of long-term hyperbaric oxygen therapy for brain injury is controversial. A *Daubert* challenge may force the plaintiff proposing a controversial treatment to establish "a reliable foundation and [that it] is relevant to the task at hand"[41] (p. 1024).

Defense counsel should keep these grounds for objecting to a life care plan in mind throughout discovery and into trial. New facts or expert opinions may arise that justify reevaluating the foundations of the plaintiff's life care plan.

Cross-Examination of the Plaintiff's Expert

Life care planning experts are increasingly used in civil litigation, and the standard that courts apply to decide whether to allow their testimony skews toward inclusion; "[s]haky but admissible evidence is to be attacked by cross-examination, contrary evidence, and attention to the burden of proof, not exclusion"[42] (p. 1024). Ultimately, the tests courts apply to admissibility are designed to find "not the correctness of the expert's conclusions but the soundness of [the expert's] methodology"[43] (p. 1318). So, while good legal arguments may exist for the exclusion of expert testimony supporting a plan, defense counsel should also be prepared to cross-examine the plaintiff's life care planning expert.

If a plaintiff's life care planner expert is allowed to testify, the expert's knowledge, education, training, or experience are relevant to the weight to be given to the expert's opinions. Some areas defense counsel should explore are whether the plaintiff's expert is state certified in rehabilitation counseling, allied health discipline, medical, or other discipline. A defendant will find it helpful also to determine whether the plaintiff's expert is a medical case manager. Often, plaintiffs will retain life care planners who have expanded their forensic practice into life care planning. Many plaintiffs' experts have never actively served as a patient advocate or coordinator of health services on behalf of an injured party. Establishing that the plaintiff's expert has done nothing more than read books and look at other life care plans in preparation for presenting a particular life care plan can be crippling to the plaintiff's case, even if the court finds the expert qualified to testify. A life care planner expert hired by the defendant to assist in preparing the defense case can assist the client by being familiar with all available training or education in the field and making defense counsel aware of any such deficiencies, including the lack of training or education that becomes apparent from a critical review of the resume presented by the plaintiff's life care expert.

Financial Bias

All retained experts are subject to certain areas of inquiry that suggest financial bias. For example, the obvious financial bias of all retained experts is that they are being paid to present opinion testimony on behalf of a party. Bias may also be demonstrated by the volume of work the expert does for either plaintiffs or defendants. If an expert does a substantial amount of work for a specific law firm, bias can potentially be shown by identifying an ongoing business relationship that the life care planner presumably would not want to jeopardize by presenting plans that would be unsupportive of the hiring firm's position.

Other opportunities for financial bias may be present with a life care planner's opinions that are not present in another expert's plan. For example, a life care plan that includes self-referrals creates the impression of impropriety and financial bias in the outcome of the case. Some life care planners are involved in rehabilitation centers that they may partly own and operate. Where the life care plan is centered on such a program, this creates the appearance of a potential financial incentive on the part of the life care planner. In some egregious cases, defense counsel can successfully establish that the life care planner has engaged in self-referral of prior plaintiffs who have received settlements or judgment awards and entered into the life care planner's own facility programs. It can be devastating to the plaintiff's case for the jury to learn that the life care planner may receive a substantial amount of the life care plan funding through payment to a medical facility which the life care planner owns or has a substantial interest.

Conflicting Recommendations

In essence, the purpose of a life care plan in a plaintiff's case should be to quantify the future care needs of the injured party and provide a number that an economist can use as the foundation for a present value analysis of economic loss. Like a physician retained only for the purpose of an independent medical examination, the life care planner should not have a role in or be part of the plaintiff's health care team. Where a life care planner goes beyond the scope of the life care planning role, there is an opportunity to demonstrate bias if recommendations from specialists are not fully considered. The life care planner who is hired by the plaintiff and ignores relevant evidence that lessens the value of the plan can be challenged for failing to account for that relevant evidence in the plan.

A defense attorney may find grounds for impeachment by cross-examining a plaintiff's life care planner on the purpose of the retention and the information the life care planner considered or failed to take into account. For example, if the plaintiff's life care planner is providing rehabilitation opinions in addition to preparing a life care plan, an opposing attorney should look for other evidence in the plaintiff's record for rehabilitation recommendations. If someone else, like a medical case manager or other rehabilitation specialist, has recommended a different, lesser course of treatment, this is an area defense counsel should be ready to explore.

A portion of a plan that is often worth investigating for the defense counsel is caregiver support. Recommendations on the appropriate level of caregiver support can vary greatly based on the individual characteristics of the patient. For example, an outside caregiver may be indicated, but if the patient will only accept a family member to provide support, then examining the life care planner on the appropriateness of allocating costs in the plan to outside caregivers maybe be worthwhile.[44] The life care planner should be prepared to explain any discrepancies between the proposed life care plan and the current care plan.

The Bases of the Opinions

The bases for an expert's opinions may be another potential area for review and, where appropriate, for possible challenges to the admissibility of evidence. Even where the evidence may be admissible, under the *Daubert* Standard, a modified standard, or the amended FRE 702, there may be a good basis for objections at trial. Expert opinions, like any other evidence, should not be admitted if it is irrelevant, if they lack foundation, go beyond the scope of the subject matter to be covered by the expert, or if they are unfair and prejudicial. The testimony may also be subject to appropriate cross-examination since, among other reasons, defense counsel may need to challenge the weight the trier of fact should give to the evidence proffered by an expert.

In discovery, especially in preparation for the deposition of the purported expert, defense counsel must establish the entirety of the work performed by the life care planner to prepare the life care plan, and should determine whether the work on the case is complete. As importantly, the deposition should include questions about any interviews conducted and any authoritative texts relied upon. A well-prepared life care expert will be able to demonstrate that they are familiar with all the relevant facts of the case and the authoritative standards applicable to the report.

Defense counsel should also determine, at the time of the deposition, that the life care planner is not attempting to interpret any of the medical, psychological, or therapeutic assessments made unless the life care planner is qualified to make such interpretations. If the inclusion of some therapy, medical examination, diagnostic testing, or other aspect of the plan requires the opinion of a physician, psychologist, or other expert, counsel should establish if such a person has been contacted to validate those aspects of the life care plan. If defense counsel can establish that the required foundations for the report were not done properly, this information can be used to challenge the expert's testimony or the admissibility of the plan. Even in cases where witnesses are allowed to testify and where their reports are admitted, this information can provide fertile ground for cross-examination and perhaps even for striking some elements of a plan for lack of proper predicate.[45]

Duplication, Generics, and Other Cost Reductions

Generally, a life care plan should include current reasonable costs for each aspect of the plan, minus the costs that the patient would have incurred anyway. In other words, has the plaintiff's life care planner considered the fixed costs that would not be relatable to the injury at issue? For example, if the injury at issue caused the patient to be wheelchair-bound, the life care plan may include costs associated with a wheelchair-compatible vehicle like a van. The patient may have needed a vehicle regardless of the injury, and if so, the appropriate cost is the difference between the cost of the ordinary vehicle and the cost of the wheelchair-accessible van. If the plan fails to account for the fixed cost of the vehicle the patient would have owned regardless of the injury, then the plan fails to provide a reasonable, realistic cost for the wheelchair-compatible van.

Other commonly encountered areas are diet and housing. Where a plaintiff's injury caused the plaintiff to need a special diet, the cost of the special diet should be offset by the normally expected food cost incurred by the plaintiff. Where group home residency is being recommended, the plaintiff's plan should include an offset for typical housing costs.

Similarly, the plan should not include multiple entries for the same type of service or item. For example, a plan might call for a home health aide and a caregiver to assist with activities of daily living and instrumental activities of daily living. However, often a home health aide can and will provide other assistance, and a separate caregiver may not be needed. The defense attorney should explore the proposed scope of services contemplated in the plan, what services are typically provided, and whether the plan improperly doubles up on the same type of service.

A plan should also consider appropriate generic drugs and alternative treatments. If a generic drug can provide the same therapeutic effect as a name-brand drug, then the generic should be considered. A defense attorney should be on the lookout for these types of errors in a life care plan, and the use of a life care planning expert as a consultant on these issues can reap significant rewards.

Application of the Collateral Source Rule

Defense counsel should also explore with the plaintiff's expert any consideration given to the availability of public programs or collateral sources in preparing the plan.[46] The collateral source rule applicable in a particular jurisdiction may impact the permissible scope of such evidence.[47] However, in most states, the collateral source rule has been modified to allow defendants to set off, from the damages to be awarded, insurance benefits offered without lien rights, and benefits provided, or that might be available, under public assistance programs. The defendant's life care planner may assist defense counsel with these issues and point out any of those matters called for in the plaintiff's plan for which there may be a government agency or other funding source not considered in the economic analysis of the plaintiff's plan.

For example, states receiving federal funds may be required to provide comparable education opportunities to severely disabled children up to age 22. The public school system also makes available those therapies that are required to further the student's educational opportunities. Therefore, the public school program is an excellent resource for cases of catastrophic injury to infants and young children. Defense counsel should explore and establish the position of the plaintiff's life care planner with respect to these public programs and be prepared to rebut the possible contention that such programs are substandard and inappropriate for the plaintiff. The failure of a plaintiff's life care planner to recognize, and consider, the availability and suitability of charitable and other publicly funded programs can cast doubt on an otherwise objectively prepared analysis and make it susceptible to challenge.

Licensing Issues

To our knowledge, no state has specific licensing requirements for persons who author life care plans. As the majority of life care planning probably involves the medicolegal context, the lack of any standardized requirements and licensure makes this area fertile ground for those persons who wish to claim expertise and wish to be retained as experts on the open market. Unlike recognized specialties that provide planned care and are subject to licensing requirements, the life care planning field is open to people from diverse backgrounds. This opens the arena to unscrupulous experts who view the life care plan as a device to market themselves in the forensic marketplace.

The long-term solution may be the creation of a national standards organization that becomes recognized by state and federal jurisdictions and lobbies for the enactment of statutory licensing. Under the current situation, defense counsel should review this issue and be prepared to point out any failure on the part of the plaintiff's expert to obtain proper certification. For example, counsel should explore and determine whether the expert has complied with applicable ethics and standards, as specified by the International Academy of Life Care Planners, which publishes *Standards of Practice* guidelines.

In the absence of required licensure, life care planners must be mindful of the limitations imposed by related and existing state licensure laws. In most states, practitioners are required to hold one or more licenses before they may prescribe or perform various therapies. Life care planners must, therefore, be mindful not to misrepresent to the client or the jury their ability to recommend various treatment modalities that the life care planner is not independently qualified to opine on as being "reasonable and necessary."

As mentioned before, the life care planner's professional background and formal training may be as a vocational rehabilitation counselor, nurse, certified case manager, mental health counselor, psychologist, occupational therapist, physical therapist, physician, or combinations of these and other professions. Thus, the ability of the life care planner to offer specific opinions for care will vary with the type of case presented and the qualifications of the life care planner. Thus, life care planners seeking to provide services in a medicolegal context should assess their own capabilities and limitations and accept cases accordingly. If this is not done properly, defense counsel should be ready to challenge the life care planners' qualifications or their work product.

Moreover, a certified case manager may be professionally qualified to opine as to future durable goods requirements and perhaps the nursing care coverage necessary for the type of injury presented. This same case manager, however, would be required to defer to a qualified healthcare provider on the issue of future surgeries and attendant complications, prescription medication, and prescribed therapies. Similarly, this life care planner should defer to orthopedists for the type of orthopedic bracing that may be required, and the various therapists involved in the care for the form and frequency of therapy provided. As the clinical care of the catastrophically injured person involves a multidisciplinary approach, the life care planner should not be hesitant to interact with, and gain insight from, these various disciplines when creating a plan. In fact, the life care planner can provide an extremely important service to a retaining attorney by expressing the limitations the planner may have to give opinions and encouraging the retaining party's use of other experts to ensure that a legally sufficient foundation is set for the admission of the life care plan and to establish its credibility.

Many life care planners are unwilling to accept their own limitations for fear that this will erode their influence and perhaps diminish their role. Such persons should look at other fields that participate in the legal system as experts. For example, economists have been called upon to render opinions concerning future economic loss in catastrophically injured cases long before the assistance provided by life care planners was available. To properly perform this assessment, the economist would frequently review the opinions of health care providers, determine the costs associated with the care required pursuant to those opinions, and extrapolate from data based upon these foundations.

The life care planner's role is to take this analysis to the next step and develop a more holistic and comprehensive approach. Historically, an economist's analysis could be unpersuasive because it was incomplete in scope. Therefore, life care planners should be able to assist legal professionals by using their experience to ascertain the probable needs associated with an individual's future care. This will ensure that the life care planner and the attorney will research and consider all aspects of care in creating the life care plan that is most appropriate for the individual. Just as most economist reports of future economic losses are predicated by facts gained from others, there is no weakness in a life care planner's reliance on information appropriately garnered from others. Such reliance, in fact, may be a necessary foundation for the arguments on whether the life care planner can testify as an expert and whether the plan prepared by such an expert will be admissible in court.

The Decision to Retain a Defense Life Care Planner

Similar to the discussion above regarding the defense retaining a life care planning expert early in the case, in a catastrophic injury or brain damage case, it may be prudent for defense counsel to retain a life care plan expert well in advance of expert disclosure deadlines. Because the life care plan often incorporates opinions from a wide variety of experts, including treating providers, medical experts retained specially for the litigation, and vocational experts, the life care plan is often one of the last expert reports to be completed. Getting a late start on an expert witness can jeopardize the ability to prepare a comprehensive defense life care plan.

To be prepared properly to rebut the plaintiff's plan and to determine whether to present a defense plan, it is vital that much of the groundwork be laid in the early portions of the discovery phase of a case. A defense life care planner can provide early assistance by suggesting the various records that should be requested and identifying persons to be deposed to make the determinations necessary to evaluate the injured party's life care needs. In most cases, the defense life care planner will not need to spend significant time or money to provide this initial assistance. Moreover, the dividends returned on this initial investment are paid in the form of easing the inevitably compressed final preparation toward trial.

Ultimately, defense counsel must exercise judgment in determining the practical interplay of the retained life care planning expert with the overall theme of the defense and the other experts. For example, if the plaintiff has no in-state experts, then the defendant's theme may be to retain only local experts on all issues in order to point out the need for the plaintiff to go to other jurisdictions to get experts to support the case. As with the selection of any expert, the overall picture of the case must not be lost, and the life care plan expert must be a good fit.

Defense Damages Evidence and the Testifying Defendant Expert

While retaining life care planning and rehabilitation experts for the defense is often beneficial in cases where the plaintiff is likely to rely on a life care plan, whether to disclose the defense experts, whether to depose the plaintiff's experts, and whether to call the defense life care planner and rehabilitation expert to testify at trial are all tactical decisions that depend heavily on individual factors. Those factors include—to name but a few—the nature of the case, the interplay between the liability and damages issues in the case, local jurisdiction rules and practices related to expert disclosures, the reasonableness of the plaintiff's damages opinions, and personal style.

Defense counsel should weigh the benefits and drawbacks of deposing the plaintiff's experts. The purpose of deposing a plaintiff's expert is, of course, to be able to prepare for the testimony at trial and line up sworn testimony to be used on cross-examination. However, reasons also exist not to depose an expert. A deposition can often offer an opportunity for an expert to correct an error or omission from the expert report or expand on the opinions offered in the report. This has the potential to weaken an otherwise strong argument to exclude the expert's opinions from trial. Deposition questioning can also spur new opinions if the expert is presented with challenges to the expert's original opinions, and there is potential that the new opinions may become admissible at trial. Additionally, the questioning of an expert in a deposition may tip off the opposing party as to the defense counsel's trial strategy.

Cases are unique, opinions differ, and trends change on how much of a damages case a defendant should put on. Arguments exist for the defense to put on limited evidence with respect to damages and instead rely on challenging the plaintiff's damages evidence and testimony through cross-examination, motions to exclude, and closing arguments. The rationale for this approach is that if the defense puts on its own evidence on damages, it may validate for the jury some or all of the plaintiff's plan, that the defendant caused the damage, or that there was damage—that is, it might bleed over into liability impressions. Additionally, just as a defendant intends to elicit substantial concessions from the plaintiff's experts on cross-examination, the plaintiff's counsel anticipates being able to reinforce much of the plaintiff's theory of the case through cross-examination of the defense expert. On the other hand, not putting on damages evidence potentially misses an opportunity to provide the jury with a reasonable set of facts upon which to base an award. The individual circumstances of the case should dictate which approach to take.

A second, and perhaps more important, factor in deciding whether to call a defense life care planner as a testifying expert is the impact of this decision on the discoverability of the expert's work and opinions. In most jurisdictions, the contributions of consulting experts who do not testify at trial are protected from disclosure by the work-product privilege. For example, under the Federal Rules, a party can discover facts known or opinions held by another party's consulting experts only upon showing "exceptional circumstances under which it is impracticable for the party to obtain facts or opinions on the same subject by other means."[48] Absent such a showing of exceptional circumstances, which is extremely rare, the expert's work is protected from discovery.

However, such protection is usually not afforded to experts expected to testify at trial. Thus, in instances where the life care planner may be called upon to testify, both the defense counsel and the life care expert should be aware that matters that would have been protected as work product, if prepared by a consulting expert, may be stripped of that protection. Notes, memoranda, research, communications, and other matters held by the consulting expert may, by the decision to have the expert testify at trial, be transformed into the discoverable file materials of a testifying expert.[49] These materials may outline a great deal of the defense theory of the case. Furthermore, under the Federal Rules, a party must automatically disclose the identity of all testifying experts, and each testifying expert must provide the opposing party with a detailed report of all the opinions the expert will testify to at trial, the reasons for those opinions, the facts and data considered, and other information.[50] The cost of disclosing these materials to the plaintiff prior to trial may outweigh the benefit of having a defense life care planner testify at trial.

Additionally, the opposing party may depose any testifying expert, and the opposing party is entitled to take that deposition after the disclosure of the expert's report.[51] Such disclosure requirements and discovery opportunities are substantial considerations in determining whether to disclose a life care expert for the defense.

In instances where the defense life care planner will testify, it is often beneficial that a physical examination of the injured party occurs or, at least, that the defense makes a motion for such an examination. Otherwise, plaintiffs' attorneys will make the often persuasive argument that the defense expert has not even seen their client. As the provision of care to severely injured persons continues to become more complex and specialized, it is essential to recognize a multidisciplinary approach and to allow the defense life care planner access to the depositions and, if possible, the actual persons involved in the care and treatment of the injured party.

In catastrophic injury cases, it is advisable for defense counsel to work with a life care planner to engage the services of the specialized physicians and therapists necessary for the overall assessment of the life care plan. Privacy protections such as HIPAA and patient–physician or other privileges that preclude defense-retained experts from meeting with the plaintiff's treating physicians and therapists may present barriers for defense experts to obtain all the information they need from treating providers. Additionally, many treating physicians and therapists do not want to become involved in litigation and therefore refuse to be informally interviewed by a defense-retained life care planner. In such situations, compiling a defense team is the only approach that will ensure a complete evidentiary foundation for a defense life care plan. Plaintiffs obviously have a distinct advantage in having access to a treating healthcare team. The defense must minimize this advantage by putting together its own team of experts and, if permitted under the laws of the relevant jurisdiction, explaining to the jury why such assembly was necessary.

Practical Considerations: The Effect on the Jury

Both plaintiffs and defendants must remember that the life care plan will not be presented in a vacuum. Issues of liability and causation can be affected by the credibility of the plaintiff's life care plan. Both plaintiff and defendant must be certain that they retain a well-qualified and knowledgeable life care planning expert who will present an objective life care plan. Some attorneys ask that a life care planner create a plan designed to be an "anchor" to the damages case. That means that the plan is designed to be unrealistically high in its costs, with the thought being that the life care plan presents the starting point for a negotiation, and a higher starting point leads to a higher compromise. Although the economic incentive to prepare an overreaching life care plan can be tempting to the plaintiff, the presentation of such a plan to the jury will often have a spillover effect on the overall view of the case. It may offend the jury and thereby swing a close liability case in favor of the defense. Defense counsel, therefore, must be prepared to take full advantage of the overreaching plaintiff's life care planner.

Conversely, the requirements of care for the injured party that are set forth in the life care plan directly affect the economic costs of the injury and indirectly affect the noneconomic losses by the life care planner's efforts at improving the injured person's quality of life. Defense counsel must, therefore, be cognizant that an attack on any aspect of the plan may be viewed as insensitive to the efforts at improving the plaintiff's quality of life. Just as the overreaching plaintiff can alienate a jury, the insensitive attack on elements of a plan for the benefit of the injured party can offend juries. Ultimately, credibility is the life care planner's most important quality, and an unreasonable life care plan can destroy the life care planner's credibility and the credibility of their client.

Conclusion

Damages in a catastrophic injury case in which the plaintiff relies upon a life care plan can be complex and nuanced, and defense counsel has many tools available to ensure that the jury is presented with an objective view of the evidence.[52] An early, proactive approach is best for addressing the issue of damages in these types of cases. Admissibility options should be explored so that opinions that lack foundational requirements are not presented to the jury. In the appropriate case, retaining expertise to help interpret the information, make suggestions, and even present counter opinions at trial on rehabilitation and life care plan issues is advised. Non-testifying defense experts playing only a consulting role can be instrumental, too, in the preparation of early discovery and effective cross-examination of the plaintiff's expert. In instances where the plaintiff's life care plan warrants, the presentation of an alternative defense life care plan, and the early involvement and careful presentation of the defense life care planner as a testifying expert, can enhance the overall credibility of the defendant's case and provide the jury with a more reasonable economic alternative.

Notes

1. Although this chapter refers generally to litigation, the same principles apply when the parties engage in any form of an alternative dispute resolution (ADR) process to resolve their differences. The life care planner can provide invaluable assistance in any ADR process and the same principles of reliability and admissibility should be considered in those settings.
2. The trier of fact is the person or body responsible for deciding the facts in a disputed matter. For example, in a jury trial of a personal injury matter, the jury is the trier of fact. That is, the jury ultimately resolves issues of fact whereas the judge answers questions of law.
3. See FRE 702.
4. See, e.g., *Estate of Petersen v. Bitters*, 954 F.3d 1164, 1171 (8th Cir. 2020) (applying Nebraska law).
5. Attorneys must appropriately familiarize themselves with the standards applicable in the specific forum where the case is being heard.
6. See, *Frye v. United States*, 54 App. D.C. 46; 293 F. 1013 (1923).

7 See generally, Riddick-Grisham, S., & Deming, *Pediatric life care planning and case management*, (2nd ed., 2011, CRC Press) for a more in-depth discussion.
8 See *Daubert v. Merrell Dow Pharmaceuticals, Inc.*, 509 U.S. 579 (1993). *Daubert* concerned the introduction of expert testimony on the causation of birth defects by the drug Bendectin that the mother took during pregnancy. The lower courts concluded that the proffered evidence provided by the plaintiffs was an insufficient foundation to allow expert testimony that Bendectin caused the injuries. Therefore, plaintiffs could not satisfy the burden of proving causation at trial.
9 This factor could still be considered but it should not be dispositive.
10 *Id.* at 596.
11 See *General Electric Co. v. Joiner*, 522 U.S. 136 (1997).
12 See *Kumho Tire Co. v. Charmichael*, 526 U.S. 137 (1999).
13 The amendments are as follows (italics):

Federal Rule of Evidence, 702. Testimony by Expert Witnesses

A witness who is qualified as an expert by knowledge, skill, experience, training, or education may testify in the form of an opinion or otherwise if *the proponent has demonstrated by a preponderance of the evidence that*:

(a) the expert's scientific, technical, or other specialized knowledge will help the trier of fact to understand the evidence or to determine a fact in issue;
(b) the testimony is based on sufficient facts or data;
(c) the testimony is the product of reliable principles and methods; and
(d) the principles and methods to the facts of the case.

14 "Preponderance of the evidence" is a common evidentiary standard. "Preponderance of the evidence" means "more likely true than not." See *Díaz-Alarcón v. Flández-Marcel*, 944 F.3d 303, 305 n.2 (1st Cir. 2019). That is, to prove something by a "preponderance of the evidence" means that the proponent of the evidence provided the court sufficient supporting information to demonstrate that the fact at issue is not only possible but is also more probable than not.
15 See full text of note at www.uscourts.gov/sites/default/files/preliminary_draft_of_proposed_amendments_-_august_2021_0.pdf, pp. 308–327.
16 *Id.*
17 For example, the Rule's requirement that the testimony "assist the trier of fact to understand the evidence or to determine a fact in issue" (see Amended FRE 702) goes primarily to relevance by demanding a valid scientific connection to the pertinent inquiry as a precondition to admissibility.
18 FRE 701.
19 FRE 702.
20 *Id.*
21 *Id.*
22 See FRE 104(a).
23 See *United States v. Mooney*, 315 F.3d 54, 62 (1st Cir. 2002).
24 *Id.*
25 FRE 702.
26 *Id.*
27 See *Jenkins v. United States*, 307 F.2d 637, 643–644 (D.C. Circuit 1962).
28 See *Burris v. Ethicon, Inc.*, 2021 U.S. Dist. LEXIS 140248, *59, 2021 WL 3190747 (determination that the plaintiff would need certain items and services held to be within the non-physician life care planner's expertise).
29 See, e.g., *Miksis v. Howard*, 106 F.3d 754, 758 (7th Cir. 1997) ("The need for a 'life plan'—in other words, a prediction of high medical costs for the remainder of plaintiff's life—was clearly foreseeable from the nature of plaintiff's injuries.").
30 FRE 702.
31 See *Burris v. Ethicon, Inc.*, 2021 U.S. Dist. LEXIS 140248, *55, 2021 WL 3190747 (citing decision in large multidistrict litigation on same subject).

32 See, e.g., *Fairchild v. United States*, 769 F. Supp. 964, 968 (W.D. La. 1991); *First Nat'l Bank v. Kansas City S. Ry.*, 865 S.W.2d 719, 738 (Mo. App. 1993); *Timmons v. Mass. Transp. Authority*, 591 N.E.2d 667, 670-71 (Mass. 1992).
33 See, e.g., *Hogland v. Town & Country Grocer of Fredericktown Mo., Inc.*, 2015 U.S. Dist. LEXIS 80493, *96, 2015 WL 3843674 (E.D. Ark. 2015).
34 See Federal Rule of Civil Procedure (FRCP) 26(b)(4).
35 See, e.g., FRCP 26(a)(2)(B).
36 See FRCP 26(a)(2)(A).
37 See FRCP 26(b)(4)(C) (providing types of communications that are protected from disclosure). Life care planners should keep in mind that their written and oral communications with counsel may be discoverable.
38 See FRCP 26(b)(4)(D).
39 See, e.g., *Yeti by Molly, Ltd. v. Deckers Outdoor Corp.*, 259 F.3d 1101, 1106–1107 (9th Cir. 2001) (concluding district court did not abuse its discretion in excluding testimony of defense expert who failed to timely provide his expert report).
40 See, e.g., *Niazi Licensing Corp. v. St. Jude Med. S.C., Inc.*, 30 F.4th 1339, 2022 U.S. App. LEXIS 9597, *31 (Fed. Cir. 2002); *Olson v. Mont. Rail Link, Inc.*, 227 F.R.D. 550, 551–553 (D. Mont. 2005) (determining defendant's failure to timely provide data underlying expert report warranted exclusion of opinions relying on that data).
41 *Elosu v. Middlefork Ranch Inc.*, 26 F.4th 1017, 1024 (9th Cir. 2022).
42 *Id.*
43 *Daubert v. Merrell Dow Pharmaceuticals*, 43 F.3d 1311, 1318 (9th Cir. 1995) ("*Daubert II*").
44 Case law on this topic differs between jurisdictions.
45 Under amended FRE 702, defense counsel should seek a motion to strike the plan and use the facts gathered during discovery to show that the proponent of the evidence has not demonstrated, by a preponderance of the evidence, that the report is admissible.
46 *See generally Cates v. Wilson*, 361 S.E.2d 734 (N.C. 1987); see also *Brewington v. United States*, 2015 WL 4511296, at *4–6 (C.D. Cal. July 24, 2015) (Affordable Care Act benefits to be considered in a determination of future medical costs). Cf. *Joerg v. State Farm Mut. Auto. Ins. Co.*, 176 So.3d 1247, 1256 (Fla., 2015) (Medicare, Medicaid, and other social legislation, are not a future benefit to be considered when determining damages for future medical costs).
47 Life care plans are subject to the same requirements for pretrial disclosure as are applied to other evidence in the particular jurisdiction, and the life care plan may be stricken for failure to comply with such pretrial discovery requirements. See *Department of Health and Rehabilitative Services v. Spivak*, 675 So.2d 241 (Fla. 4th DCA 1996).
48 FRCP 26(b)(4)(D).
49 FRCP 26(a)(2)(B).
50 FRCP 26(a)(2).
51 FRCP 26(b)(4)(A).
52 Life care planning testimony may be relevant and helpful in cases other than personal injury cases. See, e.g., *Urbanek v. Urbanek*, 484 So.2d 597 (Fla. 4th DCA 1986) (using life care testimony in a marital dissolution case to analyze the wife's changed circumstances in setting alimony amounts). Life care plans are often used to establish reserves in workers' compensation claims

Chapter 31

Special Education Law and Practices for the Pediatric Life Care Planner

Brenda Eagan-Johnson and Margaret Lockovich

Special Education Law and Practices for the Pediatric Life Care Planner

The pediatric life care planner is often tasked with understanding and navigating the complex system of special education laws and services. While federal laws protect the rights of students with disabilities, individual school districts and educational entities interpret and apply these laws very differently. In addition, parents faced with seeking special education services for a child with a newly acquired disability are often overwhelmed and undereducated about the rights that their child may have (Tarrien, 2016).

Children who experience a medical disability frequently struggle to learn and behave at school as a direct result of their diagnosis. In 2020–2021, 7.2 million children, or 15% of all public school-age students, received special education services (National Center for Education Statistics, 2022). Included in this number are children who have been seriously injured and may require educational supports throughout their academic careers. Examples of acquired medical disabilities that frequently impact learning include:

- Traumatic Brain Injury (includes concussion)
  - Common causes:
    - Abusive head trauma (Shaken Baby Syndrome)
    - Assault/abuse
    - Falls
    - Firearm
    - Motor vehicle accident (includes bicycle)
    - Pedestrian accident
    - Sports/recreation

- Non-Traumatic Brain Injury
  - Common causes:
    - Aneurysm
    - Brain tumor
    - Leukemia
    - Stroke
      - Other cancers (late-term chemotherapy/radiation effects on the brain)
    - Toxic injury due to:
      - Carbon monoxide poisoning
      - Lead poisoning
      - Mold toxicity
    - Lack of oxygen (Hypoxia/Anoxia) due to:
      - Near drowning
      - Lightning strike
      - Electric shock
      - Overdose
      - Strangulation
      - Choking
      - Cardiac event
        - Heart attack
        - Diabetic coma
        - Blood clot
    - Bilirubin encephalopathy
    - Encephalitis
    - Meningitis
    - Long-COVID-19/Neuro-COVID-19
    - PANS/PANDAS
    - Lyme Disease
    - Other viruses
    - Seizure disorder
    - Hydrocephalus
    - Opioid or alcohol addiction
- Post-Traumatic Stress Disorder (PTSD) or other mental health diagnoses
- Burns
- Spinal cord injury
- Amputations
- Diabetes
- Organ transplant
- Asthma and other chronic respiratory conditions
- Artificial Airways/Long-term mechanical ventilation
- Brachial plexus or other orthopedic injuries
- Visual impairment
- Hearing impairment
- Birth injuries such as cerebral palsy, stroke in utero

The pediatric life care planner must have knowledge of the special education process and the supports and services available to students with disabilities. This chapter provides an overview of the core components of special education laws and practices that support students with disabilities who struggle at school. Common situations that the injured child may encounter in the educational system will be explored. Additionally, the role and benefits of including an educational consultant in the life care plan will also be discussed as a safeguard to ensure that a child receives the learning supports needed as they age.

History of Special Education

Historically, the law excluded children with disabilities from attending public schools in the United States. This practice was common until the 1820s, when some states created specialized education programs for children with disabilities. Over 130 years later, the federal government began to make laws to support the creation of educational resources and training programs to better prepare teachers working with children with disabilities (England, 2011). However, children with disabilities continued to be excluded from public schools or, when included, were contained in educational settings that did not meet their needs. In 1954, a United States Supreme Court decision established that African American children had the right to free public education (*Brown v. Board of Education*, 1954). This groundbreaking decision laid the foundation for parents of children with disabilities to fight for educational rights. Two federal court cases (PARC, 1972; *Mills v. Board of Education of the District of Columbia*, 1972) challenged excluding children with disabilities from public schools without providing an alternative education suited to the child's needs. These rulings supported the right of every child to public education. They provided the basis for future federal laws that ensured the provision of special education services for children with disabilities.

In 1975, Congress passed the Education for All Handicapped Children Act, Public Law 94-142 (P.L. 94-142), to assist states and localities in protecting the rights of infants, toddlers, children, and youth with disabilities, as well as their families, in meeting their individual needs and improving their outcomes (US Department of Education [USDOE], 2022). In a 1990 reauthorization, the name of this groundbreaking law was changed to the Individuals with Disabilities Education Act (IDEA). The IDEA was last reauthorized in 2004 and renamed the Individuals with Disabilities Education Improvement Act (IDEIA). Since then, significant progress has been made toward meeting major national goals for developing and implementing effective programs and services for early intervention, special education, and related services (USDOE, 2022).

When Congress created IDEA in 1975, they promised to fund 40% of all school district special education costs. But, to date, the federal government has not paid more than 18% (National Council on Disability, 2018). Hence, school districts are placed in a difficult position where they are forced to balance the learning needs of individual students with the amount of state and local funds received, which is often not enough (National Council on Disability, 2018). The discrepancy between what students in special education require per the law and what the district has the funds to provide results in an inequitable distribution of educational resources for students from district to district.

Additionally, researchers Bonuck and Hill (2020) estimated that millions of children with medical disabilities are potentially eligible for special education services but are not receiving them. One reason is that many students have invisible disabilities (such as brain injury, asthma, diabetes, and mental health), which leads to students receiving less support than those with a visible physical disability (Magnus & Tøssebro, 2014; Schreuer & Sachs, 2014; Venville et al., 2014). Another reason is that many of these students attend schools in lower socioeconomic neighborhoods. Research findings in a 2019 study by EdBuild found that "poor, non-white school districts receive approximately $2,600 less per student than affluent white school districts" (Bonuck & Hill, 2020, p. 253), which further widens the disparity gap among students receiving special education services. These types of social determinants of health are factors that life care planners should consider when making determinations about available district supports for a child.

Current Federal Education Laws

Three federal laws provide protection for children with disabilities and ensure that they receive appropriate special education services and related services within the public school system:

(1) Section 504 of the Rehabilitation Act of 1973 (29 USC § 701),
(2) the Americans with Disabilities Act of 1990, and
(3) the Individuals with Disabilities Education Act of 2004.

Federal provisions for public education are interpreted and enacted differently by each state. Readers are strongly encouraged to consult and review individual state laws when considering Special Education services. The Office of Special Education and Rehabilitative Services (OSERS) is the governing body that oversees special education policies in the United States.

Section 504 of the Rehabilitation Act of 1973

According to the U.S. Department of Education, Office for Civil Rights (2010), Section 504 of the Rehabilitation Act is a civil rights law that prohibits discrimination based on disability. This law mandates that school districts provide a free and appropriate public education (FAPE) to qualified students who have a physical or mental impairment that substantially limits one or more major life activities [34 CFR § 104.3(j)(1)]. The key in this definition is that the medical impairment must "substantially" limit a major life function (USDOE, OCR, 2016).

Under Section 504, FAPE means providing regular or special education and related aids and services designed to meet the student's individual needs. The Section 504 regulatory provision defines a physical or mental impairment as any physiological disorder or condition, cosmetic disfigurement, or anatomical loss affecting one or more of the following body systems: neurological; musculoskeletal; special sense organs; respiratory, including speech organs; cardiovascular; reproductive; digestive; genitourinary; hemic and lymphatic; skin; and endocrine; or any mental or psychological disorder, such as intellectual disability, organic brain syndrome, emotional or mental illness, and specific learning disabilities (USDOE, OCR, 2016). The regulatory provision does not set forth an exhaustive list of specific diseases and conditions that may constitute physical or mental impairments because of the difficulty of ensuring the comprehensiveness of such a list.

Major life activities, as defined in the Section 504 regulation, include functions such as: Taking care of oneself, performing manual tasks, walking, seeing, hearing, speaking, breathing, learning, and working (USDOE, OCR, 2016). In the Amendments Act of 2008, Congress provided additional examples of general activities that are major life activities, including eating, sleeping, standing, lifting, bending, reading, concentrating, thinking, and communicating (USDOE, OCR, 2016). The Section 504 regulatory provision's list of examples of major life activities is not exhaustive. An activity or function not specifically listed can be a major life activity.

Americans With Disabilities Act of 1990

The Americans with Disabilities Act (ADA, 1990) prohibits discrimination by public entities based on disability. The ADA prohibits discrimination against individuals with disabilities in all areas of public life, including jobs, schools, transportation, and all public and private places that are open to the public. The law's purpose is to ensure that people with disabilities have the same rights and opportunities as individuals without disabilities. The ADA gives civil rights protections to individuals with disabilities like those provided based on race, color, sex, national origin, age, and religion. It guarantees equal opportunity for individuals with disabilities in public accommodations, employment, transportation, state and local government services, and telecommunications (ADA, 1990).

The ADA originally defined a disability as a "physical or mental impairment that substantially limits one or more major life activities" (USDOE, OCR, n.d., para. 18). In 2009, the Americans with Disabilities Amendment Act (ADAAA) became law. The ADAAA made several significant changes to the definition of the term "disability" which included expanding the range of limitations and not requiring these limitations to be considered severe. While the ADA does not directly govern a FAPE for children, it provides some protection to students with disabilities who attend private schools by defining reasonable accommodations.

Individuals With Disabilities Education Act of 2004 (20 USC §§1400 9d0, 2004)

The IDEA (2004) is the federal law that requires states to ensure that all eligible children with disabilities receive a FAPE. The most current version of IDEA dictates how states and public agencies provide early intervention, special education, and related services to eligible infants, toddlers, children, and youths with disabilities. This law is revised periodically through a process called re-authorization. IDEA was created with the expectation that schools will work with the student and the student's parents to develop an education plan that is comprehensive and individualized to the student's needs. IDEA states that schools must provide eligible children with specialized supports and services to address their educational needs in the least restrictive environment (LRE). The 13 disability categories recognized under IDEA (2004) are listed below (34 CFR § 300.8).

1. Autism Spectrum Disorder
2. Deaf-Blindness
3. Deafness
4. Emotional Disturbance
5. Hearing Impairment
6. Intellectual Disabilities
7. Multiple Disabilities
8. Orthopedic Impairment
9. Other Health Impairment (such as ADHD, Physical Disabilities, and Non-Traumatic Brain Injuries)
10. Specific Learning Disability (such as dyslexia, dyscalculia, dysgraphia, and other learning differences)
11. Speech or Language Impairment
12. Traumatic Brain Injury
13. Visual Impairment (including Blindness)

IDEA Part B provides services for eligible school-age children (3 to 21 years of age), while IDEA Part C provides supports for eligible children in Early Intervention (birth to 36 months of age).

Qualification for Special Education

A medical diagnosis or disability does not mean that a student will automatically qualify for special education services at school. Qualification for special education services involves meeting two essential requirements. First, the student must be identified as having a developmental delay (which only pertains to Early Intervention) or one of the 13 disability categories (outlined above) listed in IDEA. Secondly, the student must also demonstrate an educational impact and require specially designed instruction to benefit from instruction. For example, a child diagnosed by a psychiatrist with panic disorder who is then evaluated by the school and found not to need specialized instruction would not qualify for special education. However, the school could then consider whether the student qualifies for a 504 Plan.

Eligibility Criteria Varies (§ 300.100)

While Special Education eligibility is governed by IDEA, there are no definitive rules for determining who is eligible. Eligibility criteria may vary from state to state and district to district. For example, School District A provides Speech-Language support services to students who demonstrate a -1.5 standard deviation on standardized test measures. In comparison, School District B requires a -2 standard deviation to receive the same services. These differences may create a significant impact on the life care plan. The life care planner must consider factors that could impact the student in the future such as the possibility of the child changing school districts or relocating to a different state.

Key Components of Special Education

Free and Appropriate Public Education (34 CFR § 300.101)

In general, a *Free and Appropriate Public Education (FAPE)* must be available to all children residing in the United States between the ages of 3 and 21, including children with disabilities. Free appropriate public education must be made available to the eligible child no later than the third birthday. However, there may be exceptions to FAPE as each state may have individual regulations regarding the age range for services and types of services provided. The reader should always consult state law and practice when determining FAPE and special education services.

Child Find (§ 300.111)

Public schools are responsible for identifying, locating, and evaluating all children who require special education and related services. The process is called Child Find. Federal law mandates that each state must have policies and procedures in place to ensure that all children residing in the state who have disabilities (regardless of the severity) and who require special education and related services are identified, located, and evaluated. This includes children with disabilities who are homeless, migrants, wards of the state, or attending private schools (P.L. 108-446; 118 STAT. 2677). In addition, each state must employ a practical method to determine which children are receiving needed special education and related services. State governments and schools use a variety of outreach measures such as posting notices in public places, local media campaigns, providing information to local doctors and clinics, and engaging in outreach events in the community (118 STAT. 2747).

Initial Request (§ 1414(a)(1)(B))

A parent of a child with a suspected disability, a school district (also referred to in the legislation as a local education agency or LEA), or a state educational agency may initiate a request for an initial evaluation to determine if the child has a disability. Parents seeking an evaluation for special education services should submit a written request to the local school entity. Once the request is received, the district must issue a permission to evaluate to the parent within a reasonable time frame of receiving the request. Parents requesting evaluation should include the following in the written request: specific concerns with learning and/or functioning in the school setting; specific areas or services to be considered (reading, physical therapy, vision support); any medical diagnosis, outside evaluations, and any other information to support the request. A sample request for evaluation is provided in Appendix 1.

Informed Parental Consent (§ 300.300)

The parent of the child suspected of having a disability must agree to the evaluation and be provided informed consent before the initial evaluation. This consent applies to the initial evaluation only and does not provide consent for placement in special education or receipt of related services. A separate consent for services must be obtained from the parent before special education services begin.

Evaluation Process (§ 300.301)

The purpose of the evaluation is to decide the child's eligibility for special education and related services and make decisions about an appropriate educational program for the child. The evaluation should include a variety of assessment tools and strategies to gather developmental, functional, and academic information related to the child's suspected disability. These measures may include standardized tests, rating scales, observations, and parent/educator input. Evaluations completed in the private sector may also be considered. Assessment of the child with a suspected disability must include information from qualified professionals and parent(s). Assessment tools and strategies must be selected and administered without racial or cultural bias or discrimination. Assessments must be administered in the language that most likely will yield the most accurate results. No single measure may be used as the sole criterion for determining disability. If the parents disagree with the evaluation, they have the right to request an Independent Educational Evaluation (IEE) conducted outside the school district. The school district may agree to pay for the IEE. Under 34 CFR § 300.301(c)(1), the initial evaluation and determination of a student's eligibility must be completed within 60 calendar days of receipt of written parental consent.

Determination of Eligibility (§ 300.306)

Once the evaluation is complete, the evaluation team, including parents and the student, if applicable, must meet to review the evaluation results. If the child is found to be a "child with a disability," as defined by IDEA, and it is determined that the child requires specially designed instruction, that student will then be deemed eligible for special education and related services. Within 30 calendar days after a child is determined eligible, the Individualized Education Program, also referred to as Individualized Education Plan (IEP) team must meet to write an IEP for the child. The contents of an IEP are described later in this chapter. Parents have the right to challenge eligibility decisions by initiating dispute resolution procedures (mediation, due process) should they disagree with the evaluation findings.

Re-Evaluation (§ 300.303)

Children who qualify and receive Special Education services must receive a re-evaluation every three years. Students with specific disabilities may be re-evaluated every two years in some states, such as children with Intellectual Disabilities who reside in Pennsylvania. The purpose of the re-evaluation is to determine if the child continues to be a child with a disability as defined by IDEA and to determine what the child's educational needs are. Although, the parent or school team can request a re-evaluation at any time if there are concerns.

Procedural Safeguards (§ 300.121)

Procedural safeguards protect the rights of parents and children with disabilities by giving families and school systems several mechanisms to resolve their disputes. The state and school districts must provide parents with a written document detailing the rights and responsibilities of the student, parent, and educational entity under IDEA. These procedural safeguards include student rights, notification requirements, and complaint procedures.

Educational Placement (§§ 300.115–300.116)

Depending on the needs of the child, their IEP may be carried out in the regular class (with supplementary aids and services as needed), in a special class (where every student in the class is receiving special education services for some or all of the day), in a special school (approved private schools for specific disabilities), at home, in a hospital, or in another out of district setting. A school system may meet its obligation to ensure that the child has an appropriate placement available by:

- providing an appropriate program for the child on its own,
- contracting with another agency to provide an appropriate program,
- utilizing some other mechanism or arrangement consistent with IDEA for providing or paying for an appropriate program for the child.

When a school district cannot meet the needs of a student, an approved private school placement may be considered. Children with significant physical, medical, or emotional needs may benefit from receiving education services in a specialized private school setting. Approved private schools are often considered for students whose behavioral needs cannot be met in a traditional school setting. Educational placement decisions, which must include the parent, should be based on the student's needs and the school's ability to meet those individualized needs. Typically, school districts must have the opportunity to provide educational services for a student in the least restrictive environment (the local school district) before agreeing to private school placement. However, districts may also choose to place students in an approved private school without attempting to educate the student in the local school. In addition, the least restrictive environment for children who are deaf or blind is often a specialized school versus the home school district. Schools for the deaf and blind provide immersion in an environment not typically available at the public school. The life care planner should be aware that parents who enroll their children in a private school without the public school's approval (unilateral placement) risk an obligation to assume this cost as the public school is not obligated to pay for the private school under this circumstance.

Dispute Resolution (§ 300.140)

Ideally, the parents and school district work together to develop an educational plan that improves results and helps students with disabilities achieve better outcomes. However, disagreements may occur. The IDEA provides specific options for resolving these disputes, including filing a complaint with the state education agency, mediation, and due process.

State Complaint

States must establish and implement their own state complaint procedures separate from due process procedures. Differences exist between state complaints and due process regarding who can file and the subject of the complaint. A state complaint considers violation of any state or federal education law. For example, a state complaint could be filed if a child's IEP states that they will receive occupational therapy once per week and no therapy was provided for several months. Any individual or organization aware of any state or federal law violation may file a state complaint.

Mediation (§ 300.506)

Mediation is an impartial and voluntary process that brings together parties with a dispute to have confidential discussions with a qualified individual known as the mediator. The goal of mediation is for the parties to resolve the disagreement and create a legally binding written document detailing the agreed-upon terms of resolution. Mediation is typically less expensive, less time-consuming, and less adversarial than due process and civil litigation. Parents of a child with a disability have the right to refuse mediation and proceed directly to a more formal due process hearing. The individual state is responsible for costs associated with mediation.

Due Process (§ 300.508)

Due Process is a complaint that involves the identification, evaluation, educational placement, or provision of FAPE for a child with a disability. For example, a due process complaint may be filed if a child is given a disability category or educational placement that the parent does not agree with. Due process refers to a legal proceeding presided over by a hearing officer who makes decisions about a child's educational program. This process is similar to a trial, with the hearing officer acting as a judge. Attorneys represent each party, and witnesses are questioned and cross-examined. At the conclusion of the proceedings, the hearing officer issues a written decision describing the legal obligations of both parties. The decision is legally enforceable. Due process may only be filed by the parent/guardian of the student or the school district, which may file against the parent.

Delivery of Services

Individual schools, states, and the federal government have developed philosophical, legal, and ethical processes to support students with varying levels of need to ensure that students with needs that impact learning are supported (IDEA, 2006; Section 504, 1973). Before the school system provides special education and related services to the child for the first time, the parents must consent. The child begins to receive services as soon as possible after written parental permission is received.

If the parent(s) disagree with the IEP and/or placement after the student is receiving services, they may discuss their concerns with other IEP team members and try to work out an agreement. If they continue to disagree, the parents can ask for mediation, or the school can offer mediation. In addition, parents may file a complaint with the state education agency and/or request a due process hearing.

Least Restrictive Environment (§§ 300.114–300.120)

The IDEA states that children with disabilities must be educated with children who do not have disabilities to the maximum extent possible. Schools must avoid removing children with disabilities from the regular education classroom and placing them into special classes or separate schools, unless the severity of the student's disability prevents progress in the regular education setting when provided with supplementary aids and services. Children with special needs must be educated in the least restrictive environment (LRE). The LRE is not a particular place but rather a setting that meets the individual student's unique needs.

Individualized Healthcare Plan (IHP)

An Individualized Healthcare Plan (IHP) is the health component of a student's educational support plan at school overseen by the school nurse (National Association of School Nurses [NASN], 2020). The school nurse develops an IHP to support the healthcare needs of students if those needs affect the student's safe and optimal school attendance and academic performance. According to the National Association of School Nurses (2017), an IHP is a "guiding document for delivery of student-specific nursing care, illustrating the school nurse's responsibility and accountability" (para. 3). Individualized Healthcare Plans are often underutilized for students with acquired disabilities, per the authors. But, IHPs are a crucial component of an educational plan when medical issues are present that could interfere with learning or attendance (NASN, 2020). For instance, IHPs may be beneficial for students with seizures or headaches post-brain injury, medication management, need for catheterization, toileting and other self-care needs, balance, fatigue, sensory deficits, mobility issues, and pain. IHPs can be developed alone or in conjunction with 504 Plans or IEPs and should be reviewed regularly and updated as needed.

504 Plan

Not all students with a disability require specialized instruction (which would require special education via an IEP). Instead, students with disabilities in public elementary or secondary schools who qualify under Section 504 eligibility per their school team can receive a 504 Plan developed by the school team. The 504 Plan is a legally binding document (USDOE, OCR, 2016). Accommodations within the 504 Plan are determined by the school team. The accommodations provide the student *access to the curriculum* by removing barriers and allowing them the same opportunities as those without disabilities (USDOE, OCR, 2016). These accommodations do not alter the curriculum or learning expectations. A 504 Plan can also list accommodations the student can receive during school-based extracurricular activities. Although not required, the 504 Plan should be in a written format per the Office of Civil Rights (USDOE, OCR, 2016). Examples of 504 Plan accommodations include but are not limited to:

- Physical supports such as wheelchair ramps, use of an elevator, handrails, adjusting the schedule so all classes are on one floor, or allowing the student to switch classes earlier than other students.
- Adjustments to rules, policies, or procedures such as allowing a diabetic student with a brain injury to have water at their desk, allowing a student with attention deficits movement breaks during class, or allowing a student to wear sunglasses for light sensitivity.
- Learning supports such as using a calculator, math number line, written instructions, or typing versus writing by hand.
- Modifications to materials and procedures such as the use of large print, Braille, a vocal output device, an interpreter, increased time for tests or assignments, extra breaks during instruction, or testing in a separate room.

Although the Section 504 regulations do not set a specific time frame within which students with disabilities must be re-evaluated to ensure they are receiving the appropriate services, Section 504 requires schools to conduct re-evaluations periodically and before a significant change in placement. The 504 Plan should be reviewed at least annually by the school district to determine if accommodations remain appropriate and if the student's needs are being met. Any team member, including the parent, may request a review at any time if there is an educational concern or change in the student's needs. Parents should request to attend the 504 meeting. Schools are not required, but most schools do include the parents. Schools do not receive any federal or state funding for 504 Plan development or implementation. The Office of Civil Rights oversees all parent complaints pertaining to 504 Plan adherence by the school (USDOE, OCR, 2016).

Individualized Family Services Plan (§§ 303.342)

When an infant or toddler qualifies for Early Intervention services through an evaluation, an Individualized Family Services Plan (IFSP) is developed. The IFSP is a written legal document that identifies and explains the supports and services that the identified child will receive. Services are to be provided in a "natural environment," which typically includes the home or childcare setting. The IFSP contains information regarding the child's physical, cognitive, communication, self-help/adaptive, social/emotional skills, and the family's strengths and needs. Family resources, concerns, and priorities guide the development of the IFSP. Measurable outcomes or goals for the child are defined, as well as how these goals will be met and how progress will be measured. Parents and caregivers are integral to the IFSP team and encouraged to actively engage in service delivery sessions. The IFSP must be reviewed and updated at least once per year; however, any team member may request reviews more often should concerns arise.

At age three, special education supports and services change as eligible children move from Early Intervention to school-age services, which include preschool. Transition planning begins several months before a child turns three years of age. A determination as to whether the child will continue to qualify for school-aged special education services must be made. The focus of special education services also shifts at this time from Early Intervention, which focuses on helping the family meet the needs of their child, to more child-focused school-aged services. During the transition from Early Intervention to kindergarten, the IFSP is replaced by the Individualized Education Program (IEP) at this time. Life care planners must be aware that the supports and services that a child receives in Early Intervention (Part C of IDEA) will likely be different from services provided in the school-age system (Part B of IDEA).

Individualized Education Program (§ 300.324)

A school-aged child who has qualified for special education services through an evaluation is given a plan called an IEP. The IEP is a written, legally binding plan between the parent, the student, and the school that details the student's special education placement, supports, and services. An IEP is provided to qualifying students who have a disability or are gifted following an evaluation. Two qualifications must be met for a student to receive an IEP: the student must meet criteria for one of 13 disability categories defined by IDEA, and the student must require specially designed instruction to benefit from instruction. IEP team members must include parent(s) or legal guardian of the child, the student (when applicable), at least one regular education teacher, at least one special education teacher, a representative of the school district who can make decisions about the services provided, and an individual who can interpret evaluation results. Parents may also invite any outside professionals or support persons to the IEP meeting at their discretion.

The school is responsible for ensuring that the child's IEP is carried out as written. Parents receive a copy of the IEP. Each of the child's teachers and service providers has access to the IEP. Teachers and service providers are responsible for knowing and providing the identified accommodations, modifications, and supports that are stated in the IEP. The child's progress toward the annual goals and objectives must be measured according to the method and timeline detailed in the IEP. Parents must be informed of the child's progress on these goals regularly. Suppose the school does not automatically provide the parents with their child's progress monitoring data. In that case, the parents should request this documentation because school staff must track the student's progress toward meeting IEP goals and objectives throughout the academic year.

The child's IEP is reviewed by the IEP team at least once a year or more frequently if the parents or IEP team members request. If needed, the IEP may be revised. Parents, as team members, must be invited to attend these meetings. Parents can make suggestions for changes, can agree or disagree with the IEP goals, and agree or disagree with the placement. If parents do not agree with the IEP and placement, they may discuss their concerns with other members of the IEP team and try to work out an agreement. Several options include additional testing, increased data collection, an independent evaluation, mediation, or a due process hearing.

A Notice of Recommended Educational Placement (NOREP), which is also known as Prior Written Notice (PWN) in some states, is the document that the school district is required to provide to notify parents of any proposed changes (or refusal to change) to the child's special education identification or placement or the provision of FAPE. Parents may approve or disapprove of the proposed action. There is a time frame (e.g., 10 calendar days) for the parent to respond; however, the response timeline differs from state to state. Suppose the parent fails to respond within the given timeline. In that case, the district may proceed with the proposed actions (except in the initial provision of special education evaluation or services). If the parent disagrees with the proposed action, then the NOREP must be marked as such, and the parent can pursue dispute resolution.

IEP Components

While IDEA dictates what information must be included in the IEP, it does not state how this information should be presented. There are no universal IEP forms, and each state develops and uses its own IEP format.

- **Current academic and functional performance or present level of performance (PLOP).** The IEP must state how the child is currently doing in school (known as present levels of educational

performance). This information may include evaluation results, classroom tests and assignments, checklists, rating scales, and observations made by parents, teachers, related service providers, and other school staff. Current performance information should include a statement about how the child's disability affects their involvement and progress in the general curriculum.
- **Measurable annual goals (MAG).** These are goals that the child can reasonably accomplish in one year. The goals may be broken down into short-term objectives (STO) or benchmarks. Goals may be academic, address social or behavioral needs, relate to physical needs, or address other educational needs. The goals must be measurable, meaning that it must be possible to measure whether the student has achieved the goals. A sample IEP goal: Given 4th grade reading material, Jimmy will orally read at 110–115 words per minute with less than two errors during structured reading probes for five consecutive sessions.
- **Measuring progress.** The IEP must state how the child's progress will be measured and how parents will be informed of that progress. Typically, progress is reported at the same time as general education report cards are issued, which is three to four times per year.
- **Special education and related services.** The IEP must list the special education and related services to be provided to the child or on behalf of the child. This includes supplementary aids and services that the child needs. It also includes modifications (changes) to the program or supports for school personnel, such as training or professional development that will be provided to assist the child.
- **Participation with nondisabled children.** The IEP must explain the extent (if any) to which the child will not participate with nondisabled children in the regular education environment and other school activities.
- **Participation in state and district-wide tests.** Most states and districts give achievement tests to children in certain grades or age groups. The IEP must state what modifications in the administration of these tests the child will need. If a test is not appropriate for the child, the IEP must state why the test is not appropriate and how the child will be tested instead.
- **Dates and places.** The IEP must state when services will begin, how often they will be provided, where they will be provided, and how long they will last. IEPs must be reviewed annually—at a minimum.
- **Transition service needs.** Beginning when the child is age 14 (or younger when appropriate), the IEP must address post-secondary goals and include courses and supports to help the student prepare for life after graduation.

Age of Majority (§ 300.520)

When a student receiving special education supports and services reaches the age of majority, they become a legal adult. The age of majority varies per state, the details of which can be found at https://minors.uslegal.com/age-of-majority/. At the age of majority, education rights are transferred from the parent to the student. Although, in some states, only a few of the educational rights transfer. Any paperwork that the parent was required to sign in the past can now be completed and signed by the student. If a student is not capable of managing their special education needs, the school can appoint someone to represent the student, such as the parent or another individual. Beginning at least one year before the child reaches the age of majority, the IEP must include a statement that the student has been told of any rights that will transfer to him or her at that age. This statement would be needed only in states that transfer rights at the age of majority.

Case Example: 504 Plan vs. IEP

Cameron sustained an anoxic brain injury from a near drowning. His 10th grade class is required to read a novel. Although Cameron can read and comprehend the novel, he finds it difficult to read in the allotted time frame due to his slower processing speed. He also has a visual convergence insufficiency and utilizes two low-tech assistive technology tools for reading—a reading frame to highlight each sentence on the page and a colored paper filter overlay to reduce glare when reading. Cameron receives these academic accommodations via a 504 Plan which also includes additional time for reading and assignments. The accommodations that Cameron receives do not alter the curriculum; instead, they provide support to level the playing field and allow Cameron to participate in the regular education setting.

Meg is in the same 10th grade class. She also acquired an anoxic brain injury from a near drowning. Meg's disability impacts her learning in a more significant way. The general education 10th grade English curriculum is too difficult for Meg to comprehend. Therefore, she reads a book appropriate for her ability level. Meg also receives small group support from a special education teacher to ensure that she comprehends the book's key concepts. Meg requires specially designed instruction because she cannot successfully access the grade-level curriculum. Since Meg has a disability and requires adaptations to the general education curriculum, she qualifies for and receives services through an IEP.

Educational Considerations Relevant for the Life Care Planner

The following information will be significant to the Life Care planner as these areas detail the specific aids, services, and instruction that the child with a disability will receive.

Specially Designed Instruction (§ 1401(33))

Specially designed instruction (SDI) refers to instruction that meets the unique needs of a child with a disability by changing the content, methodology, and/or delivery of instruction at no cost to the parents. Instruction may be provided in the classroom, home setting, hospital, or other specialized setting. Specially designed instruction includes modification and/or adaptation to the curriculum, lessons, or instructional materials and collaboration with teachers, related service providers, or parents. Examples of SDI include a behavior plan, visual schedules, specific instructional programs such as social skills curriculum, use of a scribe or notetaker, providing audio recordings or books on tape, sensory diets, use of manipulatives, or use of visual/written prompts provided during instruction. In short, SDI can include any specific intervention or instruction unique to the child that helps them access and benefit from instruction.

Factors to Consider

Several special factors must be considered in the IEP including:

- If the child's behavior interferes with their learning or the learning of others,
- If the child is blind or visually impaired,
- If the child has communication needs,
- If the child is deaf or hard of hearing,
- If the child has limited proficiency in English,
- If the child may benefit from assistive technology devices or services.

The IEP team must consider supports and strategies to address any of these identified needs.

Related Services (§ 300.34)

A child may require any of the following related services to benefit from special education. Related services, as listed under IDEA, include (but are not limited to):

- Audiology services
- Counseling services
- Interpreting services
- Occupational therapy services
- Orientation and mobility services
- Parent counseling and training
- Physical therapy services
- Psychological counseling
- Recreation
- Rehabilitation counseling services
- School health services
- Social work services in schools
- Speech-language pathology services
- Transportation

If a child needs a particular related service to benefit from special education, the related service professional should be involved in developing the IEP.

Academic Supports: A School Team Decision

The parent should always provide community-based medical, rehabilitation, psychological, neuropsychological, or educational evaluation reports and records to the school team. Medical providers frequently recommend academic accommodations, paraprofessional support, a 504 Plan, or IEP to parents. However, these services cannot be medically prescribed, nor can medical providers require a school district to follow their recommendations. Pediatricians Lipkin et al. (2015) state, "Writing a prescription for a school to provide a particular educational service for a child would be analogous to the school requesting a certain medical evaluation or treatment from the health care provider" (p. e1656).

Instead, academic supports and services are a school-team decision, must be educationally necessary, and cannot be based on only one source for eligibility or programming (see 34 CFR § 300.304(b)(1) through 34 CFR § 300.304(b)(3)). Information provided to the school team by community providers must be considered but does not have to be used (See *Michael P. and Elizabeth G. v. Department of Education*, State of Hawaii, 57 IDELR 123, 656 F.3d 1057,1066 (9th Cir, 2011)).

Medical-Based vs. School-Based Therapy Services

Many children with disabilities require therapy services such as physical, occupational, speech, and vision services. Parents are often confused when their child qualifies for a particular therapy in the medical setting but not in the educational setting and vice versa. It is important to understand that the purpose and goals of medical-based therapies versus therapies or related services provided in the school setting are different. Medical-based services are based on a child's health and focus on rehabilitating a prior level of function or achieving a goal that will improve health and decrease the need for future medical services. A physician's order is needed to provide these services.

School-based therapies and related services focus on the child's ability to function in the educational setting, access the curriculum, and make educational progress. A child must meet the individual school district's eligibility criteria to receive these services in the school setting. Therefore, it is not unusual for a child to receive a therapy service in the medical setting and not qualify for school-based services. On the contrary, children may continue to qualify for school-based therapies long after they have been discharged from medically-based services. This reality creates a unique challenge for the life care planner in assessing what needs will be provided for and by whom. It may help the life care planner to focus on the purpose of therapies in each setting.

Supplementary Aids and Services (§ 300.42)

According to IDEA Sec. 300.42, Supplementary Aids and Services (SaS) means aids, services, and other supports that are provided in regular education classes, other education-related settings, and in extracurricular and nonacademic settings to enable children with disabilities to be educated with nondisabled children to the maximum extent appropriate in accordance with § 300.114 through § 300.116 (34 CFR § 300.42). A full range of SaS should be considered, including instructional, physical, social-behavioral, and collaboration. Examples of SaS may include but are not limited to:

- Supports to address environmental needs (preferential seating; planned seating on the bus, in the classroom, cafeteria, auditorium; modify physical room arrangement by moving furniture, lighting; locker placement; amplification; sensory room; extra set of books in each class; switch classes several minutes before the bell).
- Levels of staff support needed (weekly/quarterly/as-needed consultation; stop-in support; classroom companion; one-on-one assistance; type of personnel support: behavior specialist, health care assistant, instructional support assistant).
- Supports for adults working to support students (time for meeting/planning; co-teaching; time for parent collaboration; home/school notebook; professional development, training, and resources).
- Specialized equipment needs of the child (wheelchair; computer; software; voice synthesizer; augmentative communication device; utensils/cups/plates; restroom equipment; earbuds).
- Pacing of instruction needed (breaks; extended time; set of books at home).
- Presentation of subject matter needed (recorded lectures; cueing; repetition; sign language; primary language; paired reading and writing).
- Materials needed (scanned tests and notes into computer; shared note-taking; large print or Braille; assistive technology; colored filter paper; fidget tools).
- Assignment modification needed (e.g., shorter assignments; recorded lessons; instructions broken down into steps; allow students to record or type assignments).
- Self-management and/or follow-through needed (e.g., calendars; planner; task analysis checklist; teach study skills; graphic organizers; iPhone alarms; timed-timers; touch-base teacher for beginning and end of school day).
- Testing adaptations needed (e.g., read test to child; modify format; extend time).
- Social interaction support needed (e.g., provide a Circle of Friends; social narratives; use cooperative learning groups; teach social skills) (Kurth et al., 2019; Center for Parent Information & Resources, 2017).

Assistive Technology (§ 300.105)

Children may require assistive technology (AT) to help them access, participate, and/or respond to instruction within the classroom setting. An AT device is defined in IDEA as any item, piece of equipment, or product that is used to increase, maintain, or improve the functional capabilities of a child with a disability. Students may require AT devices and supports to communicate, write, spell, see, hear, turn a page, use a computer, or travel through the school.

Assistive Technology ranges from low-tech support (e.g., post-it notes, highlighters, filter paper, picture communication choice board, a customized pencil grip) to high-tech (e.g., software, equipment modification, smart pen, laptop, speech generating devices, note takers, or speech-to-text apps). Assistive technology also includes technical training for a child, the child's family, and school staff on using the recommended technology. It should be noted that assistive technology does not include a medical device that is implanted, such as a cochlear implant, or the maintenance of these devices.

Extended School Year (§ 300.106)

Extended school year (ESY) services are special education and related services that are provided beyond the normal school year. The district must provide ESY if a student needs these services to receive FAPE. For some students, interruptions in the school schedule, such as summer break, may result in a loss of basic skills. In addition, students may take a much longer period to regain these lost skills than their peers without disabilities. Extended school year services are designed to prevent such loss of skills. Extended school year must be considered every year for every individual student. The IEP team must consider several factors in deciding ESY services:

1. **Regression:** Does the student revert to lower level of functioning (skills or behaviors) after an interruption to school programming, such as during summer break or even weekend breaks?
2. **Recoupment:** Can the student regain the regressed skills in a reasonable amount of time, or does it take them longer than their peers?
3. **Regression/Recoupment:** Do difficulties with regression and recoupment make it unlikely that the student will maintain current skills?
4. **Mastery:** Would interruption of educational programming impact mastery of important skills?
5. **Self-sufficiency and independence:** Are the IEP goals crucial to the student's self-sufficiency and independence from caretakers?
6. **Successive interruptions:** Will successive interruptions in programming result in a student's withdrawal from the learning process?
7. **Severity of disability:** Is the student's disability severe, such as autism, emotional disturbance, severe intellectual disability, or severe multiple disabilities?

The following is an example of a student who qualifies for ESY services: Dante has an IEP with goals related to math. Dante's teacher reported that she had to reteach him many math concepts that Dante had mastered before spring break. Dante was still struggling to regain these skills six weeks after break ended. Although several students had demonstrated some regression following the break, Dante required more intensive, direct 1:1 support to relearn the skills. Because of this regression and recoupment, Dante qualified for ESY services.

Extended school year may include services such as itinerant teacher instruction, related service provider services; services contracted through community or outside agencies; take home programs; consultation; staff training; and parent training. Schools determine if students qualify for ESY services by a specific date each year. While ESY determinations must be made by district-appointed dates each year, if a parent is concerned, they should request that school staff begin to collect information on student progress toward IEP goals, especially after breaks in the school schedule (winter break). An IEP team meeting must be held to discuss ESY services and eligibility. Extended school year time frames and services are determined by individual school districts and vary from district to district and state to state. Parents should become familiar with ESY qualification requirements in their child's district. Parents have the right to request a meeting with the IEP team to review data considered when determining eligibility for ESY services. An educational consultant may be helpful in guiding parents through this process.

Transition Services (34 CFR § 361.48)

Transition refers to activities that prepare students with disabilities for adult life post-high school. In 1990, Congress decided to include mandatory transition to adulthood services in the IDEA for all students in special education. For students with disabilities, school-based transition services are needed to ensure the student is prepared to function post-high school as independently as possible.

Transition planning, per IDEA, must begin at age 14 by including a statement of transition service needs in the IEP. At 14, the school is to begin working with the student to determine their interests and future goals through a person-centered planning process. The school assists the student to investigate future career paths, consider, and draft post-secondary education and career goals, ensure coursework is on track, obtain internship and work experiences during high school, and establish linkages with adult service providers such as vocational rehabilitation.

Transition services must begin at 16 years of age (services begin at age 14 in some states). If a student is in special education, transition planning and services are mandated. The school meets annually with the student and parents to create an Individualized Transition Plan (ITP). The ITP serves as a roadmap and must include transition-related goals and services to prepare the student for post-graduation life and must be reviewed annually. Although ITPs are a federal requirement, data from the National Longitudinal Transition Study describing the transition experiences of 13,000 students found that annual transition planning discussions between school staff and students ages 17 and 18 declined to 70% (Liu et al., 2018). Therefore, the life care planner should be aware that the school district is required to create an annual transition plan in conjunction with the student who receives special education. If the school has not created an ITP for a student and the student is in high school or nearing graduation, the life care planner should consider recommending additional community-based transition-related supports and services in the life care plan to facilitate stronger post-graduation outcomes for the student.

State Vocational Rehabilitation Support for Transition

State Vocational Rehabilitation (VR) services are available to individuals with disabilities to prepare for, obtain, or maintain employment (Murray et al., 2021). Many believe the misconception that only students with an IEP qualify for this vocational support, but that is not the case. Students with disabilities who have a 504 Plan, or an IEP, may qualify for VR services. To initiate a referral, the parent or school personnel should contact their local VR agency. Typically, the VR referral is made when the student is around age 16. Although a referral can be made earlier in some states, VR counselors often do not begin providing services until the student's senior year of high school. In other states, there may be a VR wait list, so contacting the local county VR agency at an earlier age may be beneficial.

Transition to Post-Secondary Education

Approximately 1 in 10 post-secondary students has a disability (Lombardi et al., 2012). A child with a disability may pursue education and training after high school (such as community college, four-year college, or trade school), and their educational safeguards change. Parents and providers often ask if the student's high school 504 Plan or IEP transfers to the post-secondary school. The answer is no. The IDEA and FAPE protection for students ends after high school (USDOE, OCR, 2011). However, post-secondary students do still fall under the ADA, which continues to offer the student protection from being discriminated against due to their disability (USDOE, OCR, 2011). The post-secondary school must make their determination as to whether the student is a qualified individual to receive learning supports at their institution.

Almost every post-secondary school has a disability support coordinator (USDOE, OCR, 2011). Before matriculating, the student must contact the disability support office (the office name varies), and provide documentation of their medical disability, supports received in high school (504 Plan or IEP), and any updated school-based evaluations from high school or a neuropsychologist. The student's VR counselor should also be a part of this process, as both entities often work together to identify supports.

At the post-secondary level, the student must self-advocate and drive the process of securing supports, whereas in high school, that is done by the parent or school staff. Parents can, with their student's signed privacy waiver permission, participate in communication with the disability support office.

The student can request specific post-secondary accommodations and provide input, but it is up to the disability support specialist to make the final determination. For example, during high school, Yuri had a 504 Plan for deficits she experienced from a stroke. She now experiences a slower speed of processing and hemiplegia, which affects her ability to use her dominant hand. Yuri received copies of her high school teachers' lecture notes that included questions the teacher would be asking the class one day before each class. Yuri asked for the same accommodations at college. However, her disability support specialist said that Yuri's professors would not be preparing lecture notes for her each day. Instead, Yuri would receive notes from a volunteer student that the professor would identify. But the notes would not be provided until after each class session. Yuri qualified for other accommodations due to her disability that were different from what she received in high school, such as priority registration for courses each semester and a private dorm room, at a single dorm room cost. Yuri also took a reduced course load, resulting in three additional years to complete college.

Private Schools: Navigating Services (34 CFR § 200.64)

Students with disabilities enrolled by their parents in a nonpublic, private, or religious school do not have the same right to special education as students in a public school. However, the IDEA provides these students with some benefits and services through equitable participation. Equitable participation requires the public school to spend a proportionate share of IDEA funds for services for children enrolled by their parents in a private school. The public school district where the private school is located is responsible for providing these services regardless of where the child lives.

The amount and type of services that a student receives in a private school differs from what that student could receive in a public school. School districts decide how they spend funds allocated for serving private school students with disabilities. For example, the school district may choose to spend all the equitable participation funds on training private school teachers and not offer any direct services to students. Another school district may choose to only provide direct services to private school students who are eligible for speech therapy, whereas students with other needs may not receive any services. The public school district must conduct child find activities to identify children in need. They must also provide consultation and evaluation services. These costs are not typically included in the equitable participation funding.

Parents of children who attend private school and suspect their child has a disability should make a written request to their public school district for a full evaluation, including a request for any related services, such as occupational or speech therapy, that may need to be considered. The IDEA requires school districts to consider any information supplied in that request. It is helpful to include any supporting information with the request, such as private evaluations, medical diagnosis, and current academic performance is helpful. Once it is determined that the child is eligible to receive special education and/or related services, the school must develop a service plan. This plan describes the specific special education and/or related services the child will receive. Services may be provided at the private school, the public school district, or an alternate location.

A FAPE is not required for students with disabilities enrolled in a private school. Services provided in a private school are legally distinct from those provided in a public school. In addition, each state may interpret and enact policies around equitable participation differently. The reader should contact a representative from the child's public school district to learn more about services provided in private school settings.

Note that a private or religious school that accepts any federal financial assistance (such as the free and reduced lunch program) must uphold the requirements of the Rehabilitation Act of 1973. These private schools may not exclude a child with a disability if that child can be provided an appropriate education in their school, given minor adjustments or accommodations.

Common Challenges Faced by Students with Disabilities
Failure to Identify Students with Disabilities

Schools may fail to identify children with disabilities. Newly acquired 'invisible' disabilities such as traumatic brain injury, mental health issues, and behavioral concerns are often misidentified or under-identified by school staff. Hence, parent-to-school communication about their child's newly acquired disability is key. Parents may request a formal evaluation for special education and related services at any time. The request for evaluation should be in writing and include a list of concerns and any supporting documentation such as outside evaluations, medical diagnoses, and current academic performance. The school district must issue a Permission to Evaluate (PTE). Once the school district receives the signed PTE, the evaluation must be completed within 60 calendar days.

A meeting must be scheduled with the parent and the evaluation team to discuss the results and develop the IEP if necessary. Identified children must receive be reevaluated by the school every two to three years, depending on their IDEA disability category. Note that a parent of a child who already has an IEP may request a reevaluation at any time to consider new information. An example request for evaluation is provided in Appendix 1 & 2

IEP Service Delivery Issues

Once a student with a disability is identified, evaluated, and qualifies for special education and/or related services, the school must develop an IEP within 30 days. The IEP team, including the parent, is required to meet yearly. However, any team member may request an IEP meeting at any time to review progress or discuss concerns.

Some concerns regarding IEP implementation include inappropriate goals, lack of data on goals, failure to provide services/accommodations listed in the IEP, and lack of progress. A child's educational needs may frequently change depending on current medical status, changes in the home, or transitions within the school system. Reviewing IEP goals more frequently than annually is especially critical for students with an acquired brain injury who are within a few years of their injury, as skills and needs tend to fluctuate rapidly.

A child may not respond positively to the interventions planned in an IEP for various reasons. IEP team meetings are the first step in addressing these concerns and may occur as frequently as needed. If a parent is not satisfied with the results of the IEP meeting, the parent may file a complaint, request mediation, or file due process. A parent can, and should, request progress monitoring reports from their child's teachers. This data will show the student's progress toward the IEP goals and objectives.

Graduation Considerations

Sometimes, a student with a disability requires more time to master skills and knowledge for post-high school success. The IDEA supports this need by including three additional years at school for students in special education (IDEA, 2004). Students with IEPs are permitted to remain in school until the age of 21 years under IDEA (22 in some states). School districts may allow a student who turns 21 years of age during the course of the school year to remain until the year is completed. The life care planner should contact the school district special education administrator for information on graduation age considerations in a particular school district.

A school team must consider the parent's request to allow the student to remain in school for additional time. Discussions about graduation should take place during the annual IEP meeting between the student, parents, and school team (Lanford & Cary, 2000).

Pediatric Special Education Case Study

The following case study illustrates one student's school experience and the resulting school supports received, followed by proactive steps that a parent, healthcare provider, and educator can take to alleviate misidentification and inappropriate services.

Liam was five years old when he sustained a severe traumatic brain injury due to a fall. Liam was standing on a deck of a vacation rental property when the railing gave way. He fell 30 feet onto the rocky ground below. Life flight transported Liam to the closest children's hospital, where he remained in a coma for four days. In addition to Liam's traumatic brain injury, he suffered multiple broken bones which required surgical repair. Liam was hospitalized for 10 days and then transferred to an inpatient rehabilitation unit for an additional 30 days. He required physical, occupational, speech, and vision therapies. Medical staff reassured the parents that Liam would be fine because he was so young and he would likely *bounce right back*. Upon discharge, Liam continued to access therapy at his local outpatient therapy center.

Due to the hospitalization and injuries sustained, Liam missed the last four months of his preschool program. His parents noticed that he had trouble recalling previously learned academic material, such as reciting nursery rhymes, counting, and spelling his name. Additionally, Liam now had difficulty following verbal directions at home. He became easily frustrated, resulting in behavioral outbursts, crying, throwing objects, and falling to the floor. His parents assumed Liam was just a sensitive child and would grow out of the behaviors.

Liam's parents soon registered him for kindergarten. The school intake forms did not specifically ask if the child had a history of brain injury, so the parents did not report his prior injury. In addition, his parents did not want Liam to be stigmatized as having special needs at such a young age. Since Liam looked *normal*, his parents hoped that he would just acclimate to school. Prior to kindergarten starting, Liam's mother attended an open house to meet Liam's teacher. His mother shared information about his accident, as well as information about Liam's regression of pre-academic skills following the brain injury. The teacher thanked her for the information but did not report it to the principal or special education director.

Liam arrived at school on the first day and appeared confused and distraught. He cried most of the day and refused to eat his lunch. The teacher shared with Mom that Liam was "a bit upset" during the day, but assured her that "everything will be fine" and chalked it up to being a typical start of kindergarten separation. However, Liam continued to experience difficulty at school. He frequently cried, became frustrated, and refused to participate in activities. The teacher assumed that Liam's behaviors were willful and imposed restrictions on him (e.g., time out, loss of recess). Liam's behaviors continued to increase as the year progressed, while his academic performance declined. The learning gap between Liam and his peers began to grow. His parents breathed a sigh of relief when Liam graduated to first grade.

By the end of the first quarter of first grade, Liam's academic skills were falling considerably behind his peers. He struggled to read, spell, and count. The teacher referred Liam to the school's Response to Intervention (RtI) team. RtI is a tiered model that assists students who struggle at school and helps staff identify students who require special education (Alahmari, 2019). The RtI team determined that Liam qualified for informal reading support. Liam received the reading support for two nine-week cycles with little improvement.

Finally, Liam was referred for a special education evaluation in late March of his first grade year. School staff completed the evaluation and presented the recommendations to his parents in late May of the same year. Liam qualified for special education services under the IDEA Emotional Disturbance disability category. The school recommended placement for Liam in a separate supplemental support classroom for children with disabilities for 80% of his day. Liam would only participate with his regular education peers during specials and recess. Liam's parents were uncomfortable that he was removed from the regular education classroom for so much of the time but agreed to the placement, assuming his school team knew best.

During second grade, Liam's academic performance began to show positive gains, likely due to his specialized instruction. However, his behaviors also continued to increase. Daily, Liam refused to do unpreferred academic work (such as math and writing). His behaviors increased during unstructured times and times of transition (e.g., hallway, specials, recess, bathroom breaks, lunch). He screamed, cried, and hit other students. Liam also began eloping from the classroom and was now considered a flight risk. The school responded with a behavior support plan that included consequences such as denial of recess, time out, and separation from peers.

By third grade, Liam's behaviors escalated to the point that he was now considered a safety risk for himself, students, and staff. The school district recommended an outside placement at a school for students with emotional disturbance. Parents agreed to this placement as it was the only option presented by the school district. Months later, Liam's parents learned from a friend who was a special education director at another school that Liam's school should have considered other options for Liam's placement. His parents filed due process proceedings against the district to change Liam's educational placement.

Unfortunately, the scenario above is not uncommon in the public school setting. Many students with disabilities are overlooked, mislabeled, and put into less-than-ideal educational settings. These situations are not typically the result of malicious intent on the part of the school district. Rather, many factors contribute to these situations, including low socio-economic communities, lack of educational funding, under-informed parents, and overwhelmed school systems (Bonuck & Hill, 2020; DeJong et al., 2016). The responsibility of ensuring that a child receives needed special education supports and services in an appropriate placement and timely manner often falls to the parent—a parent who is typically overwhelmed and struggling to work, maintain a home, and support their child's acquired medical needs.

Several responses to Liam's experience could have prevented his negative school experience:

1. The parents could have requested an evaluation from the school district before Liam transitioned from the rehabilitation center. Depending on the state in which the child resides, this evaluation would occur through either Early Intervention or the school-age system. A timely evaluation may have resulted in Liam being identified as a child with a disability (traumatic brain injury) much sooner.
2. Information sharing between the healthcare providers and parents about the future effects of Liam's acquired disability and the possible need for special education would have been a proactive step to better prepare the parents.
3. The school district's kindergarten registration forms should have included screening questions asking parents about any prior brain injuries their child may have sustained. Liam would have been identified earlier by his school as a child who may have difficulties with learning and behavior. Liam's educational supports and services could have started in kindergarten vs. 3rd grade, likely resulting in better outcomes.
4. The parents could have shared information about Liam's traumatic brain injury with the school team prior to the school's evaluation, which would likely have increased his chances of receiving the correct disability category of "traumatic brain injury." The school's educational supports and services could target his specific disability. A lack of parent-to-school notification of an acquired injury is a nationally recognized issue (Blosser & DePompei, 2019; Canto et al., 2014) because if learning or behavior issues emerge in the future, knowing about the prior medical issue is critical for appropriate support school planning. The parents could have shared outside evaluations, therapy goals, and progress reports with the school district. The school district would have to consider this information during the evaluation and IEP planning. Information sharing of rehabilitation records also prevents the school team from administering the same cognitive standardized tests too soon, thereby impacting the validity of the assessment.
5. Parents could have challenged the school regarding providing services in the LRE. Liam was never given the opportunity to remain in regular education while receiving individualized special education supports and services. His placement in the supplemental support program appeared to result in negative emotional and social implications for Liam.
6. Parents could also have disagreed with Liam's school placement. Liam's emotionality was likely a direct result of his brain injury. Behavior planning after a brain injury differs greatly from the strategies and techniques used in a typical placement for students with behavior

issues. But parents do not always know that they have the right to disagree with the proposed IEP. For instance, in a recent study, less than 60% of parents were satisfied with their child's current IEP (DeJong et al., 2016). Before making this placement, the district did not exhaust all available supports and programs. Parents can initiate dispute resolution procedures at any time by notifying the local school district or state education department and requesting mediation or due process.

The Role of the Education Consultant in Life Care Planning

Life care planners must often consider a student's private versus public school placement, tutoring services, assistive technology, adaptive equipment, academic accommodation supports, and curriculum modifications. This is a formidable task, especially if the life care planner is not versed in the complex and frequently changing world of special education. An educational consultant can serve as a valuable resource in assisting life care planners by recommending school-related determinations, and providing insight and direction to support a child's current and future educational needs to adulthood.

Education consultants are frequently underutilized when planning for a child's current and future academic and behavioral needs from pre-kindergarten through 12th grade. It is helpful for the education consultant to demonstrate training and expertise (a) specific to the child's disability area, (b) regular and special education laws, and (c) educational pedagogy. The education consultant can provide forensic expert witness opinions, educational treatment planning, and case management. To truly navigate the nuances of local educational supports a student qualifies for that vary from region to region, collaboration between a life care planner and an education consultant (such as a brain injury education specialist) is key. An education consultant can:

(1) Evaluate to determine the clinical and functional deficits a child has due to their acquired medical disability and how these deficits impact their ability to access education, this involves formal and informal testing, and functional classroom observations.
(2) Recommend learning supports, aids, and services the child will require now until high school graduation due to their acquired medical disability.
(3) Recommend specific education and transition supports and services into adulthood for the life care plan.
(4) Provide direct support and guidance for the parents regarding how to initiate a school referral process for evaluation and obtain appropriate services.
(5) Train school staff about the educational ramifications of the child's medical disability regarding learning and behavioral accommodations, modifications, and teaching strategies.

This professional utilizes a methodology while investigating a student's cognitive, physical, socioemotional, and behavioral function at home and during the school day. The education consultant can also provide opinions and recommendations for community-based supports if there is an issue that impacts learning resulting from the medical diagnosis. Recommendations such as a referral to:

a. Pediatric physiatrist for ongoing care (because medical issues can impact learning);
b. Pediatric neuropsychologist (because cognitive processes may be impacted);
c. Psychiatrist/Psychologist (because mental health & behaviors impact learning);
d. Academic tutor (because learning is often impacted); and
e. Pediatric physical, speech, or occupational therapists (because issues within these areas often impact learning).

In addition, there are cases where it may benefit a student to have an education case manager included in the life care plan. This professional can advocate for and monitor the student's changing education needs throughout their educational career and assist in transition planning post-high school.

Questions to Ask When Developing the Life Care Plan

- What is the child's current educational placement (regular education with no support/with support, special classroom, approved private school)?
- What supports and services, if any, is the child currently receiving at school (paraprofessional/aide, adapted curriculum, accommodations, modifications, therapies, nursing services)?
- Might this child require more intensive services and supports over time? Do you foresee any future educational placement changes for this student?
- Has any testing or assessment been completed in the last 12 months (standardized testing, state/local assessments, informal rating scales/checklists)?
- How is the student progressing on their current IEP related to goals and objectives (grades, progress reports)?
- Is the student experiencing behavioral or mental health concerns (fearfulness, anxiety, refusal, defiance, lack of motivation)? Does the student have a behavior intervention plan?
- Does the student demonstrate any concerns regarding their social skills (interacting with peers appropriately, developing friendships at school)?
- Does the student engage in age-appropriate leisure activities at school (play appropriately, interests)?
- What are this student's greatest strengths and weaknesses in the school setting?
- Does the parent have any concerns regarding the school supports that their child is receiving?
- At what age will this child likely graduate from high school? (Ask both the parent and the school.)
- Do the student's teachers have prior training and experience in supporting the student's specific acquired medical disability? (If not, this should be included in the life care plan.)

Conclusion

This chapter provides an overview of the federal special education laws and practices that ensure all children with disabilities receive a FAPE. The information within this chapter details the complex nuances of special education law and the implementation variability that exists between states as well as individual school districts. School districts are required to meet standards that provide the most appropriate education, which does not always equate to the best education for each student. A life care planner is tasked to create a support plan that encompasses what a child's future learning and behavior needs may be over time due to their acquired medical disability. Yet, "professional recommendations aim at the optimum, whereas legal requirements merely demarcate the minimum" (Zirkel & Eagan Brown, 2015, p. 106). This reality fuels the variability of how school-based services are provided in different states and districts. The ever-changing world of special education is complex, confusing, and often overwhelming for parents and professionals alike. A collaborative partnership between an education consultant and a life care planner will enrich the development of the life care plan in the best interest of the child.

Glossary of Key Education Terms

Term/Acronym	Definition
ADA	Americans with Disabilities Act of 1990
AT	Assistive Technology
BIP	Behavior Intervention Plan
EI	Early Intervention
ER	Evaluation Report
ESY	Extended School Year
FAPE	Free and Appropriate Public Education
IDEA	Individuals with Disabilities Education Act of 2004
IEE	Independent Educational Evaluation
IFSP	Individualized Family Services Plan
IEP	Individualized Education Program
ITP	Individualized Transition Plan
LEA	Local Education Agency (or school district)
LRE	Least Restrictive Environment
MAG	Measurable Annual Goal
NOREP	Notice of Recommended Educational Placement
OSERS	Office of Special Education and Rehabilitative Services
PLOP	Present Levels of Performance
PWN	Prior Written Notice
RR	Reevaluation Report
SaS	Supplementary Supports and Services
SDI	Specially Designed Instruction
SEA	State Education Agency
STO	Short Term Objective
VR	Vocational Rehabilitation

References

Alahmari, A. (2019). A review and synthesis of the response to intervention (RtI) literature: Teachers' implementations and perceptions. *International Journal of Special Education*, *33*(4), 894–909.

Americans with Disabilities Act. Public Law No.101-336, 104 Stat 328 (1990), amended Public Law 110-325 (2008). www.govinfo.gov/content/pkg/STATUTE-104/pdf/STATUTE-104-Pg327.pdf

Blosser, J., & DePompei, R. (2019). *Pediatric traumatic brain injury: Proactive intervention*. Plural Publishing.

Bonuck, K., & Hill, L. A. (2020). Special education disparities are social determinants of health: A role for medical-legal partnerships. *Progress in Community Health Partnerships: Research, Education, and Action*, *14*(2), 251–257.

Brown v. Board of Education, 347 U.S. 483 (1954). https://supreme.justia.com/cases/federal/us/347/483/

Canto, A. I., Cheshire, D. J., Buckley, V. A., Andrews, T. W., & Roehrig, A. D. (2014). Barriers to meeting the needs of students with traumatic brain injury. *Educational Psychology in Practice*, *30*(1), 88–103.

DeJong, N. A., Wood, C. T., Morreale, M. C., Ellis, C., Davis, D., Fernandez, J., & Steiner, M. J. (2016). Identifying social determinants of health and legal needs for children with special health care needs. *Clinical pediatrics*, *55*(3), 272–277.

Education for All Handicapped Children Act of 1975. 20 us e 1401 Public Law 94-142 94th Congress 89 STAT. 773. https://www.govinfo.gov/content/pkg/STATUTE-89/pdf/STATUTE-89-Pg773.pdf

England, S. S. (2011). Special education law and the pediatric patient. In S. Riddick-Grisham & L. A. Deming (Eds.), *Pediatric life care planning and case management* (2nd ed., pp. 887–906). Routledge.

Individuals with Disabilities Education Improvement Act of 2004, 20 USC § 1400 et seq. (2006). https://sites.ed.gov/idea/statute-chapter-33/subchapter-i/1400

Kurth, J. A., Ruppar, A. L., McQueston, J. A., McCabe, K. M., Johnston, R., & Toews, S. G. (2019). Types of supplementary aids and services for students with significant support needs. *The Journal of Special Education*, *52*(4), 208–218.

Lanford, A. D., & Cary, L. G. (2000). Graduation requirements for students with disabilities: Legal and practice considerations. *Remedial and Special Education*, *21*(3), 152–160.

Lipkin, P. H., Okamoto, J., Norwood, K. W., Adams, R. C., Brei, T. J., Burke, R. T., Davis, B. E., Friedman, S. L., Houtrow, A. J., Hyman, S. L., Kuo, D. Z., Noritz, G. H., Turchi, R. M., Murphy, N. A., Allison, M., Ancona, R., Attisha, E., Pinto, C. D., Holmes, B., ... Young, T. (2015). The Individuals with Disabilities Education Act (IDEA) for Children With Special Educational Needs. *Pediatrics*, *136*(6), e1650–e1662. https://doi.org/10.1542/peds.2015-3409

Liu, A. Y., Lacoe, J., Lipscomb, S., Haimson, J., Johnson, D. R., & Thurlow, M. L. (2018). *Preparing for life after high school: The characteristics and experiences of youth in special education*. Findings from the National Longitudinal Transition Study 2012. Volume 3: Comparisons over time (Full report) (NCEE 2018-4007). U.S. Department of Education, Institute of Education Sciences, National Center for Education Evaluation and Regional Assistance.

Lombardi, A., Murray, C., & Gerdes, H. (2012). Academic performance of first-generation college students with disabilities. *Journal of College Student Development*, *53*, 811–826. doi:10.1353/csd.2012.0082

Magnus, E., & Tøssebro, J. (2014). Negotiating individual accommodation in higher education. *Scandinavian Journal of Disability Research*, *16*, 316–332.

Michael P. and Elizabeth G. v. Department of Education, State of Hawaii, 57 IDELR 123, 656 F.3d 1057,1066 (9th Cir, 2011).

Mills v. Board of Education of District of Columbia, 348 F. Supp. 866 (D.D.C. 1972).

Murray, A., Watter, K., McLennan, V., Vogler, J., Nielsen, M., Jeffery, S., Ehlers, S., & Kennedy, A. (2021). Identifying models, processes, and components of vocational rehabilitation following acquired brain injury: A systematic scoping review. *Disability and Rehabilitation*, 1–14. Advance online publication.

National Association of School Nurses. (2020). *Use of individualized healthcare plans to support school health services* (Position Statement). https://www.nasn.org/nasn-resources/professional-practice-documents/position-statements/ps-ihps

National Association of School Nurses. (2017). *Principles for practice: The role of individualized healthcare plans (IHPs) in care coordination for students with chronic health conditions*.

National Center for Education Statistics. (2022). *Students with disabilities*. Condition of education. U.S. Department of Education, Institute of Education Sciences. https://nces.ed.gov/programs/coe/indicator/cgg

National Council on Disability. *Broken promises: The underfunding of IDEA* [updated 2018; cited 2022 Jun 9]. https://ncd.gov/sites/default/files/NCD_BrokenPromises_508.pdf

Pennsylvania Association of Retarded Child [PARC] vs. Commonweatlh of Pennsylvania. 343 F. Supp. 279 (1972). https://law.justia.com/cases/federal/district-courts/FSupp/343/279/1691591/

Pennsylvania Department of Education. (2014). *Special education timelines*. http://pattan.net-website.s3.amazonaws.com/images/2015/04/20/SpecEd Timelns0415.pdf

Schreuer, N., & Sachs, D. (2014). Efficacy of accommodations for students with disabilities in higher education. *Journal of Vocational Rehabilitation*, *40*, 27–40.

Section 504 of the Rehabilitation Act of 1973. 29 USC § 701 et seq, (1973). www.law.cornell.edu/uscode/text/29/701

Section 504 of the Rehabilitation Act of 1973, as amended, 29 USC 794.

Supplementary aids and services. Center for Parent Information and Resources [CPIR]. (2017). www.parentcenterhub.org/iep-supplementary/

Tarrien, D. (2016). The law student as mediator IEP project: Encouraging legal services outreach in the community and empowering families. *Michigan Academician, 44*(1), 51–60.

U.S. Department of Education. (2022). A history of the Individuals with Disabilities Education Act. https://www.govinfo.gov/content/pkg/STATUTE-89/pdf/STATUTE-89-Pg773.pdf

U.S. Department of Education. (2017). Section 300.42 Supplementary aids and services. https://sites.ed.gov/idea/regs/b/a/300.42

U.S. Department of Education, Office for Civil Rights. (2010). *Guidelines for educators and administrators for implementing Section 504 of the Rehabilitation Act of 1973—Subpart D*. https://saom.memberclicks.net/assets/MACSS/MACSS_Conferences/guidelines%20for%20implementing%20504.pdf

U.S. Department of Education. (2015). *Protecting students with disabilities: Frequently asked questions about Section 504 and the education of children with disabilities*. www2.ed.gov/about/offices/list/ocr/504faq.html

U.S. Department of Education, Office for Civil Rights. (2010). *Free appropriate public education for students with disabilities: Requirements under section 504 of the Rehabilitation Act of 1973*. www2.ed.gov/about/offices/list/ocr/docs/edlite-FAPE504.html

U.S. Department of Education, Office for Civil Rights [USDOE, OCR]. (2011). *Students with disabilities preparing for postsecondary education: Know your rights and responsibilities*. www2.ed.gov/about/offices/list/ocr/transition.html

U.S. Department of Education, Office for Civil Rights [USDOE, OCR]. (2016). *Parent and educator resource guide to Section 504 in public elementary and secondary schools*. www2.ed.gov/about/offices/list/ocr/docs/504-resource-guide-201612.pdf

U.S. Health and Human Services (2006). *Your rights under Section 504 of the Rehabilitation Act*. www.hhs.gov/sites/default/files/knowyourrights504adafactsheet.pdf

Venville, A., Street, A. F., & Fossey, E. (2014). Good intentions: Teaching and specialist support staff perspectives of student disclosure of mental health issues in post-secondary education. *International Journal of Inclusive Education, 18*,1172–1188. doi:10.1080/13603116.2014.881568

Zirkel, P. A., & Eagan Brown, B. (2015). K–12 students with concussions: A legal perspective. *The Journal of School Nursing, 31*(2), 99–109.

Appendix 1
Example Parent to School Letter Request Educational Services for a Child Post-Brain Injury

January 1, 2023

Mrs. Freda Smith, Principal
Apex Elementary School
Apex, PA

Dear Mrs. Smith,
I am writing to request an evaluation for Special Education services (including speech and occupational therapies) for my daughter, Sarah, who is in the sixth grade. Sarah suffered a traumatic brain injury in July 2021 and is having considerable difficulty in school. Sarah has chronic headaches and fatigue. She has trouble with her memory, organization, and focusing on her schoolwork. Sarah's

grades are dropping in math and reading. She used to earn straight-A grades but is now struggling to pass. Sarah also is very anxious about coming to school and very worried about her grades. Sarah currently receives outpatient speech and occupational therapies, as well as counseling.

I am including a report from her neuropsychologist with testing results from January 2022. Please acknowledge receipt of this request and advise me on next steps.

Thank you for your time and consideration.

Sincerely,

Lori K.
Lori's email address
Lori's phone #
Lori's home address

Appendix 2
Example Parent to School Letter Request Educational Services for a Child Template

Date

ADD NAME, Principal,
ADD NAME, School Nurse
ADD NAME, 504 Coordinator,
ADD NAME, Special Education Coordinator (delete any
ADD SCHOOL NAME
ADD SCHOOL ADDRESS
CITY, STATE, ZIPCODE

Dear ADD NAMES,

I am writing to request that my child, STUDENT NAME, be evaluated for Special Education services including (list any specific therapies or services you want to be considered). STUDENT NAME is currently enrolled in the XX grade and is struggling to LEARN AND/OR BEHAVE.

On DATE, STUDENT NAME experienced a MEDICAL DIAGNOSIS. Since that time, STUDENT NAME has experienced difficulties FILL IN -LEARNING, BEHAVING, NAVIGATING THE SCHOOL, MEMORY, ATTENTION, CONCENTRATION, EXECUTIVE FUNCTION, MOBILITY, COMMUNICATION.

Enclosed, I have included STUDENT NAME's medical diagnosis and medical, rehabilitation, neuropsychological evaluations. Please acknowledge receipt of this request and advise me on next steps.

I would be happy to talk with you about my current concerns regarding STUDENT NAME's learning abilities. Thank you for your prompt response to my request.

Sincerely,

SIGNATURE
Parent Name
Parent Address
Parent Phone
Parent Email Address

*keep a copy of your signed, dated letter.

Chapter 32

Special Needs Planning

Benji Rubin

Special Needs Planning

Parents of children with significant disabilities must plan very differently than other parents.

They must plan for not only who will take care of their children until they are adults if they were to pass away prematurely but rather who will take care of their child for the rest of their life. Moreover, the chance that they will outlive their child with disabilities is far more likely than both parents passing away prematurely and having minor children (Farina et al., 2021). In other words, the planning is not hypothetical for some unlikely scenario but rather for the most probable outcome. Furthermore, siblings are very often essential to the process as they are most likely to be alive for most or all of the lifetime of their brother or sister with disabilities. Finally, the parents and siblings are not the only people who need to worry about "special needs planning;" it's also grandparents and sometimes other relatives that may want to leave assets to the individual with disabilities and need to ensure they do not impact their qualification for government benefits.

What Is Special Needs Planning?

Special needs planning is planning for the future of an individual with disabilities to not only ensure eligibility for government benefits they would otherwise be eligible for now or in the future, but also to ensure that they maintain eligibility for those government benefit programs for their entire lifetime. Special needs planning can be thought of as a pyramid—the base is government benefits. The goal is to not interfere with the government benefits the individual with disabilities is otherwise eligible for, so any inheritances left to them, gifts made to them, or any other financial resource they have access to will not cause them to lose their government benefit eligibility. To avoid a loss of government benefits, Special Needs Trusts (SNTs) are often used to ensure the child has a reserve fund over and above their government benefits. There are two types of SNT, and both will be discussed later in this chapter. Finally, the individual with disabilities may sometimes be able to work to some extent, which can be an additional financial resource beyond government benefits and the SNT. That said, it is important to know that earning too much money can cause a big problem for government benefits, so special needs planning should include education about all of these rules.

The cost of lifetime care and support paid for an individual with significant disabilities is often millions of dollars. The next question then is where will this money come from? First, the individual's work earnings can be a resource, but usually a limited one due to the nature of their disabilities. Second, State and Federal government benefits are often the next resource turned to. Finally, family resources can be left to a SNT, as mentioned previously.

Government Benefits 101

Understanding the primary government benefit programs that support people with special needs is a crucial part of the special needs planning process. Further, each program often has a dynamic relationship with other programs, so understanding how each program fits within the lifetime of supports the individual may need is very important as well.

Supplemental Security Income (SSI)

The first program many individuals with disabilities will apply for is Supplemental Security Income (SSI). It is effectively Social Security for someone who does not have sufficient work history to qualify for Social Security Disability Insurance (SSDI) at the time they apply for benefits. Social Security Income has both an asset and an income test. The asset test is $2,000, a limit that has not been adjusted, even for inflation, since 1989. Prior to the first month after a child turns 18, the government will include the assets of the parents in their eligibility calculation and therefore disqualifying the child. However, beginning the first month after they turn 18, the government only looks to the child's individual assets. This can include Uniform Transfer to Minor's Act Accounts (UTMA), sometimes referred to as Uniform Gift to Minor's Act (UGMA) accounts. Moreover, SSI looks back three years to see what the child had received under their Social Security number. If, for example, the child had a $10,000 UTMA account that was closed when they were 16, but then an SSI application was submitted after the child turned 18, the government will want to know what happened to the assets in that account as they will be included as a resource unless there is proof they were "spent-down" for the benefit of the individual.

The income test is still more complicated. It looks to whether the child can earn what's referred to as Substantial Gainful Activity (SGA). As of January 1, 2024, this amount is $1,470 per month (see www.ssa.gov/oact/cola/sga.html). To determine if the individual can earn this amount of money, Social Security will consider several factors. First, does the child have a current diagnosis that is considered a "listing-level impairment"? This is literally a list the Social Security Administration keeps of diagnoses—or several diagnoses that, when combined, can "equal" a listing-level impairment—to determine whether an applicant may qualify for benefits under. Assuming the claimant has a listing-level impairment or "equaled" one, the next step is to look at "functional limitations." Effectively, the individual with a disability has to prove inability to work due to their diagnosis or diagnoses. Social Security will look at documentation from medical and other professionals, including Individualized Education Programs (IEPs) and other school records for SSI qualification. They will look to factors such in the Social Security Administration's "Program Operations Manual System" (POMS) Mental Residual Functional Capacity Assessment elements as concentration, pace, and persistence in a work context (2021). The Social Security Administration considers appropriate social functioning: will challenges in terms of social interactions in a work context be a significant impediment to earning SGA? Activities of Daily Living (ADLs) are also considered to determine if those would impact earning ability, such as self-care challenges, including personal hygiene, as an example. Moreover, the government will look to whether the individual can understand, remember, and apply information in a work context or have appropriate interactions with others, adapt or manage themselves in a work contact, or have the inability to use two limbs (Social Security Administration, 2022a).

Assuming the individual qualifies under the income and asset tests, they will get approved for SSI and receive a monthly amount. The federal maximum is $841 per month as of January 1, 2022, but some states provide supplements to this amount (Social Security Administration, 2022b). This amount can be reduced in certain contexts due to work earnings, child support payments paid to their parent on their behalf, or whether someone pays food or shelter expenses for them. Current rules may reduce the federal maximum for SSI due to a third party paying food and shelter expenses, but this may be modified or eliminated in the coming years.

Social Security Disability Insurance (SSDI)

Another important program for individuals with disabilities is Social Security Disability Insurance (SSDI). To be eligible for SSDI, the individual with disabilities must qualify per the same rules as SSI about the inability to perform SGA as well as an additional requirement of sufficient recent work history. The amount of benefit the individual is entitled to is often less than the SSI amount since the claimant often has even a short work history. There is another way, however, that individuals, especially those with intellectual and developmental disabilities, may qualify for what is often a much more significant benefit under the Social Security system. It is a program called Childhood Disability Benefit (CDB) or historically referred to as Disabled Adult Child (DAC) benefit. To be eligible for this benefit, the child must be deemed disabled by SSI or SSDI prior to age 22 (the most common situation is for the child to have received SSI prior to age 22) and a parent (can be a step-parent, in some cases) is currently receiving SSDI, Social Security Retirement, or is deceased. Further, the child can never have lost that disabled "status" from age 22 until the parent begins receiving those benefits or is deceased. The amount the child is entitled to is based on the Primary Insurance Amount (PIA) of the parent. It is usually 50% when the parent is retired and 75% when the parent is deceased. If both parents are retired, the child should automatically be on the highest work record of the two parents. In most cases, the CDB benefit is significantly more than SSI, and can approach as much as $3,000 per month in today's dollars.

Medicare

If the individual with a disability has SSDI on their own work record or receives CDB benefit on a parent's work record, this will trigger eventual Medicare eligibility following a two-year waiting period. Medicare coverage is important since the individual often does not have private health insurance in most states as an adult over the age of 26, and, therefore, Medicaid is often their primary health insurance. Medicare, due to higher reimbursement rates, is much more commonly accepted by healthcare providers than Medicaid.

Medicaid

Medicaid is probably the most important government benefit program for most individuals with significant disabilities over the entirety of their lifetime. For one, if the individual lives residentially (e.g., in a group home often referred to as a Community Integrated Living Arrangement or CILA), the individual will not keep their SSI or their SSDI no matter how much they are receiving.

Instead, they will keep a Personal Needs Allowance (PNA) that in most states is less than a few hundred dollars and in some states is well under $100 per month. Further, Medicaid is much more than health insurance. The health insurance aspect of Medicaid is important, often as secondary insurance after Medicare or possibly a parent's private health insurance plan. It is especially helpful in paying for hospital and pharmacy expenses. However, since most doctors do not take Medicaid, it is, therefore, less helpful for those expenses. The most important part of Medicaid for many individuals with disabilities is the funding for Medicaid Waiver Programs.

Medicaid Waiver Programs

Historically, Medicaid only paid for institutionalized care, such as skilled-nursing facilities or institutions for people with developmental disabilities, when it was first created. However, it eventually became understood that people can be supported successfully in less restrictive environments for less money benefiting both the taxpayer as well as the individual with disabilities (Medicaid.gov). The government, therefore, waived the requirement that Medicaid only pays for institutionalized care, hence the term "Medicaid Waiver." One of the most common Medicaid Waiver programs is the Home and Community Based Services Waiver (HCBS) that each state administers differently but usually includes group homes or CILAs as one of the options it covers.

The cost of these Medicaid Waiver programs varies but, in many cases, exceeds $100,000 per person per year. The cost reflects the fact that that rate often includes not only 24/7 support (sometimes at a ratio of 1:1 or 2:1) but also including programs to create a meaningful day which increasingly includes funding for supported or customized employment as well as evenings, overnight, and weekends (see *State of the States in Intellectual and Developmental Disabilities* (11th ed.), 2017, as well as www.caseforinclusion.org/).

Each state has a different system for accessing Medicaid Waiver services depending upon when the individual has developmental disabilities, mental health challenges, or other physical disabilities, for example. Some states have a county-based system, and some states are more centralized. Families of an individual with disabilities should seek out experienced professionals that know the system in their state. There is a very large variance between states in terms of funding. Some states have multi-decade waiting lists, while others have entitlements whereby the individual automatically receives waiver services as soon as they become Medicaid eligible (often after the age of 18). Further, some states have average HCBS Waiver rates for CILAs that are less than half of other better-funded states. (see *State of the States in Intellectual and Developmental Disabilities* (11th ed.), 2017, as well as www.caseforinclusion.org/). In addition, there are Medicaid Waiver programs in many states for minor children with disabilities that do not consider parents' assets and income. Once again, it is important to engage the proper professionals in the state of residence of the individual with disabilities to learn more about qualifications in that jurisdiction.

Medicaid Requirements

Traditionally, Medicaid required that a person fit into a qualifying category. For people with disabilities, having SSI or SSDI usually meant they automatically qualified for Medicaid benefits so long as they had less than $2,000 of assets in their name. That said, over the years, Medicaid eligibility has expanded. First, many states have established Medicaid buy-in programs for individuals with disabilities that are working to a limited extent. In addition, expanded Medicaid under the Affordable Care Act (in most states) has created a new category of individuals that can qualify for Medicaid. This type of Medicaid uses a different definition of income and has no asset test.

However, this type of Medicaid often is not available to many people with disabilities for various reasons, including parental income (which is generally not a factor under traditional Medicaid rules), as well as Medicare eligibility (which also does not impact traditional Medicaid eligibility).

Special Needs Estate Planning

If an individual with disabilities receives an inheritance from their parent, grandparent, or anyone else, it will immediately jeopardize their eligibility for their important government benefits discussed above. Therefore, the individual cannot receive an inheritance directly, nor is it a good idea to leave it as a moral obligation to another relative or friend with the hope that they will use the money for the benefit of the child with special needs. The assets may be at risk even due to factors out of the control of the trusted individual due to Internal Revenue Service (IRS), creditor problems, or a divorce.

Furthermore, the individual cannot receive the funds in the form of a traditional spendthrift trust either for the lifetime of the beneficiary or until a certain age. These types of spendthrift trusts are considered "support trusts" and are, therefore, considered a resource that impacts eligibility for most important government benefits. Not only may the child lose their eligibility for crucial government benefits, but also SSI and/or Medicaid could potentially claim reimbursement for benefits previously provided to the child. If an inheritance is left incorrectly to a child with disabilities directly, then there are two main options to handle the resources discussed below, known as ABLE accounts and a First-Party SNT, respectively.

Special Needs Trusts

There are two types of Special Needs Trust (SNT) that can benefit people with special needs—both types of trust are reserve funds over and above government benefits, and both types of trust can have unlimited assets titled in their name without any impact on government benefit eligibility so long as the language of the trust follows all the state and federal law, rules, regulations and internal interpretations of those rules and regulations that SSI looks to called the Program Operations Manual System (POMS). Further, both types of SNT can own all types of assets: from inherited IRAs to brokerage accounts invested in a diversified portfolio of investments to CDs, real estate, savings and checking accounts, etc. The differences between the two SNTS, however, are crucial.

Third-Party Special Needs Trust

The most common type of SNT is a Third-Party SNT. This type of trust is created to receive lifetime gifts or inheritances from anyone in the world but the individual with disabilities themselves. Anyone can create it and/or fund it other than the individual with disabilities. Often, these trusts are established and/or funded by parents or grandparents to ensure any inheritance for their child or grandchild will not impact government benefits. As a special note, Inherited individual retirement accounts (IRAs) left by parents or grandparents directly to a Third-Party SNT receive special beneficial tax treatment in that the 10-year Required Minimum Distribution (RMD) rule that is nearly universally applied to inherited IRAs because the Secure Act that became law in 2020 will not apply. Instead of the 10-year rule, the SNT is allowed to stretch the RMDs over the lifetime of the beneficiary based on standard life tables produced by the IRS.

The best way to draft this type of SNT is to establish it as a free-standing trust established during the lifetime of the individual creating the trust (this type of trust is often referred to as an inter-vivos trust) for several reasons. First, if the parents set up the SNT, but grandparents or maybe an aunt or uncle want to leave something to the trust on their passing or make a gift during their lifetime, having a free-standing inter-vivos trust that exists ensures they have a trust to name instead to protect government benefits. Also, having one common trust that all relatives "piggyback" onto simplifies the way things will work when the beneficiary needs the SNT many years later. Furthermore, having an inter-vivos trust may also ensure that if laws, rules, or regulations, etc. change, then by its existence, the trust may be grandfathered under existing laws and rules.

It is also of crucial importance that not only the parent's estate plan references the SNT but also grandparents and sometimes even aunts and uncles reference the SNT to receive any inheritances that might benefit the beneficiary, even contingently. Therefore, it might be best for the attorney to give a "fill-in-the-blank" form to add a paragraph to the extended family's will or revocable living trust.

Yet another reason for an SNT to be done as an inter-vivos trust is it can permit parents, grandparents, or other relatives to gift money to it with the intention of impoverishing themselves to qualify for Medicaid. Normally, an individual cannot gift their assets to their family to impoverish themselves to qualify for Medicaid if they need skilled nursing care without a five-year penalty period during which they will be ineligible for Medicaid. However, there is a federally-created exception to this rule: a gift can be made by said parent or grandparent, for example, to a free-standing SNT with certain language in the trust (specific to state statute and Medicaid regulations) so that the trust will qualify as what is called a Medicaid "Sole Benefit Trust." Said gift would not be subject to the normal five-year penalty period for gifts, allowing the individual who gifted to their relative's SNT the ability to qualify immediately for Medicaid to pay for their skilled nursing care.

First-Party Special Needs Trust

The other type of SNT is a First-Party SNT, also known as a d4a Trust, an OBRA '93 Trust, and sometimes a "Payback" Trust (referred to hereinafter as a "d4A Trust"). The main reasons these trusts are established and funded are due to the failure of parents or grandparents to do proper special needs planning, leading to an inheritance being left directly to the beneficiary with disabilities or due to a medical malpractice lawsuit or other personal injury settlement. This type of trust also protects the beneficiary's eligibility for government benefits like the SNT does, but it is more restrictive in a number of ways. First, the individual must be under 65 years of age for such a Trust to be funded. Second, a d4A Trust can only be established by the individual with disabilities themselves (if they have the capacity to do so), the parents, the grandparents, the guardians, or through a court order. In other words, the people who often want to set these up (such as siblings of the individual with disabilities after their parents accidentally leave an inheritance directly to their brother or sister) cannot do so without court involvement. Also, unlike a Third-Party SNT, a d4A Trust is required to pay back the state or states from which the individual received Medicaid services during their lifetime at the time of their death before the trust can distribute the remaining assets anywhere else.

ABLE Accounts

In December 2014, Congress passed, and the President signed into law, the ABLE Act of 2014, thereby providing a new way for individuals with disabilities and their families to save without impacting government benefits (IRS, 2021). This law was amended by the Tax Cut and Jobs Act of 2017, which was effective January 1, 2018, thereby expanding the ways ABLE can be used. While it is a great new tool to have in special needs planning, "toolbox" doesn't replace the need for SNTs, nor does it cover all situations (ABLE National Resource Center, 2022).

An individual can open an ABLE account if they have a disability onset prior to the age of 26 and are eligible for SSI or SSDI because of the disability, or they are blind; or they have a medically determinable physical or mental impairment with marked, severe functional limitations that are expected to last 12 months or result in death or they have a similarly severe disability.

ABLE accounts are run by states just as 529 College Savings Plans are. Most states allow out-of-state residents to contribute to an account run by their ABLE program. There are, however, a number of restrictions no matter which state's ABLE program you choose. First, there is a maximum annual contribution limit that is tied to the annual gift tax exclusion amount ($16,000 per year as of January 1, 2023). This is a hard limit that prevents any gifts beyond a total cumulative amount (currently $17,000) from being contributed to a single ABLE account in a calendar year. Furthermore, an individual cannot have multiple ABLE accounts. If the individual does not have anyone appointed as their legal guardian, then they have full control of their ABLE account by default. Many states allow an individual in that situation to designate a parent or other relative to manage their ABLE account voluntarily. The total cumulative balance of the ABLE account also has limits. While the individual is receiving SSI, the total amount in their ABLE account cannot exceed $100,000. If they are no longer receiving SSI but rather receiving SSDI as well as possibly Medicare and Medicaid, the maximum total is different in each state but ranges from $235,000 to $550,000 (see www.ablenrc.org/what-is-able/what-are-able-acounts/). Technically there are also limitations on how the ABLE account assets may be spent, though IRS regulations on ABLE accounts are quite generous in allowing them to be used for virtually anything that would improve the individual's quality of life (see www.ablenrc.org/determining-whether-something-is-a-qualified-disability-expense-qde/). If an individual uses ABLE account assets for expenses that are not permitted, the IRS can apply a penalty as well as tax the distribution in question. There is an additional requirement that the individual must have become disabled prior to the age of 26. The definition of disability for ABLE accounts is the same as the rules for SSI and/or SSDI. Receipt of one of these government benefit programs is conclusive proof that they qualify as disabled for ABLE accounts purposes.

Finally, there is the potential issue of a "payback" to the state for what Medicaid has spent for the benefit of the beneficiary since the date the ABLE account was opened. When the ABLE Act was passed, it permitted the states to require this reimbursement, sometimes referred to as a "clawback." Following the implementation of the ABLE Act, the federal Medicaid agency (Centers for Medicare and Medicaid Services [CMS]) required that all states must enforce the payback on all Medicaid benefits provided to beneficiaries over the age of 55 as well as all Medicaid HCBS Waiver support services and Medicaid funded long-term care. Effectively, anyone with an intellectual or developmental disability who receives Medicaid would almost certainly receive services that would be subject to this payback requirement. Confusingly, many states have begun ignoring CMS requirements and are not enforcing the payback under any circumstances. Whether the federal government will continue to ignore this practice is to be determined.

Common Planning Mistakes of Special Needs Families

Special Needs Planning is very complicated if it is done well. There are many pitfalls and "traps for the unwary" when planning is not done with an expert in the field. In this section, we will begin to explore some of the places where special needs planning may unravel due to a lack of expertise guiding the family.

Poorly Drafted Special Needs Trusts

One of the most common mistakes families of individuals with disabilities will make is to find a local attorney in general practice or even a good estate planning attorney and assume they can draft a SNT containing all the provisions they would ever want or need. After all, they are an attorney or even an estate planning attorney, so they must be experts when it comes to SNTs, too. However, this is not correct. Take this simple analogy: an individual learns they need to have open-heart surgery. Their primary care physician went to medical school and did a surgery rotation just like every other doctor. That said, they would not be the appropriate doctor to operate on this patient in need of open-heart surgery. Next, the individual might seek out a surgeon to perform the operation. While the general surgeon did their residency in surgery and probably has a much better idea of how to perform surgery in general, including surgery on a heart, they still are not likely to be the best choice to perform open-heart surgery. Finally, the individual finds a heart surgeon. This doctor went to medical school just like the other two doctors. However, this doctor is differentiated not only from the primary care doctor but also from the general surgeon since following their surgery residency, they went on to a fellowship specifically in heart surgery. Just as most people would not want a primary care doctor or even a general surgeon performing open-heart surgery, so, too, they likely would not want a general practice attorney or even simply an estate planning attorney to draft their SNT, nor the rest of their estate plan that is often filled with special needs planning considerations for the family member with disabilities.

Places to find specialists:

- Special Needs Alliance: (non-profit organization of vetted attorneys who are highly specialized in the area) specialneedsalliance.org
- Academy of Special Needs Planners (for-profit company that attorneys can pay to become a member, provides education to members to become more knowledgeable) specialneedsanswers.com

There are many common mistakes that even very experienced general estate planning attorneys make when it comes to special needs planning. First, they fail to tell their client that they must submit the trust (particularly if it is funded) to SSI and/or Medicaid when they apply for benefits or within 10 days of the trust being funded if they are already on SSI and/or Medicaid. Second, for the reasons discussed above, the SNT should almost always be drafted as an inter-vivos free-standing trust rather than a testamentary trust inside of the parents' wills or revocable living trusts. Very often, an attorney that does not draft SNTs regularly will instead draft it as a testamentary trust. Third, to ensure the trust is likely to be grandfathered if laws or rules change, it is always safest to cite every law, rule, POM, and Medicaid Regulation the SNT relied on when it was established.

Fourth, SNTs will often have boilerplate language that says the trust cannot be used to pay for food, shelter, or sometimes even clothing. There is no longer any reason for an SNT to prohibit the purchase of clothing, so this language is just incorrect. Further, the restriction on the distribution of food or shelter is overly restrictive. For one thing, the rule that the provision is trying to follow (if the SNT pays for food or shelter, then the SSI benefit can be reduced by up to a maximum of one-third of the total benefit) does not impact many individuals with SNTs who are no longer on, or never even were on SSI but rather are on SSDI and/or receive CDB on a parent's work record.

For another, the reduction might be worth it if it is in the best interest of the beneficiary to take a broader view of things. There have been several statements made by officials recently suggesting they will be looking to eliminate the food restriction in the next couple of years and even possibly the housing restriction in the next five years or so.

Fifth, SNTs are often drafted, permitting the trustee to distribute money directly to the beneficiary. This language is problematic for two reasons. The first reason is if the trustee makes such a distribution, the beneficiary could see a reduction or even an elimination of their government benefits. Furthermore, even if the trustee knows not to make such a distribution, the mere fact that there is language in the document permitting it can give a reason for some Social Security offices to require monthly statements and regular "audits" to ensure that the trustee is not actually making distributions directly to the beneficiary. The proper language allows for any and all distributions for the benefit of the beneficiary but never directly to them.

Sixth, SNTs should always provide for "next generation" trustees and/or corporate trustees to ensure that the beneficiary does not outlive the people named in the SNT as trustee and successor trustee.

Seventh, flexibility to make charitable and other gifts can be very important, sometimes, the largest distributions a SNT might make each year. This language is very often missing from SNTs that are not developed by qualified attorneys.

Eighth, some states allow public pensions the parent receives during their retirement to be paid to a SNT after the retiree has died, so long as certain provisions are written into the trust. Furthermore, the U.S. Military survivor benefit pension also permits lifetime benefits to be paid to a d4A Trust in many cases when a retired member of the military is deceased. The ability for a monthly pension annuity to be paid to a SNT for the lifetime of a disabled beneficiary can mean a guaranteed income stream worth millions of dollars. Failure of the attorney to know the rules about these pensions as they relate to adult children with disabilities, as well as the special rules regarding paying them to SNTs, could result in a major loss of lifetime financial support for an individual with disabilities.

Ninth, while many SNTs will permit the trust to be modified if laws or rules change and they are not grandfathered under existing laws and rules, they often fail to provide for the possibility that the beneficiary may move to another state with different Medicaid regulations and even state laws regarding SNTs. The SNT should be drafted to allow the acting trustee to modify the trust as necessary, given any laws or rules that are different in the beneficiary's new state of residence.

Lack of Coordination of Other Estate Planning Documents

Special needs planning is not just about the SNT. For example, in many states, the will is where a parent can nominate guardians for an adult child who was found disabled. However, the language of the guardianship nomination must specifically mention the possibility of guardianship for an adult disabled child for the nomination to be effective. In addition, the parents' revocable living trusts often have boiler language in them that can accidentally interfere with government benefits for their child with disabilities, including language about what happens when the parent is incapacitated but still living, as well as many contingent provisions. Further, if there were irrevocable life insurance trusts drafted for the parents to keep the death benefits of life insurance policies out of the estate for estate tax purposes, they very often will have language that can immediately cause the individual with disabilities to lose their benefits or never qualify in the first place. Finally, the parent's powers of attorney also need additional language added to traditional statutory powers of attorney for property due to special needs planning considerations.

Failure to Change Beneficiaries

Yet another common mistake is for parents or grandparents to fail to change beneficiary designations on assets such as life insurance policies and retirement accounts. Failure to do so can partly undo even the most well-drafted special needs estate plan since the beneficiary designation bypasses any other estate planning that was done. Therefore, it is crucial that parents review every single asset to ensure the beneficiary designation is updated following the execution of a special needs estate plan.

Failure to Educate the Extended Family

Another common mistake was briefly mentioned in the introduction to this chapter. Grandparents—or, sometimes, an aunt or uncle—will choose to name their grandchild or niece or nephew with disabilities respectively as a beneficiary of their estate. Sometimes this is done via a direct beneficiary designation of a percentage of their retirement account or life insurance policy. Other times it is written into their will or revocable living trust. It is not uncommon that the grandchild or niece or nephew is named as a contingent beneficiary (if certain people are not alive, the will or trust may state the assets, or a portion of them will then be distributed to the child with disabilities). No matter how it happens, this failure can result in the immediate loss of crucial government benefits. The after-the-fact solutions to these "accidental inheritances" are often very expensive and may result in court and Medicaid involvement in approving all expenditures from the inheritance as well as a requirement that the assets left after the death of the beneficiary be used to pay back the state for Medicaid services provided during the beneficiary's lifetime.

Special Needs Divorce

When parents of a child with significant disabilities divorce, they may not realize that it is far more complicated than it is for parents of children without significant disabilities. The most common issue and concern is child support. Court-ordered child support for a child who is on means-tested government benefits such as SSI and Medicaid can reduce or, in many cases, eliminate eligibility for those programs. Most states allow child support to continue even after the age of majority so long as the child has significant disabilities. However, child support is considered a resource even if paid to the parent with whom the child is residing and will reduce the SSI payment dollar for dollar until it reaches zero and cause a "spend-down" for Medicaid before the program pays for anything. To avoid this disastrous outcome, child support payments can be court-ordered to a d4A Trust. If this is done, the child support of any value (whether it is $600 per month or $6,000 per month) will be used via the d4A Trust by the trustee for the benefit of the child without any impact on SSI or Medicaid. As of December 2021, per a senior representative from the office at the Fifth Annual Special Needs Law Institute (www.iicle.com/sni21), the Chicago region for SSA has apparently begun permitting adult child support payments to be made to an ABLE Account (so long as the monthly child support does not add up to more than the current limit of $17,000 per year) without any impact on SSI eligibility. Remember that no other SSA region is bound by a position taken by the Chicago region.

Another issue in the divorce context is life insurance to secure child support. Normally, This is not a very contentious issue as it usually requires a term life insurance policy to be in force until maybe the youngest child has finished their undergraduate degree. However, when the life insurance is securing a permanent child support order due to a child's permanent disability, then this requirement becomes much more important and costly. It requires permanent life insurance, which often costs many times more than term life insurance. If the parents are older, life insurance companies will usually set the premiums even higher. Moreover, since SSI and Medicaid do not consider life insurance, even when court ordered, to be child support, the beneficiary of the death benefit need not be the d4A Trust but rather can be a Third-Party SNT. This can be especially important if the parent with the permanent life insurance policy lives into their late 80s or 90s and, on their passing, their child with disabilities is unlikely to live more than another 10 to 15 years. If a $1,000,000 policy was paid out to a d4A Trust in that scenario, the payback to the state could loom very large, whereas if a Third-Party SNT is properly named, as is permitted, there is no concern about a payback to the state upon the child's death to wherever the trust document states it should be distributed.

Guardianship

Guardianship is very state specific. First, even the terminology can be different between states. Some states refer to all guardianships as conservatorships. Other states refer to conservatorships only in the context of a property estate in the name of the individual with disabilities and use guardianship to refer to the individual appointed to make personal decisions for the person with disabilities, such as healthcare decisions and coordinating and deciding on housing as well as services and supports provided by the government. In yet other states, the term guardianship refers to both types of arrangements but is differentiated by "guardian of the person" or "guardian of the estate," respectively. Some states have created guardianships that are tailored for individuals with intellectual and/or developmental disabilities. Most states have the same process, procedures, rules, and requirements for an 85-year-old with dementia as they do for an 18-year-old with severe autism. Whether to do a "partial" or "limited" guardianship and what that type of guardianship covers or does not cover, can again be state specific. Finally, state-specific powers of attorney may be an alternative option to a guardianship process if very specific language is added to cover the special circumstances of the Individual with disabilities. Some states are now aggressively promoting "support decision-making" forms that allow parents or other advocates to make decisions with an individual who is more independent and, therefore, can participate more in their own decisions.

Special Needs Planning Attorney's Role in the Litigation Context

Special needs planning attorneys should be brought into a personal injury or medical malpractice case for an individual who needs lifetime supports and care as soon as possible. They can help advise on many aspects of the case. They can consult on including the parents as a party to the lawsuit if possible to ensure the allocation of the amount of any potential verdict or settlement that will be subject to Medicaid reimbursement on the individual's passing is minimized. In addition, a special needs planning attorney should help protect government benefits now and in the future following a successful conclusion to the case. Moreover, they can often provide input on structured settlements given the nature of the disability, the supports they are likely to need, and the benefits that they are likely to be eligible for.

Conclusion

Families of children with special needs often struggle to keep up with the day-to-day challenge of meeting their child's current needs. The thought of planning for them as an adult after aging out of special education, or especially after the parents have both died, is often delayed continually for this reason. However, it is important that parents (and other relatives) begin planning as soon as possible. Not only because no one knows the future but also because grandparents may be doing planning while their grandchild is young that could make a big mess of government benefits after that grandparent's death. Further, there are look-back periods to worry about, as well as benefits and services (including waiver services) available to children that do not consider their parents' assets and income. All too often, a grandparent will need skilled nursing care, spend their life savings of hundreds of thousands of dollars on that care, and end up on Medicaid anyway when, had they stated the special needs planning process, they would have known of a relatively simple way to protect their life savings rather than have it all be spent down in a matter of months without any benefit to them or the rest of their family.

For all of these reasons, it is both never too early and, at the same time, never too late to begin special needs planning with the guidance of an attorney that is very experienced in special needs planning to properly draft their estate planning documents and guide them through the maze of government benefit programs and services that will be crucial for their loved one to live a full life in their community. The process is long and can be very expensive, but it is crucial to begin as soon as possible to ensure that opportunities that can be life-changing for the future of a child with special needs are not missed.

ABLE National Resource Center www.ablenrc.org/

Case for Inclusion www.caseforinclusion.org/

Equip for Equality www.equipforequality.org/

Rubin Law, A Professional Corporation www.rubinlaw.com

Social Security Administration, www.ssa.gov

Special Needs Alliance www.specialneedsalliance.org/ (National Nonprofit Organization of attorneys specializing in SNTs (membership is by invitation only)

State Health Facts, www.statehealthfacts.org

The Arc of Illinois www.thearcofil.org/

The Arc of U.S. https://thearc.org/about-us/

The Center for Medicare and Medicaid Services, www.cms.gov

U.S. Medicare, www.medicare.gov

References

ABLE National Resource Center. (2022). *History of the ABLE Act*. www.ablenrc.org/what-is-able/history-of-the-able-act/

American Association on Intellectual and Developmental Disabilities. (2017). *State of the States in intellectual and developmental disabilities* (11th ed.). www.aaidd.org/publications/bookstore-home/product-listing/state-of-the-states-in-intellectual-and-developmental-disabilities-11th-ed

Farina, M. P., Zajacova, A., Montez, J. K., & Hayward, M. D. (2021). U.S. state disparities in life expectancy, disability-free life expectancy, and disabled life expectancy among adults aged 25 to 89 years. *American Journal of Public Health*, *111*(4), 708–717. doi: 10.2105/AJPH.2020.306064

Internal Revenue Service. (2021). *ABLE accounts – tax benefit for people with disabilities*. www.irs.gov/government-entities/federal-state-local-governments/able-accounts-tax-benefit-for-people-with-disabilities#:~:text=The%20Achieving%20a%20Better%20Life,pay%20for%20qualified%20disability%20expenses.

Medicaid.gov, Centers for Medicare & Medicaid Services. (2022). *Home and community based services authorities.* www.medicaid.gov/medicaid/home-community-based-services/home-community-based-services-authorities/index.html#:~:text=Home%20and%20Community%20Based%20Services,formal%20Medicaid%20State%20plan%20option

Social Security Administration. (2021). Mental residual functional capacity assessment. *Program Operations Manual System.* https://secure.ssa.gov/poms.nsf/lnx/0424510060

Social Security Administration. (2022a). Residual functional capacity. *Program Operations Manual System.* https://secure.ssa.gov/poms.nsf/lnx/0424510000

Social Security Administration. (2022b). Supplemental Security Income (SSI) benefits. www.ssa.gov/ssi/text-benefits-ussi.htm#:~:text=Generally%2C%20the%20maximum%20Federal%20SSI,and%20%241%2C261%20for%20a%20couple.

Chapter 33

Assistive Technology, Durable Medical Equipment, and Transportation in Life Care Planning

Irmo Marini and Laura Villarreal

Medical and technological advances over the last several decades have created a vastly growing industry for items and services that, as a result, extend people's lives and improve the quality of life for individuals with severe disabilities. Computerized and robotic technology, for example, has allowed persons with low-level paraplegia to ambulate using an exoskeleton, and those who are deaf to have a cochlear implant to hear for the first time. In the interdisciplinary subspecialty of life care planning, experts need to be aware of what assistive technology (AT), durable medical equipment (DME), and vehicle modifications (VM) are available, what the cost of the items are, and the lifespan of these technologies to determine which evaluees may benefit and function more independently from these state-of-the-art aids. Before making such determinations, however, life care planners must know what technologies are available that will enhance the functional independence of individuals for whom a life care plan is being developed. The life care planner, however, must also understand many other nuances regarding the geographical regions or climate conditions (e.g., extreme cold or extreme heat) these technologies will be used in, the age and activity level of the evaluee, the severity of their disability, their other premorbid conditions such as obesity, consent or approval from the user, and the wear and tear of aids and equipment, all of which influence the equipment's maintenance and/or replacement schedules (Amsterdam, 2018; Marini et al., 2019; Rutherford-Owen & Marini, 2012). Each of these factors is addressed in this chapter, along with empirically based evidence of previously published peer studies regarding a number of these technologies. Note, however, that the wide range of AT for persons with visual impairments is extensive and beyond the scope of this chapter; therefore, the reader is directed to Chapter 28, which is devoted to visual assistive technology.

Literature Review

The peer-reviewed published literature regarding available technologies has always lagged behind the technology and marketing growth itself. Disability Expo's advertising and marketing of state-of-the-art technologies take place in different cities across the United States throughout the year. Life care planners who regularly attend these exhibitions come away with an appreciation of the technology, demonstrations of it, and the cost and contact information for its purchase. Other than these expos, medical care providers such as physical, occupational, and speech-language therapists, rehabilitation counselors, and a wide range of physician and rehabilitation nursing subspecialties have many of these technology sales representatives bring the equipment to their hospitals and clinics to demonstrate, in the hopes of drawing their business.

Technology Service Provision

The other—perhaps, most important—consultant role in this process is that of the rehabilitation technology suppliers (RTS), who specialize in medical equipment evaluations of the injured party and distribution of appropriate equipment (Amsterdam, 2018). The RTS who are most recognized are those who complete the curriculum through the Rehabilitation Engineering and Assistive Technology Society of North America (RESNA). By successfully passing the certification, the RTS earns the assistive technology supplier (ATS) title. Separately, a practitioner therapists can also become credentialed as an assistive technology practitioner (ATP) if they are a good member in standing and pass the curriculum developed by the National Registry of Rehabilitation Technology Suppliers (2003). Practitioners can then be credentialed as certified rehabilitation technology suppliers. Ideally, the ATP will evaluate and then work in tandem with the ATS to determine the appropriate equipment for the evaluee with their involvement and consent (Amsterdam, 2018; Marini et al., 2019; Scherer, 2016).

Durable Medical Equipment: Considerations

Scherer (2016) emphasizes matching the person with the technology and stresses the importance of involving the evaluee (if cognitively aware or old enough) in making equipment decisions. Specifically, Scherer describes how individuals who do not have a say in choosing equipment can often not use it or abandon it due to its bulkiness, color, weight, fatigue from using the equipment, inappropriate fit, and complexity or level of difficulty in using the equipment (see her assessment matching website www.cjsi.net). She cautions against the medical model approach and advocates for the social model of inclusion approach for such decisions. For example, some individuals with an upper or lower extremity amputation who are not consulted with prior to ordering a prosthesis may likely abandon its use if it is too heavy/bulky or ugly to use. As such, the importance of consumer input in decision-making is critical. In practice for life care planners, when equipment or aids have already been ordered and used, it is appropriate to ask the evaluee during the interview if they like the equipment, and if not, to have them evaluated by an ATS, ATP, or both, for the equipment they prefer and obtain relevant pricing.

Prior to a discussion about each of the numerous aids and technologies available for the evaluee's individualized needs, we describe other non-equipment and technology considerations that must be made, who is qualified to make such decisions within each of our own standards of practice, or when we need to consult with qualified individuals who can affirm such decisions.

Evaluee Age

In the 2011 text, *Pediatric Life Care Planning and Case Management*, Riddick-Grisham emphasizes the nuanced differences in developing life care plans for children as opposed to adults. Specifically, she addresses the growth spurts of children that must be considered and accommodated when considering mobility DME, such as the step-up approach from stroller, gait trainer, pediatric wheelchairs, to adult wheelchairs, and the overall recognition that due to these growth spurts and/or typically higher activity level of children, DME are often replaced sooner than those for adults (Amsterdam, 2018; Marini & Harper, 2006; Marini et al., 2019). This schedule can be seen in Table 33.1. Amsterdam (2018) notes that when ordering the child's wheelchair equipment, a qualified ATS or RTS will order adjustable frame pediatric wheelchairs that can be expanded with the child's growth to a certain degree. Children and teenagers with mobility impairments may also be more active and interested in sports or recreational activities that may include basketball, rugby, tennis, and recreational (beach) wheelchairs. Websites such as www.sportaid.com and www.spinlife.com offer a wide variety of these activity chairs. These high-activity specialty chairs also incur a higher rate of wear and tear, thus often needing greater maintenance and sooner replacement (Marini et al. 2019).

Amsterdam (2018) cites the increase in school athletic programs that are now inclusive of children who are wheelchair-dependent, as well as other disabilities. The integration and ongoing mainstreaming of once segregated students with disabilities into the classroom began with the initial authorization of the Education for All Handicapped Children Act (1975) and was reauthorized and supplemented several times including a name change to the Individuals with Disabilities Education Act reauthorized by Congress (2004). As such, mainstreamed students with disabilities now have greater opportunities to develop friendships with their nondisabled peers. Psychosocially and because of inclusion, far more able-bodied children have grown up with and befriended classmates with disabilities, and those friendships extend into community outings and a greater sense of normalcy and life satisfaction for those with disabilities (Marini, 2018). For many years, the Special Olympics have also included persons with various disabilities as well who compete with or without adaptive aids. In addition, there has also been an increase nationwide in playground equipment designed to hold a wheelchair, such as carousels and swings (B. Preston, personal communication, April 21, 2022).

Amsterdam (2018) specifically elaborated on those who use a wheelchair and the nuances of eventual lesser activity as one ages. Specifically, he noted ages 30 through 65 will typically see a lower activity level due to family and/or work responsibilities, spending more time indoors and mostly stationary positions, as opposed to their younger counterparts. He also opined that the 65+ age group are equally stationary and may need to progress from a manual, self-propelled, and lightweight wheelchair to a wheelchair with handles for a caregiver to push and/or alternatively a scooter or power wheelchair with a joystick.

Geographic Location and Climate

The geographical area (urban versus rural) and seasonal climatic weather conditions (extreme cold versus extreme heat) must also be considered by the life care planner in determining AT, DME, and VM decisions in terms of maintenance, wear and tear, and replacement schedules (Amsterdam, 2018; Marini & Harper, 2006; Marini et al., 2019). Marini and Harper (2006) noted how AT professionals in the northern United States often cite extreme cold with long, snow-covered winters, and snow removal measures in using sand or salt on the roads as having a deleterious erosion impact on wheelchairs, wheelchair lifts and ramps, outdoor wheelchair elevators, wheelchair bearings, and power chair computerized electronics, etc. Conversely, living in tropical conditions by oceans and beaches can equally lay waste to AT electronics, wheelchair bearings and wheels, van hydraulic lifts, and automatic fold-out ramps due to beach sand and ocean air salt corrosion on metals.

Overall, the life expectancy of these types of equipment can vary considerably if used for indoor only versus outdoor use. In short, individuals requiring AT, DME, and VM will often experience more frequent maintenance as well as earlier replacement schedules than those individuals living in more moderate climate conditions, such as in the Midwest United States, if they use their equipment outdoors as much as indoors.

Aside from weather conditions and climate, Amsterdam (2010, 2018) cites the differences in rural versus urban community living. Many sparsely populated towns can have many dirt roads, unlevel surfaces, and few, if any, local DME vendors to maintain equipment. Unmaintained dirt roads and rising waters after storms can wreak havoc on manual and power wheelchairs, once again affecting the wheel bearings, tires, and power chair electronics. Without local DME vendors to provide repairs, and because of the long travel distances to vendors in urban areas, technology users may go without repair, making them more dependent on others in the interim.

Severity of Disability and Premorbid Conditions

Severity of disability and related premorbid conditions must also be considered when deciding on AT, DME, and its maintenance, wear and tear, and replacement schedules and costs. The United States, for example, has the second-highest rate of obesity (trailing Mexico) across the globe (Romero & Marini, 2018). Amsterdam (2018) discussed the negative impact of obesity and morbid obesity regarding the accelerated wear and tear of DME, most specifically wheelchairs. He indicated that most wheelchairs come with a 250 pounds maximum weight load, noting that there are also custom bariatric wheelchair frames capable of supporting 600 and up to approximately 1,000 pounds.

Relatedly, a regular manual Hoyer lift has a maximum capacity of 400 pounds. However, Hoyer does make a bariatric lift that can carry weights anywhere from 700–1,000 pounds. These specialized lifts can cost anywhere from $1,500 to approximately $10,000 more than a regular manual lift. Similarly purposed, there are patient transfer power track ceiling lifts. The regular lifts handle approximately 440 pounds at an approximate cost of $2,750 (Medmart.com, 2002–2021). The bariatric lifts typically cost more depending on the company. These bariatric ceiling hoists must have a fortified ceiling installation, heavy-duty motor, and thick cable wiring compared to sturdy nylon fabric for the regular-weight ceiling lift.

Van hydraulic lifts like Braun have a maximum load lift of 600 pounds and typically cost upwards of about $6,500 (M. Mercado, personal communication, April 27, 2022). The life care planner, in consultation with the ATS, must not only consider the evaluee weight but also include the weight of the wheelchair as well. Wheelchair vans with a ramp are typically sturdy enough to handle higher weight capacity.

In addition to the individual's weight, consideration should be given to the evaluee's age and disability severity. Children are often rougher with their wheelchairs, regardless of whether they self-propel manually or use a power chair with a joystick. Amsterdam (2018) anecdotally noted his experience as a physical therapist where children will run into walls cutting corners that may stress the wheelchair frame. When considering disability severity, children and adults with spastic cerebral palsy who use a power chair with a joystick can also accidentally run into barriers, not due to carelessness but rather because of their spasticity. Amsterdam also discusses his experience with institutionalized hyperactive patients whom he periodically observed slamming their bodies and/or other wheelchairs into the walls. He noted that some patients with cognitive disabilities were in power wheelchairs (with a joystick) that should not really have been placed in one. In other instances, some patients would beat or try to destroy their wheelchairs with extreme behaviors.

One final consideration regarding disability severity and considering maintenance or replacement of equipment is warranted. We have discussed evaluees with severe physical disabilities that require them to always use a wheelchair for ambulation, but on the other hand, are individuals who are not totally dependent on ambulating with a wheelchair. Individuals with hemiparesis, central cord syndrome, those partially paralyzed by a stroke, and those with lower extremity amputation may only use a wheelchair outdoors or for long distances. Such individuals will typically ambulate at times, usually within their homes, using crutches or a walker, from our experience. As such, although the standard wheelchair replacement for those who ambulate solely by wheelchair is typically approximately five years before replacement, for individuals who can ambulate, their need to replace a wheelchair (except for children still growing) may be once every 7–10 years depending on their individualized use. The life care planner will need to make those determinations as well.

Equipment in the Home

Having addressed many of the issues regarding durable medical equipment, we now turn to assistive technology that can increase independence in the home. Note again that AT for persons with visual impairments is extensively covered in Chapter 28. Similarly, it is beyond the scope of this chapter to fully discuss home modifications and renovations, but it will briefly be addressed, with a greater focus on AT and other DME that is used in the home.

As an overview, there continues to be a rapidly growing market of AT devices being developed and sold to the general population, for individuals both with and without disabilities. For persons with various disabilities, AT can, and does, make them more functionally independent within the home. For those without disabilities, the technology minimizes their level of physical exertion. For example, the Roomba is a robotic vacuum that retails for approximately $180–$250. Various versions of Alexa and Google are also now in millions of homes and activate by voice to control electronics such as the television, lights, thermostat, intercom, automatic doors, and kitchen appliances. There is also a smart refrigerator that inventories and alerts the owner of what produce, beverages, etc., need to be replenished. More expensive technology that has been around for 15–20 years or so include Environmental Control Units that can be low- or high-tech and cost less than $100 to over $10,000. What becomes critically important for evaluees who depend on electricity to live safely, more functionally independent, and more convenient is that the life care planner includes a backup home generator in the event of power outages. A power outage can be life-threatening for individuals using a ventilator but is also important for non-life-threatening situations where someone with tetraplegia, for example, uses a rotating airflow mattress requiring constant electricity.

An evaluee with staircases inside (or outside) the home may benefit from a powered stair lift where a power seat is installed with track rails generally found inside two-story homes or wheelchair-accessible elevators installed near the staircase. We have observed these types of wheelchair elevators outdoors and indoors range from several feet to as high as 30+ feet. The costs of such lifts depend on the height needed, the platform configurations (straight stairwell versus spiral stairwell), and architectural safety code requirements. Depending on these factors, the elevator lift can cost anywhere from $8,000–$30,000 or more (Accessibilitypro.com, 2022).

For individuals who are deaf or hard of hearing, there are hundreds of ATs available for this population, many of which can be found on www.maxiaids.com. Of these items, there are visual safety alerts, amplifying devices, time clocks, strobe fire alarms, door knock sensors, voice-to-print phones, etc. There are also baby-signallers, motion sensors for doors and windows, vibrating alarm clocks and beds, weather alerts, paging devices, kitchen appliance alerts, and signals, etc. Most of these items on this website sell anywhere from several dollars to several thousand dollars, depending on individual needs.

The following web resources may be useful with this chapter:

Accessibilitypro.com
www.maxiaids.com
Medmart.com
Spinlife.com
Unitedaccess.com
Mobilityworks.com
Braunability.com
www.rollxvans.com
www.unitedaccess.com

Other miscellaneous AT or DME that can be ordered for the home includes electronically controlled upper cabinets on track rails and operated by a light switch, the same for a mirror or medicine cabinet in the bathroom, and voice or hand-activated sink faucets and soap dispensers. The closet or walk-in closet can also be operated by a light switch which will lower the clothing racks out and down to wheelchair level. These adaptations traditionally run from several hundred dollars to approximately $3,000, including installation.

Home Modification or Architectural Renovation

This topic could be a chapter unto itself; however, we will provide basic home modification and architectural renovation pointers that often require consideration in cases where the evaluee is partially or permanently in a wheelchair. Otherwise, the majority of visual or hearing home adaptations are typically in the form of AT and not physical alterations to the home as they are with wheelchair considerations. These are beginning points for the life care planner, but a true home renovation assessment should include consultation services from a contractor who specializes in building or renovating wheelchair-accessible homes.

For starters, all doorway widths should be a minimum of 36 inches wide or custom-made for bariatric wheelchair users. Second, floor surfaces should be wood, tile, linoleum, or some other hard surface, to avoid flooring wear and tear from wheelchair tires and minimize the energy required to navigate a wheelchair over restrictive surfaces. Third, the master bathroom or primary bathroom for the evaluee should ideally be 14' x 14' for a complete 360-degree wheelchair turnaround with space so that the wheelchair does not run into cabinets, the commode, or the shower. Ideally, there would be a roll-in shower large enough to hold what is normally a PVC shower and a commode wheelchair. Alternatively, for low-level paraplegics, the ability to pull one's wheelchair close enough to the bathtub or shower bench chair and safely transfer over to it. Fourth, hallway widths ideally should be 48 inches to allow most regular wheelchairs to turn around, as narrower hallways will require the user to either back up and turn around in an open area or go into a room down the hall to turn around and come back. Fifth, the bathroom and kitchen sinks should be open without cabinetry underneath them so the wheeler can maneuver the wheelchair under the sink. A well-designed, fully wheelchair-accessible home will also have a kitchen with wheel-under stove tops, kitchen counters, and ovens.

Additional home or architectural renovations should include the creation of level entry and exits between interior rooms of the house, as well as to the front and back door exits free from steps or doorframes as obstructions. Ideally, there will be an attached garage so the wheelchair user can get to their vehicle without having to deal with inclement weather. The garage width for wheelchair-accessible vans with the folding ramp or hydraulic lift needs to be wide enough to consider an additional 6 feet—3 feet for the ramp to extend out, and minimum 3 feet for the wheelchair to enter the vehicle via the ramp or hydraulic lift.

All light switches should be lower than usual, approximately 48 inches from the floor, for wheelchair-height access. All door handles, particularly for individuals with tetraplegia who have limited hand or finger movement, should be levers. Similarly, sink faucets should be a lever and not a round grip. For those with the highest level of tetraplegia C2–C3 who have paralysis from the neck down, automatic voice-activated door openers should be considered for maximum independence. As noted earlier, it is critically important for physically dependent individuals to have a backup generator in case of power outages for safety reasons.

Finally, it is important to note cost considerations for home modifications, which can be as low as several hundred dollars for very minor modifications, to the tens of thousands of dollars for major renovations. In some cases, individuals in existing homes or trailers may not have the capacity to be renovated, or those in rental properties may not have permission to renovate or change the structure. In those cases, renovating an existing bigger home or building one's own home should be considered with all modifications built-in in the latter instance. The U.S. Department of Veterans Affairs allots a maximum renovation for the veteran who is wheelchair dependent—approximately $101,754 for the 2022 fiscal year—to make the home accessible. Otherwise, a qualified ADA-approved home renovation contractor, when available, should be directly consulted for specific pricing and renovations needed in one's local region.

Vehicle Modification

In the not-too-distant future, self-driving vehicles will likely be set up for persons with disabilities who cannot drive, giving them greater functional independence in the community. In the interim, vehicle modifications for individuals with limited lower and/or upper extremity functional abilities afford individuals the technology needed to drive independently. A steering wheel spinner knob for someone with limited hand grip can cost as little as $15, and for someone with a C4–C5 tetraplegia to drive, modifications alone may top $60,000 or more for an elaborate computerized and voice recognition driving unit.

Allison (2018) notes a relative history of vehicle modifications starting with the Ford Econoline E-Series van in the 1980s, where the vehicle frame flooring was lowered 6 to 8 inches so the wheelchair could enter. The fuel tanks had to be moved as well. The first author, who has a C5–C6 tetraplegia with limited hand mobility, owned a 1985 Ford where all dashboard electronics were placed on the driver's door with pushbuttons. One panel was just to change gears, the other panel was for all the other electronics (e.g., air conditioning, lights, cruise control, windshield wipers). There were also two backup pumps behind the back seat if the van suddenly stalled while driving. The first allowed the driver 30 seconds of vacuum low-effort power steering to guide the vehicle off the road, while the second vacuum pump allowed the driver to safely break the zero-effort hand lever brake. These two safety backup pumps alone were over $3,000 each in 1985. Although Ford was the only initial dealer, today, several other companies, including Toyota, Honda, GM, and Chrysler all sell adaptable vehicles.

Allison (2018) also discussed the federal government safety requirements regarding fuel tank placement, crash testing, approved tie-down systems for a wheelchair, and qualifications for certified vendors to make vehicle modifications. Specifically, the U.S. Federal Motor Vehicle Safety Standards worked with the National Mobility Equipment Dealers Association (NMEDA, 2016) to ensure quality assurance to meet crash test standards for modified vehicles. Vendors adapt and sell modified vehicles that must be approved by NMEDA as certified and trained in meeting compliance standards. The life care planner would need to contact such vendors regarding vehicle modifications and costs for the life care plan, typically after an individualized evaluation of the evaluee by an occupational therapist and qualified vendor, and hopefully including the evaluee if possible.

Allison (2018, p. 801) also provided van modification resources (found under the references of this chapter) as well as key terms the life care planner should be aware of, including:

structural modifier—companies that adjust vehicle frames and alterations like Braun, Eldorado, and VMI

mobility equipment dealers—are qualified NMEDA dealers who install, sell, and service modified vehicles

driver rehabilitation specialist—an occupational therapist trained to evaluate, educate, and perform clinical or on the road evaluations

certified driver rehab specialist—a qualified individual to provide driver rehabilitation and training certified by the Association for Driver Rehabilitation Specialists.

Depending upon disability severity as well as evaluee preference, unless you do not have access to interview the evaluee, typical vehicle modifications for individuals remaining in their wheelchairs will include side entry and rear entry. The vehicle can be set up for the driver's seat to be removed to drive directly from a wheelchair. The passenger seat can be removed in the front as a passenger or behind both seats locked down in the middle. These options are for full-size and minivans (see www.rollxvans.com, www.unitedaccess.com, and www.mobilityworks.com). While vehicle purchases should not be included in the life care plan, modification for accessibility should. Such modifications vary considerably depending on disability severity and complexity of evaluee needs, as noted earlier.

There are also half-ton trucks primarily for persons with paraplegia or similar functional impairments that use the Turny driver seat, which swivels out of the driver's door and lowers to wheelchair level. The evaluee can then transfer onto the seat and electronically ascend to driving level and swerve in. The wheelchair can then be picked up by a hoist in the bed of the truck that can hold up to 350 pounds, lift it and stow the wheelchair electronically (www.braunability.com).

Allison (2018) notes that complex modifications require between 20 to 40 hours of driver training following a comprehensive occupational therapy driver evaluation by a driver rehabilitation specialist. Customization is individualized by government-approved NMEDA vendors and may take several fittings and driving trials to adjust the proper modified driving aids for persons with tetraplegia. Individuals with paraplegia may simply need a set of portable hand controls installed. The cost of this can be as little as $1,500–$18,00, with approximately one hour of installation. The Darios steering wheel is the latest state-of-the-art steering wheel with a built-in brake and accelerator priced at approximately $12,000 (www.mobilitymgmt.com). On the same website, crash test-approved wheelchair tie-downs, like the QLK-150, can safely brace a wheelchair user inside the van.

Empirical Evidence-Based Studies Related to AT, DME, and VM

There have been relatively few empirically based evidence studies relating to the maintenance and replacement values when considering AT, DME, and VM in the literature. Up until the early 1990s, expert witnesses from across disciplines could proffer unsupported and often speculated opinions solely based on their education, training, and experience. This ended with the 1993 *Daubert v. Merrill Dow Pharmaceuticals, Inc.* decision, at which point experts could be challenged and subsequently disqualified from proffering their opinions if they were unable to substantiate their opinions based on commonly accepted methodology which was scientifically valid and subjected to peer review and publication (Field, 2000; Isom & Marini, 2002).

Amsterdam (2003) cited the lack of available literature regarding replacement values of AT and DME to support the life care planner in proffering such decisions. Prior to this, life care planners had primarily relied upon their own research when speaking with ATS and RTS in obtaining costs, warranties, and relative replacement values of evaluee-specific equipment and technology needs. However, this information was limited by the number of vendors the life care planner would or could contact (Amsterdam, 2003; Deutsch & Sawyer, 2001).

Amsterdam (2003) solicited the opinions of 28 life care planners he surveyed and only received responses from 20% of them. Therefore, his findings were limited by the relatively small number of respondents, as well as the fact that these life care planners did not have the equipment expertise, like ATS or RTS would have. To date, the three most comprehensive empirically based evidence studies regarding empirical validation of AT, DME, and VM were conducted by Marini and Harper (2006), Marini et al. (2019), and Rutherford-Owen and Marini (2012).

In the 2006 study, Marini and Harper solicited the opinions of 101 AT and DME practitioners from across 45 U.S. states. Subjects were accessed through the RESNA website for certified assistive technology practitioners or were equipment suppliers with at least two years' work experience as a supplier. The authors devised a list of commonly recommended DME, which included child and adult manual and power wheelchairs, cushions, Hoyer lifts, gait trainers, environmental control units, commode chairs, hospital beds, airflow bed mattresses, sports chairs, etc. (See tables below). In addition, the researchers also included miscellaneous respiratory equipment such as nebulizers, ventilators, and oxygen concentrators regarding filter changes and replacement estimates. They obtained the median cost and range of costs for equipment/devices, as well as replacement parts as well as maintenance costs. The 2006 study also considered weather conditions on the wear and tear of certain DME when comparing northern versus southern states. The authors found no significant differences in maintenance or replacement values for all except one item, wheelchair tires, where it was found that in southern states, tires lasted approximately 16 months before requiring a change versus 12 months in the northern states.

In a follow-up duplication study expanding on the Marini and Harper (2006) study, Marini et al. (2019) surveyed 127 AT and DME sales and repair experts from across the United States for their opinions regarding maintenance, replacement, and costs of technology and equipment, along with including 11 additional items (three-wheel hand cycle, standing power tilt incline wheelchair, Clinitron gel air fluid bed, indoor wheelchair elevator, modified van replacement, Clinitron gel air bed replacements parts, indoor elevator wheelchair placement parts, folding van platform hydraulic

Table 33.1 Replacement Values

	Median Replacement Rate – 2005 (n)	Median Replacement Rate – 2019 (n)
Manual wheelchair	5 years (98)	5 years (94)
Power Wheelchair: Adult	5 years (99)	5 years (95)
Power Wheelchair: Child	4.5 years (96)	4 years (90)
Power Tilt: New Wheelchair	5 years (89)	5 years (79)
Sports Wheelchair	5 years (38)	4 years (34)
All Terrain Wheelchairs	4 years (45)	5 years (37)
Commode Shower Wheelchairs	4.6 years (87)	5 years (72)
Power Scooters for Adults	5 years (97)	5 years (86)
Power Hoyer: New Lift Replacement	7 years (65)	5 years (54)
Power Hoyer: New Sling Replacement	2 years (68)	2.5 years (46)
Manual Pump Hoyer: Hydraulic Pump Replacement	5 years (69)	3 years (41)
Power Track Ceiling Lifts: Lift Replacement	7 years (36)	9 years (17)
Power Hospital Bed: New Bed Replacement	7 years (78)	10 years (60)
Bed Mattress: ROHO	4 years (60)	3 years (43)
Bed Mattress: Power Air Flow Mattress	4 years (65)	5 years (45)
Cushions: Replacement of High/Low Profile ROHO	3 years (89)	2.5 years (43)
Cushions: Jay 2 Gel	3 years (88)	2.5 years (50)
Cushions: Cloud/Foam	2.5 years (82)	3.5 years (58)
Hydraulic Bathtub: Entire New Tublift Chair	5 years (46)	5 years (22)
Four Wheeled Walkers	4.5 years (90)	5 years (68)
Gait Trainer for Child	3 years (70)	4 years (33)
Gait Trainer for Adult	5 years (68)	5 years (37)

(Continued)

Table 33.1 (Continued) Replacement Values

	Median Replacement Rate – 2005 (n)	Median Replacement Rate – 2019 (n)
Standing Frame Manual Wheelchair	5 years (58)	5 years (50)
Oxygen (O_2) Concentrator	4 years (29)	0.5 years (75)
O_2 Concentrator Filter	4 months (34)	0.5 years (75)
Respiratory Suction Machine	5 years (27)	5 years (75)
Respiratory Suction Machine Filter	3 months (30)	0.5 years (69)
Nebulizer Machine	4.5 years (36)	5 years (105)
Nebulizer Filter	6 months (37)	0.5 years (71)
New Home Ventilator	4 years (19)	5 years (58)
Environmental Control Units: Computer Replacement	4 years (27)	5 years (10)
Environmental Control: Built-in Receiver	4.5 years (14)	3 years (8)
Power Hospital Bed: New Battery	5 years (67)	3.5 years (22)
Bed Mattress: Power Box for Air Flow	4 years (36)	3.5 years (35)
Hydraulic Bathtub: Parts for Tublift Chair	2.5 years (48)	3 years (11)
Four-Wheeled Walker Tires	2.5 years (90)	2 years (40)
Power Wheelchair for Adults: New Batteries	18 months (96)	2.5 years (59)
Power Wheelchair for Adults: New Tires	18 months (96)	2 years (55)
Power Tilt/Recline: New Batteries	13.5 months (84)	2 years (49)
Power Tilt/Recline: New Tires	14 months (82)	2 years (43)
Manual Wheelchairs: New Tires/Spokes	15 months (81)	3 years (37)
All Terrain Wheelchairs: New Batteries	18 months (38)	2 years (32)
Power Scooters: New Batteries	18 months (93)	2 years (47)
Power Scooter Tires	2 years (90)	2 years (46)
Power Hoyer New Battery	2 years (73)	2 years (40)
Power Hoyer Sling*	2 years (68)	
Manual Pump Hoyer: Replacement of Pump	5 years (69)	5 years (36)
Power Track Ceiling Lifts: New Battery	2 years (37)	3 years (16)
Power Scooters for Adults**	N/A	5 years (86)
Three-Wheeled Hand Cycle**	N/A	3 years (29)

(Continued)

Table 33.1 (Continued)   Replacement Values

	Median Replacement Rate – 2005 (n)	Median Replacement Rate – 2019 (n)
Standing Power Tilt and Recline Wheelchair **	N/A	5 years (56)
Clinitron Air Fluid Bed**	N/A	10 years (24)
Respiratory Equipment Ventilator Parts**	N/A	1.5 years (24)
Modified Van Replacement	N/A	7 years (22)
Indoor Wheelchair Elevator**	N/A	10 years (19)
Indoor Wheelchair Elevator Replacement Parts **	N/A	5 years (13)
Van Platform Lift**	N/A	5 years (10)
Van Platform Lift Replacement Parts**	N/A	3 years (10)
Van Folding Ramp**	N/A	5 years (12)
Folding Ramp Replacement Parts	N/A	3 years (12)
Clinitron Bed Replacement Parts**	N/A	3 years (14)
Power Standing Frame New Batteries*	2 years (54)	N/A
Respiratory Equipment: Ventilator Parts Changed*	6 months (15)	N/A
Sports Wheelchairs: Annual Spare Parts*	(40)	N/A
Bed Mattress: Standard*	3 years (82)	N/A
Manual Pump Hoyer: Entire Hoyer Lift*	7.5 years (68)	N/A

* Present in 2005 study.
** Present in 2019 study.

From Marini & Harper (2006), Marini et al. (2019).

lift, folding platform hydraulic lift replacement parts, van folding ramp, and folding ramp replacement parts) to the original 58 items in the 2006 study. Marini again emphasized the importance of scientifically valid empirically based evidence research on the topic as opposed to individual life care planners calling suppliers essentially to a sample size of n =1–3.

In the 2019 replication study, Marini et al. solicited 576 participants and had a 22% response rate or 127 who completed the survey from across the United States. The reader is referred to Table 33.1 for all item responses from both studies.

Overall, results between the 13-year-old studies were remarkably similar in participant responses. The additional 11 items added demonstrated that ceiling track lifts have almost a double life expectancy than Hoyer lifts, and the Clinitron low airflow mattress has approximately the same life expectancy as replacing the bed. The van life median was estimated at seven years, also mirroring the 2006 study, and the hydraulic platform lift versus the fold-out ramp is also approximately five years. The work of Rutherford-Owen and Marini (2012) is discussed in greater detail in the following section.

Follow-Up Studies regarding Purchasing AT, DME, and VM Settlement Awardees

Life care planners are sometimes asked in the course of deposition or trial if they have ever followed up with former evaluees to determine what, if any, of the life care plan recommendations were followed. There indeed have been at least five such empirically based studies completed to date.

McCollom and Crane (2001) conducted the earliest study of 10 persons with spinal cord injuries who had sustained their injuries 8–14 years prior. The original authors found 5 out of 10 participants were being evaluated annually by physicians, all 10 participants continued to require all of the supplies recommended in the life care plan, 8 out of 10 required wheelchair repairs, all 10 participants had modified vehicles, all 10 had architectural renovations made to their home, and 3 out of 10 continued with recommended educational pursuits.

Reavis (2002) similarly conducted a retrospective study of a female with a traumatic brain injury who had a life care plan developed for her 10 years earlier. At follow-up, she had continued to use case management services and other elements of the life care plan proffered by the planner.

In 2003, Casuto and Gumpel surveyed 22 families of children who had a life care plan developed to see whether the recommendations were followed. The authors concluded that for the families who were actively involved in the life care plan process, and had the requisite education to implement the life care plan, were most likely to following the recommendations in the life care plan. Areas where the life care plan was underutilized included recreation, counseling, and community services. The authors concluded that case management services were critical in guiding the process.

Marini and Miller (2007) conducted a follow-up with 10 former evaluees (five of whom participated) who had sustained a spinal cord injury and had won a settlement or jury verdict years earlier. When queried about the equipment needs recommended in their life care plans, 75% of them had purchased a van with a lift as recommended and also had hired a part or full-time home attendant, and half had built a new accessible home and purchased lifting devices.

Finally, Rutherford-Owen and Marini (2012) conducted the largest scale follow-up of 55 evaluees with spinal cord injuries who had life care plans developed for them years earlier in the course of litigation. Forty-four had reportedly received a settlement award, eight had not, and the remainder did not respond. Settlement awards ranged from $30,000 to $4.5 million, with the average being $1,653,000. Of the group who had implemented aspects of the life care plan independent of the funding source, 54% indicated their settlement amount was not enough to take care of their lifelong needs, while 25% (n=11) of respondents indicated that it was. The remaining respondents were not sure. Respondents were asked what percentage of their life care plan had been implemented, and six indicated they had not implemented any aspects of the plan, 25% or 13 had implemented approximately 1%–25% of items in the plan, eight indicated they had implemented 26%–49% of the life care plan, five indicated they had implemented 50%–74% of the plan, and 11 respondents indicated they had implemented over 75% of the recommended life care plan.

In selecting only the 36 respondents who had received a settlement or jury verdict asking the same question as above, three of them (8%) did not implement any of the life care plans, 12 (33%) indicated they had implemented approximately 1%–25% of the life care plan, eight

(22%) reported implementing 26%–49% of the plan, three had implemented 50%–74% of the plan, and 10 (28%) had implemented over 75% of the plan with their settlement or award. The seven who did not receive any settlement or award still reported implementing aspects of the life care plan. Three did not implement any of the life care plans, one had implemented 1%–25%, two had implemented 50%–74%, and one had implemented over 75% of the recommended life care plan.

Rutherford-Owen and Marini further queried respondents with settlements or awards regarding the most frequent items they had purchased, and specific to AT, DME, and VM, respondents indicated they had purchased a van with vehicle modifications (82%), a bed/mattress system (49%), power wheelchair or scooter (46.6%), manual wheelchair (42%), Hoyer or other lifting device (33.3%), made home modifications (33.3%), and purchased exercise equipment (26.7%). Twenty-four percent, or 11 out of 45, reported they had built a new wheelchair-accessible home, and three others had not purchased any of the above items recommended in the life care plan. Even among the eight respondents who did not receive any type of award, several of them still had a medical necessity to somehow purchase items recommended in the life care plan, and in five of the items (newly built home, modifying an existing home, ramp, accessible bathroom, and vehicle modifications), a higher percentage of respondents of the eight, purchased these items with some other financial support.

Overall, the comprehensive Rutherford-Owen and Marini (2012) and previously supporting studies indicate that individuals who have a spinal cord injury, with or without the finances, must find a way to obtain medically necessary as well as independent living AT, DME, and VM to safely maintain their health, be independent as possible, and enjoy some type of quality of life.

Conclusion

For evaluees with significant disabilities who require AT, DME, and VM, the life care planner needs to be meticulous in selecting the appropriate devices, ideally with the assistance of the evaluee, noting from the records what types of devices, equipment, and accommodation have already been made, and researching appropriate vendors regarding pricing. This chapter presents the numerous factors that need to be considered in this process as well as provides the reader with previously published recommendations and opinions from ATS and RTSs in the field.

References

Allison, C. D. (2018). Vehicle modifications: Useful considerations for life care planners. In R. O. Weed & D. E. Berens (Eds.), *Life care planning and case management handbook* (4th ed., pp. 799–811). CRC Press.

Amsterdam, P. (2003). Setting standards of protocol for replacement schedules of medical equipment in a life care plan. *Journal of Life Care Planning, 1*(4), 275–284.

Amsterdam, P. (2010). Medical equipment choices and the role of the rehab equipment specialist in life care planning. In R. O. Weed & D. E. Berens (Eds.), *Life care planning and case management handbook* (3rd ed., pp. 889–908). CRC Press.

Amsterdam, P. (2018). Medical equipment choices and the role of the rehab equipment specialist in life care planning. In R. O. Weed & D. E. Berens (Eds.), *Life care planning and case management handbook* (4th ed., pp. 759–785). CRC Press.

Casuto, D., & Gumpel, L. (2003). A retrospective study of pediatric life care plan outcomes: One life care planner's experience. *Journal of Life Care Planning, 2*(1), 1–56.

Daubert v. Merrill Dow Pharmaceuticals, Inc., 509 U.S. 579 (1993)

Deutsch, P. M., & Sawyer, H. W. (2001). *A guide to rehabilitation.* AHAB Press.
Education for All Handicapped Children. (1975). Available at www.govtrack.us/congress/bills/94/s6.
Field, T. (2000). *A resource for the rehabilitation consultant on the Daubert and Kumho rulings.* E & F Publication.
Individuals with Disabilities Education Act. (2004). https://ncld.org/wp-content/uploads/2014/11/IDEA-Parent Guide1.pdf
Isom, R., & Marini, I. (2002). An educational curriculum for teaching life care planning. *Journal of Life Care Planning, 1*(4), 239–264.
Marini, I. (2018). Theories of adjustment and adaptation to disability. In I. Marini, N. M. Graf, & M. J. Millington (Eds.), *Psychosocial aspects of disability: Insider perspectives and strategies for counselors* (2nd ed., pp. 133–166). Springer Publishing.
Marini, I., & Harper, D. (2006). Empirical validation of medical equipment replacement values in life care plans. *Journal of Life Care Planning, 4*(4), 173–182.
Marini, I., & Miller, E. (2007). The physical and psychosocial health status of clients with SCI awarded damages in litigation. *Journal of Life Care Planning, 5*(4), 145–158.
Marini, I., Vang, C., Antol, D. L., Mora, E., Quijino, P., Pinon, R. M., & Cuevas, S. (2019). Redux: Empirical validation of durable medical 17 equipment values in life care plans. *Journal of Life Care Planning. 17*(2) 5–17.
McCollom, P., & Crane, R. (2001). Life care plans: Accuracy over time. *The Case Manager, 12*(3), 85–87.
Metmart.com (2002–2021). https://medmartonline.com/handicare-p-440-portable-ceiling-lift
National Mobility Equipment Dealers Association. (2016). www.nmeda.com/wp-content/uploads/2016/01/QAP-103-2016-Guidelines.pdf
Reavis, S. (2002). Life care planning for successful outcomes: A ten-year study. *Journal of Life Care Planning, 1*(2), 153–156.
Rehabilitation Engineering, and Assistive Technology Society of North America. (n.d.). https:www.atia.org.
Riddick-Grisham, S., & Deming, L. (2011). The role of the life care planner in paediatric life care planning. In *Pediatric life care planning and case management* (2nd ed., pp. 49–90). CRC Press.
Romero, M. G., & Marini, I. (2018). Obesity as a disability: Medical, psychosocial, and vocational implications. In I. Marini & M. A. Stebnicki (Eds.), *The psychological and social impact of illness and disability* (pp. 443–457). Springer Publishing.
Rutherford-Owen, T., & Marini, I. (2012). Life care plan implementation among adults with spinal cord injuries. *Journal of Life Care Planning, 10*(4) 5–20.
Scherer, M. J. (2016). Assistive technology and persons with disabilities. In I. Marini & M. Stebnicki (Eds.), *The professional counselor's desk reference* (2nd ed., pp. 475–481). Springer Publishing.
US Department of Veterans Affairs. (n.d.). www.benefits.va.gov/BENEFITS/factsheets/homeloans/SAHFactsheet.pdf

Vehicle modification resources are from Allison 2018

Association for Driver Rehabilitation Specialists (ADED)—ADED was established in 1977 to support professionals working in the field of driver education, driver training, and transportation equipment modifications for persons with disabilities and persons experiencing the aging process. Through education, information dissemination, and a certification program for professionals, ADED supports these professionals so that they may better serve these individuals. The ADED stands ready to meet the professional needs of its members through educational conferences, professional development activities, and a professional certification program. The history of ADED reflects a unique blending of different professional fields into an organization dedicated to providing quality service in the field of driver rehabilitation, vehicle modifications for driving, transportation, and resources for alternative transportation.
www.aded.net
(866) 672-9466

National Mobility Equipment Dealers Association (NMEDA)—A non-profit trade association of mobility equipment dealers, driver rehabilitation specialists, and other professionals dedicated to broadening the opportunities for people with disabilities to drive or ride in vehicles modified with mobility equipment.
3327 Bearss Avenue
Tampa, FL 33618
(800) 833-0427

Adaptive Driving Alliance (ADA)—A nationwide group of vehicle-modification dealers providing van conversions, hand controls, wheelchair lifts, scooter lifts, tie-downs, conversion van rentals, paratransit, and other adaptive equipment for drivers with disabilities and passengers.
111 Stow Avenue, Ste 103
Cuyahoga Falls, OH 44221
(330) 928-7401
www.adamobility.com

National Highway Traffic Safety Administration (NHTSA)—The federal government agency authorized to regulate the manufacture of automotive adaptive equipment and modified vehicles used by persons with disabilities.
National Highway Traffic Safety Administration
1200 New Jersey Avenue, SE
Washington, DC 20590
(888) 327-4236
(800) 424-9153 (TTY)
www.nhtsa.gov

Society of Automobile Engineers (SAE)—An international organization of engineers, business executives, educators, and students who share information and exchange ideas for advancing the engineering of mobility systems.
SAE World Headquarters
400 Commonwealth Drive
Warrendale, PA 15096-0001
(724) 776–4841
www.sae.org

Chapter 34

A Personal Perspective of Life Care Planning

Various Authors

A Parent's Perspective of Navigating Medical, Legal, Educational, and Rehabilitation Systems

Anonymous Contributor
First published in Journal of Life Care Planning, Vol. 18, No. 1, (9–10)
Printed in U.S.A. All rights reserved 2020 Int'l Assoc. of Rehab Professionals

Interviewer: How did disability onset occur?

Dad: It was a birth-related injury following an otherwise healthy pregnancy. Our son's lack of oxygen at birth caused massive brain damage and he was diagnosed with hypoxic ischemic encephalopathy.

Interviewer: What was the experience of learning about the condition like?

Dad: Because the pregnancy was healthy, we did not know of his health problems until he was delivered. He was immediately taken away from us due to his seizure activity. I felt like I was in the dark, a doctor told me he was transferring him to a different hospital and asked if I wanted to go with the baby or stay with my wife. I had to instantly decide whether to go or stay. I decided to stay with my wife, who was also in shock. The baby was then transferred to a Level 1 trauma center approximately 30 minutes away. Once there, he was sedated because of his constant seizure activity. My wife remained in one hospital while my son remained at another until my wife was discharged home.

DOI: 10.4324/9781003388456-38

Interviewer: What was your inpatient experience (e.g., did you receive adequate information about the diagnosis, were you given resources to learn more)?

Dad: He was hospitalized for 12 days at the Level 1 trauma center. On the second day or so, they performed an MRI of his brain and that is when we talked to the pediatric neurologist. Based upon that conversation, I remember being told about the massive itbrain damage that my son had due to the event. The pediatric neurologist told us that he could not predict the future but that a child's brain is plastic. Remember, my son is still sedated during this entire time. The doctor told us that my son could have no motor function at all and in that situation, he would not have purposeful movement or be able to talk. In the best scenario, my son could have the ability to talk and walk but he would do all of these things with impairments. I remember asking the doctor if it was normal that my son was still sleeping and he responded that no, usually they will wake up after a day, which was very alarming to us.

Interviewer: What was the transition back home like?

Dad: We were discharged from the trauma center to our home. There was a nurse from the hospital who came to the home once a month to check on his development for the first year. We were told to return to follow up with various specialists. We also started working with an early developmental specialist right away who referred us to many services and therapists. Within the first month, because we saved his cord blood, we were able to have a transfusion in a local hospital.

Interviewer: How did you learn about resources you needed?

Dad: At the time, it seems like the people at the hospital and then the state's case manager provided us information. But when he was really young, there was not much that was recommended. As parents, we constantly tried to work with him toward developmental milestones. While we knew that he would be delayed in reaching the milestones, we did what we could to encourage him to gain control over head movement, etc. so that he would accomplish each milestone. Physical, speech, and occupational therapy services were started in the home within the first year. One of our main challenges was finding highly qualified therapists.

My wife would read online advice and stories from other parents. I do not remember her participating in those groups much, but she would read what other families were trying. Those types of forums would highlight how important it was to educate yourself about your child's disability and what resources were available. Many of those participating online would talk about being limited to only school-based resources while others would seek out summer intensive programs and other resources.

Interviewer: How did you find people to talk to about your son's health condition?

Dad: We didn't seek that out in the beginning. It was just too traumatic to talk about. We did not join support groups. We are more introverted people and did not want to relive the event.

With time, we found a national association of professionals who specialized in a speech disorder that he had, and we attended their conference. There, we were able to get information about the condition and met specialists and experts. Through that resource, we were able to find people in our region who specialized in dealing with children with this condition. We also found a local speech person there through those resources. While we used the internet, we would find that people would advertise that they work with children with this certain condition, but when we pressed them about their specialized training or experience, they did not have it. We knew from the conference and from the specialists we met there about the specialized training and what was required to be effective in this training, so we were able to differentiate between people who knew what the condition was and people who were properly trained to work with our son.

Interviewer: What was the role of your family in supporting you?

Dad: Our family members are all out of state or the country, so we had some help, but it was infrequent. My wife's mom came for 1–2 months and her sister once in a while and would do things like take my son to a movie to give us a break. My brother also came to visit for a week.

Unfortunately, family members cannot really understand. They can sympathize but they can't quite empathize. It's also hard when no one in the family offers to keep our son to afford us a break, even though they help other family members who do not have children with disabilities. Even now, it is primarily the two of us providing care. We do get some respite care now, but that is through the state, not through family members.

Interviewer: How did you find funding for what you needed? What was that experience like?

Dad: With our employment, we had good health insurance. Also, our state provides long-term care, which is not true for all states. Even with quality private health insurance that covered quite a bit, we did acquire more than $50,000 in medical debt. A lot of this was because certain (qualified) therapists and certain kinds of specialized interventions were not covered by our insurance. Again, access to highly-qualified therapists was key to seeing improvement, so we chose to pay out of pocket to receive that treatment.

Interviewer: If there was litigation as a result of the disability, what was that experience like?

Dad: I had never been engaged in litigation before. Through this I found out that lawyers did not always have the same urgency about moving the case along as I expected. Our case took approximately five years to resolve. It seemed like we were frequently reaching out to the law office and when we did, we would learn that dates had been pushed back without us knowing. I also do not feel like our lawyers prepared us for how hard the process would be and how nasty the opposing counsel could be to us. I now know that plaintiffs need to advocate for themselves even with their attorneys.

Interviewer: What was it like navigating school systems with the disability?

Dad: We had to hire an advocate to interact with the school system. Before that, we could not get the school system to provide the services that our son needed. After the advocate was hired, things moved much easier for us.

Interviewer: Critical team members who helped?

Dad: Developmental pediatricians have always followed him. I don't remember how that was started, likely through the hospital. However, these specialists are very limited in number and are always booked out in their appointments. We also had a local pediatrician who was very encouraging and warm, so she was nice to have on our team.

We would locate specialized providers and we were willing to try everything. Through this process, we have emailed and talked with two highly-regarded specialists who were engaged in various research. Both actually took time to talk with us on the telephone. I will note, however, that we did extensive research on these topics prior to contacting the researchers, so they knew (and we knew) that we were well-informed.

Interviewer: What advice would you give others who are starting in this journey?

Dad: First, I would recommend to bank cord blood and if you need it, move quickly in this intervention.

In general, we learned that you have to be an advocate for yourself and your child. Getting the right specialist is critical. If you have plateaued with a therapist or if the person is not helping your child to progress, do not be afraid to change therapists. It's hard to hurt their feelings, but if it's not working, you must change. If the therapist is not skilled, it can be a waste of time. One year with someone who knows what they are doing is better than 5 years with someone who does not know what they are doing. I will note, of course, that the place where you live does make a difference in availability of services.

In retrospect, we should have joined a support group. It would have been beneficial emotionally and we could have found other friends for our child.

We have also learned how important it is to get an advocate when navigating IEPs and the school district. The school is trying to save money and will try to do the bare minimum. Hiring an advocate is well worth it.

We also recommend trying every possible alternative therapy available. We tried many different ones and they all helped in different ways. Our son is now talking, walking, running, learning to read, and having friends. To us, he is a miracle but a miracle that took many years of hard work, dedication, love, and money investment.

A Wife's Story of Caring for Her Husband

Jasjeet Kaur
Journal of Life Care Planning, Vol 18, No 1, (19–21)
Printed in U.S.A. All rights reserved
2020 Int'l Assoc. of Rehab Professionals

Life can become very challenging when all of the sudden your loved one comes across an incident that causes him to become trapped inside his own body, unable to communicate in any possible way. The most difficult part is to watch your loved one suffer. You do all you can do to try to reduce his pain, anxiety, fear and discomfort; yet you know that cannot really help him.

My husband, Anudeep Passi, was very strong, cheerful and kind-hearted person. He was full of life and energy. We had only been married for nine months when the drowning incident changed everything for us and threw us down a sad and scary un-named road. I was expecting our first baby soon and was new to this country. Anudeep was my strength, my best friend, and my entire world. After the drowning, my husband suffered severe brain damage caused by a lack of oxygen, which left him comatose.

On the day of his injury, Anudeep was put under observation for 24 hours. I was alone with him that day and night. There was a team of doctors and nurses that watched him closely. I had a strange belief in my heart that, "He will definitely get better before our baby comes into this world and he will be by my side for the big day." After midnight, he was moved for the first time. I thought that he was finally moved into a hospital room because he had woken up. But the doctors and nurses said that his involuntary first movement was just contractions. They told me this wasn't good; however, they didn't tell me why. No one at the hospital was explaining anything to me. It was only much later that I learned, from our case manager and our attorneys, that Anudeep had irreversible brain damage.

Two weeks after our baby was born, even though Anudeep was in the same hospital, in the ICU, I was not allowed to take our baby to meet with his father because of fear of infection. After his tracheostomy and g-tube placement, my husband was moved to a subacute facility. The doctors there were very nice, and they always answered all the questions. In hindsight, I realized that I just did not know the correct questions to ask.

Unfortunately, the nurses in the subacute were very rude. Right in front of my eyes, their untrained nurses practiced IV placement on his hands and arms. Because he was in a coma and couldn't say anything, they would keep poking him again and again, resulting in bruises. When the trained nurse would come into the room to put in the IV in correctly, she would shamelessly ask the other nurse, 'Is it your first time for IV placement?', which felt very inhumane to me. The staff would put medical supplies, like syringes, suction tubes and catheters into his body. Frequently, these supplies would slide under his back and poke him. He would moan in pain and the nurses would just give him more pain medicines to make him sleep until his next turn cycle. I would watch the staff clean my husband in a very unhygienic way. They did not change gloves when they were soiled and touched him with dirty gloves while performing his care. While Anudeep was at this hospital, he had fevers all the time and he was on fever-reducing medications around the clock. Whenever I had to talk with a doctor, before signing consents regarding any planned procedures, the nurses always argued with me. He fought one infection after another, as long as he was in the hospital.

The health insurance only covered my husband's stay in the subacute facility for 100 days. My husband never responded to physical or speech therapies, but I was told he had to be discharged home or to a long-term care facility. In October of 2010, after three months had passed since his injury, he was sent home. I had no medical background at all. I was shown how to take care of him in just one day of training. My husband's employer had continued his insurance for a short-time, but then I learned he was changed over to Medi-Cal. This insurance change was very challenging. Health insurance issues were really difficult for me to understand, as I was new to the United States.

I thought that my husband should have been provided 100% care from medical professionals, however, that is not what happened. The healthcare system in the U.S. was very strange to me. Anudeep was like a newborn baby, except that he couldn't even cry. Every time he moaned in pain or looked anxious, it would pierce through my heart and drain all my energy. I was the only one who continued to manage and try to ease his pain, discomfort and anxiety.

We moved my husband into the living room of our two-story home, as there was no downstairs bedroom and no way to get Anudeep upstairs. Suddenly, the insurance company started sending their people over to pick up my husband's equipment, such as his bed and his feeding pump.

I refused to take my husband out of the bed so that they could take it. I refused to unhook his feeding pump too. They didn't even give me enough formula for one month until I could figure out another way to obtain his nutrition. I was so scared and in shock with thoughts that if they take his bed, where would he live? If they take his feeding pump, how would he get calories?

I had no knowledge of the litigation system. When the attorneys first came to my home, they were trying to discuss the case with me. I told them that I didn't want to file a lawsuit, because my husband was in coma and he could not work, so if we were to lose the case, I could not pay their fees. They explained to me if we lost, I would not have to pay them anything. That was very surprising to me. They were so kind, compassionate and helpful.

Soon these attorneys became involved in my journey. I remember that they came back to my home a second time to do the paperwork and they saw me running around, doing all of my husband's care while they tried to talk to me. They saw that his hospital bed was broken and so we had to quickly transfer him to the wheelchair. They saw how I was crying and still trying to manage everything, by myself, along with caring for my newborn son. When they saw me in that situation, they called Tracy Albee to get her involved as a case manager. She handled everything well. Finally, I had some help and the answers to all of my questions regarding my husband's health. Life started to become a little less frantic and a little more organized. Our attorneys and this case manager were like angels sent by God at that time.

Right away, Tracy talked with the insurance companies and was able to help us to keep the bed, which was fixed, and to keep the feeding pump. She arranged that the only change was to which insurance would pay for the equipment. Our attorney purchased us formula for one month as a donation, which was very expensive, until we were able to get the prescription filled out by a non-insurance physician so that Medi-Cal would pay for it. Tracy really helped to make sure all of Anudeep's needs were met.

Tracy would sit in our house for hours, going through paperwork for state disability, Social Security, medical insurance, therapies, medicines and so on. I didn't understand any of it, as I was brand new to the U.S. She helped me to understand my husband's prognosis and the expected outcome. Tracy explained to me how my husband would remain comatose for the rest of his life; what he may possibly experience regarding pain and illnesses; and how to try to prevent them. She helped the attorneys to prepare the best life care plan for my husband in his critical condition. She made me a huge binder for me to follow when I needed reminders of what to do.

Here is the list of very important steps she helped me with:

1) Find a primary care physician for my husband who could make home visits whenever necessary.
2) She found and contacted different vendors so that my husband's many types of supplies could be provided timely.
3) She gave me an emergency backup plan for any possible condition that may arise, such as getting all his medications, supplies, and clothes ready in a bag.
4) Because my husband was on an electric bed all of the time, she talked with attorneys and they purchased us a power generator in case of power outages.
5) She got us a trifold alternating pressure mattress as a backup because sometimes the primary mattress would fail, and I was fearful he would get bedsores.
6) Because my husband was comatose, Tracy called the city's fire department and listed his name with them for emergency evacuation in case of any possible natural disasters.
7) She went with us to Stanford's Neurological Research Center for consultation with neurologists and helped get my husband's name listed in case there were any possible research projects for brain regeneration that might have been successful.

8) When his skin started to breakdown, even though we had a special mattress and turned him very frequently, she helped us find a special mattress for my husband which could change his position automatically and further prevent any bedsores.
9) She helped to find nursing home health companies so that my husband could get around the clock care at home, once I could afford it.
10) She went with me to help purchase the correct van so that we could take my husband places. The first van was used and did not always meet our needs, but we were limited in funds at the time. Later, she went with me again to purchase a new and more appropriate van.
11) We eventually were able to get a modified house and she helped me to plan the set-up of his room, which included a good wheelchair; an appropriate shower chair; and a shower room with a lift transfer system in the ceiling used to transfer him from bed to chair.
12) Every time my husband had any complications, Tracy guided me over the phone, or if needed, she came to take a look at my husband and guide us accordingly.

For me, this whole situation was very challenging, but I had accepted it with an open heart. We took him to the hospital for therapies twice to three times a week. We also had to take him back and forth to doctor's appointments frequently in the beginning. I took care of him by assuming myself into his situation and did what I could do to help myself to feel comfortable. My baby's crib was on my one side and my husband in his hospital bed was on the other side. I would sleep in a recliner in the middle.

Once my husband came home, he stopped having the fevers. I took care of him all by myself for three years. It was a lot of work. I turned him every two hours; gave him water through the g-tube every three hours; gave him massages and did range of motion; and I bathed and dressed him every day. I would put him in his wheelchair for an hour and then back to the bed every day. I barely slept for those three years. I always made sure that he, and everything around him, was clean. I continued doing this for what felt like forever, even if I was sick myself. After three years, my body started wearing down, I had injured my back and I started hunching.

Finally, when the lawsuit was over, we had the opportunity to hire home care support. At first, I was very resistant. I did not think anyone would take care of Anudeep the way that I was doing it. I thought the home care nurses would be just as bad as the hospital staff had been. My mom, who lived in India, became very ill. I felt that I had to go and see her in case she was going to die. Tracy helped to find nursing companies and we hired around-the-clock care for him. We had other family in the home, but they did not provide any hands-on care, so the home health nurses took over. Once I went to India and returned to the U.S., I realized that my husband was still okay, even though it had not been me taking care of him around the clock for that two weeks.

I finally accepted the outside caregivers. I still chose to do one shift a day and we used nurses for 16 hours each day. One of the shifts was the overnight so I could finally get some consistent sleep. Even though I was told that there was enough money to have the nurses around the clock, I always worried that my husband might outlive the money and then we would be back to where we started.

Having the nurses in the house for one day shift and one night shift gave me the break that I needed and I was able to give time to my son. By this time, my son was almost four years old. He had never known what having a normal dad was like. I had to prepare him to start school and meet other children who had dads who were not living in a coma in a hospital bed.

My husband continued getting good care from nurses. I always stayed around and helped them whenever needed. This whole situation affected my career. I have a Masters Degree in Engineering. I had been looking for a job before Anudeep was injured and then afterward, I was provided good job offers. I knew that I could not accept the employment opportunities, because I was the only one to take care of and manage my husband's situation.

Of course, life and care of a loved one is the most important thing, so I am satisfied that I was there by his side all this time and I am thankful to God for blessing Anudeep with the utmost care, love, and respect he deserved.

Over time, we were able to try alternative treatments, such as acupuncture, acupressure, private physical and speech therapies, homeopathy, and Ayurveda. My husband's condition stayed the same for nine years. There was never any improvement. We would go to the emergency room on occasion, when his g-tube pulled out or when he had symptoms, such as fever and congestion. We managed to never require an admission of more than a day or two. I always felt that I, along with the home health nurses and aides, could take better care for him at home than they ever did in the hospital. Tracy used to say what a great job we were doing. He never developed any bedsores or other "unexpected" complications.

I could have never imagined any of this would have turned out to be my life. I was young and new in this country; I had no knowledge of the healthcare or health insurance systems. With the help of our attorneys, my husband received the financial help I needed for his expenses; and with our case manager's help, my husband was able to have the best possible care.

My husband passed away recently. He had survived for nine years in his coma. I am satisfied that he was surrounded by family and that he always received the love and respect as a father, husband, son, brother, and human being. We were able to provide him everything possible to ease his discomfort and we were able to try different treatments to help him. Tracy also prevented us from possible scams like stem cell treatment for brain regeneration in other countries (which is not approved by the FDA yet). She warned me by explaining the potential bad consequences that could occur for my husband's health.

After my husband's passing, Tracy introduced me to a charitable organization for patients with ALS. I was able to donate all of my husband's medical equipment and wheelchair van to this organization that will now lend it to others who have a health crisis. It felt like our tragedy was somehow turned into Anudeep's legacy. I cannot imagine how life would have been without our attorneys and our case manager.

Unfortunately, incidents happen to beautiful, innocent people that cause lifetime disabilities and painful journeys. When it happened to my family, the help from our attorneys and our case manager felt like God carried us through a path, where otherwise we would not have been able to take a single step.

My New Normal: A Mother's Story of Stroke

Anonymous Contributor
Journal of Life Care Planning, Vol. 18. No. 1 (23–28)
Printed in U.S.A. All rights reserved
2020 Int'l Assoc. of Rehab Professionals

My world took a complete turn twenty-six years ago, the day my third child was born. On that day, probably right before birth, she suffered a stroke. We didn't know that she had a stroke then. What we did know was that approximately half an hour before she entered this world, I was bleeding badly—a slow hemorrhage—and that I would need to undergo an emergency c-section.

My daughter was born that evening with Apgar scores of 2-4-6. By the time I woke from the anesthesia, I could hear her crying, but I was in a fog of pain. I honestly felt as if I had been cut in two. Attendants wheeled me to my room without my baby. Nurses told me she would be brought in soon for her first feeding. I lay awake waiting while her dad slept. When the nurse finally arrived, she said Emma had been taken to the neonatal intensive care unit because she had stopped breathing for a short time. It was just an apnea spell, I was told, but she would have to be kept there so they could "keep an eye on her." I would be able to see her in the morning. I don't know if I had ever heard of apnea spells before that night. The medical staff seemed unalarmed and reassuring every time they spoke to me, and I clung to that. But, seriously, *my baby had stopped breathing.* Sleep eluded me.

Emma was released when she was six days old, at that time we knew only that her apnea spells had been caused by infantile seizures and that for a while she would have to take Phenobarbital mixed in with milk, and she hated the stuff. Emma's release from the NICU overwhelmed me. And I was nervous. Did she need monitoring at home, in case she stopped breathing again? I was assured no, that the medicine would prevent that. Did I mention how much we had to trust these people, the doctors and the nurses who were our sole source of information? Emma's very life depended on them knowing what they were doing. She was evaluated for early intervention therapy, and we were assigned to Barbara, a pediatric occupational therapist. Barbara became my primary source of information for the next three years.

Emma was very groggy her first six months—the time she was on the Phenobarbital. She slept a lot and didn't nurse well. By the time she was two months old, I knew instinctively she was different from other babies. Then came the day when, while changing her diaper, she happily stretched out her little legs, and on an impulse, I cautiously put one hand under her head and one hand under her ankles and I slowly lifted her up. And she held that position, stiff as a board, for several long moments, like a circus trick. My heart broke. I knew then something was entirely wrong. *Babies don't do that.*

My instincts were verified by her three-month birthday when she started to reach and grab with her left hand but not with her right. Again, not at all normal. A late-night study with a book about premature babies clued me in with its discussion of possible lifelong struggles. We were talking about cerebral palsy. I was sure.

I'm certain it helped tremendously that I was not a first-time mother and that I had some resources. For one thing, I was not uneducated. I was a journalist by training, and I knew how to do research. And in my job, I worked quite a lot with scientists and researchers. Because I was comfortable interviewing scientists, I found it easy to grill medical professionals who increasingly crossed my path.

Our NICU followed up its most at-risk babies a few times after their release, and Emma was diagnosed with cerebral palsy on her first follow-up visit. The basic fact is that a diagnosis of cerebral palsy gives you no clue how global that disability might be. If there is a brain injury, that injury can affect just about anything that involves the brain, depending on where the injury lies. In addition to muscle and limb movement and coordination—the most visible part of the disability—vision, hearing, learning, emotions and behavior also might be impacted. And how much they are affected of course depends on how large the brain injury is.

But I also was reassured that Emma's affect—her cooing and smile and flirty engagement with us—was a good sign. It indicated she was not affected cognitively. The official diagnosis was right-side spastic hemiplegia—whatever damage her brain had incurred at birth was all in the left hemisphere. There were no new scans taken. The professionals simply knew because of where the deficits were. But there was very little way of knowing how severely she would be affected. That would be a waiting game. We would simply have to wait for developmental milestones to be reached. Or not.

Developmental milestones did not come quickly. She wouldn't pull herself to stand until she was 16 months, and she achieved that for the first time to peer into our new double baby stroller to get a peek at her newborn sister, who she called "Bee" (for baby). She would be nearly 22 months old before she took her first steps. And yet she had said her first word "yite," pointing at a light, at the very young age of six months, much earlier than her brothers' first words. And it was such a peculiar first word. She repeated it a number of times over several weeks, each time pointing. And then after a while, she stopped. Words like "ba" would come—and then leave again. By eighteen months, she was babbling in paragraphs—complete with hand gestures and facial expressions—but we couldn't understand a word. How I wish I'd carried around a cell phone back then with a video recorder. It was hilarious and baffling at the same time.

Shortly after Emma's second birthday, I pressed Barbara about her odd language development. She continued to speak one word at a time—or at least I could understand only one word at a time—and she was picking up new words, using them for a while, and then often dropping them from usage after a time. We also had struggled with her eating solid foods. She had no problem with pureed baby foods, but once we added a texture, she often choked and coughed and sometimes vomited it all right back up again. And she was so very thin. At two she weighed a little bit more than 25 pounds, and we were still pureeing most of her food. She used a sippy cup with so-so finesse, and we hadn't gotten rid of the bottle yet because I worried that it was what provided most of her calories and nutrition. So, she began working with a speech therapist, Marvin.

Eventually, as Emma was getting closer to her third birthday and facing her eventual release from early intervention, we drove the four hours to Riley Children's Hospital in Indianapolis to consult with a speech and language pathologist. That specialist determined that her difficulty was not rooted in her brain's language center and instead Emma had another diagnosis—oral motor dysarthria—a fancy way of saying her mouth muscles were spastic too. For example, Emma wasn't able to make pucker her lips, which explained why she still drooled. In fact, she drooled buckets, and she wore bibs twenty-four/seven in my attempt to spare her clothing. She also didn't have great tongue control.

So, for the next year we practiced sticking out our tongues and wiggling them around. We practiced making fish lips, which she and her little sister thought was hysterical. For the next several years—yes, years—every night at bath time my daughters together sucked on one little round sucker each, rolling in between their closed lips. I believe I went through several pounds of Dum-Dum suckers before we left that exercise behind us when the girls started school. But our diligence in these simple exercises paid off, and Emma was speaking so well by kindergarten that she was denied a speech therapy services.

Through my work I had been connected to the internet shortly after Emma's first birthday. Suddenly, a world of research was at my fingertips, before long I was connected with other parents—predominately mothers—of other children with various medical diagnoses. When she was about two, I had a small network of people whose children also had spastic hemiplegia. Once we found each other, we clung to each other. We had companions for this blind journey we'd never planned but found ourselves committed to. We talked about everything—family dynamics, how our kids were doing, what worried us the most. In 1996, we called ourselves Hemi-Kids and in March 2000, the IRS granted tax-exempt status to the Hemi-Kid Foundation. In the fall, we formally changed Hemi-Kids to its current name Children's Hemiplegia and Stroke Association (CHASA). I personally played no part in making any of this happen, apart from my daily participation. But I witnessed the growth of our tiny group to what has now become a global internet support group touching thousands of families every year.

For Emma, learning was rough in those early grades, even without a cognitive disability. Teachers could see she was bright and curious. Yet she struggled. She had gone to a private kindergarten for one year, but I kept her in kindergarten a second year when I moved her to public school. This put both of my daughters in the same grade, and consequently I had a good view of normal classroom learning versus struggles from the very same gene pool. By fourth grade, she was about two years behind in reading and math, and sometimes there were huge holes in her understanding of certain subjects. And then there was her social life. While she had been very popular in preschool and kindergarten, in grade school she didn't make friends the way her sister did.

Anna had been evaluated for services through the schools after early intervention ceased, but she was determined not disabled in a way that would affect her ability to learn. They said that then, but we learned differently later. She was not approved for Medicaid waiver, because she did not have a cognitive disability. From that point on she would need to get all of her therapy needs met through our medical insurance. While I had very good insurance in general, when it came to therapy, it proved to be inadequate. Any and all therapy past twenty visits per year would have to be paid out of pocket. That was for speech therapy, physical therapy *and* occupational therapy combined. Through my online friends I learned of a Canadian doctor—Karen Pape—who was using TES therapy (Therapeutic Electrical Stimulation, administered at low levels during sleep to stimulate muscle growth) and reporting good results. I found a physical therapist at Riley's Children's Hospital who was able to get Anna started with TES on her legs, and we continued that therapy until she began grade school. This involved placing electrodes up and down her right leg before bed, and then a small electrical unit in a fanny pack around her waist administered barely perceptible charges to that leg's muscles as she slept. We called it her "tickle machine." It took about fifteen minutes every night to get her set up, and she was a trooper.

Additionally, I learned about research in Louisville for children with hemiplegia studying electrical stimulation and bracing to improve hand function. Anna was accepted into that study, and for two years we made the six-hour drive each month so she could participate. That protocol began at 3-1/2 years. The study required daily exercise for 30-minute periods morning and night, a one-hour daily commitment.

These two therapies put a lot of work on my shoulders and hers, but we were doing something, hoping she would continue to improve and not go backwards. And, indeed, she didn't lose function during the remainder of her preschool years and continued to make progress developmentally. The twenty therapy sessions our health insurance *did* pay for went for occupational therapy.

Sometime between Anna's third and fourth birthday, she had begun to get anxious, and often her anxiety didn't have a particular focus. The anxiety's arrival when she was three, coincided with several other things including her release from early intervention services and the addition of therapies that involved electrical stimulation and huge daily commitments and the addition of whatever stress grade school brought. The anxiety was crippling and time-consuming and we now understand that anxiety impacts 70–80% of childhood survivors that we know. Almost all of the other CHASA moms and dads understood this, because it was going on with their kids too. And so we wonder, where does this anxiety come from? I understand that it's absolutely possible—and entirely probable—the anxiety is rooted in brain chemistry, that the original brain injury somehow causes it. Or maybe it's those the processing problems common for our sons and daughters, causing emotions like anxiety to get stuck and not move on in a way that is more typical in the average person. But I can't help but wonder. *What if the pervasive anxiety that marks our children well into their adult years has its roots in all that therapy that they endured during their formative years?*

By the beginning of grade school, I understood I would have to make some changes in my own life. I was worn ragged. I felt like I was not doing my job well, both at home and professionally. My marriage was a bust, and my husband was absent entirely from family life. At work, it seemed like I was always behind. So, I left my career—one that I adored and never intended to leave—and worked freelance from home instead. And we pulled back from all the therapies and focused on school instead.

As her parent, I made the decision to find outside therapies that were more "normal" to what other kids were doing. She participated in therapeutic horseback riding all through grade school and middle school, which she loved. Starting in middle school, we added adaptive downhill skiing. And when she started high school, she began running cross-country and track. In the summers, she competed in para track and field events, which required some travel. And we went to retreats with our CHASA group yearly. Those were the things I believe we did right. She knew other kids with disabilities like hers through CHASA—dozens and dozens of kids her own age.

But the seizure part of her story—that's the part that will puzzle me forever. At six months, Emma no longer had to take the Phenobarbital that she'd been taking since birth. An EEG at that time showed that the seizures had stopped. An EEG at her first birthday showed that time had been kind and her brain waves were completely normal. And the difference between Emma on Phenobarbital and Emma off Phenobarbital was striking. She was more alert. She began to pick up more developmental skills. And instead of just being stiff, her muscles seemed to be gaining strength. And so, at six months, with the seizures behind us, I didn't give them another thought.

Until she was ten. One night, after I had put the children in their beds and things were quiet for the night, I heard Emma moaning for maybe a minute. It wasn't long, and I was in bed, about to drift off to sleep myself. But then she was quiet, and we all slept for the night. The next day, after getting everyone dressed and fed and on the school bus for the day, I stopped to straighten Emma's room up, and I realized there was vomit in her bed and, well, all over the place. It had begun to dry, but it seemed to be everywhere—the walls, the bed, the floor and even the ceiling. I remembered her moaning, but she hadn't gotten up. She hadn't told me she had been sick. When she came home, I asked her why she hadn't told me she had been sick during the night. She said she didn't remember being sick. This should have been my clue, but I was in denial.

About a month later came the decisive day: November 5, 2004. It was a Friday. Emma had just gotten out of the bath, and I had wrapped her in a towel and sent her off to her bedroom while I helped her sister. Within seconds, I heard the moaning again. I found her in her room, on the floor on her side, choking and then vomiting prolifically. Her right side began twitching and then jerking. And her eyes rolled back and there she was in my arms having a full-blown grand mal seizure. I'd carried her back to my room and put her on the floor there. She was naked, and I yelled to my sons downstairs to call 911. Emma's lips were turning blue. The operator asked me if she was breathing, and I couldn't say.

I had struggled to get Emma's pajamas on during the seizure. For the life of me, I don't know why I thought that was important. I pulled myself away from her when the EMTs arrived to let them take over her care. Twenty minutes slipped away before they had her strapped to a gurney and took her down the stairs, into the living room and outside into the unseasonably cold air. That's when she regained consciousness. When I explained to her that she had had a seizure she denied it had ever happened. "I didn't. You dreamed it, Mama," she argued with me. She thought we were all nuts, and she was pretty unhappy about the 30-minute journey to the hospital.

When we arrived at the hospital, I called her dad. At the time we'd been separated for more than year and were nearing the finalization of our divorce. The neurologist arrived sometime after midnight. He asked for a description of what had happened. Evidently, just saying, "She had a seizure" was inadequate, because I was pressed for precise details. He didn't need many, because my description of the vomiting, convulsions, blue lips, and unconsciousness followed by confusion convinced him. Emma was admitted and an MRI was scheduled for the next day.

The MRI—her first ever—showed the brain damage that had resulted the day she was born. Seeing it was like a gut-punch. The sizable damage—about two-thirds of her left hemisphere— indicated an ischemic event, our first real confirmation that it had been a stroke. I'd always presumed that, during the placental rupture, a clot likely had traveled through the umbilicus to her brain. The MRI was the closest confirmation I'd ever have of that scenario. Emma was released the following day with a prescription for Tegretol and an appointment with a local neurologist, who while not a pediatric neurologist, did see pediatric patients.

My daughter was back in her classroom the Monday following her seizure and the day after being released from the hospital. On the days she went to school, she often spent part of the time in the office of the health aide. When Emma got off the bus in the afternoon, after a day at school, she looked ragged and spent. She cried all the time. She was tired and took naps. There were tremors, some of them going on for an hour at a time. As they increased in frequency, I didn't know whether to call them seizures or just tremors. Was it the medication making her sick, or were there underlying seizures? No one knew, least of all me.

By the middle of January, what had previously looked like tremors definitively became seizures, what I now (years later) understand to be breakthrough seizures. I had a new dilemma. I couldn't send her to school in the middle of a seizure, but should I take her in once the seizure was done? The grade school became impatient with us because of her frequent absences and tardiness. The principal actually said to me, "Look, she had a seizure. Now she's on medication. What's the problem?"

Then, in February, I stood next to the principal explaining why my daughter had missed school yet again the previous day, while Emma sat on the floor having a break-through seizure right in the school hallway. It went on a good ten minutes before I finally said, look I must take Emma to the ER now. The woman looked at me quizzically and asked me why. I had to point out that Emma was having a seizure. I wondered if I was going crazy. Why couldn't other people see what I was seeing? It wasn't even a small seizure. It was a true tonic-clonic seizure marked with huge jerking motions on her entire right side. She could not stand. She could not walk. She barely could respond to me. Yes, it had not generalized, so she was not unconscious. But her eyes were rolling back into her head and her tongue was flicking in and out of her mouth. The principal suggested I take her into the "nurse's" office. (She wasn't a nurse, but a "health aide," I had learned by that time.) The health aide asked me, "How do you know this is a seizure and not just her cerebral palsy?" I didn't even know how to answer that. I finally said, after the seizure continued another ten minutes, "Look, I'm taking her to the ER." And I picked her up and drove her there myself.

At the hospital, the seizure continued for about another 15 minutes. But the nurse admitting her told me that it wasn't a seizure, "just tremors, because she isn't unconscious." I told her, yes it is. I had to explain to her what a breakthrough seizure looks like and what it is. I don't think she was ever convinced. Once my daughter was given an IV, the seizure faded and she felt better before long. As I'm writing this, I realize this was 2005, and yet fifteen years later, when it comes to seizures, I still have this ongoing sense that other people seem completely blind to what appears obvious to me.

Because of this incident, our neurologist happily referred us to her mentor at Riley Children's Hospital—again, a four-hour drive from us—but finally I knew my daughter was getting the medical care she needed. And the new neurologist wrote the school system authorizing Emma's need for homebound education until she had better control of the seizures.

Over the next several weeks, the new neurologist switched Emma's medication to Carbatrol, believing she was having a reaction to the Tegretol. By the time she was off the Tegretol, I had my daughter back. And she was happier at home. Homebound education is only a handful of hours a week, and I had to find ways to supplement that schooling and help her stay caught up in everything. And because her sister was in the same grade, based on what she was doing in her classroom, I was able to make sure we were on target for everything else. We subscribed to Netflix and started watching documentaries about history and the end of the Civil War. We watched nature documentaries and, on the weekends, we visited museums and nature centers at nearby state parks. We also checked out all of the Newberry Award children's books—and many of the runners up as well—and that is what we read most days, usually with her listening to the audio book while following along with the printed text.

I ordered some online materials, and together we worked on penmanship. And Emma, who struggled with printing, learned she could write beautifully in cursive. Her writing assignments were to write letters to relatives, and she soon got letters back in return. Once summer came, I also ordered a math curriculum online, and we started all the way back at one plus one. By the end of fifth grade, she knew all her single-digit math facts, understood multiplication and division, and I sent her to sixth grade—middle school—almost entirely caught up with her average classmate.

Even now, I don't think I can claim credit for the remarkable progress she made in those eighteen months outside the traditional classroom. Our approach was more of an "unschool" approach. Either one of two things happened. Maybe she was having seizures all along that were interrupting her learning—subclinical seizures that we never caught. And the medication solved this. Or, maybe it was simply a matter of letting her absorb the information at her own slower pace. I don't think I did anything special except let her learn. And she did.

Emma's seizures had been completely controlled for a year when she returned to public school in sixth grade. Sixth grade was middle school—a new school building, a new principal, new teachers, an actual nurse in the building, and new friends. And she made friends, one girl in particular who became her best friend. She was invited to slumber parties and went to movies with her and this girl's other friends.

And then another shoe dropped. After six years of complete control, the seizures came back during the summer between her sophomore and junior year. And they came back with a vengeance. By early winter, she was homebound again. She had a little reprieve from the seizures in the summer, so I enrolled her back into the high school in the fall. But the same thing happened again in November, and she was home once again. This time her neurologist was not able to make them stop. Emma finished high school in homebound instruction but also in the top twenty percent of her high-achieving class—totally mainstreamed with a full diploma. Her homebound teachers were extraordinary, and they were her biggest fans. She continued to participate in concert band, which required a note from her neurologist advocating that keeping her in this one class would be helpful for her emotionally. She was not allowed to participate on sports teams, but together she and I continued to train for her para-track events. But these were lonely years.

Another heartbreak came after graduation when her sister went off to college. She and I together had decided that there was no way she'd be able to go to college with these constant breakthrough seizures. When the seizures were at their worst, she would have dozens a day. I never had a completely accurate count, because often I couldn't tell when one seizure stopped and another began. And the seizures could happen at any time of the day. Emma ended up moving into my bed, because they frequently happened in the middle of the night. We both struggled to get a full night's sleep.

I found it increasingly difficult to work, and eventually I stopped altogether, and we lived off of my 401K for a number of years. We switched to a new neurologist in Chicago, and he added another medication, Keppra, that stopped the seizures for several months. I found a job—writing for a newspaper—but within a month or two, the seizures started again. Eventually, I left that job as well. The problem was, even if I hired someone to stay with Emma during the day, the nighttime seizures were so bad I got very little sleep. And if I had to hire help around the clock, it would cost more than I could earn. And yet, as long as I had that 401K, there was no government help available to us. And once Emma was nineteen, there was no help available for someone with uncontrolled seizures anyway. Believe me, I asked—many, many times. She was an adult, she was not cognitively disabled, and she was expected to simply endure the seizures on her own while I worked. The financial consequences were devastating.

In the end, with tons of studying and monitoring both the seizures, her health and even her diet, after nearly six years of uncontrolled seizures we realized that about 90 percent of them were triggered by a food additive, monosodium glutamate. It turns out that this isn't all that unusual, but never once in all those years did anyone—doctor, nurse or even fellow seizure sufferer—ever mention this could be a cause. In fact, there are a number of food triggers, and many people seem to diminish seizures substantially by careful scrutiny of their diets. And yet, you must do a lot of reading and a lot of digging to find this mentioned anywhere in print or online.

And then—almost abruptly—the seizures stopped. She was 24 years old, and we both were battle fatigued. But they stopped. Now, as she nears her 26th birthday, Emma lives independently in her own apartment. She's been working with vocational rehab for the past year, and she's applied for her first job. She's learning to use public transportation, and her apartment is downtown and right on the bus route. She's been teaching Sunday school since she graduated from high school, and she volunteers at a local library and a Ronald McDonald House a few blocks from her apartment. And she continues to train athletically, and in the summer competes at a few para-track events in nearby states.

She went 21 months without a seizure. And then, in the time I was writing this article, she had three in one day. We don't know why. Sometimes it feels like we are stuck in some inner circle of hell. But then I remember the many people we know through CHASA and para-sports. It's never hard to think of someone else who has it worse. One family I know lost their 14-year-old son very suddenly this fall. He had a seizure and he died. And we have known a couple other kids who have passed from seizures or in surgery over the years.

But let me offer a conclusion. My biggest irritation with the medical community is that professionals don't tend to see the whole person. They work on the spasticity of the hand or the leg, or even the torso. There are exercises and stretches. There are Botox injections every three months—potentially for life—to reduce the spasticity. The orthotist fits the child with a leg brace or two to attempt to correct the gait and help the child walk more normally. And from the very beginning of awareness, this child must work harder than any other child to walk, to talk, to eat, to write, and to learn. It is a burden to family resources, eating up time and financial resources, to make the child more—what—*normal*? And then we ask, how great is normal anyway, if we also are making the child miserable?

I'll tell you what it feels like to the parent who is doing everything within her own means to give her child the best start in life, but she is wearing herself out, and money becomes tight from all the bills. All free time is taken up with the child's at-home therapy. There is that never-ending search for toys that will encourage a baby to use both hands. The search for shoes that fit over braces and for elastic waist pants for little girls who can't deal with zippers and buttons when the need to use the toilet is pressing. You're on the hunt for pediatric speech pathologists one year, TES-trained physical therapists the next, only to be hunting a few years later for a pediatric endocrinologist because it isn't normal—is it?—for a small child to develop body odor and begin to grow pubic hair when she's seven. And every single night there's the schoolwork that didn't get finished during class time.

Marriages end. Siblings get short-changed. And 401Ks get drained.

I've become exceedingly cautious regarding my expectations from medical professionals. They all want to help, and I don't question their good intentions. But I have to conclude, based on my experience, that in reality there is little we truly understand about the human body and the way each and every part of our bodies is interconnected, one piece with another. Every attempt we make to fix the body has to be considered in the context of what that effort will do to the spirit. Because, without a doubt, nothing is more disabling than unseen emotional, spiritual and psychological damage. And isn't the medical mandate to first do no harm?

What I find myself telling other parents at the beginning of this journey is this one thing: Accept your child as she is. That doesn't mean you shouldn't do the therapies or the surgeries or any other possibility offered. But first and foremost, just love your kid for the person she is. Then pace yourself. Because this is a marathon, not a sprint. Parents, take care of your spouses. Make sure one parent is not the only caregiver. And take care of yourselves.

Living with Cancer: A Story of Education

Anonymous Contributor
Journal of Life Care Planning, Vol. 18, No. 1 (33–37)
Printed in U.S.A. All rights reserved
2020 Int'l Assoc. of Rehab Professionals

By way of introduction, I am a patient who is in her 40s, who did not receive a cancer diagnosis until the cancer became metastatic. This occurred despite having sought screening and treatment for several years leading up to diagnosis. In 2020, I have a diagnosis of stage 4 cancer. Along this journey, I have learned that I am my own best advocate, to always request a copy of all test results, to always ask questions about test results and treatment options, and to request monitoring of disease progression when new symptoms appear.

Disability Diagnosis

At the time of my biopsy, I was asked by the physician where my husband or family was, and I was told they could not give me any information until I could make an appointment where my husband could accompany me to receive the initial diagnosis. That was extremely stressful because I felt like I was being told the results were bad, without the doctors directly telling me what was happening in my body.

After I had the first scan after I was diagnosed, I was told my doctor would receive the results later that day which he would share with me. However, if the results were bad, I would hear from someone before my next scheduled appointment. Being a new patient, with no background knowledge of cancer diagnosis or treatment, I heard that and thought that I understood that I was fine if no one called me sooner.

I really do not feel like I received a lot of education or preparation for learning that I had stage 4 cancer. For example, I had originally been told the cancer was stage 2B. However, when I went to a pre-chemo appointment with a friend/co-worker, I was told that my diagnosis was in fact not curable, and that I would be treated palliatively. I was not called or warned that the staging at diagnosis had changed, or that I should have someone with me for results, or even that I would be receiving results the day that I did. I thought that if the oncologist had already communicated a staging number and letter to me, that was the stage. I was unaware that it could change.

I was discouraged against conducting my own research online at my diagnosis appointment. I was told that online research was often a bad idea because every individual is different and other people's experiences online, or generalized information did not specifically apply to me. It would be better not to scare myself, but to listen to what specifically applied to me from my own doctor, which made a lot of sense to me and I did was I was told.

Acute Care Services

My initial treatment included dose dense neoadjuvant chemotherapy, a bilateral mastectomy, complete hysterectomy, oophorectomy, and palliative radiation. I requested aggressive treatment because it was very important to me to try and become "stable" as soon as I possibly could. I was told that I could possibly live for a long time, if we could keep the cancer from spreading beyond my lymph nodes and bones to my organs. After being told about my stage four diagnosis, I remember days and days of crying. I was in disbelief that over a period of four years, I had sought the opinion of a radiologist, a surgeon, and my primary care physician (whose office also treated me for my well woman exams), yet I was not diagnosed until it was "too late."

I had both the bilateral mastectomy and hysterectomy during the same surgery. While the surgeon was performing the hysterectomy and oophorectomy, he discovered my upper colon was also twisted, and he repaired that as well. When I awoke from surgery, I felt like I had been hit by a truck. I remember writhing in pain and being told that if I would stop moving around so much, that I would probably start to feel better. It was one of the worst experiences of my life. After being taken to my room, the nurse told me that I had a catheter, and it could be removed when I was ready, which I was. However, when I tried to use the bathroom, it was horribly painful and I wish that I would have left the catheter in longer. I was hospitalized for four days, and I found the nurses to be extremely kind, and the doctors treating me to be concerned and compassionate. I am very thankful that I also had a lot of support from friends, mostly newfound, through my local breast cancer support group.

Unfortunately, I did experience some complications during recovery. During the second night in the hospital, my swelled and I was horribly nauseated and in pain. I remember calling for the nurse over and over and being given injections through my IV line. I woke up the next morning and my arm was swollen with fluid because the vein where the IV was inserted had blown in the night. I don't think miserable is a strong enough word for how I felt. The nurse treating me could not access another vein because I was dehydrated, but a friend from my local support group came in while the nurse was speaking with me and she immediately asked why no one had attempted to access the power port in my chest used for chemotherapy. The nurse said she would try to find someone to do that because she was not trained to do so, and she needed sterile supplies. After the nurse left the room, my friend asked if she could pray for me, and I asked her to pray that I could throw up. She prayed for me, and I was so thankful that I was able to vomit about 5 minutes later. Shortly after that, a nurse came into my room and accessed my port to give me nausea and pain medication.

Transitioning Home

I had a six-week surgical recovery period at home, and I struggled a lot with side effects from anesthesia and pain medication. Moving around and taking care of simple tasks was painful because I did not want to take a lot of pain medication due to the side effects of nausea and constipation.

I was not offered in-home health care after surgery until a few minutes before my meeting with the anesthesiologist immediately before surgery. Given more time to plan and check on insurance benefits, I would have likely used the in-home health care assistance, but I did not have adequate time to consider it. Because of this, my husband stayed with me for the first two weeks of recovery and a good friend used her vacation time from work in order to stay with me for several days. After that, I was able to manage at home alone. I would have preferred that I was provided in-home care, so that my friend did not have to use her vacation time, but I was not given adequate time to plan for this.

When I was released to drive, I started palliative radiation for pain. I received radiation to my cervical spine, hip, and pelvis. I went to see the radiation oncologist for a consultation, and to be fitted for a mask that covered my head and neck which stopped at my shoulders. While having radiation, I was bolted to the table that was connected to the linear accelerator, used to deliver the beams to specific areas of my body. I was treated for all three areas at the first three visits. I was instructed to be nude and covered by a blanket from the waist down due to the hip and pelvis being radiated, and the need to line up the radiation beam with specific marks made at the beginning of treatment. Many people receive tattoos to mark these spots, but my team opted to use a Sharpie marker covered by a special tape and darkened at each visit. I found the first three visits to be very emotionally taxing. The room where the linear accelerator was located at did not have a traditional door, but an offset entryway, much like the entry of a public restroom. There were maintenance workers working on something in the ceiling in the hallway outside the entrance to the room, and employees using the hallway. I could hear talking and laughter while bolted to the table.

When the cervical spine portion of treatment was completed, I was uncovered from the waist down while I was still bolted to the table. I cried the entire time because I was unable to move, my face was covered, and my vision was restricted. I felt so scared and vulnerable. After the first session, the radiology tech suggested that I ask for medication to help with my anxiety, which I took for visits two and three, but it didn't make the experience any better. After visit three, my throat started to swell, my voice became hoarse, and I was unable to swallow solid food. I requested to speak with the radiation oncologist, and it was decided that I would take a break from the cervical radiation for the time being.

I continued to have pelvic and hip radiation without the mask. I developed severe diarrhea, and told the technicians, and requested to speak with the doctor. I complained repeatedly and tried to cancel several sessions. I was told the side effects were normal, to take Imodium, and that if I came to my appointments to finish, that I would be glad later because I would have then achieved the benefit of decreased hip and pelvic pain. The diarrhea became worse, and I told the technicians that I would not return until I talked to the doctor. I got an appointment to meet with the radiation oncologist, and he made an appointment for me to see a GI specialist. I also complained to the triage nurses at the cancer center, and I went in to have a nurse look at my throat. There were white spots in my throat as well as jaw swelling, so I prescribed an antibiotic for symptoms of strep throat.

The morning of my GI specialist appointment, I called a friend and asked her to drive me because I could not stand up straight. I called the radiation oncologist's office and told them that I would not be in for my appointment that day due to my symptoms. I was told that I was almost finished with the prescribed course and that the doctor wanted me to come in. When I got to the GI specialists office, I saw a nurse practitioner, who told me to go to the emergency room immediately.

I went to the emergency room, and my friend had to leave due to a prior obligation, so I called my husband at work to come and be with me. I had a CT scan, gave a stool sample, and I was given a shot of morphine for the pain, The ER doctor called the radiation oncologist's office and told them that I would not be in for my appointment. I was discharged from the emergency room several hours later and sent home. I was told to contact the cancer center in the morning. The next morning, my oncologist's nurse called and told me that I needed to be admitted to the hospital. I called my husband at work to come and take me to the hospital to check-in. I was admitted to a room with a broken toilet. It took almost 24 hours for the toilet to be repaired, and continuous changing of a plastic hat by the nurse's aide. I was on full contact precautions, meaning no one could enter my room without a gown, mask, and gloves. Unfortunately, only the daytime staff followed these procedures. When I questioned this, I was told by the night staff that they were not entering my bathroom or touching my things, so it wasn't necessary. When I told the daytime staff this, they listened, but nothing changed.

I was told that my doctor recommended that I be there for ten days (which insurance approved) but I asked to go home on day six. I was told that I had to have less than a specific number of bowel movements every 24 hours to be discharged. I met the goal on day 8, and I was able to go home. I lost over twenty pounds during my 8-day hospital stay.

After going home, I regretted my decision, as I had to clean my home with bleach, and continuously bleach my bathroom to avoid reinfection. I was home alone for about twelve hours each day, and I was very weak and struggled to take care of myself. I continued to take medication for about six weeks but relapsed due to taking antibiotics for a different infection, which caused six additional weeks of treatment. I was unable to take targeted therapy during this time.

I am currently monitored with monthly bloodwork, and quarterly scans at the cancer center in the same town where I live. I sought a second opinion after having complications after my initial treatment of chemotherapy, surgery, and a partial course of palliative radiation. Radiation was very difficult for me, and despite numerous complaints of side effects to the radiation oncologist, I became very sick with an infection that was the most miserable experience of my life.

Treatment Complications

During my cancer treatment, I have been diagnosed with Clostridioides difficile (also known as C. diff) twice. I did not get treatment for C. diff the first time it developed until it was a life-threatening situation and had difficulty getting my care team to take my concerns seriously about this complication.

I was given medication that caused me to have a compromised immune system and sent to radiation 4–5 weeks after major surgery. I had a complete hysterectomy and oophorectomy and I was then sent to have pelvic radiation for bone metastasis. At a surgical follow-up appointment, the gynecologist/surgeon told me no one cleared that with him. The hematologist/oncologist, radiation oncologist/gynecologist surgeon did not communicate with each other. This resulted in me contracting a life-threatening infection, hospitalization, and painful scar tissue that I had to have operated on later.

Critical Healthcare Team Members

I had a very good oncologist who treated me for the first two years after my diagnosis. After being told about my Stage 4 DeNovo diagnosis, my oncologist apologized to me for what I was incorrectly told about how scan results would be communicated, and she set up an appointment immediately for 7:30 am the next morning to speak with my husband and me together about my new treatment plan. I really appreciated that and I feel like she was thorough and caring. She arranged for me to see other providers, and provided referrals when necessary. She was always quick to investigate new symptoms and would ask if I wanted diagnostic tests, and noted when she believed tests were important to address disease progression or new symptoms. I appreciate that she treated me as an equally educated person, respected my input, took my concerns seriously, and that I never felt rushed during our appointments. I always knew that I could count on a response when I called her office with a concern.

Unfortunately, my oncologist left the oncology practice where I was being treated. I was assigned to a new oncologist who had a different approach, and he was more willing to "watch and wait" when I developed symptoms. I did not feel comfortable with his approach and I am currently investigating the option of changing providers.

Another important member of my treatment team was my primary care doctor. I am able to utilize my local primary care provider more quickly than my oncologist's office. I am able to call to follow-up on test results, make appointments to address side effects, to request new tests for symptoms, and to have a second set of eyes review test results with me. I have found this to be very helpful. This office does seem to want to move as quickly and efficiently as possible, so I find it necessary to have all of my concerns written down ahead of time. I do feel that I am treated with respect, that my questions and concerns are addressed, rather than quickly dismissed as if I am not able to understand the complete explanation. Like with my previous oncologist, I feel like I am treated as an educated individual who wants to learn as much as possible about my health conditions, and be part of the process when making treatment decisions. I appreciate that I am offered more than one option, and the pros and cons of each, instead of being given a prescription or referral and dismissed.

Ancillary Treatment Providers

I have received treatment for lymphedema, frozen shoulder, and deconditioning from my local physical therapy clinic. Lymphedema treatment helped me tremendously, but the frozen shoulder treatment actually made my pain worse, leading me to wonder if the person assigned to work with me had reviewed my scans and history. I was mostly given exercises to do by myself at the clinic. I expressed concern about my increased pain, but I did not feel that was taken seriously.

Because I lost a significant amount of strength and stamina, physical therapy was ordered for deconditioning. This occurred after surgeries and after I developed c-diff. Physical therapy was a very positive experience for me. My oncologist referred me to a physiotherapist, who I feel played a significant role in increasing my quality of life by listening to and addressing my concerns.

Interaction with Legal System

I became engaged in the legal process after being encouraged to have an attorney review my records by a nurse who was employed by one of my doctors. My husband and I have been fortunate that the legal team we found to assist us that has been very kind, supportive, and thorough. We appreciate the assistance that we have received in finding out what went wrong with my care.

According to the medical experts hired by my attorney, I would not have been diagnosed Stage 4 at the beginning if my past mammograms had been read correctly. I believe that if I had been offered a copy of the radiologist's report, and imaging, and had a doctor review those with me when tests were ordered, that I would have been diagnosed with cancer at a much earlier stage. I was not given that opportunity, but as a patient, I feel there is a lack of patient care in medical test reporting. The medical system where I was diagnosed, and I am being treated, does not offer these things to patients. I received a generic "all clear" form letter, and that is all. However, there remains the expectation that the radiologists will read the reports correctly. I continue to believe that if the imaging and report were reviewed with me by a medical professional at the time that the tests were ordered, the delayed diagnosis would not have occurred.

Litigation was not something I dwelled on. I tried to not dwell on the process, and to address the issues involved as they came up. I found that it was better for me to keep a list of questions as they came up, if they could wait, and then sending 5–10 questions all at the same time. I understand that I am not the only client my attorney has, and by addressing my questions like that, I would not dwell on my feelings about the delayed diagnosis all the time. It was better for me mentally to just let the attorneys do their jobs, and to not dwell on my diagnosis, or how I feel I have been wronged in my day-to-day life. I try to think of myself as someone living with cancer, rather than dying of cancer, and focusing on the litigation involved did not help me focus on the positive aspects of living my life every day. It is sometimes very hard to not be upset about what happened, but I try to live with hope and to be grateful for the time I have.

Advice for Professionals

I think it would be very valuable for the metastatic patients at my cancer center to have their own advocate or nurse navigator to assist them in finding information, making appropriate appointments and treatment, and understanding test results. Throughout this process, I have been given medication outside the standard of care guidelines, which was only corrected when I questioned it. I have had bad lab results, which have only been followed-up on after I, myself, reviewed the reports in my patient portal. I would encourage providers to set up a protocol regarding what patients are told after they have scans, when results will be communicated, and for all providers to communicate with each other.

If a hospital system or cancer center does not have the resources to monitor patients closely, they should provide medication guidelines, treatment protocols, and any other information helpful to the patient to self-monitor and have a mechanism to report issues for follow-up. I think it is very important that providers listen to patients about symptoms and run the proper tests to rule out all causes that do not include side effects.

Disability Resources

When I was initially diagnosed, the nurse navigator for my cancer center was out of town, but she left a folder for me with calendar sections, a list of reputable websites, and the phone numbers of all my providers. It was a great organizational tool that I really appreciated. This was also helpful because it gave me a place to keep the paperwork that I was given at each appointment together, so that I could refer to it when I needed to find information. The nurse navigator met me at my first oncology appointment and after I had surgery. She made sure I had her telephone number in case I had any questions.

After I had a surgery to remove as much soft tissue cancer as possible, that support went away. I have not been contacted or had anyone check on me since that time, over three years ago. This is in part because our cancer center only has one nurse navigator for all newly diagnosed patients, but that does not mean that I do not still have questions, or need support. I do understand that I can call if I need to, but now when I call the nurse navigator, I am referred to the triage nurses at the cancer center. As a stage 4 patient, I feel like any assistance I received at the beginning of my treatment has gone away.

I joined a Facebook support group for women with my diagnosis and searched the posts on the page for questions I could ask my doctor regarding treatment and to address side effects. I asked about the cancer drug and the medication for side effects that I now take, both of which I learned about from other patients. I do not know how my experience, treatment, or outcome would be different, if I was not an active part of my own care team, (always asking questions including the pros and cons of treatments) if I was not part of the online support group.

Advice for Patients

In general, my experience has been that I have people on my care team work independently of each other. I believe it would be much better for patients if these medical professionals worked together as a team for me, rather than me carrying messages and reports from each independent medical office to the next. I worry that something will fall through the cracks because I may not know the right questions to ask, or what to look for. If I was not advocating for myself, I do not believe that my care would be as thorough.

If you do not feel well as a result of a treatment, you have the power to refuse treatment until you seek another opinion, even if that only involves an appointment with your primary care doctor or a local specialist to be sure those symptoms are thoroughly investigated.

I recommend that patients get manufacturer and standard of care instructions for all medications and treatments. Ask a lot of questions, and take two copies of the questions to your appointments- one for you, which you can mark the questions off as the doctor addresses them and one for the physician. If possible, have someone with you who take notes. If I handed my list to the doctor, in my experience, my questions would not all get answered.

If you have a scan or test, ask the doctor to look at it with you and ask for a copy of the report. Take a highlighter and mark anything you do not understand and ask about it.

Keep a binder with your information in, that you take from doctor to doctor. You will be responsible for asking your doctors to communicate and for double and triple checking that they do. For example, I had gynecological surgery last summer to address the scar tissue caused having radiation too soon after surgery, and I knew from reading in my support group that I needed to take a break from targeted therapy if I was going to have any procedure that could result in infection. I proactively asked the gynecologist/surgeon if I should contact the oncologist. That was affirmed, and I called the oncologist's office. The oncologist let me know how long to hold the medication and said they expected to hear from the surgeon. On the day of surgery, the surgeon asked me what I had been told by the oncologist. The two offices never spoke to each other about my treatment or the surgery.

Most importantly ... Take the initiative to advocate for yourself, no one else will do it for you! I still do not receive a copy of images or reports unless I specifically request them. They are not offered to me. The only reason that I know that I can request them is because the nurse who initially advised me to seek legal counsel made me aware, I can request these.

Chapter 35

Life Care Planning Costing, Literature, and Summary of Resources

Mary Barros-Bailey

A portion of the cost section of the chapter is adapted from the Resources chapter by Mahina and Watson (2018) in the 4th edition of the *Life Care Planning & Case Management Handbook*.

Life Care Planning Costing, Literature, and Summary of Resources

Resources for life care planners are an important part of practice because life care planners provide services to a demographically, functionally, and medically heterogenous group of evaluees—a single source or resource does not fit all cases. Because of increased accessibility to a variety of costing, literature, and other resources year after year, this Resources chapter takes a bit of a different approach than in past editions of this text. While some resources are listed for each category, perhaps more importantly, this chapter seeks to provide life care planners with the techniques and tools to find their own resources, given the need to individualize each evaluation.

In the 'Costing' section of this chapter, some of the information is derived from Maniha and Watson (2018) in the 4th edition of the *Life Care Planning & Case Management Handbook*. In that edition, Mahina and Watson (2018) stated the following about costing approaches in life care planning:

> The life care planner with the competitive edge is the one who has a multitude of data from a variety of reputable sources rather than just the basics involved in setting up the outline for the recommendations for the life care plan. Without proper resources that are easily accessible, understandable, and updateable, the task of completing a competent, thorough, and accurate life care plan can be formidable … Using top-notch

research and providing transparent costs will help the expert during [a] deposition when asked to provide and explain the source ... The process of researching requires the life care planner to identify and define needed information and cultivate effective resources to locate the information (pp. 730–731).

We introduce a new section called critical appraisal publications as an effort to bring the life care planning community to the cutting edge of the inclusion of this emerging body of literature in the development of evidence-based life care plans. In this section, we not only provide a comprehensive bibliography of various critical appraisal literature, but also provide a case study gauged as provided life care planners with easy-to-follow instructions on how to find their own literature based on the needs of their individualized assessments.

The 'Summary of Resources' section of this chapter seeks to be a repository of resources gleaned from the various chapters in this text. The consolidation of information becomes a quick-glance repository of information for the reader.

Costing Practice and Resources

Johnson and Woodard (2022) provide a historical timeline, definitions, and literature review covering life care planning cost techniques and methods. Readers are referred to the article for contextual information about the emergence of costing functions in the life care planning process.

Definitions, Consensuses, and Standards

Fundamental definitions or updates since the publication of the Johnson and Woodard (2022) article are covered in this section.

Life Care Planning Definition

At the core of the precepts in life care planning is the definition of the practice of life care planners that posits that identified needs have associated costs (International Conference on Life Care Planning and International Academy of Life Care Planners, 1998). Johnson et al. (2022) explored the "associated cost" component of the quarter-century definition and found it repeated or inferred in more recently emerged life care planning professional or credentialing organization documents of the American Academy of Physician Life Care Planners™ as well as the American Association of Nurse Life Care Planners®/Certified Nurse Life Care Planner® credentialing board joint statement.

Costing-Relevant Consensus Statements

Furthermore, consensus statements across the field of life care planning resulted in the following (Johnson et al., 2018):

- research ... costs (#54)
- use protocols for cost research (#69)
- identify costs in life care plans that are verifiable from appropriately referenced sources; geographically specific when appropriate and available; non-discounted/market rate; more than one cost estimate, when appropriate (#85)
- gather geographically relevant and representative prices (#70)

2022 Standards of Practice by the International Academy of Life Care Planners

Most recently, practice standards (International Academy of International Academy of Life Care Planners, 2022) call for life care planners to delineate costs and produce work product by using the following standards and practice competencies (p. 18):

- Delineating costs

    This step includes methodology for determining the costs of future care recommendations.

    14. STANDARD: The life care planner uses a consistent, valid, and reliable approach to costs.

    PRACTICE COMPETENCIES

    a. Uses a consistent method to determine costs for various categories of available/needed services.
    b. Uses geographically relevant and representative costs.
    c. Identified services and products from reliable sources.
    d. Follows a consistent method for organizing and interpreting data for projecting costs.
    e. Explains the life care planning process to involved parties to obtain needed information.
    f. Cites verifiable cost data.

- Work product creation

    This step addresses communication about future care recommendations and costs.

    15. STANDARD: The life care planner communicates their opinions.

    PRACTICE COMPETENCIES:

    a. Follows a consistent method for creating the narrative component of the life care plan report.
    b. Develops and uses documentation tools for reports and cost projections.
    c. Considers classification systems (e.g., International Classification of Diseases [ICD], Current Procedural Terminology [CPT], Healthcare Common Procedure Coding System [HCPCS], International Classification of Functioning, Disability, and Health [ICF]) to provide clarity regarding care recommendations and costs.
    d. Records lack of access to pertinent information.

Therefore, the definitions, consensuses, and updated standards of practice in life care planning all suggest the importance of transparency, consistency, and methodology in costing. However, none of these documents that are fundamental to life care planning practice are prescriptive or descriptive of an agreed-upon method for gathering associated costs for the identified needs described in a life care plan. At least at this point in life care planning practice, costing methodology is left to each individual life care planner as long as the methodology meets the basic criteria outlined in practice documents.

Usual, Customary, and Reasonable (UCR) Pricing

The American Medical Association's (AMA) definition of usual, customary, and reasonable (UCR) pricing (H-385.923) has not changed since it was adopted in 2013 at their annual meeting and published in the last edition of this text (Mahina & Watson, 2018). Specifically, the AMA defines UCR policy as:

1. Our AMA adopts as policy the following definitions:
   a. "usual" fee means that fee usually charged, for a given service, by an individual physician to his[/her] private patient (i.e., his[/her] own usual fee;
   b. a fee is "customary" when it is within the range of usual fees currently charged by physicians of similar training and experience, for the same service within the same specific and limited geographical area; and
   c. a fee is "reasonable" when it meets the above two criteria and is justifiable, considering the special circumstances of the particular case in question, without regard to payments that have been discounted under governmental or private plans.
2. Our AMA takes the position that there is no relationship between the Medicare fee schedule and Usual, Customary, and Reasonable fees (AMA, 2013).

By definition, UCR does not include Medicare, insurance, or out-of-pocket costs. Also, some coverage systems do not provide for the needs that may be included within the scope of a life care plan. Therefore, as noted by Mahina and Watson (2018), "the life care planner must be careful when utilizing the medical codes and databases to not use Medicare rules for the developing of pricing in the plan" (p. 732).

Whether to use usual and customary rates and at what level to include these in a life care plan is a topic in which there is not common agreement within life care planning at this time (Allison et al., 2022; Mahina & Watson, 2018; Saltiel, 2022). Because practitioners need to ethically and responsibly include costs that will provide the probably needed services over an individual's worklife or life expectancy, it is important that if there is variability in the UCR pricing, that variability should be clear in the life care plan. This means that the life care planner should not seek the lowest or the highest cost for the item or service but select sources that account for that variability over time if research supports such variation. Note that about 65% of respondents to the Neulicht et al. (2022) practice study indicated they used cash prices when developing a life care plan, the same percentage used billed charges as well as established fee schedules, and over 92% did not use discounted rates.

Contemporary Costing Practice in Life Care Planning

Glimpses at current practice of life care planning are measured through a survey of the field occurring about every decade (Neulicht et al., 2002, 2010). In their third decennial comprehensive survey of life care planning practice, Neulicht et al. (2022) collected data about contemporary costing practices by life care planners. By permission, a preliminary reporting of some of the study's outcomes relating to costing is summarized in this chapter in the areas of general practice as well as sources and resources.

General Practice

Over 82% of life care planners routinely included cost research in their electronic or paper case files, including more than 76% who include annual and/or lifetime summaries, and nearly half (46%) relied upon others for cost research. This suggests that while life care planners find costing research sufficiently important to maintain as part of their documentation, they may not necessarily be the ones gathering the costs themselves, although they may orchestrate the effort.

A clear majority of life care planners (68%) included a specific number of cost quotes for each item (over 70% obtained more than one cost quote) with the most important factors affecting the number of costs obtained as reported by over half the respondents being: (1) how many quotes to include being the availability of the item/service in the geographical area; (2) availability of current vendor appropriate cost; (3) item or service availability whatsoever, regardless of geographical area; and (4) the nature of the item or service itself. The number of quotes requested was not asked, although Johnson and Woodard (2022) described various sources that suggest a standard to be three; Barros-Bailey et al. (2022) suggest that the N=3 was insufficient (depending on the case) in items such as attendant care that can be an expensive, but vital, service for those who need it and a more robust form of data collecting that may include confidence levels and margins of error may be more adequate. Webcrawler tools, such as CostingHelper.com, that allow life care planners to search Google Shopping for items, have beta versions of descriptive statistics outcomes that may become more common for the life care planner.

About the same rate of life care planners (67%) stated that if they had difficulty quantifying a life care plan item, they incorporated an annual allowance. In obtaining the costs quotes, more than half (55%) of life care planners used billing codes from 76% to all of the time as is consistent with the literature (Mahina, 2020).

For ancillary costs (e.g., assembly, delivery, shipping, tax), there were none that were included by the majority of life care planners with the closest being shipping as noted by about 42% of respondents. However, the highest percentage of respondents (43%) stated not including any ancillary costs at all. Similarly, there was no identified practice by the majority of life care planners to use online services for childcare, home maintenance, housekeeping, remote medical monitoring, software/apps, tutoring, or yard maintenance costs.

Finally, the vast majority of life care planners (82%) did not discount to present value the costs in the life care plan, while about 10% performed this function 76%–100% of the time.

Pre-existing Conditions

For life care plans developed in a forensic setting, items included in the life care plan are supposed to be specific to injuries associated with the incident. In querying life care planners, the 2022 decennial study found that the vast majority (76%) did not include costs for goods and services related to pre-existing conditions in the life care plan.

Attendant and Facility Care

Residential care represented an area of practice where 58% of life care planners presented more than one option 76%–100% of the time. The same percentage of life care planners included private/direct hire costs when presenting home care options. However, a clear majority of life care planners did not include additional costs for expenses such as food, utilities, supplies, etc. for live-in 24-hour care despite recent research suggesting the impact of licensing guidelines of some states, and potentially federally in the United States, which may substantially impact costing for this level of care (Barros-Bailey et al., 2022). For pediatric evaluees, 63% of life care planners consider the time a parent could be expected to perform parenting duties in the life care planner's recommendation for in-home supervision.

Considering the various categories contained in a life care plan, there was no clear majority of life care planners who used personal contacts to obtain goods and services. From 76%–100% of the time, the two areas that life care planners were most likely to use personal contacts to obtain pricing was for home care (48%) and facility care (45%). The Attendant Care Survey Methodology (ACSM) introduced in 2022 (Barros-Bailey et al.) may provide life care planners with a methodologically defensible tool to obtain such costs that often tend to be one of the largest cost items when such need is identified in a life care plan. The two areas where they were least likely to make calls to obtain costs were for home furnishings/accessories (20%) and potential complications (19%).

Architectural Accommodations and Retrofitting

For architectural or retrofitting costs, there was not a single source that the majority of life care planners used, but most of the practice split almost evenly across five of the six choices as follows:

- VA home modification benefit, 30%
- Contractor estimate/quote, 30%
- Independent home accessibility evaluator/specialist, 27%
- Architect estimate/quote, 24%
- Literature, 22%
- Rehabilitation engineer, 8%

Costing Sources and Resources

Greater than 76% of life care planners determined the following (in descending order) as sources of life care planning costs:

- Current vendors and providers, 65%
- Local vendors and providers, 64%
- Internet, 61%
- National databases with geographic adjustment, 59%
- Medical bills, 44%
- Manufacturers, 35%
- Life care planner's office cost file or database, 32%
- Price transparency data published by hospitals, 30%
- Catalogs, 18%
- National databases without geographic adjustment, 9%

Based on the sources identified as being predominant as resources, it is likely that the majority of life care planners are still reaching out and making calls to obtain pricing data for at least some of their costing tasks. Mahina and Watson (2018) proposed the use of the Area Cost Analysis Form as a data-gathering tool to detail the results of the data collection efforts. Barros-Bailey et al. (2022) also provided a form for the collection of data specific to attendant care costs. There is no standardized tool used by life care planners to record results from any specific data collection mode.

One of the newly listed sources used by nearly a third of life care planners is the Hospital Price Transparency enacted on January 1, 2021 (Centers for Medicare & Medicaid Services [CMS],

2022). The federal government of the United States now requires each hospital operating in the country to "provide clear, accessible pricing information online about the items and services they provide in two ways: (1) As a comprehensive machine-readable file with all items and services; (2) In a display of shoppable services in a consumer-friendly format" (paras. 1–3). Although CMS has a monitoring and enforcement plan, and life care planners in different areas of the country have had varied experiences accessing such cost information, just a year after the rule came into effect only 16% of hospitals were in compliance by August 2022 (PatientsRightsAdvocate.org, 2022). However, this is a source of costing that should be monitored by life care planners into the future as more hospitals come on board and the process may become standardized based on CMS criteria.

The three most used databases by life care planners were GoodRx (73%), FairHealth (54%), and American Hospital Directory (48%). There were an additional 23 private and public databases cited by life care planners in the United States while respondents in Canada indicated that none of the databases listed applied to their geographic setting. The most common categories where life care planners tended to use these databases 76%–100% of the time were aggressive medical/surgical interventions and future medical care routine (46% each); projected therapeutic modalities (45%); and acute medical interventions, projected evaluations, and medications (43% each). The least likely use of databases by life care planners were for architectural renovations (20%), home furnishings/accessories and transportation (19% each), and vocational/educational plan (15%).

As databases for a variety of life care planning needs seem to be used by a large number of life care planners, it is important that the life care planners understand some basic issues about relational database validity and reliability. Validity refers to the accuracy of the data outcome derived from the database while reliability is the consistency of the data outcome given searching the database with the same search criteria. Relational database validity is synonymous with data integrity that the life care planner may be required to answer and should, thus, seek from the database developer or publisher. Cote (2021) at Harvard Business School identified four threats to the validity of a dataset: human error, inconsistencies across formats, collection error, and cybersecurity or internal privacy breaches. Data integrity questions posed to costing databases could be in areas such as:

(1) Where and when were the data included in the database collected?
(2) What type of costing data is in the database (UCR, discounted, capped fees, etc.)?
(3) If there is a geographical adjustment, what geographical area is the benchmark and how is the adjustment validated to the area of interest?
(4) Does the database have validation studies for any inferred, smoothed, or otherwise adjusted data? (That is, what studies exist for the database verifying that the data is not wrong or misleading?)
(5) How often is the data updated?
(6) What are the data quality protocols in place to ensure there is no errors in data import or export?
(7) Is the data randomly or non-randomly collected? Specifically, what is the impetus for those contributing data to have it in the database that might skew the dataset?
(8) Does the data collected fall into a normal curve?
(9) How were outliers in the dataset handled?
(10) Are basic descriptive statistics available (e.g., Standard Error of Mean)?

Many more questions about data integrity are important for life care planners to develop as they search for costs.

Reliability refers to how consistently someone searching the database given the same criteria gets the same outcome. Remember that because there is reliability in a database does not mean there is validity as the outcome could always be the same regardless of who searches the database, but the outcome could be wrong (invalid).

Decision-Making Factors in Costing Source Selection

Over 92% of life care planners who noted the predominant factor affecting their decision-making in determining which resource(s) to use in costing cited the geographic location. Other factors noted by the majority of life care planners were the life care planner's experience with the item, service, vendor, or provider, as well as the evaluee/family preferences. Less than half of life care planners noted the following costing factors in descending order: treating physician preferences; time frames for completion of life care plan; referral source request; or other (availability of item or medical bills, billing, usual and customary practice, etc.).

Collateral Sources

It is noteworthy that half of life care planners did not identify collateral sources as a mechanism for funding in a life care plan although 31% stated this was included if required by statute or case law and another 29% included such sources when this was requested by the referral source. About one in eight life care planners performing a peer review would include collateral sources in a rebuttal report.

Life Care Planning Software

Historically, life care planning software has been of three types: (1) relational databases developed by software companies with some affiliation to the field, (2) proprietary spreadsheets, or (3) word processing tables developed by life care planners. There is not a predominant software platform that most life care planners use with new or emerging applications entering the market. To learn more about existing software, a life care planner can solicit input about current packages from online discussion boards, at professional development training sessions, or from colleagues. The life care planner new to relational database who is not developing their own spreadsheet or word processing tables is encouraged to request a free trial of the software to determine if it has the features most desired.

Critical Appraisal Literature in Life Care Planning

Critical appraisal of the literature is defined by Burls (2016) as "the process of carefully and systematically examining research to judge its trustworthiness, and its value and relevance in a particular context" (p. 2). For an in-depth discussion of critical appraisal literature, the reader could review Chapter 3 in this text or perform a simple query on a search engine. Simply put, critical appraisal literature provides a detailed and methodical review of all accessible literature located for a certain topic that meets the reviewer's selection criteria. Instead of accessing one article about one study on one topic, researchers seek all available literature on the topic of study and empirically analyze the evidence based on selected common criteria to determine the overall outcomes between studies, if possible. Such critical examination of the relevant quantitative, qualitative, or mixed methods literature is the gold standard and is often called a meta-analysis (quantitative data), meta-synthesis (qualitative data), mixed methods/research synthesis/review (quantitative + qualitative data), systematic review, or other similar terminology.

Although critical appraisal literature is fairly new to the current generation of researchers or practitioners in healthcare and other professions, in some disciplines or areas of study where there has been much research performed and a variety of systematic reviews or meta-analyses exist, another procedure to examine the evidence between all available critical appraisal reviews or analyses is called an umbrella review. Specifically, Aromataris et al. (2015) describe umbrella reviews as allowing:

> the findings of reviews relevant to a review question to be compared and contrasted. An umbrella review's most characteristic feature is that this type of evidence synthesis only considers for inclusion the highest level of evidence, namely other systematic reviews and meta-analyses … including diverse types of evidence, both quantitative and qualitative (para. 1).

An umbrella review is at the pinnacle of the critical appraisal literature gold standard. Not all topics, nor all areas of study, reach this evidence level or have the sufficient quantity or quality of research to qualify for a critical review of the literature, much less an umbrella review. The reason for this is that the field of study is nescient (e.g., life care planning) and there are insufficient numbers of studies to be methodologically examined for overarching comparisons and contrasts; another reason is that the topic could be so narrow that few researchers have examined it.

Life care planners can elevate the bar of evidence in their life care plans with the inclusion of research publications, and at the critical appraisal level whenever feasible. Beginning with the 5th edition of this text on life care planning across the lifespan, we seek to assist life care planners to meet and scale the growing trend towards aligning the individualized assessment with evidence-based practice by putting some of the critical appraisal literature at the reader's fingertips as well as providing "how to" resources to find some of this literature. The critical appraisal bibliographies included in this chapter cover the last five years before the publication of this text (2017–2022) and are on the main topics relevant to the chapters. Rather than being an all-inclusive bibliography, what is presented in this chapter is a start based on an all-database EBSCO search. Authors of specific chapters may have included critical appraisal or other literature not covered in this chapter. Therefore, the bibliographies in this chapter should not be considered all-inclusive or comprehensive as there may be reviews that are older and may be more on point to individual needs that went beyond the scope of this chapter. What is clear is that life care planners in the future will have a greater burden placed upon them to support their opinions. See discussions in other chapters regarding the new Rule 702 "preponderance of evidence" requirement for federal cases in the United States taking effect in December 2023. With greater demands placed upon life care planners to support their opinions with primary (what you collect yourself for the case, like interview information) and secondary (what someone else collected that you use for the case such as medical records, articles, etc.) evidence, familiarity with, and access to, critical appraisal or research literature is vital.

How Do Life Care Planners Find Critical Appraisal Literature?

Some life care planners may be under the impression they need to affiliate with an academic institution or pay exorbitant prices to access scholarly articles. Although that perception might have been accurate in years past, this is no longer the case.

Since 2019, life care planning students at Capital University Law School's Life Care Planning graduate certificate program have been required to join their local libraries and determine what academic databases are available to them—for free—as library members. This assignment allowed students to identify a local and accessible source to increase the evidence support in their plans once they finish their training and no longer had access to the university's library. Although a couple of students reported difficulty finding the academic databases at their local library, because these resources are sometimes buried deep into the webpages of the library's website, in 100% of the cases, students found they had access to such databases regardless of their rural or urban location or where they resided throughout the United States. Most of the time, the PDF article for the desired publication was available free through the library's research database (Academic Search Premier, EBSCO, GALE, Google Scholar, JSTOR, MEDLINE, PsycINFO, PubMed, Web of Science, etc.) that the life care planning student accessed from home/office through the library's website. If the desired publication was not available, the library could typically obtain it free for the life care planner through Interlibrary Loan (ILL) either on the day of the request or soon thereafter. Very, very rarely, a local library cannot access the desired article usually because the publication is out of print and is not owned by any of the membership libraries that are part of the network to which the library affiliates.

Beyond academic databases available for free from the local library, increasingly, using the same search method and terms, the life care planner can find critical appraisal literature through an internet browser search. The techniques used to find pinpoint accurate publications through academic research databases at your library can be used to return the same or other critical appraisal literature on a search engine. Spending 15 minutes undergoing a tutorial (e.g., YouTube, library) of effective database search techniques (e.g., Boolean) can save the life care planner hours of research time in the future through increased effectiveness and efficiency.

Critical Appraisal Literature Case Study

Kim is a life care planner who is dually credentialled as an occupational therapist and rehabilitation counselor. She is developing a life care plan for a child with a mild traumatic brain injury (mTBI) and is interested in the critical appraisal literature over the last five years for therapy outcomes and recommendations. She recently joined her local library that has the Academic Search Premier research database. She also spent less than an hour searching YouTube videos on how to use Boolean and other search techniques. Some of her favorite shortcuts include using quotation marks to delimit the searches to the terms that are precisely within the quotes or the asterisk (called a wildcard) to expand the search to terms that might have different endings to shorten her search time (e.g., disab* for disability, disabilities, disabled, etc.; orthop* for orthopedist/orthopedics). For the case of the child with mTBI, within 30 minutes of searching on the Academic Search Primer and Google, the life care planner found excellent resources. This is what Kim did:

1. CHOOSING THE DATABASE/LEVEL OF SEARCH: Choose all the databases in the Choose Databases option in Academic Search Primer/EBSCPO and went to Advanced Search.

2. SEARCH TERMS

Searching: Academic Search Premier, Show all | Choose Databases

"brain injury"	Select a Field (optional)
AND child* OR youth OR adolescent	Select a Field (optional)
AND therap*	Select a Field (optional)
AND systematic review or meta-analysis	Select a Field (optional)

This search resulted in 476 publications from 1981 through 2022, a bit too much for Kim to sift through.

3. To refine her search to more scholarly articles she could access immediately or very quickly, the life care planner further refined her search to only publications that were full text and peer-reviewed (see below), which further narrowed her selection to 145 publications from 2000 through 2022.

Limit To
- ☑ Full Text
- ☐ References Available
- ☑ Peer Reviewed

From: 2000 To: 2022 Publication Date

Within several minutes, Kim had access to the PDF copies of several articles she found helpful to her life care planning recommendations, including:

Agnihotri, S., Lynn Keightley, M., Colantonio, A., Cameron, D., & Polatajko, H. (2010). Community integration interventions for youth with acquired brain injuries: A review. *Developmental Neurorehabilitation, 13*(5), 369–382. https://doi.org/10.3109/17518 423.2010.499409

Gmelig Meyling, C., Verschuren, O., Rentinck, I. R., Engelbert, R. H. H., & Gorter, J. W. (2022). Physical rehabilitation interventions in children with acquired brain injury: A scoping review. *Developmental Medicine and Child Neurology, 64*(1), 40–48.

Kamba, G., & Plourde, V. (2022). Psychoeducational interventions and postconcussive recovery in children and adolescents: A rapid systematic review. *National Academy of Neuropsychologists, 37*(3), 568–582.

Linden, M. A., Glang, A. E., & McKinlay, A. (2018). A systematic review and meta-analysis of educational interventions for children and adolescents with acquired brain injury. *NeuroRehabilitation, 42*(3), 311–323.

Quantman-Yates, C., Cupp, A., Cunsch, C., Haley, T., Vaculik, S., & Kujawa, D. (2016). Physical rehabilitation interventions for post-mTBI symptoms lasting greater than 2 weeks: Systematic review. *Physical Therapy, 96*(11), 1753–1763. https://doi.org/10.2552/ptj.20150557

Ross, K. A., Dorris, L., & McMillan, T. (2011). A systematic review of psychological interventions to alleviate cognitive and psychosocial problems in children with acquired brain injury. *Developmental Medicine and Child Neurology, 53*(8), 692–701.

Thomas, R. E., Alves, J., Vaska Mlis, M. M., & Magalhaes, R. (2017). Therapy and rehabilitation of mild brain injury/concussion: Systematic review. *Restorative Neurology and Neuroscience, 35*(6), 643–666.

4. Buoyed by the cache of research articles found through her successful search, and understanding that each database is indexed differently or may have varied publications indexed within it, Kim opted to also do a search on the Google search engine to determine if other relevant literature could be identified. Again, using the Boolean approach she learned in her tutorial, her search terms were similar on Google as they had been on EBSCO and the search criteria looked like this:

```
← → C  ⊙ "brain injury", child* OR youth OR adolescent, therap*, "systematic review", "meta-analysis", PDF
```

In the first 100 hits, Kim found other literature that was helpful to her query:

Chan, V., Toccalino, D., Omar, S., Shah, R., & Colatonio, A. (2022). A systematic review on integrated care for traumatic brain injury, mental health, and substance use. *PLoS ONE*. https://doi.org/10.1371/journal.pone.0264116 https://journals.plos.org/plosone/article?id=10.1371/journal.pone.0264116

Department of Veterans Affairs, Department of Defense. (2016). *VA/DoD clinical practice guideline for the management of concussion-mild traumatic brain injury.* https://www.va.gov/covidtraining/docs/mTBICPGFullCPG50821816.pdf

Linden, M. A., Glang, A. E., & A. (2018). A systematic review and meta-analysis of educational interventions for children and adolescents with acquired brain injury. *NeuroRehabilitation, 42*(3), 311–323. https://doi.org/10.3233/NRE-172357. https://content.iospress.com/articles/neurorehabilitation/nre172357

Kochanek, P. M., Tasker, R. C., Carney, N., Totten, A. M., Adelson, P. D., Selden, N. R., Davis-O'Reilly, C., Hart, E. L., Bell, M. J., Bratton, S. L., Grant, G. A., Kissoon, N., Reuter-Rice, K. E., Vavilala, M. S., & Wainwright, M. S. (2019). Guidelines for the management of pediatric severe traumatic brain injury, third edition: Update of the Brain Trauma Foundation Guidelines, Executive Summary. *Neurosurgery, 84*(6), 1169–1178. https://www.biav.net/wp-content/uploads/2022/05/PD-05-Guidelines-for-the-Management-of-Pediatric-Severe-TBI-Neurosurgery-2019.0601.pdf

Kochanek, P. M., Totten, A. M., Selden, N. R., Bell, M. J., Kissoon, N., Reuter-Rice, K. E., & Wainwright, M. S. (2019). Guidelines for the management of pediatric severe traumatic brain injury, third edition: Update of the Brain Trauma Foundation Guidelines. *Pediatric Critical Care Medicine.* https://www.braintrauma.org/uploads/10/11/guidelines_pediatric3.pdf

Lumba-Brown, A., Yeates, K. O., Sarmiento, K., Breiding, M. J., Haegerich, T. M., Gioia, G. A., Turner, M., Benzel, E. C., Suskauer, S. J., Giza, C. C., Joseph, M., Broomand, C., Weissman, B., Gordon, W., Wright, D. W., Moser, R. S., McAvoy, K., Ewing-Cobbs, L.,

Duhaime, A.-C., Putukian, M., ... Timmons, S. D. (2018). Centers for Disease Control and Prevention guideline on the diagnosis and management of mild traumatic brain injury among children. *JAMA Pediatrics*. https://doi.org/10.1001/jamapediatrics.2018.2853. https://idph.iowa.gov/Portals/1/userfiles/32/Centers%20for%20Disease%20Control%20and%20Prevention%20Guideline%20on%20the%20Diagnosis%20and%20Management%20of%20Mild%20Traumatic%20Brain%20Injury%20Among%20Children.pdf

Qunatman-Yates, C. C., Hunter-Giordano, A., Shimamura, K. K., Landel, R., Alsalaheen, B. A., Hanke, T. A., & McCulloch, K. L. (2020). Physical therapy evaluation and treatment after concussion/mild traumatic brain injury: Clinical practice guidelines linked to the International Classification of Functioning, Disability, and Health from the Academic of Orthopaedic Physical Therapy, American Academic of Sports Physical Therapy, Academy of Neurologic Physical Therapy, and Academy of Pediatric Physical Therapy of the American Physical Therapy Association. *Journal of Orthopaedic & Sports Physical Therapy*, 50(4), CPG1–CPG73. https://doi.org/10.2519/jospt.2020.0301. https://www.jospt.org/https://doi.org//pdf/10.2519/jospt.2020.0301

Within her search, she also found a link to the full Thomas et al. (2017) article she had located in her EBSCO search.[1] Kim was not surprised to find so many clinical practice guidelines in her Google exploration as she knew that many of these guidelines include critical appraisal literature and are themselves often considered to be at the level of critical appraisal publications.

5. The review of search results through EBSCO and Google also identified other articles that could be helpful to other recommendations in the case. The literature not only provided Kim with support for some of the recommendations within her scopes of practice as an occupational therapist, rehabilitation counselor, and life care planner but also stimulated her with questions to ask other members of the transdisciplinary team for their input into the life care plan for greater internal validity of the life care plan.
6. Kim included a bibliography of the various articles she relied upon in an appendix and footnotes in her narrative report. When she received a subpoena for her file, she understood that for those copyrighted articles she obtained through EBSCO that were not found in the open-access Google search engine, she could only provide the reference from her bibliography but not a copy of the copyrighted article without infringing upon the copyright rights of the authors or publisher. Kim had also not provided copies of those articles to her referral source for the same copyright infringement reason. The subpoenaing party would need to either obtain the articles on their own or request the court to issue an order for copies of those materials.
7. Kim understood that when considering taking study data and applying it to her evaluee, the characteristics of the sample in the research needed to be similar to those of the person she was evaluating because the further apart those characteristics are between the individual and the study, the lower the potential for a valid application of the critical appraisal literature.

Bibliography of Critical Appraisal Literature from 2017–2022: Selected Topics

The bibliographies contained in this part of the chapter have been categorized by the areas in which they fell while performing an EBSCO/All database search. Because healthcare professionals treat individuals with a variety of different conditions, when searching the bibliographies, it would be prudent to look under both the type of individual who might treat the condition and the condition itself. If a source is not found in the bibliography, it could be that the perfect study exists but it is not at the level of critical appraisal (see Research in Life Care Planning chapter for identification of other forms of research and how they fall in the quality of evidence hierarchy). Alternatively, the perfect critical appraisal literature may exist, but it may be in a time period that is outside the five-year span searched for this chapter. Following are the individual bibliographies loosely correlated to the themes of each chapter in the text.

Care Over the Lifespan

Pediatric Care Management

Anthony, S. J., Stinson, H., Lazor, T., Young, K., Hundert, A., Santana, M. J., Stinson, J., & West, L. (2019). Patient-reported outcome measures within pediatric solid organ transplantation: A systematic review. *Pediatric Transplantation*, *23*(6), 1–15. https://doi.org/10.1111/petr.13518

Bapistella, S., Zirngibl, M., Buder, K., Toulany, N., Laube, G. F., & Weitz, M. (2021). Prophylactic antithrombotic management in adult and pediatric kidney transplantation: A systematic review and meta-analysis. *Pediatric Transplantation*, *25*(4), 1–10. https://doi.org/10.1111/petr.14021

Boerner, K. E., Green, K., Chapman, A., Stanford, E., Newlove, T., Edwards, K., & Dhariwal, A. (2020). Making sense of "somatization": A systematic review of its relationship to pediatric pain. *Journal of Pediatric Psychology*, *45*(2), 156–169. https://doi.org/10.1093/jpepsy/jsz102

Bunge, L. R., Davidson, A. J., Helmore, B. R., Mavrandonis, A. D., Page, T. D., Schuster-Bayly, T. G., & Kumar, S. (2021). Effectiveness of powered exoskeleton use on gait in individuals with cerebral palsy: A systematic review. *PloS ONE*, *16*(5), e0252193. https://doi.org/10.1371/journal.pone.0252193

Ciccia, A. H., Beekman, L., Ditmars, E., & DePompei, G. (2018). A clinically focused systematic review of social communication in pediatric TBI. *NeuroRehabilitation*, *42*(3), 331–344. https://doi.org/10.3233/NRE-172384

Cook, M. E., Braaten, E. B., & Surman, C. B. H. (2018). Clinical and functional correlates of processing speed in pediatric Attention Deficit/Hyperactivity Disorder: A systematic review and meta-analysis. *Child Neuropsychology*, *24*(5), 598–616. https://doi.org/10.1080/09297049.2017.1307952

de Cunha Menezes, E., Hora Santos, F. A., & Alves, F. L. (2017). Cerebral palsy dysphagia: A systematic review. *Revista CEFAC*, *19*(4), 565–573. https://doi.org/10.1590/1982-02160171944317

de Sena Oliveira, A. C., Athanasio, B. S., Mrad, F. C. C., Vasconcelos, M. M. A., Albuquerque, M. R., Miranda, D. M., & Simões e Silva, A. C. (2021). Attention deficit and hyperactivity disorder and nocturnal enuresis co-occurrence in the pediatric population: A systematic review and meta-analysis. *Pediatric Nephrology*, *36*(11), 3547–3559. https://doi.org/10.1007/s00467-021-05083-y

Dolbow, J. D., Dolbow, D. R., Stevens, S. L., & Hinojosa, J. (2017). Restorative effects of aquatic exercise therapies on motor, gait, and cardiovascular function in children with cerebral palsy: A review of literature. *Journal of Aquatic Physical Therapy*, *25*(1), 22–29.

Festante, F., Antonelli, C., Chorna, O., Corsi, G., & Guzzetta, A. (2019). Parent-infant interaction during the first year of life in infants at high risk for cerebral palsy: A systematic review of the literature. *Neural Plasticity*, 1–19. https://doi.org/10.1155/2019/5759694

Gaberova, K., Pacheva, I., & Ivanov, I. (2018). Task-related fMRI in hemiplegic cerebral palsy: A systematic review. *Journal of Evaluation in Clinical Practice*, *24*(4), 839–850. https://doi.org/10.1111/jep.12929

Gronski, M., & Doherty, M. (2020). Interventions within the scope of occupational therapy practice to improve activities of daily living, rest, and sleep for children ages 0–5 years and their families: A systematic review. *American Journal of Occupational Therapy*, *74*(2), 1–33. https://doi.org/10.5014/ajot.2020.039545

Hoegy, D., Bleyzac, N., Robinson, P., Bertrand, Y., Dussart, C., & Janoly-Dumenil, A. (2019). Medication adherence in pediatric transplantation and assessment methods: A systemic review. *Patient Preference & Adherence*, *13*, 705–719. https://doi.org/10.2147/PPA.S200209

Karadag-Saygi, E., & Giray, E. (2019). The clinical aspects and effectiveness of suit therapies for cerebral palsy: A systematic review. *Turkish Journal of Physical Medicine & Rehabilitation*, *65*(1), 93–110. https://doi.org/10.5606/tftrd.2019.3431

Karlsson, P., Allsop, A., Dee-Price, B.-J., & Wallen, M. (2018). Eye-gaze control technology for children, adolescents, and adults with cerebral palsy with significant physical disability: Findings from a systematic review. *Developmental Neurorehabilitation*, *21*(8), 497–505. https://doi.org/10.1080/17518423.2017.1362057

Marshall, A. N., Root, H. J., McLeod, T. C. V., & Lam, K. C. (2022). Patient-reported outcome measures for pediatric patients with sport-related injuries: A systematic review. *Journal of Athletic Training*, *57*(4), 371–384. https://doi.org/10.4085/1062-6050-0598.20

Martinie, O., Mercier, C., Gordon, A. M., & Robert, M. T. (2021). Upper limb motor planning in individuals with cerebral palsy aged between 3 and 21 years old: A systematic review. *Brain Sciences*, *11*(7), 920. https://doi.org/10.3390/brainsci11070920

Menor-Rordríguez, M. J., Sevilla Martín, M., Sánchez-García, J. C., Montiel-Troya, M., Cortés-Martin, J., & Rodríguez-Blanque, R. (2021). Role and effects of hippotherapy in the treatment of children with cerebral palsy: A systematic review of the literature. https://doi.org/10.3390/jcm10122589

Muldoon, D., Meyer, L., Cortese, J., & Zaleski, R. (2021). A literature review: Evidence base in speech-language pathology for the management of pediatric oral phase dysphagia. *Perspectives of the ASHA Special Interest Groups*, *6*(2), 444–453. https://doi.org/10.1044/2021_PERSP-19-00080

Mylonas, K. S., Repanas, T., Athanasiadis, D. I., Voulgaridou, A., Sfyridis, P. G., Bakoyiannis, C., Kapelouzou, A., Avgerinos, D. V., Tzifa, A., & Kalangois, A. (2020). Permanent pacemaker implantation in pediatric heart transplant recipients: A systematic review and evidence quality assessment. *Pediatric Transplantation*, *24*(3), 1–7. https://doi.org/10.1111/petr.13698

Nalbant, A., & Bedre, O. (2020). Essential muscle groups affected in cerebral palsy: Systematic review. *International Journal of Experimental & Clinical Anatomy*, *14*, S158.

Neugebauer, C., & Mastergeorge, A. M. (2021). The family stress model in the context of pediatric cancer: A systematic review. *Journal of Child & Family Studies*, *30*(5), 1099–1122. https://doi.org/10.1007/s10826-021-01928-0

Paprocka, J., Kaminiow, K., Kozak, S., Sztuba, K., & Emich-Widera, E. (2021). Stem cell therapies for cerebral palsy and autism spectrum disorder: A systematic review. *Brain Sciences*, *11*(12), 1–18. https://doi.org/10.3390/brainsci11121606

Poole, M., Simkiss, D., Rose, A., & Li, F.-X. (2018). Anterior or posterior walkers for children with cerebral palsy? A systematic review. *Disability and Rehabilitation: Assistive Technology*, *13*(4), 422–433. https://doi.org/10.1080/17483107.2017.1385101

Ramanandi, V. H., Parmar, T. R., Panchal, J. K., & Prabakar, M. M. (2019). Impact of parenting a child with cerebral palsy on the quality of life of parents: A systematic review of literature. *Disability, CBR & Inclusive Development, 30*(1), 57–93. https://doi.org/10.5463/DCID.v30i1.793

Rana, M., Upadhyay, J., Rana, A., Durgapal, S., & Jantwal, A. (2017). A systematic review of etiology, epidemiology, and treatment of cerebral palsy. *International Journal of Nutrition, Pharmacology, Neurological Diseases, 7*(4), 76–83. https://doi.org/10.4103/ijnpnd.ijnpnd_26_17

Rivella, C., & Vitebori, P. (2021). Executive function following pediatric stroke: A systematic review. *Child Neuropsychology, 27*(2), 209–231. https://doi.org/10.1080/09297049.2020.1820472

Szulczewski, L., Mullins, L. L., Bidwell, S. L, Eddington, A. R., & Pai, A. L. H. (2017). Meta-analysis: Caregiver and youth uncertainty in pediatric chronic illness. *Journal of Pediatric Psychology, 42*(4), 395–421. https://doi.org/10.1093/jpepsy/jsw097

Stoll, R. D., Pina, A. A., & Schleider, J. (2020). Brief, non-pharmacological interventions for pediatric anxiety: Meta-analysis and evidence base status. *Journal of Clinical Child & Adolescent Psychology, 49*(4), 435–459. https://doi.org/10.1080/15374416.2020.1738237

Tanner, K., Schmidt, E., Martin, K., & Bassi, M. (2020). Interventions within the scope of occupational therapy practice to improve motor performance for children ages 0–5 years: A systematic review. *American Journal of Occupational Therapy, 74*(2), 1–40. https://doi.org/10.5014/ajot.202

Yana, M., Tutuola, F., Westwater-Wood, S., & Kavlak, E. (2019). The efficacy of botulinum toxin A lower limb injections in addition to physiotherapy approaches in children with cerebral palsy: A systematic review. *NeuroRehabilitation, 44*(2), 175–189. https://doi.org/10.3233/NRE-18251

Elder Care Management

Asadzadeh, M., Maher, A., Jafari, M., Mohammadzadeh, K. A., & Hosseini, S. M. (2022). A review study of the providing elderly care services in different countries. *Journal of Family Medicine and Primary Care, 11*(2), 458–465. https://doi.org/10.4103/jfmpc.jfmpc_1277_21

Burkett, E., Martin-Khan, M. G., & Gray, L. C. (2017). Quality indicators in the care of older persons in the emergency departments: A systematic review of the literature. *Australasian Journal of Ageing, 36*(4), 286–298.

Chan, P., Bhar, S., Davison, T. E., Doyle, C., Knight, B. G., Koder, D., Laidlaw, K., Pachana, N. A., Wells, Y., & Wuthrich, V. M. (2021). Characteristics and effectiveness of cognitive behavioral therapy for older adults living in residential care: A systematic review. *Aging & Mental Health, 25*(2), 187–205. https://doi.org/10.1080/13607863.2019.1686457

Chau, R., Kissane, D. W., & Davison, T. E. (2019). Risk factors for depression in ong-term care: A systematic review. *Clinical Gerontologist, 42*(3), 224–237. https://doi.org/10.1080/07317115.2018.1490371

Choi, E. J., & Park, M. (2021). Preparing for the trend of aging in place: Identifying interprofessional competencies for integrated care professionals. *Journal of Korean Gerontology Nursing, 23*(3), 273–284. https://doi.org/10.17079/jkgn.2021.23.3.273

del Pino-Casado, R., Frías-Osuna, A., Palomino-Moral, P. A., Ruzafa-Martínez, M., & Ramos-Morcillo, A. J. (2018). Social support and subject burden in caregivers of adults and older adults: A meta-analysis. *PLoS ONE, 13*(1), e0189874. https://doi.org/10.1371/journal.pone.0189874

del Pino-Casado, R., Rodríguez Cardosa, M., López-Martínez, C., Ortega, V. (2019). The association between subjective caregiver burden and depressive symptoms in carers of older relatives: A systematic review and meta-analysis. *PLoS ONE, 14*(5), e0217648. https://doi.org/10.1371/journal.pone.0217648

Durand, M. J., Coutu, M. F., Tremblay, D., Sylvain, C., Gouin, M. M., Bilodeau, K., Kirouac, L., Paquette, M. A., Nastasia, L., & Coté, D. (2021). Insights into the sustainable return to work of aging workers with a work disability: An interpretative description study. *Journal of Occupational Rehabilitation, 31*, 92–106. https://doi.org/10.1007/s10926-020-09894-y

Evans, C. J., Ison, L., Ellis-Smith, C., Nicholson, C., Costa, A., Oluyase, A. O., Namisango, E., Bone, A. E., Brighton, L. J., Yi, D., Combes, S., Bajawah, S., Gao, W., Harding, R., Ong, P., Higginson, I. J., & Maddocks, M. (2019). Service delivery models to maximize quality of life for older people at the end of life: A rapid review. *Milbank Quarterly, 97*(1), 113–175. https://doi.org/10.1111/1468-0009.12373

Golding-Day, M., Whitehead, P., Radford, K., & Walker, M. (2017). Interventions to reduce dependency in bathing in community dwelling older adults: A systematic review. *Systematic Reviews, 6*, 1–6. https://doi.org/10.1186/s13643-017-0586-4

Ho, L. Y. W., & Ng, S. S. M. (2020). Non-pharmacological interventions for fatigue in older adults: A systematic review and meta-analysis. *Age & Ageing, 49*(3), 341–351. https://doi.org/10.1093/ageing/afaa019

Kalu, M. E., Maximos, M., Sengiad, S., & Del Bello-Haas, V. (2019). The role of rehabilitation professionals in care transitions for older adults: A scoping review. *Physical & Occupational Therapy in Geriatrics, 37*(3), 123–150. https://doi.org/10.1080/02703181.2019.1621419

Kurata, V. M., & Carreira, L. (2019). Influence of institutionalization in development of depression in elderly people: An integrative review. *Ciência, Cuidado e Saúde,18*(4), e42392.

Looman, W. M., Huijsman, R., & Fabbricotti, I. N. (2018). The (cost-)effectiveness of preventive, integrated care for community-dwelling frail older people: A systematic review. https://doi.org/10.1111/hsc.12571

Morelli, N., Barello, S., Mayan, M., & Graffigna, G. (2019). Supporting family caregiver engagement in the care of old persons living in hard to reach communities: A scoping review. *Health & Social Care in the Community, 27*(6), 1363–1374. https://doi.org/10.1111/hsc.12826

Murray, J., Hardicre, N., Birks, Y., O'Hara, J., & Lawton, R. (2019). How older people enact care involvement during transition from hospital to home: A systematic review and model. *Health Expectations: An International Journal of Public Participation in Health Care & Health Policy, 22*(5), 883–893. https://doi.org/10.1111/hex.12930

Nicolson, P. J. A., Sanchez-Santos, M. T., Bruce, J., Kirtley, S., Ward, L., Williamson, E., & Lamb, S. E. (2021). Risk factors for mobility decline in community-dwelling older adults: A systematic literature review. *Journal of Aging and Physical Activity, 29*, 1053–1066. https://doi.org/10.1123/japa.2020-0482

Platzer, E., Singler, K., Dovjak, P., Wirnsberger, G., Perl, A., Lindner, S., Liew, A., Roller-Wirnsberger, R. E. (2020). Evidence of inter-professional and multi-professional interventions for geriatric patients: A systematic review. *International Journal of Integrated Care, 20*(1), 1–10. https://doi.org/10.5334/ijic.4683

Ramprasad, C., Tamariz, L., Garcia-Barcena, J., Nemeth, Z., & Palacio, A. (2019). The use of tablet technology by older adults in health care settings: Is it effective and satisfying? A systematic review and meta-analysis. *Clinical Gerontologist, 42*(1), 17–26. https://doi.org/10.1080/07317115.2017.1322162

Saif-Ur-Rahman, K. M., Mamun, R., Eriksson, E., He, Y. & Hirakawa, Y. (2021). Discrimination against the elderly in health-care services: A systematic review. *Psychogeriatrics*, *21*(3), 418–429. https://doi.org/10.1111/psyg.12670

Saunders, T. J., McIsaac, T., Douillette, K., Gaulton, N., Hunter, S., Rhodes, R. E., Prince, S. A., Carson, V., Chaput, J. P., Chastin, S., Giangregorio, L., Janssen, I., Katzmarzyk, P. T., Kho, M. E., Poitras, V. J., Powell, K. E., Ross, R., Ross-White, A, Tremblay, M. S., & Healy, G. N. (2020). Sedentary behaviour and health in adults: An overview of systematic reviews. *Applied Physiology, Nutrition, and Metabolism*, *45*(10), s197–s217.

Serrano-Gemes, G., Serrano-del-Rosa, R., & Rich-Ruiz, M. (2021). Experiences in the decision-making regarding the place of care of the elderly: A systematic review. *Behavioral Sciences*, *11*(2), 1–19. https://doi.org/10.3390/bs11030014

Taylor, J., Walsh, S., Kwok, W., Pinheiro, M. B., de Oliveira, J., Hassett, L., Bauman, A., Bull, F., Tiedemann, A., Sherrington, C. (2021). A scoping review of physical activity interventions for older adults. *International Journal of Behavioral Nutrition & Physical Activity*, *18*(1), 1–14.

Tomilson, J., Cheong, V. L., Fylan, B., Silcock, J., Smith, H., Karban, K., & Blenkinsopp, A. (2020). Successful care transitions for older people: A systematic review and meta-analysis of the effects of interventions that support medication continuity. *Age and Ageing*, 558–569. https://doi.org/10.1093/ageing/afaa002

Torres-de-Araújo, J. R., Tomaz-de Lima, R. R., Ferreira-Bendassolli, M., & Costa-de Lima, K. (2018). Functional, nutritional, and social factors associated with mobility limitations in the elderly: A systematic review. *Salúd Public Mexico*, *60*, 579–585. https://doi.org/10.21149/9075

Vanderlinden, J., Boen, F., & van Uffelen, J. G. Z. (2020). Effects of physical activity programs on sleep outcomes in older adults: A systematic review. *International Journal of Behavioral Nutrition & Physical Activity*, *17*(1), 1–15. https://doi.org/10.1186/s12966-020-0913-3

Treatment and Care Specialties

Physical Medicine and Rehabilitation/Physiatry

Akkoc, Y., Ersoz, M., Cinar, E., & Gok, H. (2021). Evaluation and management of neurogenic bladder after spinal cord injury: Current practice among physical medicine and rehabilitation specialists in Turkey. *Turkish Journal of Physical Medicine and Rehabilitation*, *67*(2), 225–232. https://doi.org/10.5606/tftrd.2021.5817

Beyazova, M., Dogan, A., Kutsal, Y. G., Karahan, S., Arslan, S., Gokkaya, K. O., Toraman, F., Dincer, N., Hizmetli, S., Senel, K., Yazgan, P., Ortancil, O., Irdesel, J., Ozyemisci-Taskiran, O., Borman, P., Okumus, M., Ceceli, E., Evcik, D., Ay, S., Oztop, P., ... & Aydeniz, A. (2020). Environmental characteristics of older people attending physical medicine and rehabilitation outpatient clinics. *Central European Journal of Public Health*, *28*(1), 33–39. https://doi.org/10.21101/cejph.a5194

Borman, P. (2018). Lymphedema diagnosis, treatment, and follow-up from the viewpoint of physical medicine and rehabilitation specialists. *Turkish Journal of Physical Medicine and Rehabilitation*, *64*(3), 179–197. https://doi.org/10.5606/tftrd.2018.3539

Evcik, D., Ketenci, A., & Sindel, D. (2019). The Turkish Society of Physical Medicine and Rehabilitation (TSPMR) guideline recommendations for the management of fibromyalgia syndrome. *Turkish Journal of Physical Medicine and Rehabilitation*, *65*(2), 111–123. https://doi.org/10.5606/tftrd.2019.4815

Giacino, J. T., Katz, D. I., Schiff, N. D., Whyte, J., Ashman, E. J., Ashwal, S., Barbano, R., Hammond, F. M., Laureys, S., Ling, G., S. F., Nakase-Richardson, R., Seel, R. T., Yablon, S., Getchius, T. S. D., Gronseth, G. S., & Armstrong, M. J. (2018). Practice guidelines updated recommendations summary: Disorders of consciousness. *Archives of Physical Medicine and Rehabilitation*, 2–11. https://doi.org/10/1016/j.aprm.2018.07.001

Haldeman, S., Nordin, M., Tavares, P., Mullerpatan, R., Kopansky-Giles, D., Setlhare, V., Chou, R., Hurwitz, E., Treanor, C., Hartvigsen, J., Schneider, G., Ralph, M., Haldeman, J., Gryfe, D., Wilke, A., Brown, R., Outebridge, G., Eberspaecher, S., & Carroll, L. (2021). Distance management of spinal disorders in the COVID-19 pandemic and beyond: Evidence-based patient and clinician guides from the Global Spine Care Initiative. *Journal of Clinical Chiropractic Pediatrics*, 20(1), 3–29. https://doi.org/10.2196/preprints.25484

Paker, N., Bugdayci, D., Goksenoglu, G., Akbas, D., & Korkut, T. (2018). Recurrence rate after pressure ulcer reconstruction in patients with spinal cord injury in patient under control by a plastic surgery and physical medicine and rehabilitation team. *Turkish Journal of Physical Medicine and Rehabilitation*, 64(4), 322–327. https://doi.org/10.5606/tftrd.2018.2175

Phutrakool, P., & Pongpirul, K. (2022). Acceptance and use of complementary and alternative medicine among medical specialists: A 15-year systematic review and data analysis. *Systematic Reviews*, 11(10), 1–14. https://doi.org/10.1186/s13643-021-01882-4

Sukhov, R., Asante, A., & Ilizarov, G. (2020). Telemedicine for pediatric physiatry: How social distancing can bring physicians and families closer together. *Journal of Pediatric Rehabilitation Medicine: An Interdisciplinary Approach*, 13(3), 329-338. https://doi.org/10.3233/PRM_200747

Neurology

Rémi, J., Pollmächer, T., Spiegelhalder, K., Trenkwalder, C., & Young, P. (2019). Sleep-related disorders in neurology and psychiatry. *Deutsches Aerzteblatt International*, 116, 681–688. https://doi.org/10.3238/arztebl.2019.0681

Valliani, A. A.-A., Ranti, D., & Oermann, E. K. (2019). Deep learning and neurology: A systematic review. *Neurology & Therapy*, 8(2), 351–365. https://doi.org/10.1007/s40120-019-00153-8

Neuropsychology

Battista, P., Miozzo, A., Piccininni, M., Catricalà, E., Capozzo, R., Tortelli, R., Padovani, A., Cappa, S. F., & Logroscino, G. (2017). Primary progressive aphasia: A review of neuropsychological tests for the assessment of speech and language disorders. *Aphasiology*, 31(12), 1359–1378. https://doi.org/10.1080/0268j038.2017.1278799

Canas, A., Bordes Edgar, V., & Neumann, J. (2020). Practical considerations in the neuropsychological assessment of bilingual (Spanish-English) children in the United States: Literature review and case series. *Developmental Neuropsychology*, 45(4), 211–231. https://doi.org/10.1080/87565641.2020.1746314

González-Castañeda, H., Pineda-García, G., Serrano-Medina, A., Laura Martínez, A., Bonilla, J., & Ochoa-Ruíz, E. (2021). Neuropsychology of metabolic syndrome: A systematic review and meta-analysis. *Cogent Psychology*, 8(1), 1–33. https://doi.org/10.1080/23311908.2021.1913878

Malesci, R., Brigato, F., Di Cesare, T., Del Vecchio, V., Laria, C., De Corso, E., & Fetoni, A. R. (2021). Tinnitus and neuropsychological dysfunction in the elderly: A systematic review of possible links. *Journal of Clinical Medicine*, 10, 1–11. https://doi.org/10.3390/jcm10091881

Verberne, D. P. J., Spauwen, P. J. J., & van Heugten, C. M. (2019). Psychological interventions for treating neuropsychiatric consequences of acquired brain injury: A systematic review. *Neuropsychological Rehabilitation*, *29*(10), 1509–1542. https://doi.org/10.1080/09602011.2018.1433049

Wollman, S. C., Hauson, A. O., Hall, M. G., Connors, E. J., Stern, M. J., Stephan, R. A., Kimmel, C. L., Sarkissians, S., Barlet, B. D., & Flora-Tostado, C. (2019). Neuropsychological functioning in opioid use disorder: A research synthesis and meta-analysis. *The American Journal of Drug and Alcohol Abuse*, *45*(1), 11–25. https://doi.org/10.1080/00952990.2018.1517262

Occupational Therapy

Blas, A. J. T., Beltra, K. M. B., Martinez, P. G. V., & Yao, D. P. G. (2018). Enabling work: Occupational therapy interventions for persons with occupational injuries and diseases: A scoping review. *Journal of Occupational Rehabilitation*, *28*(2), 201–214. https://doi.org/10.1007/s10926-017-9732-z

Brown, S., Tse, T., Fortune, T., & Petrie, S. (2021). A scoping review of occupational therapy approaches to enable occupations for people living with behavioral disturbance as a result of acquired brain injury. *Open Journal of Occupational Therapy*, *9*(4), 1–10. https://doi.org/10.15453/2168-6408.1844

Cahill, S. M., & Beisbier, S. (2020). Occupational therapy practice guidelines for children and youth ages 5–21 years. *American Journal of Occupational Therapy*, *74*(4), 1–48. https://doi.org/10.5014/ajot.2020.744001

Clark, G. F., & Kingsley, K. L. (2020). Occupational therapy practice guidelines in early childhood: Birth–5 years. *American Journal of Occupational Therapy*, *74*(3), 1–23. https://doi.org/10.5014/ajot.2020.743001

Costalonga, D. A., Crozier, A. J., Stenner, B. J., & Baldock, K. L. (2020). Sport as a leisure occupation in occupational therapy literature: A scoping review. *American Journal of Occupational Therapy*, *74*(3), 1–10. https://doi.org/10.5014/ajot.2020.035949

Dancewicz, E. A., & Bissett, M. (2020). Occupational therapy interventions and outcomes measured in residential care: A scoping review. *Physical & Occupational Therapy in Geriatrics*, *38*(3), 230–249. https://doi.org/10.1080/02703181.2020.1719272

Doucet, B. M., Franc, I., & Hunter, E. G. (2021). Interventions within the scope of occupational therapy to improve activities of daily living, rest, and sleep in people with Parkinson's disease: A systematic review. *Journal of Occupational Therapy*, *75*(3), 1–32. https://doi.org/10.5014/ajot.2021.048314

Edgelow, M., Harrison, L., Miceli, M., & Cramm, H. (2020). Occupational therapy return to work interventions for persons with trauma and stress-related mental health conditions: A scoping review. *Work*, *65*(4), 821–836. https://doi.org/10.3233/WOR-203134

Fields, B. (2021). Occupational therapy interventions for older adults with chronic conditions and their care partners. *American Journal of Occupational Therapy*, *75*(6), 1–30. https://doi.org/10.5014/ajot.2021.049294

Fields, B., & Smallfield, S. (2022). Occupational therapy practice guidelines for adults with chronic conditions. *American Journal of Occupational Therapy*, *76*(6), 1–30. https://doi.org/10.5014/ajot.2022.762001

Foster, R. R., Carson, L. G., Archer, J., & Hunter, E. G. (2021). Occupational therapy interventions for instrumental activities of daily living in adults with Parkinson's disease: A systematic review. *American Journal of Occupational Therapy*, *75*(3), 1–24. https://doi.org/10.5014/ajot.2021.046581

Grace, S., Robinson, R., & Tokolahi, E. (2021). Occupational therapy interventions for persistent pain: A systematic review. *New Zealand Journal of Occupational Therapy, 68*(1), 15–22.

Gronski, M., & Doherty, M. (2020). Interventions within the scope of occupational therapy practice to improve activities of daily living, rest, and sleep for children ages 0–5 years and their families: A systematic review. *American Journal of Occupational Therapy, 74*(2), 1–31. https://doi.org/10.5014/ajot.2020.039545

Grajo, L. C., Candler, C., & Sarafian, A. (2020). Interventions within the scope of occupational therapy to improve children's academic participation: A systematic review. *American Journal of Occupational Therapy, 74*(2), 1–32. https://doi.org/10.5014/ajot.2020.039016

Hunter, E. G., Gibson, R. W., Arbesman, M., & D'Amico, M. (2017). Systematic review of occupational therapy and adult cancer rehabilitation: Part 1. Impact of physical activity and symptom management interventions. *American Journal of Occupational Therapy, 71*(2), 1–26. https://doi.org/10.5014/ajot.2017.023564

Hunter, E. G., Gibson, R. W., Arbesman, M., & D'Amico, M. (2017). Systematic review of occupational therapy and adult cancer rehabilitation: Part 2. Impact of multidisciplinary rehabilitation and psychosocial, sexuality, and return-to-work interventions. *American Journal of Occupational Therapy, 71*(2), 1–17. https://doi.org/10.5014/ajot.2017.023572

Hunter, E. G., & Rhodus, E. (2022). Interventions within the scope of occupational therapy to address preventable adverse events in inpatient and home health postacute care settings: A systematic review. *American Journal of Occupational Therapy, 76*(1), 1–12. https://doi.org/10.5014/ajot.2022.0475589

Kaldenberg, J., & Smallfield, S. (2020). Occupational therapy practice guidelines for older adults with low vision. *American Journal of Occupational Therapy, 74*(2), 1–23. https://doi.org/10.5014/ajot.2020.742003

Liu, C.-J., Chang, W.-P., & Chang, M. C. (2018). Occupational therapy interventions to improve daily living for community-dwelling older adults: A systematic review. *American Journal of Occupational Therapy, 72*(4), 1–11. https://doi.org/10.5014/ajot.2018.031252

Marik, T. L., & Roll, S. C. (2017). Effectiveness of occupational therapy interventions for musculoskeletal shoulder conditions: A systematic review. *American Journal of Occupational Therapy, 71*(1), 1–11. https://doi.org/10.5014/ajot.2017.023127

Nielsen, T. L., Petersen, K. S., Nielsen, C. V., Strøm, J., Ehlers, M. M., & Bjerrum, M. (2017). What are the short-term and long-term effects of occupation-focused and occupation-based occupational therapy in the home on older adults' occupational performance? A systematic review. *Scandinavian Journal of Occupational Therapy, 24*(4), 235–248. https://doi.org/10.1080/11038128.2016.1245357

Noyes, S., Sokolow, H., & Arbesman, M. (2018). Evidence for occupational therapy interventions with employment and education for adults with serious mental illness: A systematic review. *American Journal of Occupational Therapy, 72*(5), 1–10. https://doi.org/10.5014/ajot.2018.033068

Poole, J. L., & Siegel, P. (2017). Effectiveness of occupational therapy interventions for adults with fibromyalgia: A systematic review. *American Journal of Occupational Therapy, 71*(1), 1–10. https://doi.org/10.5014/ajot.2017.023192

Rahja, M., Comans, T., Clemson, L., Crotty, M., & Laver, K. (2018). Economic evaluations of occupational therapy approaches for people with cognitive and/or functional decline: A systematic review. *Health & Social Care in the Community, 26*(5), 635–653. https://doi.org/10.1111/hsc.12553

Raj, S. E., Mackintosh, S., Fryer, C., & Stanley, M. (2021). Home-based occupational therapy for adults with dementia and their informal caregivers: A systematic review. *American Journal of Occupational Therapy, 75*(1), 1–27. https://doi.org/10.5014/ajot.2021.040782

Rojo-Mota, G., Pedrero-Pérez, D. J., & Huertas-Hoyas, E. (2017). Systematic review of occupational therapy in the treatment of addiction: Models, practice, and qualitative and quantitative research. *American Journal of Occupational Therapy, 71*(5), 1–11. https://doi.org/10.5014/ajot.201

Smallfield, S., & Molitor, W. L. (2018). Occupational therapy interventions addressing sleep for community-dwelling older adults: A systematic review. *American Journal of Occupational Therapy, 72*(4), 1–9. https://doi.org/10.5014/ajot.2018.031211

Smallfield, S., & Molitor, W. L. (2018). Occupational therapy interventions supporting social participation and leisure engagement for community-dwelling older adults: A systematic review. *American Journal of Occupational Therapy, 72*(4), 1–8. https://doi.org/10.5014/ajot.2018.030627

Spargo, C., Laver, K., Berndt, A., Adey-Wakeling, Z., & George, S. (2021). Occupational therapy interventions to improve driving performance in older people with mild cognitive impairment or early-stage dementia: A systematic review. *American Journal of Occupational Therapy, 75*(5), 1–14. https://doi.org/10.5014/ajot.2021.042820

Tofani, M., Ranieri, A., Fabbrini, G., Bernardi, A., Pelosin, E., Valente, D., Fabbrini, A., Costanzo, M., & Galeoto, G. (2020). Efficacy of occupational therapy interventions on quality of life in patients with Parkinson's Disease: A systematic review and meta-analysis. *Movement Disorders Clinical Practice, 7*(8), 891–901. https://doi.org/10.1002/mdc3.13089

Physical Therapy

Abreu, V., Castro, S., Sousa, D., Julião, E., & Sousa, J. L. (2021). Impact of physical therapy on different types of bronchiolitis, patients, and care settings: A systematic review. *Fisioterapia e Pesquisa, 28*(4), 464–482. https://doi.org/10.1590/1809-2950/21019428042021

Alashram, A. R., Annino, G., Raju, M., & Padua, E. (2020). Effects of physical therapy interventions on balance ability in people with traumatic brain injury: A systematic review. *NeuroRehabilitation, 46*(4), 455–466. https://doi.org/10.3233/NRE-203047

Burgos-Mansilla, B., Galiano-Castillo, N., Lozano-Lozano, M., Fernández-Lao, C., Lopez-Garzon, M., & Arroyo-Morales, M. (2021). Effect of physical therapy modalities on quality of life of head and neck cancer survivors: A systematic review with meta-analysis. *Journal of Clinical Medicine, 10*, 1–18. https://doi.org/10.3390/jcm10204696

Florez-García, M., García-Pérez, F., Curbelo, R., Pérez-Porta, I., Nishishinya, B., Lozano, M. P. R., & Carmona, L. (2017). Efficacy and safety of home-based exercises versus individualized supervised outpatient physical therapy programs after total knee arthroplasty: A systematic review and meta-analysis. *Knee Surgery, Sports Traumatology, Arthroscopy, 25*, 3340–3353. https://doi.org/10.1007/s00167-016-4231-x

Fonzo, M., Sirico, F., & Corrado, B. (2020). Evidence-based physical therapy for individuals with Rett Syndrome: A systematic review. *Brain Sciences, 10*, 1–14. https://doi.org/10.3390/brainsci10070410

Fritz, N., Rao, A. K., Kegelmeyer, D., Kloos, A., Busse, M., Hartel, L., Carrier, J., & Quinn, L. (2017). Physical therapy and exercise interventions in Huntington's Disease: A mixed methods systematic review. *Journal of Huntington's Disease, 6*(3), 217–236. https://doi.org/10.3233/JHD-170260

Hoppes, C. W., Romanello, A. J., Gaudette, K. E., Herron, W. K., McCarthy, A. E., McHale, C. J., Bares, J., Turner, R., & Whitney, S. L. (2020). Physical therapy interventions for cervicogenic dizziness in a military-aged population: Protocol for a systematic review. *Systematic Reviews, 9*(1), 1–7. https://doi.org/10.1186/s13643-020-01335-4

Hugues, A., Di Marco, J., Ribault, S., Ardailon, H., Janiaud, P., Xue, Y., Zhu, J., Pires, J., Khademi, H., Rubio, L., Hernandez Bernal, P., Bahar, Y., Charvat, H., Szulc, P., Ciumas, C., Won, H., Cucherat, M., Bonan, I., Gueyffier, F., & Rode, G. (2019). Limited evidence of physical therapy on balance after stroke: A systematic review and meta-analysis. *PLoS ONE*, *14*(8), e0221700. https://doi.org/10.1371/journal.pone.0221700

Jelland, A., May, W., Zrig, A., Kalai, A., Jguirim, M., Frih, Z. B. S., & Golli, M. (2020). Intra-articular distention preceded by physical therapy versus intra-articular distention followed by physical therapy for treating adhesive capsulitis of the shoulder. *Journal of Back & Musculoskeletal Rehabilitation*, *33*(3), 443–450. https://doi.org/10.3233/BMR-181426

Li, J., Zhu, W., Gao, X., & Li, X. (2020). Comparison of arthroscopic partial meniscectomy to physical therapy following degenerative meniscus tears: A systematic review and meta-analysis. *BioMed Research International*, 1–9. https://doi.org/10.1155/2020/1709415

Ma, J., Chen, X., Xin, J., Niu, X., Liu, Z., & Zhao, Q. (2022). Overall treatment effects of aquatic physical therapy in knee osteoarthritis: A systematic review and meta-analysis. *Journal of Orthopaedic Surgery & Research*, *17*(1), 1–15. https://doi.org/10.1186/s13018-022-03069-6

Meena, R. L., Kumar, T., & Singh, S. (2022). Physical therapy in hemiplegic shoulder pain: A systematic review. *Journal of Clinical & Diagnostic Research*, *16*(4), YE0i–YE05. https://doi.org/10.7860/JCDR/2022/52483.16266

Mitchell, U. H., Helgeson, K., & Mintken, P. (2017). Physiological effects of physical therapy interventions on lumbar intervertebral discs: A systematic review. *Physiotherapy Theory & Practice*, *33*(9), 695–705. https://doi.org/10.1080/09503985.2017.1345026

Offor, N., Williamson, P. O., & Caçola, P. (2019). Effectiveness of interventions for children with developmental coordination disorder in physical therapy contexts: A systematic literature review and meta-analysis. *Journal of Motor Learning & Development*, *4*, 169–196. https://doi.org/10.1123/jmld.2015-0018

Ojha, H., Masaracchio, M., Johnston, M., Howard, R. J., Egan, W. E., Kirker, K., & Davenport, T. E. (2020). Minimal physical therapy utilization compared with higher physical therapy utilization for patients with low back pain: A systematic review. *Physiotherapy Theory & Practice*, *36*(11), 1179–1200. https://doi.org/10.1080/09503985.2019.1571135

Pieters, L., Lewis, J., Kuppens, K., Jochems, J., Bruijstens, T., Jooseens, J., & Struyf, F. (2020). An update of systematic reviews examining the effectiveness of conservative physical therapy interventions for subacromial shoulder pain. *Journal of Orthopaedic & Sports Physical Therapy*, *50*(3), 131–141. https://doi.org/10.2519/jospt.2020.8498

Prall, J., & Ross, M. (2021). The impact of physical therapy delivered ergonomics in the workplace: A narrative review. *Indian Journal of Physiotherapy & Occupational Therapy*, *15*(3), 27–36. https://doi.org/10.37506/ijpot.v15i3.16160

Rani, M., Kulandaivelan, S., Bansal, A., & Pawalia, A. (2019). Physical therapy intervention for cervicogenic headache: An overview of systematic reviews. *European Journal of Physiotherapy*, *21*(4), 217–223. https://doi.org/10.1080/21679169.2018.1523460

Rodrigues, D. L., Ledesma, A. L. L., de Oliveira, C. A. P., & Fayez, J., B. (2018). Physical therapy for posterior and horizontal canal benign paroxysmal positional vertigo: Long-term effects and recurrence: A systematic review. *International Archives of Otorhinolaryngology*, *22*(4), 455–459. https://doi.org/10.1055/s-0037-1604345

Rodríguez-Huguet, M., Vinolo-Gil, M. J., & Góngora-Rodríguez, J. (2022). Dry needling in physical therapy treatment of chronic neck pain: Systematic review. *Journal of Clinical Medicine*, *11*(9), 1–13. https://doi.org/10.3390/jcm11092370

Ruiz-González, L., Lucena-Antón, D., Salazar, A., Martín-Valero, R., & Moral-Munoz, J. A. (2019). Physical therapy in Down syndrome: Systematic review and meta-analysis. *Journal of Intellectual Disability*, *63*(8), 1041–1067. https://doi.org/10.1111/jir.12606

Soares-Macedo, F., Paz, C. C. S. C. P., Ferreira da Rocha, A., Miosso, C. J., Batista de Carvalho, H., & Menezes Mateus, S. R. (2017). New perspectives for chest physical therapy in spinal cord injury: A systematic review. *Acta Paulista de Enfermagem*, *30*(5), 546–556. https://doi.org/10.1590/1982-0194201700077

Tramontano, M., De Angelis, S., Galeoto, G., Cucinotta, M. C., Lisi, D., Botta, M., D'ippolito, M., Mornone, G., & Buzzi, M. G. (2021). Physical therapy exercises for sleep disorders in a rehabilitation setting for neurological patients: A systematic review and meta-analysis. *Brain Sciences*, *11*(9), 1–16. https://doi.org/10.3390/brainsci11091176

Zhao, Q., Dong, D., Liu, Z., Li, M., Wang, J., Yin, Y., & Wang, R. (2020). The effectiveness of aquatic physical therapy intervention on disease activity and function of ankylosing spondylitis patients: A meta-analysis. *Psychology, Health & Medicine*, *25*(7), 832–843. https://doi.org/10.1080/13548506.2019.1659984

Zhu, F., Zhang, M., Wang, D., Hong, Q., Zeng, C., & Chen, W. (2020). Yoga compared to non-exercise or physical therapy exercise on pain, disability, and quality of life for patients with chronic low back pain: A systematic review and meta-analysis of randomized controlled trials. *PLoS ONE*, *16*(9), 1–21. https://doi.org/10.1371/journal.pone.0238544

Rehabilitation Nursing

Baker, M., Pryor, J., Fisher, M. (2019). Nursing practice in inpatient rehabilitation: A narrative review (Part 1). *Australasian Rehabilitation Nurses' Association*, *22*(2), 7–21. https://doi.org/10.33235/jarna.22.2.7-21

Baker, M., Pryor, J., Fisher, M. (2019). Nursing practice in inpatient rehabilitation: A narrative review (Part 2). *Australasian Rehabilitation Nurses' Association*, *22*(3), 7–15. https://doi.org/10.33235/jarna.22.3.7-15

Wan, B., Huang, R., Xiong, W., Miao, C., & Zhang, F. (2020). Meta-analysis of clinical efficacy of postoperative rehabilitation nursing in patients with cerebral hemorrhage. *Acta Microscopica*, *29*(2), 820–829.

Vocational Rehabilitation Counseling

Al-Rashaida, M., López-Paz, J. F., Amayra, I., Lázaro, E., Martínez, O., Berrocoso, S., García, M., & Pérez, M. (2018). Factors affecting the satisfaction of people with disabilities in relation to vocational rehabilitation programs: A literature review. *Journal of Vocational Rehabilitation*, *49*, 97–115. https://doi.org/10.3233/JVR-180957

Bernstrøm, V. H., & Houkes, I. (2018). A systematic literature review of the relationship between work hours and sickness absence. *Work*, *32*(1), 84–104. https://doi.org/10.1080/02678373.2017.1394926

Black, O., Keegel, T., Sim, M., Collie, A., & Smith, P. (2018). The effect of self-efficacy on return-to-work outcomes for workers with psychological or upper-body musculoskeletal injuries: A review of the literature. *Journal of Occupational Rehabilitation*, *28*(1), 16–27. https://doi.org/10.1007/s10926-017-9697-y

Blas, A. J. T., Bletran, K. M. B., Martinez, P. G. V., & Yao, D. P. G. (2018). Enabling work: Occupational therapy interventions for persons with occupational injuries and diseases: A scoping review. *Journal of Occupational Rehabilitation*, *28*(2). 201–214. https://doi.org/10.1007/s10926-017-9732-z

Bloom, J., Dorsett, P., & McLenna, V. (2020). Vocational rehabilitation to empower consumers following newly acquired spinal cord injury. *Journal of Vocational Rehabilitation*, *53*(1), 131–144. https://doi.org/10.3233/JVR-201091

Bloom, J., McLennan, V., & Dorsett, P. (2019). Occupational bonding after spinal cord injury: A review and narrative synthesis. *Journal of Vocational Rehabilitation*, *50*(1), 109–120. https://doi.org/10.3233/JVR-180992

Brinchmann, B., Widding-Havneraas, T., Modini, M., Rinaldi, M., Moe, C. F., McDaid, D., Park, A.-L., Killackey, E., Harvey, S. B., & Mykletun, A. (2020). A meta-regression of the impact of policy on the efficacy of individual placement and support. *Acta Psychiatrica Scandinavica*, *141*(3), 206–220. https://doi.org/10.1111/acps.13129

Carlson, S. R., Morningstar, M. E., & Munandar, V. (2020). Workplace supports for employees with intellectual disability: A systematic review of the intervention literature. *Journal of Vocational Rehabilitation*, *52*(3), 251–265. https://doi.org/10.3233/JVR-201075

Carmona, V. R., Gómez-Benito, J., Heudo-Medina, T. B., & Rojo, J. E. (2017). Employment outcomes for people with schizophrenia spectrum disorder: A meta-analysis of randomized controlled trials. *International Journal of Occupational Medicine and Environmental Health*, *30*(3), 345–366. https://doi.org/10.13075/ijomeh.1896.01074

Cocchiara, R. A., Sciarra, I., D'Egidio, V., Sestilli, C., Mancino, M., Backhaus, I., Mannocci, A., De Luca, A., Frusone, F., Di Bella, O., Di Murro, F., Plameri, V., Lia, L., Pardiso, G., Aceti, V., Libia, A., Monti, M., & La Torre, G. (2018). Returning to work after breast cancer: A systematic review of reviews. *Work*, *61*(3), 463–476. https://doi.org/10.3233/WOR-182810

D'Amico, M. L., Jaffe, L. E., & Gardner, J. A. (2018). Evidence for interventions to improve and maintain occupational performance and participation for people with serious mental illness: A systematic review. *The American Journal of Occupational Therapy*, *72*(5), 1–11. https://doi.org/10.5014/ajot.2018.03332

Dean, E. E., Shogren, K. A., Hagiwara, M., & Wehmeyer, M. L. (2018). How does employment influence health outcomes? A systematic review of the intellectual disability literature. *Journal of Vocational Rehabilitation*, *49*(1), 1–13. https://doi.org/10.3233/JVR-180950

DeBaets, S., Calders, P., Schalley, N., Vermeulen, K., Vertriest, S., Van Peteghem, L., Coussens, M., Malfait, F., Vanderstraeten, G., Van Hove, G., a& Van de Velde, D. (2018). Updating the evidence on functional capacity evaluation methods: A systematic review. *Journal of Occupational Rehabilitation*, *28*(3), 418–428. https://doi.org/10.1007/s10926-017-9734-x

de Boer, A. G. E. M., Torp, S., Popa, A., Horsboel, T., Zadnik, V., Rottenberg, Y., Bardi, E., Bultmann, U., & Sharp, L. (2020). Long-term work retention after treatment for cancer: A systematic review and meta-analysis. *Journal of Cancer Survivorship*, *14*(2), 135–150. https://doi.org/10.1007/s11764-020-00862-2

Dewa, C. S., Loong, D., Trojanowski, L., & Bonato, S. (2018). The effectiveness of augmented versus standard individual placement and support programs in terms of employment: A systematic literature review. *Journal of Mental Health*, *27*(2), 174–183. https://doi.org/10.1080/09638237.2017.1322180

DiRezze, B., Viveiros, H., Pop, R., Rampton, G. (2018). A review of employment outcome measures in vocational research involving adults with neurodevelopmental disabilities. *Journal of Vocational Rehabilitation*, *49*(1), 79–96. https://doi.org/10.3233/JVR-180956

Frederick, D. E., & VanderWelle, T. L. (2019). Supported employment: Meta-analysis and review of randomized controlled trials of individual placement and support. *PLoS ONE*, *14*(2), e0212208. https://doi.org/10.1371/journal.pone.0212208

Frentzel, E., Geyman, Z., Rasmussen, J., Nye, C., Murphy, K. (2021). Pre-employment transition services for students with disabilities: A scoping review. *Journal of Vocational Rehabilitation*, *54*(2), 103–116. https://doi.org/10.3233/JVR-201123

Frutiger, M., & Borotkanics, R. (2021). Systematic review and meta-analysis suggest strength training and workplace modifications may reduce neck pain in office workers. *Pain Practice*, *21*(1), 100–131. https://doi.org/10.1111/papr.12940

Gilson, C. B., Carter, E. W., & Biggs, E. E. (2017). Systematic review of instructional methods to teach employment skills to secondary students with intellectual and developmental disabilities. *Research & Practice for Persons with Severe Disabilities*, *42*(2), 89–107. https://doi.org/10.1177/1540796917698831

Gragnano, A., Negrini, A., Miglioretti, M., & Corbière, M. (2018). Common psychosocial factors predicting return to work after common mental disorders, cardiovascular diseases, and cancers: A review of reviews supporting a cross-disease approach. *Journal of Occupational Rehabilitation*, *28*(2), 215–231. https://doi.org/10.1007/s10926-017-9714-1

Greidanus, M. A., de Boer, A. G. E. M., de Rijk, A. E., Tiedtke, C. M., Dierckx de Casterlé, B., Frings-Dresen, M. H. W., & Tamminga, S. J. (2018). Perceived employer-related barriers and facilitators for work participation of cancer survivors: A systematic review of employers' and survivors' perspectives. *Psycho-Oncology*, *27*(3), 725–733. https://doi.org/10.1002/pon.4514

Gupta, S., Jaiswal, A., Norman, K., & DePaul, V. (2019). Heterogeneity and its impact on rehabilitation outcomes and interventions for community reintegration in people with spinal cord injuries: An integrative review. *Top Spinal Cord Injury Rehabilitation*, *25*(2), 164–185. https://doi.org/10.1310/sci2502-164

Guzik, A., Kwolek, A., Druzbiki, M., & Pryzsada, G. (2020). Return to work after stroke and related factors in Poland and abroad: A literature review. *Work*, *65*(2), 447–462. https://doi.org/10.3233/WOR-203097

Harrison, J., Krieger, M., & Johnson, H. A. (2020). Review of individual placement and support employment intervention for persons with substance use disorder. *Substance Use & Misuse*, *55*(4), 636–643. https://doi.org/10.1080/10826084.2019.1692035

Harvey, K., Ockerese, T., & Fady, J. (2020). A literature review pertaining to vocational rehabilitation for people experiencing adult-acquired neurological conditions. *New Zealand Journal of Occupational Therapy*, *67*(3), 15–22.

Hellström, L., Pedersen, P., Christensen, T. N., Wallstroem, I. G., Bojesen, A. B., Stenager, E., Bejerhold, U., von Busschbach, J., Michon, H., Mueser, K. T., Reme, S. E., White, S., & Eplov, L. F. (2021). Vocational outcomes of the individual placement and support model in subgroups of diagnoses, substance, abuse, and forensic conditions: A systematic review and analysis of pooled original data. *Journal of Occupational Rehabilitation*, *31*, 699–710. https://doi.org/10.1007/s10926-021-09960-z

Hoosain, M., de Klerk, S., & Burger, M. (2019). Workplace-based rehabilitation of upper limb conditions: A systematic review. *Journal of Occupational Rehabilitation*, *29*(1), 175–193. https://doi.org/10.1007/s10926-018-9777-7

Hunter, E. G., Gibson, R. W., Arbesman, M., & D'Amico, M. (2017). Systematic review of occupational therapy and adult cancer rehabilitation: Part 2. Impact of multidisciplinary rehabilitation and psychosocial, sexuality, and return-to-work interventions. *American Journal of Occupational Therapy*, *71*(2), 1–8.

Lindsay, S., Cagliostro, E., Albarico, M., Srikanthan, & Mortaji, N. (2018). A systematic review of the role of gender in securing and maintaining employment among youth and young adults with disabilities. *Journal of Occupational Rehabilitation*, *28*(2), 232–251. https://doi.org/10.1007/s10926-017-9726-x

Lockett, H., Waghorn, G., & Kydd, R. (2018). A framework for improving the effectiveness of evidence-based practices in vocational rehabilitation. *Journal of Vocational Rehabilitation*, *49*(1), 15–31. https://doi.org/10.3233/JVR-180951

Madsen, C. M. T., Bisgaard, S. K., Primdahl, J., Christensen, J. R., & von Bülow, C. (2021). A systematic review of job loss interventions for persons with inflammatory arthritis. *Journal of Occupational Rehabilitation*, *31*(4), 866–885. https://doi.org/10.1007/s10926-021-09972-9

Magura, S., & Marshall, T. (2020). The effectiveness of interventions intended to improve employment outcomes for persons with substance use disorder: An updated systematic review. *Substance Use & Misuse*, *55*(13), 2230–2236. https://doi.org/10.1080/10826084.2020.1797810

Mani, K., Cater, B., & Hudlikar, A. (2017). Cognition and return to work after mild/moderate traumatic brain injury: A systematic review. *Journal of Prevention, Assessment, & Rehabilitation*, *58*(1), 51–62. https://doi.org/10.3233/WOR-172597

McLennan, V., Ludvik, D., Chambers, S., & Frydenberg, M. (2019). Work after prostate cancer: A systematic review. *Journal of Cancer Survivorship*, *13*(2), 282–291. https://doi.org/10.1007/s11764-019-00750-4

Meulenbroek, P., O'Neil-Pirozzi, T. M., Sohlberg, M. M., Lemoncello, R., Byom, L., Ness, B., MacDonald, S., & Phillips, B. (2022). Tutorial: The speech-language pathologist's role in return to work for adults with traumatic brain injury. *American Journal of Speech-Language Pathology*, *31*(1), 188–202. https://doi.org/10.1044/2021_AJSLP-21-00129

Momsen, A. H., Stapelfeldt, C. M., Rosbjerg, R., Escorpizo, R., Labriola, M., & Bjerrum, M. (2019). International Classification of Functioning, Disability, and Health in vocational rehabilitation: A scoping review of the state of the field. *Journal of Occupational Rehabilitation*, *29*(2), 241–273. https://doi.org/10.1007/s10926-018-9788-4

Nevala, N., Pehkonen, I., Teittinen, A., Vesala, H. T., Pörtfors, P., & Anttila, H. (2019). The effectiveness of rehabilitation interventions on the employment and function of people with intellectual disabilities: A systematic review. *Journal of Occupational Rehabilitation*, *29*(4), 773–802. https://doi.org/10.1007/s10926-019-09837-2

Nigatu, Y., Liu, Y., Uppal, M., McKinney, S., Gillis, K., Rao, S., Wang, J., & Nigatu, Y. (2017). Prognostic factors of return to work of employees with common mental disorders: A meta-analysis of cohort studies. *Social Psychiatry & Psychiatric Epidemiology*, *52*(10), 1205–1215. https://doi.org/10.1007/s00127-017-1402-0

Noyes, S., Sokolow, H., & Arbesman, M. (2018). Evidence for occupational therapy intervention with employment and education for adults with serious mental illness: A systematic review. *The American Journal of Occupational Therapy*, *72*(5), 1–10. https://doi.org/10.5014/ajot.2018.033068

O'Keefe, S., Stanley, M., Adam, K., & Lannin, N. A. (2019). A systematic scoping review of work interventions for hospitalised adults with an acquired neurological impairment. *Journal of Occupational Rehabilitation*, *29*(3), 569–584. https://doi.org/10.1007/s10926-018-9820-8

Paltrinieri, S., Fugazzaro, S., Pellegrini, M., Costi, S., Bertozzi, L., Bassi, M. C., Vicentini, M., & Mazzini, E. (2018). Return to work in European cancer survivors: A systematic review. *Supportive Care in Cancer*, *26*(9), 2983–2994. https://doi.org/10.1007/s00520-018-4270-6

Richter, D., &, H. (2019). Effectiveness of supported employment in non-trial routine implementation: Systematic review and meta-analysis. *The International Journal for Research in Social and Genetic Epidemiology and Mental Health Services*, *54*(5), 525–531. https://doi.org/10.1007/s00127-018-1577-z

Safi, F., Aniserowicz, A. N., Colquhoun, H., Stier, J., & Nowrouzi-Kia, B. (2022). Impact of eating disorders on paid or unpaid work participation and performance: A systematic review and meta-analysis protocol. *Journal of Eating Disorders*, *10*(1), 1–11. https://doi.org/10.1186/s40337-021-00525-2

Seagraves, K. (2021). Effective job supports to improve employment outcomes for individuals with autism spectrum disorder. *Journal of Applied Rehabilitation Counseling, 52*(2), 94–103. https://doi.org/10.1891/JARC-D-00017

Sundar, V. (2017). Operationalizing workplace accommodations for individuals with disabilities: A scoping review. *Work, 56*(1), 135–155. https://doi.org/10.3233/WOR-162472

Talbot, E., Völlm, B., & Khalifa, N. (2017). Effectiveness of work skills programmes for offenders with mental disorders: A systematic review. *Criminal Behaviour and Mental Health, 27*(1), 40–58. https://doi.org/10.1002/cbm.1981

Taylor, J., Avellone, L., Cimera, R., Brooke, V., Lambert, A., & Iwanaga, K. (2021). Cost-benefit analyses of employment services for individuals with intellectual and developmental disabilities: A scoping review. *Journal of Vocational Rehabilitation, 54*(2), 193–206. https://doi.org/10.3233/JVR-201130

Thomas, F., & Morgan, R. L. (2021). Evidence-based job retention interventions for people with disabilities: A narrative literature review. *Journal of Vocational Rehabilitation, 54*(2), 89–101. https://doi.org/10.3233/JVR-201122

Uyanik, H., Shogren, K. A., & Blanck, P. (2017). Supported decision-making: Implications from positive psychology for assessment and intervention in rehabilitation and employment. *Journal of Occupational Rehabilitation, 27*(4), 498–506. https://doi.org/10.1007/s10926-017-9740-z

van Bentum, J., Nicholson, J., Bale, N., & Fadyl, J. K. (2021). Supporting people experiencing a burn injury to return to work or meaningful activity: Qualitative systematic review and thematic synthesis. *New Zealand Journal of Physiotherapy, 49*(3), 134–146.

Venning, A., Oswald, T. K., Stevenson, J., Tepper, N., Azadi, L., Lawn, S., & Redpath, P. (2021). Determining what constitutes an effective psychosocial "return to work" intervention": A systematic review and narrative synthesis. *BMC Public Health, 21*(1), 1–25. https://doi.org/10.1186/s12889-021-11898-z

White, C., Green, R. A., Ferguson, S., Anderson, S. L., Howe, C., Sun, J., & Buys, N. (2019). The influence of social support and social integration factors on return to work outcomes for individuals with non-related injuries: A systematic review. *Journal of Occupational Rehabilitation, 29*(3), 636–659. https://doi.org/10.1007/s10926-018-09826-x

Wong, J., Kallish, N., Crown, D., Capraro, P., Preierweiler, R., Wafford, Q. E., Tiema-Benson, L., Hassan, S., Engel, Ed., Tamayo, C., & Heinemann, A. W. (2021). Job Accommodations, return to work, and job retention of people with physical disabilities: A systematic review. *Journal of Occupational Rehabilitation, 31*, 474–490. https://doi.org/10.1007/s10926-020-09954-3

Zafar, N., Rotenberg, M., & Rudnick, A. (2019). A systematic review of work accommodations for people with mental disorders. *Work, 64*(3), 461–475. https://doi.org/10.3233/WOR-193008

Zechen, M., Dhir, P., Perrier, L., Baylay, M., & Munce, S. (2020). The impact of vocational interventions on vocational outcomes, quality of life, and community integration in adults with childhood onset disabilities: A systematic review. *Journal of Occupational Rehabilitation, 30*(1), 1–21. https://doi.org/10.1007/s10926-019-09854-1

Physical, Mental, and Cognitive Conditions

Acquired Brain Injury

Acabchuk, R. L., Brisson, J. M., Park, C. L., Babbott-Bryan, N., Parmelee, O. A., & Johnson, B. T. (2021). Therapeutic effects of meditation, yoga, and mindfulness-based interventions for chronic symptoms of mild traumatic brain injury: A systematic review and meta-analysis. *Applied Psychology: Health and Well-Being*, *13*(1), 34–62.

Ackley, K., & Brown, J. (2020). Speech-language pathologists' practices for addressing cognitive deficits in college students with traumatic brain injury. *Journal of Speech-Language Pathology*, *29*(4), 2226–2241. https://doi.org/10.1044/2020_AJSLP-20-00079

Alsharam, A. R., Annino, G., Raju, M., & Padua, E. (2020). Effects of physical therapy interventions on balance ability in people with traumatic brain injury: A systematic review. *NeuroRehabilitation*, *46*(4), 455–466. https://doi.org/10.3233/NRE-203047

Appenteng, R., Nelp, T., Abdelgadir, J., Weledji, N., Haglund, M., Smith, E., Obiga, O., Sakita, F. M., Miguel, E. A., Vissoci, C. M., Rice, H., Vissoci, J. R. N., & Staton, C. (2018). A systematic review and quality analysis of pediatric traumatic brain injury clinical practice guidelines. *PLoS ONE*, *13*(8), e0201550. https://doi.org/10.1371/journal.pone.0201550

Brandt, A., Jensen, M. P., Søberg, M. S., Andersen, S. D., & Sund, T. (2020). Information and communication technology-based assistive technology to compensate for impaired cognition in everyday life: A systematic review. *Disability and Rehabilitation: Assistive Technology*, *15*(7), 810–824

Brownlee, N. N. M., Wilson, F. C., Curran, D. B., Lyttle, N., & McCann, J. P. (2020). Neurocognitive outcomes in adults following cerebral hypoxia: A systematic literature review. *NeuroRehabilitation*, *47*(2), 83–97. Https://doi.org/10.3233/NRE-203135

Callender, L., Brown, R., Driver, S., Dahdah, M., Collinsworth, A., & Shafi, S. (2017). Process for developing rehabilitation practice recommendations for individuals with traumatic brain injury. *BMC Neurology*, *17*, 1–6. https://doi.org/10.1186/s12883-017-0828-z

Chan, V., Tocalino, D., Omar, S., Shah, R., & Colantonio, A. (2022). A systematic review of integrated care for traumatic brain injury, mental health, and substance use. *PLoS ONE*, *17*(3), e0264116. https://doi.org/10.1371/journal.pone.0264116

Chavez-Arana, C., Catroppa, C., Carranza-Escárcega, Ed., Godfrey, C., Yáñez-Téllez, G., Prieto-Corona, B., de León, M., & Anderson, V. (2018). A systematic review of interventions in hot and cold executive functions in children and adolescents with acquired brain injury. *Journal of Psychiatric Psychology*, *43*(8), 928–942

Clasby, B., Hughes, N., Catroppa, C., & Morrison, E. (2018). Community-based interventions for adolescents following traumatic brain injury: A systematic review. *NeuroRehabilitation*, *42*(3), 345–363.

Corti, C., Oldrati, V., Oprandi, M. C., Ferrari, E., Poggi, G., Borgatti, R., Urgesi, C., & Berdoni, A. (2019). Remote technology-based training programs for children with acquired brain injury: A systematic review and a meta-analytic exploration. *Behavioral Neurology*, 1–31. https://doi.org/10.1155/2019/1346987

Cronin, H., & O'Loughlin, E. (2018). Sleep and fatigue after TBI. *NeuroRehabilitation*, *43*(3), 307–317. https://doi.org/10.3233/NRE-182484

D'Cruz, K., Douglas, J., & Serry, T. (2019). Personal narrative approaches in rehabilitation following traumatic brain injury: A synthesis of qualitative research. *Neuropsychological Rehabilitation*, *29*(7), 985–1004.

Déry, J., De Guise, E., Bussières, E. L., & Lamontagne, M. E. (2021). Prognostic factors for persistent symptoms in adults with mild traumatic brain injury: Protocol for an overview of systematic reviews. *Systematic Reviews*, *10*(1), 1–8. https://doi.org/10.1186/s13643-021-01810-6

Deschênes, P. M., Lamontagne, M. E., Gagnon, M. P., & Moreno, J. A. (2019). Talking about sexuality in the context of rehabilitation following traumatic brain injury: An integrative review of operational aspects. *Sexuality and Disability*, *37*(3), 297–314. https://doi.org/10.1007/s11 195-019-09576-5

dos Santos Silva Borges, C., & Rodrigues Neto, G. (2020). Therapeutic exercises protocols in patients with traumatic brain injury: A systematic review. *Journal of Exercise Physiology Online*, *23*(2), 71–82.

Fabio, A., Murray, A., Mellers, M., Wisniewski, S., & Bell, M. (2017). The effects of insurance status on pediatric traumatic brain injury outcomes: A literature review. *Journal of Health Disparities Research & Practice*, *10*(2), 107–120.

Gallagher, M., McLeod, H. J., & McMillan, T. M. (2019). A systematic review of recommended modifications of CBT for people with cognitive impairments following brain injury. *Neuropsychological Rehabilitation*, *29*(1), 1–21.

Gauvin-Lepage, J., Lapierre, A., & Bissonnette, S. (2021). Social participation of children and adolescents with acquired brain injury: A scoping review. *Journal of Rehabilitation*, *87*(3), 4–14.

Geber, L. H., Bush, H., Cai, C., Garfinkel, S., Chan, L., Cotner, B., & Wagner, A. (2019). Scoping review of clinical rehabilitation research pertaining to traumatic brain injury: 1990–2016. *NeuroRehabilitation*, *44*(1), 207–215.

Green, E., Huynh, A., Broussard, L., Zunker, B., Mattews, J., Hilton, C. L., & Aranha, K. (2019). Systematic review of yoga and balance: Effects on adults with neuromuscular impairment. *American Journal of Occupational Therapy*, *73*(1), 1–11.

Hill, E., Claessen, M., Whitworth, A., Boyes, M., & Ward, R. (2018). Discourse and cognition in speakers with acquired brain injury (ABI): A systematic review. *International Journal of Language & Communication Disorders*, *53*(4), 689–717.

Hill, K., & Brenner, M. (2019). Well siblings' experiences of living with a child following a traumatic brain injury: A systematic review protocol. *Systematic Reviews*, *8*(1), 1–7. https://doi.org/10.1186/s13643-019-1005-9

Hunt, C., Zahid, S., Ennis, N., Michalak, A., Masanic, C., Vaidyanath, C., Bhalerao, S., Cusimano, M. D., & Baker, A. (2019). Quality of life measures in older adults after traumatic brain injury: A systematic review. *Quality of Life Research*, *28*(12), 3137–3151. https://doi.org/10.1007/s11136-019-02297-4

Iljazi, A., Ashina, H., Al-Khazali, H. M., Lipton, R. B., Ashina, M., Schytz, H. W., & Ashina, S. (2020). Post-traumatic stress disorder after traumatic brain injury: A systematic review and meta-analysis. *Neurological Sciences*, *41*, 2737–2746. https://doi.org/10.1007/s10072-020-04458-7

Iverson, G. L., Karr, J. E., Gardner, A. J., Silverberg, N. D., & Terry, D. P. (2019). Results of scoping review do not support mild traumatic brain injury being associated with a high incidence of chronic cognitive impairment: Commentary on McInnes et al., 2017. *PLoS ONE*, *14*(9), e0218997. https://doi.org/10.1371/journal.pone.0218997

Johnson, L. W., & Hall, K. D. (2022). A scoping review of cognitive assessment in adults with acute traumatic brain injury. *American Journal of Speech-Language Pathology*, *31*, 739–756.

Khajeei, D., Smith, D., Kachur, B., & Abdul, N. (2019). Sexuality re-education program logic model for people with traumatic brain injury (TBI): Synthesis via scoping literature review. *Sexuality and Disability*, *37*(1), 41–61. https://doi.org/10.1007/s11195-018-09556-1

Laatsch, L., Dodd. J., Brown, T., Ciccia, A., Connor, F., Davis, K., Doherty, M., Linden, M., Locascio, G., Lundine, J., Murphy, S., Nagele, D., Niemeier, J., Politis, Ad., Rode, C., Slomine, B., Smetana, R., & Yaeger, L. (2020). Evidence-based systematic review of cognitive rehabilitation, emotional, and family treatment studies for children with acquired brain injury literature: From 2006–2017. *Neuropsychological Rehabilitation*, *30*(1), 130–161. https://doi.org/10.1080/09602011.2019.1678490

LaGattuta, E., Carolla, F., LoBuono, V., DeSalvo, S., Caminiti, F., Rifici, C., Alagna, A., Arcadi, F., Bramanti, A., & Marino, S. (20180). Techniques of cognitive rehabilitation in patients with disorders of consciousness: A systematic review. *Neurological Sciences, 39*(4), 641–645. https://doi.org/10.10072-017-3235-8

Li, X., Feng, Y., Xia, J., Zhou, X., Chen, N., Chen, Z., Fan, Q., Wang, H., Ding, P., & Du, Q. (2021). Effects of cognitive behavioral therapy on pain and sleep in adults with traumatic brain injury: A systematic review and meta-analysis. *Neural Plasticity,* 6552246, 1–12. https://doi.org/10.1155/2021/6552246

Li, Y., Li, Y., Li, X., Zhang, S., Zhao, J., Zhu, X., & Tian, G. (2017). Head injury as a risk factor for dementia and Alzheimer's Disease: A systematic review and meta-analysis of 32 observational studies. *PLoS ONE, 12*(1), e0169650. https://doi.org/10.1371/journal.prone.0169650

Linden, M. A., Glang, A. E., & McKinlay, A. (2018). A systematic review and meta-analysis of educational interventions for children and adolescents with acquired brain injury. *NeuroRehabilitation, 42*(3), 311–323. https://doi.org/10.3233/NRE-172357

Little, A., Byrne, C., & Coetzer, R. (2020). The effectiveness of cognitive behaviour therapy for reducing anxiety symptoms following traumatic brain injury: A meta-analysis and systematic review. *NeuroRehabilitation,* 1–16. https://doi.org/10.3233/NRE-201544

López, R. F., & Antolí, A. (2020). Computer-based cognitive interventions in acquired brain injury: A systematic review and meta-analysis of randomized controlled trials. *PLoS ONE, 15*(7), e0235510. https://doi.org/10.1371/journal.pone.0235510

Ma, Z., Dhir, P., Perrier, L., Bayley, M., & Munce, S. (2020). The impact of vocational interventions on vocational outcomes, quality of life, and community integration in adults with childhood onset disabilities: A systematic review. *Journal of Occupational Rehabilitation, 30*(1), 1–21. https://doi.org/10.1007/s10926-019-09854-1

Malá, H., & Rasmussen, C. P. (2017). The effect of combined therapies on recovery after acquired brain injury: Systematic review of preclinical studies combining enriched environment, exercise, or task-specific training with other therapies. *Restorative Neurology and Neuroscience, 35*(1), 25–64. https://doi.org/10.3233/RNN-16082

Malik, T. G., & Farooq, K. (2020). Neuroimaging in neuro-ophthalmology (systematic review). *Pakistan Journal of Ophthalmology, 36*(3), 180–189. https://doi.org/10.36351/pjo.v36i2.1026

Mani, K., Cater, B., & Hudlikar, A. (2017). Cognition and return to work after mild/moderate traumatic brain injury: A systematic review. *Work, 58*(1), 51–62.

Mantell, A., Simpson, G. K., Vungkhanching, M., Jones, K. F., Strandberg, T., & Simonson, P. (2018). Social work-generated evidence in traumatic brain injury from 1976 to 2014: A systematic scoping review. *Health & Social Care in the Community, 26*(4), 433–448. https://doi.org/10.1111/hsc.12476

Marquez, J., Weerasekara, I., & Chambers, L. (2020). Hippotherapy in adults with acquired brain injury: A systematic review. *Physiotherapy Theory and Practice, 36*(7), 779–790. https://doi.org/10.1080/09593985.2018.1494233

Marron, F., Zavatto, L., Allevi, M., Vitantonio, H. D., Millimaggi, D. F., Dehcordi, S. R., Ricci, A., & Taddei, G. (2020). Management of mild brain trauma in the elderly: Literature review. *Asian Journal of Neurosurgery, 15*(4), 809–820. https://doi.org/10.4103/ajns.AJNS_205_20

Martens, G., Laureys, S., & Thibaut, A. (2017). Spasticity management in disorders of consciousness. *Brain Sciences, 7,* 1–11. https://doi.org/10.3390/brainsci7120162

Meulenbroek, P., O'Neil-Pirozzi, T. M., Sohlberg, M. M., Lemoncello, R., Byom, L., Ness, B., MacDonald, S., & Phillip, B. (2022). Tutorial: The speech-language pathologist's role in return to work for adults with traumatic brain injury. *American Journal of Speech-Language Pathology, 3*(1), 188–202. https://doi.org/10.1044/2021_AJSLP-21-00129

Nam, J-H., & Kim, H. (2018). How assistive devices affect activities of daily living and cognitive functions in people with brain injury: A meta-analysis. *Disability and Rehabilitation: Assistive Technology*, *13*(3), 305–311. https://doi.org/10.1080/17483107.2017.1358304

O'Keefe, S., Stanley, M., Adam, K., & Lannin, N. (2019). A systematic scoping review of work interventions for hospitalised adults with an acquired neurological impairment. *Journal of Occupational Rehabilitation*, *29*(3), 569–584. https://doi.org/10.1007/s10926-018-9820-8

O'Shea, A., Frawley, P., Leahy, J. W., & Nguyen, H. D. (2020). A critical appraisal of sexuality and relationships programs for people with acquired brain injury. *Sexuality and Disability*, *38*(1), 57–83. https://doi.org/10.1007/s11195-020-09616-5

Paice, L., Aleligay, A., & Checklin, M. (2020). A systematic review of interventions for adults with social communication impairments due to an acquired brain injury: Significant other reports. *International Journal of Speech-Language Pathology*, *22*, 537–548. https://doi.org/10.1080/17549507.2019.1701082

Pan, J., Wu, J., Liu, J., Wu, J., & Wang, F. (2021). A systematic review of sleep in patients with disorders of consciousness: From diagnosis to prognosis. *Brain Sciences*, *11*(8), 1–14. https://doi.org/10.3390/brainsci11081072

Pei, Y., & O'Brien, K. H. (2021). Reading abilities post traumatic brain injury in adolescents and adults: A systematic review and meta-analysis. *American Journal of Speech-Language Pathology*, *30*, 789–816.

Perry, S. A., Coetzder, R., & Saville, C. W. N. (2020). The effectiveness of physical exercise as an intervention to reduce depressive symptoms following traumatic brain injury: A meta-analysis and systematic review. *Neuropsychological Rehabilitation*, *30(3)*, 564–578. https://doi.org/10.1080/09602011. 2018.1469417

Pertab, J. L., Merkley, T. L., Cramond, A. J., Cramond, K., Paxton, H., Wu, T. (2018). Concussion and the autonomic nervous system: An introduction to the field and the results of a systematic review. *NeuroRehabilitation*, *42*(4), 397–427. https://doi.org/10.3233/NRE-172298

Phillips, N. L., Parry, L., Mandalis, A., & Lah, S. (2017). Working memory outcomes following traumatic brain injury in children: A systematic review with meta-analysis. *Child Neuropsychology*, *23*(1), 26–66.

Ryttersgaard, T. O., Johnsen, S. P., Riis, J. O., Mogensen, P. H., & Bjarkam, C. R. (2020). Prevalence of depression after moderate to severe traumatic brain injury among adolescents and young adults: A systematic review. *Scandinavian Journal of Psychology*, *61*(2), 297–306. https://doi.org/10.1111/sjop.12587

Schlemmer, E., & Nicholson, N. (2022). Vestibular rehabilitation effectiveness for adults with mild traumatic brain injury/concussion: A mini-systematic review. *American Journal of Audiology*, *31*, 228–242.

Sharma, B., Changoor, A. T., Monteiro, L., Colella, B., & Green, R. E. A. (2019). The scale of neurodegeneration in moderate-to-severe traumatic brain injury: A systematic review protocol. *Systematic Reviews*, *8*(1), 1–5. https://doi.org/10.1186/s13643-019-1208-0

Sharma, B., Changoor, A. T., Monteiro, L., Colella, B., & Green, R. E. A. (2020). Prognostic factors for neurodegeneration in chronic moderate-to-severe traumatic brain injury: A systematic review protocol. *Systematic Reviews*, *9*(1), 1–6. https://doi.org/10.1186/s13643-020-1281-4

Shorland, J., Douglas, J., & O'Halloran, R. (2020). Cognitive-communication difficulties following traumatic brain injury sustained in older adulthood: A scoping review. *International Journal of Language & Communication Disorders*, *55*(6), 821–836. https://doi.org/10.1111/1460-6984.12560

Silveira, K., & Smart, C. M. (2020). Cognitive, physical, and psychological benefits of yoga for acquired brain injuries: A systematic review of recent findings. *Neuropsychological Rehabilitation, 30*(7), 1388–1407.

Simpson, G., Simons-Coghill, M., Bates, A., & Gan, C. (2017). What is known about sexual health after pediatric acquired brain injury: A scoping review. *NeuroRehabilitation, 41*(2), 261–280.

Stone, B., Dowling, S., & Cameron, A. (2018). Cognitive impairment and homelessness: A scoping review. *Health and Social Care in the Community, 27*, e125-e142. https://doi.org/10.1111/hsc.12682

Synnot, A., Bragge, P., Lunny, C., Menon, D., Clavisi, O., Pattuwage, L., Volovici, V., Mondello, S., Cnossen, M. C., Donoghue, E., Gruen, R. L., & Maas, A. (2018). The currency, completeness, and quality of systematic reviews of acute management of moderate to severe traumatic brain injury: A comprehensive evidence map. *PLoS ONE, 13*(6), 1–25. https://doi.org/10.1371/journal.pone.0198676

Tan, L., Zeng, L., Wang, N., Deng, M., Chen, Y., Ma, T., Zhang, L., & Lu, Z. (2019). Acupuncture to promote recovery and disorder of consciousness after traumatic brain injury: A systematic review and meta-analysis. *Evidence-Based Complementary and Alternative Medicine, 2019*. https://doi.org/10.1155/2019/5190515

Thomas, L., Lander, L., Cox, N., & Romani, C. (2020). Speech and language therapy for aphasia: parameters and outcomes. *Aphasiology, 34*(5), 603–642. https://doi.org/10.1080/02687038.2020.1712588

Thomas, R. E., Alves, J., Vaska, M., & Magalhaes, R. (2017). Therapy and rehabilitation of mild traumatic brain injury/concussion. *Restorative Neurology & Neuroscience, 35*(6), 643–666.

Unsworth, D. J., & Mathias, J. L. (2017). Traumatic brain injury and alcohol/substance abuse: A Bayesian meta-analysis comparing the outcomes of people with and without a history of abuse. *Journal of Clinical and Experimental Neuropsychology, 39*(6), 547–562. https://doi.org/10.1080/13803395.2016.1248812

Vanderbeken, I., & Kerckhofs, E. (2017). A systematic review of the effects of physical exercise on cognition in stroke and traumatic brain injury patients. *NeuroRehabilitation, 40*(1), 33–48. https://doi.org/10.3233/NRE-161388

van Dijck, J. T. J. M., Dijkman, M. D., Ophuis, R. H., de Ruiter, G. C. W., Peul, W. C., & Polinder, S. (2019). In-hospital costs after severe traumatic brain injury: A systematic review and quality assessment. *PLoS ONE, 14*(7), e0216743. https://doi.org/10.1371/journal.pone.0216743

van Dijck, J. T. J. M., Dijkman, M. D., Ophuis, R. H., de Ruiter, G. C. W., Peul, W. C., & Polinder, S. (2019). Correction: In-hospital costs after severe traumatic brain injury: A systematic review and quality assessment. *PLoS ONE, 14*(7), e0219529. https://doi.org/10.1371/journal.pone.0219529

Varghese, R., Chakrabarty, J., & Menon, M. (2017). Nursing management of adults with severe traumatic brain injury: A narrative review. *Girish Indian Journal of Critical Care Medicine, 21*(10), 684–697.

Verberne, D. P. J., Spauwen, P. J. J., & van Heugten, C. M. (2019). Psychological interventions for treating neuropsychiatric consequences of acquired brain injury: A systematic review. *Neuropsychological Rehabilitation, 29*(10), 1509–1542.

Vincy, C., Toccalino, D., Omar, S., Shah, R., & Colantonio, A. (2022). A systematic review on integrated care for traumatic brain injury, mental health, and substance use. *PLoS ONE, 17*(3), e0264116. https://doi.org/10.1371/journal.pone.0264116

Walker, L. A. S., Lindsay-Brown, A. P., & Berard, J. A. (2019). Cognitive fatigability interventions in neurological conditions: A systematic review. *Neurology and Therapy, 8*(2), 251–271.

Wong-Gonzalez, D., & Buchanan, L. (2019). A meta-analysis of task-related influences in prospective memory in traumatic brain injury. *Neuropsychological Rehabilitation*, *29*(5), 657–671. https://doi.org/10.1080/09602011.2017.1313748

Xu, G-Z., Li, Y-F., Wang, M-D., & Cao, D-Y. (2017). Complementary and alternative interventions for fatigue management after traumatic brain injury: A systematic review. *Therapeutic Advances in Neurological Disorders*, *10*(5), 229–239. https://doi.org/10.1177/1756285616682675

Zhang, J., Zhang, Y., Zou, J., & Cao, F. (2021). A meta-analysis of cohort studies: Traumatic brain injury and risk of Alzheimer's Disease. *PLoS ONE*, *16*(6), e0253206. https://doi.org/10.1371/journal.pone.0253206

Amputation

Batsford, S., Ryan, C. G., & Martin, D. J. (2017). Non-pharmacological conservative therapy for phantom limp pain: A systematic review of randomized controlled trials. *Physiotherapy Theory and Practice*, *33*(3), 173–183. https://doi.org/10.1080/09593985.2017.1288283

Blanchette, V., Brousseau-Foley, M., & Cloutier, L. (2020). Effect of contact with podiatry in a team approach context on diabetic foot ulcer and lower extremity amputation: Systematic review and meta-analysis. *Journal of Foot & Ankle Research*, *13*(1), 1–12. https://doi.org/10.1186/s13047-020-0380-8

Brooks, S. G., Atkinson, S. L., Cimino, S. R., MacKay, C., Mayo, A. L., & Hitzig, S. L. (2021). Sexuality and sexual health in adults with limb loss: A systematic review. *Sexuality & Disability*, *39*(1), 3–31. https://doi.org/10.1007/s11195-020-09665-w

Cianni, L., Bocchi, M. B., Vitiello, R., Greco, T., de Marco, D., Masci, G., Maccauro, G., Pitocco, D., & Persiano, C. (2020). Arthrodesis in the Charcot foot: A systematic review. *Orthopedic Reviews*, *12*, 64–68. https://doi.org/10.4081/or.2020.8670

Darter, B. J., Hawley, C. E., Armstrong, A. J., Avellone, L., & Wehman, P. (2018). Factors influencing functional outcomes and return-to-work after amputation: A review of the literature. *Journal of Occupational Rehabilitation*, *28*(4), 656–665. https://doi.org/10.1007/s10926-018-9757-y

Dillon, M. P., Quigley, M., & Fatone, S. (2017). A systematic review describing incidence rate and prevalence of dysvascular partial foot amputation; how both have changed over time and compare to transtibial amputation. *Systematic Reviews*, *6*, 1–16. https://doi.org/10.1186/s13643-017-0626-0

Escamilla-Nunez, R., Michelini, Al, & Andrysek, J. (2020). Biofeedback systems for gait rehabilitation of individuals with lower-limb amputation: A systematic review. *Sensors*, *20*(6), 1–26. https://doi.org/10.3390/s20061628

Fan, L., & Wu, X.-J. (2021). Sex difference for the risk of amputation in diabetic patients: A systematic review and meta-analysis. *PLoS ONE*, *16*(3), 1–16. https://doi.org/10.1371/journal.pone.0243797

Healy, A., Farmer, S., Eddison, N., Allcock, J., Perry, T., Pandyan, A., & Chockalingam, N. (2020). A scoping literature review of studies assessing effectiveness and cost-effectiveness of prosthetic and orthotic interventions. *Disability & Rehabilitation: Assistive Technology*, *15*(1), 60–66. https://doi.org/10.1080/17483107.2018.1523953

Jiang, S., Zhou, M., Xia, R., Bai, J., & Yan, L. (2021). Gabapentin for phantom limb pain after amputation in pediatric oncology: A systematic review protocol. *Systematic Reviews*, *10*(1), 1–6. https://doi.org/10.1186/s13643-020-01571-8

Limakatso, K., Bedwell, G. J., Madden, V. J., & Parker, R. (2020). The prevalence and risk factors for phantom limb pain in people with amputations: A systematic review and meta-analysis. *PLoS ONE*, *15*(10), 1–21. https://doi.org/10.1371/journal.pone.0240431

Lin, C., Liu, J., & Sun, H. (2020). Risk factors for lower extremity amputation in patients with diabetic foot ulcers: A meta-analysis. *PLoS ONE, 15*(9), 1–15. https://doi.org/10.1371/journal.pone.0239236

Liu, M., Zhang, W., Yan, Z., & Yan, X. (2018). Smoking increases the risk of diabetic foot amputation: A meta-analysis. *Experimental & Therapeutic Medicine, 15*(2), 1680–1685. https://doi.org/10.3892/etm.2017.5538

Narres, M., Kvitkina, T., Claessen, H., Droste, S., Schuster, B., Morbach, S., Rümenapf, G., Van Acker, K., & Icks, A. (2017). Incidence of lower extremity amputations in the diabetic compared with the non-diabetic population: A systematic review. *PLoS ONE, 12*(8), 1–28. https://doi.org/10.1371/journal.pone.0182081

Nawijn, F., Smeeing, D. P. J., Houwert, R. M., Leenen, L. P. H., & Hietbrink, F. (2020). Time is of the essence when treating necrotizing soft tissue infections: A systematic review and meta-analysis. *World Journal of Emergency Surgery, 15*(1), 1–11. https://doi.org/10.1186/s13017-019-0286-6

Olsson, M., Järbrink, K., Divakar, U., Bajpal, R., Upton, Z., Schmidtchen, A., & Car, J. (2019). The humanistic and economic burden of chronic wounds: A systematic review. *Wound Repair & Regeneration, 27*(1), 114–215. https://doi.org/10.1111/wrr.12683

Owolabi, E. O., Adeloye, D., Ajayi, A. I., McCaul, M., Davies, J., & Chu, K. M. 2022. Lower limb amputations among individuals living with diabetes mellitus in low- and middle-income countries: A systematic review. *PLoS ONE, 17*(4), eo266907. https://doi.org/10.1371/journal.pone.0266907

Poonsiri, J., Dekker, R., Dijkstra, P. U., Hijmans, J. M., & Geertzen, J. H. B. (2018). Bicycling participation in people with lower limb amputation: A scoping review. *BMC Musculoskeletal Disorders, 19*(1), 1–12. https://doi.org/10.1186/s12891-018-2313-2

Putko, R. M., Bedrin, M. D., Clark, D. M., Psicoya, A. S., Dunn, J. C., & Nesti, L. J. (2021). SARS-CoV-2 and limb ischema: A systematic review. *Journal of Clinical Orthopaedics and Trauma, 12*, 194–199.

Ribeiro, D., Cimino, S. R., Mayo, A. L., Ratto, M., & Hitzig, S. L. (2021). 3D printing and amputation: A scoping review. *Disability & Rehabilitation: Assistive Technology, 16*(2), 221–240. https://doi.org/10.1080/17483107.2019.1646825

ten Kate, J., Smit, G., & Breedveld, P. (2017). 3D-printed upper limb prostheses: A review. *Disability & Rehabilitation: Assistive Technology, 12*(3), 300–314. https://doi.org/10.1080/17483107.2016.1253117

Ülger, O., Yildirim Sahan, T., & Çelik, S. E. (2018). A systematic literature review of physiotherapy and rehabilitation approaches to lower-limb amputation. *Physiotherapy Theory & Practice, 34*(11), 821–834.

van Schaik, L., Geertzen, J. H. B., Dijkstra, P. U., & Dekker, R. (2019). Metabolic costs of activities of daily living in persons with a lower limb amputation: A systematic review and meta-analysis. *PLoS ONE, 14*(3), 1–24. https://doi.org/10.1371/journal.pone.0213256

Young, M., McKay, C., Williams, S., Rouse, P., & Bilzon, J. L. J. (2019). Time-related changes in quality of life in persons with lower limb amputation or spinal cord injury: Protocol for a systematic review. *Systematic Reviews, 8*(1), 1–6. https://doi.org/10.1186/s13643-019-1108-3

Blindness and Visual Impairment

Augestad, L. V. (2017). Self-concept and self-esteem among children and young adults with visual impairment: A systematic review. *Cogent Psychology, 4*(1), 1–12. https://doi.org/10.1080/23311908.2017.1319652

Dodamani, A., & Dodamani, S. (2018). Library services for the people with visual impairments in higher education: A review of the literature. *Library of Progress-Library Science, Information Technology & Computer*, *38*(1), 123–128. https://doi.org/10.5958/2320-317X.2018.00012.0

Giles, S. J., Panagioti, M., Riste, L., Cheraghi-Sohi, S., Lewis, P., Adeyemi, I., Davies, K., Morris, R., Phipps, D., Dickenson, C., Ashcroft, D., & Sanders, C. (2021). Visual impairment and medication safety: A protocol for a scoping review. *Systematic Reviews*, *10*(1), 1–6. https://doi.org/10.1186/s13643-021-01800-8

Ivy, S. E., & Ledford, J. R. (2022). A systematic review of behavioral interventions to reduce restricted or repetitive behavior of individuals with visual impairment. *Journal of Behavioral Education*, *31*, 94–122. https://doi.org/10.1007/s10864-020-09418-x

Klingenberg, O. G., Holkesvik, A. H., & Augestad, L. B. (2019). Research evidence for mathematics education for students with visual impairment: A systematic review. *Cogent Education*, *6*, 1–19. https://doi.org/10/1080/233119=86X.2019.1626322

Kroezen, M., van den Akker, N., van Genderen, M. M., & Wolkorte, R. (2020). Visual impairment and blindness in people with intellectual disabilities: A systematic review. *Optometry & Visual Performance*, *8*(3), 109–121.

Liu, C.-J., & Chang, M. C. (2020). Interventions within the scope of occupational therapy practice to improve performance of daily activities of older adults with low vision: A systematic review. *American Journal of Occupational Therapy*, *74*(1), 1–18. https://doi.org/10.5014/ajot.2019.038372

Miyauchi, H. (2020). A systematic review on inclusive education of student with visual impairment. *Education Sciences*, *10*, 1–15. https://doi.org/10.3390/educsci10110346

Miyauchi, H., & Paul, P. V. (2020). Perceptions of students with visual impairment on inclusive education: A narrative meta-analysis. *Human Research and Rehabilitation*, *10*(2), 4–25. https://doi.org/10.21554/hrr.092001

Nastasi, J. A. (2020). Occupational therapy interventions supporting leisure and social participation for older adults with low vision: A systematic review. *American Journal of Occupational Therapy*, *74*(1), 1–9. https://doi.org/10.5014/ajot.2019.038521

Schakel, W., Bode, C., Elsman, E. B. M., Aa, H. P. A., Vries, R., Rens, G. H. M. B., & Nispen, R. M. A. (2019). The association between visual impairment and fatigue: A systematic review and meta-analysis of observational studies. *Ophthalmic & Physiological Optics*, *39*(6), 399–413. https://doi.org/10.1111/opo.12647

Smallfield, S., & Kaldenberg, J. (2020). Occupational therapy interventions to improve reading performance of older adults with low vision: A systematic review. *American Journal of Occupational Therapy*, *74*(1), 1–18. https://doi.org/10.5014/ajot.2020.038380

Sorokowska, A., Sorokowski, P., Karwowski, M., Larsson, M., & Hummel, T. (2019). Olfactory perception and blindness: A systematic review and meta-analysis. *Psychological Research*, *83*, 1595–1611. https://doi.org/10.1007/s00426-018-1035-2

van der Ham, A. J., van der Aa, H. P. A., Brunes, A., Heir, T., de Vries, R., van Rens, G. H. M. B., & van Nispen, R. M. A. (2021). The development of posttraumatic stress disorder in individuals with visual impairment: A systematic search and review. *Ophthalmic & Physiological Optics*, *41*(2), 331–341.

Vervloed, M. P. J., van den Broek, E. C. G., & van Eikden, A. J. P. M. (2020). Critical review of setback in development in young children with congenital blindness or visual impairment. *International Journal of Disability, Development & Education*, *67*(3), 336–355. https://doi.org/10.1080/1034921X.2019.1588231

Brachial Plexus Injury

Cai, H., Fan, X., Feng, P., Wang, X., & Xie, Y. (2021). Optimal dose of perineural dexmedetomidine to prolong analgesia after brachial plexus blockade: A systematic review and meta-analysis of 57 randomized clinical trials. *BMC Anesthesiology, 21*(1), 1–20.

Gobets, D., Beckerman, H., DeGroot, V., Van Doorn-Loogman, M. H., & Becher, J. G. (201). Indications and effects of botulinum toxin A for obstetric brachial plexus injury: A systematic literature review. *Developmental Medicine & Child Neurology, 52*(6), 517–528. https://doi.org/10.1111/j.1469-8749.2009.03607.x

Hassan, B. S., Abbass, M. E., & Elshennawy, S. (2018). Systematic review of the effectiveness of Kinesio taping for children with brachial plexus injury. *Physiology Research International, 25,* 1–11. https://https://doi.org/g/org/10.1002/pri.1794

Héroux, J., Belley-Côté, E., Echavé, P., Loignon, M. J., Bessette, P. O., Patenaude, N., Baillargeon, J. P., & D'Aragon, F. (2019). Functional recovery with peripheral nerve block versus general anesthesia for upper limb surgery: A systematic review protocol. *Systematic Reviews, 8,* 1–7. https://doi.org/10.1186/s13643-019-1204-4

Ho, E. S., Kim, D., Klar, K., Anthony, A., Davidge, K., Borschel, G. H., Hopyan, S., Clarke, H. M., & Wright, F. V. (2019). Prevalence and etiology of elbow flexion contractures in brachial plexus birth injury: A scoping review. *Journal of Pediatric Rehabilitation Medicine: An Interdisciplinary Approach, 12,* 75–86. https://doi.org/10.3233/PRM-170511

Ho., E. S., Zuccaro, J., Klar, K., Anthony, A., Davidge, K., Borschel, G. H., Hopyan, S., Clarke, H. M., & Wright, F. V. (2019). Effectiveness of non-surgical and surgical interventions for elbow flexion contractures in brachial plexus birth injury: A systematic review. *Journal of Pediatric Rehabilitation Medicine: An Interdisciplinary Approach, 12,* 87–100. https://doi.org/10.3233/PRM-180563

Justice, D. (2018). Use of neuromuscular electrical stimulation in the treatment of neonatal brachial plexus palsy: A literature review. *The Open Journal of Occupational Therapy, 6*(3), Article 10. https://doi.org/10.15453/2168-6408.1431

Leigheb, M., Tricca, S., Percivale, I., Licandro, D., Paladini, A., Barini, M., Guzzardi, G., Grassi, F. A., Stecco, A., & Carriero, A. (2021). Diagnostic accuracy of the Magnetic Resonance Imaging in adult post-ganglionic brachial plexus traumatic injuries: A systematic review and meta-analysis. *Brain Sciences, 11,* 173. https://doi.org/10.3390/brainsci11020173

Li, M., Zhang, P., & Wei, D. (2022). Efficacy of dexamethasone versus dexmedetomidine combined with local anesthetics in brachial plexus block: A meta-analysis and systematic review. *Evidence-based Complementary & Alternative Medicine (eCAM),* 1–9. https://doi.org/10.115/2022/7996754

Mohammed, A. Q., Alhamaidah, M. F., Hussein, H. A., Alkhfaji, H., Hasan, S. R., & Roomi, A. B. (2020). Infraclavicular brachial plexus block for upper limb surgeries in adult patients: A nonsystematic review. *International Journal of Pharmaceutical Research, 12*(1), 2123–2127. Https://doi.org/10.31838/ijpr/2020.12.01.332

Pondaag, W., & Malessy, M. J. A. (2014). The evidence for nerve repair in obstetric brachial plexus palsy revisited. *BioMed Research International, 2014,* 1–11. https://dx.https://doi.org/.org/10.1155/2014/434619

Qi, W., Xu, Y, Yan, Z, Zhan, J., Lin, J., Pan, X., & Xue, X. (2021). The tight-rope technique versus clavicular hook plate for treatment of acute acromioclavicular joint dislocation: A systematic review and meta-analysis. *Journal of Investigative Surgery, 34,* 20–29. ++https://doi.org/10.1080/089411939.2019.1593559

Rezzadeh, K., Donnelly, M., Vieira, D., Daar, D., Shah, A., & Hacquebord, J. (2020). The extent of brachial plexus injury: An important factor in spinal accessory nerve to suprascapular nerve transfer outcomes. *British Journal of Neurosurgery, 34*(5), 591–594.

Sarac, C., Duijnisveld, B. J., van der Weide, A., Schoones, J. W., Malessy, M. J. A., Nelissen, R. G. H. H., & Vliet Vlieland, T. P. M. (2015). Outcomes measures used in clinical studies on neonatal brachial plexus palsy: A systematic literature review using the International Classification of Functioning, Disability, and Health. *Journal of Pediatric Rehabilitation Medicine: An Interdisciplinary Approach, 8*, 167–186. https://doi.org/10.3233/PRM-150335

Shin, H. W., Ju, B. J., Jang, Y. K., You, H. S., Kang, H., & Park, J. Y. (2017). Effect of tramadol as an adjuvant to local anesthetics for brachial plexus block: A systematic review and meta-analysis. *PLoS ONE, 12*(9), e0184649. https://doi.org/10.1371/journal.pone.0184649

Song, Z.-G., Pang, S.-Y., Wang, G.-Y., & Zhang, Z. (2021). Comparison of postoperative analgesic effects in response to either dexamethasone or dexmedetomidine as local anesthetic adjuvants: A systematic review and meta-analysis of randomized controlled trials. *Journal of Anesthesia, 35*, 270–287. https://doi.org/10.1007/s00540-021-02895-y

Thamploo, D., Bhat, D. I., Kulkarni, M. V., & Devi, B. I. (2019). Brachial plexus injury and resting-state fMRI: Need for consensus. *Neurology India, 67*(3), 679–683. https://doi.org/10.4103/0028-3886.263178

Thatte, M. R., Babhulkar, S., & Hiremath, A. (2013). Brachial plexus injury in adults: Diagnosis and surgical treatment strategies. *Annals of Indian Academy of Neurology, 16*(1), 26–33. https://doi.org/10.4103/0972-2327.107686

Wade, R. G., Takwoingi, Y., Wormald, J. C. R., Ridgway, J. P., Tanner, S., Rankine, J. J., & Bourke, G. (2018). Magnetic Resonance Imaging for detecting root avulsions in traumatic adult brachial plexus injuries: Protocol for a systematic review of diagnostic accuracy. *Systematic Reviews, 7*(1), 1–6. https://doi.org/10.1186/s13643-018-0737-2

Zhang, D., Garg, R., Earp, B., Blazar, P., Dyer, G. S. (2021). Shoulder arthrodesis versus upper trapezius transfer for traumatic brachial plexus injury: A proportional meta-analysis. *Medical Advances in Orthopedics.* https://doi.org/10.1155/2021/4445498

Burns

Hornsby, N., Blom, L., & Sengoelge, M. (2020). Psychosocial interventions targeting recovery in child and adolescent burns: A systematic review. *Journal of Pediatric Psychology, 45*(1), 15–33. https://doi.org/10.1093/jpepsy/jsz087

Mudawarima, T., Chiwaridzo, M., Jelsma, J., Grimmer, K., & Muchemwa, F. C. (2017). A systematic review protocol on the effectiveness of therapeutic exercises utilised by physiotherapists to improve function in patients with burns. *Systematic Reviews, 6*, 1–7. https://doi.org/10.1186/s13643-017-0592-6

Spronk, I., Legemate, C., Oen, I., van Loey, N., Polinder, S., & van Baar, M. (2018). Health related quality of life in adults after burn injuries: A systematic review. *PLoS ONE, 13*(5), e0197507. https://doi.org/10.1371/journal.pone.-197507

Spronk, I., Van Loey, N. E. E., Sewalt, C., Nieboer, D., Renneberg, B., Moi, A. L., Oster, C., Orwelius, L., van Barr, M. E., & Polinder, S. (2020). Recovery of health-related quality of life after burn injuries: An individual participant data meta-analysis. *PLoS ONE, 15*(1), e0226653. https://doi.org/10.1371/journal.pone.0226653

Williams, H. M., Hunter, K., Clapham, K., Ryder, C., Kimble, R., & Griffin, B. (2020). Efficacy and cultural appropriateness of psychosocial interventions for paediatric burn patients and caregivers: A systematic review. *BMC Public Health, 20*(1), 1–16. https://doi.org/10.1186/s12889-020-8366-9

Woolard, A., Hill, N. T. M., McQueen, M., Martin, L., Milroy, H., Wood, F. M., Bullman, I., & Lin, A. (2021). The psychological impact of paediatric burn injuries: A systematic review. *BMC Public Health, 21*(1), 1–27. https://doi.org/10.1186/s12889-021-12296-1

Chronic Pain

Affatato, O., Moulin, T. C., Pisanu, C., Babasieva, V. S., Russo, M., Aydinlar, E. I., Torelli, P., Chubarev, V. N., Tarasov, V. V., Schioth, H. G., & Mwinyi, J. (2021). High efficacy of onabotulinumtoxinA treatment in patients with comorbid migraine and depression: A meta-analysis. *Journal of Translational Medicine, 19*, 1–11. https://doi.org/10.1186/s12967-021-02801-w

Al Adal, S., Pourkazemi, F., Mackey, M., & Hiller, C. (2019). The prevalence of pain in people with chronic ankle instability: A systematic review. *Journal of Athletic Training, 54*(6), 662–670. https://doi.org/10.4085/1062-6050-531-17

AlMazrou, S. H., Elliott, R. A., Knaggs, R. D., & AlAujan, S. S. (2020). Cost-effectiveness of pain management services for chronic low back pain: A systematic review of published studies. *BMC Health Services Research, 20*, 1–11. https://doi.org/10.1186/s12913-020-5013-1

Allegri, N., Liccione, D., Vecchi, T., Sandrini, G., Mennuni, S., Rulli, E., Corli, O., Floriani, I., De Simone, I., Biagioli, E., Vanacore, N., Allegri, M., & Govoni, S. (2019). Systematic review and meta-analysis on neuropsychological effects of long-term use of opioids in patients with chronic noncancer pain. *Pain Practice, 19*(3), 328–343. https://doi.org/10.1111/papr.12741

Åsberg, A. N., Heuch, I., & Hagen, K. (2017). The mortality associated with chronic widespread musculoskeletal complaints: A systematic review of the literature. *Musculoskeletal Care, 15*, 104–113. https://doi.org/10.1002/msc.1156

Battista, S., Buzzatti, L., Gandolfi, M., Finocchi, C., Falsiroli, M. L., Vinceconti, A., Giardulli, B., & Testa, M. (2021). The use of Botulinum Toxin A as an adjunctive therapy in the management of chronic musculoskeletal pain: A systematic review with meta-analysis. *Toxins, 13*(9), 640. https://doi.org/10.3390/toxins13090640

Bilterys, T., Siffain, C., De Maeyer, I., Van Looveren, E., Mairesse, Ol, Nijs, J., Meeus, M., Ickmans, K., Cagnie, B., Goubert, D., Danneels, L., Moens, M., & Malfliet, A. (2021). Associates of insomnia in people with chronic spinal pain: A systematic review and meta-analysis. *Journal of Clinical Medicine, 10*(14), 3175–3175. https://doi.org/10.3390/jcm10143175

Borrella-Andrés, S., Marqués-Garcia, I., Lucha-López, M. O., Fanlo-Mazas, P., Hernández-Secorún, M., Pérez-Bellmunt, A., Tricás-Moreno, J. M. & Hidalgo-Garcia, C. (2021). Manual therapy as a management of cervical radiculopathy: A systematic review. *BioMed Research International*, 1–15. https://doi.org/10.1155/2021/9936981

Buruck, G., Tomaschek, A., Wendsche, J., Ochsmann, E., & Dörfel, D. (2019). Psychosocial areas of worklife and chronic low back pain: A systematic review and meta-analysis. *BMC Musculoskeletal Disorders, 20*, 1–16. https://doi.org/10.1186/s12891-019-2826-3

Chen, Y-J., Chen, C-T., Liu, J-Y., Shimizu Bassi, G., & Yang, Y-Q. (2019). What is the appropriate acupuncture treatment schedule for chronic pain? Review and analysis of randomized controlled trials. *Evidence-based Complementary & Alternative Medicine, x*, 1–10. https://doi.org/10.1007/s11136

Cheng, J. O. S., & Cheng, S-T. (2019). Effectiveness of physical and cognitive-behavioural intervention programmes for chronic musculoskeletal pain in adults: A systematic review and meta-analysis of randomized controlled trials. *PLoS ONE*, *14*(10), 1–30. https://doi.org/10.1371/journal.pone.0223367

Compagnoni, R., Gualtierotti, R., Luceri, F., Sciancalepore, F., & Randelli, P. S. (2019). Fibromyalgia and shoulder surgery: A systematic review and a critical appraisal of the literature. *Journal of Clinical Medicine*, *8*(10), 1–9. https://doi.org/10.3390/cm8101518

de Oliveira, N. T. B., dos Santos, I., Miyamoto, G. C., & Cabral, C. M. N. (2019). Effects of aerobic exercise in the treatment of older adults with chronic musculoskeletal pain: A protocol of a systematic review. *Systematic Reviews*, *8*(1), 1–5. https://doi.org/10.1186/s13643-019-1165-7

Dépelteau, A., Lagueux, E., Pagé, R., & Hudon, C. (2021). Occupational adaptation of people living with fibromyalgia: Systematic review and thematic synthesis. *American Journal of Occupational Therapy*, *75*(4), 1–14. https://doi.org/10.5014/ajot.2021.047134

Don, S., Voogt, L., Meeus, M., De Kooning, M., & Nijs, J. (2017). Sensorimotor incongruence in people with musculoskeletal pain: A systematic review. *World Institute of Pain*, *17*(1), 115–128. https://doi.org/10.1111/papr.12456

Duarte, R. V., Lambe, T., Raphael, J. H., Eldabe, S., & Andronis, L. (2018). Intrathecal drug delivery systems for the management of chronic noncancer pain: A systematic review of economic evaluations. *Pain Practice*, *18*(5), 666–686. https://doi.org/10.1111/papr.12650

Elibol, N., & Cavlak, U. (2019). Massage therapy in chronic musculoskeletal pain management: A scoping review of the literature. *Sports Medicine Journal*, *15*(1), 3067–3073.

Ernstzen, D. V., Louw, Q. A., & Hillier, S. L. (2017). Clinical practice guidelines for the management of chronic musculoskeletal pain in primary healthcare: A systematic review. *Implementation Science*, *12*, 1–13. https://doi.org/10.1186/s13012-016-0533-0

Faltyn, M., Cresswell, L., & Van Lieshout, R. J. (2021). Psychological problems in parents of children and adolescents with chronic pain: A systematic review and meta-analysis. *Psychology, Health & Medicine*, *26*(3), 298–312. https://doi.org/10.1080/135

Franco, J. V. A., Turk, T., Jung, J. H., Xiao, Y-T., Iakhno, S., Garrote, V., & Vietto, V. (2019). Non-pharmacological interventions for treating chronic prostatitis/chronic pelvic pain syndrome: A Cochrane systematic review. *BJU International*, *124*, 197–208. https://doi.org/10.1111/bju.14492

Fuentes-Márquez, P., Cabrera-Martos, I., & Valenza, M. C. (2019). Physiotherapy interventions for patients with chronic pelvic pai: A systematic review of the literature. *Physiotherapy Theory & Practice*, *35*(12), 1131–1138.

Garcia-Correa, H. R., Sánchez-Montoya, L. J., Daza-Arana, J. E., & Ordoñez-Mora, L. T. (2021). Aerobic physical exercise for pain intensity, aerobic capacity, and quality of life in patients with chronic pain: A systematic review and meta-analysis. *Journal of Physical Activity and Health*, *18*(9), 1126–1142. https://doi.org/10.1123/jpah.2020.0806

George, S. Z., Fritz, J. M., Silfies, S. P., Schneider, M. J., Beneciuk, J. M., Lentz, T. A., Gilliam, J. R., Hendren, S., & Norman, K. S. (2021). Clinical practice guidelines: Interventions for the management of acute and chronic low back pain: Revision 2021. *Journal of Orthopaedic & Sports Physical Therapy*, *51*(11), CPG1-CPG60. https://doi.org/10.2519/jospt.2021.0304

Geraghty, A. W. A., Maund, E., Newell, D., Santer, M., Everitt, H., Price, C., Pincus, T., Moore, M., Little, P., West, R., & Staurt, B. (2021). Self-management for chronic widespread pain including fibromyalgia: A systematic review and meta-analysis. *PLoS ONE*, *16*(7), 1–31. https://doi.org/10.1371/journal.pone.0254642

Griffin, A., Leaver, A., & Moloney, N. (2017). General exercise does not improve long-term pain and disability in individuals with whiplash-associated disorders: A systematic review. *The*

Journal of Orthopaedic and Sports Physical Therapy, 47(7), 472–480. https://doi.org/10.2519/jospt.2017/081

Griffin, H., Hay-Smith, E., & Jean, C. (2019). Characteristics of a well-functioning chronic pain team: A systematic review. *New Zealand Journal of Physiotherapy, 47*(1), 7–17. https://doi.org/10.15619/NZJP/47.1.02

Guy, L, McKinstry, C., & Bruce, C. (2019). Effectiveness of pacing as a learned strategy for people with chronic pain: A systematic review. *American Journal of Occupational Therapy, 73*(3), 1–5.

Harrison, L. E., Timmers, I., Heathcote, L. C., Fisher, E., Tanna, V., Duarte Silva Bans, T., & Simons, L. E. (2020). Parent responses to their child's pain: Systematic review and meta-analysis of measures. *Journal of Pediatric Psychology, 45*(3), 281–298. https://doi.org/10.1123/jsr.2019-0345

Heinrich, M., Steiner, S., & Bauer, C. M. (2020). The effect of visual feedback on people suffering from chronic back and neck pain: A systematic review. *Physiotherapy Theory & Practice, 36*(11), 1220–1231. https://doi.org/10.1080/09593985.2019.1571140

Hofmeister, M., Memedovich, A., Brown, S., Saini, M., Dowsett, L. E., Lozenetti, D. L., McCarron, T. L., MacKean, G., & Clement, F. (2020). Effectiveness of neurostimulation technologies for the management of chronic pain: A systematic review. *Neuromodulation, 23*(2), 150–157. https://doi.org/10.1111/ner.13020

Hruschak, V., & Cochran, G. (2018). Psychosocial predictors in the transition from acute to chronic pain: A systemic review. *Psychology, Health & Medicine, 23*(10), 1151–1167. https://doi.org/10.1080/13548506.2018.1446097

Hsu, P-C., Wu, W-T., Han, D-S., & Chang, K-V. (2020). Comparative effectiveness of botulinum toxin injections for chronic shoulder pain: A meta-analysis of randomized controlled trials. *Toxins, 12*, 1–14. https://doi.org/10.3390/toxins12040251

Johal, H., Devji, T., Chang, Y., Simone, J., Vannabouathong, C., & Bhandari, M. (2020). Cannabinoids in chronic non-cancer pain: A systematic review and meta-analysis. *Clinical Medicine Insights: Arthritis & Musculoskeletal Disorders, 13*, 1–13. https://doi.org/10.1177/1179544120906461

Joypaul, S., Kelly, F., McMillan, S. S., & King, A. (2019). Multi-disciplinary interventions for chronic pain involving education: A systematic review. *PLoS ONE, 14*(10), 1–24. https://doi.org/10.1371/journal.pone.0223306

Kichline, T., & Cushing, C. C. (2019). A systematic review and quantitate analysis on the impact of aerobic exercise on pain intensity of children with chronic pain. *Children's Health Care, 48*(2), 244–261. https://doi.org/10.1080/02739615.2018.1531756

Klotz, S. G. R., Schon, M., Ketels, G., Lowe, B., & Brunahl, C. A. (2019). Physiotherapy management of patients with chronic pelvic pain (CPP): A systematic review. *Systematic Review, 35*(6), 516–532. https://doi.org/10.1080/09593985.2018.1455251

Koechlin, H., Whalley, B., Welton, N. J., & Locher, C. (2019). The best treatment option(s) for adult and elderly patients with chronic primary musculoskeletal pain: A protocol for a systematic review and network meta-analysis. *Systematic Reviews.* https://doi.org/10.1186/s13643-019-1174-6

Kong, L., Zhou, X., Huan, Q., Zhu, Q., Zheng, Y., Tang, C., Li, J. X., & Fang, M. (2020). The effects of shoes and insoles for low back pain: A systematic review and meta-analysis of randomized controlled trials. *Research in Sports Medicine, 28*(4), 572–587. https://doi.org/10.1080/15438627.2020.1798238

Marley, J., Tully, M. A., Porter-Armstrong, A., Bunting, B., O'Hanlon, J., Atkins, L., Howes, S., & McDonough, S. M. (2017). The effectiveness of interventions aimed at increasing physical activity in adults with persistent musculoskeletal pain: A systematic review and meta-analysis. *BMC Musculoskeletal Disorders*, *18*, 1–20. https://doi.org/10.1186/s12891-017-1836-2

Miki, T., Kondo, Y., Kurakata, H., Buzasi, E., Takebayashi, T., & Takasaki, H. (2022). The effect of cognitive functional therapy for chronic nonspecific low back pain: A systematic review and meta-analysis. *BioPsychoSocial Medicine*, *16*, 1–12. https://doi.org/10.1186/s13030-022-00241-6

Moens, M., Goudman, L., & Brouns, R. (2019). Return to work of patients treated with spinal cord stimulation for chronic pain: A systematic review and meta-analysis. *Neuromodulation*, *22*(3), 253–261. https://doi.org/10.1111/ner.12797

Papaconstantinou, E., Cancelliere, C., Verville, L., Wong, J. J., Connell, G., Yu, H., Shearer, H., Timperley, C., Chung, C., Porter, B. J., Myrtos, D., Barrigar, M., & Taylor-Valsey, A. (2021). Effectiveness of non-pharmacological interventions on sleep characteristics among adults with musculoskeletal pain and a comorbid sleep problem: A systematic review. *Chiropractic & Manual Therapies*, *29*, 1–23. https://doi.org/10.1186/s12998-021-00381-6

Peck, J., Urits, I., Peoples, S., Foster, L., Malla, A., Berger, A. A., Cornett, E. M., Kassem, H., Herman, J., Kaye, A. D., & Viswanath, O. (2021). A comprehensive review of over the counter treatment for chronic low back pain. *Pain & Therapy*, *10*(1), 69–80. https://doi.org/10.1007/s40122-020-00209-w

Pocovi, N. C., de Campos, T. F., Christine Lin, C. W., Merom, D., Tiedemann, A., & Hanrock, M. J. (2022). Walking, cycling, and swimming for nonspecific low back pain: A systematic review with meta-analysis. *The Journal of Orthopaedic and Sports Physical Therapy*, *52*(2), 85–99.

Ragnarsson, S., Myleus, A., Hurtig, A. K., Sjöberg, G., Rosvall, P. A., & Petersen, S. (2020). Recurrent pain and academic achievement in school-aged children: A systematic review. *The Journal of School Nursing*, *36*(1), 61–78.

Robinson, A., McIntosh, J., Peberdy, H., Wishart, D., Brown, G., Pope, H., & Kumar, S. (2019). The effectiveness of physiotherapy interventions on pain and quality of life in adults with persistent post-surgical pain compared to usual care: A systematic review. *PLoS ONE*, *14*(12). https://doi.org/10.1371/journal.pone.0226227

Robinson, R., & Tokolahi, E. (2021). Occupational therapy interventions for persistent pain: A systematic review. *New Zealand Journal of Occupational Therapy*, *68*(1), 15–22.

Robson, E. K., Hodder, R. K., Kamper, S. J., O'Brien, K. M., Williams, A., Lee, H., Wolfenden, L., Yoong, S., Wiggers, J., Barnett, C., & Williams, C. M. (2020). Effectiveness of weight-loss interventions for reducing pain and disability in people with common musculoskeletal disorders: A systematic review with meta-analysis. *The Journal of Orthopaedic and Sports Physical Therapy*, *50*(6), 319–333. https://doi.org/10.2519/jospt.2020.9041

Saraiva, M. D., Suzuki, G. S., Lin, S. M., de Andrade, D. C., Jacob-Filho, W. & Suemoto, C. K. (2018). Persistent pain is a risk factor for frailty: A systematic review and meta-analysis from prospective longitudinal studies. *Age and Ageing*, *47*(6), 785–793. https://doi.org/10/1080/09593985.2018.1455122

Shahmahmoodi, T., Izadi Laybiby, S., Rahimi, A., Bokee, F., & Rezaeian, Z. S. (2020). Rehabilitation in subjects with chronic non-specific low back pain with sacroiliac joint origin: Protocol for a systematic review. *Ligaments & Tendons Journal*, *10*(4), 734–739. https://doi.org/10.32098/mltj.04.2020.21

Sielski, R., Rief, W., & Glombiewski, J. A. (2017). Efficacy of biofeedback in chronic back pain: A meta-analysis. *International Journal of Behavioral Medicine*, *24*, 25–41. https://doi.org/10.1007/s12529-016-9572-9

Skamagki, G., King, A., Duncan, M., & Wahlin, C. (2018). A systematic review on workplace interventions to manage chronic musculoskeletal conditions. *Physiotherapy Research International*, *23*(4), 1–16. https://doi.org/10.1002/pri.1738

Song, K-S., Cho, J. H., Hong, J-Y., Lee, J. H., Kang, H., Ham, D-W., & Ryu, H-J. (2017). Neuropathic pain related with spinal disorders: A systematic review. *Asian Spine Journal, 11*(4), 661–674. https://doi.org/10.4184/asj.2017.11.4.661

Steenstra, I., Munhall, C., Irvin, E., Oranye, N., Passmore, S., Van Eerd, D., Mahood, Q., & Hogg-Johnson, S. (2017). Systematic review of prognostic factors for return to work in workers with sub-acute and chronic low back pain. *Journal of Occupational Rehabilitation, 27*(3), 369–381. https://doi.org/10.1007/s10926-016-9666-x

Sung, S-H., Sung, A-D-M., Sung, H-K., An, T-E-B., Kim, K. H., & Park, J-K. (2018). Acupuncture treatment for chronic pelvic pain in women: A systematic review and meta-analysis of randomized controlled trials. *Evidence-based Complementary & Alternative Medicine, 2018*, 1–7. https://doi.org/10.1155/2018/9415897

Szmuda, T., Sloniewski, P., Ali, S., & Aleksandrowicz, K. (2019). Does spinal cord stimulation due to failed back surgery syndrome lead to permanent occupational disability? *Neuromodulation, 23*, 653–659. https://doi.org/10.1111/ner.13014

Tang, S. K., Tse, M. M. Y., Leung, S. F., & Fotis, T. (2019). The effectiveness, suitability, and sustainability of non-pharmacological methods of managing pain in community-dwelling older adults: A systematic review. *BMC Public Health, 19*(1), 1–10. https://doi.org/10.1186/s12889-019-7831-9

Thornton, J., Goyat, R., Dwibedi, N., Kelley, G., Thornton, D. J., & Kelley, G. A. (2017). Health-related quality of life in patients receiving long-term opioid therapy: A systematic review and meta-analysis. *Quality of Life Research, 26*(8), 1955–1967. https://doi.org/10.1007/s11136-017-1538-0

Tseli, E., Grooten, W. J. A., Stanlnacke, B. M., Boersma, K., Enthoven, P., Gerdle, B., & Ang, B. O. (2017). Predictors of multidisciplinary rehabilitation outcomes in patients with chronic musculoskeletal pain: Protocol for a systematic review and meta-analysis. *Systematic Reviews, 11*(6), 1–9. https://doi.org/10.1186/s13643-017-0598-0

Vugts, M. A. P., Joosen, M. C. W., van der Geer, J. E., Zeditz, A., M. E. E., & Vrijhoef, H. (2018). The effectiveness of various computer-based interventions for patients with chronic pain or functional somatic syndromes: A systematic review and meta-analysis. *PLoS ONE*, e0196467. https://doi.org/10.1371/journal.pone.o196467

Wong, A. Y. L., Forss, K. S., Jakobsson, J., Schoeb, V., Kumlien, C., & Borglin, G. (2018). Older adults' experience in chronic low back pain and its implications on their daily life: Study protocol of a systematic review of qualitative research. *Systematic Reviews, 7*(1). https://doi.org/10.1186/s13643-018-0742-5

Xie, G., Wang, T., Tang, X., Guo, X., Xu, Y., Deng, L., Sun, H., Ma Z, Ai, Y., Jiang, B., Li, L., Luo, W., Huang, W., Xia, Y., Zhao, H., Wang, X, Guo, Y., & Liao, J. (2020). Acupoint injection for nonspecific chronic low back pain: A systematic review and meta-analysis of randomized controlled studies. *Evidence-based Complementary & Alternative Medicine*, 1–12. https://doi.org/10.1155/2020/3976068

Deafness and Hearing Impairment

Agmon, M., Lavie, L., & Doumas, M. (2017). The association between hearing loss, postural control, and mobility in older adults: A systematic review. *Journal of the American Academy of Audiology, 28*(6), 575–588.

Alasim, K. N., & Alqraini, F. (2020). Do d/deaf and hard of hearing children need access to a spoken phonology to learn to read? A narrative meta-analysis. *American Annals of the Deaf, 164*(5), 531–545. https://doi.org/10.1353/aad.2020.0001

Almufarrij, I., Uus, K., & Munro, K. (2020). Does coronavirus affect the audio-vestibular system? A rapid systematic review. *International Journal of Audiology, 59*(7), 487–491. https://doi.org/10.1080/14992027.2020.1776406

Alsalamah, A. (2020). Using captioning services with deaf and hard of hearing students in higher education: A systematic review. *American Annals of the Deaf, 165*(1), 114–127.

Bernhard, N., Gauger, U., Romo Ventura, E., Uecker, F. C., Olze, H., Knopke, S., Hänsel, T., & Coordes, A. (2021). Duration of deafness impacts auditory performance after cochlear implantation: A meta-analysis. *Laryngoscope Investigative Otolaryngology, 6*(2), 291–301. https://doi.org/10.1002/lio2.528

Boisvert, I., Reis, M., Au, A., Cowan, R., & Dowell, R. C. (2020). Cochlear implantation outcomes in adults: A scoping review. *PLoS ONE, 15*(5), 1–26. https://doi.org/10.1371/journal.pone.0232421

Butler, L. K., Kiran, S., & Tager-Flusberg, H. (2020). Functional near-infrared spectroscopy in the study of speech and language impairment across the life span: A systematic review. *American Journal of Speech-Language Pathology, 29*(3), 1674–1701. https://doi.org/10.1044/2020_AJSLP-19-00050

Byatt, T. J., Dally, K. & Duncan, J. (2019). Systematic review of literature: Social capital and adolescents who are deaf and hard of hearing. *Journal of Deaf Studies & Deaf Education, 24*(4), 319–332. https://doi.org/10.1093/deafed/enz020

Cao, Z., Zhao, F., & Mulugeta, H. (2019). Noise exposure as a risk factor for acoustic neuroma: A systematic review and meta-analysis. *International Journal of Audiology, 58*(9), 525–532. https://doi.org/10.1080/14992027.2019.1602289

Cawthon, S. W., Fink, B., Schoffstall, S., & Wendel, E. (2018). In the rearview mirror: Social skill development in deaf youth, 1990–2015. *Americans Annals of the Deaf, 162*(5), 479–485.

Charry-Sánchez, D. J., Ramírez-Guerrero, S., Vargas-Cuellar, M. P., Romero-Gordillo, M. A., & Talero-Gutiérrez, C. (2022). Executive functions in children and adolescents with hearing loss: A systematic review of case-control, case series, and cross-sectional studies. *Salúd Mental, 45*(1), 35–49. https://doi.org/10.17711/SM.0185-3325.2022.006

Chaudhry, A., Chaudhry, D., Muzaffar, J., Crundell, G., Monksfield, P., & Bance, M. (2020). Outcomes of cochlear implantation in patients with superficial siderosis: A systematic review and narrative synthesis. *Journal of International Advanced Otology, 16*(3), 443–455. https://doi.org/10-5152/iao.2020.9037

Chaudhry, D., Chaudhry, A., Muzaffar, J., Monksfield, P., & Bance, M. (2020). Cochlear implantation: Outcomes in post synaptic auditory neuropathies: A systematic review and narrative synthesis. *Journal of International Advanced Otology, 16*(3), 411–431. https://doi.org/10.5152/iao.2020.9035

Choudhury, M., & Chavira, P. (2017). Narrative review of evidence-based intervention approaches for auditory processing disorder (APD). *Perspectives of the ASHA Special Interest Groups, 2*(2), 152–156.

Chen, Y. & Wong, L. L. N. (2017). Speech perception in Mandarin-speaking children with cochlear implants: A systematic review. *International Journal of Audiology, 56*(Suppl 2), S7-S16. https://doi.org/10.1080/14992027.2017.1300694

Chorath, K. T., Willis, M. J., Morton-Gonzaba, N., Humann, W. J., & Moreira, A. (2019). Mesenchymal stem cells for sensorineural hearing loss: Protocol for a systematic review of preclinical studies. *Systematic Reviews, 8*(1), 1–3. https://doi.org/10.1196/s13643-019-1015-7

Clarke, N. A., Hoare, D. J., & Killan, E. C. (2019). Evidence for an association between hearing impairment and disrupted sleep: Scoping review. *American Journal of Audiology, 28*(4), 1015–1024. https://doi.org/10.1044/2019_AJA-19-0026

Crowe, K., & Guiberson, M. (2019). Evidence-based interventions for learners who are deaf and/or multilingual: A systematic quality review. *American Journal of Speech-Language Pathology*, 28(3), 964–983. https://doi.org/10.1044/2019_AJSLP-IDLL-19-000

Demers, D., & Bergeron, F. (2019). Effectiveness of rehabilitation approaches proposed to children with severe-to-profound prelinguistic deafness on the development of auditory, speech, and language skills: A systematic review. *Language & Hearing Research*, 62(11), 4196–4230.

Di Stadio, A., Ralli, M., Roccamatisi, D., Scarpa, A., della Volpe, A., Cassandro, C., Ricci, G., Greco, A., & Bernitsas, E. (2021). Hearing loss and dementia: Radiologic and biomolecular basis of their shared characteristics: A systematic review. *Neurological Sciences*, 42(2), 579–588. https://doi.org/10.1007/s10072-020-04948-8

Do, B., Lynch, P., Macris, E.-M., Smyth, B., Stavrinakis, S., Quinn, S., & Constable, P. A. (2017). Systematic review and meta-analysis of the association of Autism Spectrum Disorder in visually or hearing impaired children. *Ophthalmic & Physiological Optics*, 37(2), 212–224. https://doi.org/10.1111/opo.12350

Duchesne, L., & Marschark, M. (2019). Effects of age of cochlear implantation on vocabulary and grammar: A review of the evidence. *American Journal of Speech-Language Pathology*, 28(4), 1673–1691. https://doi.org/10.1044/2019_AJSLP-18-0161

Dumanch, K. A., & Poling, G. L. (2019). Multidisciplinary evaluation and management of cortical deafness and other related central hearing impairments. *Perspectives of the ASHA Special Interest Groups*, 4(5), 910–935. https://doi.org/10.1044/2019_PERS-SIG6-2019-0002

Duncan, J., Lim, S. R., Baker, F., Flynn, T., & Byatt, T. (2019). Online and offline social capital of adolescents who are deaf or hard of hearing *Volta Review*, 119(2), 57–82. https://doi.org/10.17955/tvr.119.2.804

Eastwood, M., Biggs, K., Metcalfe, C., Muzaffar, J., Monksfield, P., & Bance, M. (2021). Outcomes of cochlear implantation in patients with temporal bone trauma: A systematic review and narrative synthesis. *Journal of International Advanced Otology*, 17(2), 162–174. https://doi.org/10.5152/JIAO.2021.9228

Fackrell, K., Potgieter, I., Shekhawat, G. S., Baguely, D. M., Sereda, M., & Hoare, D. J. (2017). Clinical interventions for hyperacusis in adults: a scoping review to assess the current position and determine priorities for research. *BioMed Research International*, 2017, 1–22. https://doi.org/10.1155/2017/2723715

Fitzpatrick, E. M., Cologrosso, E., & Sikora, L. (2019). Candidacy for amplification in children with hearing loss: A review of guidelines and recommendations. *American Journal of Audiology*, 28(4), 1025–1045. https://doi.org/10.1044/2019_AJA_19-0061

Franz, L., Frosolini, A., Parrino, D., Lovato, A., de Filippis, C., & Marioni, G. (2022). Ototoxicity of immunosuppressant drugs: A systematic review. *Journal of International Advanced Otology*, 18(2), 167–176. https://doi.org/10.5152/iao.2022.21416

Galindo Neto, N. M., Esmeraldo Áfio, A. C., de Sá Leite, S., Gomes da Silva, M., Freitag Pagliuca, L. M., & Áfio Caetano, J. (2019). Technologies for health education for the deaf: Integrative review. *Texto & Contexto Enfermagem*, 28, 1–14.

Golmohammadi, R., & Darvishi, E. (2019). The combined effects of occupational exposure to noise and other risk factors – A systematic review. *Noise & Health*, 21(101), 125–141.

Haakma, I., Janssen, M., & Minnaert, A. (2017). A literature review on the psychological needs of students with sensory loss. *Volta Review*, 116(1/2), 29–58.

Hermawati, S., & Pieri, K. (2020). Assistive technologies for severe and profound hearing loss: Beyond hearing aids and implants. *Assistive Technology*, 32(4), 182–193. https://doi.org/10.1080/10400435.2018.1522524

Hormozi, M., Ansari-Moghaddam, A., Mirzaei, R., Haghighi, J. D., Eftekharian, F., & Dehghan Haghighi, J. (2017). The risk of hearing loss associated with occupational exposure to organic solvents mixture with and without concurrent noise exposure: A systematic review and meta-analysis. *International Journal of Occupational Medicine & Environmental Health*, *30*(4), 521–535. https://doi.org/10.13075/ijomeh.1896.01024

Ibrahim, I., da Silva, S. D., Segal, B., & Zeitouni, A. (2017). Effect of cochlear implant surgery on vestibular function: Meta-analysis study. *Journal of Otolaryngology – Head & Neck Surgery*, *46*, 1–10. https://doi.org/10.1186/s40463-017-0224-0

Jaiswal, A., Aldersey, H., Wittich, W. Mirza, M., & Finalyson, M. (2018). Participation experiences of people with deafblindness or dual sensory loss: A scooping review of global deafblind literature. *PLoS ONE*, *13*(9), 1–26. https://doi.org/10.1371/journal.pone.0203772

Kalluri, S., Ahmann, B., & Munro, K. J. (2019). A systematic narrative synthesis of acute amplification-induced improvements in cognitive ability in hearing-impaired adults. *International Journal of Audiology*, *58*(8), 455–463.

Khosravipour, M., & Rajati, F. (2021). Sensorineural hearing loss and risk of stroke: A systematic review and meta-analysis. *Scientific Reports*, *11*(1), 1–11. https://doi.org/10.1038/s41598-021-89695-2

Killick, K., Macaden, L., Smith, A., Kroll, T., Stoddart, K., & Watson, M. C. (2018). A scoping review of the pharmaceutical care needs of people with sensory loss. *International Journal of Pharmacy Practice*, *26*(5), 380–386. https://doi.org/10.1111/jpp.12456

Klopfenstein, M., Bernard, K., & Heyman, C. (2020). The study of speech naturalness in communication disorders: A systematic review of the literature. *Clinical Linguistics & Phonetics*, *34*(4), 327–338. https://doi.org/10.1080/02699206.2019.1652692

Koerber, R., & Jennings, M. B. (2020). Increasing telephone accessibility for workers with hearing loss: A scoping review with recommendations. *International Journal of Audiology*, *59*(10), 727–736. https://doi.org/10.1080/14992027.2020.1753120

Lee, J., Biggs, K., Muzaffar, J., Bance, M., & Monksfield, P. (2021). Hearing loss in inner ear and systemic autoimmune disease: A systematic review of post-cochlear implantation outcomes. *Laryngoscope Investigative Otolaryngology*, *6*(3), 469–487. https://doi.org/10.1002/lio2.563

Liu, A., Wu, B., & Nunez, D. A. (2021). Motivational interviewing for hearing aid use: A systematic meta-analysis on its potential for adult patients with hearing loss. *Journal of the American Academy of Audiology*, *32*(6), 332–338. https://doi.org/10.1055/s-0041-1728755

Long, G. C., Umat, C., & Din, N. C. (2021). Socio-emotional development of children with cochlear implant: A systematic review. *Malaysian Journal of Medical Sciences*, *28*(5), 10–333. https://doi.org/10.21315/mjms2021.28.5.2

Loughran, M. T., Lyons, S., Plack, C. J., & Armitage, C. J. (2020). Which interventions increase hearing protection behaviors during noisy recreational activities? A systematic review. *BMA Public Health*, *20*(1), 1–13. https://doi.org/10.1186/s12889-020-09414-2

Luckner, J. L., & Movahedazarhoulig, S. (2019). Social-emotional interventions with children and youth who are deaf or hard of hearing: A research synthesis. *Journal of Deaf Studies & Deaf Education*, *24*(1), 1–10. https://doi.org/10.1093/deafed/eny030

Luft, P. (2018). Reading comprehension and phonics research: Review of correlational analyses with deaf and hard-of-hearing students. *Journal of Deaf Studies & Deaf Education*, *23*(2), 143–163. https://doi.org/10.1093/deafed/enx057

Magele, A., Schoerg, P., Stanek, B., Gradi, B., & Sprinzl, G. M. (2019). Active transcutaneous bone conduction hearing implants: Systematic review and meta-analysis. *PLoS ONE*, *14*(9), e0221484. https://doi.org/10.1371/journal.pone.0221484

Maharaj, S., Bello Alvarez, M., Mungul, S., & Hari, K. (2020). Otologic dysfunction in patients with COVID-19: A systematic review. *Laryngoscope Investigative Otolaryngology*, 5(6), 119201196. https://doi.org/10.1002/lio2.498

Maidment, D. W., Barker, A. B., Xia, J., & Ferguson, M. A. (2018). A systematic review and meta-analysis assessing the effectiveness of alternative listening devices to conventional hearing aids in adults with hearing loss. *International Journal of Audiology*, 57(10), 721–729. https://doi.org/10.1080/14992027.2018.1493546

Mamo, S. K., Reed, N. S., Price, C., Occhipinti, D., Pletnikova, A., Lin, F. R., & Oh, E. S. (2018). Hearing loss treatment in older adults with cognitive impairment: A systematic review. *Journal of Speech, Language & Hearing Research*, 61(10), 2589–2603. https://doi.org/10.1044/2018_JSLHR-H-18-0077

Michaud, H. N., & Duchesne, L. (2017). Aural rehabilitation for older adults with hearing loss: Impacts on quality of life – A systematic review of randomized controlled trials. *American Academy of Audiology*, 28(7), 596–609. https://doi.org/10.3766/jaaa.15090

Mohammed, S. H., Shab-Bidar, S., Abuzerr, S., Habtewold, T. D., Alizadeh, S., & Djafarian, K. (2019). Association of anemia with sensorineural hearing loss: A systematic review and meta-analysis. *BMC Research Notes*, 12(1), 1–6. https://doi.org/10.1186/s13104-019-4323-z

Myers, K., & Nicholson, N. (2021). Cochlear implant behavioral outcomes for children with auditory neuropathy spectrum disorder: A mini-systematic review. *American Journal of Audiology*, 30, 777–789. https://doi.org/10.1044/2021_AJA-20-00175

Nota Simões, P., Lüders, D., José, M. R., Romanelli, G., Lüders, V., Sampaio Santos, R., & Miranda de Araújoa, C. (2021). Musical perception assessment of people with hearing impairment: A systematic review and meta-analysis. *American Journal of Audiology*, 30(2), 458–473. https://doi.org/10.1044/2021_aja-20-00146

Rayes, H., Al-Malky, G., & Vickers, D. (2019). Systematic review of auditory training in pediatric cochlear implant recipients. *Journal of Speech, Language, and Hearing Research*, 65(5), 1574–1593. https://doi.org/10.1044/2019_JSLHR-H-18-0252

Sanders, M. E., Kant, El, Smit, A. L., & Stegeman, I. (2021). The effect of hearing aids on cognitive function: A systematic review. *PLoS ONE*, 16(12), 1–22. https://doi.org/10.1371/journal.pone.0261207

Shoham, N., Lewis, G., Favarato, G., & Cooper, C. (2019). Prevalence of anxiety disorders and symptoms in people with hearing impairment: A systematic review. *Social Psychiatry & Psychiatric Epidemiology*, 54(6), 649–860. https://doi.org/10.1007/s00127-018-1638-3

Singhal, K., Singhal, J., Muzaffar, J., Monksfield, P., & Bance, M. (2020). Outcomes of cochlear implantation in patients with post-meningitis deafness: A systematic review and narrative synthesis. https://doi.org/10.5152/iao.2020.9040

Sultan, N., Wong, L. L. N., & Purdy, S. C. (2019). Analysis of amount and style of oral interaction related to language outcomes in children with hearing loss: A systematic review (2006–2016). *Journal of Speech, Language & Hearing Research*, 62(9), 3470–3492. https://doi.org/10.1044/2019_JSLHE-L-19-0076

Thomas, R. S. (2017). Hearing loss as a risk factor for dementia: A systematic review. *Laryngoscope Investigative Otolaryngology*, 2(2), 69–79. https://doi.org/10.1002/lio2.65

Toliver-Smith, A., & Gentry, B. (2017). Investigating black ASL: A systematic review. *American Annals of the Deaf*, 161(5), 560–570.

Tseng, Y.-C., Liu, S. H.-Y., Lou, M.-F., & Huang, G.-S. (2018). Quality of life in older adults with sensory impairments: A systematic review. *Quality of Life Research*, 27(8), 1957–1971. https://doi.org/10.1007/s11136-018-1799-2

Udholm, N., Jørgensen, A. W., & Ovesen, T. (2017). Cognitive skills affect outcome of cochlear implant in children: A systematic review. *Cochlear Implants International: An Interdisciplinary Journal*, *18*(2), 63–75. https://doi.org/10.1080/14670100.2016.1273434

Verbecque, E., Marijnissen, T., De Belder, N., Van Rompaey, V., Boudewyns, A., Van de Heyning, P., Vereeck, L., & Hallemans, A. (2017). Vestibular (dys)function in children with sensorineural hearing loss: A systematic review. *International Journal of Audiology*, *56*(6), 361–381. https://doi.org/10.1080/14992027.2017.1281444

Vos, B., Noll, D., Pigeon, M., Bagatto, M., & Fitzpatrick, E. M. (2019). Risk factors for hearing loss in children: A systematic literature review and meta-analysis protocol. *Systematic Reviews*, *8*(1), 1–7. https://doi.org/10.1186/s13643-019-1073-x

Wang, B., Gould, R. L., Kumar, P., Pikett, L., Thompson, B., Costafreda, Gonzalez, S., & Bamiou, D.-E. (2022). A systematic review and meta-analysis exploring effects of third-wave psychological therapies on hearing-related distress, depression, anxiety, and quality of life in people with audiological problems. *American Journal of Audiology*, *31*(2), 487–512. https://doi.org/10.1044/2022_AJA-21-00162

Whicker, J. J., Muñoz, K., & Nelson, L. H. (2019). Parent challenges, perspectives and experiences caring for children who are deaf or hard-of-hearing with other disabilities: A comprehensive review. *International Journal of Audiology*, *58*(1), 5–11. https://doi.org/10.1080/14992027.2018.1534011

White, E. N., Ayres, K. M., Snyder, S. K., Cagliani, R. R., & Ledford, J. R. (2021). Augmentative and alternative communication and speech production for individuals with ASD: A systematic review. *Journal of Autism & Development Disorders*, *51*(11), 4199–4212. https://doi.org/10.1007/s10803-021-04868-2

Yong, M., Young, E., Lea, J., Foggin, H., Zaia, E., Kozak, F. K., & Westerberg, B. D. (2019). Subjective and objective vestibular changes that occur following paediatric cochlear implantation: Systematic review and meta-analysis. *Journal of Otolaryngology*, *48*(1), 1–10. https://doi.org/10.1186/s40463-019-0341-z

Zheng, Y., Fan, S., Liao, W., Fang, W., Xiao, S., & Liu, J. (2017). Hearing impairment and risk of Alzheimer's disease: A meta-analysis of prospective cohort studies. *Neurological Sciences*, *38*(2). https://doi.org/10.1007/s10072-016-2779-3

Zia, N., Nikookam, Y., Muzaffar, J., Kullar, P., Monksfield, P., & Bance, M. (2021). Cochlear implantation outcomes in patients with mitochondrial hearing loss: A systematic review and narrative synthesis. *Journal of International Advanced Otology*, *17*(1), 72–80. https://doi.org/10.5152/iao.2020.9226

Mental Health

Acevedo, N., Bosanac, P., Pikoos, T., Rossell, S., & Castle, D. (2021). Therapeutic neurostimulation in obsessive-compulsive and related disorders: A systematic review. *Brain Sciences*, *11*, 1–82. https://doi.org/10.3390/brainsci11070948

Amerio, A. (2019). Suicide risk in comorbid bipolar disorder and obsessive-compulsive disorder: A systematic review. *Indian Journal of Psychological Medicine*, *41*(2), 133–137. https://doi.org/10.4103/IJPSYM.IJPSYM_367_18

Angel, R., Preetha, S., & Priya, J. (2018). A systematic review of obsessive-compulsive disorder. *Drug Invention Today*, 2837–2840.

Ayano, G., Getts, K., Maravilla, J. C., & Alati, R. (2021). A systematic review and meta-analysis of the risk of disruptive behavioral disorders in the offspring of parents with severe psychiatric disorders. *Child Psychiatry & Human Development*, *52*(1). 77–95. https://doi.org/10.1007/s10578-020-00989-4

Ayano, G., Shumet, S., Tesfaw, G., & Tsegay, L. (2020). A systematic review and meta-analysis of the prevalence of bipolar disorder among homeless people. *BMC Public Health*, *20*(1), 1–10. https://doi.org/10/1186/s12889-020-08819-x

Ayano, G., Solomon, M., Tsegay, L., Yohannes, K., & Abraha, M. (2020). A systematic review and meta-analysis of the prevalence of post-traumatic stress disorder among homeless people. *Psychiatric Quarterly*, *91*(4), 1–15. https://doi.org/10.1007/s11126-020-09746-1

Barkowski, S., Schwartze, D., Strauss, B., Burlingame, G. M., & Rosendahl, J. (2020). Efficacy of group psychotherapy for anxiety disorders: A systematic review and meta-analysis. *Psychotherapy Research*, *30*(8), 965–982. https://doi.org/10.1080/10503307.1729440

Bartoli, F., Callovini, T., Calabrese, A., Cioni, R. M., Riboldi, I., Crocamo, C., & Carrà, G. (2022). Disentangling the association between ADHD and alcohol use disorder in individuals suffering from bipolar disorder: A systematic review and meta-analysis. *Brain Sciences*, *12*(1), 1–10. https://doi.org/10.3390/brainsci12010038

Bastos, R. A., Campos, L. S., Faria-Schützer, D. B., Brito, M. E., da Silva, D. R., dos Santos-Junior, A., Turato, E. R. (2022). Offspring of mothers with bipolar disorder: A systematic review considering personality features. *Revista Brasileira de Psiquiatria*, *44*(1), 94–102. https://doi.org/10.1590/1516-4446-2020-1465

Bedeschi, L. (2018). EMDR for bipolar disorder: A systematic review of the existing studies in literature. *Clinical Neuropsychiatry*, *15*(3), 222–225.

Benedict, T. M., Keenan, G., Nitz, A. J., & Moeller-Bertram, T. (2020). Post-traumatic stress disorder symptoms contribute to worse pain and health outcomes in veterans with PTSD compared to those without: A systematic review with meta-analysis. *Military Medicine*, *185*(9/10), pe1481-e1491. https://doi.org/10.1093/milmed/usaa052

Bisson, J. I., van Gelderen, M., Roberts, N. P., & Lewis, C. (2020). Non-pharmacological and non-psychological approaches to the treatment of PTSD: Results of a systematic review and meta-analysis. *European Journal of Psychotraumatology*, *11*. https://doi.org/10.1080/20008198.2020.1795361

Bortolato, B., Köhler, C. A., & Evangelou, E. (2017). Systematic assessment of environmental risk factors for bipolar disorder: An umbrella review of systematic reviews and meta-analyses. *Bipolar Disorders*, *19*, 84–96. https://doi.org/10.1111/bdi.12490

Breazeale, S., Conley, S., Gaiser, Ed., & Redeker, N. S. (2021). Anxiety symptoms after orthopedic injury: A systematic review. *Journal of Trauma Nursing*, *28*(1), 46–55. https://doi.org/10.1097/JTN.0000000000000557

Buswell, G., Haime, Z., Lloyd-Evans, B., & Billings, Jo. (2021). A systematic review of PTSD to the experience of psychosis: Prevalence and associated factors. *BMC Psychiatry*, *21*(1), 1–13. https://doi.org/10.1186/s12888-020-02999-x

Carl, E., Witcraft, S. M., Kauffman, B. Y., Gillespie, E. M., Becker, E. S., Cuijpers, P., Van Ameringen, M., Smits, J. A. J., & Powers, M. B. (2020). Psychological and pharmacological treatments for generalized anxiety disorder (GAD): A meta-analysis of randomized controlled trials. *Cognitive Behaviour Therapy*, *49*(1), 1–21. https://doi.org/10.1080/16506073.2018.1560358

Carleto, S., Maladrone, F., Berchialla, P., Oliva, F., Colombi, N., Hase, M., Hofmann, A., & Ostacoli, L. (2021). Eye movement desensitization and reprocessing for depression: A systematic review and meta-analysis. *European Journal of Psychotraumatology*, *12*(1), 1–14. https://doi.org/10.1080/20008198.1894736

Carpenter, J. K., Andrews, L. A., Witcraft, S. M., Power, M. B., Smits, J. A. J., & Hofmann, S. G. (2017). Cognitive behavioral therapy for anxiety and related disorders: A meta-analysis of randomized placebo-controlled trials. *Depression & Anxiety*, *35*, 502–514. https://doi.org/10.1002/da.22728

Chen M., Fitzgerald, H. M., Madera, J. J., & Tohen, M. (2019). Functional outcome assessment in bipolar disorder: A systematic literature review. *Bipolar Disorders*, *21*(3), 194–214. https://doi.org/10.1111/bdi.12775

Chiang, K.-J., Tsai, J.-C., Liu, D., Lin, C.-H., Chiu, H.-L., & Chou, K.-R. (2017). Efficacy of cognitive-behavioral therapy in patients with bipolar disorder: A meta-analysis of randomized controlled trials. *PLoS ONE*, *12*(5). https://doi.org/10.1371.journal.pone.0176849

Coles, A. S., Sasiadek, J., & George, T. P. (2019). Pharmacotherapies for co-occurring substance use and bipolar disorders: A systematic review. *Bipolar Disorders*, *21*(7), 595–610. https://doi.org/10.1111/bdi.12794

Cotrena, C., Damiani, B. L., Ponsoni, A., Samamé, C., Milman, S. F., & Paz Fonseca, R. (2020). Executive functions and memory in bipolar disorders I and II: New insights from meta-analytic results. *Acta Psychiatrica Scandinavica*, *141*(2), 110–130. https://doi.org/10.1111/acps.13121

Crowe, M., Eggleston, K., Douglas, K., & Porter, R. J. (2021). Effects of psychotherapy on comorbid bipolar disorder and substance abuse disorder: A systematic review. *Bipolar Disorders*, *23*(2), 141–151. https://doi.org/10.1111/bdi.12971

Cuijpers, P., van Veen, S. C., Sijbrandij, M., Yoder, W., & Cristea, I. A. (2020). Eye movement desensitization and reprocessing for mental health problems: A systematic review and meta-analysis. *Cognitive Behaviour Therapy*, *49*(3), 165–180. https://doi.org/10.1080/16506073.2019.1703801

das Neves Peixoto, F. S., Ferreira de Sousa, D., Rodrigues Pereira Luz, D. C., Barreto Vieira, N., Gonçalves Júnior, J., Alencar dos Santos, G. C., Troglio da Silva, F. C., & Rolim Neto, M. L. (2017). Bipolarity and suicidal ideation in children and adolescents: A systematic review with meta-analysis. *Annals of General Psychiatry*, *16*, 1–8. https://doi.org/10.1186/s12991-017-0143-5

de Aguiar, K. R., Cabelleira, M. D., Montezano, B. B., Jansen, K., & de Azevedo Cardoso, T. (2021). Sleep alternations as a predictor of bipolar disorder among offspring of parents with bipolar disorder: A systematic review and meta-analysis. *Trends in Psychiatry & Psychotherapy*, *43*(4), 256–269. https://doi.org/10.47626/2237-6089-2021-0256

De Crescenzo, F., Lennox, A., Gibson, J. C., Cordey, J. H., Stockton, S., Cowen, P. J., & Quested, D. J. (2017). Melatonin as a treatment for mood disorders: A systematic review. *Acta Psychiatrica Scandinavica*, *136*(6), 549–558. https://doi.org/10.1111/acps.12755

Dewa, L. H., Kalniunas, A., Orleans-Foli, S., Pappa, S., & Aylin, P. (2021). Detecting signs of deterioration in young patients with serious mental illness: A systematic review. *Systematic Reviews*, *10*(1), 1–8. https://doi.org/10.1186/s13643-021-01798-z

Di Lorito, C., Völlm, B., & Dening, T. (2018). Psychiatric disorders among older prisoners: A systematic review and comparison study against older people in the community. *Aging & Mental Health*, *22*(1), 1–10. https://doi.org/10.1080/13607863.2017.128653

Dyer, M. L., Easey, K. E., Heron, J., Hickman, M., & Munafo, M. R. (2019). Associations of child and adolescent anxiety with later alcohol use and disorders: A systematic review and meta-analysis of prospective cohort studies. *Addiction*, *114*, 968–982. https://doi.org/10.1111/add.14575

Eilert, N., Enrique, A., Wogan, R., Mooney, O., Timulak, L., & Richards, D. (2020). The effectiveness of Internet-delivered treatment for generalized anxiety disorder: An updated systematic review and meta-analysis. *Anxiety and Depression Association of America*, 196–219. https://doi.org/10.1002/da.23115

Ennis, N., Shorer, S., Shoval-Zuckerman, Y., Feedman, S., Monson, C. M., & Dekel, R. (2020). Treating posttraumatic stress disorder across cultures: A systematic review of cultural adaptations of trauma-focused cognitive behavioural therapies. *Journal of Clinical Psychology*, 76(4), 587–611. https://doi.org/10.1002/jclp.22909

Escudero, M. A. G., Gutiérrez-Rojas, L., & Lahera, G. (2020). Second Generation antipsychotics monotherapy as maintenance treatment of bipolar disorder: A systematic review of long-term studies. *Psychiatric Quarterly*, 91, 1047–1060. https://doi.org/10.1007/s1116-020-09753-2

Estrada-Prat, X., Van Meter, A. R., Camprodon-Rosanas, E., Batlle-Vila, S., Goldstein, B. I., & Birmaher, B. (2019). Childhood factors associated with increased risk for mood episode recurrences in bipolar disorder: A systematic review. *Bipolar Disorders*, 21(6), 483–502. https://doi.org/10.1111/bdi.12785

Frigerio, S., Strawbridge, R., Young, A. H. (2021). The impact of caffeine consumption on clinical symptoms in patients with bipolar disorder: A systematic review. *Bipolar Disorders*, 23(3), 241–251. https://doi.org/10.1111/bdi.12990

Gabriel, F. C., Oliveira, M., Martella, B. D. M., Berk, M., Brietzke, E., Jacka, F. N., & Felice, N. (2022). Nutrition and bipolar disorder: A systematic review. *Nutritional Neuroscience*, 1–15. https://doi.org/10.1080/1028415/x.2022.2077031

Ghahari, S., Mohammadi-Hasel, K., Malakouti, S. K., & Roshanpajouh, M. (2020). Mindfulness-based cognitive therapy for generalised anxiety disorder: A systematic review and meta-analysis. *East Asian Archives of Psychiatry*, 30(2), 52–56. https://doi.org/10.12809/eaap1885

Guan, N., Guariglia, A., Moore, P., Xu, F., & Al-Janabi, H. (2022). Financial stress and depression in adults: A systematic review. *PLoS ONE*, 17(2), 1–20. https://doi.org/10.1371.journal.pone/0264041

Gutermann, J., Schwartzkopff, L., & Steil, R. (2017). Meta-analysis of the long-term treatment effects of psychological interventions in youth with PTSD symptoms. *Clinical Child & Family Psychology Review*, 20, 422–434. https://doi.org/10.1007/s10567-017-0242-5

Haitana, T., Pitama, S., Crowe, M., Porter, R., Mulder, R., & Lacey, C. (2020). A systematic review of bipolar disorder in indigenous peoples. *New Zealand Journal of Psychology*, 49(3), 33–47.

Ham, A. J., Aa, H. P. A., Brunes, A., Heir, T., Vries, R., Rens, G. H. M. B., & Nispen, R. M. A. (2021). The development of posttraumatic stress disorder in individuals with visual impairment: A systematic search and review. *Ophthalmic & Physiological Optics*, 41(2), 331–341. https://doi.org/10.1111/opo.12784

Hediger, K., Wagner, J., Künzi, P., Haefeli, A., Theis, F., Grob, C., Pauli, E., & Gerger, H. (2021). Effectiveness of animal-assisted interventions for children and adults with post-traumatic stress disorder symptoms: A systematic review and meta-analysis. *European Journal of Psychotraumatology*, 12. https://doi.org/10.1080/20008198.2021.187913

Hoskins, M. D., Sinnerton, R., Nakamura, A., Underwood, J. F. G., Slater, A., Lewis, C., Roberts, N. P., Bisson, J. I., Lee, Matthew, & Clarke, L. (2021). Pharmacological-assisted psychotherapy for post-traumatic stress disorder: A systematic review and meta-analysis. *European Journal of Psychotraumatology*, 12. https://doi.org/10.1080/20008198.2020.1853379

Huang, T., Li, H., Tan, S., Xie, S., Cheng, Q., Xiang, Y., & Zhou, X. (2022). The efficacy and acceptability of exposure therapy for the treatment of post-traumatic stress disorder in children and adolescents: A systematic review and meta-analysis. *BMC Psychiatry*, 22(1), 1–12. https://doi.org/10.1186/s12888-022-03867-6

Huxley, P., Krayer, A., Poole, R., Prendergast, L., Aryal, S., & Warner, R. (2021). Schizophrenia outcomes in the 21st century: A systematic review. *Brain & Behavior*, 11(6), 1–12. https://doi.org/10.1002/brb3.2172

Isohanni, M., Jääskeläinen, E., Miller, B. J., Hulkko, A., Tiihonen, J., Möller, H.-J., Hartikainen, S., Huhtaniska, S., & Lieslehto, J. (2020). Medication management of antipsychotic treatment in schizophrenia – A narrative review. *Human Psychopharmacology: Clinical & Experimental, 36*, 1–12. https://doi.org/10.1002/hup.2765

Janis, R. A., Burlingame, G. M., Svien, H., Jensen, J., & Lundgreen, R. (2021). Group therapy for mood disorders: A meta-analysis. *Psychotherapy Research, 31*(3), 369–385. https://doi.org/10.1080/10503307.2020.1817603

Juruena, M. F., Young, A. H., Hodsoll, J., Lewis, G., & Veale, D. (2020). Efficacy and safety of bright light therapy for bipolar depression. *Psychiatry & Clinical Neurosciences, 74*(7), 408–410. https://doi.org/10.1111/pcn.13005

Kafes, A. Y. (2021). Behavioral intervention techniques used in the treatment of obsessive-compulsive disorder: Systematic review. *Current Approaches to Psychiatry, 13*(3), 726–738. https://doi.org/10.18863/pgy.875418

Kahn, A. M., Ahmed, R., Kotapati, V. P., Dar, S. K., Qamar, I., Jafri, A., Ibrahim, M., Kumar, P., & Begum, G. (2018). Vagus Nerve Stimulation (VNS) vs. Deep Brain Stimulation (DBS) treatment for major depressive disorder and bipolar depression: A comparative meta-analytic review. *International Journal of Medicine & Public Health, 8*(3), 119–130. https://doi.org/10.5530/ijmedph.2018.3.26

Kessing, L. V., & Andersen, P. K. (2017). Evidence for clinical progression of unipolar and bipolar disorders. *Acta Psychiatrica Scandinavica, 135*(1), 51–64. https://doi.org/10.1111/acps.12667

Kessing, L. V., Willer, I., Andersen, P. K., & Bukh, J. D. (2017). Rate and predictors of conversion from unipolar to bipolar disorder: A systematic review and meta-analysis. *Bipolar Disorders, 19*(5), 324–335. https://doi.org/10.1111/bdi.12513

Lau, P., Hawes, J., Hunt, C., Frankland, A., Roberts, G., & Mitchell, P. B. (2018). Prevalence of psychopathology in bipolar high-risk offspring and siblings: A meta-analysis. *European Child & Adolescent Psychiatry, 27*(7), 823–837. https://doi.org/10.1007/s00787-017-1050-7

Lee, Y., Brietzke, E., Cao, B., Chen, Y., Linnaranta, O., Mansur, R. B., Cortes, P., Kösters, M., Majeed, A., Tamura, J. K., Lui, L. M. W., Vinberg, M., Keinänen, J., Kisely, S., Naveed, S., Barbui, C., Parker, G., Owolabi, M., Nishi, D., Lee, J. G., ... & McIntyre, R. S. (2020). Development and implementation of guidelines for the management of depression: A systematic review. *Bulletin of the World Health Organization, 98*, 683–697H. https://doi.org/10.2471/BLT.20.251405

Lewis, C., Lewis, K., Kitchiner, N., Isaac, S., Jones, I., & Bisson, J. I. (2020). Sleep disturbance in post-traumatic stress disorder (PTSD): A systematic review and meta-analysis of actigraphy studies. *European Journal of Psychotraumatology, 11*. https://doi.org/10.1080/20008198.2020.1767349

Lewis, C., Roberts, N. P., Andrew, M., Starling, E., & Bisson, J. I. (2020). Psychological therapies for post-traumatic stress disorder in adults: Systematic review and meta-analysis. *European Journal of Pyschotraumatology, 11*. https://doi.org/10.1080/200088198.2020.1729633

Li, X., Zhu, L., Zhou, C., Liu, J., Du, H., Wang, C., & Fang, S. (2018). Efficacy and tolerability of short-term duloxetine treatment in adults with generalized anxiety disorder: A meta-analysis. *PLoS ONE, 13*(3). https://doi.org/10.1371/jornal.pone.0194501

Li, X., Zhu, L., Su, Y., & Fang, S. (2017). Short-term efficacy and tolerability of venlafaxine extended release in adults with generalized anxiety disorder without depression: A meta-analysis. *PLoS ONE, 12*(10). https://doi.org/10.1371/jornal.pone.0185865

Ljubic, N., Ueberberg, B., Grunze, H., & Assion, H.-J. (2021). Treatment of bipolar disorders in older adults: A review. *Annals of General Psychiatry, 20*(1), 1–11. https://doi.org/10.1186/s12991-021-00367-x

Lorimer, B., Kellett, S., Nye, A., & Delgadillo, J. (2021). Predictors of relapse and recurrence following cognitive behavioural therapy for anxiety-related disorders: A systematic review. *Cognitive Behaviour Therapy*, *50*(1), 1–18. https://doi.org/10.1080/16506073.2020.1812709

Mansueto, G., Cavallo, C., Palmieri, S., Ruggiero, G. M., Sassaroli, S., & Caselli, G. (2021). Adverse childhood experiences and repetitive negative thinking in adulthood: A systematic review. *Clinical Psychology & Psychotherapy*, *28*(3), 557–568. https://doi.org/10.1002/cpp.2590

Martin, A., Naunton, M., Kosari, S., Peterson, G., Thomas, J., Christenson, J. K. (2021). Treatment guidelines for PTSD: A systematic review. *Journal of Clinical Medicine*, *10*(18), 1–15. https://doi.org/10.3390/jcm10184175

Mavranezouli, I., Megnin-Viggars, O., Daly, C., Dias, S., Stockton, S., Meiser-Stedman, R., Trickey, D., & Pilling, St. (2020). Research review: Psychological and psychosocial treatments for children and young people with post-traumatic stress disorder: A network meta-analysis. *Journal of Child Psychology & Psychiatry*, *61*(1), 18–29. https://doi.org/10.1111/jcpp.13094

McKay, M. T., Cannon, M., Chambers, D., Conroy, R. M., Coughlan, H., Dodd, P., Healy, C., O'Donnell, L., & Clarke, M. (2021). Childhood trauma and adult mental disorder: A systematic review and meta-analysis of longitudinal cohort studies. *Acta Psychiatrica Scandinavica*, *143*(3), 189–205. https://doi.org/10.1111/acps.13268

Moller, C. I., Davey, C. G., Badcock, P. B., Wrobel, A. L., Cao, A., Murrihy, S., Sharmin, S., Cotton, S. M. (2022). Correlates of suicidality in people with depressive disorders: A systematic review. *Australian & New Zealand Journal of Psychiatry*, *14*, 1–20. https://doi.org/10.1177/00048674221086498

Morton, E., & Murray, G. (2019). Advancing the study of functioning in bipolar disorders—from scales to constructs. *Bipolar Disorders*, *21*(7), 662–663. https://doi.org/10.1111/bdi.12917

Naveed, S., Amray, A. N., Jahan, N., Moti-Wala, F. B., & Majeed, M. H. (2019). Psychopharmacology in pediatric mixed anxiety disorder: An evidence-based review. *Innovations in Clinical Neuroscience*, *16*(9–10), 36–43.

Oya, K., Sakuma, K., Esumi, S., Hashimoto, Y., Hatano, M., Matsuda, Y., Matsui, Y., Miyake, N., Nomura, I., Okuya, M., Iwata, N., Kata, M., Hashimoto, R., Mishima, K., Watanabe, & N., Kishi, T. (2019). Efficacy and safety of lithium and lamotrigine for the maintenance treatment of clinically stable patients with bipolar disorder: A systematic review and meta-analysis of double-blind, randomized, placebo-controlled trials with an enrichment design. *Neuropsychopharmacology Reports*, *39*(3), 241–246. https://doi.org/10.1002/npr2.12056

Perich, T., Ussher, J., Meade, T. (2017). Menopause and illness course in bipolar disorder: A systematic review. *Bipolar Disorders*, *19*(6), 434–443. https://doi.org/10.1111/bdi.12530

Potes, A., Souza, G., Nikolitch, K., Penheiro, R., Moussa, Y., Jarvis, E., Looper, K., & Rej, S. (2018). Mindfulness in severe and persistent mental illness: A systematic review. *International Journal of Psychiatry in Clinical Practice*, *22*(4), 253–261. https://doi.org/10.1080/13651501.2018.1433857

Prajapati, A. R., Wilson, J., Song, F., & Maidment, I. (2018). Second-generation antipsychotic long-acting injections in bipolar disorder: Systematic review and meta-analysis. *Bipolar Disorders*, *20*(8), 687–696. https://doi.org/10.1111/bdi.12707

Purnell, L. R., Graham, A. C. J., Bloomfield, M. A. P., & Billings, J. (2021). Reintegration interventions for CPTSD: A systematic review. *European Journal of Psychotraumatology*, *12*(1), 1–17. https://doi.org/10.1080/20008198.2021.1934789

Ratheesh, A., Davey, C., Hetrick, S., Alvarez-Jimenez, M., Voutier, C., Bechdolf, A., McGorry, P. D., Scott, J., Berk, M., & Cotton, S. M. (2017). A systematic review and meta-analysis of prospective transition from major depression to bipolar disorder. *Acta Psychiatrica Scandinavica*, *135*(4), 273–284. https://doi.org/10.1111/acps.12686

Rehman, Y., Saini, A., Huang, S., Sood, E., Gill, R., & Yanikomeroglu, S. (2021). Cannabis in the management of PTSD: A systematic review. *AIMS Neuroscience*, *8*(3), 414–434. https://doi.org/10.3934/Neuroscience.2021022

Renna, M. E., O'Toole, M. S., Spaeth, P. E., Lekander, M., & Mennin, D. S. (2017). The association between anxiety, traumatic stress, and obsessive-compulsive disorders and chronic inflammation: A systematic review and meta-analysis. *Depression & Anxiety*, *35*, 1081–1094. https://doi.org/10.1002/da.22790

Saha, S., Lim, C. C. W., Cannon, D. L., Burton, L., Bremner, M., Cosgrove, P., Huo, Y., & McGrath, J. (2021). Co-morbidity between mood and anxiety disorders: A systematic review and meta-analysis. *Depression & Anxiety*, *38*(3), 286–306. https://doi.org/10.1002/da.23113

Salloum, I. M., & Brown, E. S. (2017). Management of comorbid bipolar disorder and substance use disorders. *The American Journal of Drug and Alcohol Abuse*, *43*(4), 366–376. https://doi.org/10. 1080/00952990.2017.1292279

Sandstrom, A., Perroud, N., Alda, M., Uher, R., & Pavolva, B. (2021). Prevalence of attention-deficit/hyperactivity disorder in people with mood disorders: A systematic review and meta-analysis. *Acta Psychiatrica Scandinavica*, *143*(5), 380–391. https://doi.org/10.1111/acps.13283

Sari, O. K., & Subandi. (2021). Psychological interventions in community-based treatment of schizophrenia: A systematic narrative review. *Journal of Educational, Health, & Community Psychology*, *10*(3), 432–447.

Schneider-Thoma, J., Kapfhammer, A., Wang, D., Bighelli, I., Siafis, S., Wu, H., Hansen, W. P., Davis, J. M., Salanti, G., & Leucht, S. (2021). Metabolic side effects of antipsychotic drugs in individuals with schizophrenia during medium- to long-term treatment: Protocol for a systematic review and network meta-analysis of randomized controlled trials. *Systematic Reviews*, *10*(1), 1–9. https://doi.org/10.1186/s13643-021-01760-z

Scott, A. J., Sharpe, L., Loomes, M., & Gandy, M. (2020). Systematic review and meta-analysis of anxiety and depression in your with epilepsy. *Journal of Pediatric Psychology*, *45*(2), 133–144. https://doi.org/10.1093/jpepsy/jsz099

Shim, I. H., Bahk, W.-M., Woo, Y. S., & Yoon, B.-H. (2018). Pharmacological treatment of major depressive episodes with mixed features: A systematic review. *Clinical Psychopharmacology & Neuroscience*, *16*(4), 376–382. https://doi.org/10.9758/cpn.2018.16.376

Smith, J. R., Workneh, A., & Yaya, S. (2020). Barriers and facilitators to help-seeking for individuals with posttraumatic stress disorder: A systematic review. *Journal of Traumatic Stress*, *33*(2), 137–150. https://doi.org/10.1002/jts.22456

Snoek, A., Nederstigt, J., Ciharova, M., Sijbrandij, M., Lok, A., Cuijpers, P., & Thomaes, K. (2021). Impact of comorbidity personality disorders on psychotherapy for post-traumatic stress disorder: Systematic review and meta-analysis. *European Journal of Psychotraumatology*, *12*(1), 1017. https://doi.org/10.1080/20008198.2021.1929753

Sun, X.-N., Zhou, J.-B., & Li, N. (2021). Poor oral health in patients with schizophrenia: A meta-analysis of case-control studies. *Psychiatric Quarterly*, *92*, 135–145. https://doi.org/10.1007/s11126-020-09752-3

Szmulewicz, A., Valerio, M. P., & Martino, D. J. (2020). Longitudinal analysis of cognitive performances in recent-onset and later-life bipolar disorder: A systematic review and meta-analysis. *Journal of Bipolar Disorders*, *22*(1), 28–37. https://doi.org/10.1111/bdi.12841

Takeshima, M., Utsumi, T., Aoki, Y., Wang, Z., Suzuki, M., Okajima, I., Watanbe, N., Watanabe, K., & Takaesu, Y. (2020). Efficacy and safety of bright light therapy for manic and depressive symptoms in patients with bipolar disorder: A systematic review and meta-analysis. *Psychiatry & Clinical Neurosciences, 74*(4), 247–256. https://doi.org/10.1111/pcn.12976

Tomé, A. L., Cebriá, M. J. R., González-Teruel, A., Caronell-Asins, J. A., Nicolás, C. C., Hernández-Viadel, M. (2021). Efficacy of vitamin D in the treatment of depression: A systematic review and meta-analysis. *Actas Españolas de Psiguiatria, 49*(1), 12–23.

Tondo, L, Vásquez, G. H., & Baldessarini, R. J. (2021). Prevention of suicidal behavior in bipolar disorder. *Bipolar Disorders, 23*(1), 14–23. https://doi.org/10.1111/bdi.13017

Tsapekos, D., Seccomandi, B., Mantingh, T., Cella, M., Wykes, T., & Young, A. H. (2020). Cognitive enhancement interventions for people with bipolar disorder: A systematic review of methodological quality, treatment approaches, and outcomes. *Bipolar Disorders, 22*(3), 216–230. https://doi.org/10.1111/bdu.12848

Turan, N., & Cetintas, S. (2021). A systematic review of the effectiveness, content, and usage patterns of mobile mental health interventions on smartphone platforms for anxiety symptoms. *Journal of Evidenced-Based Psychotherapies, 21*(2), 61–80.

Velosa, J., Delgado, A., Finger, E., Berk, M., Kapczinski, F., & Azevedo Cardoso, T. (2020). Risk of dementia in bipolar disorder and the interplay of lithium: A systematic review and meta-analysis. *Acta Psychiatrica Scandinavica, 141*(6), 510–521. https://doi.org/10.1111/acps.13153

Verdolini, N., Hidalgo-Mazzei, D., Del Matto, L., Muscas, M., Pacchiarotti, I., Murru, A., Smalin, L., Aedo, A., Tohen, M., Grunze, H., Young, A. H., Carvalho, A. F., & Vieta, E. (2021). Long-term treatment of bipolar disorder type I: A systematic and critical review of clinical guidelines with derived practice algorithms. *Bipolar Disorders, 23*(4), 324–340. https://doi.org/10.1111/bdi.13040

Verdolini, N., Hidalgo-Mazzei, D., Murru, A., Pacchiarotti, I., Samalin, L., Young, A. H., Vieta, E., & Carvalho, A. F. (2018). Mixed states in bipolar and major depressive disorders: Systematic review and quality appraisal of guidelines. *Acta Psychiatrica Scandinavica, 138*(3), 196–222. https://doi.org/10.1111/acps.12896

von der Warth, R., Dams, J., Grochtdreis, T., & König, H.-H. (2020). Economic evaluations and cost analyses in posttraumatic stress disorder: A systematic review. *European Journal of Psychotraumatology, 11*, 1–20. https://doi.org/10.1080/20008198.2020.1753940

Webb, R., Ayers, S., Bogaerts, A., Jelicic, L., Pawlicka, P., Van Haeken, S., Uddin, N., Xuereb, R. B., Kolesnikova, N., & COST action CA18211_DEVoTION Team. (2021). When birth is not as expected: A systematic review of the impact of a mismatch between expectations and experiences. *BMC Pregnancy & Childbirth, 21*(1), 1–14. https://doi.org/10.1186/s12884-021-03898-z

Xiang, Y., Cuijpers, P., Teng, T., Li, X., Fan, L., Liu, X., Jiang, Y., Du, K., Lin, J., Zhou, X., & Xie, P. (2022). Comparative short-term efficacy and acceptability of a combination of pharmacotherapy and psychotherapy for depressive disorder in children and adolescents: A systematic review and meta-analysis. *BMC Phychiatry, 22*(1), 1–13. https://doi.org/10.1186/s12888-022-03760-2

Xiao, Z., Baldwin, M. M., Meinck, F., Obsuth, I., & Murray, A. L. (2021). The impact of childhood psychological maltreatment of mental health outcomes in adulthood: A protocol for a systematic review and meta-analysis. *Systematic Reviews, 10*, Article 224. https://doi.org/10.1186/s13643-021-01777-4

Yoon, S., Kim, T. D., Kim, J., & Lyoo, I. K. (2021). Altered functional activity in bipolar disorder: A comprehensive review from a large-scale network perspective. *Brain & Behavior, 11*(1), 1–18. https://doi.org/10.1002/brb3.1953

Zareifopoulos, N., Bellou, A., Spiropoulou, A., & Spiropouls, K. (2018). Prevalence of comorbid chronic obstructive pulmonary disease in individuals suffering from schizophrenia and bipolar disorder: A systematic review. *Journal of Chronic Obstructive Pulmonary Disease, 15*(6), 612–620. https://doi.org/10.1080/15412555.2019.1572730

Prosthetics

Attalah, R., Leijendekkers, R. A., Hoogeboom, T. J., & Frölke, J. P. (2018). Complications of bone-anchored prostheses for individuals with an extremity amputation: A systematic review. *PLoS ONE, 13*(8), e0201821. https://doi.org/10.1371/journal.pone.0101821

Chadwell, A., Diment, L., Micó-Amigo, M., Morgado Ramírez, D. Z., Dickinson, A., Granat, M., Kenney, L., Kheng, S., Sobuh, M., Ssekitoleko, R., & Worsley, P. (2020). Technology for monitoring everyday prosthesis use: A systematic review. *Journal of NeuroEngineering & Rehabilitation, 17*, 93: https://doi.org/10.1186/s12984-020-00711-4

Clarke, L., Dillon, M., & Shiell, A. (2019). Health economic evaluation in orthotics and prosthetics: A systematic review protocol. *Systematic Reviews, 8*. https://doi.org/10.1186/s13634-019-1066-9

Fernandes, J. C., Silva, M., & Santos, R. (2018). Components of prosthetic lower limbs for transfemoral and transtibial amputations: General prescription recommendations and literature review. *Journal of Life Care Planning, 16*(2), 11–21.

Healy, A., Farmer, S., Eddison, N., Allcock, J., Perry, T., Pandyan, A., Chockalingam, N. (2020). A scoping literature review of studies assessing effectiveness and cost-effectiveness of prosthetic and orthotic interventions. *Disability & Rehabilitation: Assistive Technology, 15*(1), 60–66. Https://doi.org/10.1080/17483107.2018.1523953

Healy, A., Farmer, S., Pandyan, A., & Chockalingam, N. (2018). A systematic review of randomised controlled trials assessing effectiveness of prosthetic and orthotic interventions. *PLoS ONE, 13*(3), e0192094. https://doi.org/10.1371/journal.pone.0192094

Luza, L. P., Ferreira, E. G., Minsky, R. C., Pires, G. K. W., & da Silva, R. (2020). Psychosocial and physical adjustments and prosthesis satisfaction in amputees: A systematic review of observational studies. *Disability and Rehabilitation: Assistive Technology, 15*(5), 582–589. https://doi.org/10.1080/17483107.2019.1602853

Tschiedel, M., Russold, M. F., & Kaniusas, E. (2020). Relying on more sense for enhancing lower limb prostheses control: A review. *Journal of NeuroEngineering & Rehabilitation, 17*. https://doi.org/10.1186/s12984-020-00726x

Spinal Cord Injury

Abbaszadeh, H. A., Niknazar, S., Darabi, S., Roozbahany, N. A., Noori-Zadeh, A., Ghoreishi, S. K., Khoramgah, M. S., & Sadeghi, Y. (2018). Stem cell transplantation and functional recovery after spinal cord injury: A systematic review and meta-analysis. *Anatomy & Cell Biology, 18*(51), 180–188. https://doi.org/10.5115/acb.2018.51.3.180

Afferi, L., Pannek, J., Burnett, A. L., Razaname, C., Tzanoulinou, S., Bobela, W., Fraga de Silva, R. A., Sturney, M., Stergiopulos, N., Cornelius, J., Moschini, M., Iselin, C., Salonia, A., Mattei, A., & Mordasini, L. (2020). Performance and safety of treatment options for erectile dysfunction in patients with spinal cord injury: A review of the literature. *Andrology, 8*(6), 1660–1673. https://doi.org/10.1111/andr.12878

Alrefaie, W. A., Salem, N. A., El Fakharanh, M. S., & El Zanaty, M. Y. (2021). Role of assistive devices on gait in patients with incomplete spinal cord injury: Systematic review. *Egyptian Journal of Hospital Medicine, 85*(2), 4075–4084. https://doi.org/10.21608/ejhm.2021.207093

Alve, Y. A., & Bontje, P. (2019). Factors influencing participation in daily activities by persons with spinal cord injury: Lessons learned from an international scoping review. *Topics in Spinal Cord Injury Rehabilitation, 25*(1), 41–61. https://doi.org/10.1310/sci2501-41

Baldassin, V., Shimizu, H. E., & Fachin-Martins, E. (2018). Computer assisted technology and associations with quality of life for individuals with spinal cord injury: A systematic review. *Quality of Life Research, 27*(3), 597–607. https://doi.org/10.1007/s11136-018-1804-9

Barbosa da Silva, J., & Soares Rodrigues, M. C. (2020). Pressure ulcers in individuals with spinal cord injury: Risk factors in neurological rehabilitation. *Rev Rene, 21*(1), 1–9. https://doi.org/10.15253/2175-6783.20202144155

Barman, A., Roy, S. S., Sasidharan, S. K., & Sahoo, J. (2021). Clinical features and prognosis of COIVD 19/SARS-CoV-2 infections in persons with spinal cord injury: A review of current literature. *Spinal Cord Series and Cases, 7*(1). https://doi.org/10.1038/s41394-021-00420-7

Bloom, J., Dorsett, P., & McLennan, V. (2019). Occupational bonding after spinal cord injury: A review and narrative synthesis. *Journal of Vocational Rehabilitation, 50*(1), 109–120. https://doi.org/10.3233/JVR-180992

Bloom, J., Dorsett, P., & McLennan, V. (2020). Vocational rehabilitation to empower consumers following newly acquired spinal cord injury. *Journal of Vocational Rehabilitation, 53*(1), 131–144. https://doi.org/10.3233/JVR-201091

Clark, J. M., & Marshall, R. (2017). Nature of the non-traumatic spinal cord injury literature: A systematic review. *Top Spinal Cord Injury Rehabilitation, 23*(4), 353–367. https://doi.org/10.1310/sci2304-353

Dixit, S., & Tedia, J. S. (2019). Effectiveness of robotics in improving upper extremity functions among people with neurological dysfunction: A systematic review. *International Journal of Neuroscience, 129*(4), 369–383. https://doi.org/10.1080/00207454.2018.1536051

Donenberg, J. G., Fetters, L., & Johnson, R. (2019). The effects of locomotor training in children with spinal cord injury: A systematic review. *Developmental Neurorehabilitation, 22*(4), 272–287. https://doi.org/10.1080/17518423.2018.1487474

Earle, S., O'Dell, L., Davies, A., & Rixon, A. (2020). Views and experiences of sex, sexuality, and relationships following spinal cord injury: A systematic review and narrative synthesis of the qualitative literature. *Sexuality and Disability, 38,* 567–595. https://doi.org/10.1007/s11195-02-09653-0

Gaspar, R., Padula, N., Freitas, T. B., de Oliveira, J. P. J., & Torriani-Pasin, C. (2019). Physical exercise for individuals with spinal cord injury: Systematic review based on the International Classification of Functioning, Disability, and Health. *Journal of Sports Rehabilitation, 28*(5), 505–516. https://doi.org/10.1123/jsr.2017-0185

Green, B. N., Johnson, C. D., Haldeman, S., Griffith, E., Clay, M. B., Kane, E. J., Castellote, J. M., Rajasekaran, S., Smuck, M., Hurwitz, E. L., Randhawa, K., Yu, H., & Nordin, M. (2018). A scoping review of biopsychosocial risk factors and co-morbidities for common spinal disorders. *PLoS ONE, 13*(6), e0197987. https://doi.org/10.1371/journal.prone.0197987

Hearn, J. H., & Cross, A. (2020). Mindfulness for pain, depression, anxiety, and quality of life in people with spinal cord injury: A systematic review. *BMC Neurology, 20*(1), 1–9. https://doi.org/10.1186/s12883-020-1619-5

Heyward, O. W., Veger, R. J. K., de Groot, S., van der Woude, L. H. V. (2017). Shoulder complaints in wheelchair athletes: A systematic review. *PLoS ONE, 12*(11), e0188410. https://doi.org/10.1371/journal.pone.0188410

Hoogenes, B., Querée, M., Townson, A., Willms, R., Eng, J. J. (2021). COVID-19 and spinal cord injury: Clinical presentation, clinical course, and clinical outcomes: A rapid systematic review. *Journal of Neurotrauma, 38*(9), 1242–1250. https://doi.org/10.1089/neu.7461

Huang, L., Zhang, Q., Fu, C., Liang, Z., Xiong, F., He, C., & Wei, Q. (2021). Effects of hyperbaric oxygen therapy on patients with spinal cord injury: A systematic review and meta-analysis of randomized controlled trials. *Journal of Back & Musculoskeletal Rehabilitation, 9*, 48. https://doi.org/10.3233/BMR-200157

Jutzeler, C. R., Bourguignon, L., Weis, C. V., Tong, B., Wong, C., Rieck, B., Pargger, H., Tschudin-Sutter, S., Egli, A., Borgwardt, K., & Walter, M. (2020). Comorbidities, clinical signs and symptoms, laboratory findings, imaging features, treatment strategies, and outcomes in adult and pediatric patients with COVID-19: A systematic review and meta-analysis. *Travel Medicine and Infectious Disease, 37*, 101825. https://doi.org/10.1016/j.tmaid.2020.101825

Kubota, T., & Kubota, N. (2021). Exacerbation of neurological symptoms and COVID-19 severity in patients with preexisting neurological disorders and COVID-19: A systematic review. *Clinical Neurology and Neurosurgery, 200*, 106349.

Naumann, K., Kernot, J., Parfitt, G., Gower, B. & Davison, K. (2021). Water-based interventions for people with neurological disability, autism, and intellectual disability: A scoping review. *Adapted Physical Activity Quarterly, 38*, 474–493. https://doi.org/10.1123/apaq.2020-0036

Raab, A. M., Mueller, G., Elsig, S., Gandevia, S. C., Zwahlen, M., Hopman, M. T. E., & Hilfiker, R. (2022). Systematic review of incidence studies of pneumonia in persons with spinal cord injury. *Journal of Clinical Medicine, 11*(1), 1–18. https://doi.org/10.3390/jcm11010211

Raguindin, P. F., Bertolo, A., Zeh, R. M., Fränkl, G., Itodo, O. A., Capossela, S., Bally, L., Minder, B., Brach, M., Eriks-Hoogland, I., Stoyanov, J., Muka, T., & Glisic, M. (2021). Body composition according to spinal cord injury level: A systematic review and meta-analysis. *Journal of Clinical Medicine, 10*(17), 1–20. https://doi.org/10.3390/jcm10173911

Rodríguez-Fernández, A., Lobo-Prat, J., & Font-Llagunes, J. M. (2021). Systematic review on wearable lower-limb exoskeletons for gait training in neuromuscular impairments. *Journal of NeuroEngineering and Rehabilitation, 18*, 22. https://doi.org/10.1186/s12984-021-00815-5

Serban, D.-E., Octavinan, D. C., Negoescu Cheregi, I., Ciobanu, V., Onose, L., Popescu, C., & Onose, G. (2020). Topical systematic and synthetic literature review regarding men sexual dysfunctions after spinal cord injury. https://doi.org/10.12680/balneo.2020.372

Shiferaw, W. S., Akalu, T. Y., Mulugeta, H., & Aynalem, Y. A. (2020). The global burden of pressure ulcers among patients with spinal cord injury: A systematic review and meta-analysis. *BMC Musculoskeletal Disorders, 21*(1), 1–11. https://doi.org/10.1186/s12891-020-03369-0

Silva, L., Lima, M. B., & Salvador, E. P. (2018). Interventions for promoting physical activity among individuals with spinal cord injury: A systematic review. *Journal of Physical Activity & Health, 15*(12), 954–959. https://doi.org/10.1123/jpah.2018-0034

Simpson, B., Villeneuve, M., & Clifton, S. (2021). Exploring well-being services from the perspective of people with SCI: A scoping review of qualitative research. *International Journal of Qualitative Studies on Health and Well-Being, 16*(1), 1–33. https://doi.org/10.1080/17482631.2021.1986922

Smith, K., Hsieh, P.-C. (2017). Sports participation and re-integration of persons with spinal cord injury. *Therapeutic Recreation Journal, 51*(1), 75–80. https://doi.org/10.18666/TRJ-2017-V51-l1-7890

Song, K.-S., Cho, J. H., Hong, J.-Y., Lee, J. H., Kang, H., Ham, D.-W., & Ryu, H.-J. (2017). Neuropathic pain related to spinal disorders: A systematic review. *Asian Spinal Journal, 11*(4), 661–674. https://doi.org/10.4184/asj.2017.11.4.661

Sousa de Andrade, V., Faleiros, F., Balestrero, L. M., Romeiro, V., & Benedita dos Santos, C. (2019). Social participation and personal autonomy of individuals with spinal cord injury. *Revista Brasileira de Enfermagem, 72*(1), 241–247. https://doi.org/10.1590/0034-7167-2018-0020

Stampas, A., Hook, M., Korupolu, R., Jethani, L., Kaner, M. T., Pemberton, E., Li, S., & Francisco, G. E. (2022). Evidence of treating spasticity before it develops: A systematic review of spasticity outcomes in acute spinal cord injury interventional trials. *Therapeutic Advances in Neurological Disorders, 15*, 1–16. https://doi.org/10.1177/17562864211070657

van der Scheer, J. W., Goosey-Tolfrey, V. L., Valentino, S. E., Davis, G. M., & Ho, C. H. (2021). Functional electrical stimulation cycling exercise after spinal cord injury: A systematic review of health and fitness-related outcomes. *Journal of NeuroEngineering and Rehabilitation, 18*(1), 1–16. https://doi.org/10.1186/s12984-021-00882-8

Wong, S., Kenssous, N., Hillier, C., Pollmer, S., Jackson, P., Lewis, S., & Saif, M. (2018). Detecting malnutrition risk and obesity after spinal cord injury: A quality improvement project and systematic review. *European Journal of Clinical Nutrition, 72*, 1555–1560. https://doi.org/10.1038/s41430-018-0194-y

Special Education

Amran, H. A., & Majid, R. A. (2019). Learning strategies for twice-expectational students. *Journal of Special Education, 33*(4), 954–976.

Bailey, J., & Baker, S. T. (2020). A synthesis of the quantitative literature on autistic pupils' experience of barriers to inclusion in mainstream schools. *Journal of Research in Special Education Needs, 20*(4), 291–307. https://doi.org/10.1111/1471-3802.12490

Crowe, K., & Guiberson, M. (2019). Evidence-based interventions for learners who are deaf and/or multilingual: A systematic quality review. *American Journal of Speech-Language Pathology, 28*(3), 964–983. https://doi.org/10.1044/2019_AJSLP-IDLL-19-0003

Cushing, L. S., Parker-Katz, M., Athamanah, L. S., Waite, S. A., & Pose, K. M. (2020). Transition trends associated with topic focus since 1990: A literature review. *Remedial and Special Education, 41*(5), 271–283. https://doi.org/10.1177/0741932519835926

Gilmour, A. F., Fuchs, D., & Wehby, J. H. (2019). Are students with disabilities accessing the curriculum? A meta-analysis of the reading achievement gap between students with and without disabilities. *Exceptional Children, 85*(3), 329–346. https://doi.org/10.1177/00144029187955830

Hott, B., Berkeley, S., Fairfield, A., & Shora, N. (2017). Intervention in school and clinic: An analysis of 25 years of guidance for practitioners. *Learning Disability Quarterly, 40*(1), 54–64. https://doi.org/10.1177/0731948716629793

Kuntz, E. M., & Carter, E. W. (2019). Review of interventions supporting secondary students with intellectual disability in general education classes. *Research and Practice for Persons with Severe Disabilities, 44*(2), 103–121. https://doi.org/10.1091/deafed/enx059

Lam, E., A., McMaster, K. L., & Rose, S. (2020). Systematic review of curriculum-based measurement with students who are deaf. *Journal of Deaf Studies and Deaf Education, 25*(4), 398–410.

Lewis, M. M., Burke, M. M., & Decker, J. R. (2021). The relationship between the Individuals with Disabilities Education Act and special needs research: A systematic review. *American Journal of Education, 127*(3), 345–368. https://doi.org/10.1086/713825

Mawene, D., & Bal, A. (2018). Factors influencing parents' selection of schools for children with disabilities: A systematic review of the literature. *International Journal of Special Education, 33*(2), 313–329.

McCoy, D., C., Yoshikawa, H., Ziol-Guest, K. M., Duncan, G. J., Schindler, H. S., Magnuson, K., Yang, R., Keopp, A., & Shonkoff, J. P. (2017). Impacts of early childhood education on medium- and long-term educational outcomes. *Educational Researcher*, *46*(8), 474–487. https://doi.org/10.3102/0013189X17737739

McKenna, J. W., Bringham, F., Garwood, J., Zurawski L., Koc, M., Lavin, C., & Werunga, R. (2021). A systematic review of intervention studies for young children with emotional and behavioral disorder: Identifying the research base. *Journal of Research in Special Educational Needs*, *21*(2), 120–145. https://doi.org/10.1111/1471-3802.12505

Metzner, F., Wichmann, M. L. Y., & Mays, D. (2020). Educational transition outcomes of children and adolescents with clinically relevant emotional or behavioural disorders: Results of a systematic review. *British Journal of Special Education*, *47*(2), 230–257. https://doi.org/10.1111/1467-8578-12310

Peterson, A. K., Fox, C. B., & Israelsen, M. (2020). A systematic review of academic discourse interventions for school-aged children with language-related learning disabilities. *Language, Speech, and Hearing Services in Schools*, *51*(3), 866–881. https://doi.org/10.1044/2020_LSHSS-19-00039

Popham, M., Counts, J., Ryan, J. B., & Katsiyannis, A. (2018). A systematic review of self-regulation strategies to improve academic outcomes of student with EBD. *Journal of Research in Special Educational Needs*, *18*(4), 239–253. https://doi.org/10.1111/1471-3802

Rogge, N., & Janssen, J. (2019). The economic cost of Autism Spectrum Disorder: A literature review. *Journal of Autism & Developmental Disorders*, *49*(7), 2873–2900. https://doi.org/10.1007/s10803-019-04014-z

Stephens, N. M., & Duncan, J. (2020). Caregiver decision-making for school placement of children who are deaf or hard of hearing and children with other disabilities: A global perspective. *Volta Review*, *120*(1), 3–20. https://doi.org/10.17955/tvr.120.1.809

Walker, V. L., Kurth, J., Carpenter, M. E., Tapp, M. C., Clausen, A., & Lockman Turner, E. (2021). Paraeducator-delivered interventions for students with extensive supports needs in inclusive school settings: A systematic review. *Research & Practice for Persons with Severe Disabilities*, *46*(4), 278–295. https://doi.org/10.1177/15407969211055127

Wilhelmsen, T., & Sørensen, M. (2017). Inclusion of children with disabilities in physical education: A systematic review of literature from 2009 to 2015. *Adapted Physical Activity Quarterly*, *34*(3), 311–337. https://doi.org/10.1123/apaq.2016.0017

Zagona, A. L., & Mastergeorge, A. M. (2018). An empirical review of peer-mediated interventions: Implications for young children with autism spectrum disorders. *Focus on Autism & Other Developmental Disabilities*, *33*(3), 131–141. https://doi.org/10.1177/1088357616671295

Assistive Technology/Durable Medical Equipment and Transportation

Aspiranti, K. B., Larwin, K. H., & Schade, B. P. (2020). iPads/tablets and students with autism: A meta-analysis of academic effects. *Assistive Technology*, *32*(1), 23–30. https://doi.org/10.1080/10400435.2018.1463575

Aydin, O, & Diken, I. H. (2020). Studies comparing augmentative and alternative communication systems (AAC) applications for individuals with autism spectrum disorder: A systematic review and meta-analysis. *Education and Training in Autism and Developmental Disabilities*, *55*(2), 119–141.

Baig, M. M., Afifi, S., SholamHosseini, H., & Mirza, F. (2019). A systematic review of wearable sensors and IoT-based monitoring applications for older adults – a focus on ageing population and independent living. *Journal of Medical Systems, 43*(8), 11–12. https://doi.org/10.1007/s10916-019-1365-7

Baldassin, V., Shimizu, H. E., & Fachin-Martins, E. (2018). Computer assistive technology and associations with quality of life for individuals with spinal cord injury: A systematic review. *Quality of Life Research, 27*(3), 597–607. https://doi.org/10.1007/s11136-018-1804-9

Barnett, D. W., Barnett, A., Nathan, A., Van Cauwenberg, J., & Cerin, E. (2017). Built environmental correlates of older adults' total physical activity and walking: A systematic review and meta-analysis. *International Journal of Behavioral Nutrition & Physical Activity, 14*, 1–24. https://doi.org/10.1186/s12966-017-0558-z

Bellagamba, D., Vionnet, L., Margot-Cattin, I., & Vaucher, P. (2020). Standardized on-road tests assessing fitness-to-drive in people with cognitive impairments: A systematic review. *PLoS ONE, 15*(5), e0233125. https://doi.org/10.1371/journal.pone.0233125

Bigras, C., Owonuwa, D. D., Miller, W. C., & Archambault, P. S. (2020). A scoping review of powered wheelchair driving tasks and performance-based outcomes. *Disability and Rehabilitation: Assistive Technology, 15*(1), 76–91. https://doi.org/10.1080/17483107.2018.1527957

Brandt, A., Hansen, E. M., & Christensen, J. R. (2020). The effects of assistive technology service delivery processes and factors associated with positive outcomes – a systematic review. *Disability and Rehabilitation: Assistive Technology, 15*(5), 590–603. https://doi.org/10.1080/17483107.2019.1682067

Brandt, A., Jensen, M. P., Søberg, M. S., Andersen, S. D., & Sund, T. (2020). Information and communication technology-based assistive technology to compensate for impaired cognition in everyday life: A systematic review. *Disability & Rehabilitation: Assistive Technology, 15*(7), 810.824. https://doi.org/10.1080/17483107.2020.1765032

Brennan-Jones, C. G., Thomas, A., Hoare, D. J., & Serada, M. (2020). Cochrane corner: Sound therapy (using amplification devices and/or sound generators) for tinnitus. *International Journal of Audiology, 59*(3), 161–165. https://doi.org/10.1080/14992027.2019.1643503

Brims, L., & Oliver, K. (2019). Effectiveness of assistive technology in improving the safety of people with dementia: A systematic review and meta-analysis. *Aging & Mental Health, 23*(8), 942–951. https://doi.org/10/1081/13607863.2018.1455805

Cistola, G., Farrús, M., & van der Meulen, I. (2021). Aphasia and acquired Reading impairments: What are the high-tech alternatives to compensate for reading deficits? *International Journal of Language Communication Disorders, 56*(1), 161–173. https://doi.org/10.1111/1460-6984.12569

Cunha Maia, J., Coutinho, J. F. V., de Sousa, C. R., Mota, F. R. N., Marques, M. B., Silva, R. R. L., & Lima, R. B. S. (2018). Assistive Technologies for demented elderly: A systematic review. *Acta Paulista de Enfermagem, 31*(6), 651–658. https://doi.org/10.1590/1982-0194201800089

Damianidou, D., Arthur-Kelly, M., Lyons, G., & Wehmeyer, M. L. (2019). Technology use to support employment-related outcomes for people with intellectual and developmental disability: An updated meta-analysis. *International Journal of Developmental Disabilities, 65*(4), 220–230. https://doi.org/10.1080/20473869.2018.1439819

Damianidou, D., Foggett, J., Wehmeyer, M. L., & Arthur-Kelly, M. (2018). Features of employment-related technology for people with intellectual and developmental disabilities: A thematic analysis. *Journal of Applied Research in Intellectual Disabilities, 32*, 1149–1162. https://doi.org/10.1111/jar.12606

Desideri, L., Lancioni, G., Malavasi, M., Gherardini, A., & Cesario, L. (2021). Step-instruction technology to help people with intellectual and other disabilities perform multistep tasks: A literature review. *Journal of Developmental and Physical Disabilities*, *33*, 857–886. https://doi.org/10.1007/s10882-020-09781-7

de Lima Barroso, B. I., Cabral Galvão, C. R., Bueno de Silva, L., & Lancman, S. (2018). A systematic review of translation and cross-cultural adaptation of instruments for the selection of assistive technologies. *Occupational Therapy International, Article ID 4984170*, 1–10. https://doi.org/10.1155/2018/4984179

El-Taher, F. E., Taha, A., Courtney, J., & Mckeever, S. (2021). A systematic review of urban navigation systems for visually impaired people. *Sensors*, *21*, 3103. https://doi.org/10.3390/s21093103

Friesen, E. L., Slattery, P., & Walker, L. (2017). Assistive technology in transition readiness assessment instruments for adolescents with physical disabilities: A scoping review. *International Journal of Adolescent Health*, *10*(3), 263–274.

Gevarter, C., & Zamora, C. (2018). Naturalistic speech-generating device interventions for children with complex communication needs: A systematic review of single-subject studies. *American Journal of Speech-Language Pathology*, *27*, 1073–1090. https://doi.org/10.1044/2018_AJSLP-17-0128

Goo, M., Maurer, A. L., & Wehmeyer, M. L. (2019). Systematic review of using portable smart devices to teach functional skills to students with intellectual disabilities. *Education and Training in Autism and Developmental Disabilities*, *54*(1), 57–68.

Hakim, R. M., Tunis, B. G., & Ross, M. D. (2017). Rehabilitation robotics for the upper extremity: Review with new directions for orthopaedic disorders. *Disability and Rehabilitation: Assistive Technology*, *12*(8), 765–771. http://dx.https://doi.org/.org/10.1080/1748107.2016.1269211

Havard, B., & Podsiad, M. (2020). A meta-analysis of wearables research in educational settings published 2016–2019. *Education Technology Research and Development*, *68*, 1829–1854. https://doi.org/10.1007/s11423-020-09789-y

Hermawati, S., & Pieri, K. (2020). Assistive technologies for severe and profound hearing loss: Beyond hearing aids and implants. *Assistive Technology*, *32*(4), 182–193. https://doi.org/1.1080/10400435.2018.1522524

Jutai, J. W., Tuazon, J. R. (2022). The role of assistive technology in addressing social isolation, loneliness, and health inequities among older adults during the COVID-19 pandemic. *Disability & Rehabilitation: Assistive Technology*, *17*(3), 248–259. https://doi.org/10.1080/17483107.2021.2021305

Kbar, G., Bhatia, A., Abidi, M. H., & Alsharawy, I. (2017). Assistive technologies for hearing, and speaking impaired people: A survey. *Disability and Rehabilitation: Assistive Technology*, *12*(1), 3–20. http://dx.https://doi.org/.org/10.3109/17483107.2015.1129456

Kim, J., & Kimm, C. H. (2017). Functional technology for individuals with intellectual disabilities: Meta-analysis of mobile device-based interventions. *The Journal of Special Education Apprenticeship*, *6*(1), 1–22.

Koester, H. H., & Arthanat, S. (2018a). Effect of diagnosis, body site, and experience on text entry rate of individuals with physical disabilities: A systematic review. *Disability and Rehabilitation: Assistive Technology*, *13*(3), 312–322. https://doi.org/10.1080/17483107.2017.1369588

Koester, H. H., & Arthanat, S. (2018b). Text entry rate of access interfaces used by people with physical disabilities: A systematic review. *Assistive Technology*, *30*(3), 151–163. https://doi.org/10.1080/10400435.2017.1291544

Lakshmi, M. S. K., Rout, A., & O'Donoghue, C. R. (2021). A systematic review and meta-analysis of digital noise reduction hearing aids in adults. *Disability and Rehabilitation: Assistive Technology*, *16*(2), 120–129. https://doi.org/10.1080/17483107.2019.1642394

Larsen, S. M., Mortensen, R. F., Kristensen, H. K., & Hounsgaard, L. (2019). Older adults' perspectives on the process of becoming users of assistive technology: A qualitative systematic review and meta-analysis. *Disability and Rehabilitation: Assistive Technology*, *14*(2), 182–193. https://doi.org/10.1080/1748107.2018.1463403

Matter, R., Haniss, M., Oderud, T., Borg, J., & Eide, A. H. (2017). Assistive technology in resource-limited environments: A scoping review. *Disability and Rehabilitation: Assistive Technology*, *12*(2), 105–114. http://dx.https://doi.org/.org/10.1080/17483107.2016.1188170

McGrath, C., Sidhu, K., & Mahl, H. (2017). Interventions that facilitate the occupational engagement of older adults with age-related vision loss: Findings from a scoping review. *Physical & Occupational Therapy in Geriatrics*, *35*(1), 3–19. http://dx.https://doi.org/.org/10.1080/02703181.2016.1267292

McNicholl, A., Casey, H., Desmond, D., & Gallagher, P. (2021). The impact of assistive technology use for students with disabilities in higher education: A systematic review. *Disability and Rehabilitation: Assistive Technology*, *16*(2), 130–143. https://doi.org/10.1080/17483107.2019.1642395

Moorcroft, A., Scarinci, N., & Meyer, C. (2019). A systematic review of the barriers and facilitators to the provision and use of low-tech and unaided AAC systems for people with complex communication needs and their families. *Disability and Rehabilitation: Assistive Technology*, *14*(7), 710–731. https://doi.org/10.1080/17483107.2018.1499135

Nam, J. H., & Kim, H. (2018). How assistive devices affect activities of daily living and cognitive functions of people with brain injury: A meta-analysis. *Disability and Rehabilitation: Assistive Technology*, *13*(3), 305–311. https://doi.org/10.1080/17483107.2017.1358304

Nerisanu, R., Nerisanu, R.-A., Maniu, I., & Neamtu, B. (2017). Cerebral palsy and eye-gaze technology, interaction, perspective, and usability: A review. *Acta Medica Transilvanica*, *22*(4), 59–62.

Pedrozo Campos Atunes, T., Souza Bulle de Oliveira, A., Hudec, R., Brusque Crocetta, T., Ferreira de Lima Antão, J. Y., de Almeida Barbosa, R. T., Guarnieri, R., Massetti, T., Garner, D. M., & de Abreu, L. C. (2019). Assistive technology for communication of older adults: A systematic review. *Aging & Mental Health*, *23*(4), 417–427. https://doi.org/10.1080/13607863.2018.1426718

Perfect, E., Jaiswal, A., & Davies, T. C. (2019). Systematic review: Investigating the effectiveness of assistive technology to enable Internet access for individuals with deafblindness. *Assistive Technology*, *31*(5), 276–285. https://doi.org/10.1080/104000435.2018.1445136

Pool, M., Simkiss, D., Rose, A., & Li, F.-X. (2018). Anterior or posterior walkers for children with cerebral palsy? A systematic review. *Disability and Rehabilitation: Assistive Technology*, *13*(4), 422–433. https://doi.org/10.1080/17483107.2017.1385101

Quamar, A. H., Schmeler, M. R., Collins, D. M., & Schein, R. M. (2020). Information communication technology-enabled instrumental activities of daily living: A paradigm shift in functional assessment. *Disability and Rehabilitation: Assistive Technology*, *15*(7), 746–753. https://doi.org/10.1080/17483107.2019.1650298

Rum, L., Sten, O., Vendrame, E., Belluscio, V., Camomilla, V., Vannozzi, G., Truppa, L., Notarantonio, M., Sciarra, T., Lazich, A., Mannini, A., & Bergamini, E. (2021). Wearable sensors in sports for persons with disability: A systematic review. *Sensors*, *21*, 1858. https://doi.org/10.3390/s21051858

Sorgini, F., Caliò, R., Carrozza, M. C., & Oddo, C. M. (2018). Haptic-assisted Technologies for audition and vision sensory disabilities. *Disability and Rehabilitation: Assistive Technology, 13*(4), 394–421. https://doi.org/10.1080/17483107.2017.1385100

Sriram, B., Jenkinson, C., & Peters, M. (2019). Informal carers' experience and outcomes of assistive technology use in dementia care in the community: A systematic review protocol. *Systematic Reviews, 8*(1), 1–6. https://doi.org/10/1186/s13643-019-1081-x

Suarez-Escobar, M., & Rendon-Velez, E. (2018). An overview of robotic/mechanical devices for post-stroke thumb rehabilitation. *Disability and Rehabilitation: Assistive Technology, 13*(7), 683–703. https://doi.org/10.1080/17483107.2018.1425746

Sundar, V. (2017). Operationalizing workplace accommodations for individuals with disabilities: A scoping review. *Work, 56*(1), 135–155. https://doi.org/10.3233/WOR-162472

Sundaram, S. A., Wang, H., Ding, D., & Cooper, R. A. (2017). Step-climbing power wheelchairs: A literature review. *Topics in Spinal Cord Injury Rehabilitation, 23*(2), 98–109. https://doi.org/10.1310/sci2302-98

Tang, K., Diaz, J., Lui, O., Proulx, L. Galle, E., & Packham, T. (2020). Do active assist transfer devices improve transfer safety for patients and caregivers in hospital and community settings? A scoping review. *Disability and Rehabilitation: Assistive Technology, 15*(6), 614–624. https://doi.org/10.1080/17483107.2019.1604822

Thordardottir, B., Fänge, A. M., Lethin, C., Gatta, D. R., & Chiatti, C. (2019). Acceptance and use of innovative assistive technologies among people with cognitive impairment and their caregivers: A systematic review. *BioMed Research International, Article ID 9196728*, 1–18. https://doi.org/10.1155/2019/9196729

Tuazon, J. R., Jahan, A., & Jutai, J. W. (2019). Understanding adherence to assistive devices among older adults: A conceptual review. *Disability and Rehabilitation: Assistive Technology, 14*(5), 424–433. https://doi.org/10.1080/17483107.2018.1493753

Wong, J., Kallish, N., Crown, D., Capraro, P., Trierweiler, R., Wafford, Q. E., Tiema-Benson, L., Hassan, S., Engel, E., Tmayo, C., & Heinemann, A. W. (2021). Job accommodations, return to work, and job retention of people with physical disabilities: A systematic review. *Journal of Occupational Rehabilitation, 31*, 474–490. https://doi.org/10.1007/s10926-020-09954-3

Yim, S. H., & Schmidt, U. (2019). Experiences of computer-based and conventional self-help interventions for eating disorders: A systematic review and meta-synthesis of qualitative research. *The International Journal of Eating Disorders, 52*, 1108–1124. https://doi.org/10.1002/eat.23142

Zeng, W., Ju, S., & Hord, C. (2018). A literature review of academic interventions for college students with learning disabilities. *Learning Disability Quarterly, 41*(3), 159–169. https://doi.org/10.1177/073194818760999

Adapted Housing

Richter, D., & Hoffmann, H. (2017). Independent housing and support for people with severe mental illness: Systematic review. *Acta Psychiatrica Scandinavica, 136*(3), 269–279. https://doi.org/10.1111/acps.12765

Lifespan, Life Expectancy, and Mortality

Agiovlasitis, S., Choi, P., Allred, A., Xu, J., & Moti, R. W. (2020). Systematic review of sedentary behaviour in people with Down syndrome across the lifespan: A clarion call. *Journal of Applied Research in Intellectual Disabilities, 33*(2), 146–159. https://doi.org/10.1111/jar.12659

Alharbi, T. A., Paudel, S., Gasevic, D., Ryan, J., Freak-Poli, R., & Owen, A. J. (2021). The association of weight change and all-cause mortality in older adults: A systematic review and meta-analysis. *Age & Ageing*, *50*(3), 697–704. https://doi.org/10.1093/ageing/afaa231

Alexandra, P., Angela, H., & Ali, A. (2017). Loneliness in people with intellectual and developmental disorders across the lifespan: A systematic review of prevalence and interventions. *Journal of Applied Research in Intellectual Disabilities*, *31*(5), 643–658. https://doi.org/10.1111/jar.12432

Amiri, S. (2020). Unemployment and suicide mortality, suicide attempts, and suicide ideation: A meta-analysis. *International Journal of Mental Health*, 1–25. https://doi.org/10.1080/00207411.2020.1859347

Åsberg, A. N., Heuch, I., & Hagen, K. (2017). The mortality associated with chronic widespread musculoskeletal complaints: A systematic review of the literature. *Musculoskeletal Care*, *15*(2), 104–113.

Axson, E. L., Ragutheeswaran, K., Sundaram, V., Bloom, C. L., Bottle, A., Cowie, M. R., & Quint, J. K. (2020). Hospitalisation and mortality in patients with comorbid COPD and heart failure: A systematic review and meta-analysis. *Respiratory Research*, *21*(1), 1–13. https://doi.org/10.1186/s12931-020-1312-7

Baron, M., Viggiani, M. T., Losurdo, G., Principi, M., Leandro, G., & Di Leo, A. (2017). Systematic review with meta-analysis: Post-operative complications and mortality risk in liver transplant candidates with obesity. *Alimentary Pharmacology & Therapeutics*, *46*(3), 236–245. https://doi.org/10.1111/apt.14139

Campbell-Enns, H. J., & Woodgate, R. L. (2017). The psychosocial experiences of women with breast cancer across the lifespan: A systematic review. *Psycho-Oncology*, *26*(11), 1711–1721. https://doi.org/10.1002/pon.4281

Catalá-López, F., Hutton, B., Page, M. J., Ridao, M., Driver, J. A., Alonso-Arroyo, A., Forés-Martos, J., Saint-Gerons, D. M., Vieta, E., Valencia, A., & Tabarés-Seisdedos, R. (2017). Risk of mortality among children, adolescents, and adults with autism spectrum disorder or attention deficit hyperactivity disorder and their first-degree relatives: A protocol for a systematic review and meta-analysis of observational studies. *Systematic Reviews*, *6*, 1–7. https://doi.org/10.1186/s13643-017-0581-9

De Paola, L., Mehta, A., Pana. T. A., Carter, B., Soiza, R. L., Kafri, M. W., Potter, J. F., Mamas, M. A., & Myint, P. K. (2022). Body mass index and mortality, recurrence, and readmission after myocardial infarction: Systematic review and meta-analysis. *Journal of Clinical Medicine*, *11*(9), 1–16. https://doi.org/10.3390/jcm11092581

Dubbelink, L. M. E. O., & Geurts, H. M. (2017). Planning skills in autism spectrum disorder across the lifespan: A meta-analysis and meta-regression. *Journal of Autism Development Disorder*, *47*(4), 1148–1165. https://doi.org/10.1007/s10803-016-3013-0

Fahey, M., Crayton, E., Wolfe, C., & Douiri, A. (2018). Clinical prediction models for mortality and functional outcome following ischemic stroke: A systematic review and meta-analysis. *PLoS ONE*, *13*(1), 1–13. https://doi.org/10.1371/journal.pone.0185402

Foroutan, F., Guyatt, G., Friesen, E., Colunga Lozano, L. E., Sidhu, A., & Meade, M. (2019). Predictors of 1-year mortality in adult lung transplant recipients: A systematic review and meta-analysis. *Systematic Reviews*, *8*, 1–5. https://doi.org/10.1186/s13643-019-1049-x

Gutral, J., Cypryanska, M., & Nezlek, J. B. (2022). Normative based beliefs as a basis for perceived changes in personality traits across the lifespan. *PLoS ONE*, *17*(2), 1–18. https://doi.org/10.1371/journal.pone.0264036

Halfpenny, R., Stewart, A., Kelly, P., Conway, E., & Smith, C. (2021). Dysphagia rehabilitation following acquired brain injury, including cerebral palsy, across the lifespan: A scoping review protocol. *Systematic Reviews*, *10*(1), 1–7. https://doi.org/10.1186/s13643-021-01861-9

Hayes, E. M. K., Neubauer, N. A., Cornett, K. M. D., O'Connor, B. P., Jones, G. R., & Jakobi, J. M. (2020). Age and sex-related decline of muscle strength across the adult lifespan: A scoping review and aggregated data. *Applied Physiology, Nutrition & Metabolism*, 45(11), 1185–1196. Https://doi.org/10.1139/apnm-2020-0081

Hazara, A. M., & Bhandari, S. (2021). Age, gender, and diabetes as risk factors for early mortality in dialysis patients: A systematic review. *Clinical Medicine & Research*, 19(2), 54–63. https://doi.org/10.3121/cmr.2020.1541

Honkaniemi, H., Bacchus-Hertzman, J., Fritzell, J., & Rostila, M. (2017). Mortality by country of birth in the Nordic countries: A systematic review of the literature. *BMC Public Health*, 17, 1–12. https://doi.org/10.1186/s12889-017-4447-9

Ida, S., Kaneko, R., Imataka, K., & Murata, K. (2019). Relationship between frailty and mortality, hospitalization, and cardiovascular diseases in diabetes: A systematic review and meta-analysis. *Cardiovascular Diabetology*, 18, 1–13. https://doi.org/10.1186/s12933-019-0885-2

Jokela, M., Airaksinen, J., Virtanen, M., Batty, G. D., Kivimäki, M., & Hakulinen, C. (2020). Personality, disability-free life years, and life expectancy: Individual participant meta-analysis of 131,195 individuals from 10 cohort studies. *Journal of Personality*, 88(3), 596–605. https://doi.org/10.1111/jopy.12513

Kabboul, N. N., Tomlinson, G., Francis, T. A., Grace, S. L., Chaves, G., Rac, V., Daou-Kabboul, T., Bielecki, J. M., Alter, D. A., & Kranhn, M. (2018). Comparative effectiveness of the core components of cardiac rehabilitation on mortality and morbidity: A systematic review and network meta-analysis.

Kim, J. Y., Steingroever, J., Lee, K. H., Oh, J. Choi, M. J., Lee, L., Larkins, N. G., Schaefer, F., Hong, S. H., Joeng, G. H., Shin, J. I., & Kronbichler, A. (2020). Clinical interventions and all-cause mortality of patients with chronic kidney disease: An umbrella systematic review of meta-analyses. *Journal of Clinical Medicine*, 9(2). https://doi.org/10.3390/jcm9020394

Lee, A., Weintraub, S., Xi, I. L., Ahn, J., & Bernstein, J. (2021). Predicting life expectancy after geriatric hip fracture: A systematic review. *PLoS ONE*, 16(12), 1–9. https://doi.org/10.1371/journal.pone.0261279

Nikolaidou, E., Kakagia, D., Kaldoudi, E., Stouras, J., Sovatzidis, A., & Tsaroucha, A. (2022). Coagulation disorders and mortality in burn injury: A systematic review. *Annals of Burns & Fire Disasters*, 25(2), 103–115.

Liyuan Peng, L. L., Peng Wang Chong, Y. L., Xi Zha, H. D., & Juaqian Fan, Y. Z. (2020). Association between vitamin D supplementation and mortality in critically ill patients: A systematic review and meta-analysis of randomized clinical trials. *PLoS ONE*, 15(12), e0243768-e0243768. https://doi.org/10.1371/journal.pone.0243768

Lui, C., Huang, C., Xie, J., Li, H., Hong, M., Chen, X., Wang, J., Wang, J., Li, Z., Wang, J., U Wang, W. (2020). Potential efficacy of erythropoietin on reducing the risk of mortality in patients with traumatic brain injury: A systematic review and meta-analysis. *BioMed Research International*, 1–9. https://doi.org/10.1155/2020/7563868

Maes, M., Qualter, P., Vanhalst, J., Van den Noortgate, W., Goossens, L., & Kandler, C. (2019). Gender differences in loneliness across the lifespan: A meta-analysis. *European Journal of Personality*, 33(6), 642–654. https://doi.org/10.1002/per.2220

Mayburd, A. L., & Baranova, A. (2019). Increased lifespan, decreased mortality, and delayed cognitive decline in osteoarthritis. *Scientific Reports*, 9(1), 1–15. https://doi.org/10.1038/s41598-019-54867-8

McGuinness, M. B., Karahalios, Ma., Finger, R. P., Guymer, R. H., & Simpson, J. A. (2017). Age-related macular degeneration and mortality: A systematic review and meta-analysis. *Ophthalmic Epidemiology*, 24(3), 141–152. https://doi.org/10.1080/09286586.2016.1259422

Nakano, J., Fukushima, T., Tanaka, T., Fu, J. B., & Morishita, S., (2021). Physical function predicts mortality in patients with cancer: A systematic review and meta-analysis of observational studies. *Supportive Care in Cancer, 29*(1), 5623–5634. https://doi.org/10.1007/s00520-021-06171-3

O'Leary, L., Hughes-McCormack, L., Dunn, K., & Cooper, S-A. (2018). Early death and causes of death of people with Down syndrome: A systematic review. *Journal of Applied Research in Intellectual Disabilities, 31*(5), 687–702. https://doi.org/10.1111/jar.12446

Owusuaa, C., Dijkland, S. A., Nieboer, D., van der Heide, A., & van der Rijt, C. C. D. (2022). Predictors of mortality in patients with advanced cancer – A systematic review and meta-analysis. *Cancers, 14*(2), 1–20. https://doi.org/10.3390/cancers14020328

Pereira Leitão Júnior, F. A., Bastos Barbosa, R. G., Diniz, J. L., Oliveira Araújo, W. C., Braga Marques, M., & Victor Coutinho, J. F. (2021). Profile and functional capacity of long-lived people: Integrative review. *Revista Enfermagem, 29*, 1–8. https://doi.org/10.12957/reuerj.2021.59737

Peterson, K., Anderson, J., Boundy, E., Ferguson, L., McCleery, E., & Waldrip, K. (2018). Mortality disparities in racial/ethnic minority groups in the Veterans Health Administration: An evidence review and map. *American Journal of Public Health, 108*(3), e1–e11. https://doi.org/10.2105/AJPH.2017.304246

Phyo, A. Z. Z., Freak-Poli, R., Craig, H., Gasevic, D., Stocks, N. P., Gonzalez-Chica, D. A., & Ryan, J. (2020). Quality of life and mortality in the general population: A systematic review and meta-analysis. *BMC Public Health, 20*(1), 1–20. https://doi.org/10.1186/s12889-02-09639-9

Pienaar, P. R., Kolbe-Alexander, T. L., van Mechelen, W., Boot, C. R. L., Roden, L. C., Lambert, E. V., & Rae, D. E. (2021). Associations between self-reported sleep duration and mortality in employed individuals: Systematic review and meta-analysis. *American Journal of Health Promotion, 35*(6), 853–865. https://doi.org/10.1177/0890117121992288

Poudel, S., Shehadeh, F., Zacharioudakis, I. M., Tansarli, G. S., Zervou, F., N., Kalligeros, M., van Aalst, R., Chit, A., & Mylonakis, E. (2019). Effect of influenza vaccination on mortality and risk of hospitalization in patients with heart failure: A systematic review and meta-analysis. *Open Forum Infectious Diseases, 6*(4), 1–8. https://doi.org/10.1093/ofid/ofz159

Prussien, K. V., Jordan, L. C., DeBaun, M. R., & Compas, B. E. (2019). Cognitive function in sickle cell disease across domains, cerebral infarct status, and the lifespan: A meta-analysis. *Journal of Pediatric Psychology, 44*(8), 948–958. https://doi.org/10.1093/jpepsy/jsz031

Rahmani, J., Roudsari, A. H., Bawadi, H., Clark, C., Paul, M., Saleisahlabadi, M., Rahimi, S. F., Goodarzi, N., & Razaz, J. M. (2022). Body mass index and risk of Parkinson, Alzheimer, dementia, and dementia mortality: A systematic review and dose-response meta-analysis of cohort studies among 5 million participants. *Nutritional Neuroscience, 25*(3), 423–431. https://doi.org/10.1080/1028415X.2020.1758888

Rosenwohl-Mack, A., Schumacher, K., Fang, M-L., & Fukuoka, Y. (2018). Experiences of aging in place in the United States: Protocol for a systematic review and meta-ethnography of qualitative studies. *Systematic Reviews, 7*(1), 1–7. https://doi.org/10.1186/s13643-018-0820-8

Schepis, T. S., Klare, D. L., Ford, J. A., & McCabe, S. E. (2020). Prescription drug misuse: Taking a lifespan perspective. *Substance Abuse: Research & Treatment, 14*, 1–28. https://doi.org/10.1177/11782218209909352

Xu, B. Y., Yan, S., Low, L. L., Vasanwala, F. F., & Low, S. G. (2019). Predictors of poor functional outcomes and mortality in patients with hip fractures: A systematic review. *BMC Musculoskeletal Disorders, 20*(1). https://doi.org/10.1186/s12891-019-2950-0

Yang, D., Robertson, J. L., Condliffe, E. G., Carter, M. T., Dewan, T., & Gnanakumar, V. (2021). Rehabilitation therapies in Rhett syndrome across the lifespan: A scoping review of human and animal studies. *Journal of Pediatric Rehabilitation Medicine*, *14*(1), 69–96. https://doi.org/10.3233/PRM-200683

Yu, N., Cheng, Y. J., Liu, L. J., Sara, J. D. S., Cao, Z. Y., Zheng, W. P., Zhang, T. S., Han, H. J., Yang, Z. Y., Yi, Z., Wang, F. L., Pan, R. Y., Huang, J. L., Wu, L. L., Ming, Z., Wei, Y. X., Ning, Y., Zhang, Y., & Zhang, M. (2017). What is the association of hypothyroidism with risks of cardiovascular events and mortality? A meta-analysis of 55 cohort studies involving 1,898,314 participants. *BMC Medicine*, *15*, 1–15. https://doi.org/10.1186/s12916-017-0777-9

Clinical Practice Guidelines

Andrade, B. F., Courtney, D., Duda, St., Aitken, M., Craig, S. G., Szatmari, P., Henderson, J., & Bennett, K. (2019). A systematic review and evaluation of clinical practice guidelines for children and youth with disruptive behavior: Rigor of development and recommendations for use. *Clinical Child & Family Psychology Review*, *22*(4), 527–548. https://doi.org/10.1007/s10567-019-00292-2

Appenteng, R., Nelp, T., Abdelgadir, J., Weledji, N., Haglund, M., Smith, E., Obiga, O., Sakita, F. M., Miguel, E. A., Vissoci, C. M., Rice, H., Vissoci, J. R. N., & Staton, C. (2018). A systematic review and quality analysis of pediatric traumatic brain injury clinical practice guidelines. *PLoS ONE*, *13*(8), 1–17. https://doi.org/10.1371/journal.pone.0201550

Barrett, E., Larkin, L., Caulfield, S., De Burca, N., Flanagan, A., Gilsenan, C., Kelleher, M., McCarthy, E., Murtagh, R., & McCreesh, K. (2021). Physical therapy management of nontraumatic shoulder problems lack high-quality clinical practice guidelines: A systematic review with quality assessment using the AGREE II checklist. *The Journal of Orthopaedic and Sports Physical Therapy*, *51*(2), 63–71. https://doi.org/10.2519/jospt.2021.9397

Bray, E. P., McMahon, N. E., Bangee, M., Al-Khalidi, A. H., Benedetto, V., Chauhan, U., Clegg, A. J., Georgiou, R. F., Gibson, J., Lane, D. A., Lip, G. Y. H., Lightbody, E., Sekhar, Al, Chatterjee, K., & Watkins, C. L. (2019). Etiologic workup in cases of cryptogenic stroke: Protocol for a systematic review and comparison of international clinical practice guidelines. *Systematic Reviews*, *8*(1), 1–5. https://doi.org/10.1186/s13643-019-1247-6

del-Rosal-Jurado, A., Romero-Galisteo, R., Trinidad-Fernández, M., González-Sánchez, M., Cuesta-Vargas, A., & Ruiz-Muñoz, M. (2020). Therapeutic physical exercise post-treatment in breast cancer: A systematic review of clinical practice guidelines. *Journal of Clinical Medicine*, *9*(4), 1–14. https://doi.org/10.3390/jcm9041239

Dhivagaran, T., Abbas, U., Butt, F. Arunasalam, L., & Chang, O. (2021). Critical appraisal of clinical practice guidelines for the management of COVID-19: Protocol for a systematic review. *Systematic Reviews*, *10*(1), 1–6. https://doi.org/10.1186/s13643-021-01871-7

Doormaal, M. C. M., Meerhoff, G. A., Vliet Vlieland, T. P. M., & Peter, W. F. (2020). A clinical practice guideline for physical therapy in patients with hip or knee osteoarthritis. *Musculoskeletal Care*, *18*(4), 575–595, 1–21. https://doi.org/10.1002/msc.1492

Ernstzen, D. V., Louw, Q. A., & Hillier, S. L. (2017). Clinical practice guidelines for the management of chronic musculoskeletal pain in primary healthcare: A systematic review. *Implementation Science*, *12*, 1–13. https://doi.org/10.1186/s13012-016-0533-0

Gabriel, F. C., de Melo, D. O., Fràguas, R. Liete-Santos, N. C., Mantovani de Silva, R. A., & Ribeiro, E. (2020). Pharmacological treatment of depression: A systematic review comparing clinical practice guideline recommendations. *PLoS ONE*, *15*(4), 1–16. https://doi.org/10.1371/journal.pone.0231700

George, S. Z., Fritz, J. M., Silfies, S. P., Schneider, M. J., Beneciuk, J. M., Lentz, T. A., Gilliam, J. R., Hendren, S., & Norman, K. S. (2021). Clinical practice guidelines: Interventions for the management of acute and chronic low back pain: Revision 2021. *Journal of Orthopaedic & Sports Physical Therapy*, *51*(11), CPG1–CPG60. https://doi.org/10.2519/jospt.2021.0304

Gerber, L. H., Deshpnde, R., Moosvi, A., Zafonte, R., Bushnik, T., Garfinkel, St., & Cai, C. (2021). Narrative review of clinical practice guidelines for treating people with moderate to severe traumatic brain injury. *NeuroRehabilitation*, 1–17. https://doi.org/.org/10.3233/nre-210024

Harris, J., Chorath, K., Balar, E., Xu, K., Naik, A., Moreira, A., & Rajasekaran, K. (2022). Clinical practice guidelines on pediatric gastroesophageal reflux disease: A systematic quality appraisal of international guidelines. *Pediatric Gastroenterology, Hepatology, and Nutrition*, *25*(2), 109–120. https://doi.org/10.5223/pghn.2022.25.2.109

Khormai, A. K., Oliveira, C. B., Maher, C. G., Bindels, P. J. E., Machado, G. C., Pinto, R. Z., Koes, B. W., & Chiarotto, A. (2021). Recommendations for diagnosis and treatment of lumbosacral radicular pain: A systematic review of clinical practice guidelines. *Journal of Clinical Medicine*, *10*(11), 1–21. https://doi.org/10.3390/jcm10112482

Lee, M., Baek, J. H., Suh, C. H., Chung, S. R., Choi, Y. J., Lee, J. H., Ha, E. J., & Na, D. G. (2021). Clinical practice guidelines for radiofrequency ablation of benign thyroid nodules: A systematic review. *Ultrasonography*, *40*(2), 256–264. https://doi.org/10.14366/usg.20015

Mehta, P., Lemon, G., Hight, L., Allan, A., Li, C., Pandher, S. K., Brennan, J., Arumugam, A., Walker, X., & Waters, D. L. (2021). A systematic review of clinical practice guidelines for identification and management of frailty. *Journal of Nutrition, Health & Aging*, *25*(3), 382–391.

Prange-Lasonder, G. B., Murphy, M. A., Lamers, I., Hughes, A.-M., Buurke, J. H., Feys, P., Keller, T., Klamroth-Marganska, V., Tarkka, I. M., Timmermans, A., & Burridge, J. H. (2021). European evidence-based recommendations for clinical assessment of upper limb in neurorehabilitation (CAULIN): Data synthesis from systematic reviews, clinical practice guidelines, and expert consensus. *Journal of NeuroEngineering and Rehabilitation*, *18*, 162. https://doi.org/10.1186/s12984-021-00951-y

Rassak, H. A., Ghader, N., Qureshi, A. A., Zafar, M., Shaijan, J. F., & Kuwari, M. A. (2021). Clinical practice guidelines for the evaluation and diagnosis of attention-deficit/hyperactivity disorder in children and adolescents: A systematic review of the literature. *Sultan Qaboos University Medical Journal*, *21*(1), e12–21. https://doi.org/10.18295/squmj.2021.21.01.003

Salas-Gama, K., Onakpoya, I. J., Coronado Daza, J., Perera, R., & Heneghan, C. J. (2022). Recommendations of high-quality clinical practice guidelines related to the process of starting dialysis: A systematic review. *PLoS ONE*, *17*(6), 1–15. https://doi.org/10.1371/journal.pone.0266202

Shrubsole, K., Worrall, L., Power, E., & O'Connor, D. A. (2017). Recommendations for post-stroke aphasia rehabilitation: An updated systematic review and evaluation of clinical practice guidelines. *Aphasiology*, *31*(1), 1–24. https://doi.org/10.1080/14647273.2017.1331048

Wiltink, L. M., White, K., King, M. T., & Rutherford, C. (2020). Systematic review of clinical practice guidelines for colorectal and anal cancer: The extent of recommendations for managing long-term symptoms and functional impairments. *Supportive Care in Cancer*, *28*(6), 2523–2532. https://doi.org/10.1007/s00520-020-05301-7

Note

1. The article was found at: https://learn.carrickinstitute.com/wp-content/uploads/2020/04/Therapy-and-rehabilitation-of-mild-brain-injury_concussion-Systematic-review.pdf

References

Allison, A., Corwin, A., Albers, M. J., White, H., & Taylor, R. H. (2022). An analysis of usual, customary, and reasonable charges in life care planning. *Journal of Life Care Planning, 20*(2), 5–19.

American Medical Association. (2013). *Definition of "usual, customary and reasonable" H-385.923*. https://policysearch.ama-assn.org/policyfinder/detail/Policy%20H-385.923%20?uri=%2FAMADoc%2FHOD.xml-0-3242.xml

Aromataris, E., Fernandez, R., Godfrey, C. M., Holly, C., Khalil, H., & Tungpunkom, P. (2015). Summarizing systematic reviews: Methodological development conduct and reporting of an umbrella review approach. *International Journal of Evidence-Based Healthcare, 13*(3), 132–140. https://doi.org/10.1097/XEB.0000000000000055

Barros-Bailey, M., Brown, S., Maxwell, A., Malloy, S., Latham, S., Thompson, A., & Donohoe, E. (2022). Attendant Care Survey Methodology (ACSM): Introducing a costing model for attendant care. *Journal of Life Care Planning, 20*(1), 5–26.

Burls, A. (2009). *What is critical appraisal? In what is this series: Evidence-based medicine.* http://www.bandolier.org.uk/painres/download/whatis/What_is_critical_appraisal.pdf

Centers for Medicare & Medicaid Services. (2022). *Hospital price transparency*. https://www.cms.gov/hospital-price-transparency

Cote, C. (2021, February 4). What is data integrity and why does it matter? *Harvard Business School Online*. https://online.hbs.edu/blog/post/what-is-data-integrity

International Academy of Life Care Planners. (2022). *Standards of practice for life care planners* (4th ed.). International Association of Rehabilitation Professionals.

International Conference on Life Care Planning and International Academy of Life Care Planners. (1998, April). *Definition of life care planning.* https://connect.rehabpro.org/lcp/about/new-item/new-item5

Johnson, C. B., Cary, J. R., & Robert, E. (2022). A comparison of the definition of a life care plan. *Journal of Life Care Planning, 20*(3), 25–44.

Johnson, C. B., Pomeranz, J. L., & Stetten, N. E. (2018). Consensus and majority statements derived from Life Care Planning Summits held in 2000, 2002, 2004, 2006, 2008, 2010, 2012, 2015, and 2017 and updated via Delphi study in 2018. *Journal of Life Care Planning, 16*(4), 15–18.

Johnson, C., & Woodard, L. (2022). Life care planning cost techniques: History, methodology, and literature review. *Journal of Life Care Planning, 20*(2), 39–57.

Mahina, A. (2020). Components of a cost/charge scenario as utilized in the life care plan. *Journal of Life Care Planning, 18*(4), 13–34.

Maniha, A., & Watson, L. L. (2018). Life care planning resources. In R. O. Weed & D. E. Berens (Eds.), *Life care planning and case management handbook* (4th ed., pp. 729–757). Routledge.

Neulicht, A., Riddick-Grisham, S., Hinton, L., Costantini, P., Thomas, R., & Goodrich, B. (2002). Life care planning survey 2009: Process, methods, and protocols. *Journal of Life Care Planning, 9*(4), 129–214.

Neulicht, A., Riddick-Grisham, S., & Goodrich, B. (2010). Life care planning survey 2001: Process, methods, and protocols. *Journal of Life Care Planning, 1*(2), 97–148.

Preston, K. (2022). Standards of practice for life care planners (4th ed.). *Journal of Life Care Planning, 20*(3), 5–20.

PatientsRightsAdvocate.org. (2022, August). *Third semi-annual hospital price transparency report*. https://www.patientrightsadvocate.org/august-semi-annual-compliance-report-2022

Saltiel (Busch), R. M. (2022). Healthcare service costing: Pricing perspectives and case studies for life care planners. *Journal of Life Care Planning, 20*(2), 21–35.

Index

Note: Page numbers in *italic* denote figures and in **bold** denote tables.

A

ABLE accounts 171–172, 888–889
Academy for Certification of Vision Rehabilitation and Education Professionals (ACVREP) 712
Academy of Special Needs Planners 890
acculturation 160–161
Achieving a Better Life Experience Act (ABLE) 171–172
acoustic immittance/impedance 427–428, *428*
acquired brain injuries 241–242, 533–561; aging with 548, 550–551; anatomy 534–539, *536*, *538*; case study 551, **551–560**; classification 539–541, **540**; cognitive problems 545–546, **546**, 548; community reintegration 548–549; comorbid mental health disorders 608; complications 543–546, **546**; consciousness disorders 241–242, 541, 916–920; costs 534; epidemiology 534; etiology 534; initial treatment 541–542; long-term impairments 547–548, 550–551; mild traumatic brain injury 347; personal perspectives 916–928; recovery 546–547, **546**; rehabilitation 269–270, 542–543, 548–551, **550**; vocational rehabilitation 549–551, **550**; *see also* neuropsychology
Active Movement Scale 742, **747**
activities of daily living (ADLs): aging and 379; amputation and 471–472; brachial plexus injuries and 755, 757, 758, 760–761; case study 397–402, **399**, *399*, **400–402**, *400*; children 187, 402–403; defined 373, 396; levels of assistance for 397; visual impairments and 706–707, 709, 712; *see also* adaptive equipment and assistive technology
actual amount paid approach 828–829
acupuncture 648
acute stress disorder 578
Adams v. Laboratory Corp. of America 805
adaptive clinical trials 82, *82*, 83
Adaptive Driving Alliance (ADA) 912
adaptive equipment and assistive technology 245–246, 248–249, 897–902; assistive listening devices 435, 902; bathing equipment 186, 381, 390, 760; brachial plexus injuries 760; children 182–188, 245, 391, 403, 760, 868–869, 899; considerations 183–185, 898–901; continuous glucose monitoring systems 714; in education settings 868–869; evaluee age 899; follow-up studies 909–910; geographic location and climate 899–900; in the home 246, 380–381, 390, 901–902; physical therapist role 390, 391, 392, 394–395, 403; replacement values 905–909, **906–908**; resources 453–460; robotic exoskeletons 246, 683–684; severity of disability and premorbid conditions 900–901; spinal cord injuries 681, 682–684; universal design 381–382; visual impairments 706, 710, 711, 713–715; *see also* hearing aids; prosthetics
admissibility of expert testimony 20, 783, 793–807; case discussion of motions to exclude 799–802; checklist **806**; *Daubert v. Merrell Dow Pharmaceuticals, Inc.* 101, 783, 793, 794–796, 815–816, 819, 837; defense attorney's perspective 836–841, 842–843; foundation and methodology 781–782, 783–785, 802–804; *Frye v. United States* 793, 794, 836–837; general acceptance test 794–795, 796, 836–837; *General Electric Co. v. Joiner* 783, 793, 796–797, 837; *Kumho Tire Co. v. Carmichael* 101, 783, 793, 797–799, 802, 837–838; plaintiff's attorney's perspective 815–817; Rule 702 amendments 782, 795–796, 798–799, 816–817, 838–839; standards of practice 804–806
adverse childhood experiences 332, 631
Affordable Care Act (ACA) 20, 803, 804, 886
age-related macular degeneration 699, 700, 702, 710
aging: with amputation 519; with brain injuries 548, 550–551; hearing loss **214**, 421, 708, 709, 711, 720; normal age-related changes 212–213, **214–215**; occupational therapy 379; with spinal cord injuries 684; visual impairments **214**, 697, 700, 701, 702, 708, 709, 711, 720; *see also* elder care management
Aging Life Care Association (ALCA) 211, 213, 220
aging services professionals 221–222
albinism 702
Allison, C. D. 903–904, 905, 911–912
Allison, L. 85
amblyopia 700
American Academy of Clinical Neuropsychology (AACN) 337, 344
American Academy of Neurology (AAN) 241–242, 364, 365
American Academy of Pediatric Neuropsychology (AAPdN) 335

1005

American Academy of Physician Life Care Planners (AAPLCP) 12, 87–88, 115–117, 127
American Association of Nurse Life Care Planners (AANLCP) 8–9, 10, 18, 21, 40, 41–42, 87–88, 113–115, 127, 784
American Bar Association (ABA) 143, 148, 339, 781
American Board for Certification in Orthotics, Prosthetics and Pedorthics (ABC) 468, 470, 472
American Board of Clinical Neuropsychology (ABCN) 334, 335, 336
American Board of Professional Neuropsychology (ABN) 335, 336
American Board of Vocational Experts (ABVE) 124, 272, 274
American Congress of Rehabilitation Medicine (ACRM) 541
American Counseling Association 109
American legal system: case law 766–767; common law system 765–767; constitutional law 767; federal court system 766, 767–768; jury trial system 766; state court systems 768–769; statutory law 767; *see also* admissibility of expert testimony; Federal Rules of Civil Procedure; Federal Rules of Evidence
American Occupational Therapy Association (AOTA) 109–110, 370–375, 382–383
American Physical Therapy Association (APTA) 389, 392
American Psychological Association (APA) 333–334, 336, 339, 624
American Speech-Language-Hearing Association (ASHA) 409, 411–414, **413**, 421, 423, 439
Americans with Disabilities Act (ADA) 171, 172, 198, 379, 381, 618, 681, 857, 871
Americans with Disabilities Act Amendment Act (ADAAA) 379, 381, 857
amputation 501–530; aging with 519; burn injuries 575, **589**; case study 521–525, **526–529**; causes 471, 502, 503; children 502–504; complications 511–513; demographics 502; functional classification levels 477, **477**; levels of 505, *505*, *506*; phantom and residual limb pain 512–513; physiatrists 240–241, 501–502, 509–510, 519–521; rehabilitation phases 505–511, **507**, **509**, **510**; vocational rehabilitation **507**, 509–510; *see also* prosthetics; prosthetists
Amsterdam, P. 899, 900–901, 905
anaplastologists 472
anatomy: brachial plexus 737–739, *738*; brain 326, 534–539, *536*, *538*; skin 571–572; spinal cord 663–665, *663*, *664*
Ancar & Ancar v. Brown & TNE Trucking 801–802
anchoring bias 812–813, 850
annuities 826–827
anosognosia 337
ANSI National Accreditation Board (ANAB) 112
antegrade continence enema (ACE) procedure 670
anticholinergics 624, 625, 626
anticonvulsants 614, 615, 625–626, 647, 673

antidepressants 512, 610, 615, 617, 620, 625, 626, 647, 653–654, 673, 680
anti-epileptic medication 176
antipsychotics 610, 614–615, 617, 621, 622, 624–625, 626, 627–628, 630
anxiety disorders *see* generalized anxiety disorder (GAD)
appellate courts 767, 768, 778
applied behavior analysis 26
Aram, D. M. 327
arbitration 786
Arnold, K. D. 35
Arthur v. Catour 829
Ashori, M. 708
assisted living programs 194
assistive listening devices 435, 902
assistive technology *see* adaptive equipment and assistive technology
assistive technology practitioner (ATP) 182, 183, 898
assistive technology supplier (ATS) 898
Association for Driver Rehabilitation Specialists (ADED) 904, 911
Association of Rehabilitation Nurses (ARN) 254
Atowa, U. C. 704
attendant care: arguments about in litigation 820–821, 827, 844, 845; brachial plexus injuries 760–761; burn injuries 577; costing 260, 939–940; spinal cord injuries 684–685
Attendant Care Survey Methodology (ACSM) 84, 260, 940
attention deficit hyperactivity disorder 326, 330
attorney work product doctrine 773, 785, 849
attorneys *see* defense attorney's perspective; plaintiff's attorney's perspective
audiology 420–442; assessment procedures 425–431, **430**; assistive listening devices 435, 902; audiological rehabilitation 431, 433–434; auditory processing disorders 434–435; billing 441–442, **441**; case study 464, **464–466**; children 422, 424–425, **425**, 429–431, **430**, **438**, 440, 442, 464, **464–466**; cochlear implants 437–438, **437–438**; code of ethics 413; communicating with individuals with hearing impairment 440–441; credentialing and qualifications 109, 412, 423; hearing aid costs 439–440; hearing aid selection and fitting 435–438, **437–438**; hearing loss causes 424–425, **425**; hearing loss impacts 420–421; intraoperative monitoring 422, 431–432; ototoxic drug therapy 433; patients and problems seen 422–423; pressure-equalizing tubes 431; roles in life care planning 442, 450–451; scope of practice 423; tinnitus management 438–439; vestibular system assessment 432–433
Audiology and Speech-Language Pathology Interstate Compact (ASLP-IC) 109, 412
auditory evoked response (AER) 429
auditory processing disorders (APDs) 434–435
Augestad, L. V. 708
augmentative and alternative communication 245

autism spectrum disorder 174, 176, 331–332, 415
autonomic dysreflexia 244, 668–669
autonomy 126, 130, 133, 134, 143
averageness measures 96–98, 100–101
axial back pain 649–651, *650*, *651*

B

Bahramfar E. 708
balance problems *see* audiology
balance system assessment 432–433
Ball, D. 812, 824
Bandura, A. 325
Barnao, M. 127–128
Barros-Bailey, M. 85, 275–276, 295
basal ganglia 535
bathroom equipment and modifications 186, 380–381, 390, 681, 760, 902–903
Bauby, J. D. 416
Beauchamp, T. L. 125–126
Beavers v. Victorian 801
Bechtol, C. O. 469
behaviorism 323, 324–325
Bell Atlantic v. Twombly 769
Bellini, J. L. 84–85
beneficence 126, 130
benefit of the bargain approach 828, 829
benzodiazepines 181, 615, 617, 625, 626, 671
Berens, D. 10
beta-blockers 618
bipolar disorder 612–616
birth injuries 329–330
birth weight 328–329, 331
bisphosphonates 676
Blackwell, T. L. 781
Bleuler, E. 622
Bonfiglio, R. 3, 6–7, 233
Bonuck, K. 855–856
botulinum toxin injections 178, 181, 182, 189, 244, 365, 547, 671, 750, 755
brachial plexus injuries 737–761; anatomy 737–739, *738*; ancillary diagnostic studies 745–746, *746*, 758; assistive devices 760; attendant care 760–761; complications 746–748; diagnosis 741–742, *742*, *743*, **744**, *744*, *747*; elbow impairments 754–755, *754*; epidemiology 739; etiology 739, **740**; forearm impairments 755, *756*; life care planning considerations 757–761; life expectancy 761; patterns of 739–741, **740**, **741**; rehabilitation 743–745, **744**, *745*, 756–757; shoulder impairments 750–754, *751*, *753*; splints 745, *745*, 750–755, *751*, *756*, 757, 758, 759; surgical intervention 748–757, *749*, *751*, *752*, *753*, *754*, 759; vocational impacts 748; wrist and hand impairments 755–756
Braille 704, 710, 711, 712, 716
brain: anatomy 326, 534–539, *536*, *538*; development 322, 326, 327; plasticity 327–328, 333; *see also* acquired brain injuries; neuropsychology

brain derived neurotrophic factor (BDNF) 331
brainstem 326, 537
Brearly, T. W. 345
Broca, P. 320
Bronfenbrenner, U. 33–34, *35*, 37
Brown v. Board of Education 855
Brown v. USA Truck, Inc. and Watkins 803–804
Brown-Henry, K. 120
Brown-Sequard syndrome 668
Bullins, S. M. 111, 708
burn injuries 569–601; case study 592–601; children 569, 570, 574, 577, 578; classification 570–571; complications 572–573, 580, **581–589**; damage assessment checklist 580, **590–592**; etiology 570; laser surgery 574–575; massage therapy 576; musculoskeletal complications 572–573, **587–589**; nutritional issues 575–576; outpatient services 577; pediatric life care plans 577; pressure garments and splints 574, 575; prevalence 569–570; prosthetics 575; psychological issues 577–578; reconstruction 574–575; recovery 573; rehabilitation 573, 576–580; severity 571; skin functions and anatomy 571–572; surgical procedures 573–575, 576; vocational rehabilitation 579–580; wound care 572
business practices, ethical considerations 148, **149**
Butters, N. 321

C

Canadian Association of Occupational Therapists (CAOT) 370–371, 372
Canadian Certified Life Care Planner (CCLCP) 111, 113
cannabis and cannabinoids 176, 181, 648
Capital University Law School 15–16
Caragonne, P. 47–48, 50–51, **68–79**, 163
cardiovascular problems: acquired brain injuries 544; age-related **214**; burn injuries 586–587; spinal cord injuries 677–678
career genograms 284
caregiver support *see* personal care assistance
case law 766–767
case management 26
case studies: acquired brain injuries 551, **551–560**; amputation 521–525, **526–529**; audiology 464, **464–466**; burn injuries 592–601; chronic pain 655–656; elder care management 223–224; mental health disorders 633–634, **635–636**; neuropsychology 347–348, **348–353**; occupational therapy 384–385; physical therapy 397–402, **399**, *399*, **400–402**, *400*, 403–404, **404–406**; rehabilitation counseling 301–305; special education 873–876; speech-language pathology 460, **461–462**; spinal cord injuries 686, **686–692**; visual impairments 722, **723–730**
Casuto, D. 89, 909
cataracts **586**, 699, 700, 701, 709
cauda equina syndromes 668
causation opinions 842–843
Cavalier, R. 125

central cord syndrome 668
cerebellum 537
cerebral cortex 326, 535
cerebral palsy 172, 173, 175, 178, 179, 182, 183, 242–243, 330, 362, 382
certification 7–8, 110–118, 120, 779–780; assistive technology suppliers and practitioners 183, 898; audiology 423; life care management 222; neurology 362; neuropsychology 335, 336; occupational therapy 372; physiatry 236; prosthetists 469–471, *470*; rehabilitation counseling 273–275; rehabilitation nurses 254, 261, 264; speech-language pathology 411–412, 413–414
Certified Care Manager (CMC) 222
Certified Life Care Planner (CLCP) 52, 111–112, 256
Certified Low Vision Therapists (CLVTs) 711
Certified Nurse Life Care Planner (CNLCP) 113–115, 256, 779
Certified Orientation and Mobility Specialists (COMS) 711, 716
Certified Physician Life Care Planner (CPLCP) 115–117, 779–780
Certified Rehabilitation Counselor (CRC) 273
Certified Rehabilitation Registered Nurse (CRRN) 254, 256
Certified Vocational Evaluation Specialist (CVE) 273–274
Chan, F. 83
Chen, Y. 710
Chi, R. 126
Child Find 858–859
child support 892–893
Childhood Disability Benefit (CDB) 885
children and adolescents: adverse childhood experiences 332, 631; amputation 502–504; birth injuries 329–330; burn injuries 569, 570, 574, 577, 578; educational impacts and rehabilitation 442, 548–549, 704, 710–711; hearing loss 424–425, **425**, 429–431, **430**, **438**, 440, 442, 464, **464**–**466**; mental health disorders 609, 612, 617, 630–631; occupational therapy 377–378; physical therapy 391, 392, 402–404, **404**–**406**; speech-language pathology assessment 414–415, **446**; spinal cord injuries 662, 665; transition planning and services 191, 288–289, 870–871; visual impairments 699, 700, 704, 710–711, 712; *see also* brachial plexus injuries; neuropsychology; pediatric life care planning; pediatric neurological conditions; special education law and practices; special needs planning
Childress, J. F. 125–126
Chinese medicine 648
Christ, S. L. 709
chronic pain 243, 645–657; axial back pain and spinal stenosis 649–652, *650*, *651*, *652*; case study 655–656; complementary medicine 648; conservative therapies 649, 653–654; costs 645; diagnostic workup 646; interventional therapies 649–652, *650*, *651*, *652*, 654–655; medications 647–648, 653–654; neuropathic pain syndromes 652–655, 672–673; opioid management 647–648; prevalence 645–646, 653; psychological considerations 647; spinal cord injuries 672–673
civil procedure *see* Federal Rules of Civil Procedure
clinical practice guidelines 32, 91–92, 164; amputation rehabilitation 506; brachial plexus injuries 748; evidence-based *82*, 83; neurology 241–242, 364–365; neuropsychology 347; prosthetics 473–474; rehabilitation counseling 276, 286; spinal cord injuries 684–685; visual impairments 710
cochlear implants 437–438, **437**–**438**
codes of ethics 127; audiology 413; cultural considerations 158–159; life care management 222; neurology 364; neuropsychology 333–334; rehabilitation counseling 273, 274; speech-language pathology 413
Cogg v. Dawson 821
cognitive behavioral therapy (CBT) 610–611, 618, 621, 627, 631, 647
cognitive development 173, 322; *see also* developmental theories
cognitive problems: acquired brain injuries 545–546, **546**, 548; burn injuries 577, 579–580; hearing loss 421
cognitive rehabilitation 335, 338
cohort studies 82, *82*
Coleman v. United States of America and Touchette 818
Collateral Source Rule 20, 783–784, 828–831, 846
College of Vocational Rehabilitation Professionals (CVRP) 274
colobomas 702
coma 541; personal perspective 916–920
Commission on Disability Examiner Certification (CDEC) 7, 18
Commission on Rehabilitation Counselor Certification (CRCC) 12, 28, 124, 159, 271, 272, 273–274
common law system 765–767
communication: with individuals with hearing impairment 440–441; multicultural and cross-cultural considerations 161–163; *see also* speech-language pathology
community reintegration: acquired brain injuries 548–549; amputation **507**, 509
competency 134, **135**–**136**
complementary and alternative medicine: children 189; chronic pain 648; neurological conditions 364
complications: acquired brain injuries 543–546, **546**; amputation 511–513; brachial plexus injuries 746–748; burn injuries 572–573, 580, **581**–**589**; spinal cord injuries 244–245, 668–680; visual impairments 720
computerized dynamic posturography (CDP) 432–433
concurrent criterion-related validity 91–92
confidentiality 140–145, **141**–**142**, **144**, **145**

consciousness disorders 241–242, 541; personal perspective 916–920
consensus 9–10, 21, 43–46; consensus and majority statements 10, 29, 44–45, 46, 64–67, 87, 159, 234, 259, 784, 936; research methods 44–46, **45**
consensus development conference 44–46, **45**
conservatorships 893
constitutional law 767
consulting experts 779, 841–842, 849
content validity 91
continuous glucose monitoring systems 714
conus medullaris syndrome 668
convergent criterion-related validity 92
Cook, D. J. 83
corneal opacity 700, 701, 709
correlations 99
cortical visual impairment 700, 701
Cosby, M. F. 158
costing 52, 259–260, 936–946; contemporary costing practice 938–940; pre-existing conditions 939; sources and resources 940–942; usual, customary, and reasonable (UCR) pricing 96, 97–98, 476, 827, 938; *see also* present value analysis of future life care needs
costs: acquired brain injuries 534; attendant and facility care 260, 939–940; bipolar disorder 616; burn injuries 570; chronic pain 645; generalized anxiety disorder 619; hearing aids 439–440; home modifications 681–682, 903, 940; major depressive disorder 611–612; obsessive-compulsive disorder 622; prosthetics 474, 476–477, 517–519; reasonableness of 827; robotic exoskeletons 684; schizophrenia 630; spinal cord injuries 681–683, 684; vehicular modifications 682–683, 903, 905
Council for the Accreditation of Counseling and Related Educational Programs (CACREP) 272–273
counseling: brachial plexus injuries 759–760; *see also* rehabilitation counseling
Counseling Compact 109
counterclaims 770
court cases: *Adams v. Laboratory Corp. of America* 805; *Ancar & Ancar v. Brown & TNE Trucking* 801–802; *Arthur v. Catour* 829; *Beavers v. Victorian* 801; *Bell Atlantic v. Twombly* 769; *Brown v. Board of Education* 855; *Brown v. USA Truck, Inc. and Watkins* 803–804; *Cogg v. Dawson* 821; *Coleman v. United States of America and Touchette* 818; *Crouch v. John Jewell Aircraft* 802; *Cuevas v. Contra Costa County* 803; *Daubert v. Merrell Dow Pharmaceuticals, Inc.* 101, 783, 793, 794–796, 815–816, 819, 837; *Dedmon v. Steelman* 829–830; *Diede v. Burlington Northern Railroad Co.* 826–827; *Fairchild v. United States* 818; *First National Bank of Fort Smith v. The Kansas City Southern Railway Co.* 814–815; *Frye v. United States* 793, 794, 836–837; *General Electric Co. v. Joiner* 783, 793, 796–797, 837; *Golden Eagle Archery v. Jackson* 811, 812; *Hale v. Gannon* 823; *Hinsdale v. N.Y., NHHRR Co.* 826; *Howell v. Hamilton Meats & Provisions, Inc.* 828–829; *John v. Friesen* 804; *Jones and Laughlin Steel vs. Pfeifer* 489; *Kent Village Associates Joint Venture v. Smith* 818–819; *Kumho Tire Co. v. Carmichael* 101, 783, 793, 797–799, 802, 819, 837–838; *McGee v. Target Corp* 800; *Marcano v. Turabo Medical Center Partnership* 820; *Marten v. State of Montana* 800; *M.D.P. v. Middleton* 800; *Mercer v. Vanderbilt University, Inc.* 826; *Mettias v. United States of America* 801; *Mills v. Board of Education of the District of Columbia* 855; *Morales-Hurtado v. Reinoso* 822–823; *Ngatuval v. Lifetime Fitness* 800; *Norwest Bank v. Kmart Corp.* 819–820; *Oram v. DeCholnoky* 820; *Pennsylvania Association of Retarded Child vs. Commonweatlh of Pennsylvania* 855; *Perez v. United States of America* 800; *Riha v. Offshore Service Vessels* 803; *Roach & Roach v. Hughes, Chicot, Chicot Sales, & Wheels* 805–806; *Sandretto v. Payson Healthcare Management, Inc.* 803; *SeaRiver Maritime, Inc. v. Pike* 819–820; *Singh v. Larry Fowler Trucking, Inc.* 811, 812; *Tarasoff v. Regents of University of California* 143; *Taylor v. Speedway Motorsports, Inc.* 804; *Tucker v. Cascade General* 802–803; *United Planters Bank v. United States* 824–825; *Vaughn v. Hobby Lobby Stores* 818; *Vaughn v. Hobby Lobby Stores, Inc.* 806; *Weston v. AKhappyTime* 829; *Worley & Worley v. State Farm Mutual Automobile Insurance Co.* 801
court systems: federal 766, 767–768; state 768–769
court-appointed experts 779
covariance 96–98
COVID-19 pandemic 8, 52, 143, 192, 197, 239, 607, 630–631
Crane, R. 89, 909
cranial complications, acquired brain injuries 543
credentialing 107–120; audiology 109, 412, 423; certification 7–8, 110–118, 120, 779–780; expert witness qualification 119–120, 780; Fellow designation 10–11, 118–119; licensure 26–27, 109–110, 120; life care management 222; neurology 362; neuropsychology 334, 335, 336; occupational therapy 109–110, 372; physiatry 236; prosthetists 469–471, *470*; qualified healthcare provider 108, 779; rehabilitation counseling 273–275; rehabilitation nurses 254, 261, 264; speech-language pathology 109, 411–412, 413–414
criterion-related validity 91–92
critical appraisal 82, 83–84
critical appraisal literature 32, *82*, 83, 161, 942–944; bibliography 947–1003; case study 944–947; finding 943–944
crossclaims 770–771
cross-culturalism *see* multicultural and cross-cultural considerations
Crouch v. John Jewell Aircraft 802
Crowley, J. 210–211
Cuevas v. Contra Costa County 803
cultural competence 161
culture *see* multicultural and cross-cultural considerations

D

damages: actual amount paid approach 828–829; anchoring bias 812–813, 850; annuities and 826–827; attachment 778; benefit of the bargain approach 828, 829; Collateral Source Rule 20, 783–784, 828–831, 846; defense challenges to 803, 824–831, 844, 845–846; defense damages evidence 848; garnishment 778; hedonic 812; non-economic 812; presenting in court 823–824; reasonable value approach 828, 829–830; reasonableness of 827; remittitur 777; replevin 778; sequestration 778; types 811–812; *see also* present value analysis of future life care needs

Daubert v. Merrell Dow Pharmaceuticals, Inc. 95, 96, 101, 783, 793, 794–796, 815–816, 819, 837, 905

day-in-the-life videos 831
decision-making, ethical 127–128
decubitus ulcers 676–677
Dedmon v. Steelman 829–830
deep vein thrombosis (DVT) 677–678
defense attorney's perspective 835–850; admissibility of expert testimony 836–841, 842–843; causation opinions 842–843; Collateral Source Rule 846; cross-examination of plaintiff's life care planner 843–847; defense damages evidence 848; defense life care planners 841–842, 847–849; deposition of plaintiff's life care planner 845, 848; effects on jury 849–850; expert disclosures 841–842, 847–849; financial bias of experts 843–844; licensing issues 846; qualifications of plaintiff's life care planner 839–841, 846–847; scope of life care planner's role in litigation 835–836; types of expert roles 841–842; *see also* plaintiff's attorney's perspective

defense life care planners 821, 827, 841–842, 847–849
Dehorter, N. 332
Del Pino, I. 332
Delphi technique 44–46, **45**
delusions 609, 613, 623
DeMaio-Feldman, D. 371
dental health: age-related issues **215**; children 177–179
Department of Veterans Affairs, US 19, 473, 506, 609–610, 681–682, 903
deposition testimony 773–774, 786–787, 845, 848, 849
depression 607; amputation and 511; hearing loss and 421; spinal cord injuries and 680; visual impairments and 708, 720; *see also* major depressive disorder
Deutsch, P. M. 3, 4–7, 11, 25, 26, 40, 47, 52, 85, 233, 282, 285, 393
developmental disorders *see* neuropsychology
developmental language disorder 327, 332
developmental psychology 26, 33–34
developmental surveillance and screening 173–174
developmental theories 322, 323–325, **324**
diabetes: amputation and 502; diabetic retinopathy 699, 700, 703, 710, 714; neuropathy 654, 655, 709, 712; spinal cord injuries and 675–676
Diede v. Burlington Northern Railroad Co. 826–827
diffuse brain injuries 540–541

Disabled Adult Child (DAC) benefit 885
disclosures 771; expert 772, 841–842, 847–849; initial 771–772; pre-trial 772
discounting *see* present value analysis of future life care needs
discovery 771, 773–774; *see also* deposition testimony; disclosures
discriminant validity 92
divergent criterion-related validity 92
divorce 892–893
dorsal root ganglion stimulation 654–655
Dravet syndrome 176
driving 245–246, 248; adolescents 187; brachial plexus injuries 760; brain injuries 548; spinal cord injuries 682–683; visual impairments 706, 715
drooling 178
dual or multiple roles 129–130, **129**
Dunn, P. 767, 769, 770, 774, 775–776, 777
durable medical equipment *see* adaptive equipment and assistive technology; hearing aids; prosthetics

E

earnings capacity analysis 294–305, **298**
ecological model 33–34, *35*, 37
ecological validity 341, 343–344
economic damages 812–813
economists 847; *see also* present value analysis of future life care needs
Edelman, L. S. 573
education, special *see* special education law and practices
education and qualifications: audiology 423; ethical issues 134–137, **137**; life care planning 6–8, 15–17, 18–19, 108, 112; mental health professionals 631–632; neurology 362; occupational therapy 371–372; physiatry 236; physical therapy 389–390; prosthetists 470–471; rehabilitation nurses 253–254; speech-language pathology 411–412, 413–414
Education for All Handicapped Children Act 855, 899; *see also* Individuals with Disabilities Education Act (IDEA)
educational impacts and rehabilitation 442, 548–549, 704, 710–711
Edwin Smith Papyrus 320
Eisele, J. A. 327
elder care management 209–224; benefits of 211–212, 222–223; care plans 218–219, **219**; case study 223–224; certification 222; methodology 213, 216–220, **217**, **219**; patients and problems seen 212–213, **214**–**215**; referral sources 220–222; resources 224–228; roles in life care planning 220; standards of practice and code of ethics 222
elder law attorneys 221
electroconvulsive therapy (ECT) 610, 633
electronic health records 210
electronystagmography 432
Elger, C. E. 330
Elliott, T. 3

employment *see* vocational impacts and rehabilitation
enculturation 160
endocrine disorders: acquired brain injuries 543; age-related **215**; spinal cord injuries 675–676
English common law 765–766
Enhanced Nurse Licensure Compact (eNLC) 109
environmental toxins 332
epidemiology: acquired brain injuries 534; bipolar disorder 612; brachial plexus injuries 739; generalized anxiety disorder 616–617; major depressive disorder 609; obsessive-compulsive disorder 619; schizophrenia 622–623; spinal cord injuries 661–663
epidural steroid injections 649–650, *650*, *651*, 654
epilepsy 175–177, 330
epileptologists 176
equipment *see* adaptive equipment and assistive technology; hearing aids; prosthetics
equitable remedies 769
Erb's palsy 739, **740**, 741, **741**
error rates 101–102
Esquenazi, A. 235–236
estate planning *see* special needs planning
ethics 88–89, 123–150; applied ethics 125; audiology 413; autonomy 126, 130, 133, 134, 143; beneficence 126, 130; business practices 148, **149**; competency 134, **135–136**; confidentiality 140–145, **141–142**, **144**, **145**; cultural considerations 132–133, **132**, 158–159; dual or multiple roles 129–130, **129**; ethical decision-making 127–128; evaluee definition 124; fees 148, **149**; fidelity 126, 133, 134, 138, 146; integrity 134, 146; justice 126, 130, 133; legal issues in forensic ethics 146, **147**; life care management 222; literature review 123–124; metaethics 125; morals vs. ethics vs. legal rules 125; neurology 364; neuropsychology 333–334; nonmaleficence 126, 130, 134, 143, 146, 472–473; normative ethics 125; peer review **49**, 50–51; principle ethics 125–126; privilege and privacy 140–143, **141–142**; professional codes of ethics 127; professional responsibility 134–137, **135–136**, **137**; prosthetists 472–473; qualifications 134–137, **137**; records 143, **144**; rehabilitation counseling 273, 274; relationships with evaluees 128–133, **129**, **131**, **132**, **133**; remote assessment 143–145, **145**; reporting violations 148–150, **150**; research and publications 83, 90–91, 146, **148**; respecting colleagues 138, **139–140**; respecting diversity 132–133, **132**; speech-language pathology 413; standards of care 124–125; termination and referral 133, **133**; values clarification 126–127; veracity 126; welfare of those served 130, **131**
Ethics Interface Panel 128
Every Student Succeeds Act (ESSA) 172, 189
evidence rules *see* Federal Rules of Evidence
evidence source model (ESM) 85
evidence-based clinical practice guidelines *82*, 83
experimental studies 82–83, *82*
expert disclosures 772, 841–842, 847–849

expert life care planners 778–788; Collateral Source Rule and 20, 783–784, 831, 846; consulting experts 779, 841–842, 849; court-appointed experts 779; defendant-retained 821, 827, 841–842, 847–849; deposition testimony 786–787, 845, 848, 849; disclosure of testimony 772, 841–842, 847–849; establishing and maintaining files 785; ethical practice 146, **147**; foundation and methodology 781–782, 783–785, 802–804; mediation and arbitration 786; qualifications 119–120, 780; report writing 782–785; retention 781; standards of practice 64, 804–806; testifying experts 779, 841, 842, 848–849; trial testimony 788; types 778–780, 841–842, 848–849; work product privilege 773, 785, 849; *see also* admissibility of expert testimony; defense attorney's perspective; plaintiff's attorney's perspective
expert witness work: audiologists 423; occupational therapists 371; prosthetists 474; rehabilitation counselors 274, 275, 292, 294; *see also* expert life care planners
extended school year 869–870
eye and ear complications, burn injuries **585–586**

F

face validity 91
Fairchild v. United States 818
FAIRHealth 97
Fairley, M. 468
false negatives 101, 102
false positives 101, 102
Federal Rules of Civil Procedure 769–778; answer 770; attachment 778; attorney work product doctrine 773, 785, 849; closing arguments 776; complaint 769; cross-examination 775–776; deposition testimony 773–774; directed verdicts 776; disclosures 771–772; discovery 771, 773–774; expert disclosures 772; garnishment 778; initial disclosures 771–772; joinder of claims and parties 770–771; jury 774–775; jury instructions 776; pre-answer motions 770; pre-trial conferences and dismissals 774; pre-trial disclosures 772; relief and appeals 777–778; replevin 778; sequestration 778; service of summons 770; trial 774–776; verdict and judgment 776–777
Federal Rules of Evidence 95–96, 119–120, 775, 781–782, 783; Rule 26 802; Rule 401 795; Rule 402 795; Rule 702 119, 781–782, 793, 795–796, 798–799, 800, 802, 804, 814, 816–817, 837, 838–839; Rule 703 822–823
fees, ethical considerations 148, **149**
Feinman, R. 794
Fellow designation 10–11, 118–119
fidelity 126, 133, 134, 138, 146
Field, T. 3, 11–12
FIG Services, Inc. 16, 117–118
financial advisors 221
financial bias of experts 843–844

First National Bank of Fort Smith v. The Kansas City Southern Railway Co. 814–815
First-Party Special Needs Trusts 888
Fitzhardinge, P. M. 329–330
Fitzhugh-Bell, K. B. 320
Flaxman, A. D. 699
focal brain injuries 540–541
forensic work: audiologists 423; ethical practice 146, **147**; occupational therapists 371; prosthetists 474; rehabilitation counselors 274, 275, 292, 294; *see also* expert life care planners
Foundation for Life Care Planning and Rehabilitation Research 11, 103
free and appropriate public education (FAPE) 189, 856, 857, 858, 869, 871, 872
Freud, S. 322, 324
Friedman, L. M. 766
Frontera, W. 235–236
Frye v. United States 793, 794, 836–837
functional capacity evaluation (FCE) 392–393
Functional Independence Measure (FIM) 241, 344, 685

G

Galen 234, 320
Gall, F. J. 320
gastrointestinal problems: acquired brain injuries 544–545; age-related **215**; children 179–180; spinal cord injuries 669–670
Geckler, C. 346
General Electric Co. v. Joiner 783, 793, 796–797, 837
generalized anxiety disorder (GAD) 616–619
genetic disorders 331
genitourinary problems: acquired brain injuries 545; age-related **215**; spinal cord injuries 244–245, 673–675
geriatric care managers *see* elder care management
Gessell, A. 322–323
Gibbs, R. L. 234
Giles, S. J. 708
Glasgow Coma Scale 539, **540**, 541
Glass, H. C. 330
glaucoma 699, 700, 701, 709–710
global alveolar hypoventilation (GAH) 671, 672
Golden Eagle Archery v. Jackson 811, 812
Goodglass, H. 321
Gopinath, B. 421
government benefits: Childhood Disability Benefit (CDB) 885; Medicaid 885–887, 888, 889, 892; Medicaid Waiver programs 886; Medicare 885; Personal Needs Allowance (PNA) 886; Social Security Disability Insurance (SSDI) 884, 885, 889; Supplemental Security Income (SSI) 884–885, 889; *see also* special needs planning
grafting: nerve 739, 750; skin 570, 573–574, **581–589**
Gross Motor Function Classification System (GMFCS) 242
guardianship 191–192, 891, 893

guide dogs 713
Guide to Rehabilitation (Deutsch & Sawyer) 5, 282, 285
Gumpel, L. 89, 909
Gunn, T. R. 108, 109, 120

H

Haidich, A. B. 83
Hale v. Gannon 823
hallucinations 609, 613, 623
Halstead, W. 320–321
Halstead–Reitan Neuropsychological Battery (HRNB) 321, 340
Hamilton, B. 282–283
Harden, T. 271, 272, 276
Harper, D. 900, 905–906
Harris, I. 371
Hastie, R. 813
hearing aids: assistive listening devices 435, 902; bone anchored devices 438; cochlear implants 437–438, **437–438**; costs 439–440; selection and fitting 435–438, **437–438**
hearing loss: age-related **214**, 421, 708, 709, 711, 720; assessment procedures 425–431, **430**; auditory processing disorders 434–435; case study 464, **464–466**; causes 424–425, **425**; children 424–425, **425**, 429–431, **430**, **438**, 440, 464, **464–466**; communicating with individuals with 440–441; impacts of 420–421; life care planning considerations 442, 450–451; ototoxic drug-induced 433; rehabilitation 431, 433–434; tinnitus management 438–439; visual impairments and 708, 709, 711, 720; *see also* audiology; hearing aids
Hebb, D. 320, 322
hedonic damages 812
Helmstaedter, C. 330
hemiplegia due to stroke 246, 683; parent's personal perspective 920–928
Hermann, B. P. 330
heterotopic ossification 545, 572, **587**, 676
Hill, L. A. 855–856
Hinsdale v. N.Y., NHHRR Co. 826
hip dysplasia 182
Hippocrates of Kos 320, 361
Home and Community Based Services Waiver (HCBS) 886
home assessment and modifications 379–382, 395, 902–903; brachial plexus injuries 760; costs 681–682, 903, 940; smart homes 246; spinal cord injuries 680–682
hormonal disorders: acquired brain injuries 543; age-related **215**; spinal cord injuries 675–676
Horner, S. M. 294
Horner's syndrome 742
Howell v. Hamilton Meats & Provisions, Inc. 828–829
Huber, S. 210–211
Huntsman, M. M. 328
hydrocephalus 544

hypomania 613
hypoxic-ischemic brain injuries 539
hypoxic-ischemic encephalopathy 330

I

individualistic and collectivistic cultures 159–160
individualized education plans (IEPs) 189, 289, 338–339, 346, 377, 711, 860, 861, 862, 863, 864–866, 867, 869–871, 873, 884
individualized family services plans (IRSPs) 863
individualized healthcare plans (IHPs) 862
Individuals with Disabilities Education Act (IDEA) 189, 198, 259, 286, 288, 346, 377, 391, 548–549, 855, 857–862, 864–872, 873, 899
infections, spinal cord injuries and 678–679
initial disclosures 771–772
Inside Life Care Planning 7, 11
Institute of Rehabilitation and Training (IRET) 16–17
Institutional Review Board (IRB) 90
instrumental activities of daily living (IADLs): aging and 379; amputation and 471–472; defined 373–374, 396–397; levels of assistance for 397; mortality and 709; *see also* adaptive equipment and assistive technology
insurance annuities 826–827
integrity 134, 146
integumentary problems: age-related **215**; burn injuries **581–585**; spinal cord injuries 676–677
International Academy of Life Care Planners (IALCP) 8–9, 10–11, 12, 18–19, 40, 42, 43, 57–64, 87–88, 118–119, 127, 234, 784, 937
International Association of Rehabilitation Professionals (IARP) 6, 8, 11, 12, 118–119, 127, 222
International Classification of Functioning, Disability, and Health (ICF) 34–37, *35*, 276, 369, 412
International Commission on Health Care Certification (ICHCC) 7–8, 52, 108, 111–113, 127, 158–159, 779, 784, 814
International Symposium on Life Care Planning 8
interpreters 162–163, 341–342, 441
Interstate Medical Licensure Compact 110
intraventricular hemorrhage 328, 362

J

Jacobs, C. 29
John v. Friesen 804
Johnson, C. 936, 939
Johnson, C. B. 10, 87, 90
Jones, N. 706–707
Jones and Laughlin Steel vs. Pfeifer 489
Journal of Life Care Planning 10, 11–12, 19, 37, **38–39**, 85, 88–89, 108, 123, 128, 164, 237–238, **238–239**
Journal of Nurse Life Care Planning 9, 123
Journal of Private Sector Rehabilitation 6
juries 766, 774–775, 776, 849–850

jury instructions 776
justice 126, 130, 133

K

Kahneman, D. 813
Kaldenberg, J. 712
Kaplan, E. 321
Karl, J. 379, 380
Katz, R. T. 237
Kaufman, A. S. 322
Keel, S. 710
Kendall, S. L. 89
Kennedy, M. R. 338
Kent Village Associates Joint Venture v. Smith 818–819
ketogenic diet 177
Khan I. 327
Kirby, A. V. 289
Kitchen, J. 3, 5, 6–7, 233
Klinger, L. 371
Klumpke palsy 739, **740**
Kraepelin, E. 622
Kreydin, E. 245
Kroezen, M. 709
Krusen, F. 235
Kulich, S. J. 126
Kumho Tire Co. v. Carmichael 101, 783, 793, 797–799, 802, 819, 837–838
Kurniawan, S. 706, 715

L

language problems *see* speech-language pathology
laser surgery 574–575
Lashley, K. S. 320
Law, C. R. 244
learning theory 324–325
least restrictive environment 197, 295, 820, 857, 860, 862
Lee, B. L. 330
legal remedies 769
legal system: case law 766–767; common law system 765–767; constitutional law 767; federal court system 766, 767–768; jury trial system 766; state court systems 768–769; statutory law 767; *see also* admissibility of expert testimony; Federal Rules of Civil Procedure; Federal Rules of Evidence
Lennox-Gastaut syndrome 176, 177
Leon-Carrion, J. 338
Leventhal B. L. 327
licensure 26–27, 109–110, 120, 846; audiology 109, 412, 423; neuropsychology 334; occupational therapy 109–110, 372; physical therapy 110; prosthetists 469, *470*; rehabilitation counseling 275; rehabilitation nurses 254; speech-language pathology 109, 412
Life Care Facts 6, 11
life care management 209–224; benefits of 211–212, 222–223; care plans 218–219, **219**; case study

223–224; certification 222; methodology 213, 216–220, **217**, **219**; patients and problems seen 212–213, **214–215**; referral sources 220–222; resources 224–228; roles in life care planning 220; standards of practice and code of ethics 222

life care planning: basic tenets 27; conferences/symposia 8; current topics of interest 17–20; definitions 4, 9, 21, 88, 936; ecological model 33–34, *35*, 37; emerging issues 51–52; evaluation framework 48, **68–79**; future 20–21; history 3–12, **13–15**; lifespan approach 26, 33–37, *35*; methodology 26–27, 28, 29–33, **30**; philosophical context 88; physiatry and 233–234; standards of practice 11, 12, 28–29, 40–43, **40**, *41*, *42*, *43*, *44*, 51, 57–64, 87–88, 127, 158, 162, 222, 784, 804–806, 937; summits 9–10, 27, 43–46, 47, 87, 159, 234, 784; training programs 6–8, 15–17, 108, 112; underlying principles 26–27; work product peer review 46–51, **49**, **68–79**; *see also* consensus; research in life care planning; scope of practice

life care planning software 940

Life Care Planning—Certified (LCP-C) 117–118

life care plans: current uses of 19–20; reliability and validity 89–92, 101–102; *see also* case studies

life expectancy 172, 190, 270; arguments about in litigation 821, 825, 826; brachial plexus injuries 761; brain injuries and 550–551; predicting 246–247; spinal cord injuries and 662, 685–686; visual impairments and 709

life insurance policies 891, 892–893

lifespan approach 26, 33–37, *35*

Lingham, G. 710

Linsell, L. 329

Lipkin, P. H. 867

lithium 610, 614, 625–626

litigation *see* admissibility of expert testimony; defense attorney's perspective; expert life care planners; Federal Rules of Civil Procedure; Federal Rules of Evidence; plaintiff's attorney's perspective

Lockley, S. W. 703, 707

longitudinal studies 82, *82*

loss of earnings capacity (LOEC) analysis 294–305, **298**

lumbar facet joint pain 650–651, *651*

Luria, A. 321, 326

lymphedema 243

M

McCollum, P. 3, 8, 11, 40–41, 89, 909

MacDonald, M. 421

McGee v. Target Corp 800

McGwin, G., Jr. 699

McKnight, Z. S. 707

macular degeneration 699, 700, 702, 706, 710

Macy, M. 34

Mahina, A. 935, 938, 940

major depressive disorder 608–612

Mallet classification 742, *743*

Manduchi, R. 706, 715

mania 613

Marcano v. Turabo Medical Center Partnership 820

Marini, I. 89–90, 900, 905–906, 909, 910

Marlow, N. 330

Marten v. State of Montana 800

Martin, B. S. 328

massage therapy, burn injuries 576

Matthews, D. J. 244

May, V. R., III 86, 87, 108, 158

M.D.P. v. Middleton 800

mediation 786

Medicaid 885–887, 888, 889, 892

Medicaid Waiver programs 886

medical equipment *see* adaptive equipment and assistive technology; hearing aids; prosthetics

medical home 190–191

Medicare 885

medications: bipolar disorder 614–615; botulinum toxin injections 178, 181, 182, 189, 244, 365, 547, 671, 750, 755; burn injuries 578; chronic pain 647–648, 653–654; epilepsy 176; errors due to visual impairments 708–709; generalized anxiety disorder 617–618; generics 845; glaucoma 709–710; major depressive disorder 610; neurological conditions 364; non-24 sleep disorder 703; obsessive-compulsive disorder 620–621; ototoxicity 433; phantom and residual limb 512; schizophrenia 622, 624–626, 630; seizures 176; sialorrhea 178; spasticity 181, 244, 547, 671; spinal cord injuries 670, 671, 673, 676, 680

medulla oblongata 539

Meier, R., III 3

mental health disorders 607–637; amputation and 511; bipolar disorder 612–616; burn injuries and 577–578; case study 633–634, **635–636**; in children and adolescence 609, 612, 617, 630–631; chronic pain and 647; comorbidity of 608; costs 611–612, 616, 619, 622, 630; generalized anxiety disorder 616–619; hearing loss and 421; life care plan checklists **632**, **637**; major depressive disorder 608–612; obsessive-compulsive disorder 619–622; prevalence 607, 608, 609, 612, 616–617, 619, 622; spinal cord injuries and 608, 680; visual impairments and 708, 720; *see also* schizophrenia

mental health professionals 631–633, **632**

Mercer v. Vanderbilt University, Inc. 826

Mertes, A. 85, 164, 271, 272, 276

meta-analyses 81, *82*, 83, 84

metabolic changes, spinal cord injuries 675–676

metaethics 125

Mettias v. United States of America 801

methodology 25–79, 83, 84, 87, 88, 97, 102, **139**, 199, 213, 260, 286, 476, 781–785, 797–821, 937

midbrain 537

mild traumatic brain injury 347

Miller, E. 909

Miller, P. H. 324–325

Mills v. Board of Education of the District of Columbia 855
minimally conscious state (MCS) 241, 541
minimally invasive lumbar decompression (MILD) procedure 651–652, *652*
Mitchell, N. 128, 379
Miyauchi, H. 704
Molnar, G. E. 235
monoamine oxidase inhibitors (MAOIs) 610
monocular vision 700
mood stabilizers 610, 614, 625–626
Moradi Rekabdarkolaee, H. 86, 87, 108, 158
Morales-Hurtado v. Reinoso 822–823
morals 125
Moschos, M. M. 708
multicultural and cross-cultural considerations 157–165; acculturation and enculturation 160–161; communication 161–163; cultural competence 161; definitions 157–158; ethics guidance 132–133, **132**, 158–159; individualistic and collectivistic cultures 159–160; interpreters 162–163; in life care planning literature 158–159; methodological framework 163–164
musculoskeletal problems: acquired brain injuries 545; brachial plexus injuries 746–748; burn injuries 572–573, **587–589**; children 180–182
music therapy 627
myringotomy 431

N

National Academy of Certified Care Managers (NACCM) 222
National Board for Certification in Occupational Therapy (NBCOT) 109–110, 372
National Highway Traffic Safety Administration (NHTSA) 912
National Longitudinal Transition Study (NLTS) 289, 870
National Mobility Equipment Dealers Association (NMEDA) 904, 905, 912
National Registry of Rehabilitation Technology Suppliers 898
Natstasi, J. A. 712
nature versus nurture 322–323
neonatal brachial plexus palsy *see* brachial plexus injuries
neonatal encephalopathy 329–330
nerve grafting 739, 750
nerve transfer surgery 750, *751*, *752*
Neulicht, A. T. 159, 780, 938–940
neurodevelopmental delays 327–329
neurogenic bladder 244–245, 674–675
neuroimaging 321
neurological conditions 362–363; age-related **215**; burn injuries and **587**; hearing loss and 424; *see also* acquired brain injuries; neuropsychology; pediatric neurological conditions; spinal cord injuries
neurology 361–367; clinical practice guidelines 241–242, 364–365; ethical issues 364; origins of 361–362;
patients and problems seen 362–363; roles in life care planning 365–366; therapies 363–364; training 362
neuromodulatory therapies 177, 654–655
neuromuscular electrical stimulation 744, 757
neuromuscular scoliosis 181, 662, 671
neuronal plasticity 328, 739
neuropathic pain syndromes 652–655, 672–673
neurophysiologic intraoperative monitoring 422, 431–432
neuropsychology 319–353; acquired disorders 329–330; attention deficit hyperactivity disorder 326, 330; autism spectrum disorder 331–332; birth injuries 329–330; brain plasticity 327–328, 333; case study 347–348, **348–353**; certification 335, 336; clinical practice guidelines 347; critical periods in development 332–333; developmental disorders 327–333; developmental language disorder 327, 332; developmental theories 322, 323–325, **324**; environmental toxins 332; genetic disorders 331; history 319–321; mild traumatic brain injury 347; nature versus nurture 322–323; neurodevelopmental delays 327–329; neuroimaging 321; neuropsychological assessment 174–175, 336–342; prematurity and birth weight 328–329, 331; questions to ask neuropsychologists 342–347; roles and scope of practice 333–335; selecting a neuropsychologist 335, 336; social learning theory 325; theoretical models of 325–326; treatment recommendations 336–339
Ngatuval v. Lifetime Fitness 800
nominal group technique 44–46, *45*
non-24 sleep disorder 703, 707
non-economic damages 812
nonmaleficence 126, 130, 134, 143, 146, 472–473
non-randomized controlled trials 82, *82*
normative ethics 125
Norwest Bank v. Kmart Corp. 819–820
Notice of Recommended Educational Placement (NOREP) 864
nurses *see* rehabilitation nurses
Nursing Licensure Compact 109
nutritional issues: age-related **214**; burn injuries 575–576; children 179–180

O

observational studies 82, *82*
obsessive-compulsive disorder (OCD) 619–622
occupational therapy 369–386; case study 384–385; children 377–378; credentialing and qualifications 371–372; home assessment 379–382; literature review 370–371; patients and problems seen 377–382; roles in life care planning 383–384; scope of practice **38–39**, 372–375, **376**; standard treatment recommendations 382–383
Occupational Therapy Licensure Compact 109–110, 372
opioids 645, 647–648
optic nerve disorders 700, 701
oral health: age-related issues **215**; children 177–179

Oram v. DeCholnoky 820
orthostatic hypotension 669
orthotics 245, 249, 471; amputation 240–241, 524; children 187–188, 189, 241, 403; myoelectric 246; occupational therapist role 382; physical therapist role 390, 394, 403; robotic exoskeletons 246, 683–684; spinal cord injuries 246, 677, 683–684; *see also* prosthetics
osteoporosis 182, 676
otoacoustic emissions (OAEs) 429
ototoxic drug therapy 433
overuse syndromes: amputation 512; spinal cord injuries 673, 679
Owen, T. 783–784

P

p values 103
pain: age-related issues **214**; brachial plexus injuries and 759; phantom and residual limb 512–513; spinal cord injuries 672–673; *see also* chronic pain
Paredes, A. M. 342
parents: children with amputations 504; personal perspectives 913–916, 920–928; *see also* special education law and practices; special needs planning
Pascal, A. 329
Patient Protection and Affordable Care Act 20, 803, 804, 886
Patterson, J. B. 781
Paul, P. V. 704
Peddle, A. 393
pediatric life care planning 171–202; audiology 422, 424–425, **425**, 429–431, **430**, **438**, 440, 442, 464, **464–466**; case studies 301–305, 403–404, **404–406**, 464, **464–466**; common diagnoses 172–173; developmental surveillance and screening 173–174; guardianship 191–192, 891, 893; hip dysplasia 182; life care plan development 194–200, *198*, **199–200**, 365–366, 577, 757–761; life expectancy 172, 190, 761; long-term living options 192–194; loss of earnings capacity (LOEC) analysis 294–305, **298**; medical equipment and assistive technology 182–188, 245, 760; medical home 190–191; musculoskeletal considerations 180–182; neuromuscular scoliosis 181, 662, 671; neuropsychological evaluation 174–175; nutritional issues 179–180; occupational therapy 377–378; oral health concerns 177–179; osteoporosis 182; personal perspectives of parents 913–916, 920–928; physiatry 237, 240, 241, 242, 243, 245; physical therapy 402–404, **404–406**; rehabilitation counseling 280–285, **283**, **284**, 286–287, 288; seizures 175–177; sialorrhea 178; spasticity and other movement disorders 180–181, 182; supported decision-making 192, 893; therapy needs 188–189; transition planning and services 191, 288–289, 870–871; typical versus atypical development 173; unique considerations 171–172; *see also* children and adolescents; special education law and practices; special needs planning
pediatric neurological conditions 362–363, 364, 365–366; cerebral palsy 172, 173, 175, 178, 179, 182, 183, 242–243, 330, 362, 382; epilepsy 175–177, 330; neuropsychological evaluation 174–175; occupational therapy 377–378; oral health concerns 177–179; seizures 175–177, 330; sialorrhea 178; therapy needs 188–189; *see also* neuropsychology
pediatric physical therapy 391, 392, 402–404, **404–406**
pediatric rehabilitation medicine 237, 240, 241, 242, 243, 245
PEEDS-RAPEL model 299–301
peer review 46–51, **49**, **68–79**
Pennsylvania Association of Retarded Child vs. Commonweatlh of Pennsylvania 855
percentiles 97–98
Perez v. United States of America 800
perinatal stroke 330; parent's personal perspective 920–928
peripheral vision 698, 701, 703
persistent vegetative state 241, 541
personal care assistance: arguments about in litigation 820–821, 827, 844, 845; brachial plexus injuries 760–761; burn injuries 577; costing 260, 939–940; spinal cord injuries 684–685
personal frequency-modulated (FM) systems 435
Personal Needs Allowance (PNA) 886
personal perspectives 913–934; living with cancer 928–934; mother's story of perinatal stroke 920–928; parent's perspective of navigating systems 913–916; wife's story of caring for husband in coma 916–920
personal sound amplification products (PSAPs) 435
Petersen, E. A. 655
Pettengill, A. 468
Pettengill, C. 468
phantom limb pain 512–513
pharmacotherapy: bipolar disorder 614–615; botulinum toxin injections 178, 181, 182, 189, 244, 365, 547, 671, 750, 755; burn injuries 578; chronic pain 647–648, 653–654; epilepsy 176; errors due to visual impairments 708–709; generalized anxiety disorder 617–618; generics 845; glaucoma 709–710; major depressive disorder 610; neurological conditions 364; non-24 sleep disorder 703; obsessive-compulsive disorder 620–621; ototoxicity 433; phantom and residual limb 512; schizophrenia 622, 624–626, 630; seizures 176; sialorrhea 178; spasticity 181, 244, 547, 671; spinal cord injuries 670, 671, 673, 676, 680
physiatry 233–250; adaptive equipment and assistive technology 245–246, 248–249; amputation 240–241, 501–502, 509–510, 519–521; brain injuries 241–242; cerebral palsy 242–243; chronic pain 243; credentialing and qualifications 236; functional considerations 245–246; history of 234–236; life expectancy opinions 246–247; lymphedema 243; patients and problems seen 239–247; pediatric

rehabilitation medicine 237; roles in life care planning 237–238, **238–239**, 247–250; scope of practice **38–39**, 236–237, **238–239**; spasticity 243–244; spinal cord injuries 244–245

physical medicine and rehabilitation (PM&R) *see* physiatry

physical therapy 389–406; case studies 397–402, **399**, *399*, **400–402**, *400*, 403–404, **404–406**; children 391, 392, 402–404, **404–406**; education and qualifications 389–390; functional capacity evaluation (FCE) 392–393; patients and problems seen 390–391; roles in life care planning 393–397, 402–403; scope of practice **38–39**, 390; service delivery 391–393; standard treatment recommendations 393

Physical Therapy Compact 110

Piaget, J. 323, **324**

Pietrafusa, N. 176

plaintiff's attorney's perspective 811–831; actual amount paid approach 828–829; admissibility of expert testimony 815–817; anchoring bias 812–813; annuities 826–827; benefit of the bargain approach 828, 829; Collateral Source Rule 828–831; day-in-the-life videos 831; defendant-retained life care planners 821, 827; defense attacks against life care planners 815, 817–823; economic valuations of life care plans 825–827; hiring a life care planning expert 813–815; present value analysis 825–826; presenting the life care planner in court 823–825; reasonable and necessary future medical costs 827; reasonable value approach 828, 829–830; role of medical providers 821–823; types of damages 811–812; *see also* defense attorney's perspective

poikilothermia 669

Pomeranz, J. L. 86, 108, 158, 783

pons 537

post-secondary education 871

post-traumatic amnesia 539

post-traumatic hypercatabolism 575–576

post-traumatic stress disorder (PTSD): burn injuries and 577–578; chronic pain and 243, 647; comorbidity of 608; guide dogs and 713; visual impairments and 708

powers of attorney 891, 893

predictive validity 91, 92

pregabalin 617–618, 649, 653, 673

prematurity 328–329, 331, 702

present value analysis of future life care needs 483–497, 815; exemplar 491–496, **491–492**, **493–495**; inflation/growth rates 486–488, **486–487**, 825; interest/discount rates 489–490, **489–490**, 825–826; life care plans as source of information 484–485; total offset method 825–826

pressure garments: burn injuries 574, 575; lymphedema 243

pressure-equalizing tubes 431

pre-trial disclosures 772

primary research 31, 84–85

principle ethics 125–126

Prior Written Notice (PWN) 864

privilege and privacy 140–143, **141–142**

probability vs. possibility 102–103

professional guidelines 88–89, 222; *see also* clinical practice guidelines

professional responsibility 134–137, **135–136**, **137**

prosthetics: burn injuries 575; children 403, 502, 503, 504; complications and 511, 512; costs 474, 476–477, 517–519; level of amputation and 505; modifications and replacements 517–519; myoelectric 246, 503, 504, 513, **514**; physical therapist role 394, 403; prescription 241, 513–517, **514**, *515*, *516*; rehabilitation phases 505, *507*, 508–509, 511, 518; *see also* orthotics

prosthetists 241, 467–478; clinical practice guidelines 473–474; credentialing and qualifications 469–471, *470*; ethical issues 472–473; patients and problems seen 471–472; resources 479–480; roles in life care planning 468, 474–478; scope of practice 469; standard treatment recommendations 473

psychiatric disorders *see* mental health disorders

psychological denial 337

psychological impacts: amputation 511; brachial plexus injuries 748; burn injuries 577–578; spinal cord injuries 608, 680; visual impairments 707–708

psychosocial development 322; *see also* developmental theories

psychotherapeutic interventions: bipolar disorder 615; children 631; chronic pain 647; generalized anxiety disorder 618; major depressive disorder 610–611; obsessive-compulsive disorder 621; schizophrenia 626–627

pulmonary embolism 678

pulmonary problems: acquired brain injuries 544; burn injuries **586**; spinal cord injuries 671–672

pulsed radiofrequency ablation 513, 651, 654

pure tone audiometry 426, *427*

Q

qualifications *see* education and qualifications

qualified healthcare providers 108, 779

R

Rabin, L. A. 340–341, 344

Rachlinski, J. J. 813

radiofrequency denervation 654

Raffa, F. 3, 4

Ramos, P. 393

Rancho Los Amigos Scale of Cognitive Functioning 241, 546, **546**

randomized controlled trials 82, *82*

reasonable value approach 828, 829–830

Reavis, S. 909

records, ethical considerations 143, **144**

recovery: acquired brain injuries 546–547, **546**; burn injuries 573

referral and termination 133, **133**
refraction errors 700, 716
Rehab Consultant, The 6, 11
rehabilitation: acquired brain injuries 542–543, 548–551, **550**; amputation 505–511, **507, 509, 510**; audiological 431, 433–434; brachial plexus injuries 743–745, *744, 745,* 756–757; burn injuries 573, 576–580; cognitive 335, 338; hearing loss 431, 433–434; visual impairments 710–716
Rehabilitation Act 198, 292, 856, 872
rehabilitation counseling 267–306; care across the lifespan 270–271; case study 301–305; contemporary role of 269–270; credentialing 273–275; definitions 271; evolution of 268–269; historical roots of 267–268; ICF Core Sets 276; interview process 284–285; loss of earnings capacity (LOEC) analysis 294–305, **298**; pediatric life care planning 280–285, **283, 284,** 286–287, 288; resources 306–310; roles in life care planning 275–276, **277**; scope of practice **38–39,** 271–273; transition planning 288–289; vocational assessment and planning **278–279,** 285–287, 290–294, **293,** 375; working in teams 276–279, 287–288
Rehabilitation Engineering and Assistive Technology Society of North America (RESNA) 183, 458, 898, 905
rehabilitation medicine *see* physiatry
rehabilitation nurses 253–264; credentialing and qualifications 253–254, 261, 264; nursing process and care plans 255–256; practice settings 254–255; research issues 257–259; roles in life care planning 256–260, **258, 261, 262–263**; scope of practice **38–39,** 257
rehabilitation technology suppliers 898
Rehabilitation Training Institute (RTI) 6, 7
Reid, C. A. 27, 111, 708
Reitan, R. 321, 325–326
relationship measures 99–101
relationships with evaluees 128–133, **129, 131, 132, 133**
reliability of life care plans 89–92, 101–102
remittitur 777
remote assessment 52, 143–145, **145**
reproduction, spinal cord injuries and 679–680
reproductive organs, age-related issues **215**
research in life care planning 30–32; application of 84–85; consensus and majority statements 87; ethical considerations 83, 90–91, 146, **148**; foundational documentation 85–88; fundamental principles 93–95; future directions 103; primary, secondary, and tertiary research 30–31, 32, 84–85; professional guidelines 88–89; rehabilitation nurses and 257–259; reliability and validity of life care plans 89–92, 101–102; role and function studies 86–87, 107–108; rules of evidence 95–96; scientific method and process 28, 93–95; standards of practice 87–88; types 81–84, *82*; *see also* statistics
residual limb pain 512–513
resources: adaptive equipment and assistive technology **453–460**; audiology **441**; bibliography of critical appraisal literature 947–1003; costing 940–942; elder care management 224–228; pediatric life care planning 207; prosthetists 479–480; rehabilitation counseling 306–310; speech-language pathology **418–420, 453–460**; vehicular modifications 911–912; visual impairments 721–722
respiratory problems: acquired brain injuries 544; burn injuries **586**; spinal cord injuries 671–672
respite care 193
reticular formation 326, 537
retinal diseases 700, 702
retinitis pigmentosa 697, 703, 706
retinopathy of prematurity 702
Riddick-Grisham, S. 3, 6–7, 12, 18, 29, 233, 899
Riha v. Offshore Service Vessels 803
Rizzo, M. 416
Roach & Roach v. Hughes, Chicot, Chicot Sales, & Wheels 805–806
robotic exoskeletons 246, 683–684
role and function studies 86–87, 107–108, 159
Roosevelt, F. D. 235
Rosenthal, M. 346
rotary chair test 432
rules of civil procedure *see* Federal Rules of Civil Procedure
rules of evidence *see* Federal Rules of Evidence
Rumrill, P. D. 84–85
Rusch, F. R. 34
Rusk, H. 235
Rutherford-Owen, T. 90, 909, 910

S

sacroiliac joint pain 650, *650*
Saito, H. 421
Sandretto v. Payson Healthcare Management, Inc. 803
Sawyer, H. 3, 5, 6, 7, 40, 282, 285
Sbordone, R. J. 335, 343–344
Schakel, W. 706
Scheb, J. M. 765–766
Scherer 898
schizophrenia 331, 622–630; costs 630; epidemiology 622–623; pharmacotherapy 622, 624–626, 630; psychosocial interventions 626–627; suicide risk 624, 628; symptoms 623–624; treatment guidelines 624; treatment refractory schizophrenia 627–628; vocational impacts 629–630
Schow, R. 434
scientific method and process 28, 93–95
scoliosis 181, 662, 671
scope of practice 37, **38–39,** 88, 107, 237–238; audiology 423; definition 28; mental health professionals 632–633, **632**; neuropsychology 333–335; occupational therapy **38–39,** 372–375, **376**; physiatry **38–39,** 236–237, **238–239**; physical therapy **38–39,** 390; prosthetists 469; rehabilitation counseling **38–39,** 271–273; rehabilitation nurses **38–39,** 257; speech-language pathology **38–39,** 412–414, **413**
SeaRiver Maritime, Inc. v. Pike 819–820

second impact syndrome 548
secondary research 30–31, 32, 84–85
seizures 175–177, 330
selective dorsal rhizotomy 181, 189, 244
selective serotonin reuptake inhibitors (SSRIs) 610, 612, 617, 620, 626
self-awareness, lack of 337
sensory complications, brachial plexus injuries 748
serotonin norepinephrine reuptake inhibitors (SNRIs) 610, 617, 647, 653–654, 673
sexual function: age-related issues **215**; spinal cord injuries and 679–680
Shahid, K. S. 712
Sharma, H. 765–766
sialorrhea 178
Simeonsson, R. J. 323
Singh v. Larry Fowler Trucking, Inc. 811, 812
skin 571–572; *see also* burn injuries; integumentary problems
skin grafting 570, 573–574, **581–589**
Skinner, B. F. 324
Slesnick, F. 294
SLP *see* speech-language pathology
Smallfield, S. 712
smart homes 246
social learning theory 325
Social Security Disability Insurance (SSDI) 884, 885, 889
Society of Automobile Engineers (SAE) 912
Sorenson, J. 26
Sorokowska, A. 710
spasticity 180–181, 182, 243–244; brain injuries and 544, 545, 547; personal perspective 920–928; spinal cord injuries and 670–671; treatment options 180–181, 201, 244, 365, 547, 670–671
special education law and practices 853–878; 504 Plans 862–863, 866, 870, 871; academic supports 867; additional years at school 873; age of majority 865; Americans with Disabilities Act (ADA) 857, 871; assistive technology 869; case study 873–876; Child Find 858–859; considerations relevant for life care planners 866–872; determination of eligibility 859–860, 872; dispute resolution 861; due process 861; educational placement 860–861; eligibility criteria 858; evaluation process 859, 872; extended school year 869–870; failure to identify students with disabilities 872; free and appropriate public education (FAPE) 189, 856, 857, 858, 869, 871, 872; graduation considerations 873; history 855–856; individualized education plans (IEPs) 189, 289, 338–339, 346, 377, 711, 860, 861, 862, 863, 864–866, 867, 869–871, 873, 884; individualized family services plans (IRSPs) 863; individualized healthcare plans (IHPs) 862; Individuals with Disabilities Education Act (IDEA) 189, 198, 259, 286, 288, 346, 377, 391, 548–549, 855, 857–862, 864–872, 873, 899; informed parental consent 859; least restrictive environment 857, 860, 862; mediation 861; medical-based vs. school-based therapy services 867–868; parental requests for evaluation 859, 872, 880–882; post-secondary education 871; private schools 871–872; procedural safeguards 860; re-evaluation 860, 872; related services 867; role of education consultant in life care planning 876–877; Section 504 of the Rehabilitation Act 856; service delivery issues 873; specially designed instruction 866; state complaint procedures 861; supplementary aids and services 868; transition services 870–871
Special Needs Alliance 890
special needs planning 883–894; ABLE accounts 171–172, 888–889; Childhood Disability Benefit (CDB) 885; common planning mistakes 889–893; divorce and child support 892–893; guardianship 191–192, 891, 893; life insurance policies 891, 892–893; Medicaid 885–887, 888, 889, 892; Medicaid Waiver programs 886; Medicare 885; Personal Needs Allowance (PNA) 886; powers of attorney 891, 893; Social Security Disability Insurance (SSDI) 884, 885, 889; special needs planning attorney's role 893; Special Needs Trusts (SNTs) 883, 887–888, 890–891, 893; Supplemental Security Income (SSI) 884–885, 889; supported decision-making 192, 893
speech audiometry 426–427
speech-language pathology 409–420; assessment process 414–417, **446**, **447**; case study 460, **461–462**; code of ethics 413; credentialing and qualifications 109, 411–412, 413–414; etiologies of communication and swallowing disorders 411; feeding safety assessment 179; life care planning checklist **448–450**; medical coding and billing 417–418, **418–420**; patients and problems seen 410–411; pediatric and adolescent assessments 414–415, **446**; resources **418–420**, **453–460**; scope of practice **38–39**, 412–414, **413**; terminology 417, **451–453**
spendthrift trusts 887
spinal cord injuries 244–245, 661–692; aging with 684; anatomy 663–665, *663*, *664*; autonomic dysfunction 244, 668–669; cardiovascular complications 677–678; case study 686, **686–692**; children and adolescents 662, 665; chronic pain 672–673; classification 244, 665–668, *667*; epidemiology 661–663; gastrointestinal complications 669–670; genitourinary complications 244–245, 673–675; home modifications 680–682; infections 678–679; integumentary complications 676–677; life expectancy and 662, 685–686; medications 670, 671, 673, 676, 680; metabolic changes 675–676; overuse syndromes 673, 679; personal care assistance needs 684–685; preservation of function by neurologic level of injury 666–668; psychological complications 608, 680; rehospitalization 661, 662, 671–672, 674, 676; respiratory complications 671–672; robotic exoskeletons 246, 683–684; sexual function and fertility 679–680; spasticity 670–671; vehicular modifications 682–683; ventilator assistance 671, 672

spinal cord stimulation 654–655
spinal stenosis 649, 651–652, *652*
splints: brachial plexus injuries 745, *745*, 750–755, *751*, 756, 757, 758, 759; burn injuries 574, 575
Spreen, O. 330
standard deviation 98–99, 100
standardized score systems 99, 100
standards of care 124–125
standards of practice 11, 12, 28–29, 40–43, **40**, *41*, *42*, *43*, *44*, 51, 57–64, 87–88, 127, 158, 162, 222, 784, 804–806, 937
State Vocational Rehabilitation (VR) services 870–871
statistics 96–103; correlations 99; covariance 96–98; error rates 101–102; false negatives 101, 102; false positives 101, 102; mean, median, and mode 96–97; measures of averageness 96–98, 100–101; measures of relationship 99–101; measures of variability 98–99, 100–101; *p* values 103; percentiles 97–98; probability vs. possibility 102–103; range 99; standard deviation 98–99, 100; standardized score systems 99, 100; T-scores 99; Z-scores 99, 100
statutory law 767
Steeper Group 473
Stern, B. 783–784
St-Pierre, D. M. 573
Suárez, P. A. 341–342
subcortical division 326
Substantial Gainful Activity (SGA) 884, 885
sudden unexpected death in epilepsy (SUDEP) 177
summits 9–10, 27, 43–46, *47*, 87, 159, 234, 784
Supan, T. J. 468
Super, D. E. 283, **283**
Supplemental Security Income (SSI) 884–885, 889
supported decision-making 192, 893
Surakka, A. 708
surgical procedures: bone anchored hearing devices 438; for brachial plexus injuries 748–757, *749*, *751*, *752*, *753*, *754*, 759; for brain injuries 541–542, 544; for burn injuries 573–575, 576, **581–589**; for chronic pain 645–646, 651–652, *652*; cochlear implants 437–438, **437–438**; for epilepsy 177; for hearing loss 437–438, **437–438**; for hip dysplasia 182; intraoperative monitoring 422, 431–432; laser surgery 574–575; myringotomy 431; nerve grafting 739, 750; nerve transfer surgery 750, *751*, *752*; for neuromuscular scoliosis 181; for residual limb pain 513; for seizures 177; selective dorsal rhizotomy 181, 189, 244; for sialorrhea 178; skin grafting 570, 573–574, **581–589**; for spasticity 181, 244, 547; for spinal cord injury complications 670, 674, 679; for spinal stenosis 651–652, *652*; tendon transfer surgery 752, *753*, 754, *754*, 755–757; therapy needs 189; tracheotomy 542, 544; for visual impairments 703, 709; *see also* amputation
Swain, T. 699
swallowing disorders *see* speech-language pathology

systematic reviews *82*, 83
Szymanski, E. M. 271

T

tapentadol 654
Tarasoff v. Regents of University of California 143
tasimelteon 703
Taylor v. Speedway Motorsports, Inc. 804
Teachers for the Visually Impaired (TVIs) 710, 716
telehealth 383
Temple, C. 328
tendon transfer surgery 752, *753*, 754, *754*, 755–757
termination and referral 133, **133**
tertiary research 84–85
testifying experts 779, 841, 842, 848–849
text-to-speech software 714–715
thalamus 535
Third-Party Special Needs Trusts 887–888, 893
Thomas Jefferson University 17
Thompson, A. 378
tinnitus management 438–439
Tofte, N. 678
topical medications 654, 673
Toronto score 742, **747**
tracheotomy 542, 544
training programs 6–8, 15–17, 108, 112
tramadol 654
transcranial magnetic stimulation 610, 618, 621, 633
transition planning and services 191, 288–289, 870–871
transportation issues: visual impairments 706, 715–716; *see also* driving; vehicular modifications and adaptive equipment
traumatic brain injuries 241, 329, 533; mild 347; *see also* acquired brain injuries
tricyclic antidepressants 512, 610, 617, 647, 653–654, 673
trust officers 221
T-scores 99
Tucker v. Cascade General 802–803
Turner, T. 86
Tversky, A. 813
tympanometry 427–428, *428*
Type I and Type II errors 101

U

Umesh, G. 83
Uniform Transfer to Minor's Act Accounts (UTMA) 884
United Planters Bank v. United States 824–825
United States Life Tables 485
universal design 381–382
unresponsive wakefulness syndrome (UWS) 241, 541
upper motor neuron syndrome 544, 545, 669
urinary tract infections (UTIs) 678–679

U.S. Supreme Court 489–490, 767–768, 769, 778, 782, 783, 795–796, 797, 798–799, 819, 837–838, 855
usual, customary, and reasonable (UCR) pricing 96, 97–98, 476, 827; revagal nerve stimulation 177

V

validity of life care plans 89–92, 101–102
valproate 614, 625–626
values clarification 126–127
van der Ham, A. J. 708
Van Handel, M. 330
variability measures 98–99, 100–101
vascular brain injuries 539
Vaughn v. Hobby Lobby Stores 818
Vaughn v. Hobby Lobby Stores, Inc. 806
vegetative state 241, 541
vehicular modifications and adaptive equipment 187, 245–246, 248, 903–905; brachial plexus injuries 760; costs 682–683, 903, 905; resources 911–912; spinal cord injuries 682–683
ventilator assistance: brain injuries 542, 544; spinal cord injuries 671, 672
Ventry, I. 421
veracity 126
Vervloed, M. P. J. 704
vesicular monoamine transporter type 2 (VMAT2) inhibitors 625, 626
Vessey, J. 282–283
vestibular evoked myogenic potentials (VEMPS) 433
vestibular system assessment 432–433
Victor, C. M. 705
video head impulse test (VHIT) 433
videonystagmography 432
virtual assessment 52, 143–145, **145**
visual acuity 698
visual field 698
visual impairments 697–731; aging and **214**, 697, 700, 701, 702, 708, 709, 711, 720; assistive technology 706, 710, 711, 713–715; Braille 704, 710, 711, 712, 716; case study 722, **723–730**; children 699, 700, 704, 710–711, 712; clinical practice guidelines 710; complications 720; definitions 698–699; etiology 699–700; example conditions 700–703; functional impacts 706–707; guide dogs 713; hearing loss and 708, 709, 711, 720; intersectionality 708–709; life care planning considerations 716–722; life expectancy and 709; medical treatments 709–710; mobility issues 712–713; prevalence 699; psychological impacts 707–708; rehabilitation 710–716; resources 721–722; transportation issues 706, 715–716; vocational impacts and rehabilitation 705, 712
vocational counseling *see* rehabilitation counseling

vocational impacts and rehabilitation: acquired brain injuries 549–551, **550**; amputation **507**, 509–510; bipolar disorder 615–616; brachial plexus injuries 748; burn injuries 579–580; generalized anxiety disorder 618–619; loss of earnings capacity (LOEC) analysis 294–305, **298**; major depressive disorder 611; obsessive-compulsive disorder 621–622; occupational therapy 374–375; rehabilitation counseling **278–279**, 285–287, 290–294, **293**, 375; schizophrenia 629–630; spinal cord injuries 662–663; transition services 870–871; visual impairments 705, 712
Voogt, R. 827
Vygotsky, L. 325

W

Wade, S. L. 347
Wang, K. 332
Watson, J. 323, 324
Watson, L. L. 935, 938, 940
Wechsler, D. 341
Weed, R. O. 3, 6–7, 9, 10, 11, 18, 29, 41, 45, 47, 233, 234, 379, 380, 468, 697–698
weight gain: amputation and 511; burn injuries and 576
Weinstein, B. 421
Wernicke, C. 320
Weston v. AKhappyTime 829
Wilkins, R. 697–698
Wilkinson, M. E. 712
Wilson, A. D. 295
Winkler, T. 3
Woodard, L. 936, 939
Woodrich, F. 781
work product peer review 46–51, **49**, **68–79**
work product privilege 773, 785, 849
World Health Organization 34, 236, 270, 276, 396, 412, 473, 506, 611, 700, 704, 705, 710
Worley & Worley v. State Farm Mutual Automobile Insurance Co. 801
wound care, burn injuries 572

Y

Yan, H. 177
Yan, Q. 210
Yin, R. K. 85
yoga 648

Z

Zapata, M. A. 707
Zhi-Han, L. 708–709
Z-scores 99, 100
Zuckerman, D. M. 700, 704, 708, 709
Zunker, V. G. 283, **283**, 284

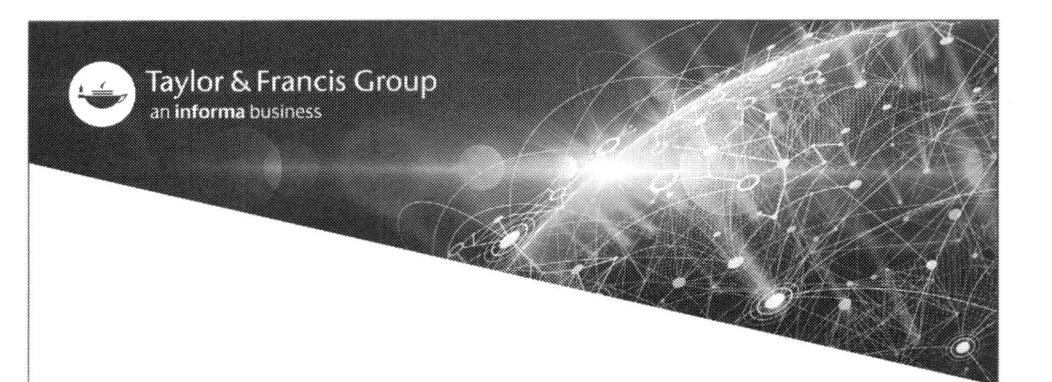

Printed in the United States
by Baker & Taylor Publisher Services